Sports Injuries

Mahmut Nedim Doral • Jon Karlsson
Editors

Sports Injuries

Prevention, Diagnosis, Treatment and Rehabilitation

Second Edition

Volume 2

With 1739 Figures and 229 Tables

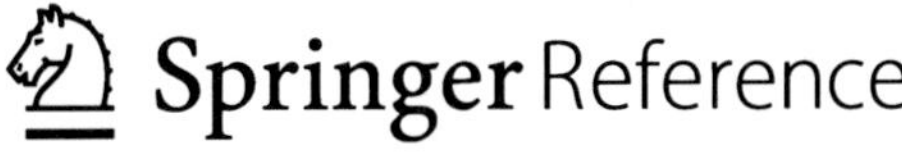

Editors
Mahmut Nedim Doral
Department of Orthopaedics
and Traumatology and Department of
Sports Medicine
Hacettepe University
Istanbul, Turkey

Jon Karlsson
Department of Orthopaedic Surgery
Sahlgrenska Academy
University of Gothenburg
Sahlgrenska University Hospital
Gothenburg, Sweden

ISBN 978-3-642-36568-3 ISBN 978-3-642-36569-0 (eBook)
ISBN 978-3-319-03953-4 (print and electronic bundle)
DOI 10.1007/978-3-642-36569-0

Library of Congress Control Number: 2015941018

Springer Heidelberg New York Dordrecht London

Printed on acid-free paper

Springer-Verlag GmbH Berlin Heidelberg is part of Springer Science+Business Media (www.springer.com)

To my mother, to my wife ESRA, to CEYLA-COŞKU, and to my grandson OZAN —Mahmut Nedim Doral

"If you think in terms of a year, plant a seed; if in terms of ten years, plant trees; if in terms of 100 years, teach the people" —Confucius

"The art of medicine consists in amusing the patient while nature cures the disease." —Voltaire

Foreword I

Looking back, the preparation of this book was an extremely exciting and long journey which started during the fifth EFOST meeting in 2008. The first edition of the book was a product of sleepless hours and the valuable effort of more than 300 scientists from all around the world. We are back with a stronger staff presenting a more comprehensive and a higher level of science to the reader. Similar to the first edition, we tried to integrate the eastern and western science in the lands of history where far eastern culture meets the west, both geographically and socioculturally.

Although we have come a long way since Watanabe performed the first arthroscopy, I believe the human body still has many unexplored mysteries forcing us to dig deeper into the vast well of science more and more every day. Each author in the book contributed their years of experience under this unified belief. It is a fact that sports traumatology and sports-related injury surgery are rising branches of orthopedics since the required performance of high-level athletes has inflated dramatically over the last decade. The fact that scientific improvements in sports traumatology is turning into a whole new sector is especially striking when one realizes the financial and global significance of just how much even one day of early recovery is vital for a team or an individual's career. Therefore, we aimed to prepare a practical guide for sports traumatologists, clinicians, and physiotherapists by gathering current concepts, treatment modalities, surgical techniques, and rehabilitation protocols together as much as possible. In addition to proved classical treatment methods, contemporary techniques and innovative ideas were provided as clear as possible for the reader. My hope is that the articles in the "Future of Sports Traumatology" section will probe the readers' imagination to create new and original ideas.

The book in your hands is the great labor of people all around the world. I am grateful to everyone who provided me with encouragement, friendship, wisdom, and patience. I have to thank first Prof. Jon Karlsson. His unbelievable and meticulous dedication to editing and preparing the index for the book in the last 3 years was extremely crucial to the success of our work.

Thereafter, I would like to express my gratitude to all national and international authors who poured their valuable experiences as well as the Springer team – Gabriele Schroeder and her coworkers.

I would like to thank my wife, Esra, my daughter, Ceyla, my son-in-law, Coşku, and my precious parents for their lifelong support. Thanks to my teachers Prof. Dr. T. Göğüs and Prof. Dr. R. Ege, who introduced Turkish orthopedics to the world, and my colleagues and my fellow scientists who trusted me.

Special thanks to my executive assistant editor, Dr. G Dönmez, and to my coworkers Dr. E. Turhan, Dr. G. Huri, and Dr. O. Bilge.

It will be the most valuable gift and the best source of motivation for me to know that this work in your hands will guide you in some way by expanding your vision.

It should not be forgotten that we orthopedic surgeons should evaluate the parts of the human body as a whole, not in components, as the human body works with dynamic and static stabilizers. For example, we focus mostly on the anterior cruciate ligament (ACL), but we should remember that there are more ligaments other than the ACL in the knee joint.

Please keep in mind that science has no religion, no language, no race, no color, and no flag. Scientific observation is the central element of the scientific method.

My deepest regards,

Istanbul, Turkey — Dr. Mahmut Nedim Doral

Foreword II

Why a new book on sports-related injuries? And don't we have enough books? And do we have enough readers for all these books?

I would like to answer these three questions simply by saying that this is a unique book. It is not only sports traumatology, arthroscopic techniques, advanced techniques and how to deal with injuries in well-equipped orthopaedic clinics. This book has it all; it is about sports, sports-related injuries, how to avoid them and how to treat them. It also covers unusual issues like extreme sports and how to deal with abdomen and chest injuries. It covers the entire athlete, not only injuries but also general health, heart conditions as well as knee injuries.

This is the main reason why this book is needed. We have worked on this project for many years now, and now we have this complete and unique book, a book that covers every aspect of the athlete's life and career. This book is therefore like no other book; it is comprehensive, and it gives the reader a broad picture of sports-related injuries and diseases, how to prevent them and how to treat them.

This is a good opportunity to thank everyone who has been involved and helped us to carry this project through. First of all, I would like to thank my co-editor, Mahmut Nedim Doral, a writer, a doctor, a researcher and a very dear friend. Second, all the Section Editors and Associate Editors and all those who have contributed with their invaluable knowledge. I would also like to thank Springer Verlag, especially Gabrielle Schröder, Vasowati Shome and Audrey Wong for their help in putting the manuscripts together. I would also like to thank those who helped me with keeping track of all chapters, authors and all corrections – Borgthór Ásgeirsson and Lára Lamb – for their invaluable help.

I hope the readers will enjoy the book!

Gothenburg, Sweden Jon Karlsson, M.D., Ph.D.

Preface I

Sports medicine and sports traumatology have gained great social importance in the last 50 years.

Prevention comes first, but improvement in the treatment of sports injuries is also of great benefit to general trauma patients with a range of common injuries and injuries caused by traffic accidents.

Competition is inherent in human nature and is a fact of life, including for reproduction and evolution in general. Civilized nations now look more towards gaining prestige via the results of individual and team sports rather than from war activities to demonstrate their actual power and might.

During the Olympic Games in the holy district of Zeus in Olympia in 824 BC, the war between the competing ancient Greek towns was stopped in favor of competition between the athletes. As the games evolved, the great event of the games was celebrated with running, jumping, throwing of discs and spears, boxing, wrestling, and chariot races.

As early as 2,500 years ago, sports medicine existed. Herodikos (or Herodicus) from Knidos (Cnidus), born in 500 BC, was famous for treating Olympionikes (Olympia Winners) in Olympian Athletes. He lived 40 years before Hippokrates (Hippocrates) of Kos.

More than 1,000 years later, fighting competitions such as knight tournaments in Europe, with fencing tournaments, archery, crossbow shooting, spear throwing, and so forth, evolved after the great wars.

With general technical developments and their evolution, all types of individual and team sports began to boom. At the same time, in parallel with the increasing number of sports injuries, sports surgery and sports medicine followed with a tremendous evolution of new knowledge and new possibilities. Technical innovations such as arthroscopy and enormous research activities due to the increased general welfare of the population as a result of financial prosperity on the one hand and better physical conditions of the population (e.g., good healthy nutrition over the whole year) on the other hand may have been responsible for this progress and improvements in the results. Fortunately, it is no longer true – as it was with our predecessors – to say "They won't come back!" when sports participants left the sportsground on a stretcher.

Competition in sports has become also a competition between nations. Thus, the overall medal ranking at the Olympic Games is the pride of nations and, in an unattended way, has been of a greater importance in the decades since World War II.

Sports medicine doctors are also heavily involved in competitions nowadays, even among themselves. Less than 40 years ago, a university professor of orthopedics stated "There is no need for sports medicine and especially sports traumatology. We do that already." How erroneous was this statement!

Look at this book! With more than 3,000 pages, it is a lexicon of sports medicine knowledge. But, there is also no doubt that the enormous increase in common sports injuries, including from the new extreme sports, brings enormous costs to the healthcare system.

Receiving the best treatment with full recovery achieved in a short period of time is important for professional athletes, players in expensive teams, recreational sportsmen, and, last but not least, the workers and their employers together with insurance companies because of the costs of injuries and flow-on economic consequences such as rents and so forth. The best, correct treatment is ultimately cheaper, especially in the long run.

The paper is patient, the Patient is not. Study, learn, and prepare the intervention you plan to perform. Do it right the first time and do not wait to learn from the complications later!

Riehen, Switzerland Werner Müller

Preface II

Sport Injury: Raising Political Awareness on a National and International Level

If you ask politicians and decision-makers about the significance of sports medicine, the reply has often more to do with anti-doping issues than actual sports injuries. The treatment and rehabilitation of injured athletes is rarely deemed a serious problem, except to those who in an athletic past may have themselves sustained an injury in training or competition. The sports doctor's daily concern for treatment–and more importantly prevention–of sports injuries is an almost entirely undiscovered country to those in a position to help most. This obscurity belies the true extent and far-reaching consequences of sports injuries that are currently near epidemic proportions. This reality was acknowledged during a recent debate on this sports injuries "epidemic" at the eighth congress of the European Federation of Sports Medicine Associations (EFSMA) in Strasbourg in September 2013. J. Kornbeck, a representative of the Sport Unit of the European Commission and European Union, mentioned that the EU policy decision-makers were simply not aware of the large-scale problem of sports injuries. Anterior cruciate ligament (ACL) injuries in particular were startlingly disproportionate in frequency and severity to the general impression of political leaders and administrators. There is a definite and pressing need to bring this subject into the political conversation. That we know many of these injuries are preventable adds to the urgency in raising awareness and creating a change for the better (Myklebust et al. 2003).

Fortunately, some forward-thinking international associations have begun to recognize the problem, and the first definitive steps are being taken in line with Van Mechelen's four-stage approach (i.e., evaluating the magnitude of the problem). The International Olympic Committee (IOC) deserves credit in driving this research forward under the auspices of Prof. Lars Engebretsen, who began to register specific types of sports injuries during the Olympic Games in 2004. Systematic data collection was limited to team sports in Athens, but by the 2008 Olympic Games of Beijing, sports injuries were being tracked in athletes across all events, and the system has become integrated into IOC policy (Junge et al. 2008). Engebretsen's data demonstrated that approximately 10 % of athletes sustained an injury while attending and competing at the Olympic Games. Similar initiatives have been undertaken in football (Champions League) (Ekstrand et al. 2013), alpine skiing (FIS World Cup), and other sports revealing comparable or even worse findings.

Injuries recorded during these events and competitions, however, represent only the tip of the iceberg. Incidence of ACL injuries, for instance, has been shown to rise significantly in populations at risk. When these and other preventable injuries are occurring in quantities that qualify them as serious public health issues, it is time to act! We in the field of sports medicine must raise public awareness of these problems, which are of great importance to the physical and psychosocial well-being of our young athletes in both professional and amateur arenas. The situation becomes especially vital when it comes to injury prevention in youth sports, where society's high duty of care has not been upheld in protecting our most precious and vulnerable citizens.

There has been a steady growth in major high-level international, continental, and global competitions for youth. Such competitions have stimulated lofty performance-oriented targets to which younger athletes can aspire. Sanctioned and overseen by various or individual international associations and federations, these events are seen as stepping stones in an athlete's development toward high-performance competitions. Unfortunately, there are no mechanisms currently in place that increase scientific knowledge of sports injuries and stimulate injury monitoring and prevention in this young population.

One example – doubtless again the tip of the iceberg – of youth sports injury may be seen in female gymnastics, one of the rare high-impact sports in which overuse injuries are as frequent if not more than acute injuries (O'Kane et al. 2011). There is a dearth of scientific literature on injuries in the sport of gymnastics. For those among us who have treated young gymnasts, the paucity of systematic injury surveillance and prevention programs in the field is surprising. We must therefore be vigilant to avoid compromising the future of young athletes not only in their development through higher levels of competition but more importantly their prospect of leading a healthy and pain-free life beyond sport. It is unacceptable that potentially preventable injury be the cause of reduced physical capacity later in life. Raising awareness of sports injuries within the greater community beyond sports and in the political arena in particular will have far-reaching benefits for citizens of all ages involved in physical activity.

The discussion has already begun, led by bodies such as the IOC and concerned members like His Royal Highness the Grand Duke Henri of Luxembourg. Curious about a visit by the former Minister of Sports to the Oslo Sports Trauma Research Centre, the Grand Duke was eager to learn more about the issue of sports injury rehabilitation and prevention. Following a tour of our newly created center in Luxembourg to gain a deeper insight into our clinical and research programs (Frisch et al. 2009; Malisoux et al. 2013), the Grand Duke determined to place current research and understanding of sports injuries onto the agenda of Luxembourg's official state visit to Norway (Fig. 1). This inclusion of sports medicine and specifically sports injuries on the agenda of an official state visit may have been a first and illustrates what easy steps can be taken by two small countries to raise awareness and initiate efforts to prevent the sports injury "epidemic" from growing. It also shows that in our roles as sports physicians and surgeons, we must not limit ourselves to

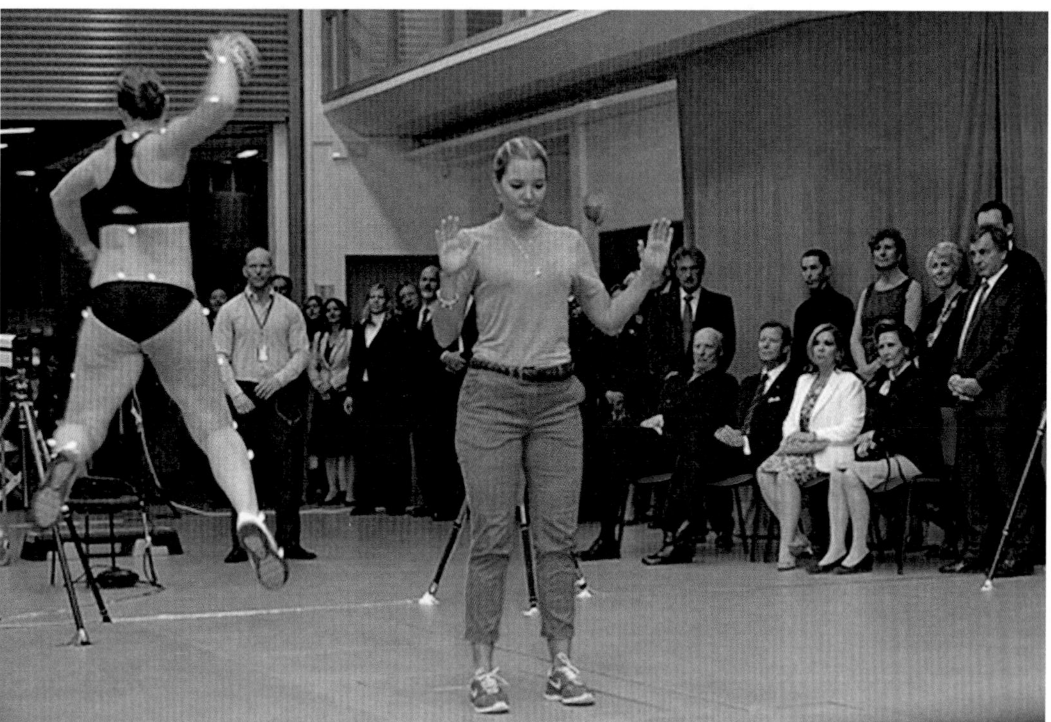

Fig. 1 Demonstration of an ACL injury prevention study with elite team handball players to the heads of state and political leaders of Luxembourg and Norway at the Oslo Sports Trauma Research Centre, Oslo, Norway in May 2011

"fixing" physical problems but become active more broadly in prevention through such professional collaboration and raising political awareness.

Therefore, gaining knowledge in the field of sports injuries, implementation of surveillance on a systematic basis, and promotion of prevention should become integral components of curricula not only in sports medicine and surgery but also in the field of sports science in general. In this regard, it is to the eminent credit of Professors Mahmut Nedim Doral and Jon Karlsson that this extensive new book catalogues the most current knowledge and up-to-date evolutions in the field of sports injury. This work of over 2,000 pages will doubtless become a milestone in orthopedic sports medicine.

Luxembourg

Romain Seil, M.D., Ph.D.
Jane Thornton, M.D., Ph.D.

References

Ekstrand J, Hägglund M, Kristenson K, Magnusson H, Waldén M (2013) Fewer ligament injuries but no preventive effect on muscle injuries and severe injuries: an 11-year follow-up of the UEFA Champions League injury study. Br J Sports Med 47:732–737

Flørenes TW, Nordsletten L, Heir S, Bahr R (2012) Injuries among World Cup ski and snowboard athletes. Scand J Med Sci Sports 22:58–66

Frisch A, Croisier JL, Urhausen A, Seil R, Theisen D (2009) Injuries, risk factors and prevention initiatives in youth sport. Br Med Bull 92:95–121

Junge A, Engebretsen L, Alonso JM, Renström P, Mountjoy M, Aubry M, Dvorak J (2008) Injury surveillance in multi-sport events: the International Olympic Committee approach. Br J Sports Med 42:413–421

Malisoux L, Frisch A, Urhausen A, Seil R, Theisen D (2013a) Injury incidence in a sports school during a 3-year follow-up. Knee Surg Sports Traumatol Arthrosc 21:2895–2900

Malisoux L, Frisch A, Urhausen A, Seil R, Theisen D (2013b) Monitoring of sport participation and injury risk in young athletes. J Sci Med Sport 16:504–508.

Myklebust G, Engebretsen L, Braekken IH, Skjølberg A, Olsen OE, Bahr R (2003) Prevention of anterior cruciate ligament injuries in female team handball players: a prospective intervention study over three seasons. Clin J Sport Med 13:71–78

O'Kane JW, Levy MR, Pietila KE, Caine DJ, Schiff MA (2011) Survey of injuries in Seattle area levels 4 to 10 female club gymnasts. Clin J Sport Med 21:486–492

Preface III

Sports medicine has made tremendous strides over the past years. This has largely been due to the renewed interest in exploring and replicating native anatomy. Take, for example, the anterior cruciate ligament (ACL); its two-bundle anatomy was described as early as 1836 by Dr. Weber Brothers in Gottingen, Germany. ACL reconstruction has been performed since the early 1900s. However, this involved mostly single-bundle reconstruction, and most techniques were rather nonanatomic. As early as 1938, Palmer proposed the idea of double-bundle reconstruction in his thesis on ACL reconstruction. However, the significance of his work was unfortunately not recognized until many years later.

In the 1980s came the transition to arthroscopic surgery. The goal was to reduce recovery time and avoid large incisions. Despite these good intentions, with the increased complexity of the procedure, the focus shifted away from anatomic reconstruction and moved toward standardized techniques to facilitate easier and more efficient graft placement. It was such techniques that led the field of sports medicine away from the teachings of Weber, Palmer, and their colleagues. Anatomy was no longer a priority.

Initially, the results of the early arthroscopic techniques were promising, but as long-term follow-up data became available, a high rate of early osteoarthritis after primary ACL reconstruction was seen. This was followed by three-dimensional imaging studies showing that these early arthroscopic techniques, although fast and efficient, failed to place the ACL graft in its anatomic location. Kinematic studies confirmed they indeed did not restore normal dynamic knee function.

These findings lead to a new movement of "going back to anatomy." Anatomic ACL reconstruction has since then gained incredible popularity. It changed the paradigm of ACL surgery and sports medicine as a whole. Anatomic ACL reconstruction restores the ACL to its native dimensions, collagen orientation, and insertion sites. The goal of *anatomic* ACL reconstruction is to replicate the knee's normal anatomy and restore its normal kinematics, all while protecting long-term knee health.

The same shift is being seen for many other procedures within orthopedic sports medicine. That is why this new book is so important. It presents the newest teachings by the leaders in our field. I commend Dr. Jon Karlsson and Dr. Mahmut Nedim Doral for putting this excellent book together.

Pittsburgh, PA, USA

Freddie H. Fu, M.D.

Distinguished Service Professor
David Silver Professor and Chairman
Division of Sports Medicine, Head Team Physician
Department of Athletics, Professor of
Physical Therapy, School of Health and
Rehabilitation Sciences, Professor of Health and
Physical Activity, School of Education
Professor of Mechanical Engineering &
Materials Science, Swanson School of Engineering
University of Pittsburgh School of Medicine and
University of Pittsburgh Medical Center

Past President, ISAKOS
(International Society of Arthroscopy
Knee Surgery and Orthopaedic Sports Medicine)

Past President, AOSSM
(American Orthopaedic Society for Sports Medicine)

Preface IV

In the past, there have been many textbooks written on sports-related injuries. However, the focus of these books was usually narrow, just focusing on the limited anatomy such as knees, upper extremities, or specific sports. Prof. Mahmut Nedim Doral and Prof. Jon Karlsson and their team created the second edition of *Sports Injuries* in a comprehensive and organized fashion covering all aspects of sports-related problems. In recent years, sports- and athletics-related problems became one of the most important and popular issues not only for athletes but also for all the population ranging from young to old generations because from infants to aged generations, almost all people at least to a certain extent are involved in athletic activities on a daily basis. In addition, therapeutically designed athletic training and rehabilitation for the disabled population also became to be known as an important issue for the general population. Epidemiological study clearly shows that sports-related injuries and problems are issues important to the entire medical care. On the basis of this issue, prevention of sports injuries and problems is very critical and is very well highlighted in this textbook. Also, highly advanced recent conservative and surgical treatment modalities are described in a timely fashion. Although sports-related problems and injuries did not draw attention until recently compared to the common orthopedic and surgical problems, it in fact started at the beginning of medicine by Hippocrates and his teacher Herodicus. Also, the issue of the dramatic increase of young physicians who became interested in sports-related problems and significant progress was seen in sports medicine–related issues in recent years. International Society of Arthroscopy, Knee and Orthopaedic Sports Medicine will celebrate its 20-year commemoration in the year 2015, and as a president of this society,

I would like to express my genuine respect to Prof. Doral, Prof. Karlsson, and all the authors who contributed to this state-of-the-art encyclopedic memorable book. I am sure that all the readers will enjoy reading this Bible-like textbook in sports medicine care.

Kobe, Japan Masahiro Kurosaka, M.D.

President of ISAKOS
(International Society of Arthroscopy
Knee and Orthopaedic Sports Medicine)

Professor and Chairman of Orthopaedic Surgery
Kobe University Graduate School of Medicine

Preface V

When I was asked to write a preface to this Second Edition, I was at the same time delighted and afraid.

Delighted, as it is always a great honour to be asked to write a preface. Afraid, because I am still wary of not being able to convey how good this whole endeavour is.

Prof. Mahmut Nedim Doral, Prof. Jon Karlsson, and their team have worked jolly hard at bettering what was already a great product. If it was ever possible, here comes the tangible truth: over 250 chapters, great authors from all the continents, and up-to-date easy-to-digest clinically relevant information. A ponderous opus, bearing witness to the work of love necessary for the careful planning and the long gestation necessary to select the topics, identify the right authors, and 'oblige' them to give their best.

It is often said that good surgeons know how to operate, better surgeons know when to operate, and outstanding surgeons know when not to operate. In this edition, much has been dedicated to the prevention of sports injuries. This, I believe, is the future, especially given the present and foreseeable conditions of healthcare even in the developed world, where cost containment and value for money are becoming an ever-pervading mantra.

Common conditions are common, and they deserve much space. Nevertheless, the book makes sure that the less-known issues which we come to face are adequately represented and that balanced opinions are given. I believe that this gives a truly global approach to sports traumatology and makes me think of this as the reference benchmark textbook for both trainees and specialists.

I can only look forward to the next edition: Knowing the editors, I am sure that they are already thinking about it!

Salerno, Italy

Nicola Maffulli, M.D., M.S., Ph.D.,
FRCP, FRCS(Orth), FFSEM

Professor of Musculoskeletal Disorders
Consultant Trauma and Orthopaedic Surgeon
University of Salerno Medical School, Salerno, Italy

Honorary Professor of Sport and Exercise Medicine
Queen Mary University of London
Barts and the London School of Medicine and
Dentistry, London, England

President, International Muscles
Ligaments and Tendons Society

Contents

Volume 1

Volume 2

Volume 3

About the Editors

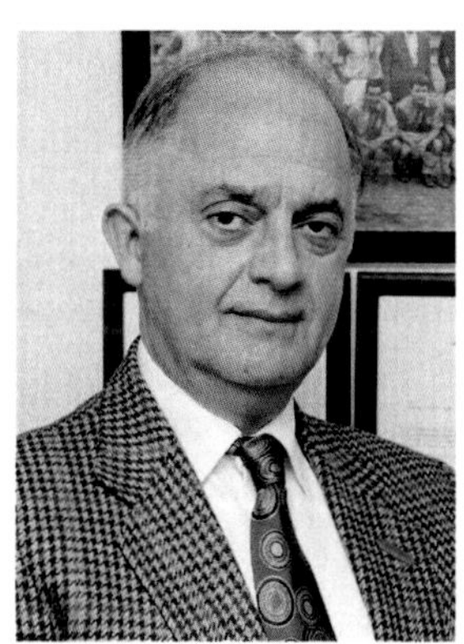

Prof. Mahmut Nedim Doral
Chief of the Department of Orthopaedics and Traumatology, Founding Chief of the Department of Sports Medicine
Hacettepe University
Istanbul
Turkey

Prof. Mahmut Nedim Doral, M.D., is internationally recognized for his expertise in orthopedic sports medicine. He has authored over 150 scientific articles in peer-reviewed journals and over 15 book chapters in internationally published books; he also acts as a referee for four national and five international journals. His last book, *Sports Injuries: Prevention, Diagnosis, Treatment and Rehabilitation*, was published by Springer in 2011. For over 30 years, Dr. Doral's major research interests have been in sports injuries and rehabilitation, arthroscopic and endoscopic surgery, basic science research in tendon injuries, and knee arthroplasty.

He is the chairman of the Department of Orthopaedics and Traumatology and the Department of Sports Medicine at the Hacettepe University Medical School.

Dr. Doral is the medical chief and health system organizer of Galatasaray Sports Club Youth Teams.

He has been the director of the Hacettepe University Sports Medicine Center since 1995. He has been board member (2003–2009), program committee member (2004–2012), and membership committee chairman (2007–2011) of the International Society of Arthroscopy, Knee Surgery & Orthopaedic Sports Medicine (ISAKOS). He is also a past member of the scientific committee of European Society of Sports Traumatology Knee Surgery and Arthroscopy (ESSKA). He currently serves in the Executive Council of the Turkish National Olympic Committee; as executive committee chair of and newsletter editor at the Asia Pacific Orthopaedic Associations; and also as newsletter editor at the European Federation of Orthopaedic Sports Traumatology (EFOST).

Dr. Doral served as president of the Turkish Society of Orthopaedics & Traumatology (TOTBID) (2010–2011). He was the past president of EFOST

(2000–2003), Asia-Pacific Knee Society (APKS/Knee Section of APOA) (2004–2006), and the Turkish Society of Sports Traumatology, Arthroscopy and Knee Surgery (2002–2004), and past chief of the Medical Committee Turkish Federation of National Basketball Team. He is the founder and past president of the Turkish Society of Sports Traumatology. He was honored as distinguished visiting professor by the University of Pittsburgh School of Engineering in 2006 and Kentucky University in 2009.

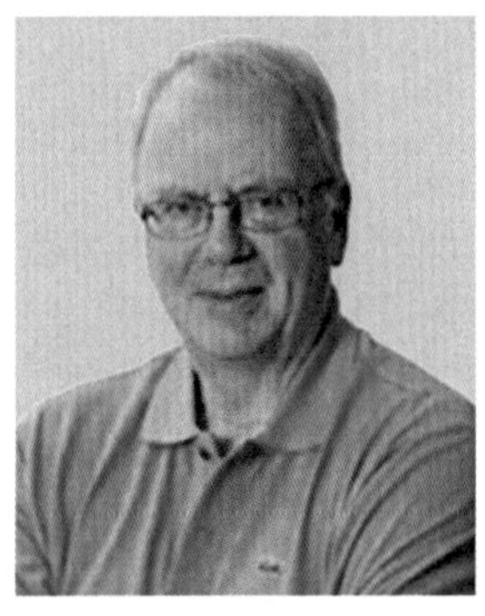

Prof. Jon Karlsson
Professor, Academic Head
Department of Orthopaedics
Sahlgrenska Academy, University of Gothenburg
Sahlgrenska University Hospital
Gothenburg
Sweden

Prof. Jon Karlsson, M.D., Ph.D., was born in Iceland, where he graduated from the medical school in Reykjavik in 1978 and moved to Gothenburg, Sweden, in 1981. He defended his Ph.D. thesis on "Chronic Lateral Ankle Instability" at the Gothenburg University in 1989 and was appointed associate professor in 1990. He has been senior consultant in the Orthopaedic Department of the Sahlgrenska University Hospital since 1991 and clinical head during 1997–2001. Since 2001, Dr. Karlsson has been the academic head at the Sahlgrenska Academy. In that capacity, he mentored 32 Ph.D. theses and was appointed chief of the orthopedic research laboratory. He is author of more than 300 peer-reviewed papers and 26 books on orthopedics and sports traumatology. He was appointed professor of orthopedics and sports traumatology in 1998. He was president of the Swedish Association of Sports Medicine in 1999–2001.

Since 2008, Dr. Karlsson has been editor-in-chief of *KSSTA* (*Knee Surgery, Sports Traumatology, Arthroscopy*), the official journal of the European Society of Sports Traumatology Knee Surgery and Arthroscopy (ESSKA). He has been program chairman of the biannual ESSKA congress for 2006, 2008, and 2010 and board member of the International Society of Arthroscopy, Knee Surgery & Orthopaedic Sports Medicine (ISAKOS) since 2005. He is currently secretary of the ISAKOS Executive Board.

Active in sports, Dr. Karlsson played basketball and is currently the caretaking physician of the Swedish soccer team IFK Gothenburg.

Co-Editors

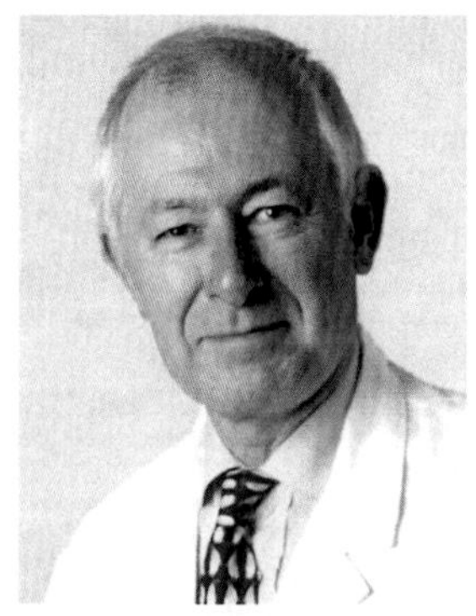

René Verdonk Faculty of Medicine, Ghent State University, Ghent, Belgium

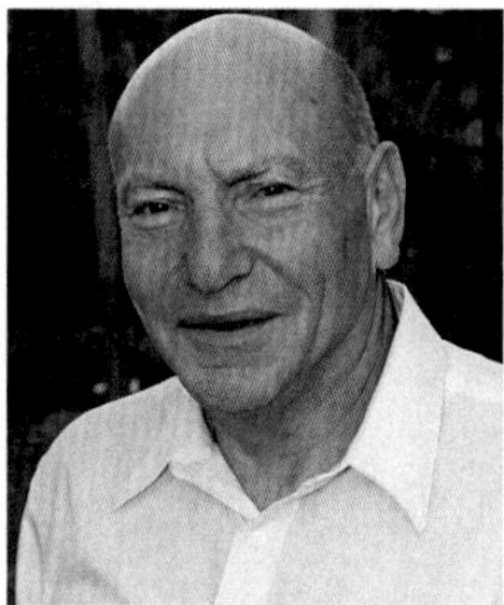

Gideon Mann Service of Sports Injuries, Department of Orthopaedic Surgery, Meir Medical Centre, Tel Aviv University, Tel Aviv, Israel

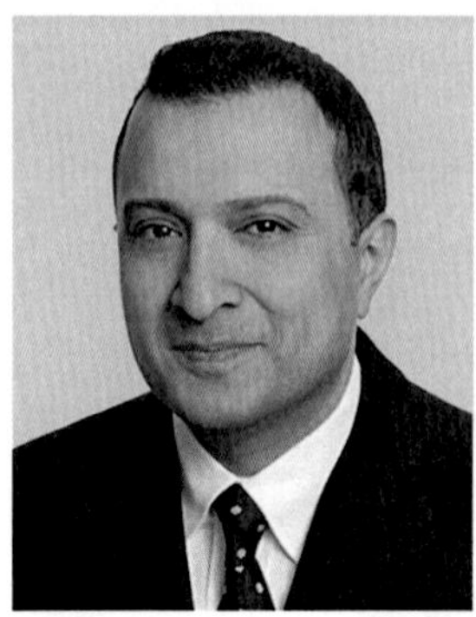

Kivanc Israel Atesok Institute of Medical Science, University of Toronto, Toronto, ON, Canada

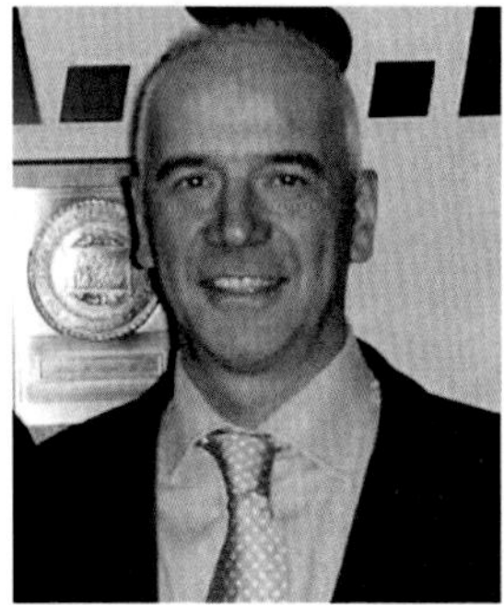

Alberto Gobbi Orthopaedic Arthroscopic Surgery International (O.A.S.I.) Bioresearch Foundation, Gobbi Onlus, Milan, Italy

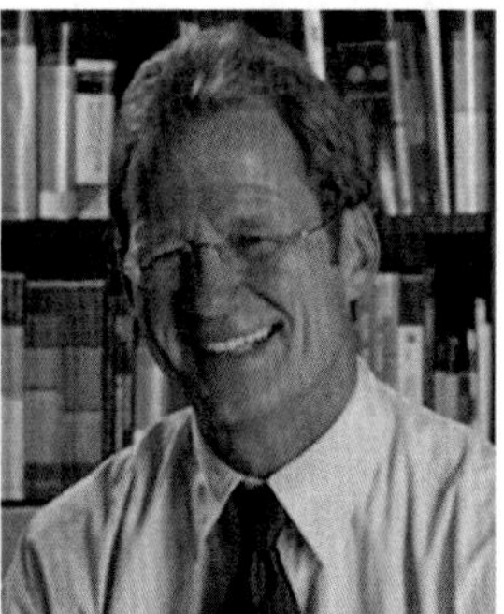

Andreas B. Imhoff Department of Orthopaedic Sports Medicine, Klinikum rechts der Isar, Technical University of Munich, Munich, Germany

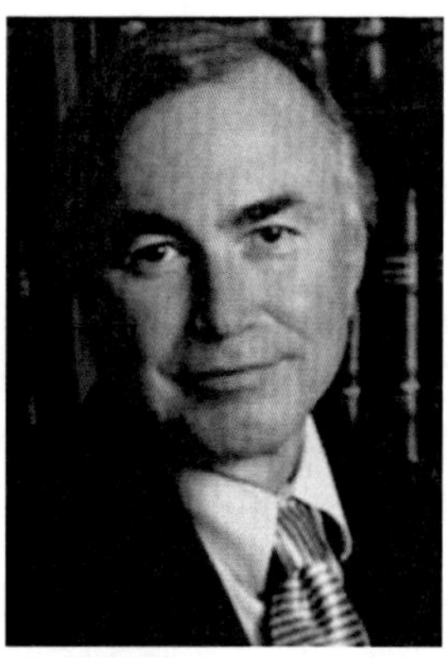

Philippe Neyret Centre Albert Trillat, Service de Chirurgie Orthopédique, Hôpital de la Croix-Rousse, University of Lyon, Lyon, France

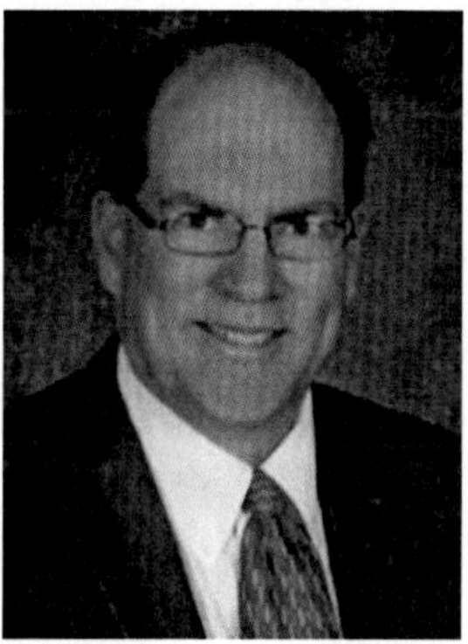

John Nyland Kosair Charities College of Health and Natural Sciences, Spalding University, Louisville, USA

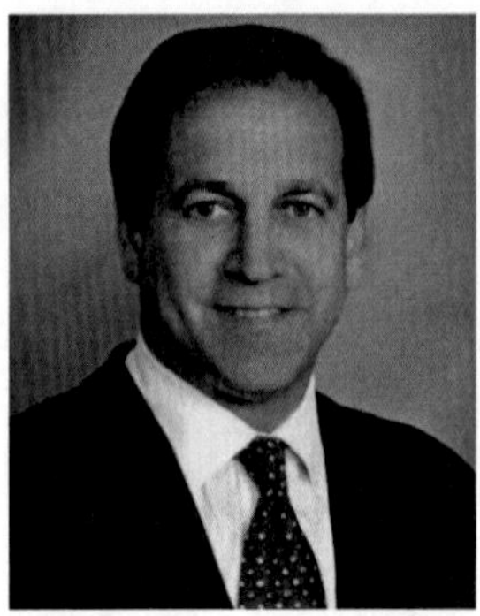

Kevin D. Plancher Orthopaedic Foundation for Active Lifestyles, Stamford, CT, USA

Plancher Orthopaedics and Sports Medicine, New York, NY, USA

Department of Orthopaedic Surgery, Albert Einstein College of Medicine, New York, NY, USA

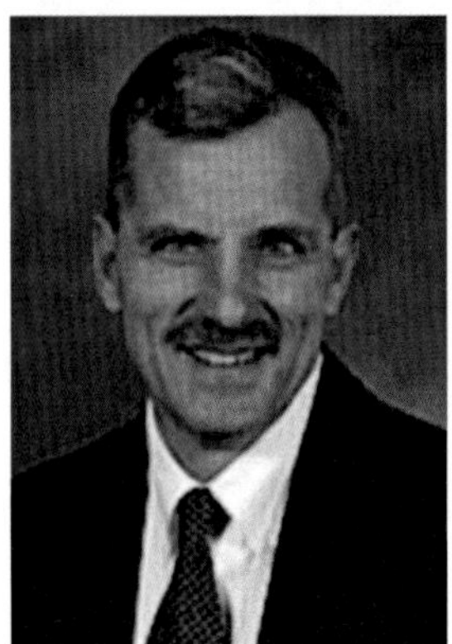

Edward M. Wojtys Department of Orthopaedic Surgery, MedSport, University of Michigan, Ann Arbor, MI, USA

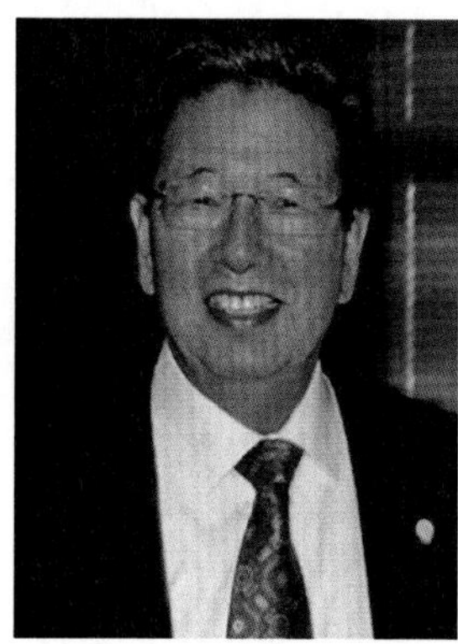

Savio L.-Y. Woo Department of Bioengineering, Musculoskeletal Research Center, Swanson School of Engineering, University of Pittsburgh, Pittsburgh, PA, USA

Executive Assistant Editor

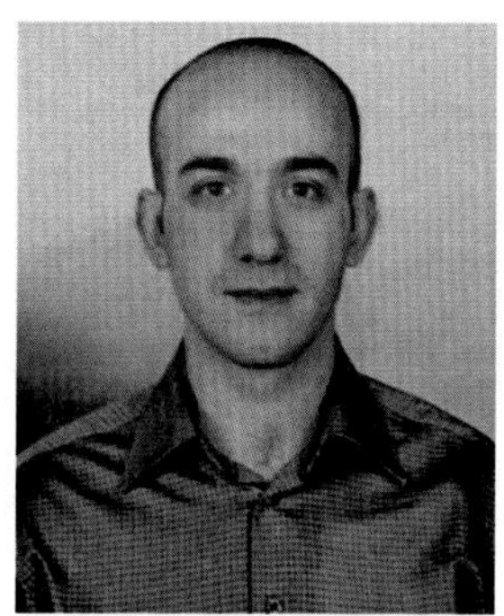

Gürhan Dönmez Faculty of Medicine, Department of Sport Medicine, Hacettepe University School of Medicine, Ankara, Sihhiye, Turkey

Assistant Editors

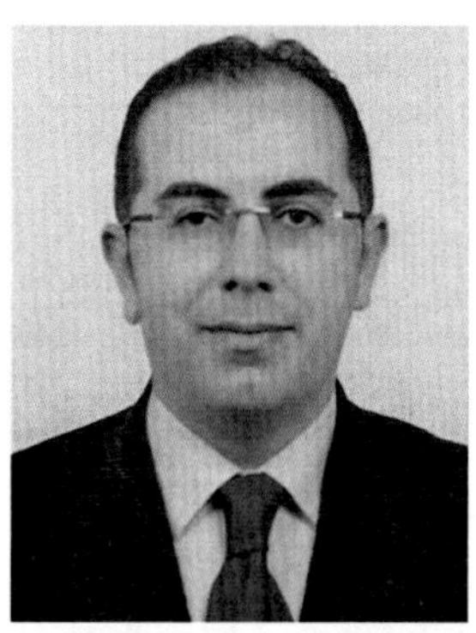

Onur Bilge Department of Orthopaedics and Traumatology, and Department of Sports Medicine, Konya NE University, Meram School of Medicine, Konya, Turkey

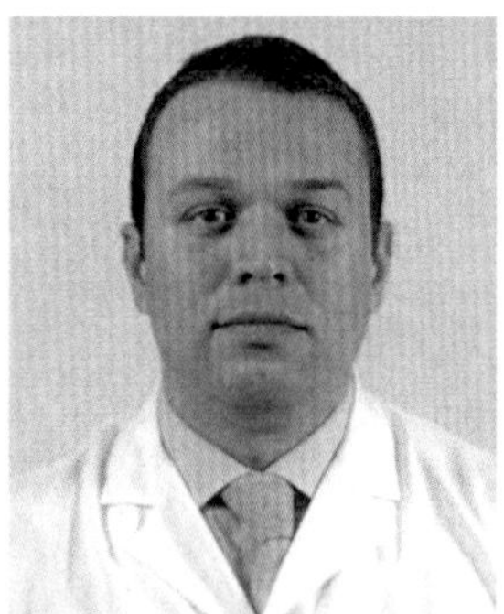

Murat Demirel Department of Orthopaedics and Traumatology, Bayındır Hospital, Ankara, Turkey

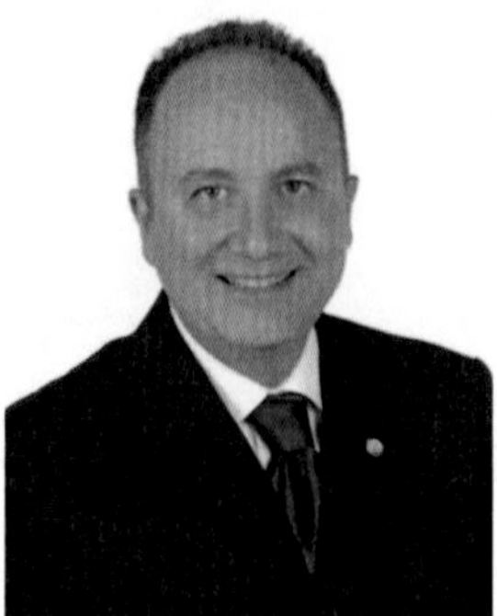

Nurettin Heybeli Department of Orthopaedic Surgery and Traumatology, Trakya University School of Medicine, Kanuni Sultan Suleyman Education and Research Hospital, Edirne, Turkey

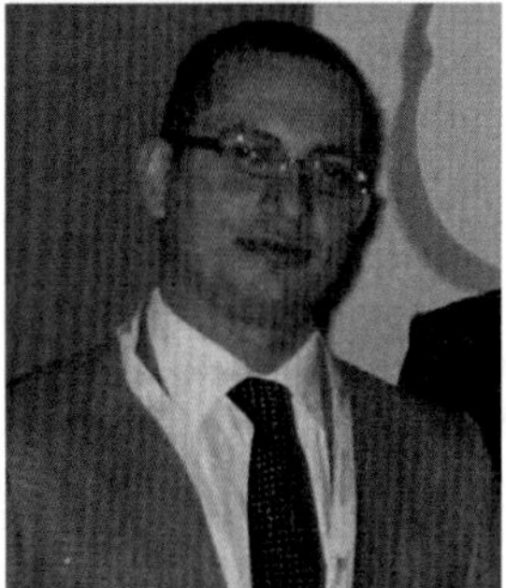

Gazi Huri Department of Orthopaedics and Traumatology, Hacettepe University, Ankara, Turkey

Division of Shoulder Surgery, Department of Orthopaedic Surgery, Johns Hopkins University, Baltimore, MD, USA

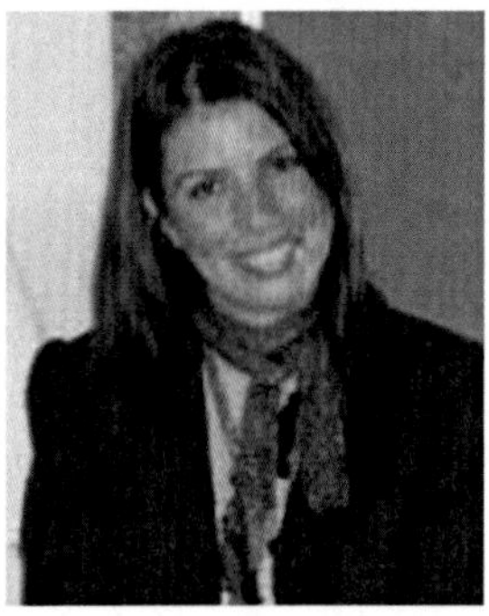

Defne Kaya Department of Physical Therapy and Rehabilitation, Faculty of Health Science, Biruni University, İstanbul, Turkey

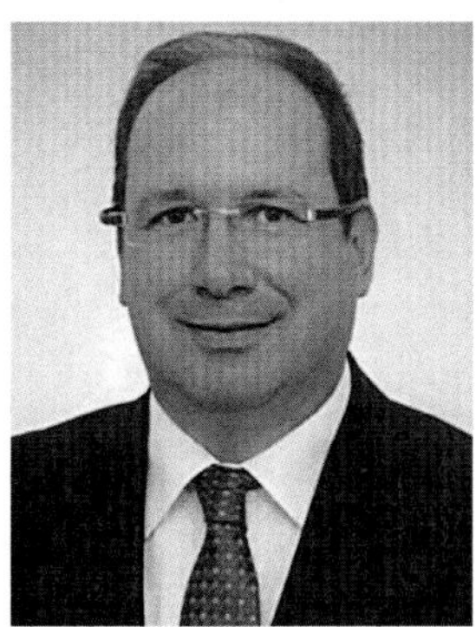

Feza Korkusuz Department of Sports Medicine, Faculty of Medicine, Hacettepe University School of Medicine, Ankara, Turkey

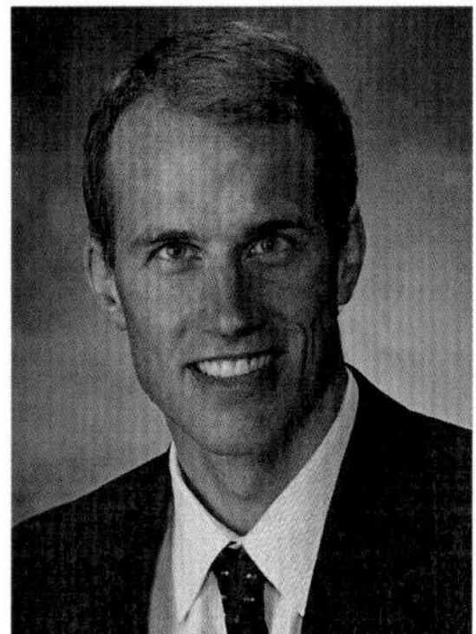

Volker Musahl Department of Orthopaedic Surgery, University of Pittsburgh Medical Center, Pittsburgh, PA, USA

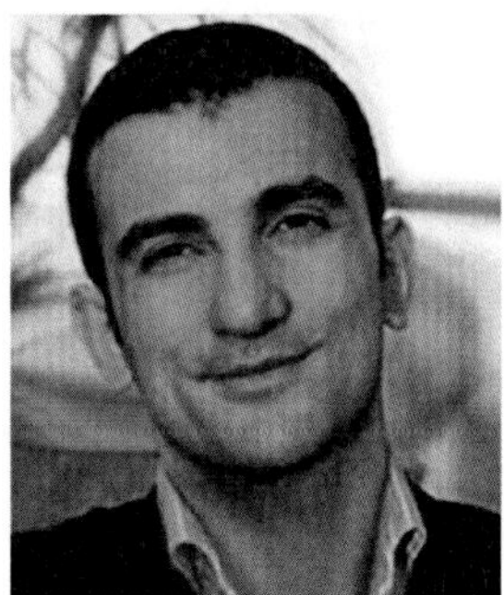

Kristian Samuelsson Department of Orthopaedics, Institute of Clinical Sciences, The Sahlgrenska Academy, University of Gothenburg, Göteborg, Sweden

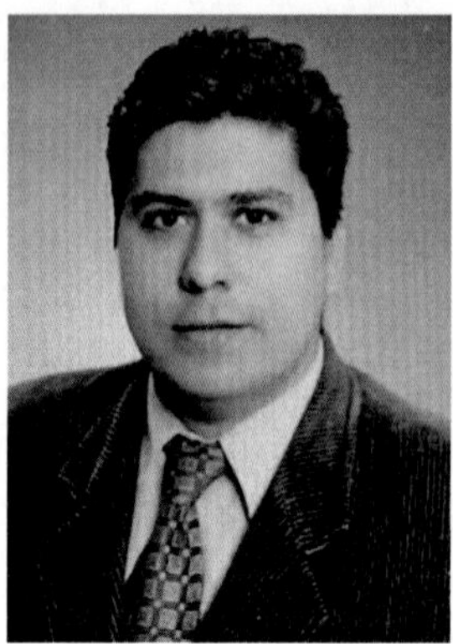

Egemen Turhan Faculty of Medicine, Department of Orthopaedics and Traumatology, Hacettepe University School of Medicine, Ankara, Sihhiye, Turkey

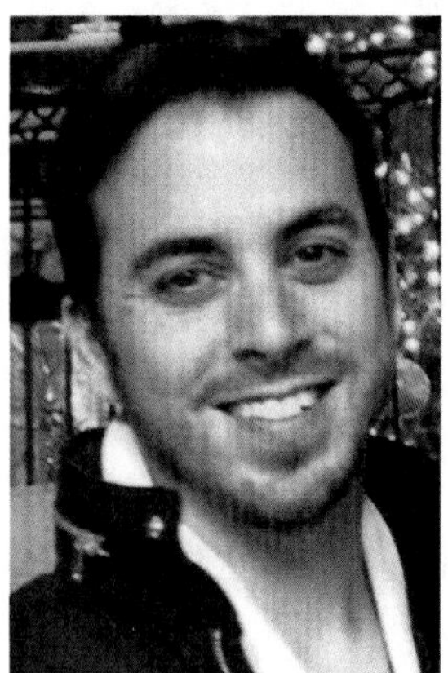

Cosku Turhan Sony Pictures Imageworks, Los Angeles, CA, USA

Section Editors

Part I: Introduction

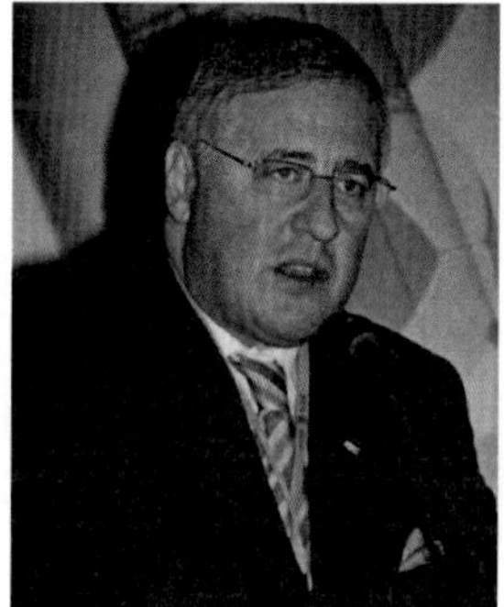

Jose Huylebroek Sports Medicine Department, Clin Parc Leopold, Brussels, Belgium

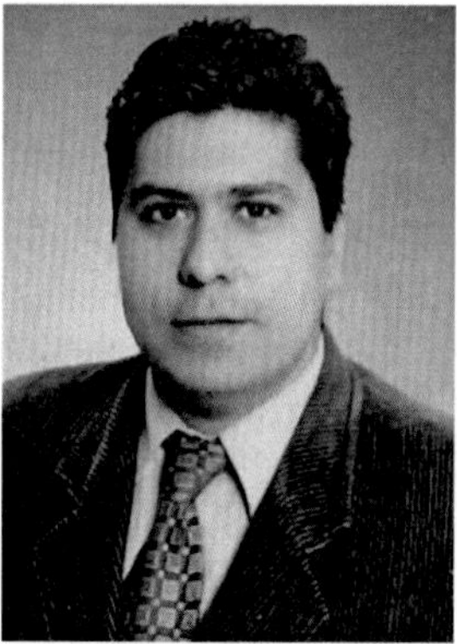

Egemen Turhan Faculty of Medicine, Department of Orthopaedics and Traumatology, Hacettepe University School of Medicine, Ankara, Sihhiye, Turkey

Part II: Shoulder Injuries

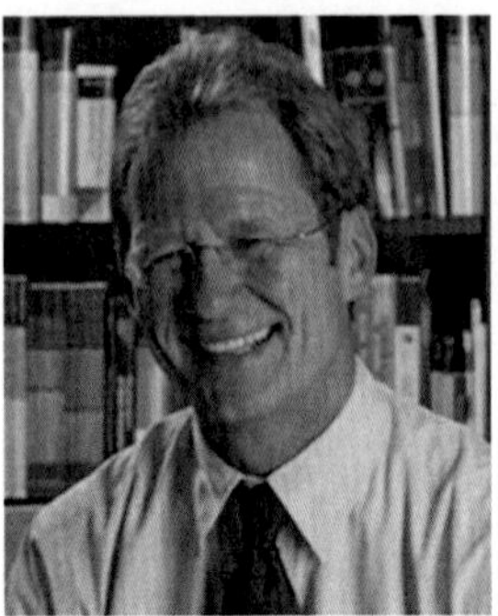

Andreas B. Imhoff Department of Orthopaedic Sports Medicine, Klinikum rechts der Isar, Technical University of Munich, Munich, Germany

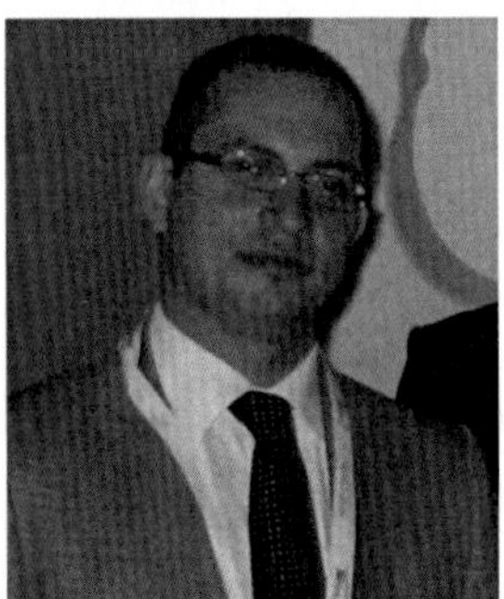

Gazi Huri Department of Orthopaedics and Traumatology, Hacettepe University, Ankara, Turkey

Division of Shoulder Surgery, Department of Orthopaedic Surgery, Johns Hopkins University, Baltimore, MD, USA

Part III: Elbow and Wrist Injuries

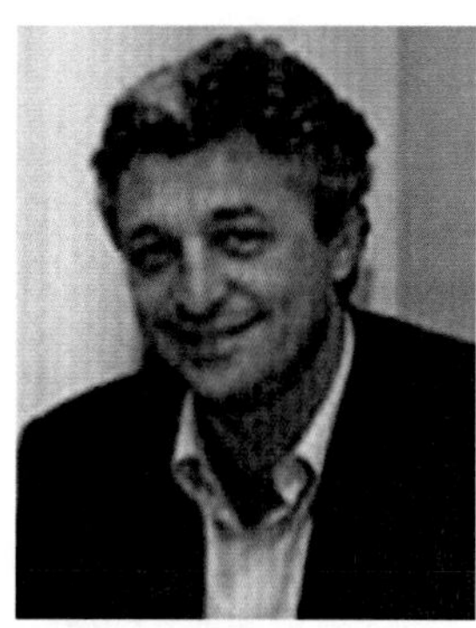

Luigi Adriano Pederzini Orthopaedic and Arthroscopic Department, New Sassuolo Hospital, Sassuolo, Modena, Italy

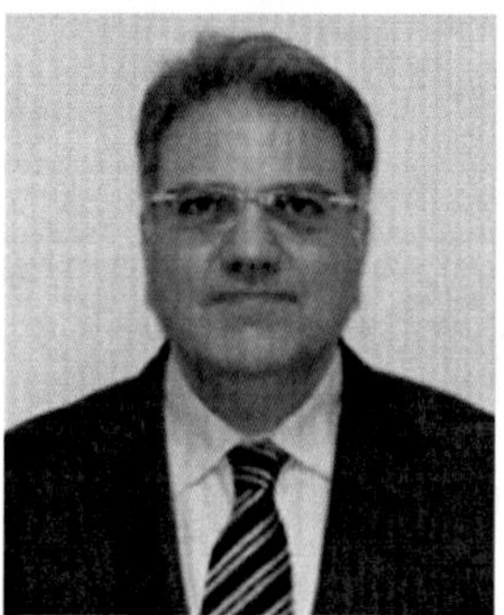

Gürsel Leblebicioğlu Faculty of Medicine, Department of Orthopaedics and Traumatology, Hacettepe University, Ankara, Turkey

Part IV: Groin and Hip Injuries

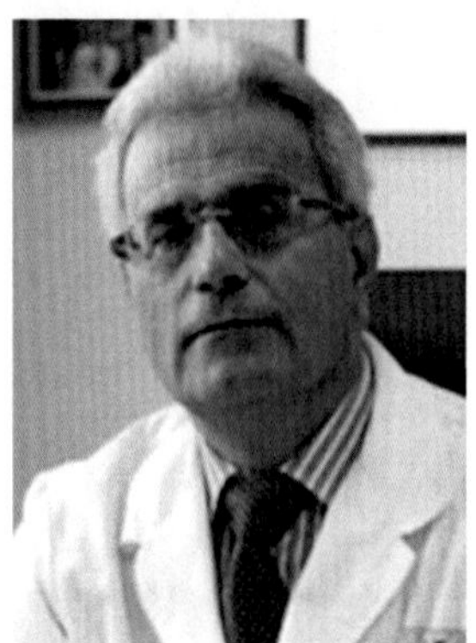

Ramón Cugat Mutualidad de Futbolistas, Real Federacion Espanola de Futbol, Barcelona, Spain

Garcia Cugat Foundation & CEU Cardenal Herrera University, Alfara del Patriarca, Valencia, Spain

Department of Orthopaedic Surgery, Sports Medicine and Trauma, Hospital Quiron Barcelona, Artroscopia gc, S.L., Barcelona, Spain

Facultad de Medicina, Universitat Internacional de Catalunya, Barcelona, Spain

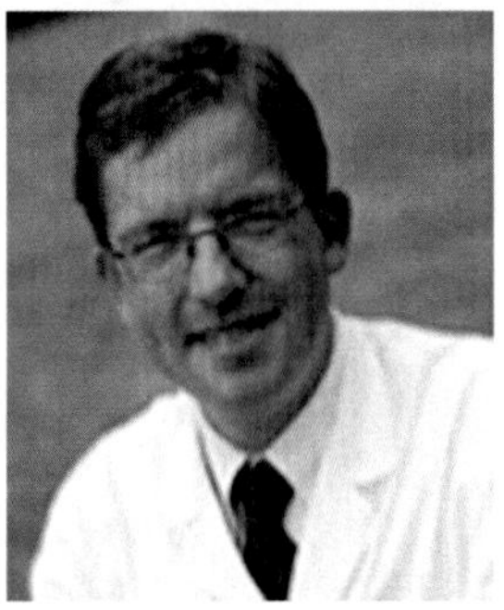

Karl F. Almqvist Department of Orthopaedic Surgery, Ghent University Hospital, Gent, Belgium

Part V: Knee Injuries

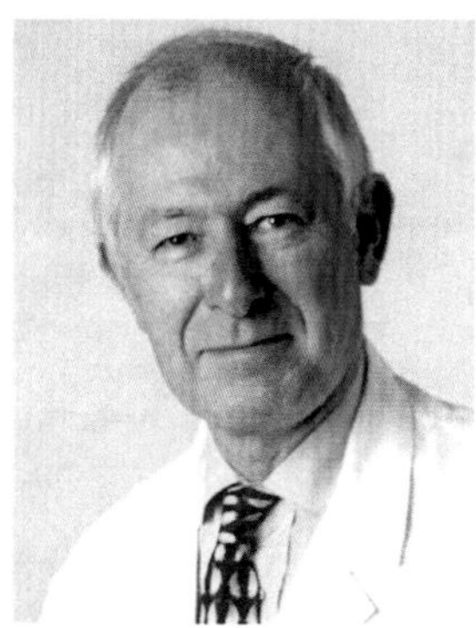

René Verdonk Faculty of Medicine, Ghent State University, Ghent, Belgium

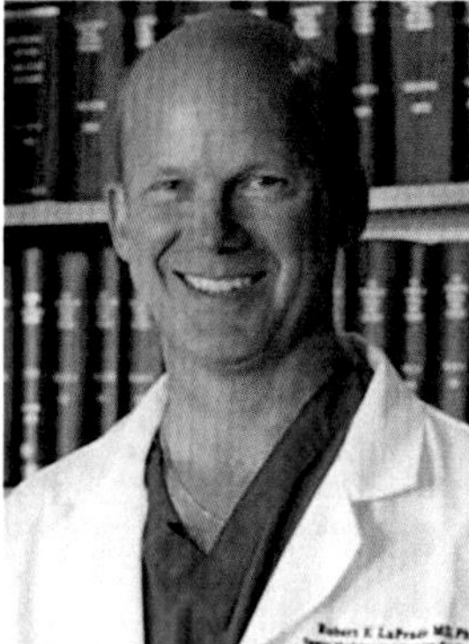

Robert F. LaPrade The Steadman Clinic and Steadman Philippon Research Institute, Vail, CO, USA

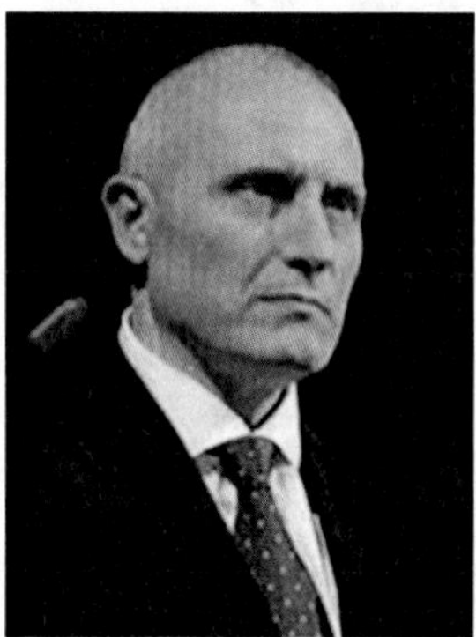

Stefano Zaffagnini Clinica Ortopedica e Traumatologica II, Laboratorio di Biomeccanica e Innovazione Tecnologica, Università di Bologna, Bologna, Italy

Part VI: Ankle Injuries

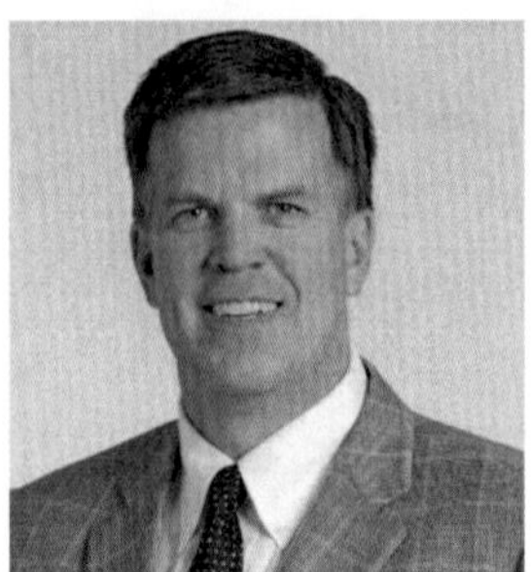

Brian G. Donley Center for Foot and Ankle Surgery, Orthopaedic Surgery, Lutheran Hospital, Cleveland, OH, USA

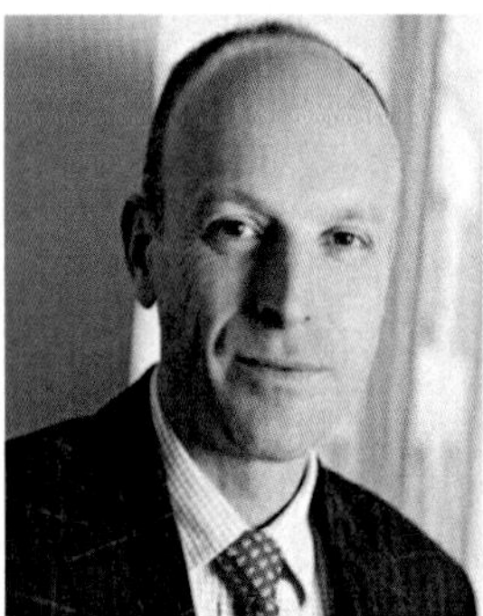

James D. Calder Department of Trauma and Orthopaedic Surgery, The Fortius Clinic, and Chelsea and Westminster Hospital, London, UK

Part VII: Cartilage Pathologies

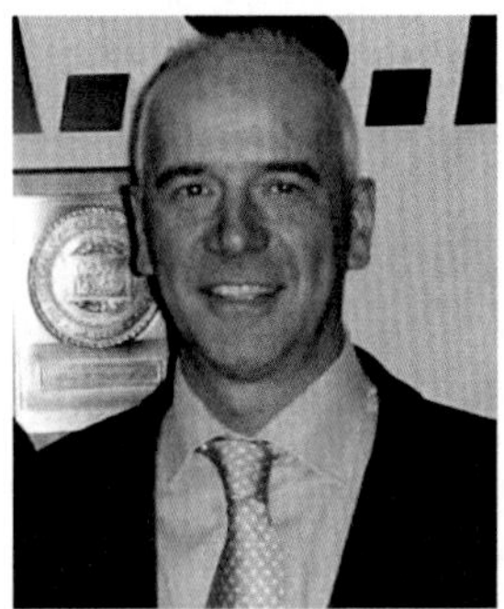

Alberto Gobbi Orthopaedic Arthroscopic Surgery International (O.A.S.I.) Bioresearch Foundation, Gobbi Onlus, Milan, Italy

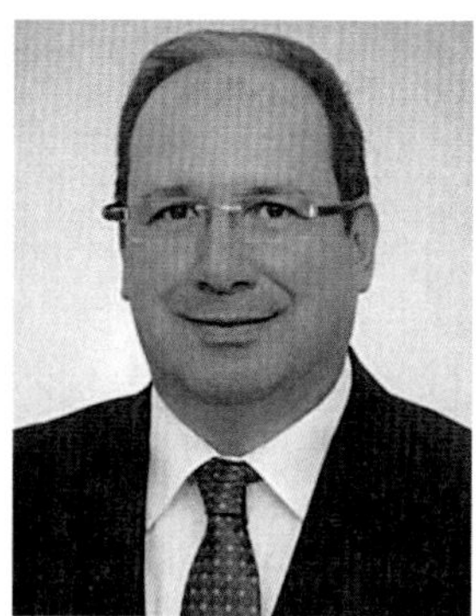

Feza Korkusuz Department of Sports Medicine, Faculty of Medicine, Hacettepe University School of Medicine, Ankara, Turkey

Part VIII: Stress Fractures

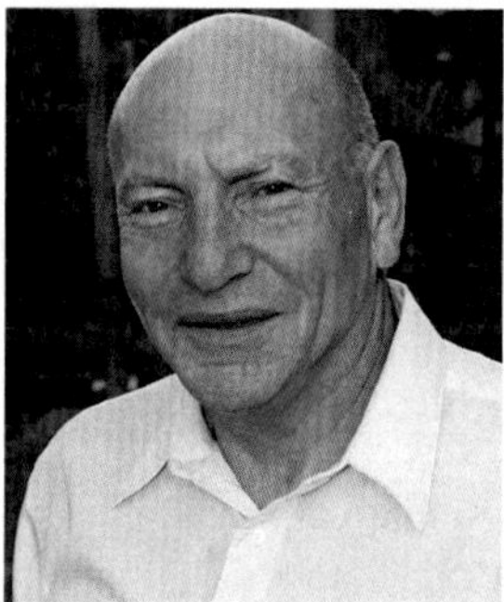

Gideon Mann Service of Sports Injuries, Department of Orthopaedic Surgery, Meir Medical Centre, Tel Aviv University, Tel Aviv, Israel

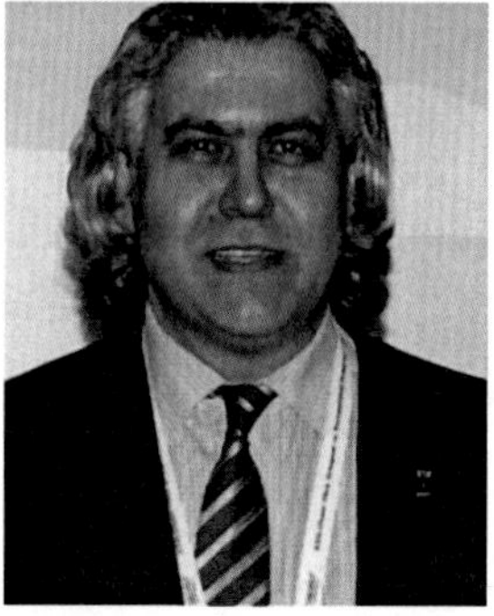

Mehmet Arazi Department of Orthopaedic Surgery and Traumatology, Farabi Klinik, Konya, Turkey

Part IX: Muscle and Tendon Injuries

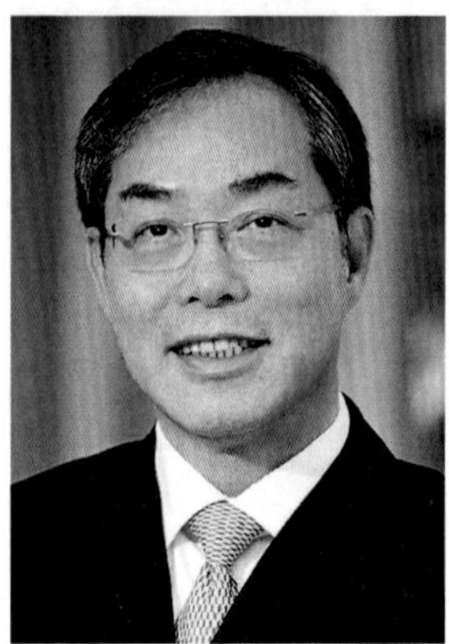

Kai-Ming Chan Department of Orthopaedics and Traumatology, The Chinese University of Hong Kong, Prince of Wales Hospital, Shatin, Hong Kong

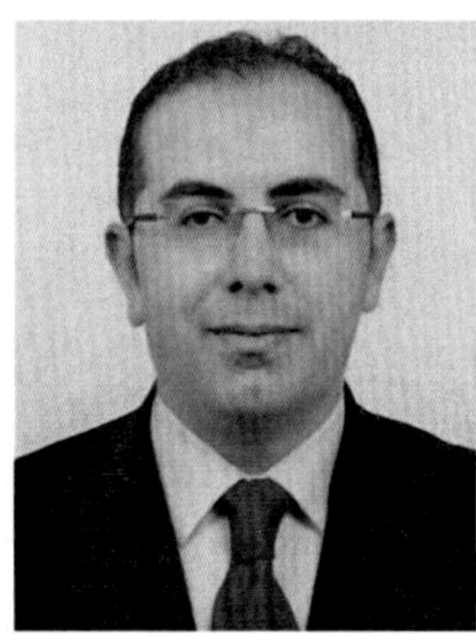

Onur Bilge Department of Orthopaedics and Traumatology, and Department of Sports Medicine, Konya NE University, Meram School of Medicine, Konya, Turkey

Part X: Osteoarthritis and Sports/Arthroplasty

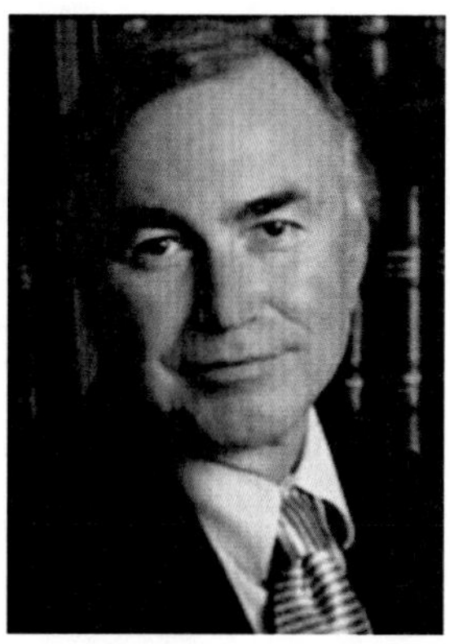

Philippe Neyret Centre Albert Trillat, Service de Chirurgie Orthopédique, Hôpital de la Croix-Rousse, University of Lyon, Lyon, France

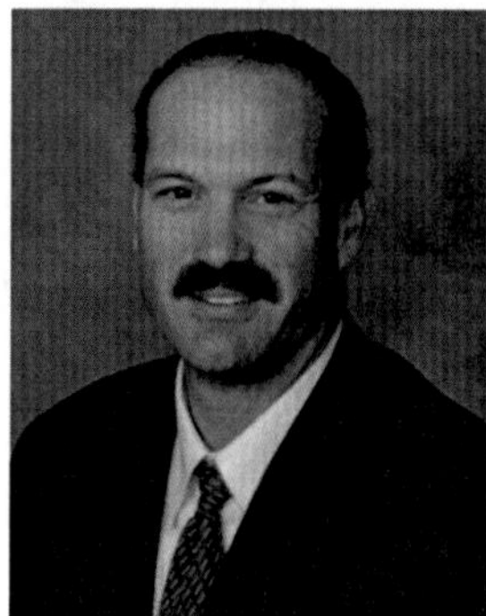

Michael D. Ries Tahoe Fracture and Orthopaedic Clinic, Carson City, NV, USA

University of California, Berkeley, Berkeley, CA, USA

Department of Orthopaedic Surgery, University of California, San Francisco, San Francisco, CA, USA

Part XI: Pediatric Sports Injuries

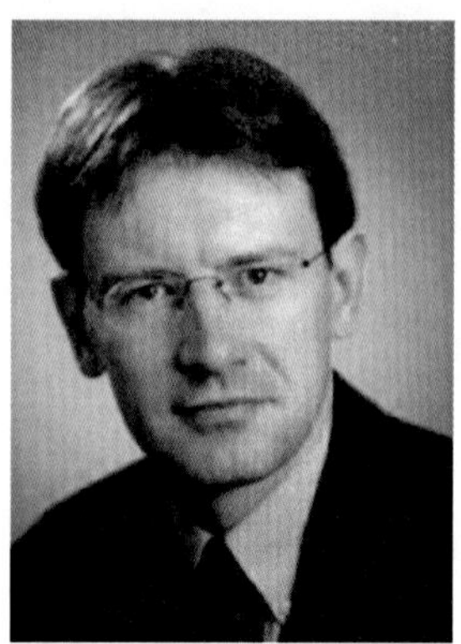

Romain Seil European Society of Sports Traumatology, Knee Surgery and Arthroscopy (ESSKA); Département de l'Appareil Locomoteur, Centre Hospitalier de Luxembourg, Clinique d' Eich; Luxembourg Olympic Medical Center, and Sports Medicine Research Laboratory, CRP-Santé, Strassen, Luxembourg

Orthopaedic Surgery, University of Saarland, Homburg/Saar, Germany

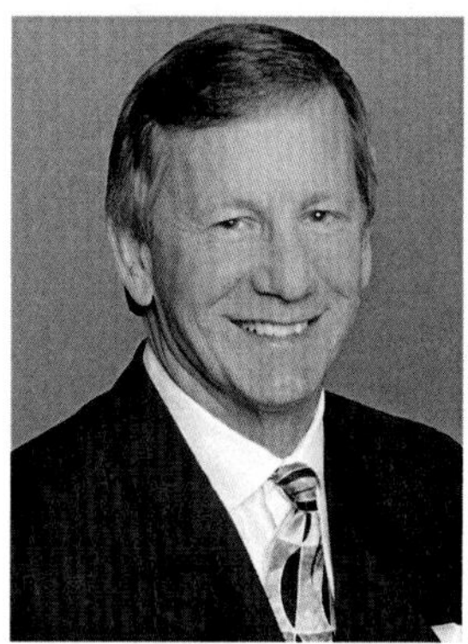

Allen F. Anderson Tennessee Orthopaedic Alliance, Nashville, TN, USA

Part XII: Sport-Specific Injuries

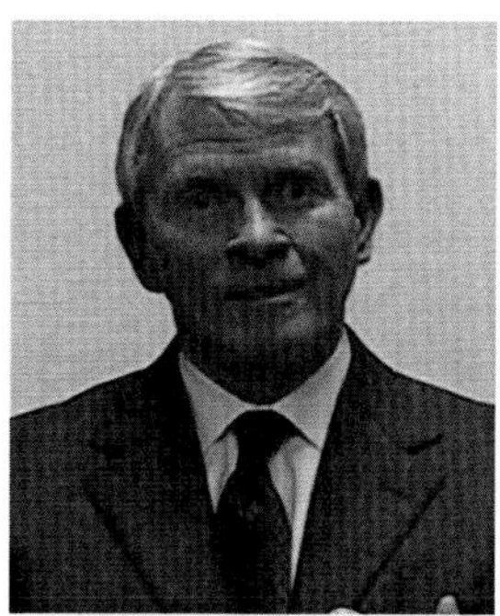

Terry L. Whipple American Self, Plastic Surgery and Orthopaedics, PLC, and Orthopaedic Research of Virginia, Richmond, VA, USA

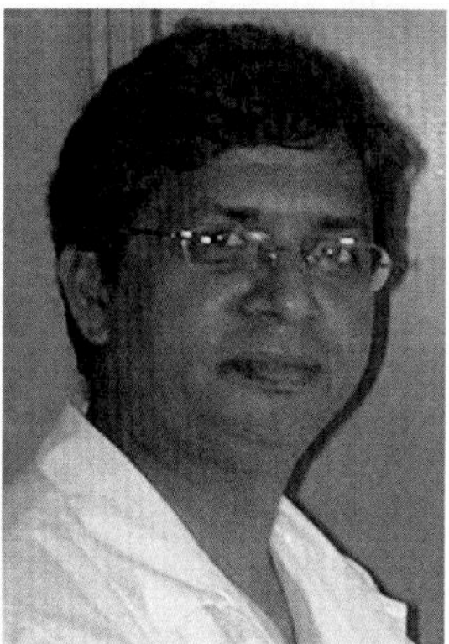

Chakra Raj Pandey Department of Orthopaedics and Traumatology, Grande International Hospital and Medicare National Hospital and Research Centre, Kathmandu, Nepal

Part XIII: Extreme Sports and Motorsport Injuries

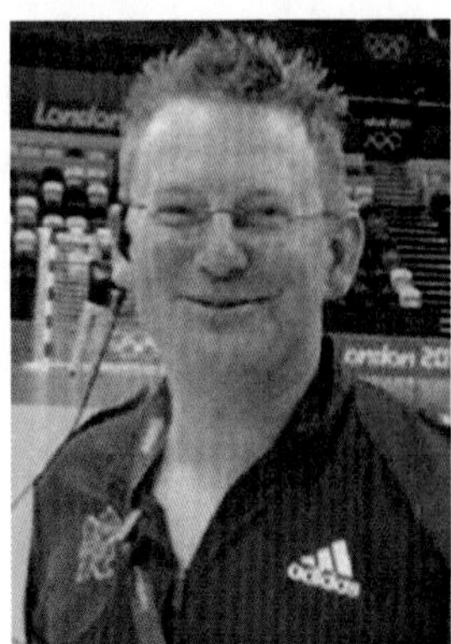

Michael R. Carmont The Princess Royal Hospital, Shrewsbury and Telford NHS Trust, Telford, United Kingdom

Northern General Hospital, Sheffield Teaching Hospitals NHS Foundation Trust, Sheffield, United Kingdom

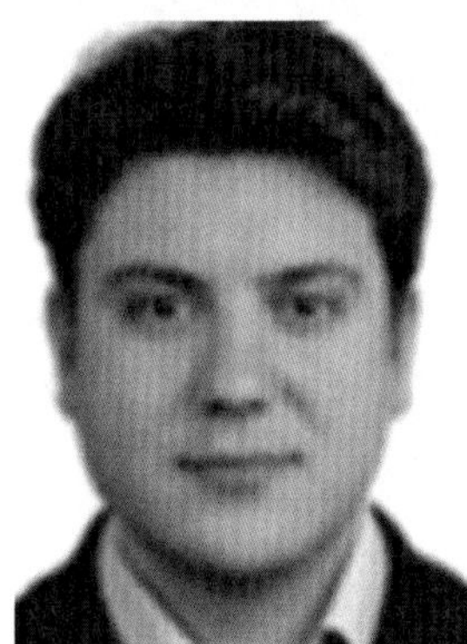

Fatih Küçükdurmaz Department of Orthopaedics and Traumatology, Bezmialem Vakif University, Istanbul, Turkey

Part XIV: The Field of Play and Pitchside Management of Sports Emergencies

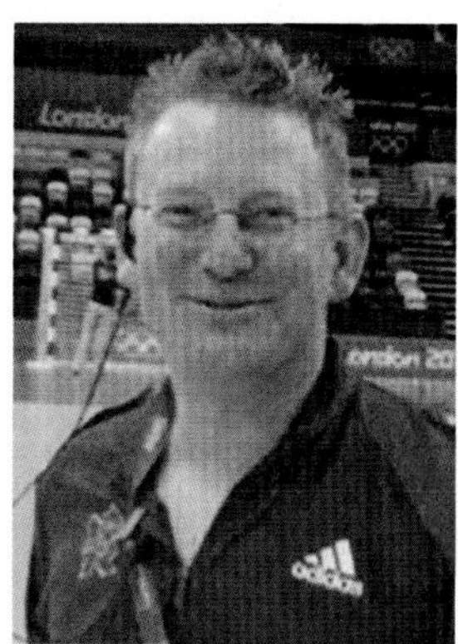

Michael R. Carmont The Princess Royal Hospital, Shrewsbury and Telford NHS Trust, Telford, United Kingdom

Northern General Hospital, Sheffield Teaching Hospitals NHS Foundation Trust, Sheffield, United Kingdom

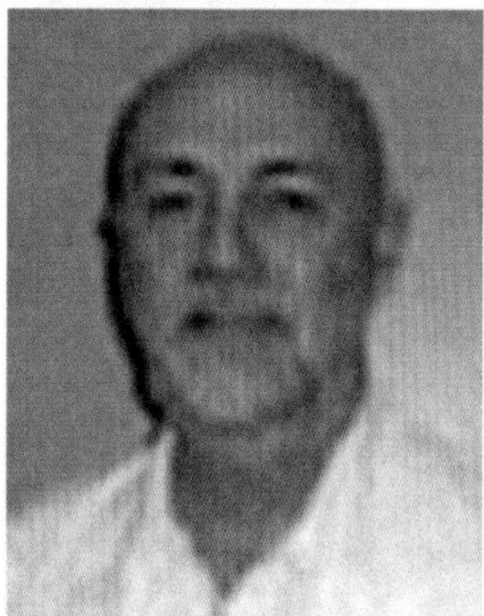

David McDonagh The Princess Royal Hospital, Shrewsbury and Telford NHS Trust, Telford, United Kingdom

Northern General Hospital, Sheffield Teaching Hospitals NHS Foundation Trust, Sheffield, United Kingdom

Department of Emergency Medicine, University Hospital Trondheim, Trondheim, Norway

Medical Commission Fédération Internationale de Bobsleigh et de Tobogganing (FIBT), OSKP, St. Olavs Hospital, Trondheim, Norway

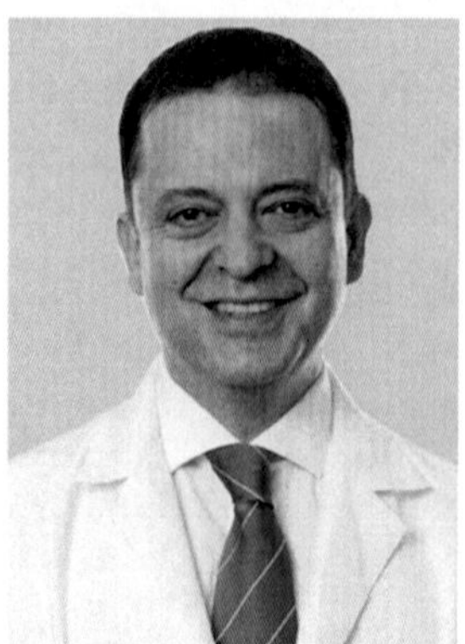

Ahmet Alanay Department of Orthopaedics and Traumatology, Acibadem University Faculty of Medicine, Acibadem Comprehensive Spine Center, Acibadem Maslak Hospital, Maslak, Istanbul, Turkey

Part XV: Future of Sports Traumatology

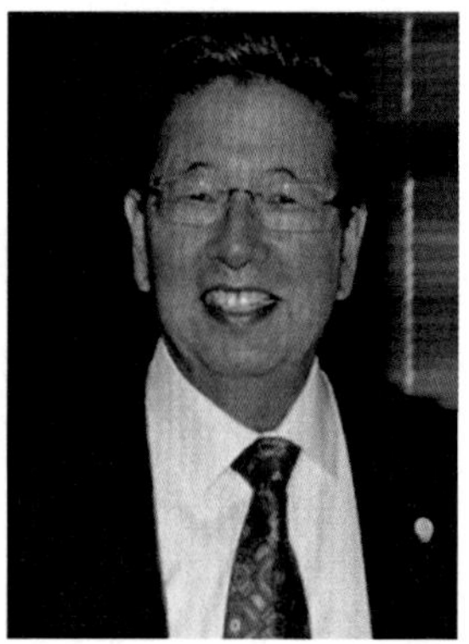

Savio L.-Y. Woo Department of Bioengineering, Musculoskeletal Research Center, Swanson School of Engineering, University of Pittsburgh, Pittsburgh, PA, USA

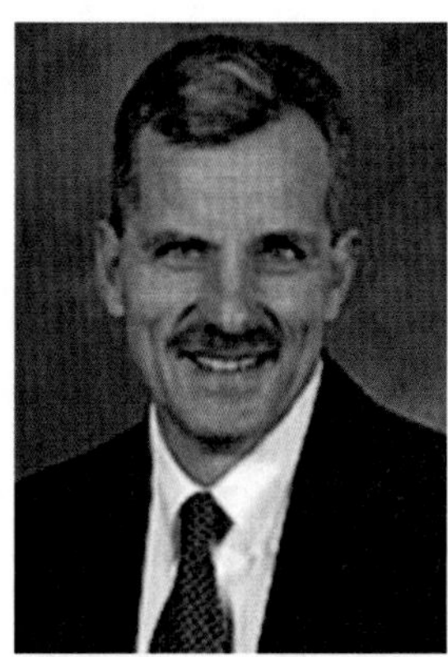

Edward M. Wojtys Department of Orthopaedic Surgery, MedSport, University of Michigan, Ann Arbor, MI, USA

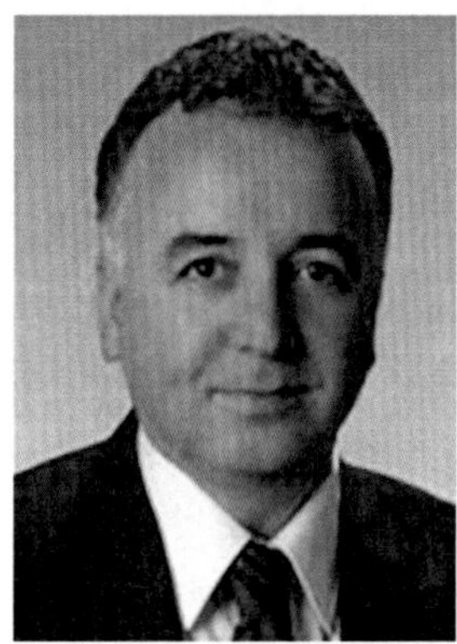

Mehmet Aşık Department of Orthopaedics and Traumatology, Faculty of Capa, Istanbul University, Istanbul, Turkey

Part XVI: Industry and Orthopedic Sports Medicine

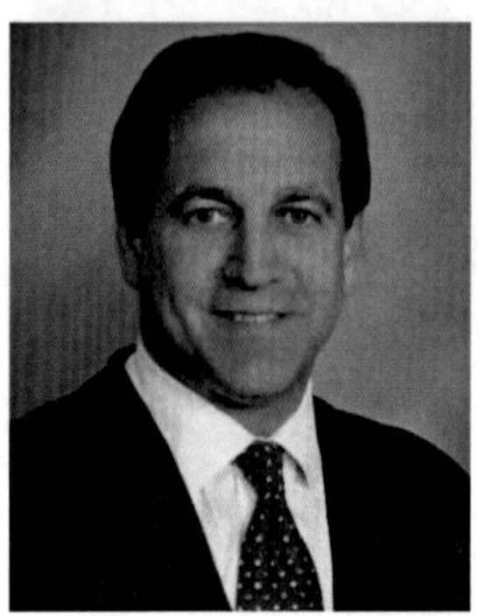

Kevin D. Plancher Orthopaedic Foundation for Active Lifestyles, Stamford, CT, USA

Plancher Orthopaedics and Sports Medicine, New York, NY, USA

Department of Orthopaedic Surgery, Albert Einstein College of Medicine, New York, NY, USA

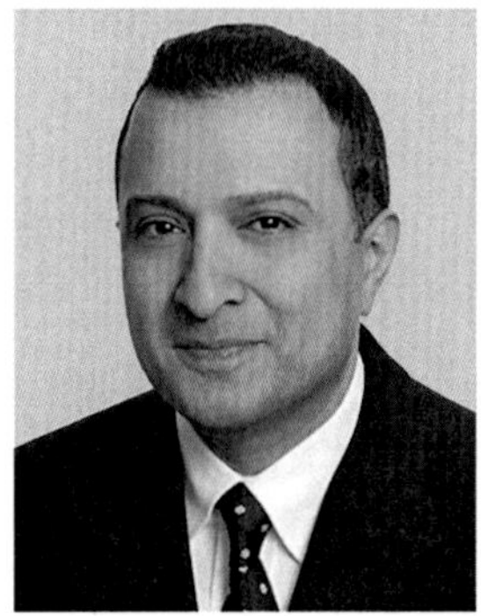

Kivanc Israel Atesok Institute of Medical Science, University of Toronto, Toronto, ON, Canada

Part XVII: Miscellaneous

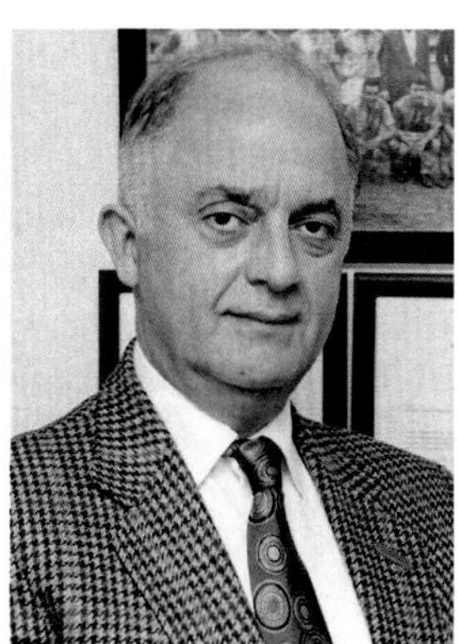

Mahmut Nedim Doral Department of Orthopaedics and Traumatology and Department of Sports Medicine, Hacettepe University, Istanbul, Turkey

Contributors

Emrah Açan Department of Orthopedic Surgery, Dokuz Eylül University, İzmir, İnciraltı, Turkey

Paul W. Ackermann Karolinska Institute, Department of Molecular Medicine and Surgery, Karolinska University Hospital, Stockholm, Sweden

Sait Ada Orthopaedics and Traumatology, EMOT Hospital, İzmir, Turkey

Grzegorz Adamczyk Department of Orthopedics, Centrum Medyczne Gamma, Warsaw, Poland

Filon Aganthagelidis Blue Cross, Euromedica Clinic, Orthopaedic Department, Thessaloniki, Greece

Olcay Akdeniz Department of Orthopedic Surgery, Dokuz Eylül University, İzmir, İnciraltı, Turkey

Ibrahim Akkawi Istituto Ortopedico Rizzoli, Bologna, Italy

Bülent Aksoy Bahçeşehir University, Istanbul, Turkey

Mehmet Cemalettin Aksoy Faculty of Medicine, Department of Orthopedics and Traumatology, Sihhiye, Ankara, Turkey

Kemal Aktuğlu Department of Orthopaedics Surgery and Traumatology, Ege University Hospital, Izmir, Turkey

Ahmet Alanay Department of Orthopaedics and Traumatology, Acibadem University Faculty of Medicine, Acibadem Comprehensive Spine Center, Acibadem Maslak Hospital, Maslak, Istanbul, Turkey

Eduard Alentorn-Geli Department of Orthopaedic Surgery and Traumatology, Parc de Salut Mar, Hospital del Mar & Hospital de l'Esperança, Universitat Autonoma de Barcelona (UAB), Barcelona, Spain

Erkan Alkan Department of Orthopaedics and Traumatology, Hacettepe University, Ankara, Turkey

Karl F. Almqvist Department of Orthopaedic Surgery, Ghent University Hospital, Gent, Belgium

Faik Altintas Orthopaedics and Traumatology Department, Yeditepe Medical Faculty, Kozyatagi, Istanbul, Turkey

Pedro Álvarez Chair of Medicine and Regenerative Surgery, Garcia Cugat Foundation & CEU Cardenal Herrera University, Alfara del Patriarca, Valencia, Spain

Facultad de Medicina y Ciencias de la Salud, Universitat Internacional de Catalunya, Barcelona, Spain

Mutualidad de Futbolistas, Real Federacion Espanola de Futbol, Barcelona, Spain

Department of Orthopaedic Surgery, Sports Medicine and Trauma, Hospital Quiron Barcelona, Artroscopia gc, S.L., Barcelona, Spain

Facultad de Medicina, Universitat Internacional de Catalunya, Barcelona, Spain

Jeffrey Alwine Plancher Orthopaedics and Sports Medicine, New York, NY, USA

Orthopaedic Foundation, Stamford, CT, USA

Konstantinos Anagnostakos Department of Orthopedic Surgery, Saarland University, Homburg (Saar), SL, Germany

Georgoulis D. Anastasios Department of Trauma and Orthopaedic Surgery, University of Ioannina, Ioannina, Greece

Daniel Andernord Vårdcentralen Gripen, Karlstad, Sweden

Primary Care Research Unit, County Council of Värmland, Karlstad, Sweden

Department of Orthopaedics, Institute of Clinical Sciences, The Sahlgrenska Academy, University of Gothenburg, Göteborg, Sweden

Colin J. Anderson Department of Orthopedic Surgery, School of Medicine, University of Colorado, Aurora, CO, USA

Nihal Apaydin Department of Anatomy, Ankara University Medicine Faculty, Sihhiye, Ankara, Turkey

Paulo Araujo Department of Biomechanics, Medicine and Rehabilitation of Locomotor System – Ribeirao Preto Medical School – São Paulo University, Brazil, São Paulo, Brazil

Mehmet Arazi Department of Orthopaedic Surgery and Traumatology, Farabi Klinik, Konya, Turkey

Elizabeth A. Arendt Department of Orthopaedic Surgery, University of Minnesota, Minneapolis, MN, USA

Oscar Ares Chair of Medicine and Regenerative Surgery, Garcia Cugat Foundation & CEU Cardenal Herrera University, Alfara del Patriarca, Valencia, Spain

Department of Orthopaedic Surgery, Sports Medicine and Trauma, Hospital Quiron Barcelona, Artroscopia gc, S.L., Barcelona, Spain

Facultad de Medicina, Universitat Internacional de Catalunya, Barcelona, Spain

Orthopaedic Surgery and Trauma, Hospital Clínic de Barcelona, Barcelona, Spain

Serdar Arıtan Biomechanics Research Group, Faculty of Sport Sciences, Hacettepe University, Ankara, Turkey

Asbjørn Årøen Oslo Sports Trauma Research Center, The Norwegian School of Sport Sciences, Oslo, Norway

Department of Orthopaedic Surgery, Akershus University Hospital, Lørenskog, Norway

Claudio Ascani Orthopaedics and Traumatology, Azienda Sanitaria Roma C, Rome, Italy

Mehmet Aşik Department of Orthopaedics and Traumatology, Faculty of Capa, Istanbul University, Istanbul, Turkey

Carl M. Askling The Swedish School of Sport and Health Sciences and the Section of Orthopaedics and Sports Medicine, Department of Molecular Medicine and Surgery, Karolinska Institutet, GIH, Stockholm, Sweden

Ata Can Atalar Department of Orthopaedics and Traumatology, Istanbul University, Istanbul Medical Faculty, Fatih, Istanbul, Turkey

Erdoğan Atasoy Department of Surgery, Kleinert Kutz and Associates Hand Care Center, University of Louisville School of Medicine, Louisville, KY, USA

Özgür Ahmet Atay Faculty of Medicine, Department of Orthopaedics and Traumatology, Hacettepe University, Ankara, Sihhiye, Turkey

Filiz Ateş Biomedical Engineering Institute, Boğaziçi University, Çengelköy, Istanbul, Turkey

Kivanc Israel Atesok Institute of Medical Science, University of Toronto, Toronto, ON, Canada

Etobicoke, ON, Canada

Aravind Athiviraham The Joseph Barnhart Department of Orthopaedic Surgery, Baylor College of Medicine, Houston, TX, USA

Halil Murat Aydın BMT Calsis Health Technologies Co., Sarayköy, Ankara, Turkey

Environmental Engineering Department & Bioengineering Division and Center for Bioengineering, Hacettepe University, Ankara, Turkey

Sedat Tolga Aydoğ Sports Medicine Center, Acibadem Fulya Hospital, İstanbul, Turkey

Egemen Ayhan Orthopaedics and Traumatology Department, Liv Hospital, Istanbul, Turkey

Selim Ayhan Department of Neurosurgery, Malatya State Hospital, Malatya, Turkey

Ülkü Aypar Department of Anesthesiology and Reanimation, Hacettepe University School of Medicine, Ankara, Sihhiye, Turkey

Mehmet Ayvaz Faculty of Medicine, Department of Orthopedics and Traumatology, Hacettepe University, Ankara, Sihhiye, Turkey

Klaus Bak Department of Orthopaedic Surgery, Division of Shoulder and Elbow Surgery, Copenhagen University Herlev, Herlev, Denmark

Emin Bal Orthopaedics and Traumatology, EMOT Hospital, İzmir, Turkey

J. R. Ballesteros Departamento de Anatomía y Embriología Humana. Facultad de Medicina., Universidad de Barcelona, Barcelona, Spain

Servicio de Cirugía Ortopédica y Traumatología, Hospital Clínic de Barcelona, Barcelona, Spain

Adad Baranto Department of Orthopaedics, Institute of Clinical Sciences at the Sahlgrenska Academy, University of Gothenburg and Sahlgrenska University Hospital, Gothenburg, Sweden

A. Barg Orthopaedic Department, University Hospital Basel, Basel, Switzerland

Wael Barsoum Department Orthopedic Surgery & Sports Health, Cleveland Clinic Foundation, Garfield Heights, OH, USA

Güray Batmaz Department of Orthopadics and Traumatology, Hacettepe University, Ankara, Sihhiye, Turkey

Cem Bayram Nanotechnology and Nanomedicine Division, Hacettepe University, Institute of Graduate Studies in Science, Ankara, Turkey

Alp Bayramoglu Faculty of Medicine, Department of Anatomy, Acibadem University School of Medicine,

Philippe Beaufils Orthopaedic Department, Versailles Hospital, Le Chesnay, France

Christoph Becher Department of Orthopedic Surgery, Hannover Medical School, Hannover, Germany

Roland Becker Klinik für Orthopädie und Unfallchirurgie, Städtische Klinikum Brandenburg, Hochstrasse, Brandenburg an der Havel, Germany

Knut Beitzel Department of Orthopaedic Sports Medicine, Technical University Munich, Munich, Germany

Şenol Bekmez Department of Orthopaedics and Traumatology, Dr. Sami Ulus Training and Research Hospital, Ankara, Altindag, Turkey

Joseph Bellapianta Orthopaedic Foundation, Stamford, CT, USA

Plancher Orthopaedics and Sports Medicine, New York, NY, USA

Francesco Benazzo Clinica Ortopedica e Traumatologica, Fondazione IRCCS Policlinico San Matteo di Pavia, Università degli Studi di Pavia, Pavia, Italy

Mark A. Bergin University of Pittsburgh, Pittsburgh, PA, USA

Graziano Bettelli Shoulder and Elbow Unit, Istituto Ortopedico Rizzoli, Bologna, Italy

Clayton C. Bettin Department of Orthopaedic Surgery and Biomedical Engineering, University of Tennessee – Campbell Clinic, Memphis, TN, USA

Tahsin Beyzadeoglu Orthopaedics and Traumatology, Beyzadeoglu Sports Medicine Clinic, Istanbul, Turkey

Physiotherapy and Rehabilitation, Halic University, Istanbul, Turkey

Mohit Bhandari Division of Orthopaedic Surgery, McMaster University, Hamilton, ON, Canada

Elcil Kaya Bicer Faculty of Medicine, Department of Orthopedics and Traumatology, University of Ege, Bornova, Izmir, Turkey

Roland M. Biedert Orthopedics & Sport Traumatology, Sportclinic Villa Linde AG, Swiss Olympic Medical Center Magglingen-Biel, Biel, Switzerland

F. Erkal Bilen Head of Shoulder and Elbow Unit, Orthopaedic Surgery, Istanbul Memorial Hospital, Istanbul, Marmara, Turkey

Onur Bilge Department of Orthopaedics and Traumatology, and Department of Sports Medicine, Konya NE University, Meram School of Medicine, Konya, Turkey

Tommaso Bonaninga II Clinica Ortopedica e Traumatologica, Istituto Ortopedico Rizzoli, Bologna, Italy

Michel Bonnin Centre Orthopédique Santy, Lyon, France

Mats Börjesson Astrand laboratory, Swedish School of Sports and Health Sciences (GIH), Stockholm, Sweden

Department of Cardiology, Karolinska University Hospital, Stockholm, Sweden

Itamar Botser Orthopedic Sports Medicine, Stanford Sports Medicine, Stanford University, Redwood City, CA, USA

Achilleas Boutsiadis Stavroupoli Thessaloniki, Greece

David J. Bozentka University of Pennsylvania, Philadelphia, PA, USA

Murat Bozkurt Department of Orthopaedics and Traumatology, Yildirium Beyazit University, Faculty of Medicine, Ankara, Turkey

Department of Orthopedics and Traumatology, Ankara Atatürk Training and Research Hospital, Ankara, Turkey

Daniel N. Bracey Department of Orthopaedic Surgery, Wake Forest School of Medicine, Medical Center Boulevard, Winston–Salem, NC, USA

Molecular Medicine and Translational Science Program, Medical Center Boulevard, Wake Forest University, Winston–Salem, NC, USA

Jefferson Brand Fellowship-Trained Sports Medicine Specialist, Heartland Orthopedic Specialists, Alexandria, MN, USA

Sepp Braun Department of Orthopaedic Sports Medicine, Klinikum rechts der Isar, Technical University of Munich, Munich, Germany

Jonathan T. Bravman Department of Orthopaedics, Division of Sports Medicine and Shoulder Surgery, University of Colorado, Aurora, CO, USA

Mats Brittberg Cartilage Research Unit, University of Gothenburg, Region Halland Orthopaedics, Kungsbacka Hospital, Kungsbacka, Sweden

Charles H. Brown Jr. International Knee and Joint Centre, Abu Dhabi, United Arab Emirates

Peter U. Brucker Department of Orthopaedic Sports Medicine, Klinikum rechts der Isar, Technical University of Munich, Munich, Germany

Danilo Bruni II Clinica Ortopedica e Traumatologica, Istituto Ortopedico Rizzoli, Bologna, Italy

Stefan Buchmann Department of Orthopaedic Sports Medicine, Klinikum rechts der Isar, Technical University of Munich, Munich, Germany

Kadir Büyükdoğan Faculty of Medicine, Department of Orthopaedics and Traumatology, Hacettepe University School of Medicine Ankara, Sihhiye, Turkey

Paolo Cabitza Dipartimento di Scienze Biomediche per la Salute, Università degli Studi di Milano, IRCCS Policlinico San Donato, Milano, Italy

David N. M. Caborn JPG – Shea Orthopaedic Group, Orthopedic Surgery, University of Louisville, Kentucky OneHealth, Louisville, KY, USA

Angelo Cacchio Department of Health Sciences, University of L'Aquila, L'Aquila, Italy

Murat Menderes Caglar Sportomed Physical Therapy and Rehabilitation Center, Istanbul, Turkey

Omur Caglar Faculty of Medicine, Department of Orthopaedics and Traumatology, Hacettepe University, Ankara, Sihhiye, Turkey

E. Lyle Cain American Sports Medicine Institute, Andrews Sports Medicine and Orthopaedic Center, Birmingham, AL, USA

James D. Calder Department of Trauma and Orthopaedic Surgery, The Fortius Clinic, and Chelsea and Westminster Hospital, London, UK

Michael J. Callaghan Centre for Rehabilitation Science, University of Manchester, Manchester, UK

Vincenzo Campana Department of Orthopaedics, Catholic University of Rome, Rome, RM, Italy

Gian Luigi Canata Centre of Sports Traumatology, Koelliker Hospital, Institute of Sports Medicine, Torino, Italy

Arnold I. Caplan Department of Biology, Skeletal Research Center, Case Western Reserve University, Cleveland, OH, USA

Silvio Carminati Dipartimento di Scienze Biomediche per la Salute, Università degli Studi di Milano, IRCCS Policlinico San Donato, Milano, Italy

Michael R. Carmont The Princess Royal Hospital, Shrewsbury and Telford NHS Trust, Telford, UK

Northern General Hospital, Sheffield Teaching Hospitals NHS Foundation Trust, Sheffield, UK

Alessandro Castagna Shoulder and Elbow Service, IRCCS Humanitas Institute, Rozzano, Milano, Italy

Unit for Surgery of the Shoulder, Istituto Clinico Humanitas, Rozzano, Milano, Italy

Danilo S. Catelli School of Human Kinetics, University of Ottawa, Ottawa, ON, Canada

Ibrahim Fatih Cengiz 3B's Research Group – Biomaterials, Biodegradables and Biomimetics, Headquarters of the European Institute of Excellence on Tissue Engineering and Regenerative Medicine, University of Minho, Taipas, Guimarães, Portugal

ICVS/3B's – PT Government Associated Laboratory, Guimarães, Portugal

Eugenio Cesari Shoulder and Elbow Service, IRCCS Humanitas Institute, Rozzano, Milano, Italy

Kai-Ming Chan Department of Orthopaedics and Traumatology, The Chinese University of Hong Kong, Prince of Wales Hospital, Shatin, Hong Kong

Chih-Hsiang Chang Department of Orthopaedic Surgery, Chang Gung Memorial Hospital at Linkou, College of Medicine, Chang Gung University, Taoyuan, Taiwan

Harman Chaudhry Division of Orthopaedic Surgery, McMaster University, Hamilton, ON, Canada

Chih-Hwa Chen Department of Orthopaedic Surgery, Taipei Medical University Hospital, School of medicine, College of Medicine, Taipei Medical University, Taipei, Taiwan

Connie Chen Department of Bioengineering, Musculoskeletal Research Center, Swanson School of Engineering, University of Pittsburgh, Pittsburgh, PA, USA

Franck Chotel Department of Pediatric Orthopaedic Surgery, Lyon University Hospital for Mother and Children, Université Claude Bernard Lyon, Bron, Luxembourg

Akin Cil Department of Orthopaedics, Division Head Shoulder, Elbow and Sports Medicine, Truman Medical Centers, Sports Medicine Section, University of Missouri-Kansas City, Kansas City, MO, USA

Steven B. Cohen Department of Orthopedic Surgery, Thomas Jeffersonv University/Rothman Institute, Philadelphia, PA, USA

Brian J. Cole Department of Orthopaedic Surgery, Cartilage Restoration Center at Rush, Rush University Medical Center, Chicago, IL, USA

Michael Collins Department of Orthopaedic Surgery, University of Pittsburgh School of Medicine, Pittsburgh, PA, USA

Philippe Colombet Centre de Chirurgie Orthopédique et Sportive, Bordeaux-Mérignac, Mérignac, France

Naama Constantini Department of Orthopedic Surgery, The Hadassah-Hebrew University Medical Center, Jerusalem, Israel

Marco Conti Shoulder and Elbow Service, IRCCS Humanitas Institute, Rozzano, Milano, Italy

Myles R. J. Coolican Consultant Orthopaedic and Trauma Surgeon, Sydney Orthopaedic Research Institute, Chatswood, NSW, Australia

Department of Orthopaedic Surgery, Royal North Shore Hospital, Sydney, NSW, Australia

Ann Cools Department of Rehabilitation Sciences and Physiotherapy, Ghent University, Ghent, Belgium

Alessandro Corradini Department of Orthopaedic Clinic, University of Modena, Modena, Italy

Charles T. Crellin Department of Orthopedics, CU Sports Medicine, University of Colorado, Aurora, CO, USA

Ricardo Cuellar Hospital Universitario Donostia, San Sebastian, Spain

Ramón Cugat Mutualidad de Futbolistas, Real Federacion Espanola de Futbol, Barcelona, Spain

Garcia Cugat Foundation & CEU Cardenal Herrera University, Alfara del Patriarca, Valencia, Spain

Department of Orthopaedic Surgery, Sports Medicine and Trauma, Hospital Quiron Barcelona, Artroscopia gc, S.L., Barcelona, Spain

Facultad de Medicina, Universitat Internacional de Catalunya, Barcelona, Spain

Liang R. Cui Department of Orthopaedic Surgery, University of Pittsburgh Medical Center, Pittsburgh, PA, USA

Xavier Cuscó Chair of Medicine and Regenerative Surgery, Garcia Cugat Foundation & CEU Cardenal Herrera University, Alfara del Patriarca, Valencia, Spain

Department of Orthopaedic Surgery, Sports Medicine and Trauma, Hospital Quiron Barcelona, Artroscopia gc, S.L., Barcelona, Spain

Ziad Dahabreh Clinical Knee Fellow in Knee Surgery, Sydney Orthopaedic Research Institute, Chatswood, NSW, Australia

Miquel Dalmau-Pastor Department of Pathology and Experimental Therapeutics (Human Anatomy Unit), University of Barcelona, Laboratory of Arthroscopic and Surgical Anatomy, L'Hospitalet de Llobregat, Barcelona, Spain

Niel P. Davis Royal Cornwall Hospital, Truro, Cornwall, UK

Francesco de Boccard Official F1H2O Racing Medical Consultant, Torino, Italy

Artur Pereira de Castro DESPORSANO Sports Clinic, Lisboa, Portugal

Peter A. J. de Leeuw Department of Orthopaedic Surgery, Academic Medical Center, University of Amsterdam, DE, Amsterdam, The Netherlands

Kristof De Mey Department of Rehabilitation Sciences and Physiotherapy, Ghent University, Ghent, Belgium

Marieke M. de Vaal Department of Orthopaedic Surgery, Ziekenhuis Amstelland, Amstelveen, AM, The Netherlands

Francisco Serrano Sáenz de Tejada Hospital Asepeyo, Coslada, Madrid, Spain

Caroline Debette Centre Albert Trillat, Service de Chirurgie Orthopédique, Hôpital de la Croix-Rousse, University of Lyon, Lyon, France

Masataka Deie Department of Orthopaedic Surgery, Hiroshima University, Hiroshima, Japan

David Dejour Department of Knee Surgery & Sports Traumatology, Lyon-Ortho-Clinic; Clinique de la Sauvegarde, Lyon, France

Demetris Delos Department of Orthopedic Surgery, Hospital for Special Surgery, New York, NY, USA

Burak Demirağ Department of Orthopaedics and Traumatology, Uludağ University Faculty of Medicine, Bursa, Turkey

Murat Demirel Department of Orthopaedics and Traumatology, Bayındır Hospital, Ankara, Turkey

Mehmet Demirhan Department of Orthopedics and Traumatology, Koc University School of Medicine, Istanbul, Turkey

Gokhan Demirkiran Faculty of Medıcıne, Department of Orthopaedıcs and Traumatology, Hacettepe Unıversıty, Ankara, Sihhiye, Turkey

Emir Baki Dcnkbaş Faculty of Science, Chemistry Department, Hacettepe University, Ankara, Turkey

Pierre d'Hemecourt Division of Sports Medicine, Boston Children's Hospital, Boston, MA, USA

Pieter d'Hooghe Department of Orthopaedic Surgery, Aspetar Orthopaedic and Sports Medicine Hospital, Doha, Qatar

Jorge Díaz Heredia Unidad de Hombro y Codo, Hospital Universitario Ramón y Cajal, Madrid, Spain

Ugur Dilicikik Department of Sports Medicine, Kanuni Sultan Süleyman Education and Research Hospital, Istanbul, Turkey

Giotis Dimitrios Department of Trauma and Orthopaedic Surgery, University of Ioannina, Ioannina, Greece

Alexander C. Disch Spine Unit Center for Musculoskeletal Surgery, Charité – University Hospital Berlin, Berlin, Germany

Metin Dogan Department of Orthopedics and Traumatology, Ankara Atatürk Training and Research Hospital, Ankara, Turkey

Eran Dolev Orthopedic Department, Meir Medical Centre, Kfar Saba, Israel

Brian G. Donley Center for Foot and Ankle Surgery, Orthopaedic Surgery, Lutheran Hospital, Cleveland, OH, USA

Gürhan Dönmez Faculty of Medicine, Department of Sport Medicine, Hacettepe University School of Medicine, Ankara, Sihhiye, Turkey

Mahmut Nedim Doral Department of Orthopaedics and Traumatology and Department of Sports Medicine, Hacettepe University, Istanbul, Turkey

A. S. M. Dunn Plancher Orthopaedics and Sports Medicine, New York, NY, USA

Orthopaedic Foundation, Stamford, CT, USA

Ceyda Kanli Dursun Department of Periodontology, Faculty of Dentistry, Hacettepe University, Ankara, Turkey

Erhan Dursun Department of Periodontology, Faculty of Dentistry, Hacettepe University, Ankara, Turkey

Victoria B. Duthon Division of Orthopaedic Surgery, Department of Surgery, University Hospital of Geneva, Geneva, Switzerland

John Eggers Truman Medical Centers, University of Missouri Kansas City, Kansas City, MO, USA

Kenneth A. Egol Department of Orthopaedic Surgery, New York University Hospital for Joint Diseases, New York, NY, USA

Triantafyllidi Eleni Department of Trauma and Orthopaedic Surgery, University of Ioannina, Ioannina, Greece

Madi El-Haj Department of Orthopaedics, Hadassah Hebrew University Hospital, Jerusalem, Israel

Michael Ellman Department of Orthopedic Surgery, Rush University Medical Center, Chicago, IL, USA

Nurzat Elmalı Department of Orthopaedics and Traumatology, Dr. Lütfi Kırdar Kartal Education and Research Hospital, İstanbul, Turkey

Meric Enercan Istanbul Spine Center, Florence Nightingale Hospital, Sisli/Istanbul, Turkey

Lars Engebretsen Department of Sports Medicine and Oslo Sports Trauma Research Center, Norwegian School of Sport Sciences, Oslo, Norway

IOC Medical & Scientific Department, Lausanne, Switzerland

Department of Orthopaedic Surgery, Oslo University Hospital, Oslo, Norway

Cenk Ermutlu Department of Orthopaedics and Traumatology, İstanbul Training and Research Hospital, İstanbul, Turkey

Lucio S. Ernlund Knee and Shoulder Institute, Curitiba, PR, Brazil

Cem Zeki Esenyel Department of Orthopedics and Traumatology, Vakif Gureba Training and Research Hospital, Fatih, Istanbul, Turkey

Iris Eshed Orthopedic Department, Meir Medical Centre, Kfar Saba, Israel

Department of Diagnostic Imaging, Sheba Medical Center, Tel Hashomer, Israel

João Espregueira-Mendes 3B's Research Group – Biomaterials, Biodegradables and Biomimetics, Headquarters of the European Institute of Excellence on Tissue Engineering and Regenerative Medicine, University of Minho, Taipas, Guimarães, Portugal

Clínica Espregueira–Mendes F.C. Porto Stadium – FIFA Medical Centre of Excellence, Porto, Portugal

Orthopedic Department, Centro Hospitalar Póvoa de Varzim, Vila do Conde, Portugal

ICVS/3B's – PT Government Associated Laboratory, Braga/Guimarães, Portugal

Orthopaedic Department, Hospital S. Sebastião, Feira, Portugal

Mustafa Kürşat Evrenos Department of Plastic and Reconstructive Surgery, Celal Bayar University School of Medicine, Manisa, Turkey

Nicola Fabbri Department of Orthopaedic Surgery, Memorial Sloan Kettering Cancer Center, New York, NY, USA

Martin Fahlström Department of Clinical Sciences, Professional Development, Rehabilitation Medicine, Umeå University, Umeå, Sweden

Kathryn F. Farraro Department of Bioengineering, Musculoskeletal Research Center, Swanson School of Engineering, University of Pittsburgh, Pittsburgh, PA, USA

Lutul Farrow Cleveland Clinic Sports Health Center, Garfield Heights, OH, USA

Margarida Fernandes FIFA Medical Centre of Excellence, Clínica Espregueira-Mendes F.C. Porto Stadium, Porto, Portugal

Paulo Renato Fernandes Saggin Instituto de Ortopedia e Traumatologia de Passo Fundo, Passo Fundo, RS, Brazil

Giuseppe Filardo Biomechanics Laboratory, Istituto Ortopedico Rizzoli, Bologna, Italy

Aharon S. Finestone Foot and Ankle Unit, Orthopaedics Department, Assaf HaRofeh MC, Zerifin, Israel

Alex Finsterbush Unit of Sports Medicine, Department of Orthopedics, Hadassah University Hospital, Jerusalem, Israel

Jonquil R. Flowers Department of Bioengineering, Musculoskeletal Research Center, Swanson School of Engineering, University of Pittsburgh, Pittsburgh, PA, USA

Freddie H. Fu Department of Orthopaedic Surgery, University of Pittsburgh School of Medicine, Pittsburgh, PA, USA

Sai-Chuen Bruma Fu Department of Orthopaedics and Traumatology, The Chinese University of Hong Kong, Prince of Wales Hospital, Shatin, Hong Kong

Isabella Fusaro Physical Therapy and Rehabilitation Unit, Istituto Ortopedico Rizzoli, Bologna, Italy

Michele Gagliardi University of Bologna, Bologna, Italy

Theodore J. Ganley Orthopaedic Surgery, The Children's Hospital of Philadelphia, Philadelphia, PA, USA

Montserrat García-Balletbó Chair of Medicine and Regenerative Surgery, Garcia Cugat Foundation & CEU Cardenal Herrera University, Alfara del Patriarca, Valencia, Spain

Department of Orthopaedic Surgery, Sports Medicine and Trauma, Hospital Quiron Barcelona, Artroscopia gc, S.L., Barcelona, Spain

Department of Regenerative Medicine Hospital Quiron Barcelona, WGB Bioregeneracion, Barcelona, Spain

Miguel García Navlet Hospital Asepeyo, Coslada, Madrid, Spain

Raffaele Garofalo Shoulder and Elbow Service, IRCCS Humanitas Institute, Rozzano, Milano, Italy

Louise E. Gartner National University Hospital, Singapore

Celeste Geertsema Sports Medicine, Aspetar Orthopaedic and Sports Medicine Hospital, Doha, Qatar

Andrew Geeslin School of Medicine, Western Michigan University, Kalamazoo, MI, USA

Christos S. Georgiou Department of Orthopaedic Surgery, University Hospital of Patras, Rio, Greece

Anastasios D. Georgoulis School of Medicine, Department of Orthopedics, University of Ioannina, Ioannina, Greece

Matteo Ghiara Clinica Ortopedica e Traumatologica, Fondazione IRCCS Policlinico San Matteo di Pavia, Università degli Studi di Pavia, Pavia, Italy

Alessio Giai Via Department of Orthopaedics and Traumatology, University of Rome "Tor Verata", Rome, Italy

Alberto Gobbi Orthopaedic Arthroscopic Surgery International (O.A.S.I.) Bioresearch Foundation, Gobbi Onlus, Milan, Italy

Nevzat Selim Gokay Esenyurt University School of Health, Istanbul, Turkey

Alper Gokce Nisantasi University School of Health, Istanbul, Turkey

Pau Golanó Laboratory of Arthroscopic and Surgical Anatomy, Human Anatomy & Embriology Unit, Department of Pathology and Experimental Therapeutics (c/Feixa Llarga s/n (Campus Bellvitge)), University of Barcelona, L'Hospitalet de Llobregat, Barcelona, Spain

School of Medicine, Department of Orthopaedic Surgery, University of Pittsburgh, Pittsburgh, PA, USA

M. Mustafa Gomberawalla Feinberg School of Medicine, Department of Orthopaedic Surgery, Northwestern University, Chicago, IL, USA

Zsigmond Göndöcs Hungarian Ambulance Service, Budapest, Hungary

Laszlo Gorove Hungarian Air Ambulance Nonprofit Ltd., Budaörs, Budapest, Hungary

Lars-Petter Granan Oslo Sports Trauma Research Center, The Norwegian School of Sport Sciences, Oslo, Norway

Department of Physical Medicine and Rehabilitation, Oslo University Hospital, Oslo, Norway

Mathilde Gras Institut de la Main, Clinique Jouvenet, Paris, France

Alberto Grassi II Clinica Ortopedica e Traumatologica, Istituto Ortopedico Rizzoli, Bologna, Italy

Lovorka Grgurevic Laboratory for Mineralized Tissues, Center for Translational and Clinical Research, School of Medicine, University of Zagreb, Zagreb, Croatia

Michael J. Griesser Performance Orthopaedics and Sports Medicine, Clinton Memorial Hospital, Wilmington, OH, USA

Taner Güneş School of Medicine, Department of Orthopedics, Gaziosmanpasa University, Tokat, Turkey

Ashish Gupta Clinique Générale d'Annecy, Alps Surgery Institute, Annecy, France

Safa Gursoy Department of Orthopaedics, Ankara Ataturk Training and Research Hospital, Ankara, Turkey

Karen Gustafson Department of Orthopedics, CU Sports Medicine, University of Colorado, Aurora, CO, USA

Ugur Haklar Orthopaedics and Traumatology Department, Bahcesehir University Medical Faculty, Liv Hospital, Istanbul, Turkey

Bruce Hamilton High Performance Sport NZ, Millennium Institute of Sport and Health, Auckland, New Zealand

Azmi Hamzaoglu Istanbul Spine Center, Florence Nightingale Hospital, Sisli/Istanbul, Turkey

Jonathan Hanson Broadford hospital Skye, Broadford, Skye, Scotland, UK

Onur Hapa Department of Orthopedic Surgery, Dokuz Eylül University, İzmir, İnciraltı, Turkey

Hasan Havitçioğlu Department of Orthopedic Surgery, Dokuz Eylül University, İzmir, İnciraltı, Turkey

Jennifer Heda KARL STORZ GmbH & Co. KG, Tuttlingen, Germany

Bryan C. Heiderscheit Department of Orthopedics and Rehabilitation, University of Wisconsin-Madison, Madison, WI, USA

Eva Lisa Heinrichs Tissue Therapies Europe, Tissue Therapies Europe Ltd – Global Med Affairs, Daresbury Cheshire, UK

Iftach Hetsroni Department of Orthopedic Surgery, Meir Medical Centre, Kfar Saba, Israel

Sackler Faculty of Medicine, Tel Aviv University, Tel Aviv, Israel

Laszlo T. Hetzman Hungarian Air Ambulance Nonprofit Ltd., Budaörs, Budapest, Hungary

Nurettin Heybeli Department of Orthopaedic Surgery and Traumatology, Trakya University School of Medicine, Kanuni Sultan Suleyman Education and Research Hospital, Edirne, Turkey

Stefan Hinterwimmer Department of Orthopaedic Sports Medicine, Klinikum rechts der Isar, Technische Universität München, München, Germany

Marcus Hofbauer Department of Trauma Surgery, Medical University of Vienna, Vienna, Austria

Yuichi Hoshino Department of Orthopaedic Surgery, Kobe Kaisei Hospital, Kobe, Japan

Joel Huleatt The Steadman Clinic and Steadman Philippon Research Institute, Vail, CO, USA

Gazi Huri Department of Orthopaedics and Traumatology, Hacettepe University, Ankara, Turkey

Division of Shoulder Surgery, Department of Orthopaedic Surgery, Johns Hopkins University, Baltimore, MD, USA

Waqas M. Hussain ORA Orthopedics, Moline, IL, USA

Yoon S. Hyun Division of Shoulder Surgery, The Department of Orthopaedic Surgery, The Johns Hopkins University, Baltimore, MD, USA

Francesco Iacono Codivilla-Putti Research Centre, Bologna, Italy

Andreas B. Imhoff Department of Orthopaedic Sports Medicine, Klinikum rechts der Isar, Technical University of Munich, Munich, Germany

Cansel Işıklı Nanotechnology and Nanomedicine Division, Hacettepe University, Institute of Graduate Studies in Science, Ankara, Turkey

BMT Calsis Health Technologies, Çankaya, Ankara, Turkey

Susan N. Ishikawa Department of Orthopaedic Surgery and Biomedical Engineering, University of Tennessee – Campbell Clinic, Memphis, TN, USA

Alan Ivkovic Department of Orthopaedic Surgery, University Hospital Sveti Duh, Zagreb, Croatia

Matthias Jacobi Orthopadie am Rosenberg, St. Gallen, SG, Switzerland

Roland Jakob Department of Orthopaedic Surgery, Hopital Cantonal, Fribourg, Switzerland

Laith Miguel Jazrawi Department of Orthopaedic Surgery, New York University Hospital for Joint Diseases, New York, NY, USA

Mislav Jelic Department of Orthopaedic Surgery, Clinical Hospital Center, School of Medicine, University of Zagreb, Zagreb, Croatia

Kevin Jiang Department of Orthopaedic Surgery, University of Pittsburgh, Pittsburgh, PA, USA

Henrique Jones Department of Orthopedic Surgery, Knee and Sports Traumatology, Montijo Orthopaedic Clinic, Lusofona University, Lisbon, Portugal

Eralp Kacmaz Albert Trillat Center, Lyon North Univerity, Lyon, France

Saygin Kamaci Department of Orthopaedics and Traumatology, Hacettepe University, Sihhiye, Ankara, Turkey

Fatih Karaaslan Department of Orthopedics, Bozok University Medical Faculty, Yozgat, Turkey

Mustafa Karahan Department of Orthopedics and Traumatology, Faculty of Medicine, Acibadem University, Maltepe, Istanbul, Turkey

Nazim Karalezli Department of Orthopaedics and Traumatology, Department of Sports Medicine, Konya Necmettin Erbakan University, Meram Faculty of Medicine, Ankara, Turkey

Yiğitcan Karanfil Department of Sports Medicine, Faculty of Medicine, Hacettepe University School of Medicine, Ankara, Turkey

Sinan Karaoğlu Department of Orthopaedics and Traumatology, Memorial Kayseri Hospital, Kayseri, Turkey

Dimitrios Karataglis Blue Cross, Euromedica Clinic, Orthopaedic Department, Thessaloniki, Greece

Jon Karlsson Department of Orthopaedic Surgery, Sahlgrenska Academy, University of Gothenburg, Sahlgrenska University Hospital, Gothenburg, Sweden

Georgios Karnatzikos Orthopaedic Arthroscopic Surgery International (O.A.S.I.) Bioresearch Foundation, Gobbi Onlus, Milan, Italy

Defne Kaya Department of Physical Therapy and Rehabilitation, Faculty of Health Science, Biruni University, İstanbul, Turkey

Murat Kayalar Orthopaedics and Traumatology, EMOT Hospital, İzmir, Turkey

Robi Kelc Department of Orthopaedic Surgery, University Medical Center Maribor, Maribor, Slovenia

Eran Keltz Orthopedic Surgery Department, Rambam Health Care Campus, Haifa, Israel

Nicholas I. Kennedy Steadman Philippon Research Institute, Vail, CO, USA

Gino M. M. J. Kerkhoffs Department of Orthopaedic Surgery, Academic Medical Center, University of Amsterdam, DE, Amsterdam, The Netherlands

Mauricio Kfuri Department of Biomechanics, Medicine and Rehabilitation of Locomotor System – Ribeirao Preto Medical School – São Paulo University, Brazil, São Paulo, Brazil

Fahmi Yousef Khan Department of Medicine, Hamad General Hospital, Doha, Qatar

Kwang E. Kim Department of Bioengineering, Musculoskeletal Research Center, Swanson School of Engineering, University of Pittsburgh, Pittsburgh, PA, USA

Seung-Ho Kim Department of Orthopaedic Surgery, Madi Hospital, Gangnam-gu, Seoul, South Korea

Daniel G. Kipnis Center for Teaching and Learning and Scott Memorial Library, Thomas Jefferson University, Philadelphia, PA, USA

Mininder Singh Kocher Division of Sports Medicine, Harvard Medical School, Boston Children's Hospital, Boston, MA, USA

Pradeep Kodali HMC Doctors, Sugar Land, TX, USA

Hideyuki Koga Department of Joint Surgery and Sports Medicine, Graduate School of Medical Science, Tokyo Medical and Dental University, Bunkyo–ku, Tokyo, Japan

Department of Orthopaedic Surgery, Tokyo Medical and Dental University Hospital, Bunkyo–ku, Tokyo, Japan

Ismet Koksal Social Security Institution, Balgat/Ankara, Turkey

Elizaveta Kon Biomechanics Laboratory, NaBi Laboratory, Istituto Ortopedico Rizzoli, Bologna, Italy

Eiji Kondo Department of Advanced Therapeutic Research for Sports Medicine, Hokkaido University, Graduate School of Medicine, Sapporo, Hokkaido, Japan

George M. Kontakis Department of Orthopaedics and Trauma, University Hospital of Heraklion, Heraklion, Crete, Greece

Sebastian Kopf Section Sports Traumatology & Arthroscopy, Center for Musculoskeletal Surgery, Charité – University Medicine Berlin, Berlin, Germany

Feza Korkusuz Department of Sports Medicine, Faculty of Medicine, Hacettepe University School of Medicine, Ankara, Turkey

Gamze Torun Köse Department of Genetics and Bioengineering, Yeditepe University, Faculty of Engineering and Architecture, Istanbul, Turkey

Eugene Kots Department of Diagnostic Radiology, Meir Medical Center, Kfar Saba, Israel

Antonios Kouzelis Department of Orthopaedic Surgery, University Hospital of Patras, Rio, Greece

Lutfu Ozgur Koyuncu Department of Orthopaedics and Traumatology, American Hospital, Istanbul, Turkey

Ryan J. Krupp Division of Sports Medicine, Department of Orthopaedic Surgery, University of Louisville, Louisville, KY, USA

SportsHealth Program, Norton Orthopaedic Specialists, Louisville, KY, USA

Fatih Küçükdurmaz Department of Orthopaedics and Traumatology, Bezmialem Vakif University, Istanbul, Turkey

Christina Kunec Department of Orthopaedic Surgery, University of Pittsburgh School of Medicine, Pittsburgh, PA, USA

Fabiano Kupczik Cajuru University Hospital – PUCPR, Curitiba, PR, Brazil

Nuri Hünkar Kutlu BMT Calsis Health Technologies Co., Sarayköy, Ankara, Turkey

Joanna Kvist Division Physiotherapy, Department of Medical and Health Sciences, Linköping University, Linköping, Sweden

Polyvios Kyritsis Orthopaedic and Sports Medicine Hospital, Aspetar, Doha, Qatar

Dnyanesh G. Lad Orthopaedic Arthroscopic Surgery International (O.A.S.I) Bioresearch Foundation, Gobbi Onlus, Milan, Italy

Laurent Lafosse Clinique Générale d'Annecy, Alps Surgery Institute, Annecy, France

Thibault Lafosse Clinique Générale d'Annecy, Alps Surgery Institute, Annecy, France

Kah Weng Lai Sydney Orthopaedic Research Institute, Chatswood, NSW, Australia

Department of Orthopaedic Surgery, National University Hospital, Singapore, Singapore

Christopher M. LaPrade Department of BioMedical Engineering, Steadman Philippon Research Institute, Vail, CO, USA

Mario Lamontagne School of Human Kinetics, University of Ottawa, Ottawa, ON, Canada

Department of Mechanical Engineering, University of Ottawa, Ottawa, ON, Canada

Werner Müller Department of Orthopaedic Surgery, University of Basel, Basel, Switzerland

Philippe Landreau Orthopaedic and Sports Medicine Hospital, Aspetar, Doha, Qatar

Robert F. LaPrade The Steadman Clinic and Steadman, Philippon Research Institute, Vail, CO, USA

Chris Larson Minnesota Orthopedic Sports Medicine Institute at Twin Cities Orthopedics, Edina, MN, USA

Kerstin Lautemann KARL STORZ GmbH & Co. KG, Tuttlingen, Germany

Lior Laver Department of Orthopaedic Surgery, Sports Medicine Unit, "Meir" Medical Center and Tel–Aviv University Hospital, Kfar–Saba, Israel

Department of Orthopaedic Surgery, Division of Sports Medicine, Duke University Medical Center, Durham, NC, USA

Gürsel Leblebicioğlu Faculty of Medicine, Department of Orthopaedics and Traumatology, Hacettepe University, Ankara, Turkey

Chian-Her Lee Department of Orthopaedic Surgery, Taipei Medical University Hospital, School of Medicine, College of Medicine, Taipei Medical University, Taipei, Taiwan

Yee Han Dave Lee Department of Orthopedic Surgery, Changi General Hospital, Singapore

Andreas Lenich Department of Orthopaedic and Sports Medicine, Klinikum Rechts der Isar/University of Munich, Munich, Germany

Martin Leonhard KARL STORZ GmbH & Co. KG, Tuttlingen, Germany

L. Scott Levin University of Pennsylvania, Philadelphia, PA, USA

Tommy Lindau Pulvertaft Hand Centre, Kings Treatment Centre, Royal Derby Hospital, Derby, UK

M. Llusa Facultad de Medicina, Universidad de Barcelona, Barcelona, Spain

Department of Orthopaedic Surgery, Sports Medicine and Trauma, Hospital Quiron Barcelona, Hospital Quiron Barcelona, Barcelona, Spain

Sverre Løken Orthopaedic Department, Oslo University Hospital, Oslo, Norway

Oslo Sports Trauma Research Center, The Norwegian School of Sport Sciences, Oslo, Norway

Nicola Lopomo II Clinica Ortopedica e Traumatologica, Istituto Ortopedico Rizzoli, Bologna, Italy

Olaf Lorbach Department of Orthopedic Surgery, Saarland University, Homburg (Saar), SL, Germany

Stephan Lorenz Department of Orthopaedic Sports Medicine, Klinikum rechts der Isar, Technische Universität München, München, Germany

Joseph Lowe Head (Emeritus) Sports Injury Unit, Division of Orthopaedic Surgery, Hadassah Medical Center, Hebrew University School of Medicine, Jerusalem, Israel

Jose Luis Ávila Hospital Maz, Zaragoza, Spain

Sébastien Lustig Centre Albert Trillat, Service de Chirurgie Orthopédique, Hôpital de la Croix-Rousse, University of Lyon, Lyon, France

T. Sean Lynch Department of Orthopaedic Surgery, Feinberg School of Medicine, Northwestern University, Chicago, IL, USA

Jay D. Mabrey Department of Orthopaedic Surgery, Baylor University Medical Center, Dallas, TX, USA

Kenneth G. W. Mackinlay Division of Sports Medicine, Department of Orthopaedic Surgery, University of Louisville, Louisville, KY, USA

Annelies Maenhout Department of Rehabilitation Sciences and Physiotherapy, Ghent University, Ghent, Belgium

Nicola Maffulli Department of Musculoskeletal Disorders, School of Medicine and Surgery, University of Salerno, Salerno, Italy

Barts and the London School of Medicine and Dentistry, Centre for Sports and Exercise Medicine, Mile End Hospital, Queen Mary University of London, London, UK

Robert A. Magnussen Department of Orthopaedics, Sports Health and Performance Institute, The Ohio State University, Columbus, OH, USA

Francesc Malagelada Barts and The London NHS Trust, London, UK

Gideon Mann Service of Sports Injuries, Department of Orthopaedic Surgery, Meir Medical Centre, Tel Aviv University, Tel Aviv, Israel

Sandeep Mannava Department of Orthopaedic Surgery, Wake Forest School of Medicine, Medical Center Boulevard, Winston-Salem, NC, USA

Giulia Mantovani School of Human Kinetics, University of Ottawa, Ottawa, ON, Canada

Salih Marangoz Orthopaedics and Traumatology, Koc University, School of Medicine, Sarıyer, Istanbul, Turkey

Maurilio Marcacci II Clinica Ortopedica e Traumatologica, Istituto Ortopedico Rizzoli, Bologna, Italy

Niv Marom Department of Orthopedic Surgery, Meir University Hospital Medical Center, Kfar-Saba, Israel

Maria Carmen Marongiu Department of Orthopaedic Clinic, University of Modena, Modena, Italy

Frank Martetschläger Department of Orthopaedic Sports Medicine, Technical University of Munich, Munich, Germany

Robert G. Marx Foster Center for Clinical Outcome Research, Hospital for Special Surgery, New York, NY, USA

Weill Medical College of Cornell University, New York, NY, USA

Philippe Masouye Department of Anesthesia, Intensive Care and Pharmacology, University Hospital of Geneva, Geneva, Switzerland

Christophe L. Mathoulin Institut de la Main, Clinique Jouvenet, Paris, France

Charalampos Matzaroglou Department of Orthopaedic Surgery, University Hospital of Patras, Rio, Greece

Brett W. McCoy Southwest Orthopaedics Inc., Parma, OH, USA

Paul McCrory The Florey Institute of Neuroscience and Mental Health, University of Melbourne, Melbourne Brain Centre – Austin Campus, Heidelberg, VIC, Australia

David McDonagh The Princess Royal Hospital, Shrewsbury and Telford NHS Trust, Telford, UK

Northern General Hospital, Sheffield Teaching Hospitals NHS Foundation Trust, Sheffield, UK

Department of Emergency Medicine, University Hospital Trondheim, Trondheim, Norway

Medical Commission Fédération Internationale de Bobsleigh et de Tobogganing (FIBT), OSKP, St. Olavs Hospital, Trondheim, Norway

Edward G. McFarland Division of Shoulder Surgery, The Department of Orthopaedic Surgery, The Johns Hopkins University, Baltimore, MD, USA

Omer Mei-Dan Orthopedics Department, Sports Devision, Hip Preservation Service, University of Colorado Medical School, Boulder, CO, USA

Jurdan Mendiguchía Department of Physical Therapy, Zentrum Rehab and Performance Center, Barañain, Navarre, Spain

Jacques Menetrey Swiss Olympic Medical Center, Division of Orthopaedic Surgery, Department of Surgery, HUG, University Hospital of Geneva, Geneva, Switzerland

Faculty of Medicine, University of Geneva, Geneva, Switzerland

Max Michalski Department of Biomedical Engineering, Steadman Philippon Research Institute (SPRI), Vail, CO, USA

Giuseppe Milano Department of Orthopaedics, Catholic University of Rome, Rome, RM, Italy

Charles Milgrom Department of Orthopaedics, Hadassah University Hospital, Jerusalem, Israel

Anthony Miniaci Department Orthopedic Surgery & Sports Health, Cleveland Clinic Foundation, Garfield Heights, OH, USA

Emily Monroe Department of Orthopaedic Surgery, Northwestern University, Chicago, IL, USA

Jill Monson University Orthopaedic Therapy Center, Minneapolis, MN, USA

Alberto Monteiro Clínica Espregueira-Mendes F.C. Porto Stadium, FIFA Medical Centre of Excellence, Porto, Portugal

Valencia Mora Mora Unidad de Hombro y Codo, Hospital Universitario Ramón y Cajal, Madrid, Spain

M. R. Morro Facultad de Medicina, Universidad de Barcelona, Barcelona, Spain

Giulio Maria Marcheggiani Muccioli II Clinica Ortopedica e Traumatologica, Istituto Ortopedico Rizzoli, Bologna, Italy

Bart Muller Department of Orthopaedic Surgery, University of Pittsburgh, Pittsburgh, PA, USA

Department of Orthopaedic Surgery, Academic Medical Center, University of Amsterdam, Amsterdam, NH, Netherlands

Raman Mundi Division of Orthopaedic Surgery, McMaster University, Hamilton, ON, Canada

Takeshi Muneta Department of Joint Surgery and Sports Medicine, Graduate School of Medical Science, Tokyo Medical and Dental University, Bunkyo–ku, Tokyo, Japan

Department of Orthopaedic Surgery, Tokyo Medical and Dental University Hospital, Bunkyo–ku, Tokyo, Japan

Christopher D. Murawski Department of Orthopaedic Surgery, University of Pittsburgh School of Medicine, Pittsburgh, PA, USA

G. Andrew Murphy Department of Orthopaedic Surgery and Biomedical Engineering, University of Tennessee – Campbell Clinic, Memphis, TN, USA

D. Andrew Murray SportScotland Institute of Sport, Stirling, UK

Volker Musahl Department of Orthopaedic Surgery, University of Pittsburgh Medical Center, Pittsburgh, PA, USA

Division of Sports Medicine, Orthopaedic Surgery, University of Pittsburgh, Pittsburgh, PA, USA

Gregory D. Myer Division of Sports Medicine, Cincinnati Children's Hospital Medical Center, Cincinnati, OH, USA

Grethe Myklebust Department of Sports Medicine, Oslo Sport Trauma Research Center, Norwegian School of Sport Sciences, Norwegian University of Sport and Physical Education, Oslo, Norway

Norimasa Nakamura Department of Orthopaedics, Osaka Health Science University, Osaka, Japan

Department of Rehabilitation Science, Osaka University Center for Advanced Medical Engineering and Informatics, Osaka, Japan

Sven Nebelung Universitätsklinikum Aachen, Klinik für Orthopädie, Aachen, Germany

Wolfgang Nebelung Marienkrankenhaus Düsseldorf Kaiserswerth, Düsseldorf, Germany

Jeffrey J. Nepple Associate Professor Department of Orthopaedic Surgery, Washington University School of Medicine, St. Louis, MO, USA

Philippe Neyret Centre Albert Trillat, Service de Chirurgie Orthopédique, Hôpital de la Croix-Rousse, University of Lyon, Lyon, France

K. C. Geoffrey Ng Department of Mechanical Engineering, University of Ottawa, Ottawa, ON, Canada

Fabio Nicoletta Orthopaedic and Arthroscopic Department, New Sassuolo Hospital, Formigine, MO, Italy

Paschos K. Nikolaos Department of Trauma and Orthopaedic Surgery, University of Ioannina, Ioannina, Greece

Department of Biomedical Engineering, University of California, Davis, CA, USA

Katarina Nilsson-Helander Department of Orthopaedics, Kungsbacka Hospital, Kungsbacka, Sweden

Marco Nitri Biomechanics Laboratory, Sports Traumatology Department, Istituto Ortopedico Rizzoli, Bologna, Italy

John Nyland Kosair Charities College of Health and Natural Sciences, Spalding University, Louisville, USA

Meir Nyska Department of Orthopaedic Surgery, Meir Medical Center, Jerusalem, Israel

The Sackler School of Medicine, Tel-Aviv University, Kfar Saba, Israel

Luke O'Brien Howard Head Sports Medicine, Vail, CO, USA

Mitsuo Ochi Department of Orthopaedic Surgery, Hiroshima University, Hiroshima, Japan

Andrew Ockuly Orthopaedic Surgery, St. Mary's Medical Center, Blue Springs, MO, USA

Kerstin Oestreich Department of Peadiatric Plastic Surgery, Birmingham Childrens Hospital, Birmingham, UK

Bruno Ohashi Center for Orthopaedics and Traumatology of Brasilia, Brasilia, DF, Brazil

Francesco Oliva Department of Orthopaedics and Traumatology, University of Rome "Tor Verata", Rome, Italy

Joaquim Miguel Oliveira 3B's Research Group – Biomaterials, Biodegradables and Biomimetics, Headquarters of the European Institute of Excellence on Tissue Engineering and Regenerative Medicine, University of Minho, Taipas, Guimarães, Portugal

ICVS/3B's – PT Government Associated Laboratory, Braga/Guimarães, Portugal

FIFA Medical Centre of Excellence, Clínica Espregueira–Mendes F.C. Porto Stadium, Porto, Portugal

Nicklas Olsson Department of Orthopaedics, Institute of Clinical Sciences at Sahlgrenska Academy, University of Gothenburg, Göteborg, Sweden

Ayberk Onal Orthopedics and Traumatology, Yeditepe University Hospital, Istanbul, Turkey

David Ou-Yang Department of Orthopaedic Surgery, University of Minnesota, Minneapolis, MN, USA

Levent Mete Özgürbüz BMT Calsis Health Technologies Co., Sarayköy, Ankara, Turkey

Turhan Ozler Orthopaedics and Traumatology Department, Yeditepe Medical Faculty, Kozyatagi, Istanbul, Turkey

Hakan Özsoy Memorial Ankara Hospital, Department of Orthopaedics and Traumatology, Ankara, Turkey

Haluk H. Öztekin Private Center for Orthopaedics and Traumatology, İzmir, Turkey

Volkan Öztuna Department of Orthopaedics Surgery and Traumatology, Mersin University School of Medicine, Mersin, Turkey

Hans H. Paessler Center of Knee and Foot Surgery, Atos-Klinik, Heidelberg, Germany

G. Pagensteert Orthopaedic Department, University Hospital Basel, Basel, Switzerland

F. Di Palma Orthopaedic and Arthroscopic Department, New Sassuolo Hospital, Sassuolo, Modena, Italy

Ezequiel Palmanovich Orthopedic Department, Meir Medical Centre, Kfar Saba, Israel

Chakra Raj Pandey Department of Orthopaedics and Traumatology, Grande International Hospital and Medicare National Hospital and Research Centre, Kathmandu, Nepal

Pericles Papadopoulos 1st Orthopaedic Department, Aristotelian University of Thessaloniki, "G. Papanikolaou" General Hospital, Exohi Thessaloniki, Greece

Brian S. Parsley The Joseph Barnhart Department of Orthopaedic Surgery, Baylor College of Medicine, Houston, TX, USA

Nikolaos K. Paschos Sports Medicine, University of Ioannina, Ioannina, Greece

School of Medicine, Department of Orthopedics, University of Ioannina, Ioannina, Greece

J. Paul Orthopaedic Department, University Hospital Basel, Basel, Switzerland

Christopher J. Pearce Department of Trauma and Orthopaedic Surgery, Jurong Healthcare (Alexandra Hospital), Singapore

Yong Loo Lin School of Medicine, Singapore

Luigi Adriano Pederzini Orthopaedic and Arthroscopic Department, New Sassuolo Hospital, Sassuolo, Modena, Italy

Albert Martin Pendleton Pediatric Orthopedic Associates, Children's Hospital of Atlanta, Atlanta, GA, USA

Hélder Pereira 3B's Research Group – Biomaterials, Biodegradables and Biomimetics, Headquarters of the European Institute of Excellence on Tissue Engineering and Regenerative Medicine, University of Minho, Taipas, Guimarães, Portugal

ICVS/3B's – PT Government Associated Laboratory, Guimarães, Portugal

Clínica Espregueira–Mendes F.C. Porto Stadium – FIFA Medical Centre of Excellence, Porto, Portugal

Orthopedic Department, Centro Hospitalar Póvoa de Varzim, Vila do Conde, Portugal

Rogério Pereira FIFA Medical Centre of Excellence, Clínica Espregueira-Mendes F.C. Porto Stadium, Porto, Portugal

Wolf Petersen Department for Orthopaedic and Trauma Surgery, Martin Luther Hospital, Berlin, Grunewald, Germany

Kalojan Petkin Clinique Générale d'Annecy, Alps Surgery Institute, Annecy, France

Stephanie C. Petterson Orthopaedic Foundation, Stamford, CT, USA

Marc J. Philippon Center for Outcomes-Based Orthopaedic Research, Steadman Philippon Research Institute, Vail, CO, USA

Sérgio R. Piedade Orthopaedic and Traumatology Department of FCM/UNICAMP, Univerisdade Estadual de Campinas, Campinas, Brazil

Bas A. C. M. Pijnenburg Department of Orthopaedic Surgery, Ziekenhuis Amstelland, Amstelveen, AM, The Netherlands

Marco Pisaniello Dipartimento di Scienze Biomediche per la Salute, Università degli Studi di Milano, IRCCS Policlinico San Donato, Milano, Italy

Kevin D. Plancher Orthopaedic Foundation for Active Lifestyles, Stamford, CT, USA

Plancher Orthopaedics and Sports Medicine, New York, NY, USA

Department of Orthopaedic Surgery, Albert Einstein College of Medicine, New York, NY, USA

Sourav K. Poddar Department of Orthopedics, CU Sports Medicine, University of Colorado, Aurora, CO, USA

Gary G. Poehling Department of Orthopaedic Surgery, Wake Forest School of Medicine, Medical Center Boulevard, Winston-Salem, NC, USA

Amy E. Pohlman Division of Orthopaedic Surgery, Cincinnati Children's Hospital Medical Center, Cincinnati, OH, USA

Andrew Pountney Emergency Medicine and Pre Hospital Care, Mid Yorkshire Hospitals NHS Trust, Wakefield, UK

M. Prandini Orthopaedic and Arthroscopic Department, New Sassuolo Hospital, Sassuolo, Modena, Italy

Lluís Puig-Verdié Department of Orthopaedic Surgery and Traumatology, Parc de Salut Mar, Hospital del Mar & Hospital de l'Esperança, Universitat Autonoma de Barcelona (UAB), Barcelona, Spain

Nicola Pujol Orthopaedic Department, Versailles Hospital, Le Chesnay, France

Vincenza Ragone Dipartimento di Scienze Biomediche per la Salute, Università degli Studi di Milano, IRCCS Policlinico San Donato, Milano, Italy

Filippo Randelli Dipartimento di Scienze Biomediche per la Salute, Università degli Studi di Milano, IRCCS Policlinico San Donato, Milano, Italy

Pietro Randelli Department of Medical Surgical Sciences, University of Milano, IRCCS Policlinico San Donato, Milan, Italy

Matthew T. Rasmussen Department of BioMedical Engineering, Steadman Philippon Research Institute, Vail, CO, USA

Giovanni Francesco Raspugli Orthopedics and Traumatology Specialization School, Laboratory of Biomechanics and Technology Innovation, Bologna, Italy

Frank Reichwein Marienkrankenhaus Düsseldorf Kaiserswerth, Düsseldorf, Germany

Rui Luís Reis Clínica Espregueira–Mendes F.C. Porto Stadium, FIFA Medical Centre of Excellence, Porto, Portugal

Orthopaedic Department, Hospital de S. Sebastião, Feira, Portugal

ICVS/3B's – PT Government Associated Laboratory, Braga/Guimarães, Portugal

3B's Research Group – Biomaterials, Biodegradables and Biomimetics, Headquarters of the European Institute of Excellence on Tissue Engineering and Regenerative Medicine, University of Minho, Taipas, Guimarães, Portugal

David R. Richardson Department of Orthopaedic Surgery and Biomedical Engineering, University of Tennessee – Campbell Clinic, Memphis, TN, USA

Michael D. Ries Tahoe Fracture and Orthopaedic Clinic, Carson City, NV, USA

University of California, Berkeley, Berkeley, CA, USA

Department of Orthopaedic Surgery, University of California, San Francisco, San Francisco, CA, USA

Pedro Luís Ripoll Ripoll y De Prado Sport Clinic -FIFA Medical Centre of Excellence, Murcia, Spain

Marta Rius Orthopaedic Surgery, Artroscopia G.C., Fundación García–Cugat. Hospital Quirón Barcelona (Spain), Universitat Internacional de Catalunya, Barcelona, Spain

García–Cugat Foundation for Biomedical Research, Barcelona, Spain

Pedro Costa Rocha Department of Orthopedic Surgery, Portuguese Air Force Hospital, Lisbon, Portugal

Andrew J. Roche Department of Trauma and Orthopaedic Surgery, The Fortius Clinic, London, UK

Thomas Rogers Department of Orthopaedic Surgery, Division of Sports Medicine, University of Louisville, Louisville, KY, USA

Harald P. Roos Skåne University Hospital, Lund, Sweden

Department of Orthopedics, Lund University, Lund, Sweden

Stefano Marco Paolo Rossi Clinica Ortopedica e Traumatologica, Fondazione IRCCS Policlinico San Matteo di Pavia, Università degli Studi di Pavia, Pavia, Italy

Roberto Rotini Shoulder and Elbow Unit, Istituto Ortopedico Rizzoli, Bologna, Italy

René-Christopher Rouchy Department of Orthopaedic Surgery and Sport Traumatology, Grenoble South Teaching Hospital, Grenoble, Échirolles, France

Claudio Rovesta Department of Orthopaedic Clinic, University of Modena, Modena, Italy

Miguel Ángel Ruiz Ibán Unidad de Hombro y Codo, Hospital Universitario Ramón y Cajal, Madrid, Spain

Marc R. Safran Department of Orthopaedic Surgery, Stanford University School of Medicine, Redwood City, CA, USA

Orthopedic Sports Medicine, Stanford Sports Medicine, Stanford University, Redwood City, CA, USA

Matthew Salzler Department of Orthopaedic Surgery, University of Pittsburgh, Pittsburgh, PA, USA

Gonzalo Samitier Clinique Générale d'Annecy, Alps Surgery Institute, Annecy, France

Kristian Samuelsson Department of Orthopaedics, Institute of Clinical Sciences, The Sahlgrenska Academy, University of Gothenburg, Göteborg, Sweden

Sukeshrao Sankineni Sports Medicine, OASI Bioresearch Foundation Gobbi NPO, Orthopaedic Arthroscopic Surgery International, Milan, Italy

E. Delli Sante Orthopaedic and Arthroscopic Department, New Sassuolo Hospital, Sassuolo, Modena, Italy

Dominique Saragaglia Department of Orthopaedic Surgery and Sport Traumatology, Grenoble South Teaching Hospital, Grenoble, Échirolles, France

Mustafa Fevzi Sargon Faculty of Medicine, Department of Anatomy, Hacettepe University, Ankara, Turkey

Fatma Saricaoglu Department of Anesthesiology and Reanimation, Hacettepe University School of Medicine, Ankara, Sihhiye, Turkey

Alkis Saridis Department of Orthopaedic Surgery, University Hospital of Patras, Rio, Greece

Eric J. Sarkissian Orthopaedic Surgery, Stanford University Medical Center, Palo Alto, CA, USA

Iskender Sayek Emeritus, Hacettepe University School of Medicine, Ankara, Sihhiye, Turkey

Bruno Sbrissia Cajuru University Hospital – PUCPR, Curitiba, PR, Brazil

Bernd Volker Scheer Team Axarsport, Alicante, Spain

Sven Scheffler Sporthopaedicum, Charite Universitatsmedizin, Berlin, Germany

Tuvia Schlesinger The Sheri and Arnold Schlesinger Radiation Protection Information, Training and Research Center, Ariel University, Ariel, Israel

J. Paul Schroeppel Department of Orthopedics and Sports Medicine, University of Kansas Medical Center, Kansas, KS, USA

Fabio Valerio Sciarretta Orthopedic Department, Clinica Nostra Signora della Mercede, Rome, Italy

Anthony J. Scillia New Jersey Orthopaedic Institute, Wayne, NJ, USA

Tommaso Scuccimarra Orthopaedic and Arthroscopic Department, New Sassuolo Hospital, Pescara, Italy

Roberto Seijas Chair of Medicine and Regenerative Surgery, Garcia Cugat Foundation & CEU Cardenal Herrera University, Alfara del Patriarca, Valencia, Spain

Department of Orthopaedic Surgery, Sports Medicine and Trauma, Hospital Quiron Barcelona, Barcelona, Spain

Facultad de Medicina y Ciencias de la Salud, Universitat Internacional de Catalunya, Barcelona, Spain

Romain Seil European Society of Sports Traumatology, Knee Surgery and Arthroscopy (ESSKA); Département de l'Appareil Locomoteur, Centre Hospitalier de Luxembourg, Clinique d' Eich; Luxembourg Olympic Medical Center, and Sports Medicine Research Laboratory, CRP-Santé, Strassen, Germany

Orthopaedic Surgery, University of Saarland, Homburg/Saar, Germany

Tarik Ait Si Selmi Centre Orthopédique Santy, Lyon, France

Gernot Seppel Department of Orthopaedic Sports Medicine, Klinikum rechts der Isar, Technical University of Munich, Munich, Germany

Elvire Servien Centre Albert Trillat, Service de Chirurgie Orthopédique, Hôpital de la Croix-Rousse, University of Lyon, Lyon, France

Adnan Sevencan Department of Sports Medicine/Department of Orthopaedics of Osmangazi, Eskişehir Osmangazi University Hospital, Eskişehir, Turkey

Ronen Sever Department of Pediatric Orthopedics, Dana Children's Hospital, Tel Aviv Medical Center, Tel Aviv, Israel

Gabriele Severini Facoltà di Medicina e chirurgia, Università Cattolica del Sacro Cuore, Rome, RM, Italy

Aksel Seyahi Department of Orthopedics and Traumatology, Koc University School of Medicine, Istanbul, Turkey

Thorsten M. Seyler Department of Orthopaedic Surgery, Wake Forest School of Medicine, Medical Center Boulevard, Winston–Salem, NC, USA

Molecular Medicine and Translational Science Program, Medical Center Boulevard, Wake Forest University, Winston–Salem, NC, USA

Teresa Sforza Physical Therapy and Rehabilitation Unit, Istituto Ortopedico Rizzoli, Bologna, Italy

David Shepherd Centre Orthopédique Santy, Lyon, France

Rainer Siebold HKF – Specialized Hip–Knee–Foot Surgery, Center for Hip, Knee and Foot Surgery, ATOS Hospital Heidelberg, Heidelberg, Germany

Institute for Anatomy and Cell Biology, Ruprecht–Karls University Heidelberg, Heidelberg, Germany

Cecilia Signorelli II Clinica Ortopedica e Traumatologica, Istituto Ortopedico Rizzoli, Bologna, Italy

Karin Grävare Silbernagel Department of Physical Therapy, University of Delaware, Newark, DE, USA

Luís Duarte Silva Clínica Espregueira–Mendes F.C. Porto Stadium, FIFA Medical Centre of Excellence, Porto, Portugal

Orthopedic Department ULS–Guarda, Guarda, Portugal

Joana Silva-Correia 3B's Research Group – Biomaterials, Biodegradables and Biomimetics, Headquarters of the European Institute of Excellence on Tissue Engineering and Regenerative Medicine, University of Minho, Taipas, Guimarães, Portugal

ICVS/3B's – PT Government Associated Laboratory, Guimarães, Portugal

Einar Andreas Sivertsen Orthopaedic Department, Martina Hansen's Hospital, Sandvika, Norway

Sam G. G. Smedberg Helsingborg/Ängelholm Hospital, Helsingborg, Sweden

Lund University, Lund, Sweden

Helsingborg, Sweden

Eduardo Sanchez Sãnchez Alepuz Unión de Mutuas, Valencia, Spain

Torbjørn Soligard IOC Medical & Scientific Department, Lausanne, Switzerland

Sergi Sastre Solsona Hospital Clinic, Barcelona, Spain

Ioannis V. Sperelakis Department of Orthopaedics and Trauma, University Hospital of Heraklion, Heraklion, Crete, Greece

Jack Spittler Department of Orthopedics, CU Sports Medicine, University of Colorado, Aurora, CO, USA

Ioannis M. Stavrakakis Department of Orthopaedics and Trauma, University Hospital of Heraklion, Heraklion, Crete, Greece

Kathrin Steffen Department of Sports Medicine, Oslo Sport Trauma Research Center, Norwegian School of Sport Sciences, Norwegian University of Sport and Physical Education, Oslo, Norway

IOC Medical & Scientific Department, Lausanne, Switzerland

David R. Steinberg University of Pennsylvania, Philadelphia, PA, USA

Regina Stern KARL STORZ GmbH & Co. KG, Tuttlingen, Germany

Susanna Stignani K. Physical Therapy and Rehabilitation Unit, Terme di S.Petronio–Antalgik, Bologna, Italy

PhysioMedica, Faenza, Italy

Shouldertech, Forlì, Italy

Tahir Sadık Sügün Orthopaedics and Traumatology, EMOT Hospital, İzmir, Turkey

Hakkı Sur Faculty of Medicine, Department of Orthopedics and Traumatology, University of Ege, Bornova, Izmir, Turkey

Cuneyt Tamam Department of Orthopaedic Surgery, Wake Forest School of Medicine, Medical Center Boulevard, Winston-Salem, NC, USA

Seval Tanrıkulu Faculty of Medicine, Department of Orthopaedics and Traumatology, Hacettepe University, Ankara, Turkey

Stephen Targett Sports Medicine Department, Qatar Orthopaedic and Sports Medicine Hospital, Doha, Qatar

Michael A. Terry Department of Orthopaedic Surgery, Feinberg School of Medicine, Northwestern University, Chicago, IL, USA

Giulia Tesei Biomechanics Laboratory, Istituto Ortopedico Rizzoli, Bologna, Italy

Darin D. Tessier Brookwood Sports Medicine, Birmingham, AL, USA

Onur Tetik Department of Orthopedics and Traumatology, Koc University, School of Medicine, İstanbul, Turkey

Hajo Thermann HKF – Specialized Hip-Knee-Foot Surgery, Centre for Hip, Knee and Foot Surgery, ATOS Clinic Center Heidelberg, Sports Traumatology, Heidelberg, Germany

Roland Thomeé Sahlgrenska Academy, Institute of Neuroscience and Physiology Section of Health and Rehabilitation, Unit of Physiotherapy, University of Gothenburg, Göteborg, Sweden

Konstantinos E. Tilkeridis Department of Orthopaedics, General University Hospital, Democritus University of Thrace, Alexandroupolis, Greece

Scott M. Tintle Walter Reed National Military Medical Center, Bethesda, MD, USA

Rozi Dzoleva Tolevska University Clinic for Orthopaedic Surgery, Skopje, Republic of Macedonia

Marc Tompkins Department of Orthopedic Surgery, University of Minnesota, Minneapolis, MN, USA

Massimo Tosi Orthopaedic and Arthroscopic Department, New Sassuolo Hospital, Campogalliano, MO, Italy

Emanuele Tripoli Orthopaedic and Arthroscopic Department, New Sassuolo Hospital, Sassuolo, Modena, Italy

R. Shane Tubbs Pediatric Neurosurgery, Children's Hospital, Birmingham, AL, USA

Akın Turgut Department of Sports Medicine/Department of Orthopaedics of Osmangazi, Eskişehir Osmangazi University Hospital, Eskişehir, Turkey

Egemen Turhan Faculty of Medicine, Department of Orthopaedics and Traumatology, Hacettepe University School of Medicine, Ankara, Sihhiye, Turkey

Cosku Turhan Sony Pictures Imageworks, Los Angeles, CA, USA

Tekin Kerem Ulku Orthopaedics and Traumatology Department, Camlica Erdem Hospital, Istanbul, Turkey

Cagatay Ulucay Orthopaedics and Traumatology Department, Yeditepe Medical Faculty, Kozyatagi, Istanbul, Turkey

Burkay Utku Department of Sports Medicine, Faculty of Medicine, Hacettepe University School of Medicine, Ankara, Turkey

Akın Üzümcügil Faculty of Medicine, Department of Orthopaedic Surgery and Traumatology, Hacettepe University, Ankara, Sıhhiye, Turkey

Filiz Üzümcügil Department of Anesthesiology and Reanimation, Hacettepe University School of Medicine, Ankara, Sihhiye, Turkey

V. Valderrabano Orthopaedic Department, University Hospital Basel, Basel, Switzerland

Michel P. J. van den Bekerom Department of Orthopaedic Surgery, Onze Lieve Vrouwe Gasthuis, Amsterdam, HM, The Netherlands

Caroline van der Zee Department of Plastic, Reconstructive & Hand Surgery, Onze Lieve Vrouwe Gasthuis, Amsterdam, The Netherlands

Carola F. van Eck Department of Orthopaedic Surgery, University of Pittsburgh Medical Center, Pittsburgh, PA, USA

Frederik J. T. van Oosterom Department of Plastic, Reconstructive & Hand Surgery, Medisch Centrum Alkmaar, Alkmaar, Netherlands

Wouter van Zuuren Medisch Centrum Alkmaar, Alkmaar, JD, The Netherlands

J. C. Vasconcelos FIFA Medical Centre of Excellence, Clínica Espregueira-Mendes F.C. Porto Stadium, Porto, Portugal

Jordi Vega Hospital Quiron, Barcelona, Spain

Giulia Venieri Biomechanics Laboratory, Istituto Ortopedico Rizzoli, Bologna, Italy

Peter Verdonk Antwerp Orthopaedic Center, Monica Hospitals Antwerpen, Antwerpen, Belgium

Department of Orthopaedic Surgery and Traumatology, Ghent University Hospital, Ghent, Belgium

René Verdonk Faculty of Medicine, Ghent State University, Ghent, Belgium

Anne L. Versteeg Department of Orthopaedics Surgery, University Medical Center Utrecht, Utrecht, The Netherlands

Athanasios N. Ververidis Department of Orthopaedics, General University Hospital, Democritus University of Thrace, Alexandroupolis, Greece

Diana Villegas Alpha Orthopaedics, Inc., Hayward, CA, USA

Manuel Virgolino Department of Orthopedic Surgery, Portuguese Air Force Hospital, Lisbon, Portugal

Sotirios Vlachoudis High School of Special Education of Thessaloniki, Sports and Physical Education, Thessaloniki, Greece

Matjaz Vogrin Department of Orthopaedic Surgery, University Medical Center Maribor, Maribor, Slovenia

Lisa Marie Geheb Vopat Division of Sports Medicine, Boston Children's Hospital, Boston, MA, USA

Andreja Vukasovic Department of Histology and Embryology, School of Medicine, University of Zagreb, Zagreb, Croatia

Slobodan Vukicevic Laboratory for Mineralized Tissues, Center for Translational and Clinical Research, School of Medicine, University of Zagreb, Zagreb, Croatia

Department of Anatomy, School of Medicine, University of Zagreb, Zagreb, Croatia

Abhijeet L. Wahegaonkar Institute for Orthopedics & Rehabilitation, Pune, India

Department of Orthopedics and Traumatology, B.V.D.U. Medical College & Hospitals, Pune, India

Garth N. Walker University of Pittsburgh Medical Center, Pittsburgh, PA, USA

Eric J. Wall Division of Orthopaedic Surgery, Cincinnati Children's Hospital Medical Center, Cincinnati, OH, USA

James Ward Department of Orthopaedic Surgery, University of Pittsburgh Medical Center, Pittsburgh, PA, USA

Yoram A. Weil Department of Orthopaedic Surgery, Orthopaedic Trauma Service, Hadassah Hebrew University Hospital, Jerusalem, Israel

Jeff Wera Division of Sports Medicine, Department of Orthopaedic Surgery, University of Louisville, Louisville, KY, USA

Robert P. Wessel Division of Sports Medicine, Department of Orthopaedic Surgery, University of Louisville, Louisville, KY, USA

Olof Westin Department of Orthopaedics, Institute of Clinical Sciences, The Sahlgrenska Academy, University of Gothenburg, Göteborg, Sweden

Department of Orthopaedics, Sahlgrenska University Hospital, Mölndal, Sweden

Rumeal Whaley Department of Orthopaedic Surgery, Division of Sports Medicine, University of Louisville, Louisville, KY, USA

Terry L. Whipple American Self, Plastic Surgery and Orthopaedics, PLC, and Orthopaedic Research of Virginia, Richmond, VA, USA

Patrick W. Whitlock Department of Orthopaedic Surgery, Division of Pediatric Orthopedics Cincinnati Children's Hospital Medical Center, University of Cincinnati, Cincinnati, OH, USA

Erik Witvrouw Orthopaedic and Sports Medicine Hospital, Aspetar, Doha, Qatar

Megan Wolf Department of Orthopaedic Surgery, University of Pittsburgh School of Medicine, Pittsburgh, PA, USA

Theodore S. Wolfson Department of Orthopaedic Surgery, New York University Hospital for Joint Diseases, New York, NY, USA

Savio L.-Y. Woo Department of Bioengineering, Musculoskeletal Research Center, Swanson School of Engineering, University of Pittsburgh, Pittsburgh, PA, USA

Moshe Yaniv Department of Pediatric Orthopedics, Dana Children's Hospital, Tel Aviv Medical Center, Tel Aviv, Israel

Kazunori Yasuda Department of Sports Medicine and Joint Surgery, Hokkaido University, Graduate School of Medicine, Sapporo, Hokkaido, Japan

Duygu Yazgan Aksoy Internal Medicine, Endocrinology and Metabolism, Department of Internal Medicine, Acıbadem University, Oran, Ankara, Turkey

Mustafa Yel Department of Orthopaedics and Traumatology, Department of Sports Medicine, Konya Necmettin Erbakan University, Meram Faculty of Medicine, Konya, Turkey

Caglar Yilgor Faculty of Medicine, Department of Orthopaedics and Traumatology, Hacettepe University, Ankara, Sihhiye, Turkey

Ibrahim Yilmaz ClinPharm, Tekirdag State Hospital, Turkish Republic Ministry of Health, Tekirdag, Turkey

Patrick Yoon Department of Orthopaedic Surgery, University of Minnesota, Minneapolis, MN, USA

Department of Orthopaedic Surgery, Hennepin County Medical Center, Minneapolis, MN, USA

Simon W. Young Department of Orthopaedic Surgery, Stanford University School of Medicine, Redwood City, CA, USA

Altug Yucekul Department of Orthopedics and Traumatology, Faculty of Medicine, Hacettepe University, Ankara, Turkey

Can A. Yucesoy Biomedical Engineering Institute, Boğaziçi University, Çengelköy, Istanbul, Turkey

Inci Yuksel Department of Physical Therapy and Rehabilitation, Faculty of Health Science, Hacettepe University, Ankara, Samanpazari, Turkey

Shu-Hang Patrick Yung Department of Orthopaedics and Traumatology, The Chinese University of Hong Kong, Prince of Wales Hospital, Shatin, Hong Kong

Stefano Zaffagnini Clinica Ortopedica e Traumatologica II, Laboratorio di Biomeccanica e Innovazione Tecnologica, Università di Bologna, Bologna, Italy

Eva Zeisig Department of Surgical and Perioperative Sciences, Orthopeadics, Umeå University, Umeå, Sweden

Part V

Knee Injuries

Anterior Cruciate Ligament Augmentation in Partial Ruptures

64

Rainer Siebold and Philippe Colombet

Contents

Abstract

The anatomical double-bundle concept changed the understanding of assessing and treating partial anterior cruciate ligament (ACL) tears. The diagnosis of a symptomatic anteromedial (AM) bundle or posterolateral (PL) bundle tear is a combination of the patient's history and complaints, the clinical examination, the magnetic resonance imaging (MRI) findings, and – of greatest importance – the arthroscopic evaluation. An ACL augmentation is performed similar to a "traditional" single-bundle reconstruction technique. It is technically more demanding because of the aim to preserve remnants and – consequently – a restricted arthroscopic visualization. Potential advantages are increased stability and better proprioception, allowing for faster rehabilitation and return to sports. However, clinical results have to be followed up closely in the long-term to investigate if there are any disadvantages for patients.

ACL Augmentation in Partial Ruptures

A partial ACL tear is a frequent injury to the knee, but only about 5–15 % of patients show persistent symptoms of pain, swelling, and instability during activities of daily living (ADL) or sports and may require surgery (Ochi et al. 2006; Siebold and Fu 2008; Ochi et al. 2009; Colombet et al. 2010; Borbon et al. 2011). The majority of partial tears are AM bundle ruptures. Ochi et al. found a

R. Siebold (✉)
HKF – Specialized Hip–Knee–Foot Surgery, Center for Hip, Knee and Foot Surgery, ATOS Hospital Heidelberg, Heidelberg, Germany

Institute for Anatomy and Cell Biology, Ruprecht–Karls University Heidelberg, Heidelberg, Germany
e-mail: rainer.siebold@atos.de

P. Colombet
Centre de Chirurgie Orthopédique et Sportive, Bordeaux-Mérignac, Mérignac, France
e-mail: philippe.colombet5@wanadoo.fr

M.N. Doral, J. Karlsson (eds.), *Sports Injuries*,
DOI 10.1007/978-3-642-36569-0_86

symptomatic partial tear in 10 % of ACL cases; of these 7.5 % had an AM bundle tear (Ochi et al. 2006).

A systematic literature review on the natural history of partial ACL tears including 12 articles was performed by Pujol et al. (2012). In all studies, the initial diagnosis was reconfirmed by an arthroscopy. The authors reported that nonsurgical treatment of partial tears was good over the medium term, especially if patients limited their sports activity. However, the greater the functional instability, the more frequent was residual pain. Laxity did progress over time, with a positive pivot-shift test emerging in 25 %. Similar findings were observed by Bak et al. (1997). They evaluated the natural history of 34 patients with partial ACL tears and conservative treatment. Five years after the initial injury, 73 % had a negative Lachman test with an instrumented side-to-side difference of less than 2 mm. Only 62 % had a good or excellent knee function, and a significant decline in activity was seen (Bak et al. 1997). The authors recommend nonsurgical treatment only in nonathletic low-demanding patients without meniscal lesions. In addition to a specific rehabilitation program, the patient has to be followed until the return to full sport activity.

In case of recurrent symptoms, an ACL augmentation should be considered. The idea of such surgery is to preserve intact ACL remnants and to reconstruct only insufficient (elongated or ruptured) parts of the ACL. This usually involves reconstructing the AM or PM fibers (Adachi et al. 2000; Buda et al. 2006; Ochi et al. 2006; Sonnery-Cottet and Chambat 2007; Siebold and Fu 2008; Ochi et al. 2009; Sonnery-Cottet et al. 2010). An ACL augmentation may also be a "central" reconstruction while preserving the surrounding intact fibers.

There might be several arguments to save ACL fibers and remnants. Deie et al. showed in an experimental study that ACL fibers may have the capacity to produce collagen (Deie et al. 1995). The resection of remnants of intact fibers may therefore be counterproductive. The ACL remnants may also add biomechanical strength in the immediate postoperative period to the reconstruction, while the graft strength depends primarily on the fixation device. Crain et al. found different types of ACL remnants, which add differently to stability (Crain et al. 2005). ACL remnants which scarred to the roof of the notch (8 %) or to the lateral wall of the notch (12 %) or the medial aspect of the lateral femoral condyle (20 %) contributed to anterior stability and therefore act as a biomechanical restraint against anterior translation. Liu et al. (2002) designed a computer model to simulate different levels of AM and PL bundle tears (Liu et al. 2002). Their results demonstrated that the degree of anterior instability was related to the amount of partial ACL disruption and remnants. The conclusion of both studies was that the augmentation may be protected by the intact ACL fibers while the graft is in the healing process. This may allow an accelerated rehabilitation program and an earlier return to sports activity.

Preserving the residual portion of the ACL may also partially maintain its blood supply, providing a support for the healing process of the graft. The vascularization of the human native ACL was investigated by Dodds et al. (Dodds and Arnoczky 1994). They described a vascularized synovial envelope around the intact ACL and periligamentous vessels penetrating the ligament transversely and anastomosing with a longitudinal network of endoligamentous vessels. The authors also showed that the tibial and femoral parts of the ACL have a greater vascular density and the proximal part has greater vascularity compared to the distal part. In an animal study by Bray et al., standardized partial injuries were surgically induced to the anterior cruciate ligament in rabbits (Bray et al. 2002). Four months after injury, the ACL was dissected and compared to a control group. The results showed direct injury induced a significant increase in blood flow and vascular volume. The time interval for maturity and remodeling, following arthroscopically assisted ACL reconstruction, was described by Falconiero et al. (1998). Superficial and deep biopsy specimens at different intervals from 3 to 120 months after ACL reconstruction were examined under light microscopy in 48 patients. The authors concluded that revascularization and ligamentization occur over a 12-month period following autogenous ACL reconstruction, with peak maturity evident after 1 year.

By the 12-month period, the graft maturity resembles that of a normal ACL. Additionally, two of the four parameters observed, vascularity and fiber pattern, showed significant evidence that maturity may occur at an earlier time ranging from 6 to 12 months.

Several excellent studies also provided information on the proprioceptive innervation of the ACL and its benefit when retaining ACL remnants. In 1984 Schultz et al. described mechanoreceptors that resemble Golgi tendon organs beneath the synovial membrane of the ACL (Schultz et al. 1984). They gave the first detailed description of mechanoreceptors in the human ACL and suggested that they may have an important proprioceptive function. In 1987 Schutte et al. reported that the human ACL is extensively innervated and that neural elements comprise approximately about 1 % of the area of the ligament (Schutte et al. 1987).

Surgeons should also consider preserving ACL remnants as an important source of reinnervation for the ACL graft. Several studies have showed that by saving remnants, postoperative knee proprioception and joint position sense can be improved. These may allow a faster and saver return to sports. Several tests were developed in recent years to measure proprioception at the knee joint. The joint position sense test was described by Co et al. (1993) and Corrigan et al. (1992), the threshold to detect passive motion by Barrack et al. (1990), and the latency of reflex hamstring contraction by Beard et al. (1993).

Adachi et al. (2002) measured the correlation between the number of mechanoreceptors and the accuracy of joint position sense in 29 knees and reported that the proprioceptive function of the ACL was correlated to the number of mechanoreceptors in the ACL. Interestingly, the authors also found mechanoreceptors in patients having a long interval between the ACL injury and the surgery. These findings were reconfirmed by Georgoulis et al., who investigated the presence of neural mechanoreceptors in the ACL remnants from 17 patients 3 months to 3.5 years after injury (Georgoulis et al. 2001). They noted free neural ends in all 17 patients. In patients with an ACL remnant adapted to the posterior cruciate ligament (PCL), mechanoreceptors exist even 3 years after injury. Ochi et al. found somatosensory evoked potentials in about 50 % of the investigated ACL remnants as confirmation that the original sensory neurons were preserved to some extent in the ACL remnants (Adachi et al. 2002). Denti et al. (1994) and Barrack et al. (1990) reconfirmed these findings for bone–patellar tendon bone grafts which were reinnervated 3–6 months postoperatively in animals.

Finally, intact remnants may serve as a guide for orientation and the point of reference for a proper anatomical placement of the bone tunnels as described by Siebold and Fu (2008) and others. On the other hand, intact femoral remnants can restrict the visualization of the intercondylar notch, which makes orientation and correct bone tunnel placement even more difficult. Therefore, especially when performing an ACL augmentation, intraoperative fluoroscopy may be a wise decision to control anatomical bone tunnel placement (Siebold and Fu 2008).

Diagnosis

Dejour et al. demonstrated that a preoperative evaluation of different types of ACL tears showed differences between complete and partial ACL tears (Dejour et al. 2013). The combination of clinical tests and stress radiographs produced threshold values that distinguished complete from partial tears. The authors examined 300 consecutive ACL-deficient patients with isolated ACL tears with the Lachman test, the pivot-shift test, stress radiographs, and MRI. The injury was reconfirmed arthroscopically. The results showed that a pivot-shift test of 0–1+ was strongly related to partial tears and instrumented anterior laxity was significantly less for partial tears compared to a complete ACL tear (5.2 mm versus 9.1 mm). Partial ACL tears with functional remaining fibers had a pivot-shift test of 0–1+ and less than 4 mm in stress radiographs (sensitivity 0.76, specificity 0.90), whereas partial ACL tears with nonfunctional fibers had a positive pivot-shift test and an anterior stress radiograph of 4–9 mm (sensitivity 0.56, specificity 0.92). A positive pivot-shift test and an anterior stress radiograph of more than 9 mm were recorded in complete ACL tears (sensitivity 0.88, specificity 0.96). MRI results revealed overlapping results between complete and partial ACL tears.

Surgical Technique

The surgery starts with an examination under anesthesia including two essential tests: the Lachman test and the pivot-shift test. The latter is much more pertinent under anesthesia (Bach et al. 1988). The pivot-shift test may be negative or a glide, which is one of the characteristics of an ACL partial tear (Panisset et al. 2008).

The surgery itself is quite similar than a standard procedure for ACL reconstruction with some differences in the graft choice, notch cleaning, tunnels positions, and drilling. Saving ACL fibers in the notch decreases the arthroscopic vision of bony landmarks and may increase the risk for surgical errors, especially in tunnel positioning.

The patient setting is classic with a leg holder or not, depending on the surgeon's preference. The portals remain the same; an anterolateral arthroscopic portal is performed close to the patellar tendon and an anteromedial instrument portal 15 mm medial to the patellar tendon. Some authors propose to do a third low anteromedial portal to facilitate PL bundle reconstruction (Siebold and Fu 2008). The augmentation requires a perfect visualization of the intercondylar notch, so the surgery may be started with the knee close to extension (20° of flexion). This position provides the largest space of the anterior part of the intercondylar notch. It is recommended to not harm the fat pad as much as possible because of postoperative scaring; instead, for better tibial visualization of the tibial ACL insertion, bring the knee close to extension. In this situation, the ruptured AM bundle fibers may be seen far anterior, which is usually not easily visualized when the knee is flexed to 90°.

The next diagnostic step is to assess the remaining intraligamentous ACL fibers. On the tibial side, it may be easier as explained above. Moreover, usually the ACL rupture occurs on the femoral side of the ACL. There may be two different situations: either one bundle was torn and the remaining bundle was intact or stretched or both bundles were torn and the ruptured fibers formed some scar tissue and adhered to the PCL or to the femoral condyle. It is difficult to give the perfect advice for the wide range of partial ACL lesions; therefore, a thorough knowledge of the anatomical ACL footprints is required (Colombet et al. 2006). It is helpful to shift portals and to place the arthroscope in the anteromedial portal to improve visualization on the lateral side of the intercondylar notch. The shaver is helpful for better visualization of the remnants, too. However, care should be taken to not be too aggressive on the residual fibers. A non-motorized instrument may be recommended which decreases the risk of damaging the remnants.

The next step now is to assess the mechanical properties of the remnants by using a probe. Is has to be decided if the remnants are of any value for anterior or rotational stability. Therefore, the knee can be placed in the figure-of-four position (Sonnery-Cottet and Chambat 2007), in which situation the PL fibers are tight and can be better tested with a probe. A measurement may also be recommended to match the graft size to the size of the remnants and to the size of the intercondylar notch. Some cases of extension deficit caused by Cyclops lesions have been reported in ACL augmentation (Sonnery-Cottet et al. 2009).

After identifying the exact injury pattern of the ACL, femoral and tibial tunnel positioning has to be performed. A careful cleaning of the AM or PL footprint with a curette or a low-frequency shaver is recommended. Tunnel drilling requires specific conditions. On the femoral side, it may be safer to drill the tunnel from outside-in using a specific aimer. However, most surgeons may use an inside-out drilling technique, which requires careful (slow) drilling so as to not damage the remnants. A good alternative is to dilate the femoral tunnel, which reduces the risk of damage to the remnants. On the tibial side, care should be taken when the drill reaches the tibial plateau, so the drill speed has to be reduced when the cortical bone of the tibial plateau is close. The authors advise to use intraoperative fluoroscopy to control and to document bone tunnel positioning, especially with restricted arthroscopic visualization.

Graft Selection

It can be systematic according to the surgeon's experience. Such a procedure may be easier when using a none-bone block graft. Hamstring grafts are widely used for such reconstructions (Adachi et al. 2000; Siebold and Fu 2008; Ochi et al. 2009; Sonnery-Cottet et al. 2010). When using a bone-tendon-bone graft, it may be difficult to manage the graft passage through the remnants and the intercondylar notch. The intercondylar notch should not be overstuffed. A 7–8 mm graft may be the ideal size (Buda et al. 2006; Sonnery-Cottet et al. 2009). The use of a double- or triple-stranded semitendinosus graft may be the perfect size, leaving the gracilis tendon in situ.

Specificities for Missing Bundle

Anteromedial bundle reconstruction represents the large majority of cases (Ochi et al. 2006; Panisset et al. 2008; Sonnery-Cottet et al. 2009), and debridement must be done carefully to avoid any damage of PL bundle. Siebold et al. (Siebold and Fu 2008) recommend to set the tibial drill guide to 60°, and the tunnel will start 1.5 cm medial to the anterior tibial tuberosity. The tibial insertion of the AM bundle is in the anteromedial aspect of the native ACL footprint in front of the intact PL fibers. Three to four millimeter of native AM stump should be preserved to enhance healing and to seal the internal aperture of the tibial tunnel to avoid the penetration of joint fluid inside the tunnel. Femoral AM tunnel positioning is more difficult because the femoral AM footprint is located deep in the notch behind the intact PL fibers. Bony landmarks are not easy to find. The posterior outlet of the intercondylar notch roof and the posterior aspect of the lateral condyle can be used to navigate. A small socket for AM drilling should be debrided with a low-frequency shaver or with radiofrequency. After marking of the selected position with an awl tip, the tunnel position should be controlled with the arthroscope and by fluoroscopy. Then the K-wire can be brought in place through a low anteromedial portal and is over drilled according to the graft size. An alternative is to drill the femoral tunnel in an outside-in fashion.

In contrast, PL bundle reconstruction is easier on the femur and more difficult on the tibia because the tibial PL footprint is situated posterior to the AM bundle. Inside the joint, the landmarks are between the AM bundle insertion and the PCL. On the femur, the tunnel must be placed close to the cartilage and just in front of the AM bundle. Siebold (Siebold and Fu 2008) proposed to mark the position with an awl 5 mm posterior to the shallow articular cartilage of the lateral femoral condyle at 90° of knee flexion and then drill in 130° of flexion through a low anteromedial portal. It is important to be careful with the medial femoral condyle to not damage the articular cartilage. Alternatively an outside-in guide or a dilator can be used to prevent any cartilage damage.

Graft Fixation

Many authors (Adachi et al. 2000; Siebold and Fu 2008; Ochi et al. 2009) use a suspensory fixation such as Endobutton® system (Smith and Nephew, Andover, MA) for femoral graft fixation and an absorbable interference screw on the tibial side. However, the fixation is not specific and it is related to the technique used. The PL bundle has to be fixed close to extension at 10–20° of flexion and the AM bundle in 70–80° of flexion. A fixation around 20° of flexion can be advised. Before final tibial fixation, the ACL graft has to be conditioned by cycling loading. It is recommended to arthroscopically assess the behavior of the graft all along flexion to correct any soft tissue impingement of the original or new ACL fibers.

Clinical Results

Clinical results of AM or PL bundle augmentation were first described by Adachi et al. (2000). They compared 40 patients in which they performed a selective reconstruction of the AM or PL bundles to a group of patients with complete ACL reconstruction. The ACL augmentation group demonstrated significantly better anteroposterior stability than the ACL reconstruction group. The side-to-side difference of anterior displacement, as measured by the KT-2000 arthrometer, was significantly improved to an average of 0.7 mm in the augmentation group compared to 1.8 mm in the reconstruction group. The final inaccuracy of joint position sense of the augmentation group was 0.7°, while that of the reconstruction group was 1.7°, which also showed a significant difference.

Buda et al. evaluated the midterm MRI appearance of 28 partial ACL tear augmentations with quadrupled distally inserted hamstrings and over-the-top fixation while preserving the intact ACL bundle (Buda et al. 2006). The mean score for the International Knee Documentation Committee (IKDC) knee examination form at 15–40 months of follow-up was 93.8. Twenty-five patients were rated as clinically excellent, three as fair. A correlation was noted between the clinical and MRI results: the graft was not visible or continuous with high-intensity areas and the mean decrease in the tunnel section area was 3 % in the three cases rated as fair. The graft appeared continuous and low intensity and the reduction in tibial tunnel section area was 30 % in the cases with excellent clinical results. The residual part of the ACL was still recognizable in 79 % of cases. The tibial hamstring attachment appeared normal in 93 % of cases. The authors concluded that excellent results correlated with a decrease in tunnel size and normal graft appearances on MRI. The poor results showed that the graft was not visible or not continuous, with high-intensity areas and intraligamentous cystic formation within the tunnel.

Sonnery-Cottet et al. performed 36 augmentations in a series of 256 ACL reconstructions using outside-in drilling (Sonnery-Cottet et al. 2010). They reported excellent results for the IKDC (97 % A or B) and an instrumented side-to-side laxity of 0.8 mm at a mean of 24 months after surgery. In two patients with larger graft diameters, they had to perform an arthrolysis caused by a cyclops lesion. These authors also reported on a retrospective multicenter study of 168 AM bundle augmentations (Sonnery-Cottet et al. 2012). At an average of 26 months postoperatively, the IKDC and Lysholm scores had improved significantly and the anterior laxity had a 1.1 mm side-to-side difference.

Similar findings were reported by Siebold and Fu (2008). They used an autologous doubled or tripled semitendinosus tendon graft for augmenting the AM or PL fibers and also observed a significant improvement in the objective and subjective IKDC, the Cincinnati Knee Score, and the KT-1000 side-to side difference from preoperation to follow-up.

Another retrospective study was performed by Abat et al. including 28 patients after ACL augmentation using 20 triple semitendinosus grafts and eight quadruple hamstring grafts (Abat et al. 2013). The authors concluded that the technique provided excellent functional scores with normalized stability (average 0.6 mm side-to-side difference) and a return to previous level of activity at 2.5 years follow-up.

Pujol et al. reported on a prospective randomized study comparing 29 AM bundle reconstructions to 25 anatomic single-bundle ACL reconstructions (Pujol et al. 2012). The only significant finding at preliminary 1-year follow-up was a better control of anterior laxity for AM bundle compared to a complete ACL reconstruction (1.2 vs. 1.9 mm).

Second look arthroscopies 1 year after ACL augmentation were performed by Ohsawa et al. to evaluate the morphology of the preserved remnants (Ohsawa et al. 2012). In each of 19 cases, the authors found taut and preserved remnants with an acceptable synovial coverage. Clinical results at an average of 40 months reconfirmed the arthroscopic impression and showed an instrumented anterior laxity of 2.0 mm for AM and 1.0 mm for PL reconstructions.

A systematic review on the management of partial ACL tears, including ten peer-reviewed articles including 634 patients, reconfirmed the encouraging results of ACL augmentation but criticized the current evidence as being too weak to support the routine use of augmentation in clinical practice (Papalia et al. 2014).

Conclusions

An ACL augmentation is performed similar to a "traditional" single-bundle reconstruction technique. It is technically more demanding because of the aim to preserve remnants and – consequently – a restricted arthroscopic visualization. Potential advantages are increased stability and better proprioception, allowing for faster rehabilitation and return to sports. However, clinical results have to be followed up closely in the long-term to investigate if there are any disadvantages for patients

References

Abat F, Gelber PE, Erquicia JI et al (2013) Promising short-term results following selective bundle reconstruction in partial anterior cruciate ligament tears. Knee. doi:10.1016/j.knee.2013.05.006

Adachi N, Ochi M, Uchio Y et al (2000) Anterior cruciate ligament augmentation under arthroscopy. A minimum 2-year follow-up in 40 patients. Arch Orthop Traum Surg 120(3–4):128–133

Adachi N, Ochi M, Uchio Y et al (2002) Mechanoreceptors in the anterior cruciate ligament contribute to the joint position sense. Acta Orthop Scand 73(3):330–334

Bach BR Jr, Warren RF, Wickiewicz TL (1988) The pivot shift phenomenon: results and description of a modified clinical test for anterior cruciate ligament insufficiency. Am J Sports Med 16(6):571–576

Bak K, Scavenius M, Hansen S et al (1997) Isolated partial rupture of the anterior cruciate ligament. Long-term follow-up of 56 cases. Knee Surg Sports Traumatol Arthrosc 5(2):66–71

Barrack RL, Buckley SL, Bruckner JD et al (1990) Partial versus complete acute anterior cruciate ligament tears. The results of nonoperative treatment. J Bone Joint Surg Br 72(4):622–624

Beard DJ, Kyberd PJ, Fergusson CM et al (1993) Proprioception after rupture of the anterior cruciate ligament. An objective indication of the need for surgery? J Bone Joint Surg Br 75(2):311–315

Borbon CA, Mouzopoulos G, Siebold R (2011) Why perform an ACL augmentation? Knee Surg Sports Traumatol Arthrosc 20(2):245–251

Bray RC, Leonard CA, Salo PT (2002) Vascular physiology and long-term healing of partial ligament tears. J Orthop Res 20(5):984–989

Buda R, Ferruzzi A, Vannini F et al (2006) Augmentation technique with semitendinosus and gracilis tendons in chronic partial lesions of the ACL: clinical and arthrometric analysis. Knee Surg Sports Traumatol Arthrosc 14(11):1101–1107

Co FH, Skinner HB, Cannon WD (1993) Effect of reconstruction of the anterior cruciate ligament on proprioception of the knee and the heel strike transient. J Orthop Res 11(5):696–704

Colombet P, Robinson J, Christel P et al (2006) Morphology of anterior cruciate ligament attachments for anatomic reconstruction: a cadaveric dissection and radiographic study. Arthroscopy 22(9):984–992

Colombet P, Dejour D, Panisset JC et al (2010) Current concept of partial anterior cruciate ligament ruptures. Orthop Traumatol Surg Res 96(8 Suppl):S109–S118

Corrigan JP, Cashman WF, Brady MP (1992) Proprioception in the cruciate deficient knee. J Bone Joint Surg Br 74(2):247–250

Crain EH, Fithian DC, Paxton EW et al (2005) Variation in anterior cruciate ligament scar pattern: does the scar pattern affect anterior laxity in anterior cruciate ligament-deficient knees? Arthroscopy 21(1):19–24

Deie M, Ochi M, Ikuta Y (1995) High intrinsic healing potential of human anterior cruciate ligament. Organ culture experiments. Acta Orthop Scand 66(1):28–32

Dejour D, Ntagiopoulos PG, Saggin PR et al (2013) The diagnostic value of clinical tests, magnetic resonance imaging, and instrumented laxity in the differentiation of complete versus partial anterior cruciate ligament tears. Arthroscopy 29(3):491–499

Denti M, Monteleone M, Berardi A et al (1994) Anterior cruciate ligament mechanoreceptors. Histologic studies on lesions and reconstruction. Clin Orthop Relat Res 308:29–32

Dodds JA, Arnoczky SP (1994) Anatomy of the anterior cruciate ligament a blueprint for repair and reconstruction. Arthroscopy 10(2):132–139

Falconiero RP, DiStefano VJ, Cook TM (1998) Revascularization and ligamentization of autogenous anterior cruciate ligament grafts in humans. Arthroscopy 14(2):197–205

Georgoulis AD, Pappa L, Moebius U et al (2001) The presence of proprioceptive mechanoreceptors in the remnants of the ruptured ACL as a possible source of re-innervation of the ACL autograft. Knee Surg Sports Traumatol Arthrosc 9(6):364–368

Liu W, Maitland ME, Bell GD (2002) A modeling study of partial ACL injury: simulated KT-2000 arthrometer tests. J Biomech Eng 124(3):294–301

Ochi M, Adachi N, Deie M, et al. (2006) Anterior cruciate ligament augmentation procedure with a 1-incision technique: anteromedial bundle or posterolateral bundle reconstruction. Arthroscopy 22(4):463 e461–465

Ochi M, Adachi N, Uchio Y et al (2009) A minimum 2-year follow-up after selective anteromedial or posterolateral bundle anterior cruciate ligament reconstruction. Arthroscopy 25(2):117–122

Ohsawa T, Kimura M, Kobayashi Y et al (2012) Arthroscopic evaluation of preserved ligament remnant after selective anteromedial or posterolateral bundle anterior cruciate ligament reconstruction. Arthroscopy 28(6): 807–817

Panisset JC, Duraffour H, Vasconcelos W et al (2008) Clinical, radiological and arthroscopic analysis of the ACL tear. A prospective study of 418 cases. Rev Chir Orthop Reparatrice Appar Mot 94(8 Suppl):362–368

Papalia R, Franceschi F, Zampogna B, et al (2014) Surgical management of partial tears of the anterior cruciate ligament. Knee Surg Sports Traumatol Arthrosc. PMID: 23263259 22(1):154–165

Pujol N, Colombet P, Cucurulo T et al (2012) Natural history of partial anterior cruciate ligament tears: a systematic literature review. Orthop Traumatol Surg Res 98(8 Suppl):S160–S164 [Review]

Schultz RA, Miller DC, Kerr CS et al (1984) Mechanoreceptors in human cruciate ligaments. A histological study. J Bone Joint Surg Am 66(7):1072–1076

Schutte MJ, Dabezies EJ, Zimny ML et al (1987) Neural anatomy of the human anterior cruciate ligament. J Bone Joint Surg Am 69(2):243–247

Siebold R, Fu FH (2008) Assessment and augmentation of symptomatic anteromedial or posterolateral bundle tears of the anterior cruciate ligament. Arthroscopy 24(11):1289–1298

Sonnery-Cottet B, Chambat P (2007) Arthroscopic identification of the anterior cruciate ligament posterolateral bundle: the figure-of-four position. Arthroscopy 23(10):1128 e1121–1123

Sonnery-Cottet B, Barth J, Graveleau N et al (2009) Arthroscopic identification of isolated tear of the posterolateral bundle of the anterior cruciate ligament. Arthroscopy 25(7):728–732

Sonnery-Cottet B, Lavoie F, Ogassawara R et al (2010) Selective anteromedial bundle reconstruction in partial ACL tears: a series of 36 patients with mean 24 months follow-up. Knee Surg Sports Traumatol Arthrosc 18(1):47–51

Sonnery-Cottet B, Panisset JC, Colombet P et al (2012) Partial ACL reconstruction with preservation of the posterolateral bundle. [Multicenter Study]. Orthop Traumatol Surg Res 98(8 Suppl):S165–S170

Anterior Cruciate Ligament Graft Selection and Fixation

65

Daniel Andernord, Olof Westin, Jon Karlsson, and Kristian Samuelsson

Contents

D. Andernord (✉)
Vårdcentralen Gripen, Karlstad, Sweden

Primary Care Research Unit, County Council of Värmland, Karlstad, Sweden

Department of Orthopaedics, Institute of Clinical Sciences, The Sahlgrenska Academy, University of Gothenburg, Göteborg, Sweden
e-mail: daniel.andernord@gmail.com

O. Westin
Department of Orthopaedics, Institute of Clinical Sciences, The Sahlgrenska Academy, University of Gothenburg, Göteborg, Sweden

Department of Orthopaedics, Sahlgrenska University Hospital, Mölndal, Sweden
e-mail: olof.westin@me.com

J. Karlsson
Department of Orthopaedic Surgery, Sahlgrenska Academy, University of Gothenburg, Sahlgrenska University Hospital, Gothenburg, Sweden
e-mail: jon.karlsson@telia.com

K. Samuelsson
Department of Orthopaedics, Institute of Clinical Sciences, The Sahlgrenska Academy, University of Gothenburg, Göteborg, Sweden
e-mail: kristian@samuelsson.cc

M.N. Doral, J. Karlsson (eds.), *Sports Injuries*,
DOI 10.1007/978-3-642-36569-0_94

Abstract

Today, a primary anterior cruciate ligament reconstruction is commonly performed by selecting an ipsilateral tendon autograft from the patient undergoing reconstruction. The bone-patellar tendon-bone autograft with metal interference screw fixation was once the gold standard for this type of procedure. Modern advancements have however introduced a diversity of options with different grafts and fixation techniques to choose from. Today, a doubled or quadrupled hamstring tendon autograft with cortical suspensory fixation to the femur and interference screw fixation to the tibia is widely adopted as a first choice for anterior cruciate ligament reconstruction. However, certain situations such as multi-ligament injuries and revision surgery often necessitate other considerations.

Graft Selection

Autografts

Bone-Patellar Tendon-Bone

Historically, the bone-patellar tendon-bone (BPTB) autograft was considered the gold standard for anterior cruciate ligament (ACL) reconstructions. The use of the patellar tendon autograft dates back to the early 1960s when Dr. Jones published his landmark paper (Jones 1963) on a new surgical technique for ACL reconstruction. Jones used the central one-third of the patellar ligament but left the ligament attached to the tibial tubercle. A decade later, it was concluded that the still distally attached patellar tendon autografts were simply too short to enable an anatomical insertion (Artmann and Wirth 1974). Franke published the first results from clinical case series which laid the foundation for the modern free bone-patellar tendon-bone autograft (Franke 1976). The BPTB autograft has withstood the test of time by producing favorable long-term follow-up success rates as well as allowing for early return to sporting activities. Theoretically, the success is attributable to the presence of bone plugs in both ends that facilitate graft fixation and osseointegration (Andersson et al. 2009; Samuelsson et al. 2009). The latter is an important factor in the healing process and rehabilitation, which explains selection of a BPTB autograft in elite athletes where return to sports is important. Orthopedic surgeons can employ the press-fit technique, which allows for fixation without interference screws or other fixation devices. In fact, this technique provides equal pullout strength and stiffness compared with hardware techniques (Widuchowski et al. 2012), leading to several advantages. First, there is no hardware to interfere with future diagnostic imaging. Second, there is no locus minoris resistentiae to make way for bacteria. Third and fourth, it is associated with less cost and easier future revision procedures. In addition, long-term results after ACL reconstruction with press-fit BPTB autografts show excellent outcome even after 15 years of follow-up (Widuchowski et al. 2012). Another advantage of the BPTB autograft is the possibility to assess graft size via MRI. This aids orthopedic surgeon in preoperative planning. Also, advocates of the BPTB autograft argue that it yields less postoperative side-to-side knee joint laxity compared with the hamstring tendon (HT) autograft. However, this is not a reflection of the scientific literature (Andersson et al. 2009; Samuelsson et al. 2009). In fact, a systematic review (Samuelsson et al. 2009) of randomized controlled clinical trials published the last 15 years revealed that the BPTB autograft was associated with more postoperative general knee pain and kneeling pain, although this appears to disappear over time. Furthermore, harvest-site morbidity includes anterior knee pain, quadriceps weakness, potential patella fracture, and risk of patella tendon rupture. Harvest-site morbidity of the anterior aspect of the knee is an important consideration in patients with high demands on satisfactory kneeling abilities in sporting or occupational activities. A further disadvantage of the BPTB autograft is that it cannot be used for double-bundle reconstruction due to anatomical properties. Finally, there is some concern regarding the higher incidence of graft failures and osteoarthritis associated with the BPTB autograft compared with the HT autograft (Leys et al. 2012). Consequently, the BPTB autograft has lost its position as the preferred graft choice and is now considered secondary to the HT autograft.

Quadriceps Tendon

The quadriceps tendon (QT) autograft, with its many advantages and few complications, is presumably an underestimated resource in ACL reconstruction. The aforementioned issues with the BPTB autograft prompted surgeons to turn their attention elsewhere (Blauth 1984; Fulkerson and Langeland 1995). The QT autograft possesses important similarities with the BPTB autograft with possible preoperative MRI planning to assess graft dimensions and, more importantly, bone attachment possibilities. The QT autograft can also be harvested with or without a patellar bone block. However, there are also some important differences; it is substantially thicker. In fact, it is often twice the size of the BPTB autograft. Hence, the cross-sectional area is considerably larger, giving it appealing biomechanical properties. Also, the anatomical structure, with the rectus femoris and vastus intermedius portions, enables single-bundle and double-bundle reconstruction, respectively (Noyes et al. 1984). It is also associated with less anterior knee pain and numbness compared with the BPTB autograft (Geib et al. 2009). The larger cross-sectional area has also proven to be an excellent aid in patients undergoing revision surgery, who might have enlarged bone tunnels.

Hamstring Tendon

The hamstring tendon (HT) autograft is another excellent graft choice. Over the past decade, it has grown in popularity, making it the number one choice for most surgeons and patients. Today, more than 98 % of all primary ACL reconstructions in Sweden are performed with an HT autograft (The Swedish National Knee Ligament Register 2013). In the USA, it accounts for 44 % (Magnussen et al. 2010). The HT autograft is associated with less donor-site morbidity compared with the BPTB autograft. Also, the HT autograft is stronger and stiffer compared with the BPTB autograft (Noyes et al. 1984) and has proven its versatility in both single-bundle and double-bundle reconstructions. However, there are some important disadvantages to consider, which mainly correlate to the soft tissue-to-bone fixation methods (Samuelsson et al. 2009). Soft tissue-to-bone fixation results in longer healing time compared with bone-to-bone fixation, even though it does not affect postoperative knee laxity. Studies also suggest a greater incidence of bone tunnel widening with HT autografts compared with BPTB autografts. The clinical importance of this finding is unclear, and it is not associated with increased postoperative knee laxity or inferior patient-reported outcome (Andersson et al. 2009; Samuelsson et al. 2009). In addition, patients tend to develop weakness in deep knee flexion and internal rotation, although this weakness disappears over time. The latter is probably not applicable to patients where both the semitendinosus tendon and the gracilis tendon (STG autografts) are harvested. In fact, this group of patients faces slower recovery and longer rehabilitation and shows additional deficits on internal rotation (Samuelsson et al. 2009). These deficits are attributed to the gracilis' important role in knee flexion at higher angles as well as in internal rotation. Hence, using only the ST autograft is preferable. There are numerous studies that are concerned with the question of the optimal graft selection – a debate that has been persistent throughout the last decades. The reality is, however, more complicated than a simple yes or no when it comes to graft selection. Different grafts merely represent different characteristics and mechanical properties. In terms of clinical outcome, there appears to be no clinically relevant differences between the two main competitors – the BPTB autograft and the HT autograft (Andersson et al. 2009; Samuelsson et al. 2009). In conclusion, both BPTB autografts and HT autografts are viable options for ACL reconstruction with equal long-term outcome.

Allografts

The most commonly used allografts are the patellar tendon, the Achilles tendon, and the tibialis anterior tendon. Theoretically, the use of allografts in ACL reconstruction is very appealing because of a markedly shortened operating time and no postoperative harvest-site morbidity affecting the flexor or extensor apparatus around the knee (Samuelsson et al. 2013). ACL reconstruction with allografts was restricted at first because of issues with potential disease transmission, inferior tensile properties, and low availability. Today, this is no longer a concern owing to improved sterilization techniques and increased supply to accommodate the growing demand. Allografts actually re-vascularize after integration and since harvest-site morbidities are avoided, the allograft is an appealing choice to elite athletes, where only minor decreases in muscle strength and range of motion can make all the difference between winning and losing. Unfortunately, studies have shown a prolonged healing time – the allograft-bone interface will not be as competent as the autograft-bone alternative – and an increased risk of graft failure, especially among young athletes (Carey et al. 2009; Maletis et al. 2013). Allografts are, however, very useful in situations where no other options are readily available, such as revision surgery, elderly patients, and injuries with multiple ligament involvement. With a constantly increasing interest from the orthopedic community, accompanied by new surgical indications, allografts hold a promising future.

Synthetic Grafts

Synthetic grafts were once thought to be the future of ACL reconstruction, with ideal graft properties: a custom-made, off-the-shelf product without any donor-site morbidity or time-consuming harvest. Several clinical attempts have been carried out trying to find the perfect synthetic graft (silk, silver wire, Teflon®, polyester, carbon fibers, the polypropylene ligament augmentation device, and Gore-Tex®) (Samuelsson et al. 2013). Unfortunately, neither has proven to be the success that was hoped for. Graft failure remains the principal adverse event associated with synthetic materials (Moyen and Lerat 1994; Grontvedt et al. 1996; Murray and Macnicol 2004). Today, synthetic grafts are only considered for experimental settings and are not intended for clinical use on ACL-deficient patients.

Graft Fixation

The bone-graft interface is often considered a weak link after ACL reconstruction, predisposing the construct to early failure. In order to overcome this problem, a wide range of different fixation techniques and materials have been developed over the last few decades.

Metal Interference Screws

Metal interference screws have been a popular choice ever since Kurosaka et al. (1987) brought them to wider attention with a cadaveric study in the late 1980s. Interference screws quickly became the gold standard together with the BPTB autograft. This technique was further developed by Pinczewski et al. (1997), by demonstrating evidence of true osseointegration with collagen fiber continuity between bone and graft, after ACL reconstruction with an HT autograft and a round-headed interference screw (RCI). These qualities made the RCI screw universally suitable for all soft tissue-to-bone fixations. Hill (Hill et al. 2005) introduced another technique, using a staple inserted distally to the tibial screw, below the tibial tunnel aperture. However, this technique has not been widely adopted due to kneeling pain following this type of fixation. The main disadvantage of the interference screws is the aperture fixation, which might alter graft kinematics by pressing the graft to one side of the bone tunnel wall, thereby preventing 360° bone-to-tendon interface (Andersson et al. 2009).

Bioabsorbable Interference Screws

There are principally two types of bioabsorbable screws on the market; these are either made from poly-L-lactic acid (PLLA) or polyglyconate. Their popularity has grown over the last decade, especially in HT autograft fixation to the tibia. As the name suggests, the screws are eventually absorbed into the bone although this takes considerably longer than one might expect. With no metal in the knee, future MRIs are not affected and future knee surgery is more convenient by not having to remove the previous fixation material. Bioabsorbable screws can also be used in conjunction with a type of plastic bead sewn to the graft to prevent the graft from slipping inside the bone tunnel (Kocabey et al. 2004). A systematic review (Andersson et al. 2009) compared clinical results of bioabsorbable and metal interference screws and reported comparable clinical outcome. Some disadvantages were reported, such as tunnel widening and screws breaking on insertion.

Cortical Suspensory Fixation

The cortical suspensory technique, which was introduced in the early 1990s, fixates the ligament graft with a suture loop to a flipping button located at the aperture level, most commonly on the femoral side (Andersson et al. 2009). Its use has increased along with the rising popularity of HT autografts. Initially designed only to anchor the HT autograft at the femoral tunnel aperture, adaptations were made to use it with the patellar tendon autograft as well (Andersson et al. 2009). Cortical suspensory fixation creates a long 360° bone-to-tendon interface, promoting adequate osseointegration. It is also useful for single-bundle and double-bundle reconstructions. An important disadvantage is a fixation farther from the joint line, which has been suspected to induce graft micro-mobility, thereby causing bone tunnel widening during loading (Andersson et al. 2009).

Cross-Pins

The final fixation technique discussed in this chapter is the use of cross-pins. Cross-pins enable graft fixation in closer proximity of the knee joint line, which is thought to counteract the aforementioned graft mobility inside the bone tunnel. Cross-pins also exhibit high failure loads and cause minimal bone tunnel widening. Transtibial bone tunnel drilling together with cross-pin fixation was once considered the gold standard in ACL reconstruction, but this has changed after the introduction of transportal bone tunnel drilling. However, guidelines are only available for the use of cross-pins in conjunction with a transtibial access. Numerous studies on ACL reconstruction, with either HT or BPTB autografts, comparing cross-pins with cortical suspensory fixation as well as interference screws, have shown comparable clinical outcome (Harilainen and Sandelin 2009; Stengel et al. 2009; Price et al. 2010).

A weak link or not, it remains to be proven that specific fixation techniques can significantly reduce the risk of early revision surgery (Andernord et al. 2014).

Cross-References

- ▶ Anterior Cruciate Ligament Injuries and Surgery: Current Evidence and Modern Development
- ▶ Anterior Cruciate Ligament Reconstruction with Autologous Quadriceps Tendon
- ▶ Allografts in Anterior Cruciate Ligament Reconstruction
- ▶ Different Techniques of Anterior Cruciate Ligament Reconstruction: Guidelines
- ▶ State of the Art in Anterior Cruciate Ligament Surgery

References

Andernord D, Bjornsson H, Petzold M, Eriksson BI, Forssblad M, Karlsson J, Samuelsson K (2014) Surgical predictors of early revision surgery after anterior cruciate ligament reconstruction: results from the Swedish national knee ligament register on 13,102 patients. Am J Sports Med. doi:10.1177/0363546514531396

Andersson D, Samuelsson K, Karlsson J (2009) Treatment of anterior cruciate ligament injuries with special reference to surgical technique and rehabilitation: an assessment of randomized controlled trials. Arthrosc J Arthrosc Relat Surg 25(6):653–685. doi:10.1016/j.arthro.2009.04.066

Artmann M, Wirth CJ (1974) Is the length of the patellar ligament sufficient for the repair of the anterior cruciate ligament? A roentgenologic analysis (author's transl). Arch Orthop Unfallchir 79(2):149–152

Blauth W (1984) 2-strip substitution-plasty of the anterior cruciate ligament with the quadriceps tendon. Unfallheilkunde 87(2):45–51

Carey JL, Dunn WR, Dahm DL, Zeger SL, Spindler KP (2009) A systematic review of anterior cruciate ligament reconstruction with autograft compared with allograft. J Bone Joint Surg Am 91(9):2242–2250. doi:10.2106/JBJS.I.00610

Franke K (1976) Clinical experience in 130 cruciate ligament reconstructions. Orthop Clin North Am 7(1):191–193

Fulkerson JP, Langeland R (1995) An alternative cruciate reconstruction graft: the central quadriceps tendon. Arthrosc J Arthrosc Relat Surg 11(2):252–254

Geib TM, Shelton WR, Phelps RA, Clark L (2009) Anterior cruciate ligament reconstruction using quadriceps tendon autograft: intermediate-term outcome. Arthrosc J Arthrosc Relat Surg 25(12):1408–1414. doi:S0749-8063(09)00516-7 [pii] 10.1016/j.arthro.2009.06.004

Grontvedt T, Engebretsen L, Benum P, Fasting O, Molster A, Strand T (1996) A prospective, randomized study of three operations for acute rupture of the anterior cruciate ligament. Five-year follow-up of one hundred and thirty-one patients. J Bone Joint Surg Am 78(2):159–168

Harilainen A, Sandelin J (2009) A prospective comparison of 3 hamstring ACL fixation devices–Rigidfix, BioScrew, and Intrafix–randomized into 4 groups with 2 years of follow-up. Am J Sports Med 37(4):699–706. doi:10.1177/0363546508328109

Hill PF, Russell VJ, Salmon LJ, Pinczewski LA (2005) The influence of supplementary tibial fixation on laxity measurements after anterior cruciate ligament reconstruction with hamstring tendons in female patients. Am J Sports Med 33(1):94–101

Jones KG (1963) Reconstruction of the anterior cruciate ligament. A technique using the central one-third of the patellar ligament. J Bone Joint Surg Am 45:925–932

Kocabey Y, Nawab A, Caborn DN, Nyland J (2004) Endopearl augmentation of bioabsorbable interference screw fixation of a soft tissue tendon graft in a tibial tunnel. Arthrosc J Arthrosc Relat Surg 20(6):658–661

Kurosaka M, Yoshiya S, Andrish JT (1987) A biomechanical comparison of different surgical techniques of graft fixation in anterior cruciate ligament reconstruction. Am J Sports Med 15(3):225–229

Leys T, Salmon L, Waller A, Linklater J, Pinczewski L (2012) Clinical results and risk factors for reinjury 15 years after anterior cruciate ligament reconstruction: a prospective study of hamstring and patellar tendon grafts. Am J Sports Med 40(3):595–605. doi:10.1177/0363546511430375

Magnussen RA, Granan LP, Dunn WR, Amendola A, Andrish JT, Brophy R, Carey JL, Flanigan D, Huston LJ, Jones M, Kaeding CC, McCarty EC, Marx RG, Matava MJ, Parker RD, Vidal A, Wolcott M, Wolf BR, Wright RW, Spindler KP, Engebretsen L (2010) Cross-cultural comparison of patients undergoing ACL reconstruction in the United States and Norway. Knee Surg Sports Traumatol Arthrosc Off J ESSKA 18(1):98–105. doi:10.1007/s00167-009-0919-5

Maletis GB, Inacio MC, Desmond JL, Funahashi TT (2013) Reconstruction of the anterior cruciate ligament: association of graft choice with increased risk of early revision. Bone Joint J 95-B(5):623–628. doi:10.1302/0301-620X.95B5.30872

Moyen B, Lerat JL (1994) Artificial ligaments for anterior cruciate replacement. A new generation of problems. J Bone Joint Surg Br 76(2):173–175

Murray AW, Macnicol MF (2004) 10–16 year results of Leeds-Keio anterior cruciate ligament reconstruction. Knee 11(1):9–14. doi:10.1016/S0968-0160(03)00076-0 S0968016003000760 [pii]

Noyes FR, Butler DL, Grood ES, Zernicke RF, Hefzy MS (1984) Biomechanical analysis of human ligament grafts used in knee-ligament repairs and reconstructions. J Bone Joint Surg Am 66(3):344–352

Pinczewski LA, Clingeleffer AJ, Otto DD, Bonar SF, Corry IS (1997) Integration of hamstring tendon graft with bone in reconstruction of the anterior cruciate ligament. Arthrosc J Arthrosc Relat Surg 13(5):641–643

Price R, Stoney J, Brown G (2010) Prospective randomized comparison of endobutton versus cross-pin femoral fixation in hamstring anterior cruciate ligament reconstruction with 2-year follow-up. ANZ J Surg 80(3):162–165. doi:10.1111/j.1445-2197.2009.05128.x

Samuelsson K, Andersson D, Karlsson J (2009) Treatment of anterior cruciate ligament injuries with special reference to graft type and surgical technique: an assessment of randomized controlled trials. Arthrosc J Arthrosc Relat Surg 25(10):1139–1174. doi:10.1016/j.arthro.2009.07.021

Samuelsson K, Andersson D, Ahlden M, Fu FH, Musahl V, Karlsson J (2013) Trends in surgeon preferences on anterior cruciate ligament reconstructive techniques. Clin Sports Med 32(1):111–126. doi:10.1016/j.csm.2012.08.011

Stengel D, Casper D, Bauwens K, Ekkernkamp A, Wich M (2009) Bioresorbable pins and interference screws for fixation of hamstring tendon grafts in anterior cruciate ligament reconstruction surgery: a randomized controlled trial. Am J Sports Med 37(9):1692–1698. doi:10.1177/0363546509333008

The Swedish National Knee Ligament Register (2013) Annual report 2012. http://www.aclregister.nu

Widuchowski W, Widuchowska M, Koczy B, Dragan S, Czamara A, Tomaszewski W, Widuchowski J (2012) Femoral press-fit fixation in ACL reconstruction using bone-patellar tendon-bone autograft: results at 15 years follow-up. BMC Musculoskelet Disord 13:115. doi:10.1186/1471-2474-13-115

Anterior Cruciate Ligament Injuries and Surgery: Current Evidence and Modern Development

66

Raman Mundi, Harman Chaudhry, and Mohit Bhandari

Contents

Abstract

Anterior cruciate ligament injuries are among the most common orthopedic injuries affecting young and active patients. Several variations in surgical techniques exist to treat these injuries. Autografts have shown comparable results to nonirradiated allografts with respect to clinical stability, functional outcomes, and failure rates. Several randomized trials have been published comparing the double-bundle and single-bundle techniques. Pooled analysis of such studies shows the two techniques produce comparable functional outcomes, but suggest the double-bundle technique leads to superior clinical stability. There are several options for graft fixation, including interference screw, cross-pin, and cortical fixation. Despite a proliferation in fixation devices, there remains a lack of evidence to endorse any one technique exclusively. Postoperative protocols also remain varied, and current evidence has not supported the use of bracing or outpatient physiotherapy compared to home physiotherapy. The findings of future high-quality randomized trials have the potential to strengthen current reviews and inform clinical practice guidelines, to ensure that the practice of ACL reconstruction surgery remains "evidence based" and on par with emerging knowledge.

R. Mundi (✉) • H. Chaudhry • M. Bhandari
Division of Orthopaedic Surgery, McMaster University, Hamilton, ON, Canada
e-mail: raman.mundi@medportal.ca; harman.chaudhry@medportal.ca; bhandam@mcmaster.ca

M.N. Doral, J. Karlsson (eds.), *Sports Injuries*,
DOI 10.1007/978-3-642-36569-0_102

Introduction

Anterior cruciate ligament (ACL) ruptures represent one of the most common orthopedic conditions afflicting young and active patients. With an estimated incidence of 200,000 per year, over 100,000 ACL reconstructions are performed annually in the United States alone and have become the sixth most commonly performed orthopedic procedure (Prodromos et al. 2008; Lyman et al. 2009; Tiamklang et al. 2012). From its origins as a primary repair procedure using silk suture, to the modern-day double-bundle reconstruction technique, ACL surgery has evolved considerably over the past century and has been touted as one of the most successful orthopedic procedures today (Ayeni et al. 2013; Samuelsson et al. 2013).

Given the high functional demands of patients who typically sustain ACL injuries, even relatively "minor" improvements in surgical outcomes can have potentially profound implications on patient satisfaction and quality of life. Despite cementing its success as a proven method for restoring knee stability, new techniques and devices are continuously being put forward in an attempt to further improve outcomes for ACL reconstructive surgery. Owing to this, several aspects of ACL reconstruction remain equivocal and continue to be shrouded in controversy (Prodromos et al. 2008).

Four salient issues of current contention include (i) graft selection (autograft vs. allograft), (ii) double-bundle versus single-bundle technique, (iii) graft fixation, and (iv) postsurgical rehabilitation. This chapter will explore the arguments around each of these issues and discuss the most recent, high-quality clinical evidence informing these debates. The chapter will conclude with a discussion of issues holding particular importance to future research trials on ACL reconstruction outcomes.

Graft Selection

The ideal graft choice for ACL reconstructive surgery is one that has rapid incorporation, a minimal failure rate, low donor site morbidity, and a high level of safety. Although the ideal graft does not exist, there are several options available to orthopedic surgeons, with each carrying certain benefits and shortcomings (Jost et al. 2011).

Among autografts, bone-patellar tendon-bone (BPTB) grafts were historically the gold standard for ACL reconstruction (Samuelsson et al. 2013). Bone plugs at both ends of the graft optimize fixation and osseointegration while the graft is relatively easy to harvest. However, patellar tendon grafts have been associated with poor donor site morbidity, resulting in anterior knee pain, pain with kneeling, and quadriceps weakness. The most commonly used graft today remains the quadruple hamstrings tendon autograft. The multiple bundles provide strength and a large graft size to enhance graft incorporation, while there is less donor site morbidity compared to the patellar tendon graft (Ayeni et al. 2013; Samuelsson et al. 2013).

In a 2011 Cochrane review, Mohtadi et al. analyzed nineteen randomized and quasi-randomized trials directly comparing the outcomes of patellar tendon and hamstrings tendon ACL reconstruction. These trials spanned across ten countries and collectively recruited 1,748 patients with a mean age ranging from 21.5 to 32 years. This meta-analysis found no significant difference between the two autografts in terms of functional outcomes (hop test), activity participation (Tegner score, Lysholm score), and re-rupture rates (2.6 % PT vs. 3.3 % HT). However, the patellar tendon autograft demonstrated superior clinical stability, as determined by the KT-arthrometer (analyzed as mean difference), Lachman, and Pivot shift tests. Pooled analysis also demonstrated a statistically significant difference in extension deficit and a trend towards decreased extension strength for the patellar tendon group, whereas hamstring grafts were associated with a significant loss in flexion strength and a trend towards a flexion deficit. Ultimately, the authors deemed there is insufficient evidence to provide a clinical recommendation for either type of autograft. In large part, this was attributed to the methodological flaws of current trials, as only four studies had an adequate method of randomization, two had adequate allocation concealment, and only two had blinded outcome assessors (Mohtadi et al. 2011).

The debate surrounding graft selection in ACL reconstruction surgery has primarily centered on the use of autografts compared to allografts, with each having purported benefits over the other (Prodromos et al. 2008). Although the quadruple hamstring tendon autograft remains the current gold standard, the use of allografts has risen considerably in certain centers over the past several years (Jost et al. 2011). Common allograft options include the patellar tendon, Achilles tendon, and tibialis anterior tendon. Allografts have the benefit of reducing operative time and eliminating donor site morbidity, but incorporate slower and carry the risks of disease transmission (Hu et al. 2013). Although irradiated allografts have demonstrated higher rates of failure compared to autografts, nonirradiated allografts have shown more promise (Borchers et al. 2009; Mariscalco et al. 2013).

Two independent systematic reviews have recently been published comparing the outcomes of autograft to nonirradiated allograft. Hu and colleagues evaluated nine prospective studies, with five of the studies comparing BPTB autograft to BPTB allograft and the remaining four evaluating soft-tissue autograft to soft-tissue allograft. They found no significant difference between autograft and allograft with respect to clinical stability (KT-arthrometer, Lachman, and Pivot shift), objective International Knee Documentation Committee (IKDC) score, Lysholm and Tegner scores, and graft failure. In a subgroup analysis, however, it was demonstrated that BPTB autografts had statistically significant better Tegner scores compared to BPTP allograft. Although all studies were prospective in nature, only four were randomized trials and none of them were of high methodological quality (Hu et al. 2013).

These findings have been supported by the review from Mariscalco et al. Their review also identified nine studies. However, three of these studies were different from the abovementioned review and included both prospective and retrospective studies. The pooled analyses demonstrated no significant difference between autograft and nonirradiated allograft with respect to clinical stability (Lachman, Pivot shift) and graft failure. Although a pooled analysis for patient-reported functional scores was not done, none of the individual studies found a significant difference in such scores (Tegner, Lysholm, subjective IKDC, Cincinnati scores) (Mariscalco et al. 2013).

Current evidence does not substantiate the use of one graft type over the other, both among autografts and when comparing autograft to nonirradiated allograft. As highlighted by the above reviews, there remains a need for methodologically robust randomized trials to elucidate the true efficacy of the various graft types.

Double-Bundle Versus Single-Bundle Technique

The immediate goal of anatomic ACL surgery is to restore the native ACL anatomy and normal knee biomechanics (Muller et al. 2013). Recognizing the complimentary functions of the anteromedial and posterolateral bundles of the ACL during flexion and extension of the knee, respectively, the double-bundle technique has garnered much attention. Specifically, the double-bundle technique attempts to recreate both functional bundles, and it has been argued this technique better restores the rotational stability of the knee offered by the native posterolateral bundle (Prodromos et al. 2008; Samuelsson et al. 2013). However, the double-bundle technique remains a technically demanding procedure, which inevitably raises concern, as the most common cause for ACL reconstruction failure is improper bone tunnel placement (Prodromos et al. 2008). Furthermore, double-bundle reconstruction is not tantamount to "anatomic" reconstruction. Anatomic reconstruction requires the functional restoration of the ACL to its native dimensions, orientation, and insertions sites, which can be met with success or failure with both the double-bundle and single-bundle techniques (Muller et al. 2013).

In a 2012 Cochrane review, 17 randomized trials were identified that compared the outcomes of double-bundle reconstruction to single-bundle reconstruction in young, active adults with ACL ruptures. In a pooled analysis of nine trials, there was no significant difference between the two techniques for subjective functional outcomes (subjective IKDC score, Lysholm score, Tegner activity score) or adverse events (graft failure, infection). However, the double-bundle technique resulted in significantly better return to pre-injury level of activity and clinical stability (IKDC examination, KT-arthrometer, Pivot shift). Given the severe methodological flaws and risk of bias in the included trials, the authors concluded there is insufficient evidence to determine the relative effectiveness of the double-bundle versus single-bundle techniques and advocated for large, high-quality, randomized trials with long-term follow-up (Tiamklang et al. 2012).

The debate on the double-bundle versus single-bundle technique remains a highly active one, as three randomized trials have been published since this recent review. In a trial of 103 patients by Ahldén et al., there was no significant difference between the two techniques at 2-year follow-up for all outcomes, including measures of clinical stability (Lachman, KT-arthrometer, pivot shift), functional outcomes (one-legged hop test, square hop test), and subjective functional outcomes (Lysholm score, Tegner score, Knee Injury and Osteoarthritis and Outcome Score (KOOS)) (Ahldén et al. 2013). Hussein and colleagues carried out a larger randomized trial comparing three techniques in 281 patients – anatomical double-bundle, anatomical single-bundle, and conventional single-bundle reconstructions. The anatomic double-bundle technique was associated with significantly improved clinical stability (KT-arthrometer and pivot shift) but similar subjective functional outcomes (Lysholm score, subjective IKDC score) when compared to the anatomic single-bundle technique (Hussein et al. 2012). Finally, in the randomized trial of 108 patients by Zhang et al., the double-bundle group demonstrated significantly superior rotational stability, but no difference from the single-bundle group with respect to anteroposterior laxity (KT-arthrometer, Lachman test) or subjective functional outcomes (Lysholm score, Tegner score, KOOS score) (Zhang et al. 2013).

In large part, the outcomes of these trials remain consistent with the findings of the Cochrane review in that the double-bundle and single-bundle techniques produce similar subjective functional outcomes. However, they provide discrepant results in regard to the clinical stability offered by each technique. As a potential explanation for these conflicting findings, the trials varied in their operative techniques (anatomic vs. transtibial femoral tunnel drilling), fixation devices used, rehabilitation protocols, and study methodology. Furthermore, the majority of studies provided results at a 2-year follow-up. The long-term outcomes of the double-bundle versus single-bundle techniques have yet to be determined. Summaries of newly emerging meta-analyses comparing these techniques can be found at OrthoEvidence, an online source that provides pre-appraised summaries of the latest orthopedic evidence (www.myorthoevidence.com).

Fixation Devices

With the rise in popularity of soft-tissue autografts and allografts, a wide variety of fixation devices have been developed for ACL reconstruction (Samuelsson et al. 2013). Unfortunately, there is no consensus as to which fixation device is optimal (Prodromos et al. 2008).

The interference screw fixation technique has been deemed the gold standard, particularly when used with a patellar tendon autograft. Two primary options for interference screw fixation include metallic screws or bioabsorbable screws, with the latter having the advantage of eliminating interference with subsequent MRI examinations and simplifying potential revision surgery (Samuelsson et al. 2013). In a meta-analysis of ten randomized trials comparing metallic to bioabsorbable screw fixation in single-bundle ACL reconstruction, there was no significant difference demonstrated between the two fixation methods in terms of clinical stability (KT-arthrometer, pivot shift), functional scores (IKDC score, Lysholm score), or infection rates. The trials varied, however, in the type of graft utilized and their reported rehabilitation protocols (Shen et al. 2010).

Cortical fixation and cross-pin fixation remain two alternative techniques utilized for graft fixation. Although cortical fixation devices are suitable for many types of reconstruction technique due to the lengthened bone-tendon interface, they allow for increased motion of the graft within the tunnel and may result in tunnel widening (Samuelsson et al. 2013). Cross pins offer fixation closer to the joint which theoretically offers a more stable fixation compared to cortical fixation, although evidence to support this is lacking (Prodromos et al. 2008).

Colvin et al. performed a systematic review of eight prospective trials, including six randomized trials, comparing interference femoral screw fixation to noninterference (cortical and cross-pin) fixation for hamstring tendon autograft ACL reconstruction. Pooled analysis showed no significant difference in failure rates or IKDC scores between the two groups. However, the authors acknowledged the limitations of their analysis given the small number of identified trials, the small sample sizes of the trials, the lack of reporting of clinical stability outcomes, and the variation in tibial fixation devices used (Colvin et al. 2011).

Despite the proliferation of fixation devices utilized for graft fixation in ACL surgery, there remains a paucity of high-quality evidence in the form of large, randomized trials to definitely establish which fixation devices are associated with improved clinical outcomes.

Rehabilitation Protocol

Rehabilitation after ACL reconstruction is a multifaceted and prolonged intervention, lasting anywhere from 3 months to a year postoperatively. Rehabilitation protocols focus on regaining full range of motion, strength, and functionality of the knee through a series of progressive step-wise exercises and other miscellaneous interventions.

There is a fair amount of debate surrounding the optimal rehabilitation protocol, with each component – from the immediate postoperative period to the point where unrestricted physical activity is permissible – coming under investigation at some point. Indeed, given the extent of clinical equipoise, standard rehabilitation protocols vary greatly around the world (Cook et al. 2008).

Three systematic reviews have comprehensively evaluated the current state of the literature pertaining to rehabilitation protocols following ACL reconstruction. Wright and colleagues have collected and analyzed all the relevant clinical trial evidence to 2005 (Wright et al. 2008a, b), while Kruse and colleagues have done the same for the period of 2005–2010 (Kruse et al. 2012). The evidence for and against various rehabilitation protocol components is drawn from these comprehensive reviews.

Interventions that can be employed in the immediate postoperative period to improve outcomes have been investigated. Postoperative bracing has universally been shown to be of no additional benefit following ACL reconstruction. Theoretically, postoperative bracing was thought to improve knee stability (by preventing varus/valgus stress), improve desired knee range of motion (i.e., flexion-extension arc), and provide a sense of stability (both physically and psychologically). However, a total of 18 randomized controlled trials that have been published through to 2010 have almost unanimously failed to demonstrate a benefit between use and nonuse, as well as between various protocols for use and types of braces. Based on these findings, postoperative bracing appears to have a limited role in ACL rehabilitation. Continuous Passive Motion (CPM) devices have also been evaluated in the postoperative period. These devices cyclically range a patient's knee with the aim of more rapidly regaining full knee range of motion. Despite early enthusiasm, these devices have not been shown to be of any benefit.

There has been no evidence to suggest a difference in outcome based on the setting in which rehabilitation occurs. Clinical trials employing home-based rehabilitation protocols either following a standardized, but shortened, physiotherapy regimen or involving minimal supervision have not demonstrated superiority. The one trial, and its follow-up publication, which demonstrated superiority of home-based physiotherapy in terms of ACL-specific quality of life had a number of patients that were lost to follow-up (Grant et al. 2005; Grant and Mohtadi 2010). Therefore, evidence supporting the superiority of home-based rehabilitation is presently lacking. Home-based rehabilitation may be equivalent to standard outpatient physiotherapy, but larger trials with non-inferiority designs are needed to corroborate these findings.

Several investigators have attempted to accelerate the rehabilitation protocol, a particularly pertinent topic for highly motivated athletes desiring a faster return to competitive sport. A total of seven trials evaluating revised protocols have attempted to complete postoperative rehabilitation more quickly through earlier weight-bearing, range of motion, and strengthening exercises. Interventions in these trials typically compare standard 5–6-month protocols to protocols involving shortened timelines achieved by beginning strengthening immediately or aggressively (e.g., eccentric strengthening beginning 2–3 weeks postoperatively). While demonstrating that these protocols are in some cases significantly more effective (and in other cases likely no less effective), the sample sizes and outcomes of these studies are not powered to evaluate the safety of these protocols (Johnson and Beynnon 2012). Larger, adequately powered clinical trials will be needed to ensure the safety of early aggressive rehabilitation.

Other "nontraditional" interventions have largely been of minimal benefit, if any. Water-based, psychological, and neuromuscular therapies have been shown to be of possible benefit, but should only be included in the context of more conventional elements of rehabilitation protocols (i.e., range of motion and strengthening). Supplementations with oral vitamins E and C were shown to have no impact on recovery, while intra-articular hyaluronic acid injection at postoperative week 8 demonstrated some benefits in a single trial. These, and other nonconventional interventions, will require further investigations to allow for definitive conclusions.

Conclusions

Orthopedic surgeons performing ACL reconstructive surgery are confronted with an array of options for several aspects of the procedure. Current practices are exceedingly variable, which in part may be attributable to the lack of high-quality clinical research to elucidate the relative efficacy of these advancements. This variability in practice was highlighted in a recent international survey on trends in ACL surgery, which involved 261 surgeons across 57 countries. In terms of graft choice, hamstring tendon and patellar tendon autograft were the most frequently preferred, with 63 % and 26 % of surgeons listing these as their first preference, respectively. An anteromedial arthroscopic approach to drilling the femoral tunnel was preferred by 68 % of surveyed surgeons, whereas the transtibial approach was used by 31 %. Two-thirds (67 %) of surveyed surgeons use the single-bundle technique and the preferred method of fixation was highly variable, including the Endo-button (40 %), bioabsorbable interference screw (34 %), metallic interference screw (12 %), and Rigidfix (10 %) (Chechik et al. 2013).

As concluded by several of the systematic reviews discussed in this chapter, there remains a need for large, high-quality, randomized controlled trials to further elucidate which techniques, devices, and protocols lead to better and safer long-term outcomes after ACL reconstruction. Future trials must ensure robust methodology, including an adequate method of randomization, the preservation of allocation concealment, balanced surgeon experienced in all treatment arms, and the implementation of blinded outcome assessors, among other design issues. The use of expertise-based randomize trials can ensure balanced surgeon skill and avoid the ethical dilemma of participating surgeons performing a procedure against personal preference. In this design, patients are randomized to a particular surgeon (instead of a procedure) and that surgeon is responsible for performing only the surgical technique of their preference.

The findings of future high-quality randomized trials have the potential to strengthen current reviews and inform clinical practice guidelines, to ensure that the practice of ACL reconstruction surgery remains "evidence based" and on par with emerging knowledge.

References

Ahldén M, Senert N, Karlsson J et al (2013) A prospective randomized study comparing double- and single-bundle techniques for anterior cruciate ligament reconstruction. Am J Sports Med 41:2484 [Epub ahead of print]

Ayeni OR, Evaniew N, Ogilvie R et al (2013) Evidence-based practice to improve outcomes of anterior cruciate ligament reconstruction. Clin Sports Med 32(1):71–80

Borchers JR, Pedroza A, Kaeding C (2009) Activity level and graft type as risk factors for anterior cruciate ligament graft failure: a case-control study. Am J Sports Med 37(12):2362–2367

Chechik O, Amar E, Khashan M et al (2013) An international survey on anterior cruciate ligament reconstruction practices. Int Orthop 37(2):201–206

Colvin A, Sharma C, Parides M et al (2011) What is the best femoral fixation of hamstring autografts in anterior cruciate ligament reconstruction?: a meta-analysis. Clin Orthop Relat Res 469(4):1075–1081

Cook C, Nguyen L, Hegedus E et al (2008) Continental variations in preoperative and postoperative management of patients with anterior cruciate ligament repair. Eur J Phys Rehabil Med 44(3):253–261

Grant JA, Mohtadi NG (2010) Two- to 4-year follow-up to a comparison of home versus physical therapy-supervised rehabilitation programs after anterior cruciate ligament reconstruction. Am J Sports Med 38(7):1389–1394

Grant JA, Mohtadi NG, Maitland ME et al (2005) Comparison of home versus physical therapy-supervised rehabilitation programs after anterior cruciate ligament reconstruction: a randomized controlled trial. Am J Sports Med 33:1288–1297

Hu J, Qu J, Xu D et al (2013) Allograft versus autograft for anterior cruciate ligament reconstruction: an up-to-date meta-analysis of prospective studies. Int Orthop 37(2):311–320

Hussein M, van Eck CF, Cretnik A et al (2012) Prospective randomized clinical evaluation of conventional single-bundle, anatomic single-bundle, and anatomic double-bundle anterior cruciate ligament reconstruction. Am J Sports Med 40(3):512–520

Johnson RJ, Beynnon BD (2012) What do we really know about rehabilitation after ACL reconstruction?: commentary on an article by L.M. Kruse, MD, et al.: "rehabilitation after anterior cruciate ligament reconstruction. A systematic review". J Bone Joint Surg 94(19):e14, 1-2

Jost PW, Dy CJ, Robertson CM et al (2011) Allograft use in anterior cruciate ligament reconstruction. HSS J 7(3):251–256

Kruse LM, Gray B, Wright RW (2012) Rehabilitation after anterior cruciate ligament reconstruction. J Bone Joint Surg 94(19):1737–1748

Lyman S, Koulouvaris P, Sherman S et al (2009) Epidemiology of anterior cruciate ligament reconstruction: trends, readmissions, and subsequent knee surgery. J Bone Joint Surg Am 91(10):2321–2328

Mariscalco MW, Magnussen RA, Mehta D et al (2013) Autograft versus nonirradiated allograft tissue for anterior cruciate ligament reconstruction: a systematic review. Am J Sports Med 42:492 [Epub ahead of print]

Mohtadi NG, Chan DS, Dainty KN et al (2011) Patellar tendon versus hamstring tendon autograft for anterior cruciate ligament rupture in adults. Cochrane Database Syst Rev 9:CD005960

Muller B, Hofbauer M, Wongcharoenwatana J et al (2013) Indications and contraindications for double-bundle ACL reconstruction. Int Orthop 37(2):239–246

Prodromos CC, Fu FH, Howell SM et al (2008) Controversies in soft-tissue anterior cruciate ligament reconstruction: grafts, bundles, tunnels, fixation, and harvest. J Am Acad Orthop Surg 16(7):376–384

Samuelsson K, Andersson D, Ahldén M et al (2013) Trends in surgeon preference on anterior cruciate ligament reconstructive techniques. Clin Sports Med 32(1):111–126

Shen C, Jiang SD, Jiang LS et al (2010) Bioabsorbable versus metallic interference screw fixation in anterior cruciate ligament reconstruction: a meta-analysis of randomized controlled trials. Arthroscopy 26(5):705–713

Tiamklang T, Sumanont S, Foocharoen et al (2012) Double-bundle versus single-bundle reconstruction for anterior cruciate ligament rupture in adults. Cochrane Database Syst Rev 11:CD008413

Wright RW, Preston E, Fleming BC et al (2008a) A systematic review of anterior cruciate ligament reconstruction rehabilitation: part I: continuous passive motion, early weight bearing, postoperative bracing, and home-based rehabilitation. J Knee Surg 21(3):217–224

Wright RW, Preston E, Fleming BC et al (2008b) A systematic review of anterior cruciate ligament reconstruction rehabilitation: part II: open versus closed kinetic chain exercises, neuromuscular electrical stimulation, accelerated rehabilitation, and miscellaneous topics. J Knee Surg 21(3):225–234

Zhang Z, Gu B, Zhu W et al (2013) Double-bundle versus single-bundle anterior cruciate ligament reconstructions: a prospective, randomized study with 2-year follow-up. Eur J Orthop Surg Traumatol 24:559 [Epub ahead of print]

Anterior Cruciate Ligament Injuries with Concomittant Meniscal Pathologies

67

Yuichi Hoshino, Matthew Salzler, Kevin Jiang, and Volker Musahl

Contents

Y. Hoshino
Department of Orthopaedic Surgery, Kobe Kaisei Hospital, Kobe, Japan
e-mail: you.1.hoshino@gmail.com

M. Salzler • K. Jiang
Department of Orthopaedic Surgery, University of Pittsburgh, Pittsburgh, PA, USA
e-mail: salzlermj@upmc.edu; jiangkn@upmc.edu

V. Musahl (✉)
Department of Orthopaedic Surgery, University of Pittsburgh Medical Center, Pittsburgh, PA, USA

Division of Sports Medicine, Orthopaedic Surgery, University of Pittsburgh, Pittsburgh, PA, USA
e-mail: musahlv@upmc.edu

M.N. Doral, J. Karlsson (eds.), *Sports Injuries*,
DOI 10.1007/978-3-642-36569-0_88

Abstract

Meniscal tears are present in conjunction with anterior cruciate ligament (ACL) injuries in approximately half of the cases. The menisci serve many important functions in the knee. Specifically in regard to the ACL-injured knee, the lateral meniscus plays a role in rotational loading. It is frequently damaged by the subluxation of the lateral compartment at the time of the ACL rupture. The medial meniscus is a secondary stabilizer to anterior tibial translation and is often torn over time due to accumulated mechanical stress from abnormal knee kinematics in the ACL-deficient knee. With these important functions, meniscal pathology could worsen the already abnormal laxity of the ACL-deficient knee. Surgical treatment aims to preserve as much meniscal structure as possible while removing unstable flaps through meniscectomy or stabilize the meniscus through repair. Loss of normal meniscus function leads to increased articular cartilage degeneration, osteoarthritis (OA), and worse clinical outcomes. Therefore, to improve knee stability and long-term outcomes, meniscal pathology must be carefully considered in the management of patients with ACL ruptures.

Introduction

Meniscal tears commonly occur in conjunction with anterior cruciate ligament (ACL) injuries. Recent studies have found up to 35–61 % of ACL ruptures have meniscal pathology (Granan et al. 2009; Slauterbeck et al. 2009; Rotterud et al. 2013). Reports differ on the relative frequency of medial versus lateral meniscal tears in the ACL-injured knee. Rotterud et al. reported on a large cohort of patients with ACL injuries from the Scandinavian registry and found a 43 % incidence of meniscal injuries including 20 % medial meniscus, 14 % lateral meniscus, and 8 % both (Rotterud et al. 2013). A retrospective study by Slauterbeck et al. of 1,209 patients with ACL ruptures revealed 52 % had isolated lateral meniscal tears compared to 26 % with isolated medial meniscus tears (Slauterbeck et al. 2009).

The etiology and pathology are different between medial and lateral meniscal injuries. This is due to differing tibial plateau morphology, tibiofemoral movement, mobility of the menisci, and meniscal function in the separate knee compartments (see "► Chap. 72, Anatomy and Biomechanics of the Knee"). The loss of these important functions of the menisci can lead to increased knee instability in the ACL-deficient knee. Studies have shown preservation of meniscal structure during ACL reconstruction through meniscal repair rather than meniscectomy leads to better clinical outcomes (Shelbourne and Carr 2003; Shelbourne and Dersam 2004). Meniscal repairs performed in conjunction with ACL reconstruction have been found to have higher success rates than those repairs performed in isolation (Warren 1990). However, repair may not always be possible due to the morphology of the tear. Also healing of the repair can depend on timing of surgery. Therefore, diagnosis, surgical timing, and preoperative planning of meniscal pathology are important factors to consider in patients with ACL injuries in order to better clinical outcomes of surgical reconstruction.

Biomechanical Effects of Concomitant Meniscal and ACL Injuries

The actual incidence of the meniscus tear associated with the ACL injury is different between medial and lateral meniscus depending on the time after the initial injury. This could be attributed to the different injury mechanisms for meniscal tears in medial and lateral compartments (Fig. 1). Lateral meniscal tears tend to occur at the time of ACL injury or during instability episodes

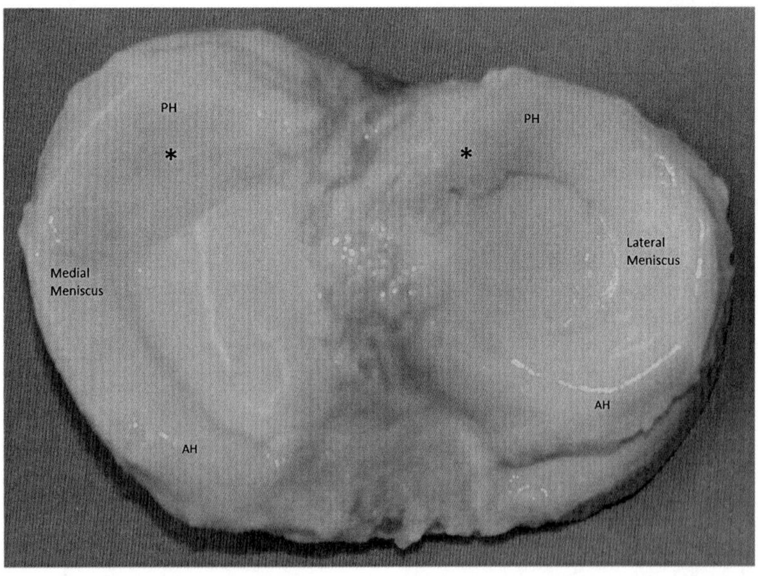

Fig. 1 Photograph of a tibial plateau demonstrating the medial and lateral menisci with *'s identifying the most common location of tears seen in conjunction with ACL injuries. *AH* anterior horn, *PH* posterior horn

Table 1 Demonstration of the biomechanical effects with deficiency of the medial or lateral meniscus

Deficiency	Anterior drawer	Lachman	Pivot shift	Contact pressures
Medial meniscus	↑↑	↑↑	↑	↑
Lateral meniscus	↑	↑	↑↑	↑

of an ACL-deficient knee secondary to the traumatic subluxation of the tibia on the femur. This pathologic tibiofemoral movement in the lateral compartment that is specific to ACL injury is called the pivot shift phenomenon. It is also the source of the sensation of knee instability which patients often describe as "giving way" or "buckling" of the knee (Galway and MacIntosh 1980). This abnormal movement can be reproduced by the pivot shift test during clinical evaluation of ACL insufficiency (Galway et al. 1972). In the pivot shift test, when an ACL rupture is present, the tibia is anteriorly subluxed with internal rotation and knee extension. In this position, the iliotibial band acts as an extensor and keeps the tibia anteriorly subluxed. When a valgus and axial force is applied while moving from extension into flexion, the iliotibial band changes from an extensor to a flexor at 30° and helps reduce the subluxation resulting in a clunk. The clinical grading of the pivot shift test, which could be graded as glide (+), clunk (++), or gross (+++), is based on the magnitude of the lateral compartment subluxation and reduction (Bedi et al. 2010).

The posterior portion of the lateral meniscus can trapped and damaged between lateral femoral condyle and posterior edge of the lateral tibial plateau during the subluxation of the tibia at the time of ACL injury (Matsumoto 1990). This also leads to the typical bone bruise pattern seen on MRI, middle third of the lateral femoral condyle and posterior third of the lateral tibial plateau (Viskontas et al. 2008). Due to the high impaction stress transferred through the lateral compartment at the time of the ACL injury, further mechanical damage apart from lateral meniscal tears such as osteochondral impaction injuries can be seen.

The medial meniscus acts as a secondary stabilizer with the ACL to anterior translation of the tibia. In an ACL-deficient knee, abnormal tibiofemoral motion leads to increased stress transferred to the medial meniscus. In contrast to the gross instability episodes associated with lateral meniscal injuries, medial meniscal injuries in the ACL-injured knee occur over time due to the accumulated effects of this transferred stress especially during walking and pivoting with axial rotation (Andriacchi and Dyrby 2005; Ristanis et al. 2005; Fuentes et al. 2011; Lam et al. 2011). Unlike the obvious subluxation in the pivot shift phenomenon, patients are often unaware of the difference from normal knee kinematics. Along with increased stress on the medial meniscus, the altered tibiofemoral motion during daily activity also results in increased joint contact forces. In a computer simulation study, Andriacchi et al. (2006) demonstrated abnormal rotation in the ACL-deficient knees that were associated with larger contact stresses in the medial compartment when compared to intact knees (Andriacchi et al. 2006). Therefore, although this abnormal knee motion may be asymptomatic for the patients, the associated increased contact pressures in the medial compartment may lead to increased wear of articular cartilage and OA in the long term.

Medial and lateral meniscal tears are caused by differing mechanisms with ACL injury. They also have different biomechanical effects on the knee stability when they occur concomitantly with ACL deficiency (Table 1). It is well known that the medial meniscus functions as a secondary restraint to anterior tibial translation in the ACL-deficient knee. Medial meniscal deficiency leads to increased anterior tibial translation against isolated anterior tibial loading (Allen et al. 2000; Papageorgiou et al. 2001). This increased translation was found to be purely an anterior motion in the anterior-posterior plane. This abnormal anterior tibial translation can be successfully reduced by the ACL reconstruction; however, studies have shown higher stresses are transferred to implanted grafts in knees with medial meniscal tears compared to ones with intact medial menisci (Allen et al. 2000; Papageorgiou et al. 2001).

In regard to the lateral meniscus, Musahl et al. (2010) examined the biomechanical effect of lateral meniscal tears in ACL-deficient knees using a cadaveric ACL injury model; they found that the removal of the lateral meniscus in the ACL-deficient knee increased anterior tibial translation which was induced by applying a rotational force of pivot shift test (Musahl et al. 2010a). Therefore, from the biomechanical point of view, the medial meniscus functions against pure anterior tibial loading, such as in clinical Lachman test or anterior drawer test, whereas the lateral meniscus contributes to stability against rotational loading in the pivot shift test. Knowledge of the ways in which a medial and/or a lateral meniscal tear affects the knee kinematics and stability in the ACL-deficient knee can improve the clinician's understanding of physical examination findings and, in conjunction with imaging, can potentially improve diagnosis of meniscal pathology in the setting of an ACL injury.

Morbidity of Meniscal Injuries in ACL-Deficient Patients

The menisci function in shock absorption, joint stability, and greater than 50 % of load transmission through either compartment. ACL injury alone already increases the likelihood of developing OA in the knee. Loss of the meniscus and its function leads to further transfer of stress to articular cartilage with accelerated degeneration to OA (see "► Chap. 72, Anatomy and Biomechanics of the Knee"). A time-dependent increase of medial meniscal tears in ACL-deficient knees has been reported as well. Millet et al. demonstrated as much as a threefold increase of meniscus tears in the chronic ACL injury case at more than 6 weeks after injury (36 %) compared to acute cases (11 %) (Millett et al. 2002). Also, Yoo et al. compared MRIs of knees with ACL injury in the acute and chronic phases 6 months apart and found worse meniscus status in 42 % of their patients (Yoo et al. 2009). These degenerative changes were mostly seen in the medial meniscus.

The menisci and ACL are codependent on each other in terms of function. Cadaver studies have shown a 33–50 % increase in stress on a graft used for ACL reconstruction after meniscectomy (Papageorgiou et al. 2001). Loss of meniscal function could increase failure rates and worsen functional results as well as knee stability after ACL reconstruction (Trojani et al. 2011). Therefore, meniscal surgery during ACL reconstruction should attempt to preserve or repair the meniscus when possible to maximize its functional potential and decrease future morbidity.

Treatment for Meniscal Injuries During ACL Reconstruction

Preoperative identification of meniscal tears via physical examination and magnetic resonance imaging (MRI) is important to make a surgical plan. However, intraoperative inspection and probing may reveal meniscal tears that were not shown on MRI or have developed in the interim between preoperative imaging study and actual surgery. After identification of a meniscal tear during the ACL reconstruction, the surgeon must determine the type and location of the meniscus tear to make an operative plan. Tears in the peripheral area, or in the red-red zone, have high potential for healing by suture repair, whereas tears in the central region, or in the white-white zone, have limited blood supply for healing so that meniscectomy is often indicated in most of such cases (see "► Chaps. 77, Arthroscopic Repair of the Meniscus Tears" and "► 97, Meniscectomy"). Studies have found improved healing rates with earlier surgical repair of meniscal tears (Tengrootenhuysen et al. 2011). There is debate as to whether meniscal repair and ACL reconstruction should be staged; however, it is generally accepted that they should be performed concurrently.

Meniscal tears present at the time of ACL reconstruction often require surgical intervention with either meniscectomy or meniscal repair. Similar to surgeries for isolated meniscal tears, meniscal repair in conjunction with ACL reconstruction often has better outcomes and less pain than meniscectomy for large repairable tears such as medial or lateral bucket-handle tears (Shelbourne and Carr 2003; Shelbourne and

Dersam 2004). As described above, the meniscus has a significant impact on the knee stability secondary to the ACL. Thus, meniscectomy in addition to the ACL reconstruction is shown to lead to higher rates of OA, increased laxity, and higher rates of ACL graft rupture compared to the ACL reconstruction without meniscectomy (Hertel et al. 2005; Salmon et al. 2006; Nakata et al. 2008). Judging from the previously reported evidence, meniscal tears with the ACL injury should be surgically repaired to maintain the anatomic structure as much as possible. However, not all the meniscal tears are amenable to repair; in such cases meniscectomy is often performed. In reality, when performed in conjunction with ACL reconstruction, meniscectomy is more often performed than meniscal repair (Noyes and Barber-Westin 2012). An analysis of the American Board of Orthopaedic Surgeons (ABOS) database revealed that only about 15 % of ACL reconstructions were performed in conjunction with meniscus repair by orthopedic surgeons in the USA (Musahl et al. 2010b). Choice of surgery for the meniscus tear depends on the site and type of the lesion, but there are no established objective criteria. Surgeons must subjectively determine whether the meniscus tear is repairable or not, except for obvious cases. Those inexperienced in meniscal repair might avoid the repair procedure by judging a lesion as unrepairable. As a result, there are probably a fewer number of the meniscus repair cases than indicated in conjunction with the ACL reconstruction. However, as surgical techniques of meniscal repair surgery improve and surgeon experience expands, the number of meniscal repair cases will increase in the future.

Although maintenance of meniscal structure and function is a key goal in treatment of ACL injury with concomitant meniscus pathology, there are certain types of meniscal tears that may not require any surgical treatment at all. Shelbourne et al. reported that some lateral meniscal tears in conjunction with the ACL injury can be left in situ or treated by a simple abrasion and trephination without risk of further progression of the tear. These include posterior horn tears, stable radial flap tears, or peripheral or posterior third tears that do not extend further than 1 cm in front of the popliteus tendon (Shelbourne and Gray 2012). In order to maintain anatomic meniscus structure as much as possible, these types of meniscal tears should be properly identified intraoperatively and treated accordingly.

As compared with leaving a tear in situ or performing a meniscectomy, the goal of a meniscal repair is to prevent the abnormal knee laxity that can be found in ACL-reconstructed knees seen with meniscectomy (Petrigliano et al. 2011). Thus, though meniscal repair requires additional surgical effort, time, cost, and possibly an additional incision, it is worthwhile for repairable tears, especially in younger patients. The alternatives to early surgical repair for the large meniscal tear, which should not be excised, are poor and involve meniscus reconstruction using collagen implants or meniscus allografts (see "▶ Chaps. 89, Human Meniscus: From Biology to Tissue Engineering Strategies," "▶ 95, Meniscal Allografts: Indications and Results," "▶ 98, Meniscus Reconstruction Using a New Collagen Meniscus Implant" and "▶ 96, Meniscal Substitutes: Polyurethane Meniscus Implant: Technique and Results"). Although those meniscus substitutions are still developing, clinical outcome following meniscus reconstruction is inferior to meniscus repair and usually influenced by concomitant procedures and development of early OA (Yoldas et al. 2003; Elattar et al. 2011).

Surgical Techniques

Operative techniques and indications of the meniscectomy and the meniscal repair in conjunction with ACL reconstruction are similar to those for the isolated meniscal tears (see "▶ Chaps. 77, Arthroscopic Repair of the Meniscus Tears" and "▶ 97, Meniscectomy"). Varus or valgus force while placing the knee in different ranges of motion may be necessary to properly perform meniscal surgery. Therefore, meniscal pathology should be surgically addressed first to prevent unnecessary stress on an ACL graft. Also bleeding after ACL tunnel drilling may worsen visualization necessary for meniscectomy or meniscal repair. The goal of meniscectomy is to remove any unstable portion of the meniscus tear leaving behind a smooth and stable rim without losing any viable meniscal tissue.

Meniscal repair techniques include inside-out, outside-in, and all-inside techniques (see "▶ Chap. 77, Arthroscopic Repair of the Meniscus Tears"). While outcomes and failure rates are similar across all techniques, the inside-out technique remains the gold standard (Nepple et al. 2012). Meniscal repair should begin with debridement to clean margins along with rasping of the healing edges. With the inside-out technique, sutures are placed through the torn meniscus using a needle cannula under arthroscopic visualization. Sutures are passed on either side of the tear, brought out through the capsule, and tied down to the capsule through a skin incision. With outside-in techniques, a needle is placed through the meniscus from the outside and sutures are shuttled through the needle with a wire. Use of inside-out and outside-in techniques is limited in repair of posterior portions of the meniscus due to the neurovascular structures. All-inside techniques are then preferred where implant devices with suture penetrate the meniscus on either side of the tear leaving anchors outside the posterior capsule. Sliding knots are then used to secure the meniscal tear.

When meniscal repair is performed in conjunction with ACL reconstruction, augmentation of the repair may not be necessary due to the intra-articular bleeding already present from drilling of bone tunnels. Techniques such as trephination (puncturing the meniscus through the periphery with a spinal needle at the repair site), placement of fibrin clot, and platelet-rich plasma injection all bring elements of autologous blood to the repair site. No clinical studies exist to show efficacy of these augmentation techniques for meniscal repair in the setting of ACL reconstruction.

Rehabilitation

Postoperative rehabilitation of ACL reconstruction with meniscectomy does not differ significantly from that of ACL reconstruction alone (see "▶ Chap. 117, Structured Rehabilitation Model with Clinical Outcomes After Anterior Cruciate Ligament Reconstruction"). The need for meniscal repair is not always predictable; therefore, it is important that the patient is informed of possible need for significant limitations involved with the rehabilitation of an ACL reconstruction with meniscal repair. In the first 4 weeks, patients are made partial weight bearing with a brace locked in extension and knee flexion is restricted from 0° to 60° during therapy. Range of motion and weight bearing are then progressed along with strengthening; however, pivoting and cutting exercises which place stress on the repaired meniscus are restricted for the first 4–5 months. Thereafter, patients are progressed through standard ACL rehabilitation protocols with stepwise introduction of sport-specific activities and finally return to competition by 6–9 months depending on return to play criteria (see "▶ Chap. 117, Structured Rehabilitation Model with Clinical Outcomes After Anterior Cruciate Ligament Reconstruction").

Outcomes of Meniscal Surgery in the ACL-Injured Knee

Meniscal repairs performed in conjunction with ACL reconstruction have higher success rates compared to meniscus repair performed in isolation (Warren 1990). This can be attributed to several factors present in the ACL-injured knee. Postoperative hemarthrosis is usually present with ACL reconstruction and surrounds the repaired meniscus with fibrin clot, which contains important growth factors that may contribute to improved healing. Meniscal tears in conjunction with ACL injury are generally acute tears in previously normal meniscus as compared to tears that involve degenerative changes.

Meniscal resection in combination with ACL reconstruction is associated with worsened long-term outcomes when compared with isolated ACL reconstruction; however, the extent of these clinical implications is not fully understood. Limited data is available on the short-term clinical outcomes on the effect of concomitant meniscal surgery with ACL reconstruction. Rotterud et al. conducted a large cohort study to compare the clinical results, such as patient-reported

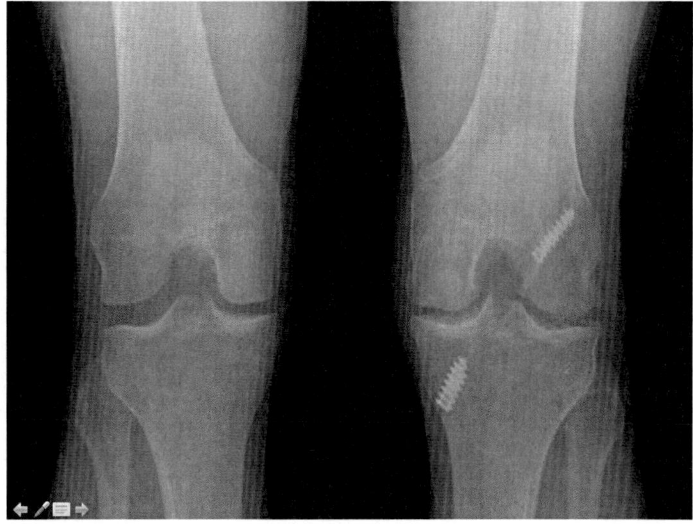

Fig. 2 Radiograph of a knee status post ACL reconstruction with Fairbanks changes, medial joint space narrowing, and early OA

outcome, between ACL reconstruction with and without concomitant meniscal surgery at 2 years after operation, and found no difference between groups (Rotterud et al. 2013). Though meniscal surgery may not impact such clinical outcomes, it does affect postoperative rehabilitation program, especially when the meniscus was repaired, which might lead to short-term patient satisfaction. The addition of a meniscus repair to the ACL reconstruction is typically accompanied with delays or increased restrictions in postoperative weight bearing, range of motion, and time of return to pivoting sports (Barber and Click 1997). The recovery to the sports activity after the ACL reconstruction is normally allowed 6–9 months after the operation. Consequently, the strict postoperative rehabilitation immediately after the ACL reconstruction surgery might affect short-term satisfaction of the patients.

Radiographic findings of OA are often observed in long-term, more than 5 years, follow-up of patients after ACL reconstruction. However, meniscectomy at the time of ACL reconstruction is associated with increased radiographic changes of OA (Fig. 2) (Cohen et al. 2007; Magnussen et al. 2009). In addition to long-term radiographic changes, meniscal surgery at or before the time of ACL reconstruction has been associated with poor clinical outcomes scores at long-term follow-up (Cohen et al. 2007; Kowalchuk et al. 2009; Shelbourne and Gray 2009; Spindler et al. 2011). Shelbourne et al. demonstrated that worse long-term, more than 10 years, clinical outcomes after the ACL reconstruction were observed in the patients with deficit in the range of motion and additional meniscus surgery (Shelbourne and Gray 2009). Kowalchuk et al. could not find a significant impact from the medial meniscectomy on the long-term clinical outcome using multivariate logistic regression analysis (Kowalchuk et al. 2009). The long-term radiographic and clinical effects of meniscal surgery in conjunction with ACL reconstruction could have multiple potential explanations, including a more significant impact on the knee joint at the time of injury which causes additional structural damages such as chondral injury, additional collateral ligament tears, and posterolateral corner injury (see "▶ Chap. 149, Epidemiology of Cartilage Injuries").

Summary

Meniscal tears are present in >50 % in ACL-injured knees. The lateral meniscus is frequently injured acutely at the time of the ACL rupture, while the medial meniscus is often secondarily injured due to accumulated stress from abnormal knee kinematics in ACL-deficient knees. Biomechanically, the medial meniscus functions as a secondary restraint to anterior tibial translation, while the lateral meniscus is an important secondary restraint to rotatory loads during the pivot shift test. Preservation of meniscal structure and function through meniscal repair when possible leads to improved knee kinematics with ACL reconstruction. Healing rates are improved when meniscal repairs are performed in conjunction with ACL reconstruction; however, rehabilitation will be more limited in the short term possibly leading to worse short-term clinical outcomes. In the long term, meniscus preservation is associated with less radiographic findings of OA and therefore better clinical outcomes. Therefore, the goal of treatment of ACL injuries with concomitant meniscal pathologies should be to create a stable knee while preserving meniscal structure and function.

Cross-References

- ▶ Anatomy and Biomechanics of the Knee
- ▶ Arthroscopic Repair of the Meniscus Tears
- ▶ Epidemiology of Cartilage Injuries
- ▶ Human Meniscus: From Biology to Tissue Engineering Strategies
- ▶ Meniscal Allografts: Indications and Results
- ▶ Meniscal Substitutes: Polyurethane Meniscus Implant: Technique and Results
- ▶ Meniscectomy
- ▶ Meniscus Reconstruction Using a New Collagen Meniscus Implant

References

Allen CR, Wong EK, Livesay GA et al (2000) Importance of the medial meniscus in the anterior cruciate ligament-deficient knee. J Orthop Res 18(1):109–115

Andriacchi TP, Dyrby CO (2005) Interactions between kinematics and loading during walking for the normal and ACL deficient knee. J Biomech 38(2):293–298

Andriacchi TP, Briant PL, Bevill SL et al (2006) Rotational changes at the knee after ACL injury cause cartilage thinning. Clin Orthop Relat Res 442:39–44

Barber FA, Click SD (1997) Meniscus repair rehabilitation with concurrent anterior cruciate reconstruction. Arthroscopy 13(4):433–437

Bedi A, Musahl V, Lane C et al (2010) Lateral compartment translation predicts the grade of pivot shift: a cadaveric and clinical analysis. Knee Surg Sports Traumatol Arthrosc 18(9):1269–1276

Cohen M, Amaro JT, Ejnisman B et al (2007) Anterior cruciate ligament reconstruction after 10 to 15 years: association between meniscectomy and osteoarthrosis. Arthroscopy 23(6):629–634

Elattar M, Dhollander A, Verdonk R et al (2011) Twenty-six years of meniscal allograft transplantation: is it still experimental? A meta-analysis of 44 trials. Knee Surg Sports Traumatol Arthrosc 19(2):147–157

Fuentes A, Hagemeister N, Ranger P et al (2011) Gait adaptation in chronic anterior cruciate ligament-deficient patients: pivot-shift avoidance gait. Clin Biomech (Bristol, Avon) 26(2):181–187

Galway HR, MacIntosh DL (1980) The lateral pivot shift: a symptom and sign of anterior cruciate ligament insufficiency. Clin Orthop Relat Res (147):45–50

Galway R, Beaupre A, MacIntosh D (1972) Pivot shift: a clinical sign of symptomatic anterior cruciate insufficiency. J Bone Joint Surg (Br) 54:763–764

Granan LP, Forssblad M, Lind M et al (2009) The Scandinavian ACL registries 2004–2007: baseline epidemiology. Acta Orthop 80(5):563–567

Hertel P, Behrend H, Cierpinski T et al (2005) ACL reconstruction using bone-patellar tendon-bone press-fit fixation: 10-year clinical results. Knee Surg Sports Traumatol Arthrosc 13(4):248–255

Kowalchuk DA, Harner CD, Fu FH et al (2009) Prediction of patient-reported outcome after single-bundle anterior cruciate ligament reconstruction. Arthroscopy 25(5):457–463

Lam MH, Fong DT, Yung PS et al (2011) Knee rotational stability during pivoting movement is restored after anatomic double-bundle anterior cruciate ligament reconstruction. Am J Sports Med 39(5): 1032–1038

Magnussen RA, Mansour AA, Carey JL et al (2009) Meniscus status at anterior cruciate ligament reconstruction associated with radiographic signs of osteoarthritis at 5- to 10-year follow-up: a systematic review. J Knee Surg 22(4):347–357

Matsumoto H (1990) Mechanism of the pivot shift. J Bone Joint Surg (Br) 72(5):816–821

Millett PJ, Willis AA, Warren RF (2002) Associated injuries in pediatric and adolescent anterior cruciate ligament tears: does a delay in treatment increase the risk of meniscal tear? Arthroscopy 18(9):955–959

Musahl V, Citak M, O'Loughlin PF et al (2010a) The effect of medial versus lateral meniscectomy on the stability of the anterior cruciate ligament-deficient knee. Am J Sports Med 38(8):1591–1597

Musahl V, Jordan SS, Colvin AC et al (2010b) Practice patterns for combined anterior cruciate ligament and meniscal surgery in the United States. Am J Sports Med 38(5):918–923

Nakata K, Shino K, Horibe S et al (2008) Arthroscopic anterior cruciate ligament reconstruction using fresh-frozen bone plug-free allogeneic tendons: 10-year follow-up. Arthroscopy 24(3):285–291

Nepple JJ, Dunn WR, Wright RW (2012) Meniscal repair outcomes at greater than five years: a systematic literature review and meta-analysis. J Bone Joint Surg Am 94(24):2222–2227

Noyes FR, Barber-Westin SD (2012) Treatment of meniscus tears during anterior cruciate ligament reconstruction. Arthroscopy 28(1):123–130

Papageorgiou CD, Gil JE, Kanamori A et al (2001) The biomechanical interdependence between the anterior cruciate ligament replacement graft and the medial meniscus. Am J Sports Med 29(2):226–231

Petrigliano FA, Musahl V, Suero EM et al (2011) Effect of meniscal loss on knee stability after single-bundle anterior cruciate ligament reconstruction. Knee Surg Sports Traumatol Arthrosc 19(Suppl 1):S86–S93

Ristanis S, Stergiou N, Patras K et al (2005) Excessive tibial rotation during high-demand activities is not restored by anterior cruciate ligament reconstruction. Arthroscopy 21(11):1323–1329

Rotterud JH, Sivertsen EA, Forssblad M et al (2013) Effect of meniscal and focal cartilage lesions on patient-reported outcome after anterior cruciate ligament reconstruction: a nationwide cohort study from Norway and Sweden of 8476 patients with 2-year follow-up. Am J Sports Med 41(3):535–543

Salmon LJ, Russell VJ, Refshauge K et al (2006) Long-term outcome of endoscopic anterior cruciate ligament reconstruction with patellar tendon autograft: minimum 13-year review. Am J Sports Med 34(5):721–732

Shelbourne KD, Carr DR (2003) Meniscal repair compared with meniscectomy for bucket-handle medial meniscal tears in anterior cruciate ligament-reconstructed knees. Am J Sports Med 31(5):718–723

Shelbourne KD, Dersam MD (2004) Comparison of partial meniscectomy versus meniscus repair for bucket-handle lateral meniscus tears in anterior cruciate ligament reconstructed knees. Arthroscopy 20(6):581–585

Shelbourne KD, Gray T (2009) Minimum 10-year results after anterior cruciate ligament reconstruction: how the loss of normal knee motion compounds other factors related to the development of osteoarthritis after surgery. Am J Sports Med 37(3):471–480

Shelbourne KD, Gray T (2012) Meniscus tears that can be left in situ, with or without trephination or synovial abrasion to stimulate healing. Sports Med Arthrosc 20(2):62–67

Slauterbeck JR, Kousa P, Clifton BC et al (2009) Geographic mapping of meniscus and cartilage lesions associated with anterior cruciate ligament injuries. J Bone Joint Surg Am 91(9):2094–2103

Spindler KP, Huston LJ, Wright RW et al (2011) The prognosis and predictors of sports function and activity at minimum 6 years after anterior cruciate ligament reconstruction: a population cohort study. Am J Sports Med 39(2):348–359

Tengrootenhuysen M, Meermans G, Pittoors K et al (2011) Long-term outcome after meniscal repair. Knee Surg Sports Traumatol Arthrosc 19(2):236–241

Trojani C, Sbihi A, Djian P et al (2011) Causes for failure of ACL reconstruction and influence of meniscectomies after revision. Knee Surg Sports Traumatol Arthrosc 19(2):196–201

Viskontas DG, Giuffre BM, Duggal N et al (2008) Bone bruises associated with ACL rupture: correlation with injury mechanism. Am J Sports Med 36(5):927–933

Warren RF (1990) Meniscectomy and repair in the anterior cruciate ligament-deficient patient. Clin Orthop Relat Res (252):55–63

Yoldas EA, Sekiya JK, Irrgang JJ et al (2003) Arthroscopically assisted meniscal allograft transplantation with and without combined anterior cruciate ligament reconstruction. Knee Surg Sports Traumatol Arthrosc 11(3):173–182

Yoo JC, Ahn JH, Lee SH et al (2009) Increasing incidence of medial meniscal tears in nonoperatively treated anterior cruciate ligament insufficiency patients documented by serial magnetic resonance imaging studies. Am J Sports Med 37(8):1478–1483

Anterior Cruciate Ligament Reconstruction with Autologous Quadriceps Tendon

68

Onur Tetik, Gürhan Dönmez, and Mahmut Nedim Doral

Contents

Abstract

The quadriceps tendon (QT) has recently become an acceptable graft option for primary and revision anterior cruciate ligament (ACL) reconstructions. It offers good biomechanical strength, a large cross-sectional area, and an appropriate length. Patients who participate in pivoting and high valgus stress activities and sports and who have a concomitant medial collateral ligament (MCL) injury are the best candidates for a *QT graft*. It may also be used for patients with patella baja, Osgood–Schlatter's disease sequelae, and patellar tendinitis. The surgical technique is demanding and has a learning curve, but with meticulous surgery, complications are rare. The QT is a reasonable alternative for *ACL reconstruction* and could be an important graft source for primary *ACL reconstruction* in the future.

Introduction

Anterior cruciate ligament tears, which are a common musculoskeletal injury, are being treated with the ligament reconstruction in increasing numbers. It is clear that a perfect graft for *ACL reconstruction* does not exist. Because of this, the surgeon must be familiar with all varieties of possible graft choices. Graft selection is an important decision for optimal outcomes following reconstruction, and there are several graft options, such as autografts, allografts, and synthetic grafts,

O. Tetik (✉)
Department of Orthopedics and Traumatology, Koc University, School of Medicine, İstanbul, Turkey
e-mail: onurtetik@yahoo.com

G. Dönmez
Faculty of Medicine, Department of Sport Medicine, Hacettepe University School of Medicine, Ankara, Sihhiye, Turkey
e-mail: gurhan@hacettepe.edu.tr; gdonmez_1805@yahoo.com

M.N. Doral
Department of Orthopaedics and Traumatology and Department of Sports Medicine, Hacettepe University, Istanbul, Turkey
e-mail: mndoral@gmail.com; ndoral@hacettepe.edu.tr

M.N. Doral, J. Karlsson (eds.), *Sports Injuries*,
DOI 10.1007/978-3-642-36569-0_90

available for the *ACL reconstruction* (West and Harner 2005).

Most of the primary *ACL reconstructions* are performed with using either bone–patellar–bone (BPTB) or hamstring autografts, but there is still a search for the ideal graft option (Duquin et al. 2009). The most important reason for this is donor (harvest) site morbidities. These morbidities can be grouped into anterior knee pain and discomfort resulting from decreased function, including range of motion and muscular strength; local discomfort caused by numbness, tenderness, or an inability to kneel; and late tissue reaction at the donor site (Franceschi et al. 2008).

One of the alternative techniques to the most common two grafts is the QT autograft, which has long been reported as an ACL graft option (Santori et al. 2004). Quadriceps tendon grafts have been utilized less frequently than other types of autografts, but because of low donor-site morbidity reported, there has been recent popularization of this graft (De Angelis and Fulkerson 2007).

History of the QT

Blauth reported his technique for harvesting the central third of the QT with patellar bone block at one end in 1984 (Blauth 1984). Then Staubli published his series about QT reconstruction in 1997 (Staubli 1997). In the original technique, the *QT graft* was composed of both tendon and a patellar bone block. In 1999, Fulkerson modified this technique by only using the QT without a bone block to decrease the risk of the patellar fracture (Fulkerson 1999).

Properties of the QT Autograft

Anatomically the quadriceps tendon consisted of three layers. The rectus femoris (RF) tendon is present at the most surface layer. The middle layer consists of the vastus lateralis (VL) and medialis (VM) tendons, and the deep layer is the vastus intermedius (VI) tendon. The strength and size of the quadriceps come from the VL and VI tendons, which were overlapped and were firmly connected. The narrowest width of the RF was reported to be 15.3 mm, and the narrowest point is 4.8 mm proximal to the upper end of the patella. The average length of the RF is 27.3 cm (Iriuchishima et al. 2012). The entire quadriceps tendon may be used as an ACL graft, but VL and VI tendons show different fiber directions so that the strength of the quadriceps tendon is questionable (Iriuchishima et al. 2012).

The quadriceps tendon attaches to a broad and profound area of the proximal pole of the patella, whereas the PT originates superficially from the anterior aspect of the patellar apex (Staubli et al. 1999). The amount of fibrocartilage is significantly greater in the attachment zone of the QT compared to the PT (Evans et al. 1990). This may suggest that *QT graft* may be a more physiologic graft choice because of the angulation between the ligament and the bone during knee movements.

The sagittal angle between the axis of the QT and the patella changes by approximately 30° during flexion–extension of the knee, which may result in a better range of motion after an *ACL reconstruction*. This angle remains unchanged for the PT origin (Eijden et al. 1987). These anatomical and biomechanical properties of the *QT tendon* reveal that *QT tendon* is a good alternative to the other autograft sources.

The quadriceps tendon has four layers that were oriented longitudinally and obliquely. The biomechanical strength, large cross-sectional area, appropriate length, and the advantage of having a bone plug on one end are the advantages of the QT (Brand et al. 2000). Anterior knee pain has been reported to be less with this graft compared with a BPTB graft (Theut et al. 2003).

In Staubli et al. study, *QT graft* and BPTB grafts were compared. The mean *QT graft* lengths averaged 87 ± 9.7 mm for the right knee and 85.2 ± 8.4 mm for the left knee without the bone block. The tendinous part of the patellar tendon was on average 51.6 ± 6.9 mm in the right knee and 52.2 ± 4.8 mm in the left knee. The cross-sectional area of a 10 mm wide *QT graft* averaged 64.4 ± 8.4 mm^2. This value was greater when compared with the patellar tendon (36.8 ± 5.7 mm^2). These anatomical studies reveal that the

Table 1 Comparison of tensile loads and load to failure of grafts according to Woo's, Noyes', and West's studies

A	Tensile loads			
	Intact ACL	10 mm *QT graft*	BPTB graft	
	2,160 ± 157 N	2,173 ± 618 N	1,953 ± 325 N	
B	Load to failure			
	Hamstring	Patella	Quadriceps	Normal
	4,090 N	2,977 N	2,352 N	1,725–2,160 N

quadriceps tendon is thicker, longer, and wider than the patellar tendon (Staubli et al. 1999).

The ultimate tensile loads of the intact ACL, 10 mm *QT graft*, and BPTB graft are 2,160 ± 157 N, 2,173 ± 618 N, and 1,953 ± 325 N, respectively, which means that the QT is biomechanically an option to the other choices (Woo et al. 1991). The quadriceps tendon is thicker and wider than the patella tendon. One can obtain a quadriceps tendon graft for *ACL reconstruction* with a volume, which is 50 % larger than a bone–patellar tendon–bone graft of similar width (Fulkerson and Langeland 1995).

The early physical findings of hamstring, patellar tendon, and quadriceps tendon *ACL reconstructions* were prospectively compared by Joseph and colleagues, and they reported that the quadriceps free tendon group achieved knee extension earlier than the patellar tendon group, and QT group required less pain medication postoperatively than the other two groups (Joseph et al. 2006). The central quadriceps tendon was reported to be as strong after graft harvest as the patellar tendon when testing to failure in cadaveric knees (Adams et al. 2006). Also in another study, there was a significant influence of bone plug length on the stability of the press-fit fixation technique. If graft harvest generates bone plugs of 15 mm length, knee flexion should be limited to 60° during the first 3 weeks of postperative period. Biomechanically loading characteristics when tested to ultimate failure with a rising load angle using a 25 mm length patellar bone plug were comparable for the quadriceps tendon with bone plug and a traditional bone–patellar tendon–bone construct. According to that study, the biomechanical characteristics of QTPB grafts are comparable to BPTB grafts in femoral press-fit fixation technique (Dargel et al. 2006).

Biomechanical and cadaveric studies showed that the normal ACL's cross-sectional area was 44 mm^2 and an ultimate load to failure was 1,725–2,160 N (Noyes et al. 1984). This load to failure was highest when the ACL was intact in its anatomical position (Woo et al. 1991). The QT provides a thicker graft than other two common autograft options with an adequate load to failure in cadaveric models (West and Harner 2005). In comparison, the BPTB autograft, four-strand hamstring graft, and QT graft have different cross-sectional areas (35, 53, and 62 mm^2, respectively), while the greatest is the QT. All autografts (hamstring 4,090 N, patella 2977 N, quadriceps 2,352 N) have a greater load to failure than the native ACL (Table 1).

Mulford et al. (2012) have reported that 81–95 % of patients had a normal Lachman test and 80–95 % a normal pivot shift test compared with the 76–100 % and 81–100 % following a PT graft and 64–100 % and 72–100 % following a hamstring graft, respectively. They also reported that the IKDC scores were A and B (normal and nearly normal) in 88 % compared with the A and B in 91.6 % of reconstructions using PT and in 90.7 % of hamstring grafts. The mean Lysholm score was 91 points for QT reconstruction, whereas it was 91–93 and 80–94, respectively, following PT and hamstring *ACL reconstructions* (Mulford et al. 2012) (Table 2).

Evidence from anatomic, cryosectional, and structural properties analyses has reported that the QT graft can be a valuable and versatile adjunct for the *ACL reconstruction* (Staubli et al. 1996). The multilayer structure of the QT allows this graft to be split, on one end into two separate tails, which makes it a good option for a double-bundle repair. It may be used with one side tunnel with bone block and the other side for

Table 2 Lachman, pivot-shift, IKDC, and Lysholm scores comparison of three graft options according to Milford

	QT	PT	Hamstring
Lachman %	81–95	76–100	64–100
Pivot shift %	80–95	81–100	72–100
IKDC A–B	88 %	91.6 %	90.7 %
Lysholm	91	91–93	80–94

double-bundle tunnels for split tails of the QT (Caborn and Chang 2005).

The properties of QT autograft are as follows:

- Harvesting is easy after one has an initial learning curve.
- The graft can be obtained with or without a patellar bone block.
- In revision operations, the diameter can often be sufficient to accommodate an expanded tibial tunnel.
- Donor-site problems have been reported to be than the patellar tendon.
- Biomechanical characteristics are good.
- Cross-sectional area is larger when compared to the PT.
- Quadriceps inhibition after the harvest is usually less.
- The residual strength of the extensor mechanism has been reported to be less impaired compared to PT graft (Fulkerson and Langeland 1995; Morgan et al. 1995; Staubli et al. 1996; Noronha 2002; Adams et al. 2006; Chen et al. 2006).

The QT autograft is an alternative to BPTB, especially in patients who need to kneel frequently or who require deep flexion of the knee. However, the best fixation method still has to be decided (Fulkerson and Langeland 1995; Morgan et al. 1995; Staubli et al. 1996; Theut et al. 2003).

Harvesting the central third of the QT does not affect the function of the extensor mechanism as much compared with the bone–tendon–bone autografts (Pigozzi et al. 2004). Biomechanically, Fulkerson tested both the native intact QT and the residual QT after harvest and had a statistically higher strength at failure than the corresponding patellar tendon construct (Fulkerson 1999).

Harvesting the quadriceps tendon autograft is not difficult and obtaining this graft can be safe, but surgeons should be aware of the anatomy of the proximal patella with a curved proximal surface, dense cortical bone, and closely adherent suprapatellar pouch. Donor-site morbidity has been reported to be minimal with QT graft. The quadriceps–patellar bone graft is sufficiently large and strong, and it can achieve good ligament function after reconstruction (Chen et al. 2006).

Patient Selection

Patients, who participate in pivoting and high valgus stress activities and sports, who have a concomitant MCL injury, whose jobs require kneeling or long periods of knee flexion, could be treated with *QT graft*. With using this graft, the medial stabilizers are spared. It may also be used for patient with patella baja, Osgood–Schlatter's disease sequelae, and patellar tendinitis, and it can also be used for ACL revision surgeries and multiple knee ligament injuries. A poorly motivated female patient where postoperative quadriceps weakness is a potential problem may be a relative contraindication. When the QT is used for revision surgery, the results also have been acceptable (Garofalo et al. 2006).

In one study after follow-up for more than 36 months, simultaneous arthroscopically assisted reconstruction of both ACL and PCL using hamstring and quadriceps autografts for restoring knee stability were reported to be effective and safe. Harvesting the QT autograft was reportedly easy during arthroscopic surgery for PCL reconstruction, and the affixed sutures of the tendinous end of the quadriceps tendon–patella construct pass easily from the tibial tunnel through the joint to the femoral tunnel, while the bone plug remains within the tibial tunnel. In this study the ACL reconstruction portion of the procedure had a more predictable outcome than the PCL reconstruction (Lo et al. 2009).

Surgical Technique

A suprapatellar incision, about 5 cm long, is performed. Skin flaps are raised, the fascia over the tendon is incised, and the entire width of the QT is exposed. The central portion of the tendon with a patellar bone block is harvested with the careful dissection to the joint. The deep synovium of the suprapatellar pouch should not be violated during the tendon harvesting to prevent fluid leakage during the *arthroscopy*. If the pouch is opened, subcutaneous fluid distention, decrease in the operative vision, and adhesions between tendon and anterior femur may occur (Woo et al. 1991). Bending the knee over 120° may provide a satisfactory arthroscopic view. If any violation occurs, clamping or suturing the defect will decrease the leakage.

The midportion one cm width of the QT is harvested longitudinally until the superior end of the patella distally (Fig. 1). After freeing the tendon, a 25 mm long, 10 mm wide, and 5 mm thick bone block is harvested from the proximal patella (Fig. 2). During the bony harvest, one should keep in mind that the proximal part of the patella is oblique and short, and oblique harvesting of the patella should be avoided. After the graft is harvested, the defect can be filled with bone chips from the tibial tunnel drilling if available. During the learning curve, the harvesting incision may be extended longer for less complications and operation time.

The free end of the QT is stitched with #5 Ethibond (Ethicon, Somerville, NJ) sutures to facilitate graft passage (Fig. 3). Then, the diameter of the tendinous part of the graft is measured. The patellar bone plug should be 25 mm long, 10 mm wide, and 5 mm thick. In general, the tendon portion is 70–80 mm long, 10 mm wide, and 5–6 mm thick. The tendon of that size allows an easy passage of an 11 mm diameter template. After the graft preparation, the tibial footprint is prepared in the usual fashion, such as stump protection and limited notchplasty if needed, for a single-bundle reconstruction. The tibial tunnel is placed in slightly posteriorly to the central part of the residual ACL footprint.

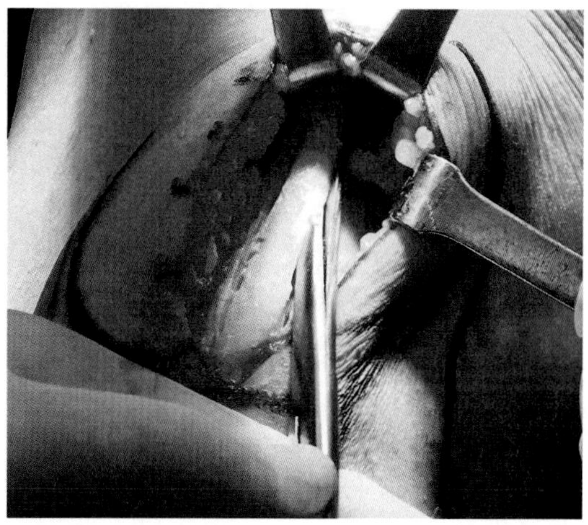

Fig. 1 Midportion of the QT of 1 cm width was dissected longitudinally till the superior end of the patella distally

The tibial drill guide is adjusted to a 55° angle, and the tibial tunnel is reamed starting from a 6 mm diameter and end up to a 10 mm reamer. Femoral and tibial tunnels are drilled 1 mm smaller than the desired size and are enlarged with appropriately sized dilators. After drilling the femoral and tibial tunnels, the bone plug is pulled with the sutures into the femoral socket through the anteromedial portal, and the free tendon end is pulled into the tibial tunnel with the grasping forceps holding the sutures at the end of the tendinous part. Both sides can be fixed with a 9 mm tricalcium phosphate interference screw (Mega fix, Karl Storz GmbH). The tension, stability, and impingement of the graft are checked after the fixation is completed (Fig. 4). Comparison of preoperative and postoperative X-rays from a revision case of a nonfunctioning ACL repair that was performed with a QT autograft is shown in (Fig. 5).

Rehabilitation

The rehabilitation protocol is similar to the hamstring graft reconstruction rehabilitation. The rehabilitation program is started before surgery with patient education and achieving full ROM and if possible complete reduction of

Fig. 2 After freeing the tendon proximally, 25 mm long, 10 mm wide, and 5 mm thick bone block is freed from the patella

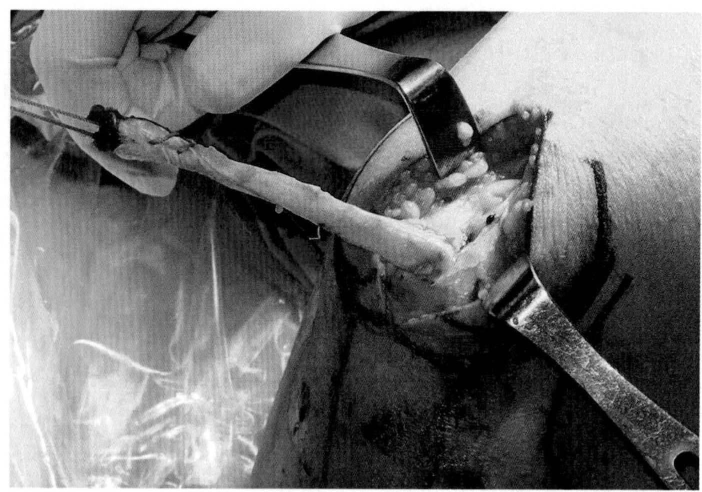

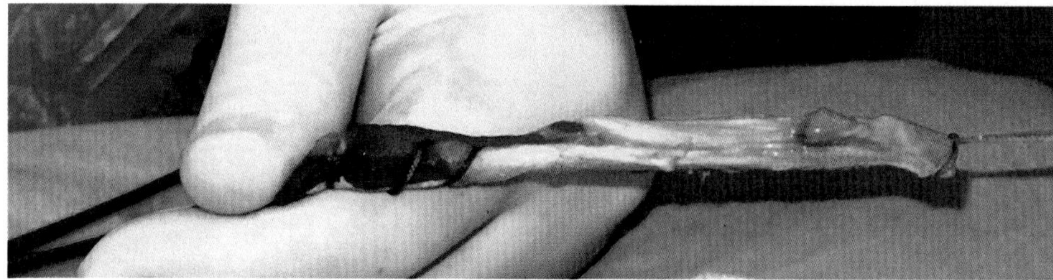

Fig. 3 Free end of the QT is stitched with the #5 Ethibond sutures and also another #5 Ethibond is passed through the bony end of the graft to facilitate graft passage

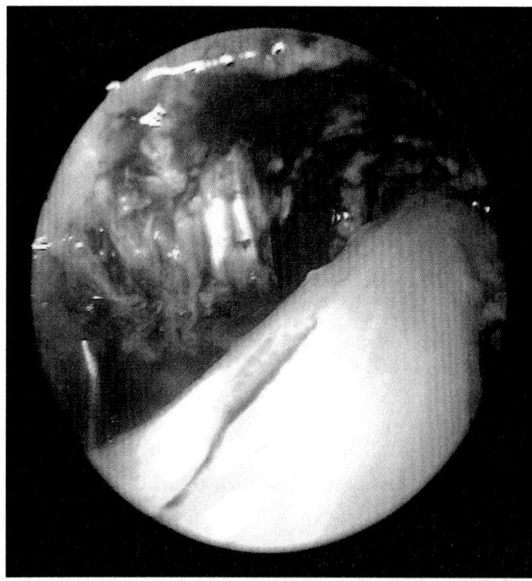

Fig. 4 The tension of the graft is checked with the probe

intra-articular inflammation and swelling before surgery to avoid arthrofibrosis.

On the first postoperative day, the swelling and pain are tried to be controlled to limit muscular inhibition and atrophy. Weight bearing is allowed the next day with crutches, and full passive extension, early initiation of quadriceps, and hamstring activity should be obtained at first week. Early open chain exercises that may theoretically shear or tear the weak immature ACL graft are avoided. Rehabilitation programs should involve functional testing and functional sport-specific training prior to return to sport.

Our rehabilitation program following *ACL reconstruction* with QT autograft is composed of five main phases:

Phase 1 (first 2 weeks) is the maximal protection phase. The active range of motion (AROM)

0–90° within 10 days, active quadriceps contraction, full weight bearing on crutches without knee brace, edema control, graft protection, and wound healing are the aims of this phase. Achieving full extension is important during phase 1. During the first 2–3 weeks, early rehabilitation exercises may appear difficult in some patients having suprapatellar pain and tenderness causing major discomfort.

Phase 2 (3–6 weeks) is the medium protection phase. The goals of this phase are full AROM equal to nonsurgical knee, normal gait without assistive device, and independent activities of daily living.

Phase 3 (7–12 weeks) is the minimum protection and strengthening phase. The goals are good strength of the quadriceps at the operative site with equal quadriceps muscle girth. Single-leg squats to 60° with good form should be performed by the end of this phase.

Phase 4 (12–20 weeks) is the progressive strengthening phase. The goals during this phase are pain-free running, landing, and jumping with the uninvolved limb dominating effort and gaining at least 75 % of the uninvolved knee in jump tests.

Phase 5 (20–26 weeks) is the return to sports phase and aims at least 85 % of the uninvolved knee in jumping tests. Single-leg squats, 20 repetitions to 60° of knee flexion, should be performed during this phase in addition to single-leg stance at least 60 s (Berker et al. 2009).

Results

Patient satisfaction, knee joint function, and donor-site morbidity differ for *QT graft* from other autograft choices. The BPTB graft is better according to the IKDC scores, whereas functional parameters such as Lysholm and Noyes scores report comparable results. The donor-site morbidity was reported to be significantly less with QT grafts than the BPTB grafts. The QT may be a preferable graft source for patients who load the knee joint and who participate in activities with deep knee function. Also, the QT may be an alternative for revision ACL surgery when the patella tendon already was harvested (Gorschewsky et al. 2007).

The use of the QT as a graft choice for ACL reconstruction has been reported to provide acceptable clinical outcomes (Howe et al. 1991; Kaplan et al. 1991; Staubli 1997; Chen et al. 1999; Kim et al. 2001; Theut et al. 2003). From these outcome analyses, the average Lysholm knee scores were 93 points at the final assessment compared to preoperatively 61 points. During strenuous or moderate activities, minimal pain and swelling were reported for 91 % of the patients after reconstruction, and moreover, during that activities 85 % of the patients did not display partial giving way of their reconstructed knee, and 91 % of the patients reported no full giving way according to IKDC guideline. Less than 5 mm ligament laxity postoperatively with KT-1000 arthrometer tests was observed in 94 % of the patients. The average anterior displacement preoperatively and postoperatively was 11.88 ± 1.09 mm and 1.74 ± 1.80 mm, respectively (Chen et al. 2006).

Satisfactory results with QT reconstruction were reported with improved Lysholm scores in which 94 % of the patients were graded A or B with a median laxity of 2 mm postoperatively. Extension peak torque of the quadriceps muscle recovered to 82 % and 89 % of that of the contralateral knee at 180°/s at 1 year and 2 years after surgery, respectively. The patellar congruence angle and Insall–Salvati ratio did not show any significant change after QT usage (Lee et al. 2004).

In one study, most patients recovered to 80 % or more of extensor and flexor muscle strength (94 % and 91 %, respectively). In this study, only 56 % of the patients could recover over 90 % of extensor muscle strength and 50 % of the patients over 90 % of flexor muscle strength compared to the normal side, but the reason for it was explained with the sources of the patients, which included only 47 % (16 of 34 patients) of professional and recreational athletes (Chen et al. 2006).

Bone tunnel enlargement was observed in 37 % of patients in Segawa's study. Enlargement occurred in 25 % of the femoral tunnels and 30 %

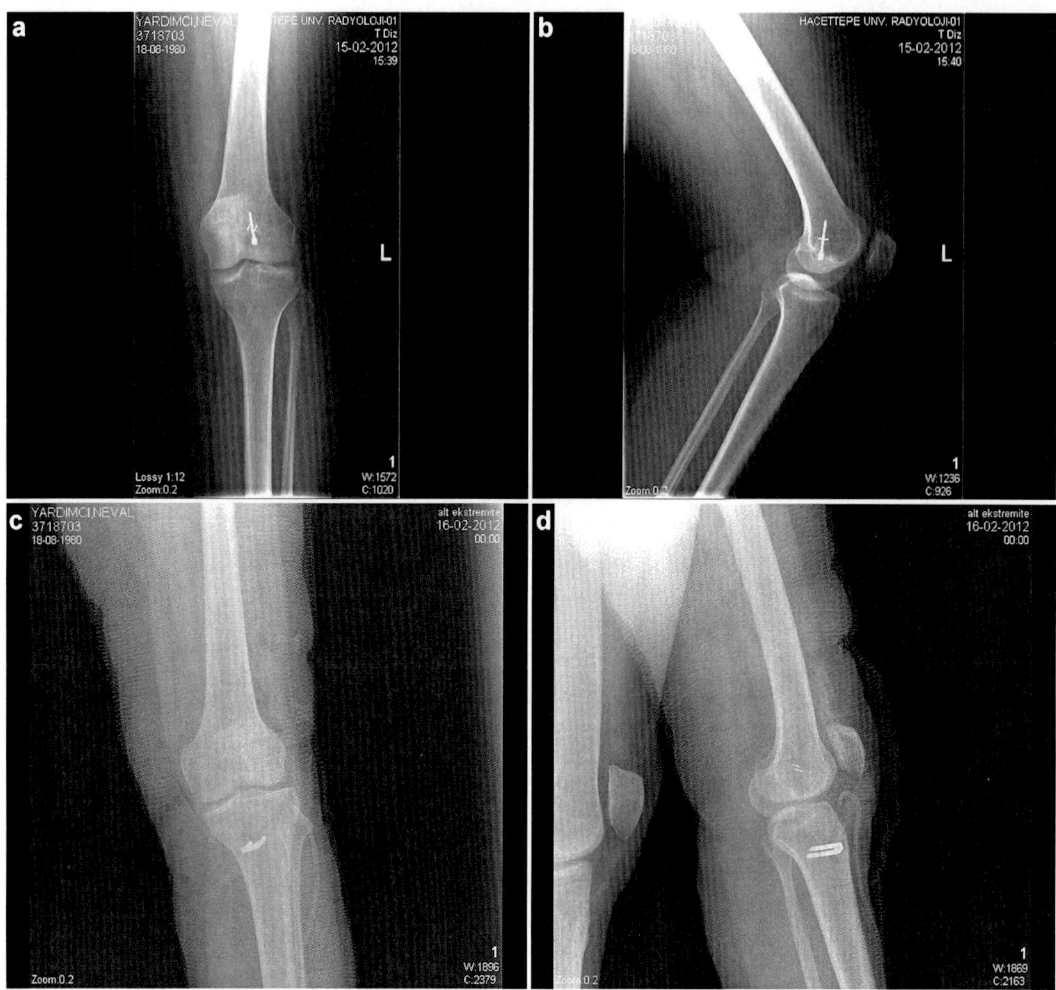

Fig. 5 (**a**) Preoperative AP X-ray of a revision case of a nonfunctioning ACL repair. (**b**) Preoperative lateral X-ray of a revision case of a nonfunctioning ACL repair. (**c**) Postoperative AP X-ray. (**d**) Postoperative lateral X-ray

of the tibial tunnels. Enlargement of both tunnels occurred in 18 % of the knees (Segawa et al. 2001). In Chen et al. study with bone–quadriceps tendon graft, tunnel expansion with more than 1 mm was only found in two (6 %) tibial tunnels (Chen et al. 2006).

Discussion

Patellar, hamstring, and quadriceps tendon are three autologous graft choices currently mainly used for *ACL reconstruction*. Clinical studies have not revealed any major differences in clinical outcomes among these grafts regardless of fixation technique yet. Mostly, other factors, such as graft harvest morbidity and complications, are more important when comparing different grafts.

The QT bone or *QT graft* is gaining popularity because of high reported rates of chronic patellofemoral problems with patellar tendon grafts. Any solutions such as suturing the tendon gap or bone grafting the patellar defect do not reduce anterior knee problems and kneeling complaints to treat this frustrating morbidity (Shino et al. 1993, Breitfuss et al. 1996).

In one study, no patients had signs or symptoms of patellofemoral pain at minimum 2-year follow-up evaluation, which is an important advantage in comparison to central third patellar tendon reconstructions. There was no case of quadriceps tendon rupture following harvest of the central quadriceps tendon (Theut et al. 2003).

Because a perfect graft for *ACL reconstructions* does not exist, the surgeon must be familiar with all varieties of possible graft choices. With understanding the anatomy of the proximal patella, which includes a curved proximal surface, dense cortical bone, and a closely adherent suprapatellar pouch, graft harvesting becomes easier. The quadriceps tendon autograft is usually not difficult to harvest and surgeons can obtain and use this graft safely.

Cross-References

- ▶ Anterior Cruciate Ligament Graft Selection and Fixation
- ▶ Anterior Cruciate Ligament Injuries and Surgery: Current Evidence and Modern Development

References

Adams DJ, Mazzocca AD, Fulkerson JP (2006) Residual strength of the quadriceps versus patellar tendon after harvesting a central free tendon graft. Arthroscopy 22(1):76–79

Berker N, Canbulat N, Demirhan M (2009) Ön Çapraz Bağ Rekonstrüksiyonları. In: Omuz Dirsek Diz Ayakbileği Rehabilitasyon Protokolleri.,1st edn. Nobel Tıp Kitabevi, İstanbul, pp113–124

Blauth W (1984) Die zweizügeligeersatzplastik des vorderenkreuzbandesaus der quadricepssehne (2-strip substitution-plasty of the anterior cruciate ligament with the quadriceps tendon). Unfallheilkkunde 87:45–51

Brand J Jr, Hamilton D, Selby J, Pienkowski D, Caborn DN, Johnson DL (2000) Biomechanical comparison of quadriceps tendon fixation with patellar tendon bone plug interference fixation in cruciate ligament reconstruction. Arthroscopy 16:805–812

Breitfuss H, Frohlich R, Povacz P, Resch H, Wicker A (1996) The tendon defect after anterior cruciate ligament reconstruction using the mid third patellar tendon—a problem for the patellofemoral joint? Knee Surg Sports Traumatol Arthrosc 3(4):194–198

Caborn DN, Chang HC (2005) Single femoral socket double-bundle anterior cruciate ligament reconstruction using tibialis anterior tendon: description of a new technique. Arthroscopy 21(10):1273

Chen CH, Chen WJ, Shih CH (1999) Arthroscopic anterior cruciate ligament reconstruction with quadriceps tendon patellar bone autograft. J Trauma 46:678–682

Chen CH, Chuang TY, Wang KC (2006) Arthroscopic anterior cruciate ligament reconstruction with quadriceps tendon autograft: clinical outcome in 4–7 years. Knee Surg Sports Traumatol Arthrosc 14(11): 1077–1085

Dargel J, Schmidt-Wiethoff R, Schneider T et al (2006) Biomechanical testing of quadriceps tendon-patellar bone grafts: an alternative graft source for press-fit anterior cruciate ligament reconstruction? Arch Orthop Trauma Surg 126(4):265–270

De Angelis JP, Fulkerson JP (2007) Quadriceps tendon–a reliable alternative for reconstruction of the anterior cruciate ligament. Clin Sports Med 26:587–596

Duquin T, Wind W, Fineberg M, Smolinski R, Buyea C (2009) Current trends in anterior cruciate ligament reconstruction. J Knee Surg 22(1):7–12

Evans EJ, Benjamin M, Pemberton DJ (1990) Fibrocartilage in the attachment zones of the quadriceps tendon and patellar ligament of man. J Anat 171:155–162

Franceschi F, Longo UG, Ruzzini L, Papalia R, Maffulli N, Denaro V (2008) Quadriceps tendon-patellar bone autograft for anterior cruciate ligament reconstruction: a technical note. Bull NYU Hosp Jt Dis 66(2):120–123

Fulkerson J (1999) Central quadriceps free tendon for anterior cruciate ligament reconstruction. Oper Tech Sports Med 7(4):195–200

Fulkerson JP, Langeland R (1995) An alternative cruciate reconstruction graft: the central quadriceps tendon. Arthroscopy 11(2):252–254

Garofalo R, Djahangiri A, Siegrist O (2006) Revision anterior cruciate ligament reconstruction with quadriceps tendon-patellar bone autograft. Arthroscopy 22(2):205–214

Gorschewsky O, Klakow A, Putz A, Mahn H, Neumann W (2007) Clinical comparison of the autologous quadriceps tendon (BQT) and the autologous patella tendon (BPTB) for the reconstruction of the anterior cruciate ligament. Knee Surg Sports Traumatol Arthrosc 15:1284–1292

Howe JG, Johnson RJ, Kaplan MJ, Fleming B, Jarvinen M (1991) Anterior cruciate ligament reconstruction using quadriceps patellar tendon graft. Part I. Long-term follow-up. Am J Sports Med 19:447–457

Iriuchishima T, Shirakura K, Yorifuji H, Fu FH (2012) Anatomical evaluation of the rectus femoris tendon and its related structures. Arch Orthop Trauma Surg 132:1665–1668

Joseph M, Fulkerson J, Nissen C et al (2006) Short-term recovery after anterior cruciate ligament reconstruction: a prospective comparison of three autografts. Orthopedics 29(3):243–248

Kaplan MJ, Howe JG, Fleming B, Johnson RJ, Jarvinen M (1991) Anterior cruciate ligament reconstruction using quadriceps patellar tendon graft. Part II. A specific sport review. Am J Sports Med 19:458–462

Kim DW, Kim JO, You JD, Kim SJ, Kim HK (2001) Arthroscopic anterior cruciate ligament reconstruction with quadriceps tendon composite autograft. Arthroscopy 17:546–550

Lee S, Seong SC, Jo H, Park YK, Lee MC (2004) Outcome of anterior cruciate ligament reconstruction using quadriceps tendon autograft. Arthroscopy 20(8):795–802

Lo YP, Hsu KY, Chen LH, Wang CJ, Yeh WL, Sheng Chan Y, Chen WJ (2009) Simultaneous arthroscopic reconstruction of the anterior and posterior cruciate ligament using hamstring and quadriceps tendon autografts. J Trauma 66:780–788

Morgan CD, Kalmam VR, Grawl DM (1995) Isometry testing for anterior cruciate ligament reconstruction revisited. Arthroscopy 11(6):647–659

Mulford JS, Hutchinson SE, Hang JR (2012) Outcomes for primary anterior cruciate reconstruction with the quadriceps autograft: a systematic review. Knee Surg Sports Traumatol Arthrosc 21(8):1882–1888

Noronha JC (2002) Reconstruction of the anterior cruciate ligament with quadriceps tendon. Arthroscopy 18(7):E37

Noyes F, Butler D, Grood E, Zernicke R, Hefzy M (1984) Biomechanical analysis of human ligament grafts used in knee ligament repairs and reconstructions. J Bone Joint Surg Am 66:344–352

Pigozzi F, Di Salvo V, Parisi A (2004) Isokinetic evaluation of anterior cruciate ligament reconstruction: quadriceps tendon versus patellar tendon. J Sports Med Phys Fitness 44(3):288–293

Santori N, Adriani E, Pederzini L (2004) ACL reconstruction using Quadriceps Tendon. Orthopedics 27(1):31–35

Segawa H, Omori G, Tomita S, Koga Y (2001) Bone tunnel enlargement after anterior cruciate ligament reconstruction using hamstring tendons. Knee Surg Sports Traumatol Arthrosc 9:206–210

Shino K, Nakagawa S, Inoue M, Horibe S, Yoneda M (1993) Deterioration of the patellofemoral articular surfaces after anterior cruciate ligament reconstruction. Am J Sports Med 21(2):206–211

Staubli HU (1997) The quadriceps tendon–patellar bone construct for ACL reconstruction. Sports Med Arthrosc Rev 5:59–67

Staubli HU, Schatzmann L, Brunner P, Rincon L, Noite LP (1996) Quadriceps tendon and patellar ligament: cryosectional anatomy and structural properties in young adults. Knee Surg Sports Traumatol Arthrosc 4:100–110

Staubli HU, Schatzmann L, Brunner P, Rincon L, Nolte LP (1999) Mechanical tensile properties of the quadriceps tendon and patellar ligament in young adults. Am J Sports Med 27:27–34

Theut PC, Fulkerson JP, Armour EF, Joseph M (2003) Anterior cruciate ligament reconstruction utilizing central quadriceps free tendon. Orthop Clin North Am 34(1):31–39

van Eijden TMGJ, de Boer W, Kouwenhoven E, Verburg J, Weijs WA (1987) Forces acting on the patella during maximal voluntary contraction of the quadriceps femoris muscle at different knee flexion/extension angles. Acta Anat 129:310–314

West RV, Harner CD (2005) Graft selection in anterior cruciate ligament reconstruction. J Am Acad Orthop Surg 13:197–207

Woo SL, Hollis JM, Adams DJ, Lyon RM, Takai S (1991) Tensile properties of the human femur anterior cruciate ligament-tibia complex: the effects of specimen age and orientation. Am J Sports Med 19:217–225

Allografts in Anterior Cruciate Ligament Reconstruction

69

Antonios Kouzelis, Christos S. Georgiou, Alkis Saridis, and Charalampos Matzaroglou

Contents

Abstract

Allograft indications in anterior cruciate ligament reconstruction have recently expanded from revision cases and multiligament knee injuries to their routine use in some primary reconstructions. The surgeon making the decision will need to consider certain issues before employing an allograft: the potential for disease transmission, the possible immunogenic reactions, the procurement and sterilization protocols followed and their impact on graft strength and performance, and finally the cost implications. In this chapter the question of whether the advantages of the allograft use outweigh these risks and costs is being explored. This subject is of great importance as more anterior cruciate ligament reconstructions are performed and allograft sources become more readily available.

Introduction

Although the anterior cruciate ligament (ACL) is a common athletic injury and a large number of ACL reconstructions, with an estimated number of 175,000–200,000 in the USA (Hettrich et al. 2013), are performed annually, there still remains a considerable amount of controversy over whether an autograft or an allograft should be used. Allografts were in the past reserved for revision cases or for multiligament injuries, when the autologous tissue was not sufficiently

A. Kouzelis (✉) • C.S. Georgiou • A. Saridis • C. Matzaroglou
Department of Orthopaedic Surgery, University Hospital of Patras, Rio, Greece
e-mail: akouzelis@yahoo.gr; csgeorgiou@gmail.com; alkisaridis@hotmail.com; orthopatras@yahoo.gr

M.N. Doral, J. Karlsson (eds.), *Sports Injuries*,
DOI 10.1007/978-3-642-36569-0_95

available. Today, however, they are increasingly being used for some routine primary ACL reconstructions, especially in the USA (Granan et al. 2012). Various allograft tissue types exist, but the most commonly used are bone–patellar tendon–bone (BTB), hamstrings, quadriceps, Achilles tendon, and anterior tibialis tendon grafts.

Reconstruction with autografts has increased benefits of faster incorporation and no risk of immunologic rejection or disease transmission but leads to potential donor site morbidity, including anterior knee pain, patellar tendinitis or even late patellar tendon rupture, patella fracture, knee flexion weakness, altered quadriceps function, and saphenous nerve injury (Hu et al. 2013; Lamblin et al. 2013). Allografts have the main advantage of eliminating donor site morbidity but also the benefits of providing multiple grafts, shorter operative times, smaller incisions and improved cosmesis, less postoperative pain, and potentially faster rehabilitation (Siebold et al. 2003; Barrera et al. 2011; Hu et al. 2013). Unfortunately, however, allografts have the major disadvantages of potential disease transmission, possible immunogenicity, and slower maturation and increased costs (Barrera et al. 2011; Lamblin et al. 2013). To reduce the potential of disease transmission, gamma irradiation was extensively used in the past for allograft secondary sterilization (Hu et al. 2013). However, many published studies have indicated that gamma irradiation significantly decreases the biomechanical properties and structure of allografts in a dose-dependent pattern. Although the potential for disease transmission remains the main concern, the improved donor screening and modern processing and sterilization techniques have allowed a decrease in the use of high-dose gamma irradiation. According to the modern standards of the tissue banks, low-dose irradiation is limitedly used for the terminal tissue sterilization after graft procurement and before packaging.

In this chapter the incorporation process of the allografts in ACL reconstruction will be discussed and the effect of the various sterilization techniques in allograft stability. A review of the current evidence in the literature, which refers to the use of allografts, in terms of immunologic reactions and disease transmission, and their clinical performance, is also included.

Special Considerations with Allografts in ACL Reconstruction

Allograft Incorporation

Due to obvious technical difficulties in biopsies, the knowledge about graft healing process in human subjects is limited. It appears that after ACL reconstruction, the intra-articular region of the tendon graft first begins its incorporation process to the new environment (Scheffler et al. 2008). As reported the incorporation process (ligamentization) of an ACL graft consists of four phases: initial avascular necrosis, revascularization, cellular repopulation, and finally remodeling (Falconiero et al. 1998). During ligamentization, revascularization plays a key role by acting as a prerequisite for the other phases (Li et al. 2012). Graft revascularization is present as early as 3 weeks after operation and increases in prevalence over the next 5 weeks (Li et al. 2012). Simultaneously the intra-tunnel graft incorporation is taking place, which develops either by bone-to-bone or by tendon-to-bone healing (Scheffler et al. 2008). The whole process for autografts appears to last up to 12 months, although this is not a rule (Falconiero et al. 1998). In the case of allografts, however, the maturation process takes longer. Shino et al. (1988), after an arthroscopic and histological study of the remodeling process of human allogenic tendons, found that complete remodeling occurs by 18 months (Shino et al. 1988). Malinin et al. (2002), however, investigated entire retrieved ACL allografts and observed that the central portions of the grafts remained acellular even at 2 years postoperatively. They postulated that the complete remodeling and cellular replacement might require 3 years or longer (Malinin et al. 2002). The inferior allograft maturity at 2 years postoperatively in comparison to autograft tendons in ACL reconstruction was also confirmed by MRI cohort studies (Li et al. 2012). However, this delay in allograft maturation has not been reflected to the clinical outcomes, as will be demonstrated in the relevance section.

Processing, Decontamination, and Their Effects on Allografts

Allografts are either used as non-sterilized fresh-frozen or cryopreserved tissue or are processed with different sterilization techniques prior to implantation. Every sterilization method contributes changes to the biomechanical features of grafts. Non-sterilized fresh-frozen allografts appear to be the strongest (Guo et al. 2012). They require meticulous serological screening of the donor and the donor's graft tissue to exclude the possibility of an infection. Even so the danger of a viral infection exists due to the time window in which the virus is undetectable (Scheffler et al. 2005). Reports from the Centers for Disease Control and Prevention on disease transmission after ACL fresh-frozen allograft reconstructions (Centers for Disease Control and Prevention 2001), the most unfortunate that of a 23-year-old man's death from Clostridium sordellii contamination (Kainer et al. 2004), have led to the implementation of graft sterilization methods (Yanke et al. 2013). Except from donor screening, the first step of the effort to stop disease transmission is aseptic recovery. Aseptic recovery minimizes the initial risk of contamination by infectious agents introduced when removing tissues from donors. Preventing the introduction of infectious agents during recovery and processing may obviate the requirement of sterilization. It does not however remove the existing bioburden in the tissue. Antibiotic soaks can effectively reduce bacterial concentration on the surface of grafts, but they are unable to penetrate and have no effect on viruses (Eastlund 2006).

Two types of sterilization have become most accepted for musculoskeletal tissue allografts: chemical sterilization, utilizing ethylene oxide gas, and ionizing radiation, gamma or electron beam. Ethylene oxide gas sterilization, although an effective method, is no longer used for allografts because the associated breakdown products, such as ethylene chlorhydrin, may cause chronic synovitis (Jackson et al. 1990) or even graft failure by dissolution (Roberts et al. 1991). On the contrary sterilization with peracetic acid–ethanol solution seems safe and not to affect biomechanical properties (Scheffler et al. 2005). Gamma irradiation is a secondary sterilization method preferred by many tissue banks. Non-spore-forming bacteria are susceptible to up to 0.5 Mrad of irradiation. Yeasts and molds require doses of approximately 0.8 Mrad, while bacterial spores may require up to 2.1 Mrad (Yanke et al. 2013). Viruses, and most importantly HIV, have been reported to require doses up to 4 Mrad. The latter is based on studies that assume that HIV is present in high levels (Fideler et al. 1994). However, after donor screening and tissue disinfection, the risk that HIV is present in an allograft is low (Hernigou 2000). It has been estimated theoretically to be between 1 in 600,000 (Buck et al. 1989) and 1 in 1,667,000 (Centers for Disease Control and Prevention 1995). Taking into account that the objective is to achieve a probability of 1 in 1,000,000, that virus is present before implantation, and that 0.4 Mrad of irradiation is required to reduce the population by 1 log cycle (Conway et al. 1991), a dose range of 1–2 Mrad is efficient in eradicating the virus after donor screening and tissue disinfection (Moore 2012). Low-dose (1.0–1.2 Mrad) gamma irradiation decreases BTB graft stiffness by 20 %, but it does not affect maximum load, maximum stress, elongation, strain at maximum stress, or other cyclic parameters (Yanke et al. 2013). This and other studies (Samsell and Moore 2012) indicate that treatment below 2–2.5 Mrad have minimal impact on biomechanical properties of the tendons. Parameters as irradiation temperature, dose range, and prior tissue treatment rather than the target dose alone seem to play a significant role (Samsell and Moore 2012). On the other hand, it is an old knowledge that using more than 3 Mrads for allograft sterilization to kill viral pathogens affects the biomechanical properties of the tissue (Fideler et al. 1994), by reducing crosslink density and by causing fragmentation of collagen (McGuire and Hendricks 2009). The use of such irradiation levels produces an estimated 25 % or 35 % reduction in strength for fresh-frozen or freeze-dried

BTB grafts, respectively, and with accurate nonanatomic surgical technique or improper rehabilitation can lead to graft failures (Buck et al. 1990). Such high doses are, however, unnecessary with tissue banking standards that include donor screening, aseptic procurement and processing, antibiotic decontamination, and terminal sterilization with low-dose irradiation before packaging. Tissue banks that perform terminal sterilization do so at 1–2.5 Mrad; the addition of cross-linking and scavenging methods would have potentially even greater protective effect (Seto et al. 2008). Another option instead of gamma radiation is to use electron beam, which allows improved control of dose application and shorter irradiation times. High-energy electrons cause in this case chemical changes similar to gamma irradiation. However, significant decrease in structural properties remains a problem with high doses, although the potential of fractionation of radiation dosages is promising (Hoburg et al. 2011).

Commonly accepted allograft storage methods used include cryopreservation, fresh freezing, and lyophilization (McGuire and Hendricks 2009). Cryopreservation maintains viable tissues and cells by cryoprotected freezing but adds expenses (McGuire and Hendricks 2009). Lyophilization or freeze-drying includes freezing the tissue and then dehydrating it under high vacuum at a low temperature. Freeze-drying of allografts has been shown to reduce antigenicity of grafts and minimize the effect of free radicals because both antigens and radicals are less active at these conditions (Woo et al. 1986; Hoburg et al. 2011). As is shown also in the next chapter, there is growing evidence that the process of freeze-drying may decrease the risk of viral transmissions. Before freeze-drying, allografts go through multiple ethyl alcohol washes, which also may contribute to these properties. Freeze-drying cannot achieve terminal sterilization and thus eliminate the risk of disease transmission, but it may reduce risk of graft-to-host reactions without compromising graft structure (Hoburg et al. 2011).

The BioCleanse (Regeneration Technologies, Alachua, FL) is another sterilization process that is currently under discussion. It is considered safe since it has passed FDA approval for use on soft tissue grafts, but adds significant expense to the procedure (McGuire and Hendricks 2009). It uses a pressure chamber, where a repeated cycle of chemical sterilants and detergent washes followed by vacuum removal of the residues takes place. This method is reportedly effective against a broad range of viruses, including enveloped and nonenveloped RNA and DNA viruses. A study, comparing BioCleanse-treated BTB allografts with untreated controls identified no significant biomechanical differences between them (Jones et al. 2007).

It is obvious however that as the processing techniques vary among different tissue banks and until a uniform system would be established, surgeons should become familiar with them and ask their supplier how exactly the graft they intend to use was processed (McGuire and Hendricks 2009).

Immunogenicity and Disease Transmission

Cellular-mediated and humoral immune responses have been reported in the literature with allograft tissue (Harner and Fu 1993; McGuire and Hendricks 2009). In the past tunnel enlargement has been associated with the use of allograft tissue for ACL reconstruction (Wilson et al. 2004; Bach et al. 2005). A subclinical immune response was postulated responsible for this difference (Fahey and Indelicato 1994). However, allogenic tissue processing and decontamination with the removal and neutralization of antigens by washing and freezing processes significantly decrease immunogenicity (Bach et al. 2005; McGuire and Hendricks 2009). No significant local or systemic immune responses affecting graft healing or clinical outcome have been recorded in a number of studies comparing autografts and frozen allografts (Arnoczky et al. 1986; McGuire and Hendricks 2009). Wilson et al. (2004) reviewed the literature regarding tunnel enlargement after ACL surgery and stated, "Based on the current literature, it is difficult to conclude that there was an increased risk of tunnel lysis with allograft tissue as compared to autograft." Sporadic cases of acute synovitis after surgery with fresh-frozen allografts have been also recorded, without serious consequences or need for reoperation (Guo et al. 2012). There is no mention of these conditions in the meta-analyses (Prodromos et al. 2007; Krych et al. 2008; Carey et al. 2009; Foster et al. 2010; Tibor et al. 2010; Hu et al. 2013; Kraeutler et al. 2013; Lamblin et al. 2013) that evaluate the use of allografts in ACL reconstruction. Consequently, it seems that recipient immune reactions have limited or benign effects on clinical outcome. Tissue typing and host immunosuppression, both common processes with solid organ transplantation, seem unnecessary for tendon allografts (McGuire and Hendricks 2009).

Although the risk is relatively low, allograft tissue-related viral transmission is an acknowledged subject of concern (McGuire and Hendricks 2009). With proper donor screening and serology testing, the estimated HIV risk is lower than 1:1,600,000 (Buck et al. 1989; McGuire and Hendricks 2009). There have been only three documented HIV cases in the literature as a consequence of frozen allograft tissue implantation from a HIV-positive donor (Simonds et al. 1992). Four patients received fresh-frozen allografts and three of these patients tested positive for HIV. Two patients received fresh-frozen femoral head allografts, and the third patient received a fresh-frozen BTB allograft for ACL reconstruction. None of the 42 recipients of freeze-dried grafts obtained from this donor became infected with HIV (Simonds et al. 1992). No freeze-dried allograft recipient was transformed to HCV positive in another case of a HCV-infected donor in the literature (Tugwell et al. 2005). In contrast, from the eight patients who received cryopreserved or fresh-frozen tendon–bone, four were tested positive for HCV. Freeze-drying and the washes used with it may have fundamental differences with the other graft storage options as cryopreservation and freezing. It seems that freeze-drying process has contributed to the prevention of viral disease transmission at least in these two cases (McGuire and Hendricks 2009).

The propensity for bacterial infections with fresh-frozen allografts has been emphasized by the Centers for Disease Control and Prevention (Centers for Disease Control and Prevention 2001; Kainer et al. 2004). This has led some to consider routine intraoperative cultures of allograft tissue before implantation. Positive routine cultures in ACL allografts have a reported incidence of 5.7–13.25 % (Fowler et al. 2011). In a retrospective study of 115 cases (Fowler et al. 2011), no patient with a culture-positive allograft developed a clinical infection postoperatively, whereas in another study of 247 patients (Guelich et al. 2007), 67 % grew organisms of high pathogenicity and 33 % of low pathogenicity, but the two cases of septic arthritis had negative intraoperative cultures. Routine preimplantation culture of soft tissue allografts thus cannot be recommended given the lack of correlation with clinical infection. Antibiotic treatment is not indicated only with the presence of a positive preimplantation allograft culture. In contrast, clinical signs of septic arthritis should be aggressively treated (Fowler et al. 2011). It is worth noticing that no difference in the infection rate between autografts and allografts (irrespective of the method of processing) has been recognized in the available meta-analyses. Furthermore, Maletis et al. (2013b) after a prospective cohort study of 10,626 cases from the Kaiser Permanente Anterior Cruciate Ligament Reconstruction Registry found no difference in the incidence of infection between allografts and BTB autografts (Maletis et al. 2013b).

What Is the Clinical Evidence?

Since the first description by Shino et al. in 1984 (Shino et al. 1984; Siebold et al. 2003) of the replacement of the ACL by an allogenic tendon graft, numerous case series were reported, and over 50 comparative studies have evaluated the clinical results of allografts and autografts in the past 30 years. Some studies have shown comparable success with both autograft and allograft tissues (Rihn et al. 2006) in ACL reconstruction, whereas other studies have found an unacceptable increased failure rate (Pallis et al. 2012). It appears that how irradiation affects clinical outcomes is dependent not only on the target dose but also on the specific use, the accuracy of surgical technique, and the patient compliance to the rehabilitation instructions. Most of these publications, however, are low-quality, underpowered studies, or different graft sterilization techniques have been used in those studies. To our knowledge only eight systematic reviews of the clinical outcomes of allograft versus autograft for ACL reconstruction have been published so far; five of them were conducted over 3 years ago, between 2007 and 2010 (Prodromos et al. 2007; Krych et al. 2008; Carey et al. 2009; Foster et al. 2010; Tibor et al. 2010), and three (Prodromos et al. 2007; Krych et al. 2008; Tibor et al. 2010) identified differences in laxity in favor of autografts. Specifically, the study by Prodromos et al. (2007) is also the only meta-analysis in the literature that compares irradiated with nonirradiated allografts, showing worse outcome for the former. However, all these findings are either inconclusive (Krych et al. 2008) or compromised by methodological limitations (Prodromos et al. 2007; Samsell and Moore 2012) and by the limited availability of comparative clinical trials (Tibor et al. 2010).

Since 2010 several studies have been published adding data and making the previous systematic reviews obsolete. This new knowledge has been presented in meta-analysis from three recent studies (Hu et al. 2013; Kraeutler et al. 2013; Lamblin et al. 2013). In the best designed study, Hu et al. (2013) systematically reviewed all the level I and II prospective studies that evaluated the clinical outcomes of BTB autograft versus BTB allograft and soft tissue autograft versus soft tissue allografts for primary ACL reconstruction. The analysis excluded studies that included gamma-irradiated allografts. Nine studies, with 410 patients in the autograft and 408 patients in the allograft group, were determined to be appropriate. Hu et al. (2013) found no significant differences between allograft and autograft on the outcomes of instrumented laxity measurements, Lachman test, pivot shift test, objective International Knee Documentation Committee (IKDC) Scores, Lysholm scores, and clinical failures. However, a subgroup analysis of Tegner scores involving only BTB grafts reported a statistical difference in favor of autografts. The authors concluded that there was insufficient evidence to identify which of the two types of grafts was significantly better for ACL reconstruction, though the subgroup analysis indicated that reconstruction with BTB autograft might allow patients to return to higher levels of activity in comparison with BTB allograft (Hu et al. 2013). In another recent meta-analysis, this time reviewing studies with level of evidence from I to III, Lamblin et al. (2013) compared autografts again with nonirradiated but also nonchemically treated allografts. The authors excluded also those studies that compared BTB with soft tissue grafts. With a similar pool size as the analysis by Hu et al. (2013), they found no significant differences between autografts and allografts in Lysholm scores, IKDC scores, Lachman examinations, pivot shift testing, KT-1000 measurements, or failure rates. Lamblin et al. (2013) concluded that the results after autograft ACL reconstruction are comparable to those using nonchemically processed nonirradiated allograft tissue. Still none of these newer studies have stratified outcomes according to age or other confounding variables such as activity level. Furthermore the minimum follow-up set at the eligibility criteria was 2 years in both of them.

The third and the most recent of the 2013 meta-analysis compared BTB autografts and allografts and has the largest pool of 5,182 patients (Kraeutler et al. 2013). In order to increase the power of the analysis, the authors have included heterogenous data that are both comparative and non-comparative studies with different surgical techniques and both irradiated and nonirradiated allografts. Outcomes on subjective IKDC, Lysholm, Tegner, single-legged hop, and KT-1000 arthrometer were statistically significant in favor of autografts. Reflecting the methodological limitations, the return to preinjury activity level (in contrast to the Hu et al. (2013) study), overall IKDC, pivot shift, and anterior knee pain were significant in favor of allografts, although allograft BTB demonstrated a threefold increase in rerupture rates. There was no significant difference between the two groups for Cincinnati Knee scores. The authors advocated the use of BTB autografts based on graft rupture, knee laxity, and overall patient satisfaction, but they have also stressed the need of more high-quality randomized controlled trials with specified age and activity level to draw reliable conclusions (Kraeutler et al. 2013).

The Scandinavian national ACL registries, that is, the Danish, the Swedish, and the oldest Norwegian, generate also useful data about ACL reconstructions. No association between graft failure and use of allografts has been revealed after a prospective cohort study of 12,193 primary ACL reconstructions performed between 2005 and 2010 of the Danish knee ligament reconstruction registry. On the contrary, the use of allograft tissue for the revision procedure resulted in a higher risk of re-revision (Lind et al. 2012). A 2012 cross-sectional ACL reconstruction registry comparison between the Norwegian Knee Ligament Registry (NKLR) with 11,217 patients registered and the US Kaiser Permanente Anterior Cruciate Ligament Reconstruction Registry (KP ACLRR) with 11,050 patients has shown that between 2005 and 2010 in the NKLR, allograft was used less (0.2 % vs. 41 %) for primary ACL reconstructions than in the KP ACLRR. A similar distribution of graft usage was found in the revision cohorts (Granan et al. 2012). In contrast with the USA where allografts are widely used in ACL reconstruction, a similar approach of the Scandinavian surgeons to patients seems to exist as shown also by the Swedish registry. The 2010 annual report depicts a scarce use of allografts in primary reconstructions with figures up to 30 per year and a relatively larger scale use in revision surgery and multiple ligament reconstructions (Swedish ACL Register 2011). With so small numbers any statistical correlation is not possible. In the USA, however, the Multicenter Orthopaedic Outcomes Network (MOON) after a prospective study of 980 patients has found that the use of allografts compared with autografts in ACL reconstruction is a risk factor for subsequent surgery (Hettrich et al. 2013). Kaeding et al. (2011) from the same consortium have found that both graft type and patient age are significant predictors of graft failure. The odds of graft rupture with an allograft reconstruction were four times higher than those of autograft reconstructions. For each 10-year decrease in age, the odds of graft rupture increased 2.3 times. Patients in the age group of 10–19 years had the highest percentage of graft failures (Kaeding et al. 2011). These associations were also confirmed by a recent retrospective cohort study of 9,817 primary ACL reconstructions from the KP ACLRR (Maletis et al. 2013). In terms of clinical performance based on IKDC and Knee Injury and Osteoarthritis Outcome Score (KOOS) results at two and six postoperatively, a MOON cohort study of 448 patients has also found that the use of allografts is a predictor of worse outcome (Spindler et al. 2011). As far as the question which allograft is best, to the best of our knowledge, the only study to date is that of Siebold et al., who have compared fresh-frozen patellar versus Achilles tendon allografts for primary ACL reconstruction. The Achilles tendon-bone allograft seemed to be advantageous as its failure rate was 4.8 % compared to the 10.4 % rerupture rate of the patellar tendon allografts. On the contrary, no significant difference between the two groups was found in subjective (as assessed by Cincinnati Knee Score and Lachman, pivot shift, and varus/valgus stress tests) and objective (assessed by KT-1000 arthrometer testing, IKDC, and Cincinnati Sports Activity Score) clinical outcomes (Siebold et al. 2003).

Cross-References

- ▶ Anterior Cruciate Ligament Graft Selection and Fixation
- ▶ Anterior Cruciate Ligament Injuries and Surgery: Current Evidence and Modern Development
- ▶ Combined Anterior and Posterior Cruciate Ligament Injuries
- ▶ Costs and Safety of Allografts
- ▶ Graft Remodeling and Bony Ingrowth After Anterior Cruciate Ligament Reconstruction
- ▶ Perioperative and Postoperative Anterior Cruciate Ligament Rehabilitation Focused on Soft Tissue Grafts
- ▶ Revision Anterior Cruciate Ligament Reconstruction

References

Arnoczky SP, Warren RF, Ashlock MA (1986) Replacement of the anterior cruciate ligament using a patellar tendon allograft. An experimental study. J Bone Joint Surg Am 68(3):376–385

Bach BR Jr, Aadalen KJ, Dennis MG et al (2005) Primary anterior cruciate ligament reconstruction using fresh-frozen, nonirradiated patellar tendon allograft: minimum 2-year follow-up. Am J Sports Med 33(2):284–292

Barrera Oro F, Sikka RS, Wolters B et al (2011) Autograft versus allograft: an economic cost comparison of anterior cruciate ligament reconstruction. Arthroscopy 27(9):1219–1225

Buck BE, Malinin TI, Brown MD (1989) Bone transplantation and human immunodeficiency virus: an estimate of risk of acquired immunodeficiency syndrome (AIDS). Clin Orthop 240:129–136

Buck BE, Resnick L, Shah SM et al (1990) Human immunodeficiency virus cultured from bone. Implications for transplantation. Clin Orthop 251:249–253

Carey JL, Dunn WR, Dahm DL et al (2009) A systematic review of anterior cruciate ligament reconstruction with autograft compared with allograft. J Bone Joint Surg Am 91(9):2242–2250

Centers for Disease Control and Prevention (CDC) (1995) Case-control study of HIV seroconversion in health-care workers after percutaneous exposure to HIV-infected blood – France, United Kingdom, and United States, January 1988–August 1994. MMWR Morb Mortal Wkly Rep 44(50):929–933

Centers for Disease Control and Prevention (CDC) (2001) Unexplained deaths following knee surgery–Minnesota, 2001. MMWR Morb Mortal Wkly Rep 50(48):1080

Conway B, Tomford W, Mankin HJ et al (1991) Radiosensitivity of HIV-1–potential application to sterilization of bone allografts. AIDS 5(5):608–609

Eastlund T (2006) Bacterial infection transmitted by human tissue allograft transplantation. Cell Tissue Bank 7(3):147–166

Fahey M, Indelicato PA (1994) Bone tunnel enlargement after anterior cruciate ligament replacement. Am J Sports Med 22(3):410–414

Falconiero RP, DiStefano VJ, Cook TM (1998) Revascularization and ligamentization of autogenous anterior cruciate ligament grafts in humans. Arthroscopy 14(2):197–205

Fideler BM, Vangsness CT Jr, Moore T et al (1994) Effects of gamma irradiation on the human immunodeficiency virus. A study in frozen human bone-patellar ligament-bone grafts obtained from infected cadavera. J Bone Joint Surg Am 76(7):1032–1035

Foster TE, Wolfe BL, Ryan S et al (2010) Does the graft source really matter in the outcome of patients undergoing anterior cruciate ligament reconstruction? An evaluation of autograft versus allograft reconstruction results: a systematic review. Am J Sports Med 38(1):189–199

Fowler JR, Truant AL, Sewards JM (2011) The incidence of and clinical approach to positive allograft cultures in anterior cruciate ligament reconstruction. Clin J Sport Med 21(5):402–404

Granan LP, Inacio MC, Maletis GB et al (2012) Intraoperative findings and procedures in culturally and geographically different patient and surgeon populations: an anterior cruciate ligament reconstruction registry comparison between Norway and the USA. Acta Orthop 83(6):577–582

Guelich DR, Lowe WR, Wilson B (2007) The routine culture of allograft tissue in anterior cruciate ligament reconstruction. Am J Sports Med 35(9):1495–1499

Guo L, Yang L, Duan XJ et al (2012) Anterior cruciate ligament reconstruction with bone-patellar tendon-bone graft: comparison of autograft, fresh-frozen allograft, and γ-irradiated allograft. Arthroscopy 28(2):211–217

Harner CD, Fu FH (1993) The immune response to allograft ACL reconstruction. Am J Knee Surg 6:45–46

Hernigou P (2000) Allograft sterility as exemplified by human immunodeficiency virus and sterilization by irradiation. J Arthroplasty 15(8):1051–1058

Hettrich CM, Dunn WR, Reinke EK et al (2013) The rate of subsequent surgery and predictors after anterior cruciate ligament reconstruction: two- and 6-year follow-up results from a multicenter cohort. Am J Sports Med 41(7):1534–40

Hoburg A, Keshlaf S, Schmidt T et al (2011) Fractionation of high-dose electron beam irradiation of BPTB grafts provides significantly improved viscoelastic and structural properties compared to standard gamma irradiation. Knee Surg Sports Traumatol Arthrosc 19(11):1955–1961

Hu J, Qu J, Xu D et al (2013) Allograft versus autograft for anterior cruciate ligament reconstruction: an up-to-date meta-analysis of prospective studies. Int Orthop 37(2):311–320

Jackson DW, Windler GE, Simon TM (1990) Intraarticular reaction associated with the use of freeze-dried, ethylene oxide-sterilized bone-patella tendon-bone allografts in the reconstruction of the anterior cruciate ligament. Am J Sports Med 18(1):1–10 (discussion 10–11)

Jones DB, Huddleston PM, Zobitz ME et al (2007) Mechanical properties of patellar tendon allografts subjected to chemical sterilization. Arthroscopy 23(4): 400–404

Kaeding CC, Aros B, Pedroza A et al (2011) Allograft versus autograft anterior cruciate ligament reconstruction: predictors of failure from a MOON prospective longitudinal cohort. Sports Health 3(1):73–81

Kainer MA, Linden JV, Whaley DN et al (2004) Clostridium infections associated with musculoskeletal-tissue allografts. N Engl J Med 350(25):2564–2571

Kraeutler MJ, Bravman JT, McCarty EC (2013) Bone-patellar tendon-bone autograft versus allograft in outcomes of anterior cruciate ligament reconstruction: a meta-analysis of 5182 patients. Am J Sports Med 41(10):2439–48

Krych AJ, Jackson JD, Hoskin TL et al (2008) A meta-analysis of patellar tendon autograft versus patellar tendon allograft in anterior cruciate ligament reconstruction. Arthroscopy 24(3):292–298

Lamblin CJ, Waterman BR, Lubowitz JH (2013) Anterior cruciate ligament reconstruction with autografts compared with non-irradiated, non-chemically treated allografts. Arthroscopy 29(6):1113–1122

Li H, Tao H, Cho S et al (2012) Difference in graft maturity of the reconstructed anterior cruciate ligament 2 years postoperatively: a comparison between autografts and allografts in young men using clinical and 3.0-T magnetic resonance imaging evaluation. Am J Sports Med 40(7):1519–1526

Lind M, Menhert F, Pedersen AB (2012) Incidence and outcome after revision anterior cruciate ligament reconstruction: results from the Danish registry for knee ligament reconstructions. Am J Sports Med 40(7):1551–1557

Maletis GB, Inacio MC, Desmond JL et al (2013a) Reconstruction of the anterior cruciate ligament: association of graft choice with increased risk of early revision. Bone Joint J 95-B(5):623–628

Maletis GB, Inacio MC, Reynolds S et al (2013b) Incidence of postoperative anterior cruciate ligament reconstruction infections: graft choice makes a difference. Am J Sports Med 41(8):1780–5

Malinin TI, Levitt RL, Bashore C et al (2002) A study of retrieved allografts used to replace anterior cruciate ligaments. Arthroscopy 18(2):163–170

McGuire DA, Hendricks SD (2009) Allograft tissue in ACL reconstruction. Sports Med Arthrosc 17(4):224–233

Moore MA (2012) Inactivation of enveloped and non-enveloped viruses on seeded human tissues by gamma irradiation. Cell Tissue Bank 13(3):401–407

Pallis M, Svoboda SJ, Cameron KL et al (2012) Survival comparison of allograft and autograft anterior cruciate ligament reconstruction at the United States Military Academy. Am J Sports Med 40(6):1242–1246

Prodromos C, Joyce B, Shi K (2007) A meta-analysis of stability of autografts compared to allografts after anterior cruciate ligament reconstruction. Knee Surg Sports Traumatol Arthrosc 15(7):851–856

Rihn JA, Irrgang JJ, Chhabra A et al (2006) Does irradiation affect the clinical outcome of patellar tendon allograft ACL reconstruction? Knee Surg Sports Traumatol Arthrosc 14(9):885–896

Roberts TS, Drez D Jr, McCarthy W et al (1991) Anterior cruciate ligament reconstruction using freeze-dried, ethylene oxide-sterilized, bone-patellar tendon-bone allografts. Two year results in thirty-six patients. Am J Sports Med 19(1):35–41

Samsell BJ, Moore MA (2012) Use of controlled low dose gamma irradiation to sterilize allograft tendons for ACL reconstruction: biomechanical and clinical perspective. Cell Tissue Bank 13(2):217–223

Scheffler SU, Scherler J, Pruss A et al (2005) Biomechanical comparison of human bone-patellar tendon-bone grafts after sterilization with peracetic acid ethanol. Cell Tissue Bank 6(2):109–115

Scheffler SU, Unterhauser FN, Weiler A (2008) Graft remodeling and ligamentization after cruciate ligament reconstruction. Knee Surg Sports Traumatol Arthrosc 16(9):834–842

Seto A, Gatt CJ Jr, Dunn MG (2008) Radioprotection of tendon tissue via crosslinking and free radical scavenging. Clin Orthop Relat Res 466(8):1788–1795

Shino K, Kawasaki T, Hirose H et al (1984) Replacement of the anterior cruciate ligament by an allogeneic tendon graft. J Bone Joint Surg (Br) 66(5):672–681

Shino K, Inoue M, Horibe S et al (1988) Maturation of allograft tendons transplanted into the knee. An arthroscopic and histological study. J Bone Joint Surg (Br) 70(4):556–560

Siebold R, Buelow JU, Bös L et al (2003) Primary ACL reconstruction with fresh-frozen patellar versus Achilles tendon allografts. Arch Orthop Trauma Surg 123(4):180–185

Simonds RJ, Holmberg SD, Hurwitz RL et al (1992) Transmission of human immunodeficiency virus type 1 from a seronegative organ and tissue donor. N Engl J Med 326(11):726–732

Spindler KP, Huston LJ, Wright RW et al (2011) The prognosis and predictors of sports function and activity at minimum 6 years after anterior cruciate ligament reconstruction: a population cohort study. Am J Sports Med 39(2):348–359

Swedish ACL Register (2011). Annual report 2011. https://www.artroclinic.se/info/rapport2011en.pdf. Accessed 17 Jun 2013

Tibor LM, Long JL, Schilling PL et al (2010) Clinical outcomes after anterior cruciate ligament reconstruction: a meta-analysis of autograft versus allograft tissue. Sports Health 2(1):56–72

Tugwell BD, Patel PR, Williams IT et al (2005) Transmission of hepatitis C virus to several organ and tissue recipients from and antibody-negative donor. Ann Intern Med 143(9):648–654

Wilson TC, Kantaras A, Atay A et al (2004) Tunnel enlargement after anterior cruciate ligament surgery. Am J Sports Med 32(2):543–549

Woo SL, Orlando CA, Camp JF et al (1986) Effects of postmortem storage by freezing on ligament tensile behavior. J Biomech 19(5):399–404

Yanke AB, Bell R, Lee A, Kang RW et al (2013) The biomechanical effects of 1.0 to 1.2 Mrad of gamma irradiation on human bone-patellar tendon-bone allografts. Am J Sports Med 41(4):835–840

Allografts in Posterior Cruciate Ligament Reconstructions

70

Luís Duarte Silva, Hélder Pereira, Alberto Monteiro, Artur Pereira de Castro, Sérgio R. Piedade, Pedro Luís Ripoll, Joaquim Miguel Oliveira, Rui Luís Reis, and João Espregueira-Mendes

Contents

Abstract

Posterior cruciate ligament (PCL) injuries are often associated with other ligament lesions. Multiligament reconstructions require an important quantity of grafts and often determine the need for cadaver allografts during the surgical repair procedures. Herein, the fundamentals of allografts that have been currently used for PCL reconstructions are overviewed. The main issues to be considered when surgeons choose this therapeutic option are also discussed.

L.D. Silva (✉)
Clínica Espregueira–Mendes F.C. Porto Stadium, FIFA Medical Centre of Excellence, Porto, Portugal

Orthopedic Department ULS–Guarda, Guarda, Portugal
e-mail: luisduartesilva1985@gmail.com

H. Pereira • J. Espregueira-Mendes
3B's Research Group – Biomaterials, Biodegradables and Biomimetics, Headquarters of the European Institute of Excellence on Tissue Engineering and Regenerative Medicine, University of Minho, Guimarães, Taipas, Portugal

ICVS/3B's – PT Government Associated Laboratory, Braga/Guimarães, Portugal

Clínica Espregueira–Mendes F.C. Porto, Stadium – FIFA Medical Centre of Excellence, Porto, Portugal

Orthopedic Department, Centro Hospitalar Póvoa de Varzim, Vila do Conde, Portugal
e-mail: heldermdpereira@gmail.com; jem@espregueira.com; joaoespregueira@netcabo.pt

A. Monteiro
Clínica Espregueira–Mendes F.C. Porto Stadium, FIFA Medical Centre of Excellence, Porto, Portugal
e-mail: albertohmonteiro@gmail.com

A.P. de Castro
DESPORSANO Sports Clinic, Lisboa, Portugal
e-mail: arturpcastro@hotmail.com

S.R. Piedade
Orthopaedic and Traumatology Department of FCM/UNICAMP, Univerisdade Estadual de Campinas, Campinas, Brazil
e-mail: sergiopiedade@terra.com.br

M.N. Doral, J. Karlsson (eds.), *Sports Injuries*,
DOI 10.1007/978-3-642-36569-0_111

Introduction

The low frequency of PCL and PCL-based multiligament knee injuries is responsible for several limitations in clinical studies. Similarly, a delay in basic science and clinical research exists when compared to other ligament injuries (Fanelli et al. 2010). However, it has been stated that the incidence of lesions of this “forgotten” ligament could not be correctly established overtime. In fact, it might be somewhat higher than previously thought (Miller et al. 1993). Controversy still exists considering conservative versus surgical treatment (Shelbourne et al. 1999; Rosenthal et al. 2012).

Clinical diagnosis and grading is not considered an easy task even when leaded by experienced surgeons. Given the need to couple image with function for correct classification, stress radiography (Fig. 1) techniques have been attempted (Garavaglia et al. 2007; Menetrey et al. 2007; Levy and Stuart 2012). Recent developments from Porto School have allowed dynamic and functional evaluation in the same MRI imaging protocol (Espregueira-Mendes et al. 2012). A device has been developed which enables MRI imaging while posterior stress is put in the tibia at different knee flexion angles and foot rotation (Fig. 2).

The best graft source for posterior cruciate ligament (PCL) reconstruction is also debated and it can include autografts, allografts, and synthetic ligaments (Rosenthal et al. 2012). In the multiligament-injured knee, a combination of autograft and some source of allograft (e.g., allograft Achilles tendon, allograft BPTB, anterior tibialis) is often required (Fanelli and Edson 2002; Adler 2013). The alternative for synthetic ligament is under intense research, but still in the early beginning of clinical testing for the last-generation implants (Brunet et al. 2005). Some gender-specific features have been reported concerning PCL, similarly to what has been found in anterior cruciate ligament repair (Jung et al. 2011; Collins et al. 2013). A superior reduction of posterior tibial laxity in female patients compared with male patients has been reported, indicating that possible gender-related differences exist after PCL surgery (Jung et al. 2011). In that study, matching parameters included number/type of reconstructed ligaments, revision/primary surgery, autograft/allograft use, preoperative tibial displacement, time interval from injury to surgery, follow-up interval, and age. It is advisable that all these factors are considered in the final option of the graft chosen for the PCL reconstruction.

Allogeneic and autogeneic tissues have unique advantages and disadvantages, but knowledge remains limited about the performance of one versus the other. No appreciable clinical differences between allograft and autograft PCL reconstruction have been reported (Hudgens et al. 2013). Despite the paucity of data comparing

P.L. Ripoll
Ripoll y De Prado Sport Clinic -FIFA Medical Centre of Excellence, Murcia, Spain
e-mail: pedrolripoll@gmail.com

J.M. Oliveira
3B's Research Group – Biomaterials, Biodegradables and Biomimetics, Headquarters of the European Institute of Excellence on Tissue Engineering and Regenerative Medicine, University of Minho, Taipas, Guimarães, Portugal

ICVS/3B's – PT Government Associated Laboratory, Braga/Guimarães, Portugal

FIFA Medical Centre of Excellence, Clínica Espregueira–Mendes F.C. Porto Stadium, Porto, Portugal
e-mail: miguel.oliveira@dep.uminho.pt

R.L. Reis
Clínica Espregueira–Mendes F.C. Porto Stadium, FIFA Medical Centre of Excellence, Porto, Portugal

Orthopaedic Department, Hospital de S. Sebastião, Feira, Portugal

ICVS/3B's – PT Government Associated Laboratory, Braga/Guimarães, Portugal

3B's Research Group – Biomaterials, Biodegradables and Biomimetics, Headquarters of the European Institute of Excellence on Tissue Engineering and Regenerative Medicine, University of Minho, Guimarães, Taipas, Portugal
e-mail: rgreis@dep.uminho.pt

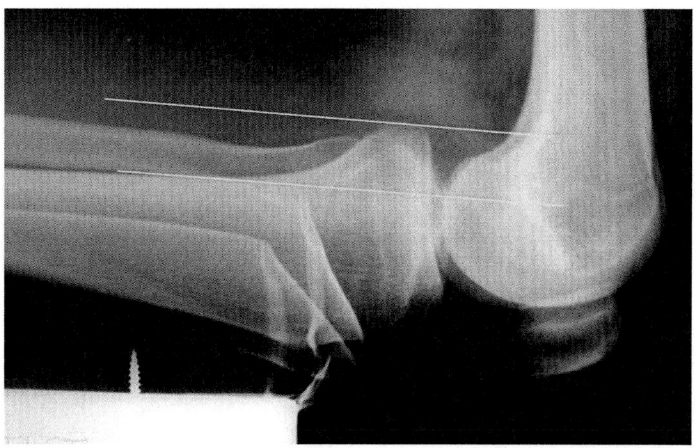

Fig. 1 Posterior stress x-ray obtained using load of the body (in addition to gravity)

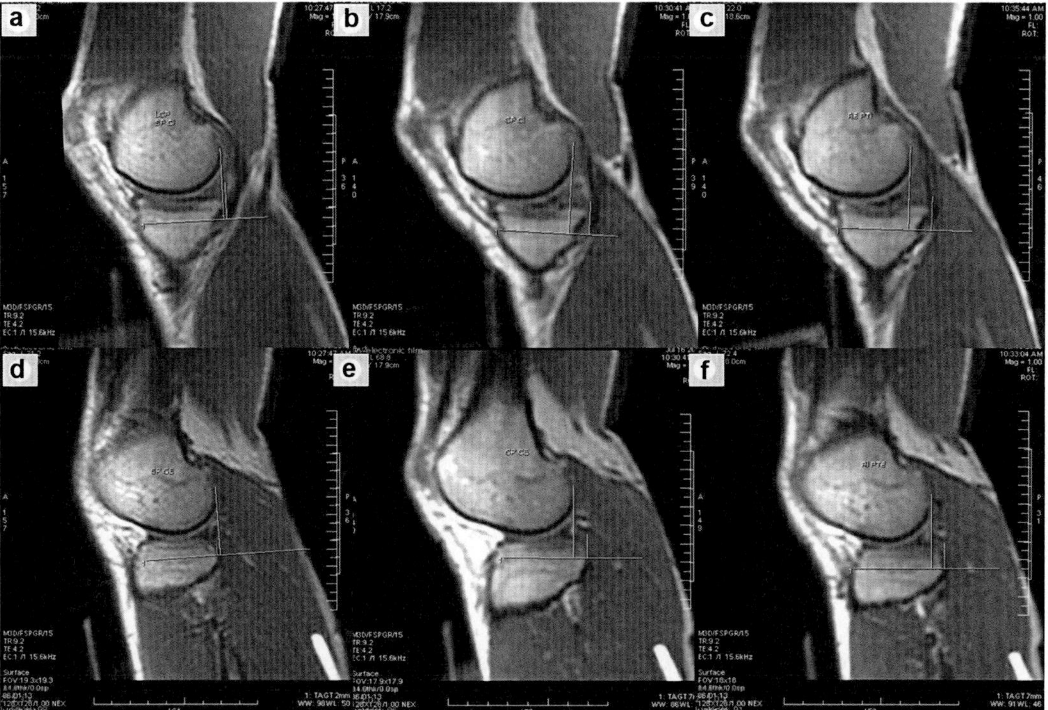

Fig. 2 Standard protocol evaluation of MRI with Porto-knee testing device (*PKTD*) of a PCL rupture at 30° of flexion. Sagittal view with foot in neutral position without load application correspondent to medial (**a**) and lateral compartments (**d**). Result after posterior load applications correspondent to medial (**b**) and lateral compartments (**e**). Notice the lines enabling objective measurement of the amount of posterior translation between bony landmarks in mm. Image correspondent to load after maximum external foot rotation in medial compartment (**c**) and after maximum internal foot rotation in lateral compartment (**f**)

allogeneic and autogeneic PCL reconstruction, satisfactory clinical and functional results have been obtained with both graft sources (Hudgens et al. 2013).

In addition to the increasing understanding of knee ligament biology and biomechanics, the technical advancements in allograft tissue, surgical instrumentation, and fixation methods have

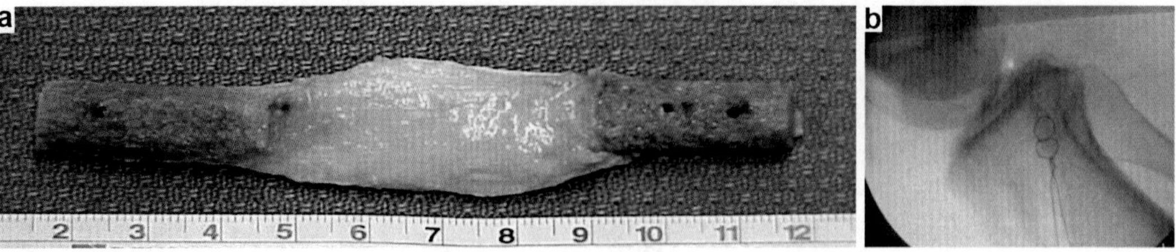

Fig. 3 Tailored patellar tendon allograft in table: length measurement prior to implantation (**a**). Intraoperative fluoroscopy image to control adequate position of patellar tendon graft during arthroscopic single-bundle PCL reconstruction (**b**)

been improving the clinical outcomes in PCL reconstruction and PCL-based multiligament knee surgery (Fanelli et al. 2010). Improved surgical techniques and postoperative rehabilitation methods have also contributed to this positive progress. PCL reconstruction in general improves both subjective patient outcomes and return to sport (Voos et al. 2012), although stability and knee kinematics may not return completely to normal (Voos et al. 2012).

Athletic population presents an additional challenge according to the different sports-specific demands (Margheritini et al. 2002). Preoperative decision concerning the surgical technique is critical concerning the choice of the graft. This will determine several aspects including the required length, fixation, or method to passage tendon grafts through tunnels (soft tissue alone, soft tissue with bone block in one of the endings, or soft tissue bone block in both extremities). Furthermore, the technique to prepare a graft also depends if a single- or double-bundle technique will be used. Recent laboratory and cadaveric studies have suggested that double-bundle reconstructions of the posterior cruciate ligament could better restore normal knee kinematics as compared to single-bundle reconstructions, although such difference could not be demonstrated by clinical outcomes (Voos et al. 2012).

It has been reported that arthroscopic single-bundle PCL reconstruction (Fig. 3) produces satisfactory return of function and decrease in symptoms (Sekiya et al. 2005). In that study, all patients improved laxity of at least 1 grade.

When compared with chronic reconstructions, acute reconstructions showed statistically significant better Activities of Daily Living Scale (ADLS) and Sports Activities Scale (SAS) scores (Sekiya et al. 2005).

Many authors favor double-bundle reconstructions which have also been described by all-inside technique (Yoon et al. 2005; Slullitel et al. 2012). Both the single-bundle and the double-bundle PCL reconstruction surgical techniques using allograft tissue provide successful results in the PCL-based multiligament-injured knee when evaluated with stress radiography, arthrometer measurements, and knee ligament rating scales (Fanelli et al. 2012).

A recent systematic review concluded that the superiority of single-bundle or double-bundle posterior cruciate ligament reconstruction remains uncertain (Kohen and Sekiya 2009). Harner's group proposed that adapting the PCL reconstruction technique to the individual injury pattern will probably provide a reconstruction that better replicates the natural biomechanics of the native knee, thereby improving functional outcomes (Chhabra et al. 2006).

Reconstruction of the PCL using the tibial inlay fixation (Fig. 4) (either open or arthroscopic) has been reported as an alternative to the transtibial tunnel technique, being the preferred method for several authors (Cooper and Stewart 2004; Piedade et al. 2006). The arguments behind this choice include the attempt to avoid the "killer turn" and graft laxity with cyclic loading.

Outcomes of isolated PCL reconstructions performed with a mixed graft (hamstrings autograft plus tibialis anterior allograft tendon) presented superior results to those using solely an Achilles tendon allograft in terms of functional knee scores, posterior stability, and the graft appearance. The use of allograft alone in that

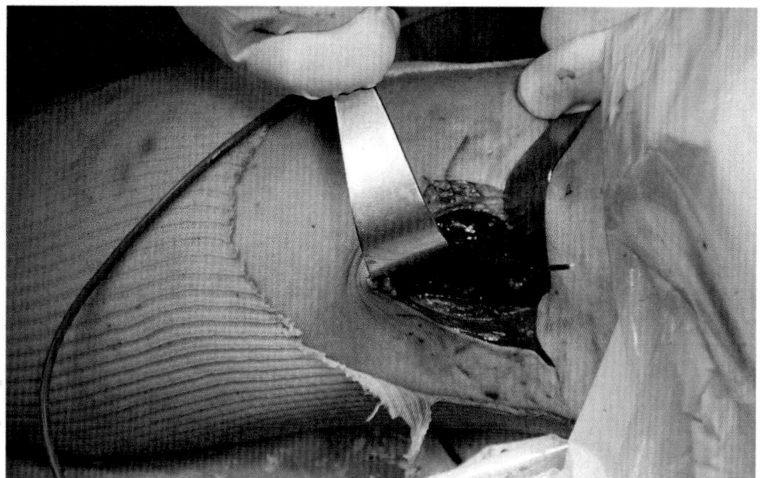

Fig. 4 Posterior approach for inlay PCL reconstruction

series presented a relatively higher rate of partial re-tear and less synovialization in the femoral aperture area (Yang et al. 2012). This might be explained by superior biologic features of fresh autografts as compared to allografts. However, deeper insights on the matter are still required.

Considerations on Allografts

In order to avoid the morbidity associated to harvesting of autografts, particularly when an important amount of tissue is necessary, the possibility of allograft (tissue transplantation from a different donor) has been considered (Malinin 1993; Robertson et al. 2006).

Autografts have the advantage of presenting no pitfalls concerning rejection or disease transmission, a relatively easy availability, and inherent lower cost (Wang et al. 2004). The main disadvantages relate to limitations in graft "size" and the limited amount of tissue available for harvesting. Frequently an additional incision is required, and thus, inherent morbidity, "donor site pain," and increased surgical time and infection must be considered (Wang et al. 2004).

The use of an adequate allograft will impair the issue of harvesting-related morbidity. The disadvantages of allografts include: increased costs, possibility of poor biological performance and disease transmission (although this aspect has fallen in parallel with better tissue banks and last-generation methods), and graft rejection or failure (James 1953; Lord et al. 1988; Simonds et al. 1992; Kainer et al. 2004; Wang et al. 2004). Concerning PCL reconstruction, one can find conflicting data in literature which makes the decision even more difficult between allograft and autograft. One study reported that in functional results and clinical outcomes, the results can be the same but complications were greater in autografts (Wang et al. 2004). Another study reported inferior capability with progressive attenuation of the allograft (Bullis and Paulos 1994), but there are also animal studies that reported that autografts may never approach normal ligament characteristics (Bosch and Kasperczyk 1992; Kasperczyk et al. 1993).

Some researchers report that the conflicting results may be due to the surgical technique and not only to the type of graft used (Montgomery et al. 2013).

Other important factors that surgeons should be aware of include: (i) tissue bank regulation, (ii) tissue procurement/donor screening, (iii) graft harvesting and processing, (iv) sterilization, and (v) storage.

Tissue bank regulation and tissue procurement vary according to local/country laws. One must consider that these differences and legal issues determine the availability of allograft tissue and secondarily influence the technical experience and therapeutic method choice in a given region (Kraft et al. 1992; Joyce 2005; MTF 2005).

The selection of a potential allograft donor is currently subject to strict epidemiological, clinical, and laboratory rules (Vangsness et al. 2003).

Laboratory tests include, among others, pathological agents such as HIV, hepatitis B, and C, human T-lymphocyte virus (HTLV), and syphilis.

Epidemiological and clinical questions include general health information (long-term steroid therapy, blood transfusion, cancer, active infection or recent infection, history of organ/tissue transplantation, acupuncture, body piercing, etc.). Travel risk (determined by local criteria) and behavioral risk assessments are also important aspects to be considered (Robertson et al. 2006; U.S. Department of Health and Human Services 2007).

Graft harvest is an important step and must comply with well-defined criteria. Harvesting process should be "aseptic," but this term does only refer to the technique used during the process because it does not eliminate the risk of the tissue being already contaminated. In some cases, antimicrobial solutions (antiseptics and/or antibiotics) are used to prevent infectious disease transmission (Robertson et al. 2006). To increase security, every stage requires written documentation and control (Vangsness et al. 2003).

Allograft Processing

Graft processing requires sterile laboratory conditions, and it aims to ensure that maximum use is made of donor tissue by trimming, sizing, and splitting, if required. It also intends to minimize antigenicity within the tissue and ensure that the graft material is free from bacterial and viral contamination while minimizing damage to its structural integrity (Hansen and Shaffer 2001; Robertson et al. 2006). Implantable medical devices are sterilized to reach a sterility assurance level (SAL) of 10^{-6}. However, sterilization in musculoskeletal tissue presents different challenges when compared to nonorganic material. The biomechanical properties of allografts are altered by radiation (Rasmussen et al. 1994; Fideler et al. 1995). Gases and liquids used as sterilizers may not have adequate tissue penetration. Musculoskeletal tissues may have a vast number of organisms in contrast with plastics or metals and the tissue itself can protect the microorganisms.

The current methods of sterilization include ethylene oxide or gamma irradiation (Vangsness et al. 2003).

Gamma irradiation has the capability to destroy bacteria and virus. However, as recently demonstrated, an increased dose of radiation which can alter biomechanical properties of the tissues is necessary (Fideler et al. 1994; Rasmussen et al. 1994; Fideler et al. 1995; Mariscalco et al. 2013). Gamma irradiation has a virucidal and bactericidal effect both by direct alteration of nucleic acids leading to genome destruction and by the production of free radicals (Robertson et al. 2006). Freeze-dried grafts require higher doses of irradiation because such grafts have relatively lower content of water from which the free radicals are generated. Accordingly to dose, radiation should destroy infective agents, including bacteria, bacterial spores, viruses, and prions without causing structural damage to the allograft. Gamma irradiation induces dose-dependent damage to collagen. A minimum dose of 35 kGy is required to eliminate HIV in tissue. Several tissue banks use gamma irradiation in doses ranging from 10 to 25 kGy in order to obtain a compromise between sterilization and damaging the structural integrity of the graft (Vangsness et al. 2003). Cyclic loading experiments have demonstrated that even low-dose irradiation (20 kGy) can lead to increased elongation of the graft and a decreased load to failure compared with nonirradiated controls (Curran et al. 2004).

Ethylene oxide (EtOx) has a limited ability to penetrate tissue (Prolo et al. 1980) and has been associated with intra-articular synovial and immune reactions (Jackson and Simon 1990) and a high rate of mechanical failure (Roberts et al. 1991). EtOx applied in a gaseous state with inert diluents such as carbon dioxide has been widely used in the sterilization of biological tissue (Curran et al. 2004; Robertson et al. 2006). The main concerns regarding the use of EtOx in tendon allografts include the degree of bone penetration that may be achieved by the gas, and reports of graft dissolution, persistent synovial effusion, and a poor clinical outcome (Jackson and Simon 1990; Roberts et al. 1991). Persistent effusions in the knee have been reported in patients receiving allograft treated with EtOx for up to 14 months following graft implantation due to the presence of toxic reaction products within allograft and synovium (Jackson and Simon 1990).

New sterilization methods are being studied such as electron irradiation (Hoburg et al. 2011) and microwave (Singh and Singh 2012).

Bacterial decontamination of the surface of a given graft may be achieved by immersion in an antibiotic solution with minimal damage to tissue properties.

The concerns related to deep bacterial, viral, or prion infection should be addressed by a combination of harvesting under aseptic conditions, donor screening, bacterial testing, and controlled processing. In grafts which are obtained by processes not fulfilling these criteria, sterilization by gamma irradiation or EtOx can be used. However, for composite tendon allografts, the possibility of deleterious effects caused by the sterilization processes on all elements of the graft must be considered.

The complexity and difficulties in obtaining adequate viral elimination using sterilization methods should help to bear in mind the importance of having a thorough program of donor screening.

Allograft Storage

The main options concerning storage methods are fresh transplantation, freeze-drying, and deep-freezing/cryopreservation.

Fresh transplantation occurs generally until 24 days after the allograft harvesting. It has been recognized even in meniscus transplantation that this possibility favors the biologic conditions of a given graft (Monllau et al. 2010). However, besides limitations in donor screening and graft processing, it would be by far the most expensive in terms of organization and logistic requirements for surgery. In contrast with the use of fresh-frozen or cryopreserved grafts, a strict time-schedule from harvest moment to transplantation is mandatory. This type of graft can produce an undesired immunologic response. Therefore, all the previously exposed fresh allografts are not currently used in ligament reconstruction surgery.

Fresh-frozen processed graft material may be stored for three up to 5 years, prior to use (Gelber et al. 2008; Sun et al. 2011; Guo et al. 2012; Lawhorn et al. 2012). Fresh-frozen allograft is frozen after its harvest. After being washed in an antibiotic solution, it is cooled to −70/−80 °C. This type of graft produces a minor immunologic response than fresh allograft.

Freeze-dried allograft undergoes a process called lyophilization. After being washed in an antibiotic solution and cooled to −70 °C, it is dehydrated by reducing the surrounding pressure to allow the frozen water in the material to sublimate directly from the solid phase to the gas phase (Vangsness et al. 2003). The water content is reduced to <5 %. This type of graft produces almost no immunologic response.

Cryopreservation is a process to preserve whole tissues, or any other substances susceptible to damage caused by chemical reactivity or time when cooling to very low temperatures. At low temperatures, the deleterious enzymatic or chemical activity which might cause damage to the tissue is impaired (Suhodolcan et al. 2013). Deep-freezing (up to −180 ºC) is then the most used method, allowing tissue storage up to 5 years. This process destroys all cells which, apparently, has low clinical relevance (Vangsness et al. 2003). Cryopreservation methods aim to reach low temperatures without causing further damage caused by the formation of ice during freezing. Traditional cryopreservation has relied on coating the material to be frozen with a class of molecules termed cryoprotectants. New methods are constantly being investigated due to the inherent toxicity of several cryoprotectants.

The importance of strict adherence to protocols is illustrated by reports of clostridium septicum infection following anterior cruciate ligament reconstruction, which has been related to graft contamination during processing in tissue bank (Barbour and King 2003).

Allografts in Posterior Cruciate Ligament Repair

The surgical techniques in PCL reconstruction are multiple and present several variables including: (i) inlay, (ii) all-inside, (iii) single or double bundle, (iv) single or multiple strains, and (v) a variety of graft options (Fanelli et al. 2010).

As aforementioned, there is no consensus regarding graft choice in PCL reconstruction (Robertson et al. 2006). Several studies that compare allografts and autografts in isolated PCL reconstructions using specific techniques revealed similar clinical, functional, knee scores as well as instrumented testing results (Wang et al. 2004; Ahn et al. 2005). Some authors prefer mainly the use of allograft (Peter MacDonald 2009).

Others begin the approach with autograft in isolated lesions, using ipsilateral quadriceps tendon-patellar bone autograft or allografts as a secondary option. These consider allografts as their first option in combined ligament lesions, in order to avoid further aggression to an already compromised knee joint (Noyes and Barber-Westin 2011).

For others, the main options using allograft are the Achilles tendon (Dennis et al. 2004; Peter MacDonald 2009) and bone-patellar tendon-bone (Noyes and Barber-Westin 2011). The other most referred grafts includes: (i) tibial posterior, (ii) tibial anterior, and (iii) mixed grafts.

Achilles tendon allograft is one of the most appreciated choices due to its favorable properties, namely, strong, tendon graft with bone block (Kim et al. 2012; Noh et al. 2012), ample graft length, large amount of graft material, and easier passage of soft tissue end (Ahn et al. 2005; Irrgang et al. 2006). To retrieve the Achilles tendon it is necessary a large paratendinous incision until musculotendinous junction is identified. It is necessary to dissect the tendon from the muscular fibers for obtaining a graft with the maximum possible length (Service 2004).

Because of the aforementioned properties, it has become increasingly popular and there are several articles describing different applications such as double-bundle inlay technique (Dennis et al. 2004), double-bundle augmentation (Yoon et al. 2005), tibial inlay using endoscopic techniques (Kim et al. 2004a; Kim and Park 2005), and single-bundle and double-bundle "all-inside" (Yoon et al. 2011).

Bone-patellar tendon-bone (BPTB) allograft is another popular choice (Noyes and Barber-Westin 2011). The bone contact in both ends of the graft increases the chance of bone-to-bone healing but can also present length mismatch problems (Figs. 3 and 5) (Farrow and Bergfeld 2009). Some new options have been proposed for double-bundle reconstructions, such as bifid BPTB allograft (Whiddon and Sekiya 2005). The BPTB unit is harvested with the objective of the distal block reaching (3.5 cm long and 2 cm wide). Precautions must be taken into account to avoid fracture of bone blocks. In multiligament reconstructions of the knee, one single complete

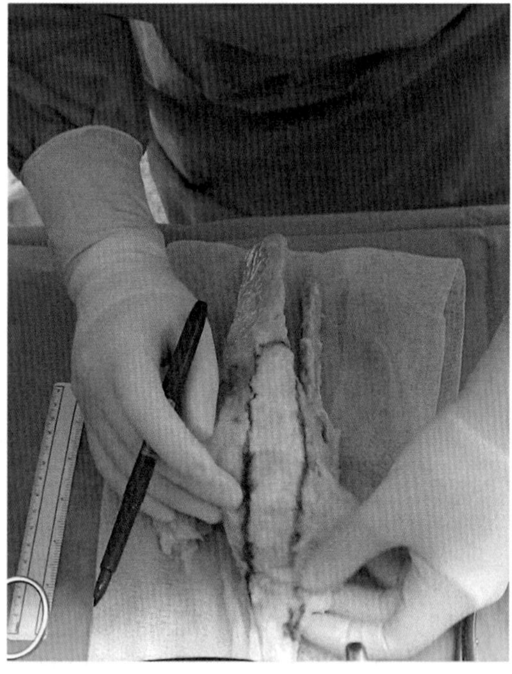

Fig. 5 Extensor mechanism allograft for multiligament knee reconstruction

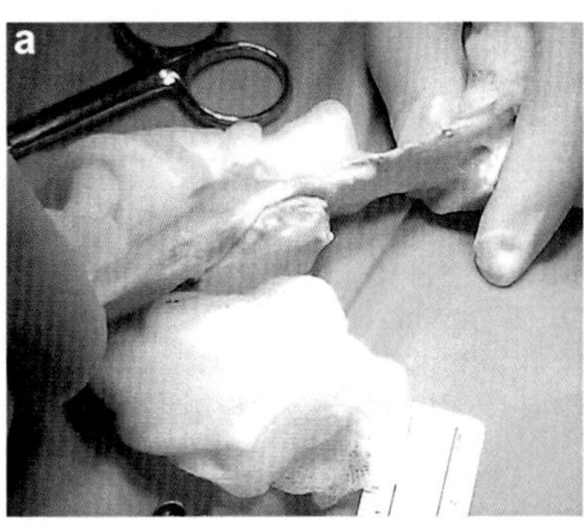
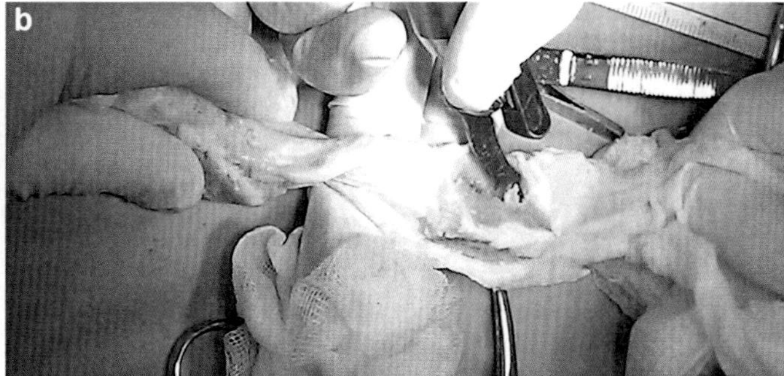

Fig. 6 In table preparation of a patellar tendon allograft (**a**). Bone blocks are being tailored to match specific patient needs (**b**)

extensor apparatus graft will enable the use of both BPTB and quadriceps tendon allografts (Figs. 5 and 6).

Tibialis anterior is another allograft that has been investigated as an option for the reconstruction of the PCL and has already different double-bundle surgical techniques (Min et al. 2011; Daniel Slullitel et al. 2012). Tibialis posterior may also be used in double-bundle procedures with three strands (Kim et al. 2004b). These two tendons were also used in combination, in a double-double-bundle reconstruction with two femoral and two tibial tunnels (Makino et al. 2006).

There are also cases in which autograft and allograft can be mixed such as tibialis anterior with hamstring in a single-bundle surgical technique (Yang et al. 2012).

Conclusions

With the advances in processing techniques, sterilization, and storage, it is possible now to obtain high-quality and safer allografts. Increased quality and experience in tissue banks as a result of the cooperation with orthopedic surgeons have greatly improved the possibility of allograft clinical application. However, there are no consensus and different legislations conditioning its use. Novel insights are arising from basic science research (possibility to augment biologic capacity of allografts) besides tissue engineering and regenerative medicine (possibility to overcome the need for cadaver allografts). These advances promise to favor conditions for ligament repair in the future.

Cross-References

▸ Allografts in Anterior Cruciate Ligament Reconstruction
▸ Combined Anterior and Posterior Cruciate Ligament Injuries
▸ Posterior Cruciate Ligament Reconstruction: New Concepts

References

Adler GG (2013) All-inside posterior cruciate ligament reconstruction with a GraftLink. Arthrosc Tech 2: e111–e115

Ahn JH, Yoo JC, Wang JH (2005) Posterior cruciate ligament reconstruction: double-loop hamstring tendon autograft versus Achilles tendon allograft–clinical results of a minimum 2-year follow-up. Arthroscopy 21:965–969

Barbour SA, King W (2003) The safe and effective use of allograft tissue–an update. Am J Sports Med 31:791–797

Bosch U, Kasperczyk WJ (1992) Healing of the patellar tendon autograft after posterior cruciate ligament reconstruction–a process of ligamentization? An experimental study in a sheep model. Am J Sports Med 20:558–566

Brunet P, Charrois O, Degeorges R, Boisrenoult P, Beaufils P (2005) Reconstruction of acute posterior cruciate ligament tears using a synthetic ligament. Rev Chir Orthop Reparatrice Appar Mot 91:34–43

Bullis DW, Paulos LE (1994) Reconstruction of the posterior cruciate ligament with allograft. Clin Sports Med 13:581–597

Chhabra A, Kline AJ, Harner CD (2006) Single-bundle versus double-bundle posterior cruciate ligament reconstruction: scientific rationale and surgical technique. Instr Course Lect 55:497–507

Collins JE, Katz JN, Donnell-Fink LA, Martin SD, Losina E (2013) Cumulative incidence of ACL reconstruction after ACL injury in adults: role of age, sex, and race. Am J Sports Med 41:544–549

Cooper DE, Stewart D (2004) Posterior cruciate ligament reconstruction using single-bundle patella tendon graft with tibial inlay fixation: 2- to 10-year follow-up. Am J Sports Med 32:346–360

Curran AR, Adams DJ, Gill JL, Steiner ME, Scheller AD (2004) The biomechanical effects of low-dose irradiation on bone-patellar tendon-bone allografts. Am J Sports Med 32:1131–1135

Daniel Slullitel HG, Ojeda V, Seri M (2012) Double-bundle "all-inside" posterior cruciate ligament reconstruction. Arthrosc Tech 1:141–148

Dennis MG, Fox JA, Alford JW, Hayden JK, Bach BR Jr (2004) Posterior cruciate ligament reconstruction: current trends. J Knee Surg 17:133–139

Espregueira-Mendes J, Pereira H, Sevivas N, Passos C, Vasconcelos JC, Monteiro A et al (2012) Assessment of rotatory laxity in anterior cruciate ligament-deficient knees using magnetic resonance imaging with Porto-knee testing device. Knee Surg Sports Traumatol Arthrosc 20:671–678

Fanelli GC, Edson CJ (2002) Arthroscopically assisted combined anterior and posterior cruciate ligament reconstruction in the multiple ligament injured knee: 2- to 10-year follow-up. Arthroscopy 18:703–714

Fanelli GC, Beck JD, Edson CJ (2010) Current concepts review: the posterior cruciate ligament. J Knee Surg 23:61–72

Fanelli GC, Beck JD, Edson CJ (2012) Single compared to double-bundle PCL reconstruction using allograft tissue. J Knee Surg 25:59–64

Farrow LD, Bergfeld JA (2009) Posterior Cruciate Ligament reconstruction: Single Bundle Tibial Inlay Technique. In: Gill TJ (ed) Arthroscopic techniques of the knee: a visual guide. SLACK incorporated, Thorofare, pp 171–188

Fideler BMVCJ, Moore T et al (1994) Effects of gamma irradiation on the human immunodeficiency virus. A study in frozen human bone-patellar ligament-bone grafts obtained from infected cadavera. J Bone Joint Surg Am 76(7):1032–1035

Fideler BM, Vangsness CT Jr, Lu B, Orlando C, Moore T (1995) Gamma irradiation: effects on biomechanical properties of human bone-patellar tendon-bone allografts. Am J Sports Med 23:643–646

Garavaglia G, Lubbeke A, Dubois-Ferriere V, Suva D, Fritschy D, Menetrey J (2007) Accuracy of stress radiography techniques in grading isolated and combined posterior knee injuries: a cadaveric study. Am J Sports Med 35:2051–2056

Gelber PE, Gonzalez G, Lloreta JL, Reina F, Caceres E, Monllau JC (2008) Freezing causes changes in the meniscus collagen net: a new ultrastructural meniscus disarray scale. Knee Surg Sports Traumatol Arthrosc 16:353–359

Guo L, Yang L, Duan XJ, He R, Chen GX, Wang FY et al (2012) Anterior cruciate ligament reconstruction with bone-patellar tendon-bone graft: comparison of autograft, fresh-frozen allograft, and gamma-irradiated allograft. Arthroscopy 28:211–217

Hansen JM, Shaffer HL (2001) Sterilization and Preservation by Radiation Sterilization, In: Block SS (ed) Disinfection, sterilization, and preservation, 5th edn. Lippincott, Williams & Wilkins, Philadelphia, pp 729–746

Hoburg A, Keshlaf S, Schmidt T, Smith M, Gohs U, Perka C et al (2011) Fractionation of high-dose electron beam irradiation of BPTB grafts provides significantly improved viscoelastic and structural properties compared to standard gamma irradiation. Knee Surg Sports Traumatol Arthrosc 19:1955–1961

Hudgens JL, Gillette BP, Krych AJ, Stuart MJ, May JH, Levy BA (2013) Allograft versus autograft in posterior cruciate ligament reconstruction: an evidence-based systematic review. J Knee Surg 26:109–115

Irrgang JJ, West R, Sahasrabudhe A, Harner C (2006) Rehabilitation after Posterior Cruciate Ligament Reconstruction. In : Manske RC (ed) Postsurgical Orthopedic Sports Rehabilitation: Knee & Shoulder. Elsevier Health Sciences, Missouri, pp 245–256

Jackson DW WG, Simon TM (1990) Intraarticular reaction associated with the use of freeze-dried, ethylene oxide-sterilized bone-patella tendon-bone allografts in the reconstruction of the anterior cruciate ligament. Am J Sports 18:1–11

James JI (1953) Tuberculosis transmitted by banked bone. J Bone Joint Surg Br 35-B:578

Joyce MJ (2005) Safety and FDA regulations for musculoskeletal allografts: perspective of an orthopaedic surgeon. Clin Orthop Relat Res 22–30

Jung TM, Lubowicki A, Wienand A, Wagner M, Weiler A (2011) Knee stability after posterior cruciate ligament reconstruction in female versus male patients: a prospective matched-group analysis. Arthroscopy 27:399–403

Kainer MA, Linden JV, Whaley DN, Holmes HT, Jarvis WR, Jernigan DB et al (2004) Clostridium infections associated with musculoskeletal-tissue allografts. N Engl J Med 350:2564–2571

Kasperczyk WJ, Bosch U, Oestern HJ, Tscherne H (1993) Staging of patellar tendon autograft healing after posterior cruciate ligament reconstruction. A biomechanical and histological study in a sheep model. Clin Orthop Relat Res 286:271–282

Kim SJ, Park IS (2005) Arthroscopic reconstruction of the posterior cruciate ligament using tibial-inlay and double-bundle technique. Arthroscopy 21:1271

Kim SJ, Choi CH, Kim HS (2004a) Arthroscopic posterior cruciate ligament tibial inlay reconstruction. Arthroscopy 20(Suppl 2):149–154

Kim SJ, Park IS, Cheon YM, Ryu SW (2004b) Double-bundle technique: endoscopic posterior cruciate ligament reconstruction using tibialis posterior allograft. Arthroscopy 20:1090–1094

Kim SJ, Bae JH, Lim HC (2012) Comparison of Achilles and tibialis anterior tendon allografts after anterior cruciate ligament reconstruction. Knee Surg Sports Traumatol Arthrosc 22:135–41

Kohen RB, Sekiya JK (2009) Single-bundle versus double-bundle posterior cruciate ligament reconstruction. Arthroscopy 25:1470–1477

Kraft J, Alexander LA, Rowlands DT Jr (1992) Tissue transplantation. Quality assurance in the banking and utilization of musculoskeletal allografts. Physician Assist 16(49–50):3–6

Lawhorn KW, Howell SM, Traina SM, Gottlieb JE, Meade TD, Freedberg HI (2012) The effect of graft tissue on anterior cruciate ligament outcomes: a multicenter, prospective, randomized controlled trial comparing autograft hamstrings with fresh-frozen anterior tibialis allograft. Arthroscopy 28:1079–1086

Levy BA, Stuart MJ (2012) Treatment of PCL, ACL, and lateral-side knee injuries: acute and chronic. J Knee Surg 25:295–305

Lord CF, Gebhardt MC, Tomford WW, Mankin HJ (1988) Infection in bone allografts. Incidence, nature, and treatment. J Bone Joint Surg Am 70:369–376

Makino A, Aponte Tinao L, Ayerza MA, Pascual Garrido C, Costa Paz M, Muscolo DL (2006) Anatomic double-bundle posterior cruciate ligament reconstruction using double-double tunnel with tibial anterior and posterior fresh-frozen allograft. Arthroscopy 22(684):e1–e5

Malinin T (1993) Allografts for the reconstruction of the cruciate ligaments of the knee: procurement, preservation, and storage. Sports Med Arthrosc Rev 1:31–41

Margheritini F, Rihn J, Musahl V, Mariani PP, Harner C (2002) Posterior cruciate ligament injuries in the athlete: an anatomical, biomechanical and clinical review. Sports Med 32:393–408

Mariscalco MW, Magnussen RA, Mehta D, Hewett TE, Flanigan DC, Kaeding CC (2013) Autograft versus nonirradiated allograft tissue for anterior cruciate ligament reconstruction: a systematic review. Am J Sports Med 42:492–499

Menetrey J, Garavaglia G, Fritschy D (2007) Definition, classification, rationale and treatment for PCl deficient knee. Rev Chir Orthop Reparatrice Appar Mot 93:5S70–5S73

Miller MD, Johnson DL, Harner CD, Fu FH (1993) Posterior cruciate ligament injuries. Orthop Rev 22:1201–1210

Min BH, Lee YS, Lee YS, Jin CZ, Son KH (2011) Evaluation of transtibial double-bundle posterior cruciate ligament reconstruction using a single-sling method with a tibialis anterior allograft. Am J Sports Med 39:374–379

Monllau JC, González-Lucena G, Gelber PE, Pelfort X (2010) Allograft meniscus transplantation: a current review. Tech Knee Surg 9:107–113

Montgomery SR, Johnson JS, McAllister DR, Petrigliano FA (2013) Surgical management of PCL injuries: indications, techniques, and outcomes. Curr Rev Musculoskelet Med 6:115–123

MTF (2005) Allograft safety and ethical considerations. Proceedings of the fourth symposium sponsored by the Musculoskeletal Transplant Foundation. September 2003. Edinburgh, Scotland, United Kingdom. Clin Orthop Relat Res 435:2–117

Noh JH, Roh YH, Lee K, Lee JS (2012) Achilles tendon allograft with its bony attachment to repair rupture and extensive degeneration of the heel cord. Acta Orthop Belg 78:678–680

Noyes FR, Barber-Westin S (2011) Decision Making and Surgical Treatment of Posterior Cruciate Ligament Ruptures. In: Scott WN, Insall JN, Scuderi GR (eds) Insall and Scott Surgery of the Knee, 5th edn. Elsevier/Churchill Livingstone

Peter MacDonald DW (2009) Technical considerations in posterior cruciate ligament reconstruction. A Canadian perspective. Oper Tech Sports Med 17:156–161

Piedade SR, Munhoz RR, Cavenaghi G, Miranda JB, Mischan MM (2006) Knee P.C.L. reconstruction: a tibial bed fixation ("INLAY") technique. Objective and subjective evaluation of a 30-cases series. Acta Ortop Bras 14:92–96

Prolo DJ, Pedrotti PW, White DH (1980) Ethylene oxide sterilization of bone, dura mater, and fascia lata for human transplantation. Neurosurgery 6:529–539

Rasmussen TJ, Feder SM, Butler DL, Noyes FR (1994) The effects of 4 Mrad of gamma irradiation on the initial mechanical properties of bone-patellar tendon-bone grafts. Arthroscopy 10:188–197

Roberts TS, Drez D Jr, McCarthy W, Paine R (1991) Anterior cruciate ligament reconstruction using freeze-dried, ethylene oxide-sterilized, bone-patellar tendon-bone allografts. Two year results in thirty-six patients. Am J Sports Med 19:35–41

Robertson A, Nutton RW, Keating JF (2006) Current trends in the use of tendon allografts in orthopaedic surgery. J Bone Joint Surg Br 88:988–992

Rosenthal MD, Rainey CE, Tognoni A, Worms R (2012) Evaluation and management of posterior cruciate ligament injuries. Phys Ther Sport 13:196–208

Sekiya JK, West RV, Ong BC, Irrgang JJ, Fu FH, Harner CD (2005) Clinical outcomes after isolated arthroscopic single-bundle posterior cruciate ligament reconstruction. Arthroscopy 21:1042–1050

Service SNBTSST (2004) Standard Operating Procedure TSD 290 03 Tendon donor referral and retrieval from multi-organ donors. p. Nation

Shelbourne KD, Davis TJ, Patel DV (1999) The natural history of acute, isolated, nonoperatively treated posterior cruciate ligament injuries. A prospective study. Am J Sports Med 27:276–283

Simonds RJ, Holmberg SD, Hurwitz RL, Coleman TR, Bottenfield S, Conley LJ et al (1992) Transmission of human immunodeficiency virus type 1 from a seronegative organ and tissue donor. N Engl J Med 326:726–732

Singh R, Singh D (2012) Sterilization of bone allografts by microwave and gamma radiation. Int J Radiat Biol 88:661–666

Slullitel D, Galan H, Ojeda V, Seri M (2012) Double-bundle "all-inside" posterior cruciate ligament reconstruction. Arthrosc Tech 1:e141–e148

Suhodolcan L, Brojan M, Kosel F, Drobnic M, Alibegovic A, Brecelj J (2013) Cryopreservation with glycerol improves the in vitro biomechanical characteristics of human patellar tendon allografts. Knee Surg Sports Traumatol Arthrosc 21:1218–1225

Sun K, Zhang J, Wang Y, Xia C, Zhang C, Yu T et al (2011) Arthroscopic reconstruction of the anterior cruciate ligament with hamstring tendon autograft and fresh-frozen allograft: a prospective, randomized controlled study. Am J Sports Med 39:1430–1438

U.S. Department of Health and Human Services FaDA, Center for Biologics Evaluation and Research (2007) Guidance for industry: eligibility determination for donors of human cells, tissues, and cellular and tissue-based products

Vangsness CT Jr, Garcia IA, Mills CR, Kainer MA, Roberts MR, Moore TM (2003) Allograft transplantation in the knee: tissue regulation, procurement, processing, and sterilization. Am J Sports Med 31:474–481

Voos JE, Mauro CS, Wente T, Warren RF, Wickiewicz TL (2012) Posterior cruciate ligament: anatomy, biomechanics, and outcomes. Am J Sports Med 40:222–231

Wang CJ, Chan YS, Weng LH, Yuan LJ, Chen HS (2004) Comparison of autogenous and allogenous posterior cruciate ligament reconstructions of the knee. Injury 35:1279–1285

Whiddon DR, Sekiya JK (2005) Double-bundle posterior cruciate ligament reconstruction with a bifid bone-patellar tendon-bone allograft. Oper Tech Sports Med 13(4):233–240

Yang JH, Yoon JR, Jeong HI, Hwang DH, Woo SJ, Kwon JH et al (2012) Second-look arthroscopic assessment of arthroscopic single-bundle posterior cruciate ligament reconstruction: comparison of mixed graft versus achilles tendon allograft. Am J Sports Med 40:2052–2060

Yoon KH, Bae DK, Song SJ, Lim CT (2005) Arthroscopic double-bundle augmentation of posterior cruciate ligament using split Achilles allograft. Arthroscopy 21:1436–1442

Yoon KH, Bae DK, Song SJ, Cho HJ, Lee JH (2011) A prospective randomized study comparing arthroscopic single-bundle and double-bundle posterior cruciate ligament reconstructions preserving remnant fibers. Am J Sports Med 39:474–480

Alternative Techniques for Double-Tunnel Anatomic Anterior Cruciate Ligament Reconstruction

71

Stefano Zaffagnini, Alberto Grassi, Giulio Maria Marcheggiani Muccioli, Tommaso Bonaninga, Cecilia Signorelli, Nicola Lopomo, Danilo Bruni, and Maurilio Marcacci

Contents

S. Zaffagnini (✉)
Clinica Ortopedica e Traumatologica II, Laboratorio di Biomeccanica e Innovazione Tecnologica, Università di Bologna, Bologna, Italy
e-mail: s.zaffagnini@biomec.ior.it; stefano.zaffagnini@unibo.it

A. Grassi • G.M.M. Muccioli • T. Bonaninga • C. Signorelli • N. Lopomo • D. Bruni • M. Marcacci
II Clinica Ortopedica e Traumatologica, Istituto Ortopedico Rizzoli, Bologna, Italy
e-mail: alberto.grassi@ior.it; marcheggianimuccioli@me.com; t.bonanzinga@gmail.com; c.signorelli@biomec.ior.it; n.lopomo@biomec.ior.it; d.bruni@biomec.ior.it; m.marcacci@biomec.ior.it

M.N. Doral, J. Karlsson (eds.), *Sports Injuries*,
DOI 10.1007/978-3-642-36569-0_93

Abstract

This chapter presents a nonanatomical double-bundle ACL reconstruction technique. The reconstruction is performed using hamstring tendons that are harvested, maintaining intact the tibial insertion. The anteromedial bundle is restored placing the graft in the "over-the-top" position, while the posterolateral bundle is replaced retrieving the graft from a femoral tunnel. Graft fixation is obtained using metal staples.

Hundreds of patients have been treated with this technique during the last 10 years, including athletes with high functional requests. Furthermore, in vivo analysis of knee kinematic confirmed the effectiveness of the technique.

Introduction

Numerous surgical procedures including different graft selections have been proposed for anterior cruciate ligament (ACL) reconstruction. The literature revealed a remarkable lack of consensus which could be considered the best technique in terms of postoperative stability, patient safety, and prevention of osteoarthritis.

In 2003, Marcacci et al. developed an original technique that includes the advantages of a double-bundle (DB) reconstruction and the simplicity of the over-the-top position as well (Marcacci et al. 2003). This technique allows the ACL reconstruction without the inherent risks associated with drilling four tunnels and it does not need any extra surgical tools. Given that, the proposed technique shows conservative advantages to patients and economic benefits to the National Health Service.

Surgical Technique

The ACL reconstruction is performed with the patient placed in a supine position under general or spinal anesthesia. A tourniquet is recommended. Usually a medial suprapatellar portal is used for the water inflow, while an anterolateral portal is commonly used for the arthroscope and an anteromedial portal for instruments. Arthroscopic evaluation and eventually treatment of meniscal or cartilage lesion is performed as usual. When the ACL lesion is confirmed, the tibial insertion area and the intercondylar notch are prepared. Notchplasty is performed only in chronic cases to avoid impingement of the graft. Any soft tissues in the posterior part of the roof represent a possible obstruction for the "over-the-top" position, and they need to be carefully removed.

Graft Harvesting

With the patient's leg placed in a figure-of-four position, a 3 cm transverse incision is created over the pes anserinus, which is located following the hamstring tendons distally to their attachment to the anteromedial part of the tibia. Then a fascial incision parallel to the orientation of the pes tendons is made. Both the gracilis and semitendinosus tendon are released from the surrounding soft tissue and fascial attachments. The tendons are harvested using a blunt tendon stripper (Acufex, Microsurgical, Mansfield, MA). This procedure is performed while maintaining firm tension distally on the tendon and holding the knee joint at more than 90° of flexion. Dissecting the distal attachment of semitendinosus from the adjacent gracilis tendon allows to increase the length of the graft of around 1–2 cm.

To ensure the neurovascular supply, the tibial insertions of both tendons are preserved (Fig. 1).

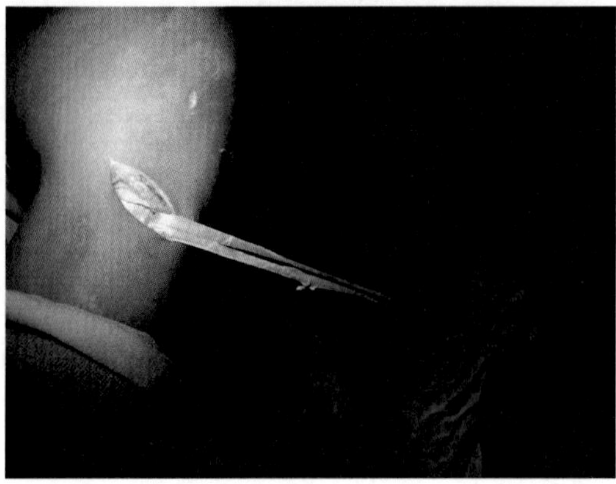

Fig. 1 Hamstring tendons are harvested maintaining the distal insertion intact

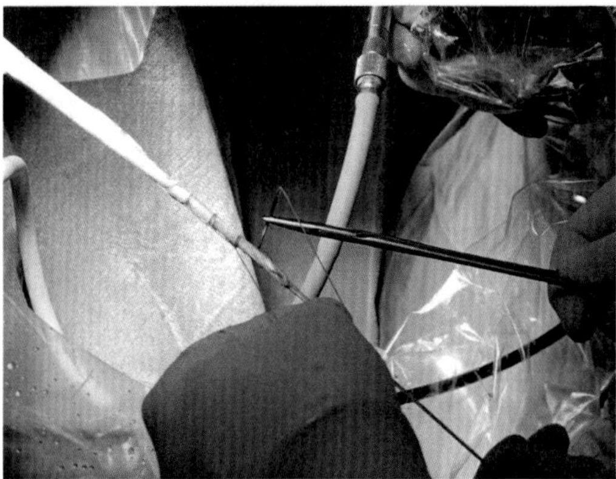

Fig. 2 The gracilis and semitendinosus tendons are tightly sutured together at the free end

The harvested tendons are sutured together using three nonabsorbable sutures. Particular attention must be paid to fix the suture to the free proximal tendon ends (Fig. 2).

Tunnel Creation

Tibial Tunnel

Under arthroscopic visualization, a guide pin is inserted on the medial aspect of the tibia through the graft harvesting incision. It is directed to the medial posterior part of the ACL tibial insertion. The tibial tunnel is performed according to the ligament diameter (usually 7–8 mm). The remaining debris are removed. The sharp edges of the bone tunnels are smoothed by a motorized shaver. After that, under arthroscopic visualization and passing through the tibial tunnel, a wire loop passer is inserted into the notch and brought out from the anteromedial portal.

Femoral Tunnel

The femoral tunnel is performed holding the knee at 90° of flexion (or less). A guide pin is inserted on the medial wall of the lateral condyle, approximately 5 mm anterior to the "over-the-top" position. After that, the knee is flexed at 130° and the guide pin advanced until passing the femoral cortex immediately above the edge of the lateral femoral condyle. A reamer is inserted along to the guide pin to create a 7 mm tunnel. Osseous debris is removed and the edge smoothed using a shaver.

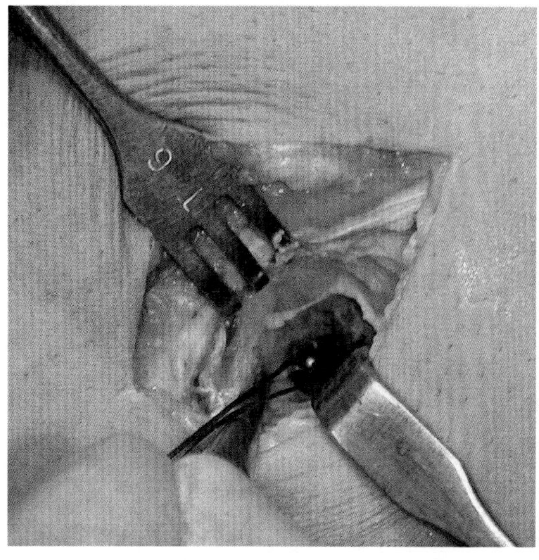

Fig. 3 The tip of the clamp is pushed through the thin posterior layer of knee capsule, reaching the posterior space previously prepared

ACL Reconstruction

Anteromedial Bundle

Holding the knee at 90° of flexion and the foot externally rotated, a 3–5 cm longitudinal incision is made immediately above the lateral femoral condyle and through the iliotibial band. The lateral aspect of the thigh is dissected with electrocautery and scissors to reach the lateral intermuscular septum. The septum inserts into the lateral femoral condyle and separates the vastus lateralis muscle from the lateral head of the gastrocnemius muscle. When the septum has been clearly identified, it is possible to reach the posterior aspect of the joint capsule passing over this structure. It is possible to identify the correct position of the "over-the-top" passage by manually feeling the posterior tubercle of the lateral femoral condyle. A curved Kelly clamp is passed from the anteromedial portal into the notch with the tip placed as proximal as possible and keeping the contact with the posterior part of the capsule. After palpating the tip of the clamp from the lateral side of the femur just posteriorly to the intermuscular septum, the tip itself is pushed through the thin posterior layer of knee capsule, reaching the posterior space previously prepared (Fig. 3).

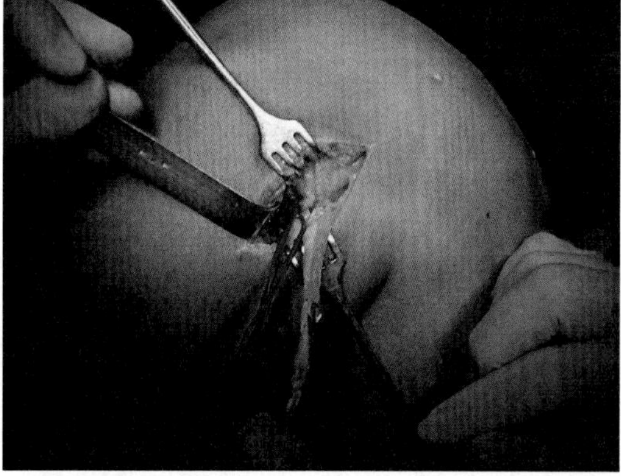

Fig. 4 The anteromedial bundle is replaced placing the graft in the "over-the-top" position. The knee is bent to 130°

Thus, a suture loop is placed into the tip of the clamp. It is retrieved from the anteromedial portal and placed into the wire loop that was previously inserted in the same portal. Pulling the wire from the tibial side brings the suture loop at the bottom of the tibial tunnel and out from the tibial incision. The suture is tied on the free end of the graft and pulled through the knee joint. The graft is then retrieved from the lateral incision, restoring the anteromedial bundle (Fig. 4).

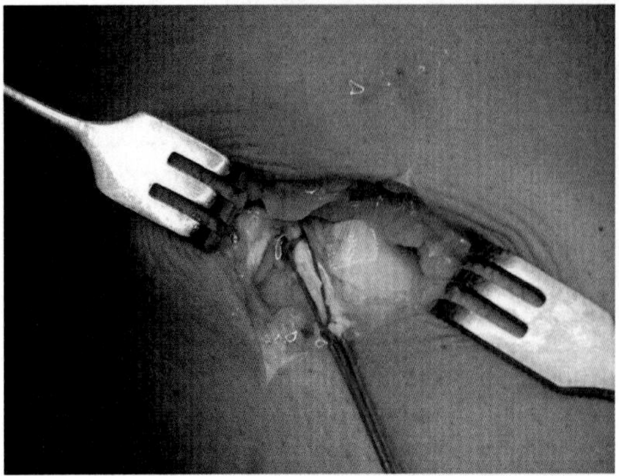

Fig. 5 The graft exits through the tibial tunnel at the same incision as the tendon harvesting

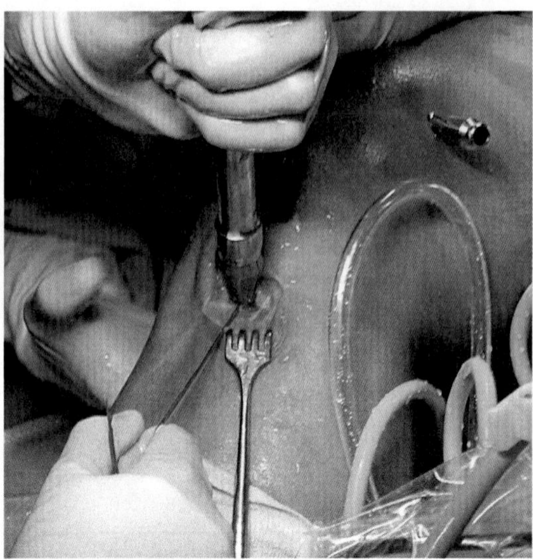

Fig. 6 One metal staple is used to secure the graft to the anteromedial aspect of the tibia

Posterolateral Bundle

A suture loop is introduced into the joint through the anteromedial portal using a suture passer. The loop is then pushed into the femoral tunnel under arthroscopic view. At this point the exit on the lateral aspect of the femoral shaft is reached, and the suture loop needs to be pulled out from the lateral incision. The other side of the suture loop is be pulled down through the tibial tunnel. This latter is performed using a grasper and under arthroscopic control. The suture on the free end of the semitendinosus and on the gracilis tendon grafts is passed a second time around the suture previously inserted into the femoral tunnel and coming out of the lateral incision. The suture is then pulled through the femoral tunnel, the knee joint, and the tibial tunnel to retrieve the graft from the tibial incision (Fig. 5). After that the posterolateral bundle is restored.

Graft Fixation

Once both bundles are restored, the graft is tensioned and the joint cycled 20 times. This allows to check the isometry of the neoligament, the capacity of flexion-extension, and the restoration of knee laxity.

Successively the combined graft is tensioned and secured to the femur with two metal staples placed on the lateral side of the condyle and to the anteromedial aspect of the tibia with an additional metal staple (Fig. 6).

The iliotibial tract defect is then closed, taking care to prevent lateral tilt and patellar compression. The medial fascia over the pes anserinus is left open.

Features of the Technique

Analogously to a DB ACL reconstruction, this technique aims to better replicate the kinematic behavior of both anteromedial and posterolateral bundles of a native ACL when compared to a single-bundle technique. The first "over-the-top" passage restores the anteromedial bundle while the second passage through the femoral tunnel restores the posterolateral bundle (Fig. 7).

The use of hamstring grafts allows different architectural reconstructions due to their length and versatility. Moreover, the recent literature confirms the structural and mechanical validity of this choice, especially when it is used for a double-bundle reconstruction (Simonian et al. 1997; Hamada et al. 1998; Brahmabhatt et al. 1999; Hoher et al. 2000). Furthermore, this graft choice avoids the frequent complications that usually come with a patellar tendon reconstruction such

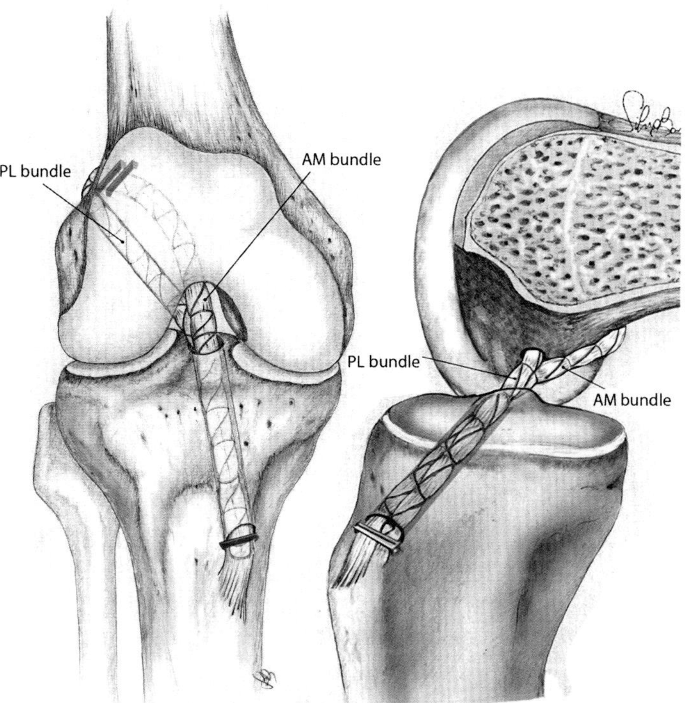

Fig. 7 Final appearance of the nonanatomical double-bundle reconstruction on antero-posterior and lateral view

as anterior knee pain, knee stiffness, and extensor apparatus deficit (Lipscomb et al. 1982; Wilk et al. 1991; Lephart et al. 1993; Shino et al. 1993; Kleipool et al. 1994; Natri et al. 1996; Muneta et al. 1998; Sachs et al. 1989). These complications can be serious drawbacks for athletes, especially for soccer players. Moreover, the preservation of the tendon tibial insertions maintaining both innervation and vascularization of these structures (Zaffagnini et al. 2003) could improve the neoligamentization process.

With regard to the position of the graft, the "over-the-top" approach guarantees a safe posterior position for the anteromedial bundle. Although both experimental and clinical studies have confirmed the validity of an "over-the-top" positioned graft (Brower et al. 1992), the nonanatomical location of the anteromedial bundle could represent a restriction to the effectiveness of this technique. Nevertheless, drilling only one femoral tunnel reduces the risk of tunnel misplacement and simplifies the revision surgery in case of failure.

The second passage within the femoral and tibial tunnel allows a rigid fixation of the graft on the femur reproducing a *bone bridge*. Thus, expensive fixation devices can be safely replaced by this fixation method.

Following this reconstruction technique, the two bundles are positioned in a more anatomic fashion with respect to the classic single-bundle reconstruction that has been proved to not restore rotational stability (Zaffagnini et al. 2004). The different sizes of the tibial and femoral tunnel allow a better distribution and positioning of the tendon in the tibial insertion, providing a wider insertion and better press-fit tendon fixation inside the tunnel.

During the procedure, the most complicated step is to find the correct location of the exit point for the femoral tunnel. This point should be on the lateral cortex, not far from the posterior condyle edge and very close to the "over-the-top" location. Thus, the graft results to be isometric avoiding the risk that the back side of the graft does not enter into the tibial tunnel.

Despite previous technical, anatomical, and biomechanical considerations, at the state of the art, it is still not possible to identify the gold-standard ACL reconstruction technique. This is probably due to the high variability of the knees involved and different levels of evidence of the numerous studies in the scientific literature (Meredick et al. 2008).

Clinical Results

Hundreds of patients have been successfully treated with this original double-bundle technique since 2003. Forty patients have been prospectively evaluated at an 8-year minimum follow-up. The group, with a mean age of 27 ± 9 years, underwent surgical reconstruction after 8.9 ± 10.4 months after ACL injury. Twenty-two patients (55 % of the total) underwent partial meniscectomy as well. All patients were evaluated with subjective and objective IKDC score, Tegner Activity scale, and KT-2000 arthrometer. Radiographic evaluation of osteoarthritis (OA) was performed using the IKDC score.

At 8-year minimum follow-up, the patients presented 88 ± 9 points at subjective IKDC score and a Tegner Activity level that reached the median pre-injury value of 6 points. Furthermore 89 % of the patients were classified as A, 10 % as B, and 1 % as C according to the objective IKDC score. Knee laxity evaluation showed 90 % of knees with negative pivot-shift test, 7 % with +, 3 % with ++, and 0 % with +++. Moreover, the objective evaluation with KT-2000 arthrometer revealed a side-to-side difference of the manual maximum displacement test of 1.1 ± 1.9 mm. Regarding osteoarthritis process, only 15 % of the reconstructed knees presented an IKDC grade of B and C. Revision surgery due to meniscal lesion was performed in 4 % of the patients.

Positive outcomes of this ACL reconstruction technique were reported also in young, active, and high-demanding athletes. A group of 21 male professional soccer players, with a mean age of 22.9 ± 5.4 years, were prospectively followed for 12 months after ACL reconstruction. Ten required meniscectomy, while three underwent meniscal suture as well. Clinical evaluation using the KOOS and Tegner scores showed a progressive improvement during the 3-month, 6-month, and 12-month follow-up (Fig. 8). All patients

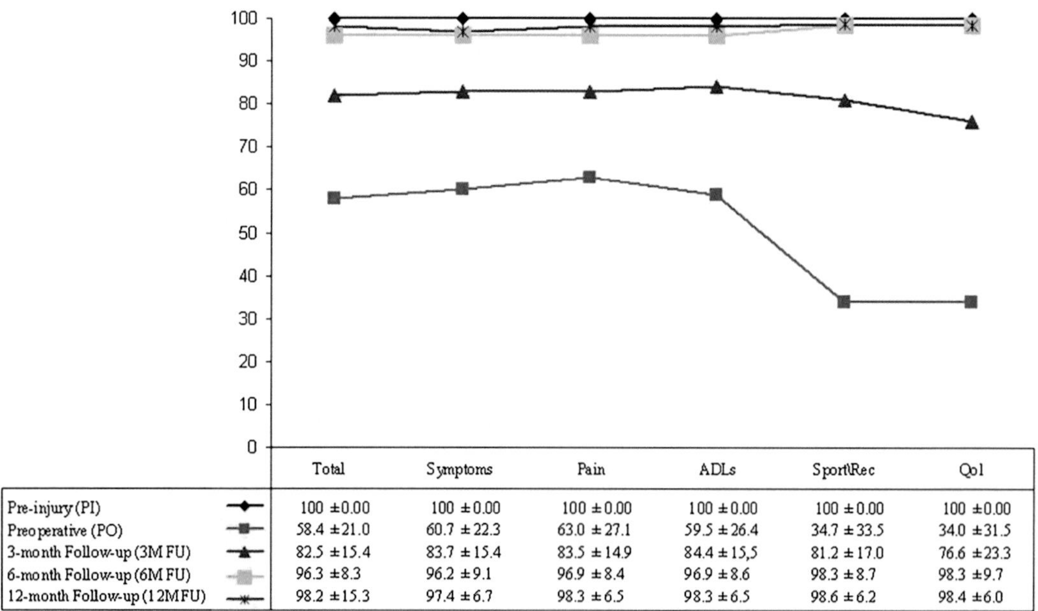

	Total	Symptoms	Pain	ADLs	Sport\Rec	Qol
Pre-injury (PI)	100 ±0.00	100 ±0.00	100 ±0.00	100 ±0.00	100 ±0.00	100 ±0.00
Preoperative (PO)	58.4 ±21.0	60.7 ±22.3	63.0 ±27.1	59.5 ±26.4	34.7 ±33.5	34.0 ±31.5
3-month Follow-up (3M FU)	82.5 ±15.4	83.7 ±15.4	83.5 ±14.9	84.4 ±15,5	81.2 ±17.0	76.6 ±23.3
6-month Follow-up (6M FU)	96.3 ±8.3	96.2 ±9.1	96.9 ±8.4	96.9 ±8.6	98.3 ±8.7	98.3 ±9.7
12-month Follow-up (12MFU)	98.2 ±15.3	97.4 ±6.7	98.3 ±6.5	98.3 ±6.5	98.6 ±6.2	98.4 ±6.0

Fig. 8 Clinical evaluation using the KOOS score

presented the same pre-injury value of KOOS score already 6 months after surgery and restoration of baseline Tegner Activity level at the final follow-up. The mean time to return to play soccer was 169 ± 49 days, while the first official match was played 186 ± 52 days after surgery. Several athletes have been able to return to complete sport activity already 4 months after ACL reconstruction.

Quantitative Evaluation with a Navigation System

In addition to the good clinical results, biomechanical analysis has confirmed the efficacy of the presented technique. The biomechanical analysis included 26 consecutive patients that underwent ACL reconstruction in the Rizzoli Orthopaedic Institute with an isolated anterior cruciate ligament injury. In 13 patients the original reconstruction technique was performed while the remainder were treated with a classical anatomical double-bundle reconstruction (two tibial tunnels and two femoral tunnels required). Standard clinical static laxity test and pivot-shift tests were quantified before and after the ACL reconstruction using a navigation system for intraoperative kinematic assessment. Specifically, concerning the clinical static laxity tests, the joints were passively taken, at the maximum load, through: varus/valgus (VV) rotation at 0° and 30° of flexion, anterior-posterior (AP) translation at 30° and 90° of flexion, and internal-external (IE) rotation at 30° and 90° flexion. The quantitative analysis considered both the anterior-posterior displacement and the whole rotation of the tibial plateau. Concerning the dynamic laxity test, the lateral tibial plateau compartment (in anterior-posterior direction) with respect to the flexion-extension angles was assessed. The displacement of the lateral tibial plateau compartment during the pivot-shift test was also evaluated, according to Lopomo et al. (2010). Lastly, the posterior acceleration reached by the lateral tibial plateau compartment was calculated according to Zaffagnini et al. (2012). The value given by the differences between pre- and post-reconstruction test results was defined as reduction of laxity. Reliability of the navigation system for the clinical laxity tests was previously analyzed by the authors (Martelli et al. 2007; Lopomo et al. 2009, 2010). In both study groups, comparison between pre- and postsurgery conditions has shown significant differences ($P < 0.05$) at any considered laxity parameters. Considering the postoperative

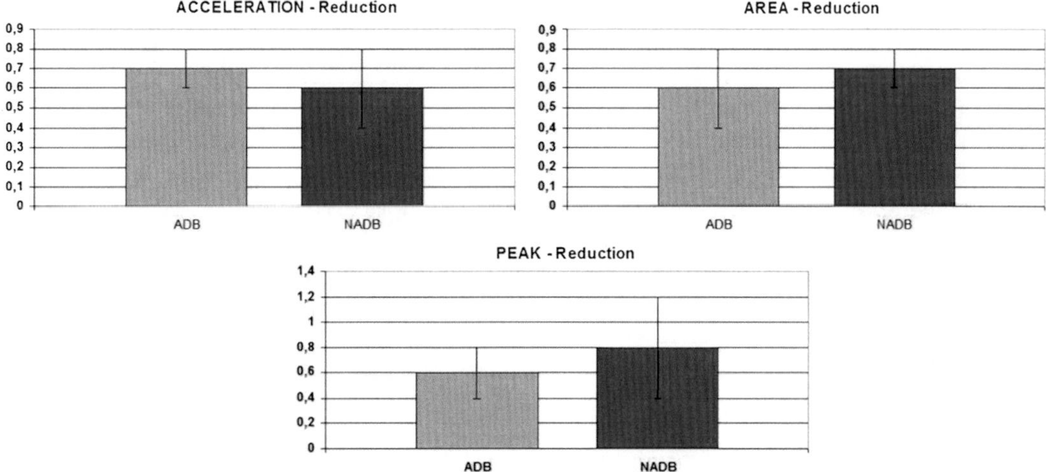

Fig. 9 Global amount of acceleration, area and peaks reduction of the lateral tibial plateau during pivot-shift test. Differences between the groups were not statistically significant

condition, the values did not differ for the most part between the two groups.

Postoperatively, the only statistically significant differences found refer to the anterior-posterior tibial plateau displacement. The group that underwent this reconstruction shows a lower value concerning both medial ($P = 0.003$) and lateral ($P = 0.04$) compartment when compared with the other group during the internal-external rotation at 30° of flexion. Moreover, for what concerns the pivot-shift test, the two study groups showed no statistically significant differences with respect to the dynamic laxity parameters (Fig. 9). Though, when compared with the standard DB-group, this technique showed a slightly higher area and peak reduction as well.

In conclusion the presented technique of nonanatomical double-bundle reconstruction can be considered a good option with respect to standard anatomical DB reconstruction that reduces the risk of technical errors during the surgical procedure but guarantees satisfactory results.

Cross-References

- ▶ Anterior Cruciate Ligament Graft Selection and Fixation
- ▶ Anterior Cruciate Ligament Injuries and Surgery: Current Evidence and Modern Development
- ▶ Different Techniques of Anterior Cruciate Ligament Reconstruction: Guidelines
- ▶ Double-Tunnel Anatomic Anterior Cruciate Ligament Reconstruction
- ▶ Soccer and Associated Sports Injuries
- ▶ State of the Art in Anterior Cruciate Ligament Surgery

References

Brahmabhatt V, Smolinski R, McGlowan J et al (1999) Double stranded hamstring tendons for anterior cruciate ligament reconstruction. Am J Knee Surg 12:141–145

Brower RS, Melby A III, Askew MJ et al (1992) In vitro comparison of over-the-top and through-the-condyle anterior cruciate ligament reconstruction. Am J Sports Med 20:567–574

Hamada M, Shino K, Tomoki M et al (1998) Cross-sectional area measurement of the semitendinosus tendon for anterior cruciate ligament reconstruction. Arthroscopy 14:696–701

Hoher J, Scheffler SU, Withrow JD et al (2000) Mechanical behavior of two hamstring graft constructs for reconstruction of the anterior cruciate ligament. J Orthop Res 18:456–461

Kleipool AE, van Loon T, Marti RK (1994) Pain after use of the central third of the patellar tendon for cruciate ligament reconstruction: 33 patients followed 2–3 years. Acta Orthop Scand 65:62–66

Lephart SM, Kocher MS, Arner CD et al (1993) Quadriceps strength and functional capacity after anterior cruciate ligament reconstruction: patellar tendon autograft versus allograft. Am J Sports Med 21:738–743

Lipscomb AB, Johnston RK, Snyder RB et al (1982) Evaluation hamstring muscle strength following use of semitendinosus and gracilis tendon to reconstruct the anterior cruciate ligament. Am J Sports Med 10:340–342

Lopomo N, Bignozzi S, Martelli S et al (2009) Reliability of a navigation system for intra-operative evaluation of antero-posterior knee joint laxity. Comput Biol Med 39:280–285

Lopomo N, Zaffagnini S, Bignozzi S et al (2010) Pivot-shift test: analysis and quantification of knee laxity parameters using a navigation system. J Orthop Res 28:164–169

Marcacci M, Molgora AP, Zaffagnini S et al (2003) Anatomic double-bundle anterior cruciate ligament reconstruction with hamstrings. Arthroscopy 19:540–546

Martelli S, Lopomo N, Bignozzi S et al (2007) Validation of a new protocol for navigated intraoperative assessment of knee kinematics. Comput Biol Med 37:872–878

Meredick RB, Vance KJ, Appleby D et al (2008) Outcome of single-bundle versus double-bundle reconstruction of the anterior cruciate ligament: a meta-analysis. Am J Sports Med 36:1414–1421

Muneta T, Sekiya I, Ogiuchi T et al (1998) Effects of aggressive early rehabilitation on the outcome of anterior cruciate ligament reconstruction with multi-strand semitendinosus tendon. Int Orthop 22:352–356

Natri A, Jarvinen M, Latuala K et al (1996) Isokinetic muscle performance after anterior cruciate ligament surgery. Int J Sports Med 17:223–228

Sachs RA, Daniel DM, Stone ML et al (1989) Patellofemoral problems after anterior cruciate ligament reconstruction. Am J Sports Med 17:760–765

Shino K, Nakagawa S, Inoue M et al (1993) Deterioration of patellofemoral articular surface after anterior cruciate ligament reconstruction. Am J Sports Med 21:206–211

Simonian PT, Harrison SD, Cooley WJ et al (1997) Assessment of morbidity of semitendinosus and gracilis tendon harvested for ACL reconstruction. Am J Knee Surg 10:54–59

Wilk KE, Keirns MA, Andrews JR et al (1991) Anterior cruciate ligament reconstruction rehabilitation: a six-month follow-up of isokinetic testing in recreational athletes. Isokinet Exerc Sci 1:36–43

Zaffagnini S, Golano P, Farinas O et al (2003) Vascularity of the pes anserinus: anatomic study. Clin Anat 16:19–24

Zaffagnini S, Martelli S, Acquaroli F (2004) Computer investigation of ACL orientation during passive range of motion. Comput Biol Med 34:153–163

Zaffagnini S, Signorelli C, Lopomo N et al (2012) Anatomic double-bundle and over-the-top single-bundle with additional extra-articular tenodesis: an in vivo quantitative assessment of knee laxity in two different ACL reconstructions. Knee Surg Sports Traumatol Arthrosc 20:153–159

Anatomy and Biomechanics of the Knee

72

Werner Müller

Contents

W. Müller (✉)
Department of Orthopaedic Surgery, University of Basel, Basel, Switzerland
e-mail: w.u.mueller@gmail.com

M.N. Doral, J. Karlsson (eds.), *Sports Injuries*,
DOI 10.1007/978-3-642-36569-0_66

Abstract

This chapter of anatomy and biomechanics of the knee is guided by my proper experience through precise critical learning by doing knee ligament surgery and studying anatomy of the ligaments from 1970 on in a first phase by doing the operations following the general scientific evolution until 1974. After the unsatisfactory outcomes with these types of operations, published and practiced in the 1960s and 1970s, which did rarely restore a knee to the expected full function, Prof. Arthur von Hochstetter from the Basel University Anatomy Institute showed me the key to understand knee ligament kinematics by the work of Alfred Menschik (Mechanik des Kniegelenkes 112:481–495, 1974; Mechanik des Kniegelenkes 113:388–400, 1975; Biometrie, das Konstruktionsprinzip des Kniegelenks, des Hüftgelenks der Beinlänge und der Körpergrösse. Springer, Berlin/Heidelberg/New York/London/Paris/Tokyo1985). The crossed four-bar link system with the cruciate ligaments is the central pivot gear of knee motion determining the anatomic position of the peripheral ligaments for their cofunction. The menisci are parts of the enlarged central pivot with a longer lever arm from the axis of rotation—the important controllers and stabilizers of the rotation next to the cruciate ligaments towards the periphery. Some of the peripheral ligaments like MCL or LCL are primary stabilizers against varus–valgus rotation as well as IR and ER. Some of the ligaments are connected with tendons to be actively reinforced and tightened in critical positions when the ligaments are at risk and need help by muscular force as actively dynamized ligaments.

Introduction

First of all, each knee you have to consider needs your full attention and a precise examination. You have to follow up the results of all decisions you made for nonoperative and operative treatment, especially the results of your operative procedures.

With the aim to improve the results for a perfect restitution, I asked the patient regularly what could still be better.

"Good results come from experience and experience comes from bad results, but not everyone has to make the same mistakes again"!

Learning by doing – the learners curve!

We must learn from the experiences, but often we get experience only when we would have needed it already before.

The most dangerous day for a patient in the OR is the day after a congress! The proposed new operative techniques seemed easy to be performed, but without the experience of the author they end often in a primary failure.

Historical Passage

How was the actual state of the art when I started with knee ligament surgery in 1960?

Future needs' origin: learning from the past.

Lorenz Böhler in 1932 put the knees with complex ligament lesions up to 12 weeks in plaster.

Mandic (1959) took the multiruptured menisci totally out of the unstable subluxing knees.

On the other hand, Tavernier warned already in 1927 to take the menisci out and showed how to suture menisci back to the peripheral wall.

In 1960 as a young resident, I had to put ligament-injured knees for two times 6 weeks in plaster. They were then quite stable but with all the well-known difficulties. It was hard to get the correct function back because all the synovial folds, also around the patella and under the menisci, were scarred and glued together. The knees were stable but with restricted mobility in all six degrees of freedom. Very often, patellar atrophy and even dystrophy were a serious factor of lasting pain.

The Period of the Bad Experiences

Anyhow, the cruciate ligaments were already known as being important for the stabilization of the knee.

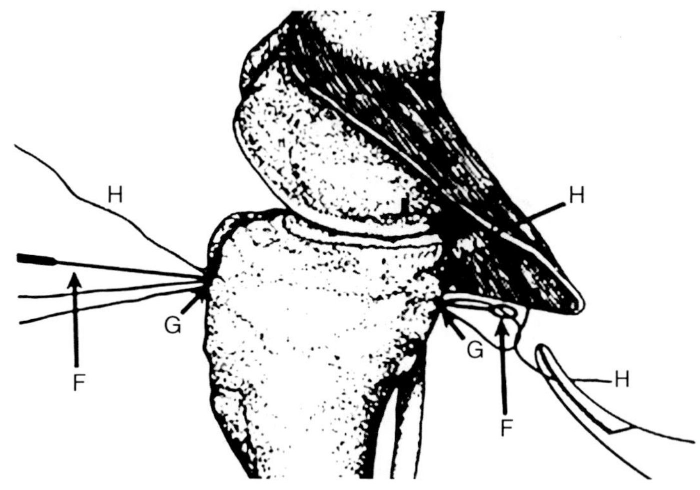

Fig. 1 Typ of O'Donoghue Operation Nr 2 for complex anteromedial instability. The whole capsulo-ligamentous part of the medial joint side is detached from the tibia, the meniscus is excised and its wall is fixed with transosseous sutures 2 cm distal to the joint line back to the tibia (Journal of Bone and Joint Surgery American, July, 1973, 55, 5, Reconstruction for Medial Instability of the Knee, Odonoghue, 941–955. http://jbjs.org/)

Reconstructions were done with ligamentum patellae like zur Verth in Wittek 1935 and quite some others as also Kenneth Jones in 1963.

In the mid 1960s, we did all types of published intra-articular and extra-articular reconstructions, e.g., with semitendinosus tendons like Lindemann (1950).

At the end of the operations, still on the OR table, these knees were quite stable, and we were of best hope for a good result, but after 4 months p. o. (post operative) subluxation was present again.

As a consequence, we changed to these cruel peripheral interventions like the Don O'Donoghue (1973) second procedure from 1973, taking down the whole medial capsular ligament complex from the tibial head far back close to the PCL. The medial meniscus was completely excised and its insertion area refixed about 2 cm distal to the joint line with transosseous sutures from the back to the front of the tibial head (Fig. 1).

McIntosh operations were done with rerouting an important strip of the ITT system around the lateral collateral ligament. The flexed knee was then fixed in external rotation within a plaster. I did Slocum's (Slocum and Larson 1968) pes anserinus transfer for better controlling actively the external rotation to prevent the subluxation (Fig. 2).

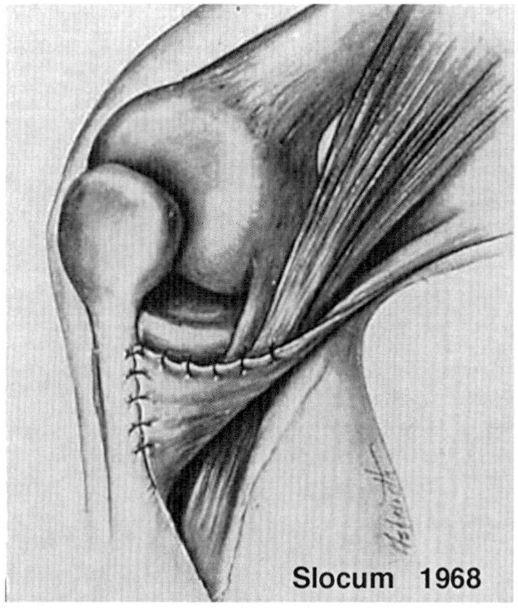

Fig. 2 The Slocum pes anserinus transposition to reinforce internal rotation against anterior subluxation (Journal of Bone and Joint Surgery American, March, 1968, 50, 2, Pes anserinus transplantation, Slocum, 226–242. http://jbjs.org/)

But all the functional results of these procedures have been far away from being sufficient. This rotational subluxation still reappeared. "When I pivot, my knee shifts" the patients claimed.

The next step of the positive experiences here was the successful treatment of complex

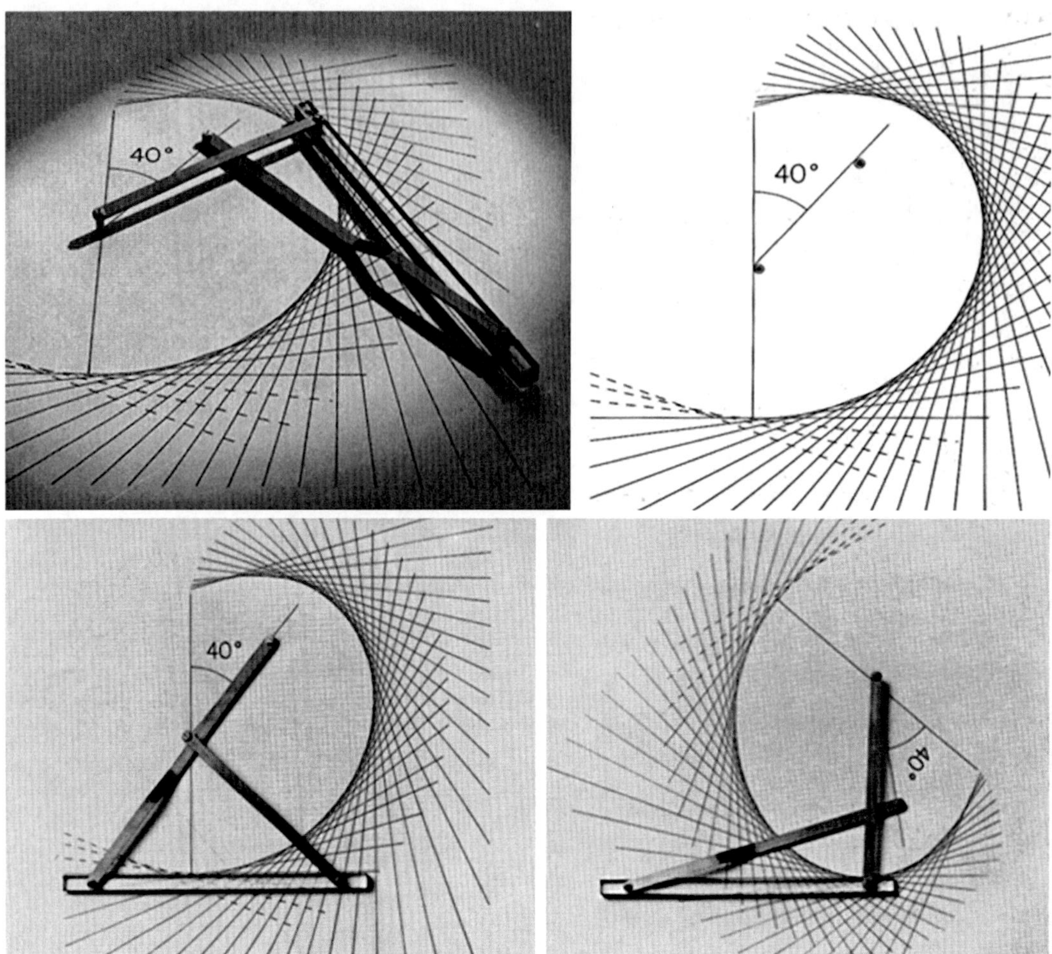

Fig. 3 Model of a four bar link system with a condylar *curve*. The four bar link system of the cruciates is the gear of the knee motion for the rolling and gliding of the femur on the tibia

intra-articular fractures with the AO internal fixation method. When an anatomic reconstruction of the joint fragments was achieved, a perfect function of this joint could be expected.

Why did this not work with the knee ligaments and the soft tissue reconstructions?

Were the specific kinematic laws for the ligament function around the knee not known? Did one miss the specific functional fine structure in the anatomy of the knee ligaments?

Was Carl Henschen's "intelligence of the tissues" disturbed with our procedures, so that they could not cooperate to heal as they should? (Carl Henschen, Prof. of Surgery University of Basel 1926–1947 in Basel).

The Four-Bar Link System

The revelation came to me in 1974 by our anatomy Prof. Arthur von Hochstetter (Anatomisches, Institut der Universität Basel), who gave me the first small papers of Alfred Menschik about the ligament kinematics of the knee with the cruciate ligament gear, the crossed four-bar link system, and the controlled rolling gliding system. It was published in 1974 in "Mechanik des Kniegelenkes."

This has immediately changed the thinking about the behavior of soft tissue structures under the law of kinematic principles. In each ligament, a fine-tuned system of the fiber arrangement could now be detected (Fig. 3).

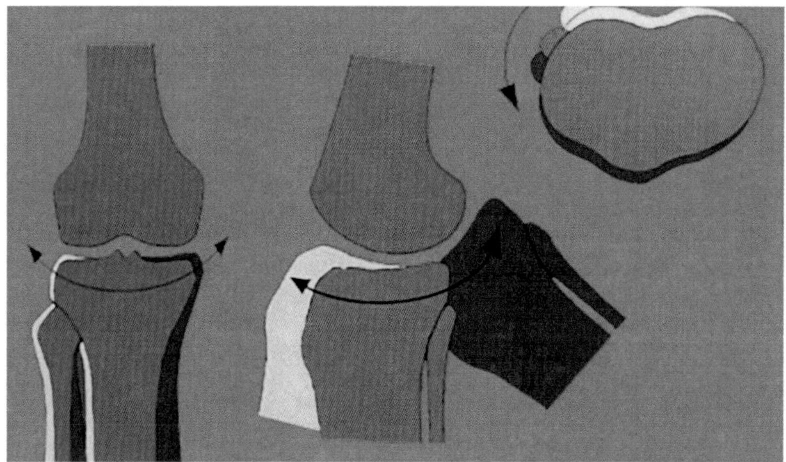

Fig. 4 The three rotations:, extension-flexion, internal-external and varus-valgus

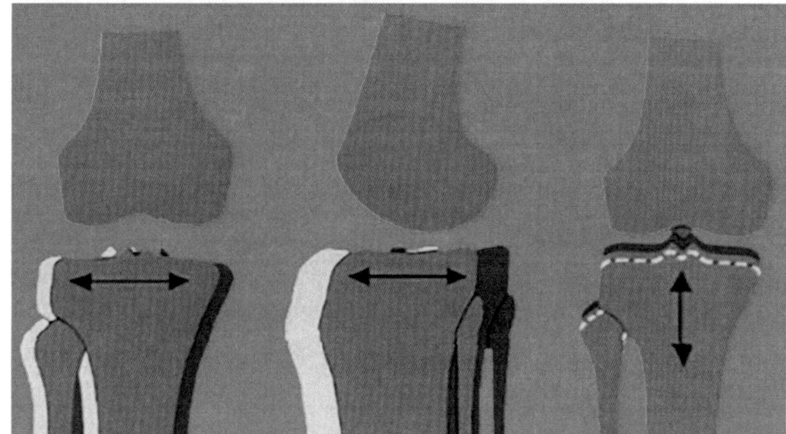

Fig. 5 The three translations: medio-lateral, antero-posterior and compression-distraction

Biomechanics in a Joint with Six Degrees of Freedom and with Migrating Axes

The former anatomists called the knee joint a trochoginglymos, which means a hinge gliding on a surface, a gliding hinge.

The six degrees of freedom are

Three rotations: extension–flexion, internal–external, and varus–valgus (Fig. 4).

Three translations: mediolateral, anteroposterior, and compression–distraction (Fig. 5)

All these six freedoms of motion are simultaneously involved in the complex function within the envelope of motion.

Biomechanics, mechanics in the knee joint, cannot be compared with the mechanics of an engine, e.g., a steam engine of a locomotive because in the knee, the guiding elements are not stiff metallic bars but elastic collagen ligament structures stressed in multiple directions.

Adalbert Kapandji, the author of the well known physiology of the joints in a biomechanical aspect (Ref.: Kapandji IA (1970) The physiology of the joints vol II. Churchill Livingstone, Edinburgh, London) said, when he was asked once in an interview article in a SICOT Bulletin some years ago about biomechanics: "You said biomechanics… ? It's 'fuzzy' mechanics!!" because it is not Industrial mechanics, but mechanics for living structures.

Therefore, it is better to use the term *kinematics* of the knee joint. Kinematics describes the motion

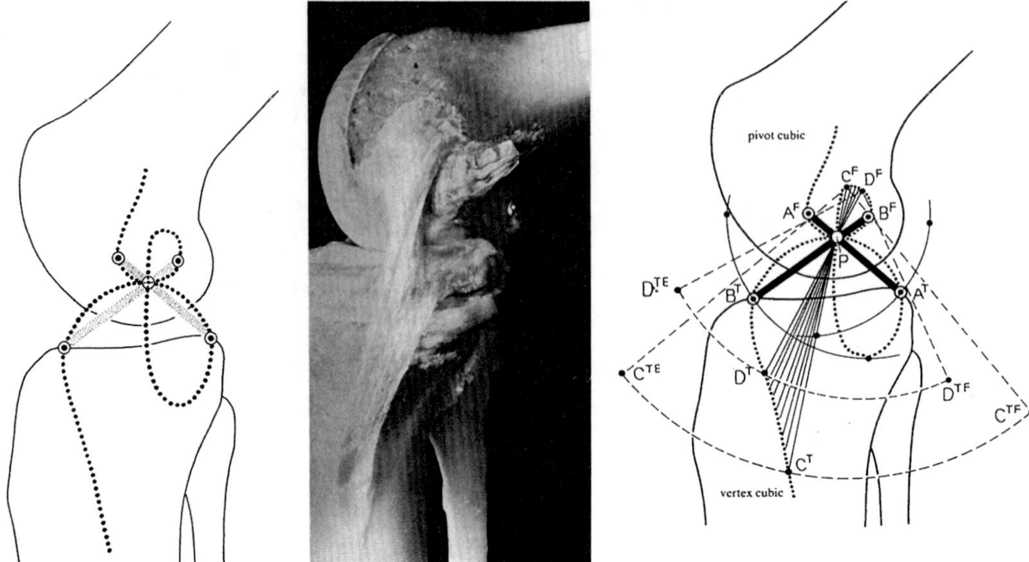

Fig. 6 The Burmester curve given by the four bar link gear system determines here the position of the medial collateral ligament. It can follow the motion with a minimum of length change

of a point or of a body which moves, e.g., on a circle, guided by a pendulum of constant length. In case of the knee, the living joint, there is no stiff pendulum but guidelines depending on the crossed four-bar link system of the cruciates and of the Burmester curve (1888), which is a mathematical third-order curve given by the crossed four bars. This Burmester curve designs the only possible position of the peripheral ligaments so that they can follow the motion with a minimum of length change (Fig. 6).

These New Kinematic Principles from 1974 and the Pivot Shift

How is the connection between these principles and the reason for the spontaneous instability with the subluxation and the shift? This was now the question! By the time the enlightenment came, the explanation was: If the anterior cruciate is ruptured, the lateral condyle is not anymore kept in its controlled rolling gliding motion and just rolls too far back to an abnormal contact point back on the tibial plateau. When the tightened ITT system in flexion crosses the femoral condylar axis, then the posteriorly subluxed lateral condyle snaps forward into the position which corresponds to the femorotibial contact point at this degree of flexion for the normal rolling–gliding motion (Fig. 7).

The Knee Subluxes and Shifts

The first description of the pathophysiology of the pivot shift was in Müller 1977.

By this pathological rolling back of the condyles, the menisci get squeezed, especially the posterior horn on the medial side with the posterior oblique ligament, the POL being stretched. On the lateral side, the whole capsulopopliteal complex gets displaced backward (See Figs. 20 and 24).

The Central Pivot and the Enlarged Central Pivot

The cruciates function as central pivot, leading as a gear, and the menisci around them act with their capsular attachments as a peripheral force

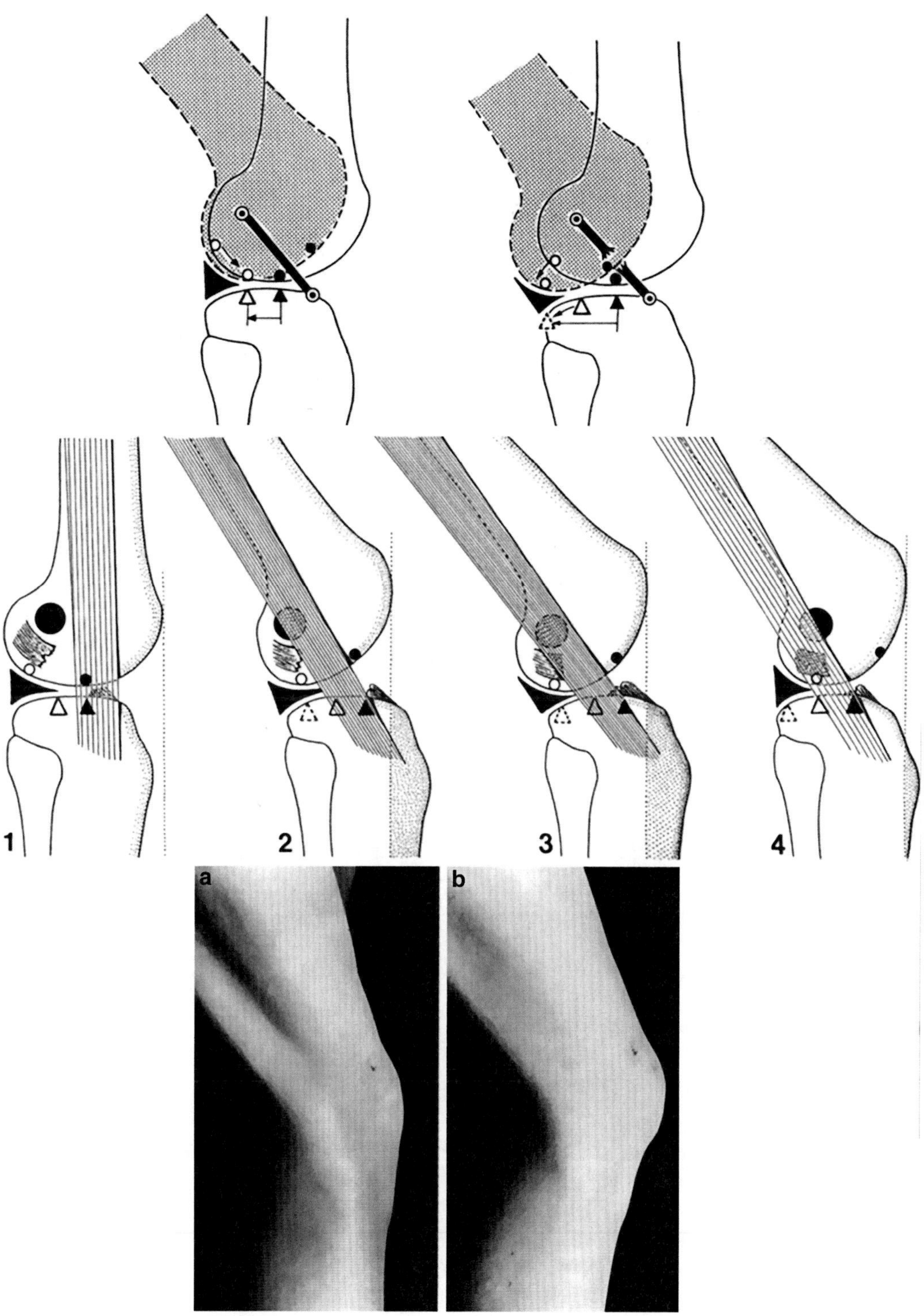

Fig. 7 When I pivot my knee shifts.! When the ACL is ruptured the lateral condyle rolls too far back, subluxes, tightens the ITT and snaps, when the ITT passes the condylar axis, back to the position which corresponds to the position of the normal roll-glide process

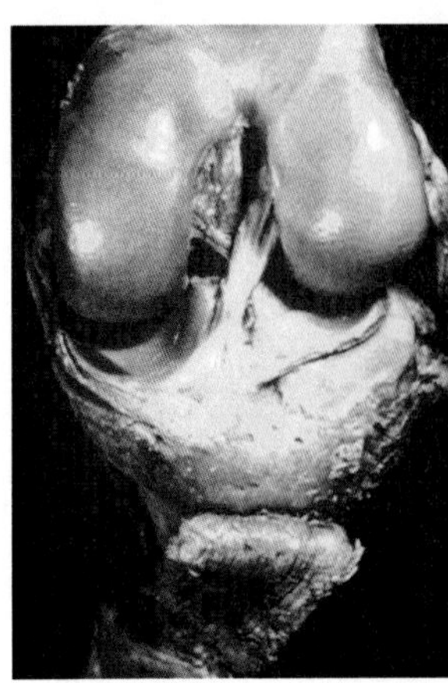
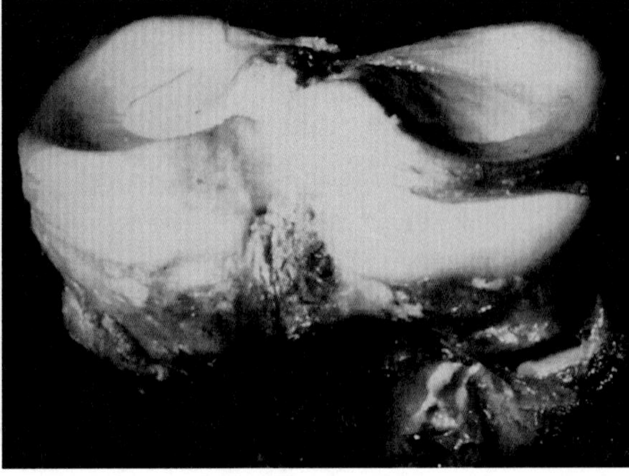

Fig. 8 The central pivot ACL and PCL which form together with the two menisci the "enlarged" central pivot. Both menisci insert on and around the intercondylar eminence and have fiber connections with ACL and PCL. Notice also the gliding area for the posterior horn of the medial meniscus on the tibial plateau (Courtesy A.von Hochstetter)

controlling and as a sustaining brake system, functioning then as the enlarged central pivot (Fig. 8).

From No-Metry to Iso-Metry to Anatomo-Metry

Now, we had also the explanation for the fragments of broken wire sutures in the ACL reconstructed knees.

The sutures were not in so-called isometric positions too far forward on the lateral condyle and would limit the flexion or had to break. That's what happened. The same happened also in so many ACL reconstructed knees with a position of the ACL too far anterior on the lateral condyle with insufficient results needing revision due to the recurrent shift subluxation (Fig. 9).

With these facts, it was demonstrated that ligaments and sutures have to be placed along the most isometric lines as the guides given by the kinematic laws. It was also evident that the whole amount of mechanically needed fibers could not stay on the most isometric line because there was not enough room for them all on it.

The Ingenious System of the Progressive Recruitment of Fibers During Action

For the ACL, this means that in knee flexion, the position of the ACL is almost horizontal. The lever arm to resist against anterior translation is much longer, and less fibers have to be in function for the mechanical need against anterior translation forces. In knee extension, the ACL is more vertical and its lever arm therefore evidently shorter. All fibers are now recruited to withstand the load and to fulfill together the function of controlling the increased mechanical demand (Fig. 10).

The Automatic End Rotation and the ACL

The automatic end rotation, this external rotation of the tibia, tightens up also the rotation controlling posterolateral fibers. This part is the posterolateral bundle of the ACL (See Fig. 20).

From now on, we knew that we had to reconstruct the ACL in a kinematically correct anatomic position.

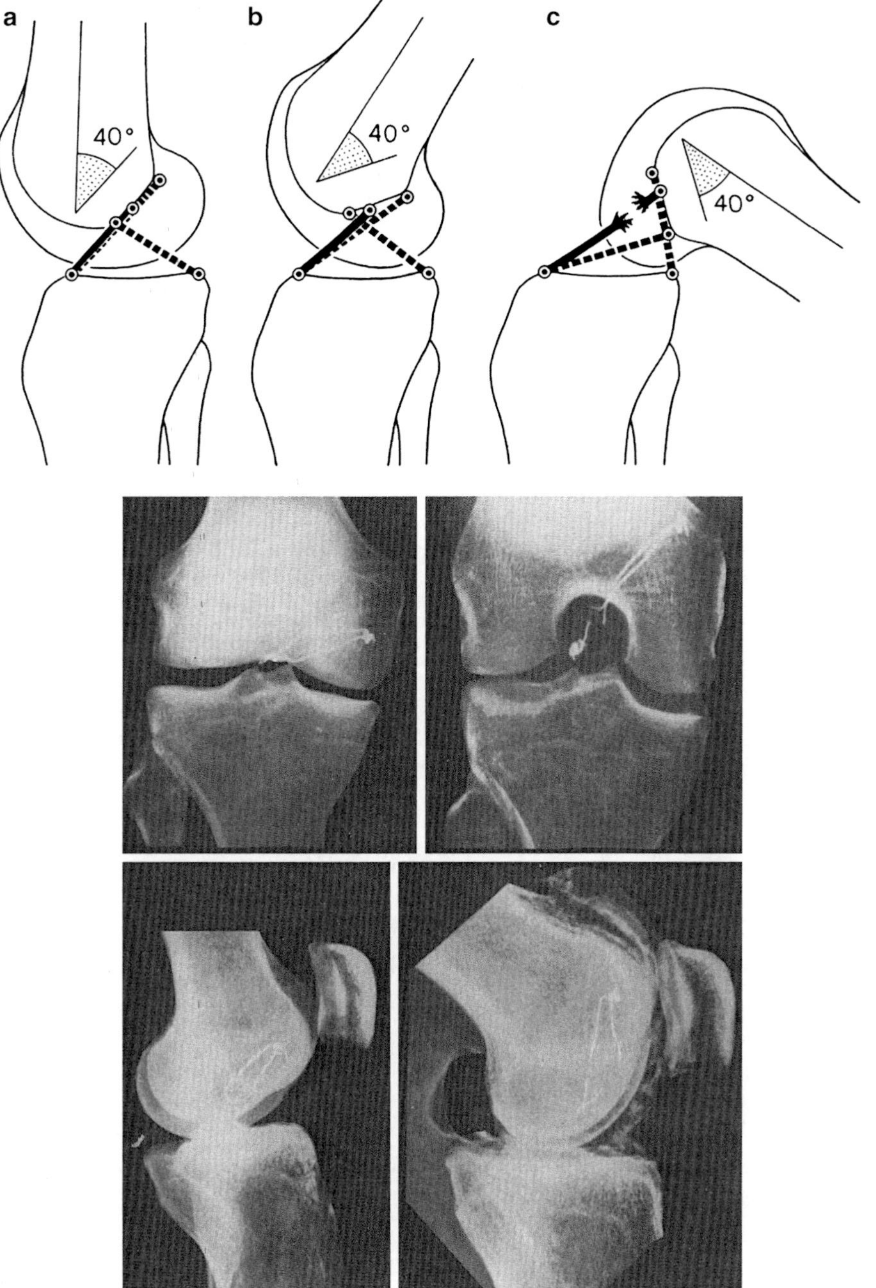

Fig. 9 The schematic isometry shows an anterior cruciate ligament inserted too far forward. It will break like the visible wires in the x-rays in a case with a post op. failure, or at least it will be elongated and be insufficiant

But were sutures alone sufficient?

In some cases, yes, when a proximal rupture could be fixed back to freshened bone and when one could back it up and sustain the fixed ACL by retightening the secondary peripheral restraints, the posterior horn of the medial meniscus with the POL and for the lateral side the ITT Kaplan fibers (Lobenhoffer et al. 1978)

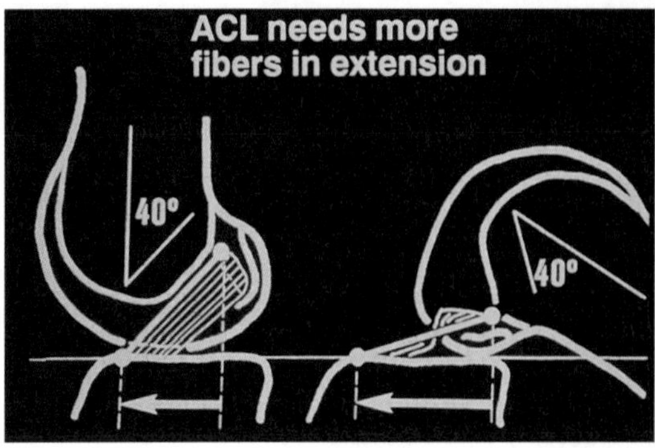

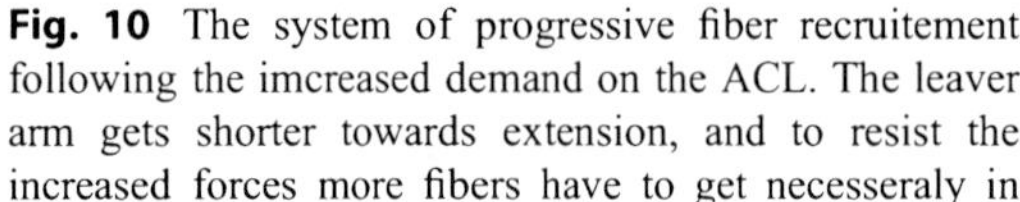

Fig. 10 The system of progressive fiber recruitement following the imcreased demand on the ACL. The leaver arm gets shorter towards extension, and to resist the increased forces more fibers have to get necesseraly in action to hold against anterior translation. Vice versa the PCL needs more resisting fibers in knee flexion (Courtesy N. Friederich)

and the popliteal meniscal junction (see also Figs. 11, 12, and 23).

ACL Reconstruction

But how to reconstruct a dilacerated ACL?

Years before, we did reconstructions (Lindemann, etc.) with semitendinosus. In the meanwhile, we learned that all the pes anserinus tendons together were strong internal rotators and therefore important active protectors of the posteromedial corner and the ACL.

That's why the patellar tendon was then preferred as replacement structure (zur Verth/Wittek (1935); Brückner and Brückner 1972 etc.)

Could a free patellar tendon graft survive and be revascularized in due time?

For our first reconstructions with the patellar tendon, the graft was left distally attached to the tibia to maintain the anterior longitudinal artery on the graft. But by this technique, problems were encountered with the length of the graft. To compensate length, the galea aponeurotica was used with bony chips of the patella and was pulled through a trough over the top. Additional transosseus sutures fixed it to the anatomic ACL insertion site of the lateral condyle.

Clancy showed then a method to leave the graft pediculated on the vascularizing Hoffa pedicle. It worked well for the vascularity, but it led to too much adhesions disturbing the function.

Drobny et al. (1986, 1990) from our team could do sheep experiments with pediculated and free grafts in the AO labs of Davos. Contrary to other experiments done at this time, Drobny knew exactly where to place "isometric" and anatomically correct ACL replacement grafts. Very astonishingly, he found revascularization also in the free grafts already after 2 weeks. Obviously, the intelligence of tissues could cooperate and help when the healing cells could work under kinematically normal anatomic conditions.

How Many Bundles, This Was Now the Question

One bundle, two bundles, two bundles with an intermediate third bundle or six to ten fiber "bundles" as Dorothe Mommersteeg (1995, 1996) demonstrated? Or even no bundles as Arnoczky, Kennedy, and Odensten wrote before? This was then the question (See also Figs. 13 and 14).

Appel and Gradinger showed 1989 in a not well-propagated German paper that the ACL fiber system does not show isolated bundles. They found in 50 knees a fiber architecture similar to folding trellis (Scherengitter). With that, they are closer to the findings of Mommersteeg (Fig. 14).

We stayed finally with the one-bundle reconstruction. A small 10 × 10 × 5 mm rectangular patellar bone block was taken to be placed

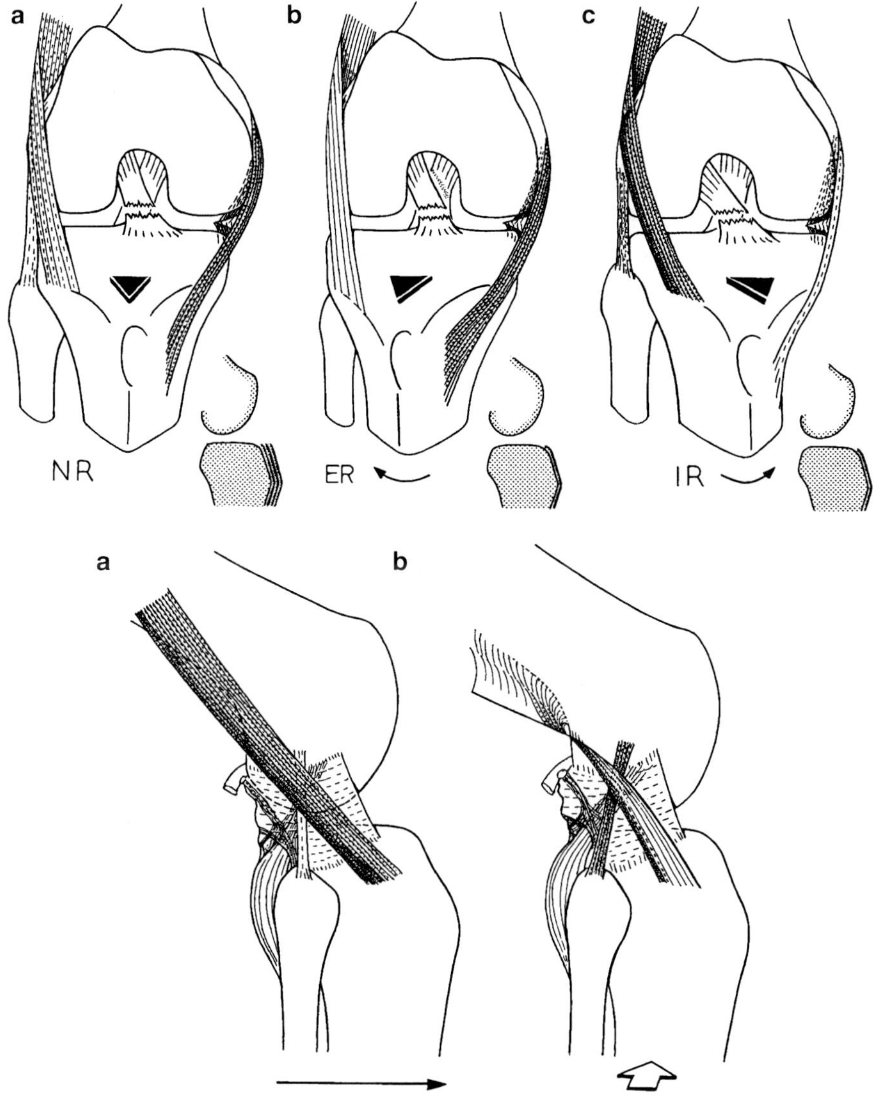

Fig. 11 The secondary restraints to be considered in cases of ACL injuries from Müller (1982)

centered in the oblique ACL footprint behind and parallel to the transition line on the lateral condyle just snug fit with the surface so there was a fan-shaped insertion without kinking off the graft fibers over a round hole (see Fig. 13 iso-anatomic). At the tibial side, the tunnel exit was slightly enlarged posteriorly to an oval shape, so that the tightened graft could choose its best position in knee flexion within the original shape of the cashew nut–like footprint of the tibia without kinking over the tunnel rim.

This description mimics the normal anatomy of the ACL on its femoral and tibial insertion. The experimental anatomical studies of Friederich and O'Brien (1989) about the most isometric guidelines and the amount of length change during extension and flexion of the fiber trajectory outside the given most isometric position showed also that there was no possibility for functioning fibers to insert ventral of the transition line on the femoral condyle and ventral of the transition line on the tibia. They found also that fiber positions away from the most isometric line and the

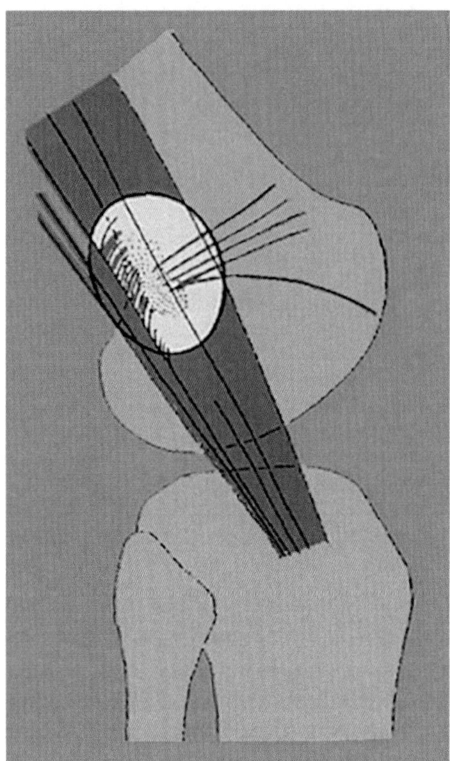

Fig. 12 The Kaplan fiber connection between distal ITT and the femoral crest which forms an important anterolateral dynamised stabilizer (From Müller 1982)

consecutive length change during extension is more forgiving on the tibial insertion side than on the femoral insertion side (Fig. 15).

The Menisci and the Five Peripheral Ligaments

The menisci form a mobile containment on the tibial plateau adapting to the rolling–gliding and rotating femoral condyle (see Fig. 8). This meniscal motion during internal and external rotation at 90° flexion can nicely be seen and followed on an open MRI (Schneider U, Orthop Surgeon and Elsig JP, Radiologist Zürich), which allows this imaging (Figs. 16, 17, and 18).

The menisci are generally fixed to the capsular periphery, where Biedert (2000) of our team found a very rich innervation with free nerve endings, important for the proprioception of the rotational control in knee stabilization.

The medial posterior horn is strongly fixed to the POL and is in the posteromedial corner an important secondary corestraint to the ACL and with its parallel orientation to the PCL also a corestraint for the PCL (Fig. 19).

The Kinematic Difference of the Two Compartments

The Medial Compartment, the Stable Compartment

The medial compartment is tightly fixed between the two strongest ligaments, the PCL and the medial collateral ligament system, including the POL with the meniscus. Therefore, there is less rotation excursion on this side, and the axis of internal–external rotation stays in this medial compartment.

The automatic end rotation instead occurs when the anteromedial segment of the medial condyle turns in; this motion is guided by a different axis staying back in the lateral compartment on the tibia below the ACL insertion (Fig. 20).

The Lateral Compartment, the More Mobile, the Swinging Compartment

The axis of the internal–external rotation stays in the medial compartment; therefore, the medial compartment has less rotational excursion, while the lateral compartment has to move with much more rotational excursion.

The Dynamized Ligaments of the Lateral Compartment

As a consequence, this lateral compartment cannot have a bone-to-bone ligament between femur and tibia because of too much length change during extension–flexion and external–internal rotation. Therefore, the LCL goes from the femur to the fibula. The proximal tibiofibular joint allows the necessary adaption for the needed length change (Fig. 21).

And additionally, the biceps tendon passes before it ends on the tibia and fibula around the distal end of the LCL and tightens the LCL up in positions where it is too loose. This also is an

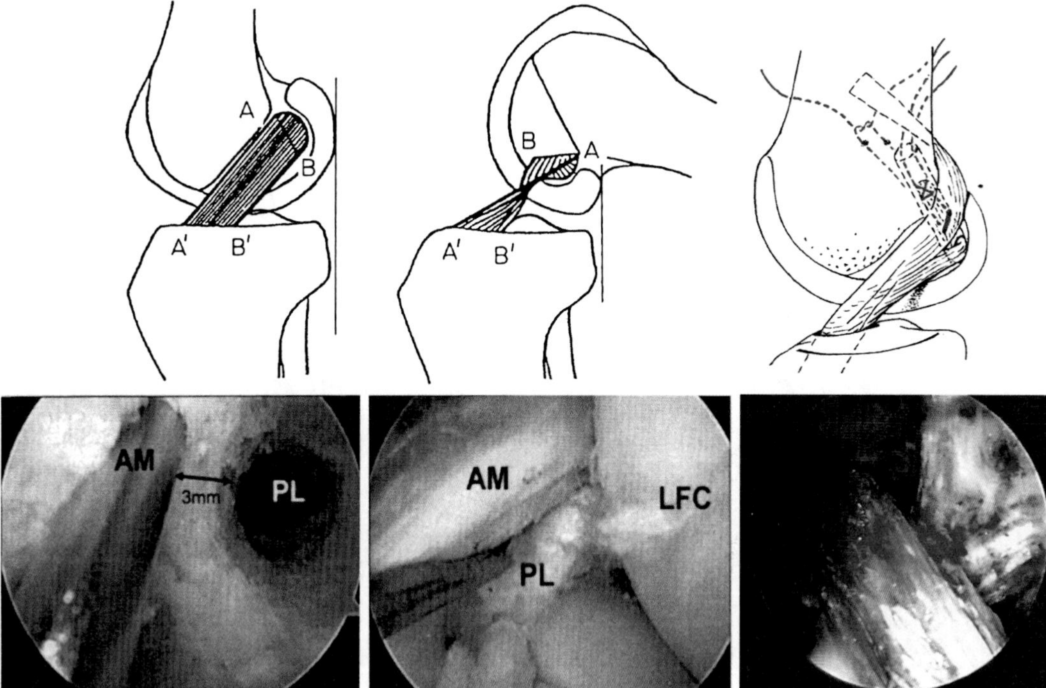

Fig. 13 How many bundles to replace the fan shaped ACL (modified after Girgis 1975 and Jakob/Stäubli 1990)) Two bundles (Müller 1982, Fu 2007) Iso-anatomic one bundle (Courtesy M. Arnold)

example of a typically dynamized ligament. The deep portion of the biceps tendon ends on the tibia below the meniscus above Gerdy's tubercle at a spot where also the Segond fragment gets avulsed and where the Segond ligament, starting behind and slightly above the LCL from the femur, is ending on the anterolateral tibia. This Segond ligament is also connected as stabilizer with the meniscus (Claes : antero lateral ligament ALL).

The popliteus system with its three tendon expansions is as well a main dynamically stabilizing complex for the stability of the lateral compartment. The muscle directs one of its tendons into the posterior wall of the lateral meniscus. The second tendon bifurcates to the fibula to maintain as so-called popliteofibular ligament the angulation of the third tendon, the politeus tendon, which goes up, passing under the LCL to its insertion slightly ventral and distal to the femoral LCL insertion. When this second tendon, the so-called politeofibular ligament, is ruptured and does not anymore maintain the angulation for the popliteus tendon, then this popliteus tendon gets straightened; that means it is relatively lengthend by about 1 cm. Therefore, more a-p rotation of the tibia is the consequence of progressing anterolateral rotational instability.

The popliteus muscle with its belly on the medial back side of the proximal tibia reaches with its popliteus tendon diagonally over the lateral joint line to the femur and is itself an important internal rotator.

Its aponeurosis behind the tibia is interwoven with spreaded tendon fibers from the fifth end of the semimembranosus tendon creating a link for the proprioception between the posteromedial and the posterolateral stabilizers (Fig. 22).

The same dynamization can be found in the ITT system as anterolateral stabilizer. Its Kaplan fibers starting distal from the femoral crest integrated then in the ITT down to Gerdy's tubercle are a femorotibial dynamic ligamentous junction, which is actively sustained by the forces of m.

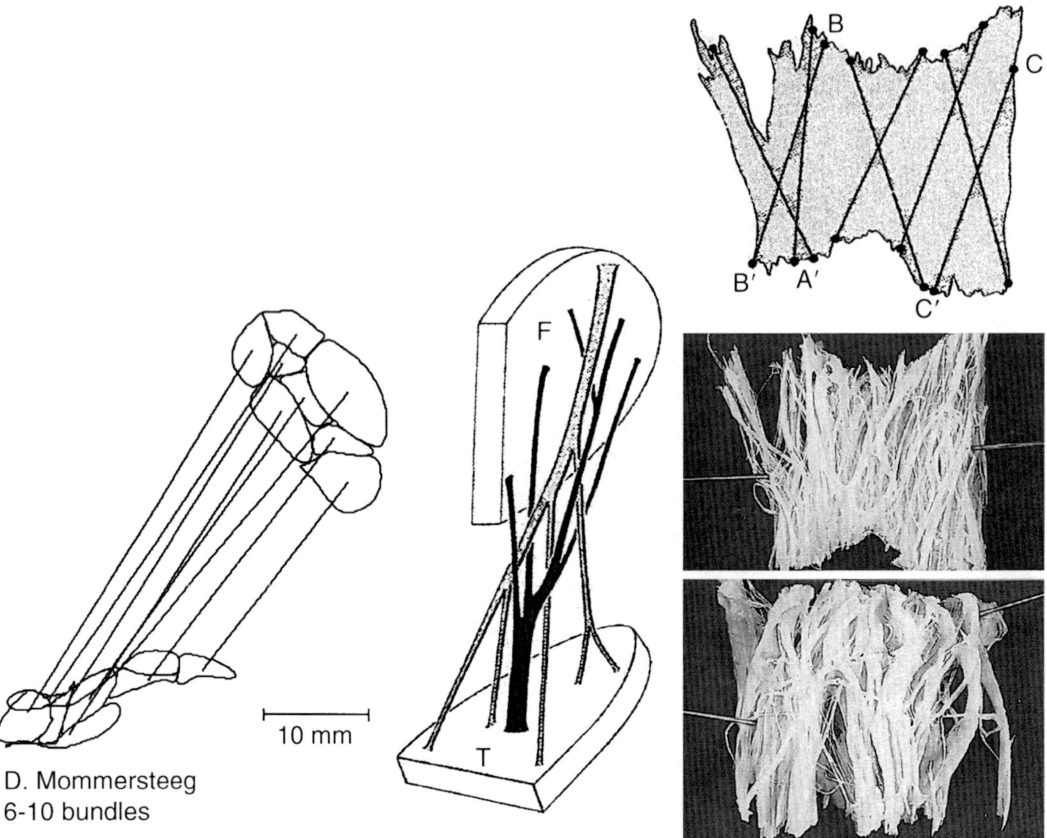

Fig. 14 How many bundles in the ACL architectrural structure? Mommersteeg et al. in 1995 could distinguish 6–10 bundles. Appel and Gradinger found 1989 a structure of folding trellis (© Dorethe Mommersteeg)

tensor fasciae latae and m. glutaeus maximus with their insertion pulling powerfully on the ITT (Lobenhoffer et al. 1978).

The lateral meniscus is dynamized as well. The popliteus muscle, as mentioned above, directs its first tendon to insert widely in the posterior horn of the meniscus, pulling this one back from the over-rolling condyle in fast flexion with IR.

A second tendon as described above bifurcates and is directed to the fibular head and has to maintain the functionally important angle of the third tendon, the well-known popliteus tendon. If this popliteofibular ligament as mentioned before is ruptured or cut, the popliteus tendon looses its angulation, straightens, and gets longer, allowing with 1 cm more length quite some important degrees more of a-p rotation of the tibial plateau. This stresses the lateral meniscus additionally and distends the meniscotibiopopliteofibular fascicles (Stäubli and Birrer 1990, restraints helping to control excessive rotation. They get at risk and are involved when the popliteofibular ligament is ruptured. These fascicles have to leave a passage, the hiatus popliteus, for the tendon on its way up to the femur because of the local motion difference between the meniscus and the tendon. In chronic lateral a-p instabilities, the normally 10–12 mm long hiatus gets twice or more as long as normal (Fig. 23).

The popliteus system is an important secondary restraint to PCL due to its parallel orientation to it. Indirectly, it is a secondary restraint to ACL as well because it is a helpful internal rotator and meniscus stabilizer too.

On the medial side instead, the less rotating side, the posterior horn of the meniscus is firmly

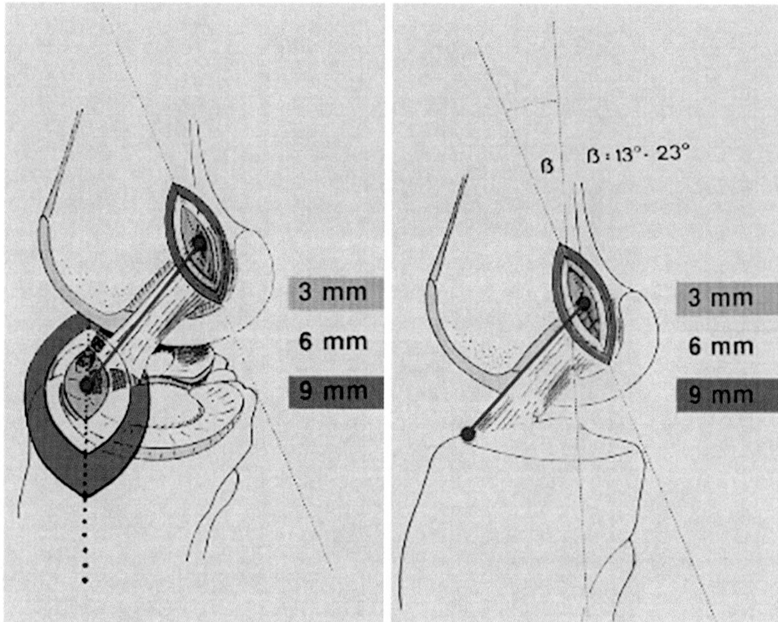

Fig. 15 The most isometric guide line for the ACL with the transition line and the zones of length change when the correct placement for the graft is missed. Evidently the tibial side is more forgiving (Courtesy N. Friederich, W. O'Brien)

fixed to the POL because the kinematic laws allow this important junction. Like this, the posterior horn of the medial meniscus forms with the POL a strong posteromedial stabilizer.

Together, they are effective corestraints to ACL and PCL (Fig. 19).

The Five Principal Peripheral Ligaments

Menschik has demonstrated the cruciate gear which determines also the anatomic position of the five peripheral ligaments and ligamentous structures.

Combined with the crossed four-bar link system, there is the mentioned Burmester curve. It is mathematically a third-order curve. This curve passes as a kind of a double sling through all the four endpoints of the bars and through the crossing point of the bars. The proximal part of the curve is the pivot cubic, and the distal part is the vertex cubic. The theoretic position for a ligament, e.g., the MCL, starts in the pivot cubic sling and goes through the crossing point P to the free ending part of the vertex cubic and shows, e.g., the possible position of the MCL. The five ligaments have such a position in the Burmester curve and can so follow the motion without important length change (Fig. 24).

But keep in mind that Kapandji spoke of "fuzzi mechanics," because all the lines are not stiff lines, just the "idea" of the construction plan; the theoretical mathematical principle is given by them. The medial side with the less rotational swing shows better the corresponding anatomy to this kinematic law (See Fig. 7).

On the medial capsular ligament complex, we can observe also nicely the system of the progressive fiber recruitment toward extension when more force for the resistance against valgus is necessary.

The Individuality of the Knees and Their Curves

The crossed four-bar link curves are different when the length relation of the bars ACL and PCL is different. An ACL can be relatively longer or shorter in relation to the PCL. Then, the length relations between the ACL and the PCL are different. This explains also the individual different shapes of the femoral condyles.

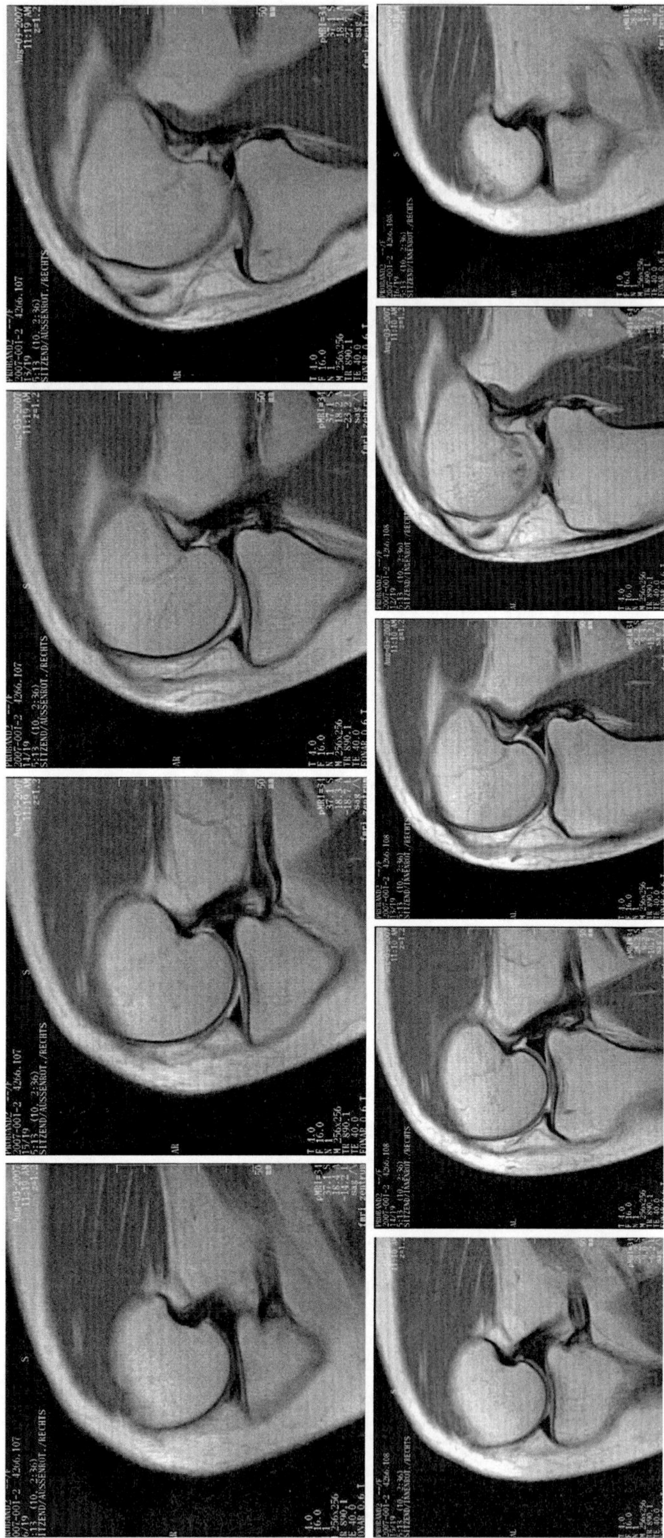

Fig. 16 MRI showing the medial compartment with the meniscus, cuts at 90° flexion from medial to central. *Above* in external rotation with the meniscus pushed backwards. *Below* in internal rotation with the meniscus staying behind and the condyle moved forward. Observe the spaces between condylus and meniscus (Courtesy Urs Schneider U, Orthop Surgeon and Elsig JP, Radiologist Zürich)

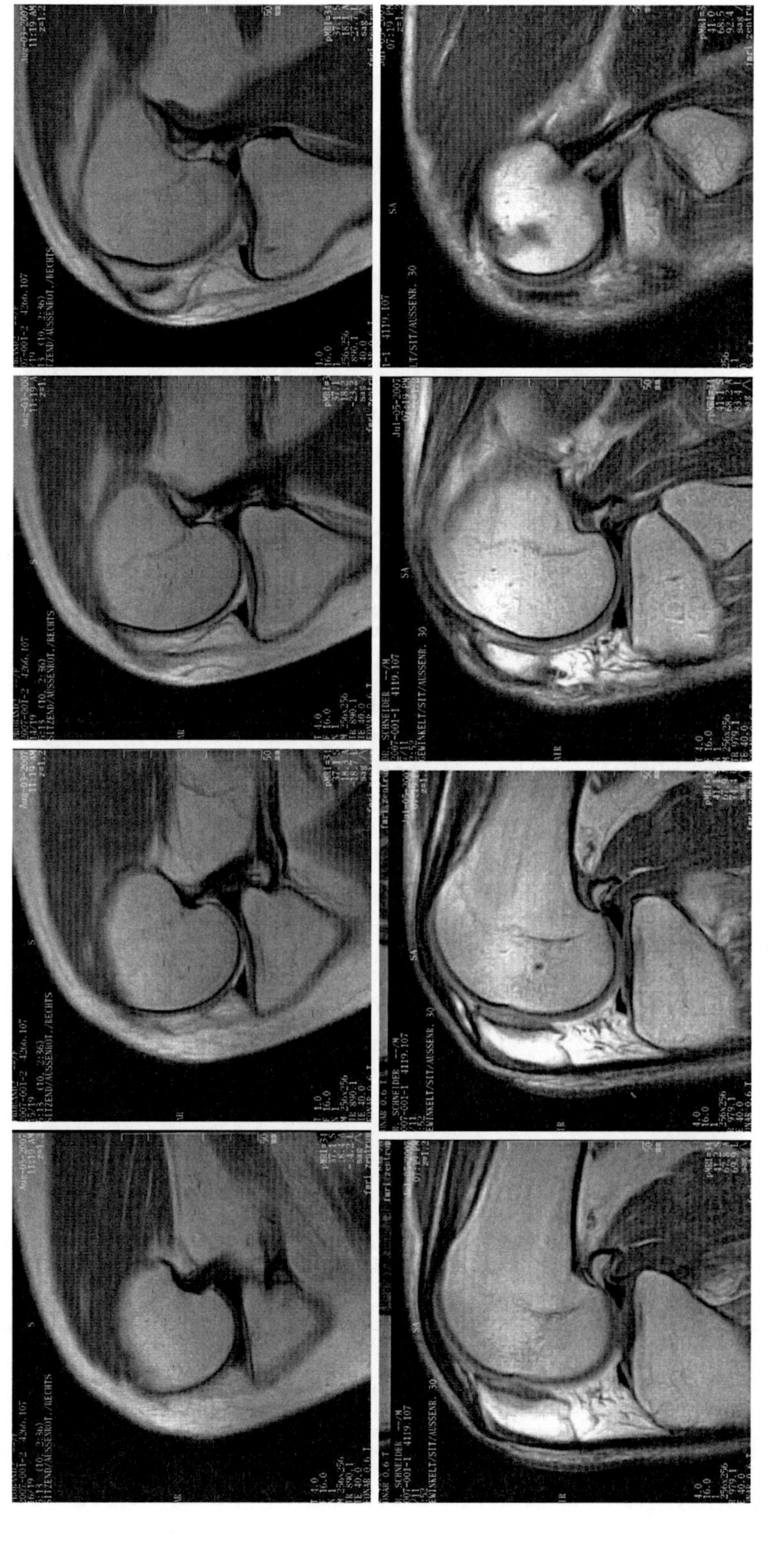

Fig. 17 Medial and lateral compartment with the menisci at 90° flexion in external rotation. Cuts from medial to lateral. *Above*: the medial meniscus is pushed postero-medially backwards. *Below*: the lateral meniscus vice versa is pushed antero-laterally forward (Courtesy Schneider U, Orthop Surgeon and Elsig JP, Radiologist Zürich)

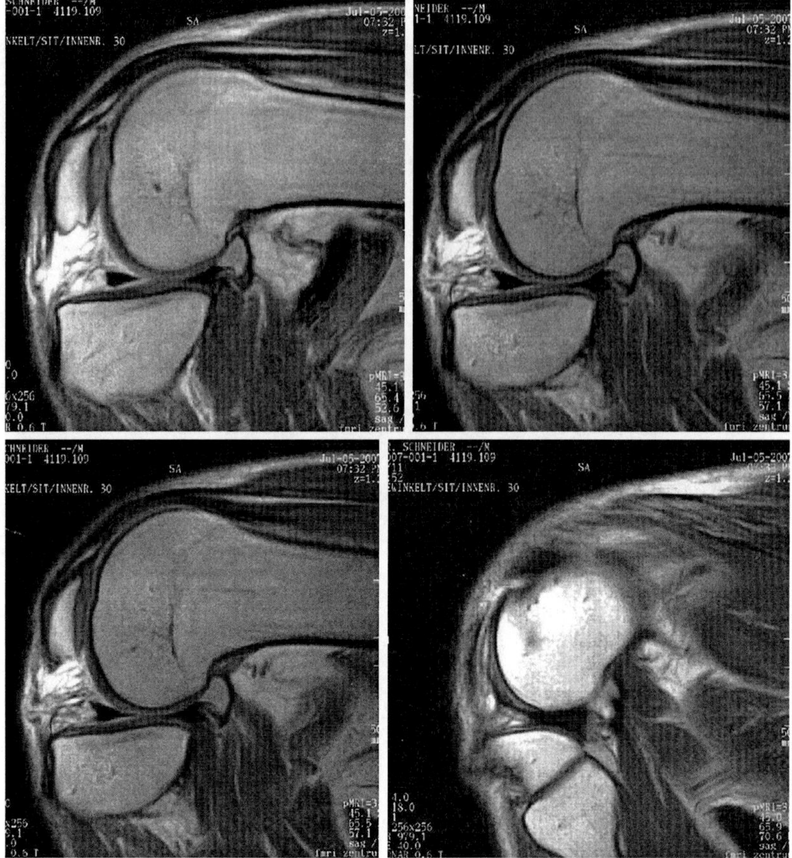

Fig. 18 Lateral compartment with the meniscus at 90° flexion and internal rotation. Cuts from central to lateral. Notice also the changing configuration of the tibial plateau from the center to the posteriror slope towards the fibula (Courtesy Schneider U, Orthop Surgeon and Elsig JP, Radiologist Zürich)

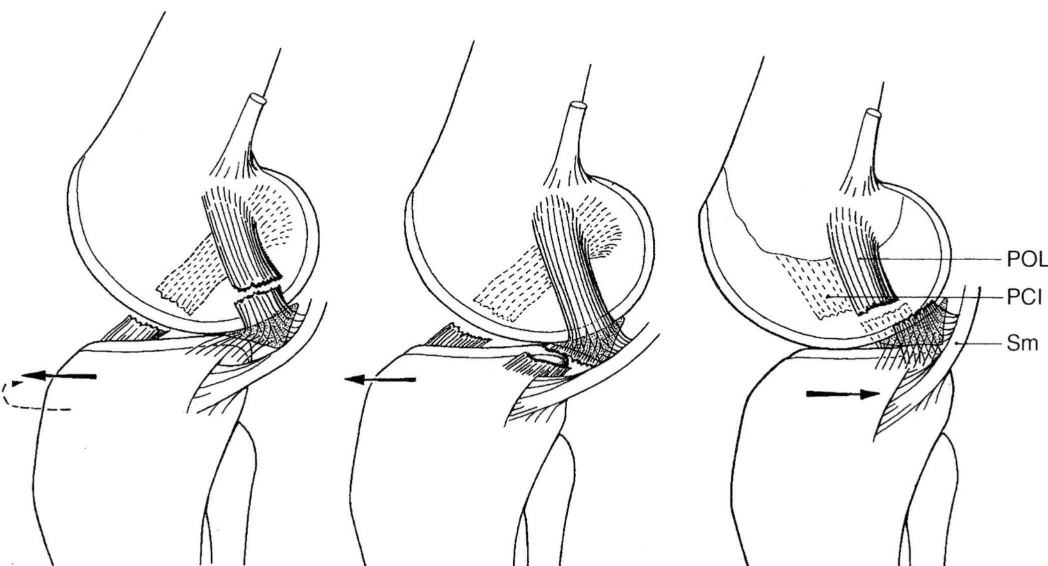

Fig. 19 The posterior horn of the medial meniscus is well fixed together with the POL. The schematic drawings demonstrate very well how this functional component is a co-restraint to ACL and PCL (From W. Müller the Knee)

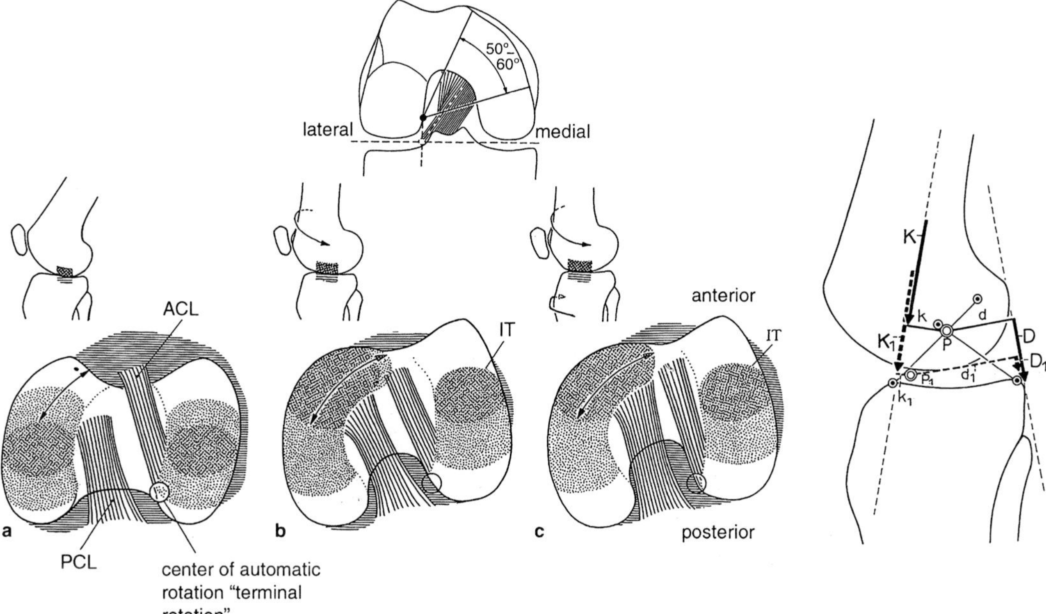

Fig. 20 Schematic illustration of the automatic rotation. On the *left*: the two condyles are at 20° flexion still in a mid position. Then towards extension, the lateral condyle reaches sulcus terminalis, (*IT* impressio terminalis) and the medial condyle rolls further in with its additional segment. Thus the tibia rotates out and vice versa the femur in. The contact point gets to a most anterior position on the tibia. The leaver arm for the posterior capsule acting against hyperextension gets so longer and the forces to resist get stronger (From W. Müller the Knee)

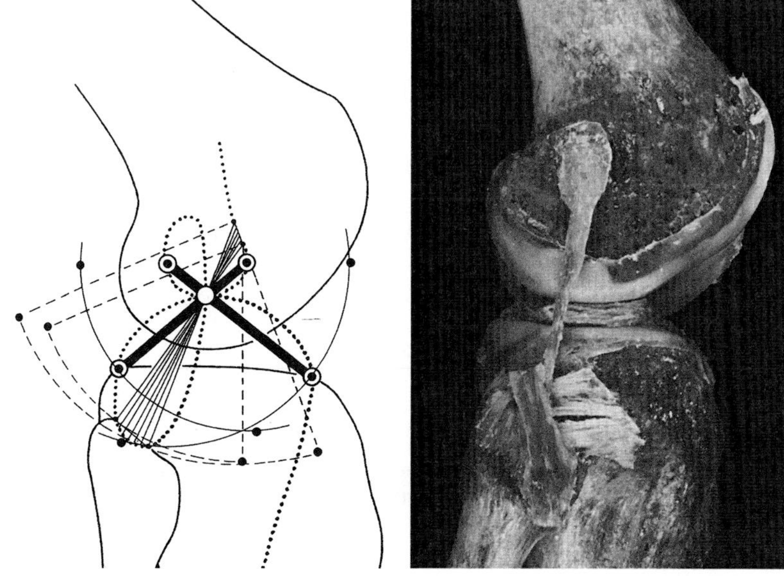

Fig. 21 The lateral compartment with the position of the LCL from femur to fibula. It fits quite well within the theoretic Burmester curve (From W. Müller the Knee)

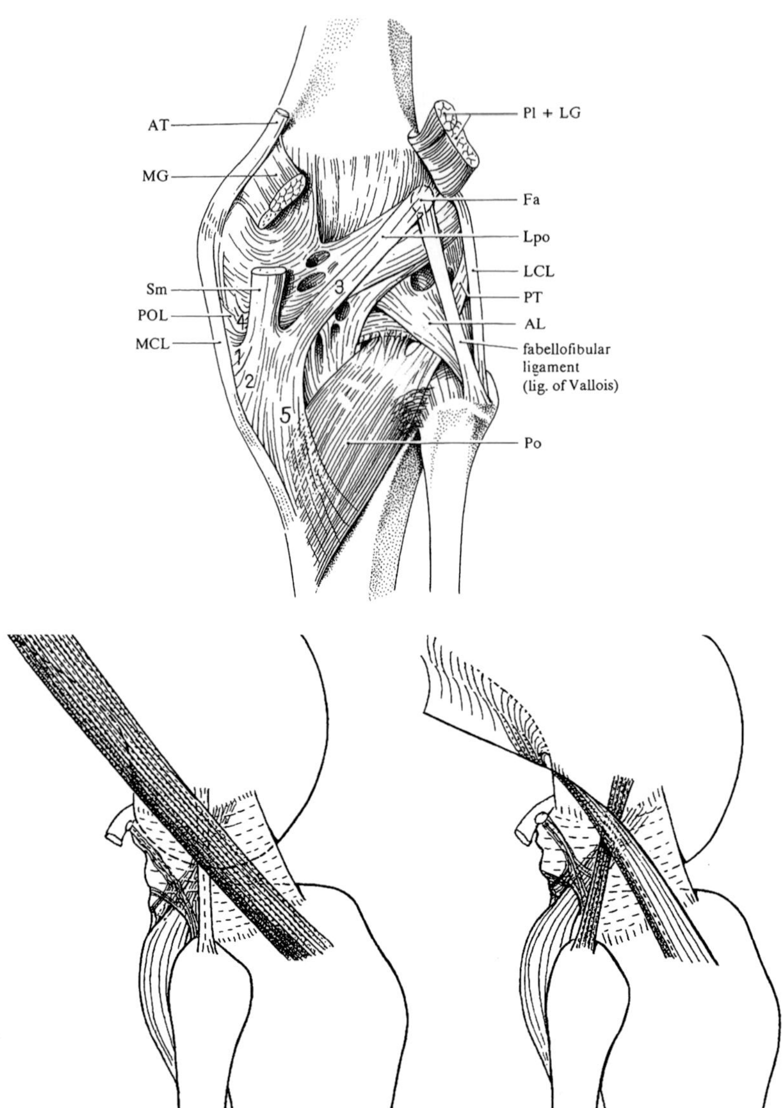

Fig. 22 The dynamized posterior and lateral capsulo-ligamentous structures. The Semimembranosus with its five tendon expansions, the ITT with the Kaplan fibers and especially the popliteus system (From W. Müller the Knee)

In each case also, the shape of the Burmester curve will be individually different.

The Burmester Curve and the Tendon Insertion Sites

The principle that no collagenous tissue should be shortened or elongated over a certain amount during knee motion brings also the tendon insertions close to positions on the Burmester curve (see Fig. 24).

It is to remember that the cruciates in the center as central pivot get tightened and are at risk in internal rotation. The peripheral ligaments, vice versa, are at risk in external rotation. Therefore, the periphery needs help by powerful internal rotators. The pes anserinus tendons insert on the tibia directly in front of and parallel to the LCM on the Burmester curve. Like the ligament, they are antivalgus restraints in extension, and in flexion, they become internal rotators to protect the MCL complex against external rotation.

The most important and strongest protector against valgus and external rotation is the

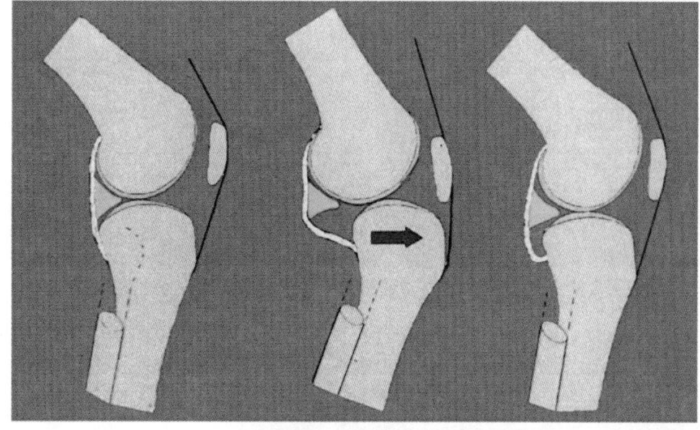

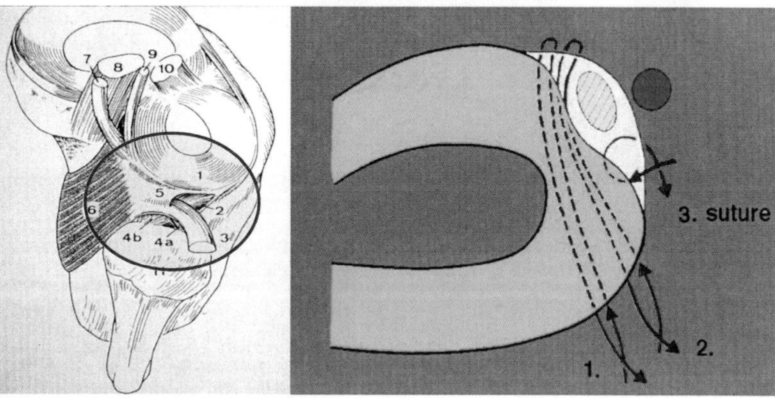

Fig. 23 The postero-lateral menisco-popliteal stability by the fascicle complex is distended after antero-lateral pivot shift dislocation. The hiatus politeus is in chronic situations elongated and can be reduced by sutures (Courtesy H.U. Stäubli (center) and We Müller)

semimembranosus with its insertion close to the POL on the tibia and with its five tendon arms, two to the tibia, one to the POL-medial meniscus, one as lig. popliteum obliquum (oblique popliteal ligament) to the fabella, and the fifth into the aponeurosis of the popliteus muscle. It controls the posteromedial stability from an ideal position in all directions. In extension, the pars directa goes to the posterior tibial crest stabilizing against valgus. In flexion, the pars reflexa passing under the MCL is best positioned for protective internal rotation (see Fig. 22).

The Importance of the Semimembranosus in Serious Medial Ligament Injuries and Instabilities

For many years, there were problems in stabilizing chronic medial valgus instabilities until we recognized in fresh medial dislocations that the two main tendons, the pars directa and the pars reflexa of the semimembranosus, have been torn away from the tibia. After successful refixations in the fresh knee dislocations, it is mandatory also in chronic instability cases to find these two tendon tips and to refix them. The stability results improved clearly from then on!

Importance and Function of Hoffa's Fat Pad and of the Plicae

Last but not least, Hoffa's fat pad has to be mentioned (Fig. 25).

During extension and flexion of the knee, the form of the intra-articular volume is very much changing. Hoffa's soft and remodeling soft tissue cushion and the movable plicaes are filling spontaneously the opening gaps during extension and flexion. Therefore, only a few drops of intra-articular synovial fluid are necessary. Without Hoffa's fat pad and without the plicae, the knee could only function with quite an amount of synovial fluid to compensate and fill the changing spaces, which means

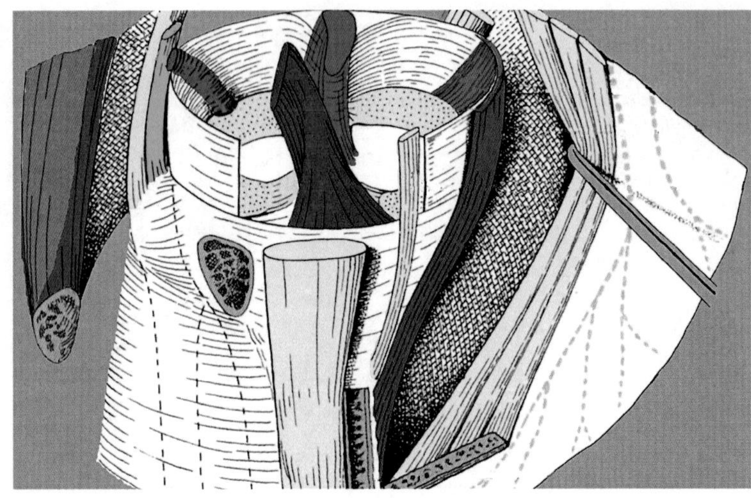

Fig. 24 This overall picture illustrates the central pivot ACL/PCL enlarged with the menisci. The POL (*violet*) as the medial and together with the popliteus (*darkgreen*) as the lateral corner stabilizer, MCL (*brown*), LCL (*lightgreen*), IIT detached with Gerdy's tubercle and all the tendons in *yellow* (Modified from Müller We Das Kniee 1982)

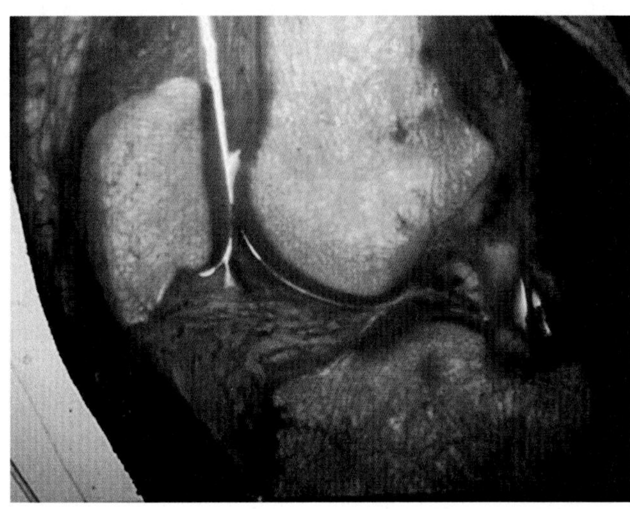

Fig. 25 The patella and Hoffa's fat pad with the inner vessel fine structure and with the space filling plicae. The quadriceps tendon in continuity with the praepatellar galea aponeurotica and the patellar tendon act together as anterior dynamic tension band protecting the patella from fatigue fracture by being continuously bent under tension

always with some effusion. The function without effusion is necessary for two important reasons:

First of all, it maintains the vacuum in the joint, which functions as first line of defense against any deformation before the ligaments are put at a higher risk for rupture. The rich innervated synovial layer gives order for the muscular reactions.

Second, a full efficient proprioception works only when the synovial layers are in tight contact with the bony surfaces of the femur to recognize the momentary position of the joint and to give the specific orders to the moving and stabilizing muscle forces.

This is the reason why the athletes should never be allowed to go back to sports as long as they do not have a dry joint. With effusion, they are still at risk for an early reinjury.

Furthermore, the Hoffa and its retropatellar plicae keep the space open between the patellar tendon and the front of the tibia behind the tendon and allow the tendon's necessary gliding. Closing adhesions between the tendon and the tibia front shorten the free-functioning proximal rest of the tendon and are responsible for a deficit of 5° of extension or even more! This is in addition often one of the main reasons for a post-traumatic or a postoperative anterior knee pain.

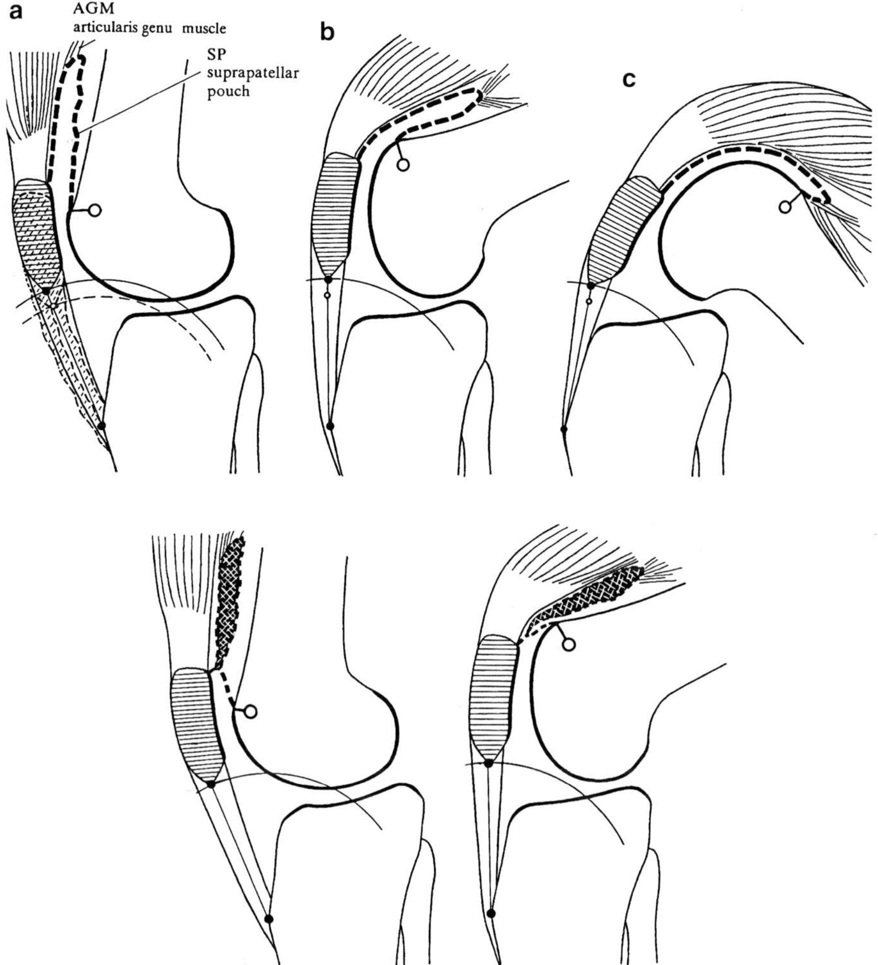

Fig. 26 The suprapatellar recessus, the pouch, has to be completly open for an undisturbed patello-femoral function. A closed recessus due to fibrosis still allows about 80° of flexion

Then, remember that ¾ of the dorsal patellar tendon part gets the blood supply from the Hoffa vessels. It is important to know when post-traumatic or postoperative shrinking contraction of the patellar tendon is a complication after damaged blood supply. This is probably also the reason of some known spontaneous patellar tendon ruptures after TKA implantations.

The Patello-Femoral Function

After the look into the Hoffa and peripatellar plicae function, now we move to the patellofemoral function (Fig. 26).

The patella must be free for riding and gliding on the trochlea. This means that the suprapatellar recessus, the so-called pouch, has to be open and free from adhesions. The same is necessary for all the surrounding plicae. The patella must be able to glide freely in all directions, in mediolateral and proximal–distal directions as well as in rotation in front of the trochlea or above it. Therefore, this motion has to be brought back immediately postoperatively by active exercises with the muscular play as well as sustained with moving the patella passively in the described directions by the patient or by the physiotherapist (Fig. 27).

There are two components of the patellofemoral function: first, the anatomic condition of the

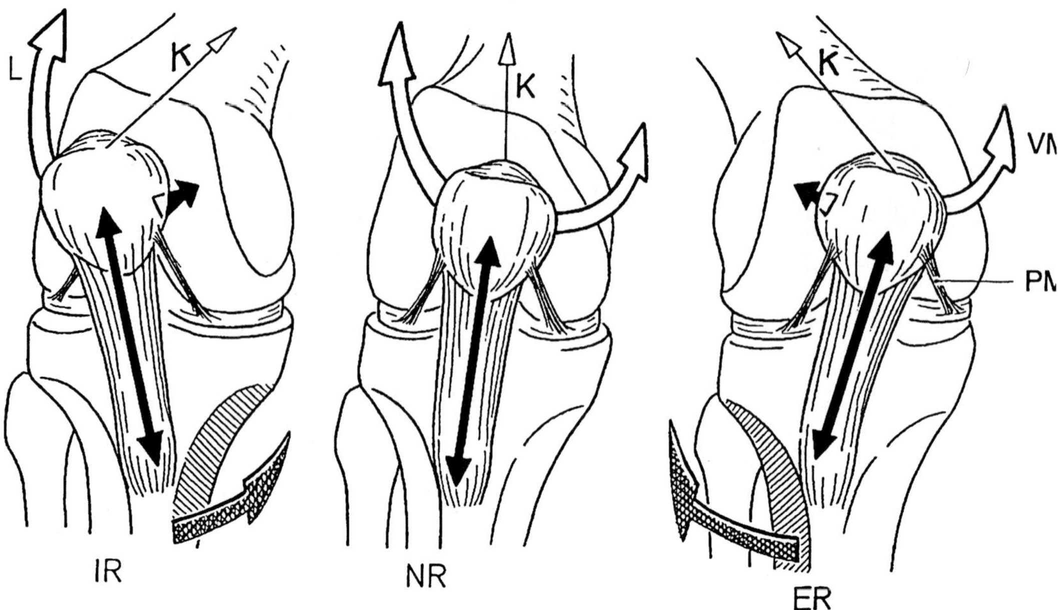

Fig. 27 The patello-femoral joint in dynamic action. The patella needs a free play to act with and to react to the forces and constraints (From Müller: Das Knie 1982)

trochlea femoris and of the patella as a sesamoid bone in the deceleration–extensor mechanism. The second component is the dynamic part with the patella guidance by all the muscles reaching over the knee joint. The quadriceps's four parts and pes anserinus, biceps, and all the iliotibial muscles react on proprioceptive inputs from the joint positions in all the six degrees of freedom with eccentric quad action under load from extension to flexion and vice versa concentric from flexion active to extension. The input of the corresponding tensions in the ligaments and tendons around the knee as well as from the position signals of the richly innervated menisci is also mandatory for the guidance.

Conclusion

This is how I came to understand the complex function of the knee.

It is now self-understanding that in this overall explanation of knee anatomy and function, many points can be stuffed with scientific details, but this fundamental basis and these given elements of functional anatomy and kinematics can guide us to understand the important basic principles to which the individual knee has its solution in its proper anatomy.

References

Appel M, Gradinger R (1989) Die Architektur des Kreuzbandaufbaus. Praktische Sport-Traumatologie und Sportmedizin 1:12–16, W.Zuckschwerdt Verlag München, Bern/Wien/San Francisco

Appel M, Hawe W, Gradinger R (1989) Topographische Anatomie der Kreuzbandinsertionen unter dem Gesichtspunkt der Kreuzbandplastik. Praktische Sport-Traumatologie und Sportmedizin 1:19–23, W. Zuckschwerdt Verlag München, Bern/Wien/San Francisco

Arnold MP (2004) Spotlight on crucial details in anterior cruciate ligament surgery, about tension, position and twist. Ponsen and Looijen, Wageningen

Biedert R (2000) Free nerve endings in the medial and posteromedial capsuloligamentous complexes: occurrence and distribution. KSSTA 8:68–72

Böhler L (1932) Technik der Knochenbruchbehandlung Verl. Wilhelm Maudrich, Wien

Brückner H, Brückner H (1972) Bandplastiken im Kniebereich nach dem Baukastenprinzip. Zentralbl Chir 97:65–77

Burmester (1888) Lehrbuch der Kinematik. Leipzig

Drobny T, Müller W, Wentzensen A, Perren SM (1986) Patellar tendon graft with a fat pad pedicle for anterior cruciate ligament reconstruction. In: Trickey EL, Hertel P (eds) Surgery and arthoscopy of the knee. Springer, Berlin/Heidelberg/New York/Tokyo, pp 181–191

Drobny Th, Müller We, Munzinger U, Perren SM (1990) Das Hoffa-gestielte Patellarsehnentransplantat als Ersatz für das vordere Kreuzband: Eine tierexperimentelle Untersuchung. In: Jakob RP, Stäubli HU (Hrsg) Kniegelenk und Kreuzbänder. Springer, Berlin/Heidelberg/New York

Friederich N, O'Brien WR (1989) Anterior curuciate ligament fiber tension patterns during knee motion. In: Proceedings of the 6th ISK congress American Journal of Sports Medicine, vol 17, p 699

Girgis FG, GirgisF G, Marshall JL, Monajem ARS (1975) The cruciate ligaments of the knee. Clin Orthop 106:216–231

Jones KG (1963) Reconstruction of the anterior cruciate ligament. JBJS (Am) 45:925–932

Lindemann K (1950) Über den plastischen Ersatz der Kreuzbänder durch gestielte Sehnenverpflanzungen

Lobenhoffer P, Posel P, Witt S, Piehler J, Wirth CJ (1978) Distal femoral fixation of the iliotibial tract. Arch Orthop Trauma Surg 106:285–290

Mandic V (1959) Experimental investigations of knee menisci regeneration in dogs. Reconstr Surg Traumatol 11:200–207, Verlag Karger, Basel, New York, 1969

Menschik A (1974) Mechanik des Kniegelenkes Teil 1. Z Orthop 112:481–495

Menschik A (1975) Mechanik des Kniegelenkes Teil 2. Z Orthop 113:388–400

Menschik A (1987) Biometrie, das Konstruktionsprinzip des Kniegelenks, des Hüftgelenks der Beinlänge und der Körpergrösse. Springer, Berlin/Heidelberg/New York/London/Paris/Tokyo

Mommersteeg TJ, Kooloos JG, Blankevoort L et al (1995) The fibre bundle anatomy of human cruciate ligaments. J Anat 187:461–471

Mommersteeg TJ, Blankevoort L, Huiskes R et al (1996) Characterization of the mechanical behavior of human knee ligaments. J Biomech 29:151–60

Müller W (1977) Verletzungen der Kreuzbänder. Zentralbl Chir 102:974–981

Müller W (1982) Das Knie, Form, Funktion und ligamentäre Wiederherstellung. Springer, Heidelberg/Berlin/NewYork

Müller W (1983) The knee, form, function and ligament reconstruction. Springer, Heidelberg/Berlin/NewYork

O'Donoghue DM (1973) Reconstruction of medial instability of the knee. JBJS (Am) 55:941–955

Slocum DB, Larson RL (1968) Pes anserinus transplantation. JBJS 50:226–242

Stäubli HU, Birrer S (1990) The popliteus tendon and its fascicles at the popliteal hiatus: gross anatomy and functional arthoscopic evaluation with and without anterior cruciate ligament deficiency. J Arthosc 6(3):209–220

Tavernier L (1927) Pathologie des Ménisques du genou. Rapport Mouchet A, Tavernier L

Wittek A (1935) Kreuzbandersatz aus dem lig.patellae (nach zur Verth). Schweiz Med Wochenschr 65:103–104

Anteromedial Knee Instability

73

Gian Luigi Canata

Contents

Abstract

The medial side of the knee should not be overlooked in combined anteromedial instabilities. There is a wide consensus on functional rehabilitation for grade I and II medial collateral ligament (MCL) injuries. Grade III injuries can also be treated nonsurgically with early functional rehabilitation using a knee brace. Persistent symptomatic valgus laxity is treated surgically. Patellar tendon (BPTB) is preferred as an anterior cruciate ligament (ACL) substitute to save the medial active restraints, but ACL reconstruction alone may be not enough in combined anteromedial laxities. Medial ligament surgery reduces stress on the reconstructed ACL. Stability can be regained with autografts, allografts, or anatomic repairs addressing the MCL and posterior oblique ligament (POL). In chronic laxities satisfactory results with stability restoration can be achieved with an anatomic tissue-sparing technique avoiding more invasive surgery.

Introduction

The MCL complex is the most commonly damaged ligamentous stabilizer of the human knee (Heitmann et al. 2013). The goal in knee ligament injuries is the restoration of anatomy and stability. Instability can lead to a damage of the secondary structures: cartilage and menisci. The ACL is a primary knee stabilizer and many techniques have

G.L. Canata (✉)
Centre of Sports Traumatology, Koelliker Hospital, Institute of Sports Medicine, Torino, Italy
e-mail: studio@ortosport.it; canata@ortosport.it

M.N. Doral, J. Karlsson (eds.), *Sports Injuries*,
DOI 10.1007/978-3-642-36569-0_115

been developed in order to reconstruct ACL tears. In some cases the medial side is involved resulting in an anteromedial instability. For adequate treatment, the classification and exact knowledge about concomitant injuries are important. There are several dynamic and static medial compartment stabilizers. The dynamic stabilizers are the pes anserinus (sartorius, gracilis, and semitendinosus), semimembranosus, and vastus medialis obliquus. The static stabilizers are the capsuloligamentous complex: MCL, deep MCL, and POL. The MCL is the primary stabilizer against valgus stress with a different action in the arc of movement: 25° knee flexion, 78 % restraining force against valgus stress; 5° knee flexion, 57 %. In extension, ACL and POL are important restraints (Inoue et al. 1987; Griffith et al. 2009; Wijdicks et al. 2009). The ACL is a primary stabilizer and represents 21 % resistance to valgus stress. Integrity of the posteromedial corner (PMC) is important. A synergistic action of the posteromedial complex (PMC) and ACL is well known (Muller 1983). Acute MCL lesions usually heal without surgery (Indelicato 1995; Reider 1994, 1996). The best results are seen with early range of motion and no repair (Millet et al. 2003; Halinen et al. 2006). These results reinforce the clinical importance of early mobilization in the MCL-injured knee. In grade III MCL injuries, there is a high frequency of associated ACL injuries (Fetto and Marshall 1978). Controversies still exist in the management of acute combined ACL and MCL injuries: according to some authors, ACL reconstruction is sufficient to restore the knee stability (Shelbourne and Nitz 1990; McCarroll et al. 1994), whereas some others advocate a repair of both ACL and MCL (Fetto and Marshall 1978; Tibor et al. 2011). The current trend consists in a less aggressive treatment of the medial laxity with a great effort to improve ACL reconstruction (Millett et al. 2004). Vigorous competitive sports need medial stability, and medial laxity implies a larger load on ACL in chronic anteromedial instability (Canata et al. 2012). In the context of a multiligamentous injury or complex instability, the majority of authors suggest an operative stabilization. An adequate initial treatment of acute medial knee tears is of great importance, as the management of chronic instability can be challenging. Injuries to the PMC may not heal without surgical repair or reconstruction, particularly when part of a multiple ligament injury (Hughston and Eilers 1973; Warren and Marshall 1979; Fanelli et al. 2010).

Residual laxities remain when ACL reconstruction is performed in patients with combined ACL and MCL lesions, and raise the question of addressing the medial knee ligaments when grade II residual laxity is found (Zaffagnini et al. 2007). Surgical treatment is considered when the patient presents a valgus laxity in the affected knee versus the contralateral knee on physical examination, associated with a compromised function, as well as stress radiographs that are consistent with an incompetent MCL (Miyamoto et al. 2009; LaPrade et al. 2010). Many surgical techniques are described: reattachment, reefing, advancement, augmentation, and dynamic transfers with satisfactory results in 70–82 % (Lind et al. 2009; Coobs et al. 2010; Laprade and Wijdicks 2011).

Either allograft or autograft reconstructions of both the MCL and PMC can be successful. Successful elimination of anteromedial rotary instability is the key to successfully treating PMC injuries (Kim et al. 2008). In 1983, Werner Muller reported that anatomical repair was better than the pes plasty and stressed on the importance of the dynamic medial stabilizers (Muller 1983). A mini-invasive medial ligamentous plasty can be associated with ACL reconstruction when the medial compartment is still lax after ACL graft fixation (>5 mm) (Canata et al. 2012).

Evaluation

The medial side is evaluated in 30° of flexion and in full extension. The test for MCL injury is valgus stress testing with the knee in 30° of flexion. The amount of joint line opening is compared to the contralateral knee. Medial side injuries are subjectively defined by the amount of joint line opening: grade I, <5 mm of medial joint line opening; grade II, 5–10 mm of joint line opening; and grade III, >10 mm of joint line opening (Miyamoto et al. 2009). Examination of the amount of tibial rotation is performed at 90° of flexion. The anteromedial drawer test assesses the amount of increased external rotation due to a medial knee injury. Rotational abnormalities due to posterolateral injuries are evaluated with the dial test at 30° of flexion (isolated posterolateral injuries) and 90° of flexion (combined posterolateral and PCL injuries) (Laprade and Wijdicks 2012). Valgus stress testing should then be performed with the knee in full extension to test the integrity of both the MCL and the POL. Increased joint opening in full extension means POL injury and a possible concomitant cruciate ligament injury. Valgus stress radiographs provide a reliable measure of medial compartment gapping even if they cannot differentiate between meniscofemoral- and meniscotibial-based injuries. A grade III medial collateral ligament injury should be suspected with greater than 3.2 mm medial gapping compared to the contralateral knee at 20° of flexion and gapping also in full extension (Laprade et al. 2010).

Radiographic evaluation of a knee with a chronic MCL injury may show calcification in the proximal origin of the ligament. This heterotopic bone is called a Pellegrini-Stieda lesion (Miyamoto et al. 2009).

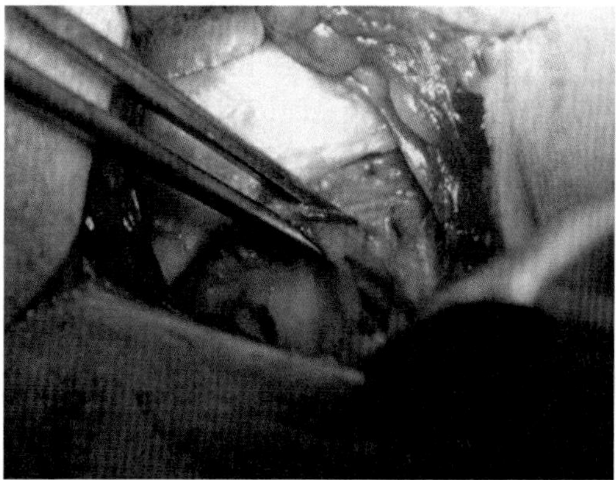

Fig. 1 Laxity of the medial compartment after ACL fixation

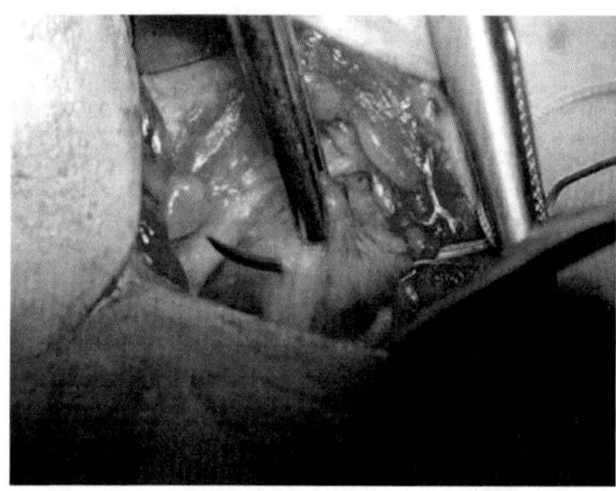

Fig. 2 Sutures with nonabsorbable material are made

Techniques

Arthroscopic ACL reconstruction can be performed with different techniques. Patellar tendon grafts are usually preferred in these cases to save the medial active stabilizers. Medial ligament reconstruction can be made with autografts or allografts addressing the MCL and the POL if needed (Kim et al. 2008; Miyamoto et al. 2009; Coobs et al. 2010; Tibor et al. 2011; Laprade and Wijdicks 2012) (Fig. 1). A plasty avoiding any harvesting can be done with a short longitudinal incision over the medial femoral epicondyle. A simple medial ligaments' plasty is then performed suturing the MCL and POL to the femoral epicondyle with figure-of-eight stitches and restoring the medial ligaments' tension (Canata et al. 2012) (Figs. 2, 3, 4 and 5). Same ACL rehabilitation is allowed.

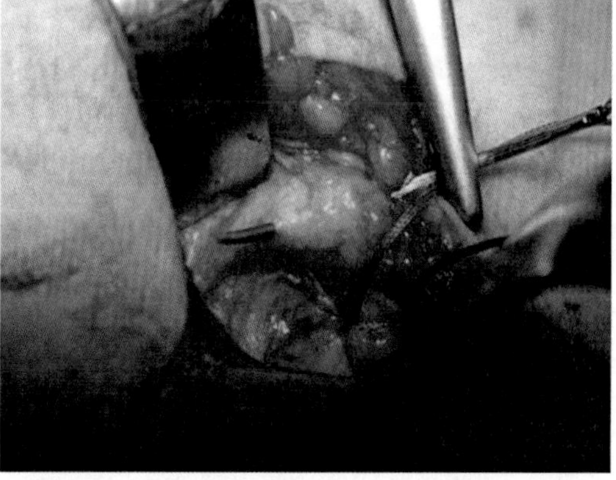

Fig. 3 The lax medial tissue is tightened up to the epicondyle

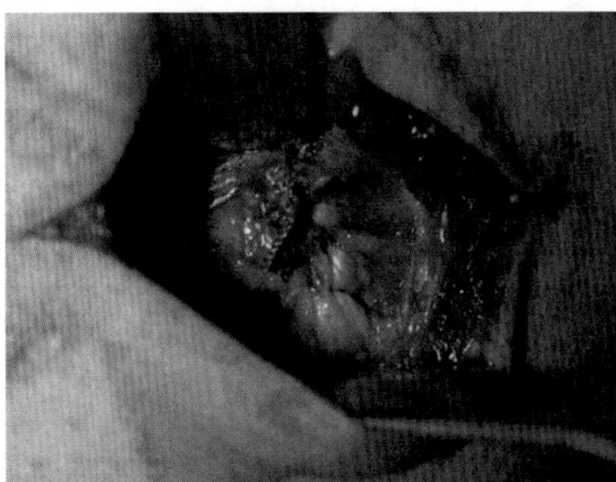

Fig. 4 Sutures at the end

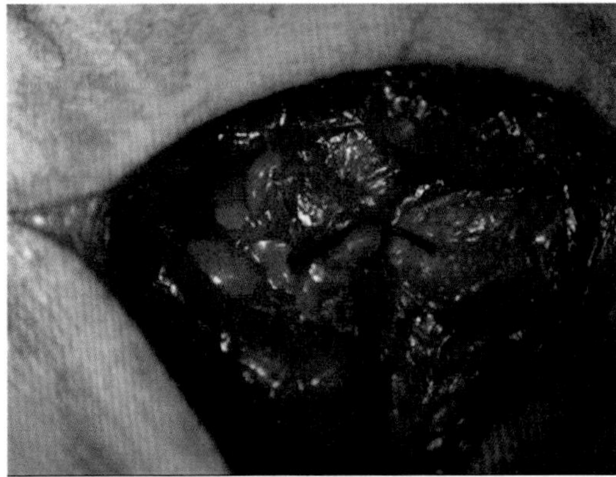

Fig. 5 Suture of the retinaculum

Discussion

There is a wide consensus on functional rehabilitation for grade I and II MCL injuries. Grade III injuries can also be treated nonsurgically with early functional rehabilitation using a knee brace. Persistent symptomatic valgus laxity is treated surgically. For combined ACL and MCL injuries, the current techniques are aimed at a less aggressive treatment of medial laxity, but in grade III medial injuries, both the MCL and POL are damaged with a substantial increase of medial laxity and external rotation. Usually the ACL is reconstructed after 6 weeks of brace wear and ROM exercises but the medial side should not be neglected. Intraoperatively, the knee is placed under a valgus stress after the ACL has been reconstructed. Patellar tendon grafts are often preferred to save the medial active restraints, but ACL reconstruction alone may not be enough. If medial laxity persists on intraoperative physical examination (>5 mm at either 0° or 30° and abnormal external tibial rotation), then the MCL injury should be treated surgically (Stannard 2010; Canata et al. 2012). Medial ligamentous plasty reduces stress on the reconstructed ACL. In literature a higher failure rate is described in medial collateral repairs compared to reconstructions in knees with multiple ligament injuries (Stannard 2010). On the other end positive results were reported in avulsion repairs (Owens et al. 2007; Laprade and Wijdicks 2011). Nakamura found that in chronic distal lesions, a proximal repair could not stabilize the medial compartment due to poor-quality scarring: in these cases a reconstructive technique should be used (Nakamura et al. 2003). Anatomical techniques can restore near normal stability (Coobs et al. 2010). In grade III medial injuries techniques addressing both the MCL and the POL should be preferred (Lind et al. 2009). A biomechanical study did not find any significant difference between anatomic MCL augmented repairs and anatomic MCL reconstructions when tested at time zero (Wijidicks et al. 2013). Stability can be regained with several techniques utilizing autografts, allografts, or anatomic repairs. Satisfactory results with stability restoration can, nevertheless, be achieved using an anatomic tissue-sparing technique avoiding more invasive surgery

Cross-References

- ▶ Anterior Cruciate Ligament Graft Selection and Fixation
- ▶ Anterior Cruciate Ligament Injuries and Surgery: Current Evidence and Modern Development
- ▶ Anteromedial Knee Instability
- ▶ Different Techniques of Anterior Cruciate Ligament Reconstruction: Guidelines

- ▶ Double-Tunnel Anatomic Anterior Cruciate Ligament Reconstruction
- ▶ Measuring In Vivo Joint Motion and Ligament Function: New Developments
- ▶ State of the Art in Anterior Cruciate Ligament Surgery

References

Canata GL, Chiey A, Leoni T (2012) Surgical technique: does mini-invasive medial collateral ligament and posterior oblique ligament repair restore knee stability in combined chronic medial and ACL injuries? Clin Orthop Relat Res 470(3):791–797

Coobs BR, Wijdicks CA, Armitage BM, Spiridonov SI, Westerhaus BD, Johansen S, Engebretsen L, Laprade RF (2010) An in vitro analysis of an anatomical medial knee reconstruction. Am J Sports Med 38(2):339–347

Fanelli GC, Stannard JP, Stuart MJ, MacDonald PB, Marx RG, Whelan DB, Boyd JL, Levy BA (2010) Management of complex knee ligament injuries. J Bone Joint Surg Am 92(12):2235–2246

Fetto JF, Marshall JL (1978) Medial collateral ligament injuries of the knee: a rationale for treatment. Clin Orthop Relat Res 132:206–218

Griffith CJ, Wijdicks CA, LaPrade RF, Armitage BM, Johansen S, Engebretsen L (2009) Force measurements on the posterior oblique ligament and superficial medial collateral ligament proximal and distal divisions to applied loads. Am J Sports Med 37(1):140–148

Halinen J, Linpahl J, Hirvensalo E et al (2006) Operative and nonoperative treatments of medial collateral ligament rupture with early ACL reconstruction: a prospective randomized study. Am J Sports Med 34(7):1134–1140

Heitmann M, Preiss A, Giannakos A, Frosch KH (2013) Acute medial collateral ligament injuries of the knee: diagnostics and therapy. Unfallchirurg 116(6):497–503. doi:10.1007/s00113-013-2371-8

Hughston JC, Eilers AF (1973) The role of the posterior oblique ligament in repairs of acute medial (collateral) ligament tears of the knee. J Bone Joint Surg Am 55(5):923–940

Indelicato PA (1995) Isolated medial collateral ligament injuries in the knee. J Am Acad Orthop Surg 3(1):9–14

Inoue M, McGurk-Burleson E, Hollis JM, Woo SL (1987) Treatment of the medial collateral ligament injury. I: the importance of anterior cruciate ligament on the varus-valgus knee laxity. Am J Sports Med 15(1):15–21

Kim SJ, Lee DH, Kim TE, Choi NH (2008) Concomitant reconstruction of the medial collateral and posterior oblique ligaments for medial instability of the knee. J Bone Joint Surg Br 90(10):1323–1327

Laprade RF, Wijdicks CA (2011) Surgical technique: development of an anatomic medial knee reconstruction. Clin Orthop Relat Res 470(3):806–814

Laprade RF, Wijdicks CA (2012) The management of injuries to the medial side of the knee. J Orthop Sports Phys Ther 42(3):221–233

LaPrade RF, Bernhardson AS, Griffith CJ, Macalena JA, Wijdicks CA (2010) Correlation of valgus stress radiographs with medial knee ligament injuries: an in vitro biomechanical study. Am J Sports Med 38(2):330–338

Lind M, Jakobsen BW, Lund B, Hansen MS, Abdallah O, Christiansen SE (2009) Anatomical reconstruction of the medial collateral ligament and posteromedial corner of the knee in patients with chronic medial collateral ligament instability. Am J Sports Med 37(6): 1116–1122

McCarroll JR, Shelbourne KD, Porter DA, Rettig AC, Murray S (1994) Patellar tendon graft reconstruction for midsubstance anterior cruciate ligament rupture in junior high school athletes. An algorithm for management. Am J Sports Med 22(4):478–484

Millet PJ, Johnson B, Carlson J et al (2003) Rehabilitation of the arthrofibrotic knee. Am J Orthop 32:531–538

Millett PJ, Pennock AT, Sterett WI, Steadman JR (2004) Early ACL reconstruction in combined ACL-MCL injuries. J Knee Surg 17:94–98

Miyamoto RG, Bosco JA, Sherman OH (2009) Treatment of medial collateral ligament injuries. J Am Acad Orthop Surg 17(3):152–161

Muller W (1983) The knee. Form, function and ligament reconstruction. Springer, Berlin Heidelberg

Nakamura N, Horibe S, Toritsuka Y, Mitsuoka T, Yoshikaua H, Shino K (2003) Acute Grade III medial collateral ligament injury of the knee associated with anterior cruciate ligament tear: the usefulness of magnetic resonance imaging in determining a treatment regimen. Am J Sports Med 31:261–267

Owens BD, Neault M, Benson E, Busconi BD (2007) Primary repair of knee dislocations: results in 25 patients (28 knees) at a mean follow-up of four years. J Orthop Trauma 21:92–96

Reider B (1994) Treatment of isolated medial collateral ligament injuries in athletes with early functional rehabilitation. A five-year follow-up study. Am J Sports Med 22(4):470–477

Reider B (1996) Medial collateral ligament injuries in athletes. Sports Med 21(2):147–156

Shelbourne KD, Nitz P (1990) Accelerated rehabilitation after anterior cruciate ligament reconstruction. Am J Sports Med 18(3):292–299

Stannard JP (2010) Medial and posteromedial instability of the knee: evaluation, treatment, and results. Sports Med Arthrosc 18(4):263–268. doi:10.1097/JSA.0b013e3181eaf713

Tibor LM, Marchant MH Jr, Taylor DC, Hardaker WT Jr, Garrett WE Jr, Sekiya JK (2011) Management of medial-sided knee injuries, part 2: posteromedial corner. Am J Sports Med 39(6):1332–1340

Warren LF, Marshall JL (1979) The supporting structures and layers on the medial side of the knee: an anatomical analysis. J Bone Joint Surg Am 61(1):56–62

Wijdicks CA, Griffith CJ, LaPrade RF, Spiridonov SI, Johansen S, Armitage BM, Engebretsen L (2009) Medial knee injury: part 2, load sharing between the posterior oblique ligament and superficial medial collateral ligament. Am J Sports Med 37(1):1771–1776

Wijdicks CA, Michalski MP, Rasmussen MT, Goldsmith MT, Kennedy NI, Lind M, Engebretsen L, Laprade RF (2013) Superficial medial collateral ligament anatomic augmented repair versus anatomic reconstruction: an in vitro biomechanical analysis. Am J Sports Med. 41(12):2858–2866

Zaffagnini S, Bignozzi S, Martelli S, Lopomo N, Marcacci M (2007) Does ACL reconstruction restore knee stability in combined lesions? An in vivo study. Clin Orthop Relat Res 454:95–99

Arthrofibrosis of the Knee

74

Ugur Haklar, Egemen Ayhan, Tekin Kerem Ulku, and Sinan Karaoğlu

Contents

U. Haklar (✉)
Orthopaedics and Traumatology Department, Bahcesehir University Medical Faculty, Liv Hospital, Istanbul, Turkey
e-mail: dr.haklar@superonline.com

E. Ayhan
Orthopaedics and Traumatology Department, Liv Hospital, Istanbul, Turkey
e-mail: egemenay@yahoo.com

T.K. Ulku
Orthopaedics and Traumatology Department, Camlica Erdem Hospital, Istanbul, Turkey
e-mail: keremulku@gmail.com

S. Karaoğlu
Department of Orthopaedics and Traumatology, Memorial Kayseri Hospital, Kayseri, Turkey
e-mail: sinankaraoglu@hotmail.com

M.N. Doral, J. Karlsson (eds.), *Sports Injuries*,
DOI 10.1007/978-3-642-36569-0_100

Abstract
Arthrofibrosis is the abnormal proliferation of fibrous tissue in a joint with an unclear etiopathogenesis that leads to loss of motion, pain, muscle weakness, swelling, and functional limitation. The incidence of knee arthrofibrosis varies from 0 % to 57 % depending on the severity of injury. In the knee, arthrofibrosis may present as a localized form (cyclops lesion, infrapatellar contracture syndrome, patellar clunk syndrome, localized intra-articular scarring) or it may present as a generalized stiffness. A thorough patient history and a systematic evaluation of the knee are vital. The initial treatment is aggressive physical therapy. Arthroscopic debridement combined with manipulation under anesthesia is preferred after 6 weeks of failed conservative treatment. A comprehensive arthroscopic arthrolysis and careful postoperative rehabilitation are the hallmarks for successful outcomes.

Introduction

Synovium is the important tissue of the synovial joints that provides synovial fluid. The synovial fluid lubricates the joints and by this way articular surfaces can smoothly slide on each other. For normal motion, the joints should be free of adhesions. Loss of motion is one of the most devastating complications that may be seen after any kind of knee surgery.

Gait analysis studies have reported that 67° of knee flexion is required in the swing phase of walking, 83° to ascend stairs, 90° to descend stairs, and 93° to rise from a standard chair (Laubenthal et al. 1972). Even a 5–10° loss of extension can cause a noticeable limp during ambulation with the increased incidence of patellofemoral symptoms (Sachs et al. 1989). Extension deficits of >20° result in significant limb-length discrepancy. Loss of motion disrupts normal knee kinematics and the knee joint becomes prone to progressive degenerative changes.

Arthrofibrosis is an abnormal proliferation of fibrous tissue in a joint that can lead to loss of motion, pain, muscle weakness, swelling, and functional limitation. Its presentation may be localized or as a generalized fibrosis or capsulitis presenting with severe stiffness. In 1982, Sprague et al. (1982) was first to describe the pathoanatomic classification of motion loss. They classified the "fibroarthrosis" in three groups: *group 1*, discrete bands or a single sheet of adhesions traversing the suprapatellar pouch; *group 2*, complete obliteration of the suprapatellar pouch and peripatellar gutters with masses of adhesions; and *group 3*, multiple bands of adhesions or complete obliteration of the suprapatellar pouch with extracapsular involvement with bands of tissue from proximal patella to anterior femur. Subsequently, many authors have described arthrofibrosis as limited range of motion (ROM) from intra-articular and extra-articular fibrosis after surgery (Hughston 1985; Paulos et al. 1987; Harner et al. 1992; Fisher and Shelbourne 1993; Cosgarea et al. 1994; Shelbourne et al. 1996).

The incidence of knee stiffness has been reported to vary from 0 % to 57 % depending on the severity of injury (Magit et al. 2007). Therefore, the exact incidence of motion loss is hard to ascertain because the incidence is less common with single-ligament, low-energy injuries than with high-energy, multiligament injuries. However, despite the relatively high incidence of arthrofibrosis for some injuries, the precise etiopathogenesis is unclear.

Etiology and Pathogenesis

The plausible etiology of arthrofibrosis is multifactorial, involving a combination of mechanical and biologic factors (Magit et al. 2007). Risk factors include severe injuries like knee dislocations and multiligament injuries, immobility duration before surgery, timing of surgery, surgical technical errors, prolonged immobilization, delayed postoperative physical therapy, infection, and complex regional pain syndrome (CRPS) (O'Brien et al. 1995; Noyes and Barber-Westin 1997; Magit et al. 2007). Extra-articular stiffness may be caused by femoral fractures, muscular fibrosis and contracture, or heterotopic ossification. Also, genetic predisposition was proposed to be a factor in the etiology. One study found that patients with arthrofibrosis were more likely to have HLA-Cw*08 and less likely to have HLA-Cw*07 or DQB1*06 allelic groups (Skutek et al. 2004).

For the pathogenesis of arthrofibrosis, a stimulus such as a traumatic event (intra-articular fracture, injury to extensor mechanism), an intra-articular/ligament knee surgery, a knee arthroplasty, and an infection may lead to an excessive inflammatory reaction that progresses to arthrofibrosis. Normally, healing occurs through a sequence of coordinated events. The healing response is initiated by the clotting cascade, which results in the migration of inflammatory cells and proliferation of fibroblasts at the site of injury. This is followed by the release of cytokines, growth factors, and reactive oxygen and nitrogen species (ROS/RNS) (Poli and Parola 1997; Cochrane and Ricardo 2003; Baran et al. 2004). Once the healing process comes to an end, the majority of the inflammatory cells undergo apoptosis, the tissue heals, and the release of mediators ceases. In arthrofibrosis, the normal resolution of the inflammatory reaction in tissue repair fails, resulting in a persistent inflammation of the synovial tissue. Besides the deregulation of inflammatory cytokines, there is an upregulation of transforming growth factor-β (TGF-β) and platelet-derived growth factor (PDGF), triggering an irreversible tissue fibrosis via the transformation of fibroblasts (Watson et al. 2010). Additionally, vascular endothelial growth factor is proposed to be released after injury to the infrapatellar fat pad leading to vascular ingrowth and scarring (Ushiyama et al. 2003).

TGF-β plays a key role in the pathogenesis of arthrofibrosis and is a potent mediator of extracellular matrix protein synthesis (Ihn 2002; Freeman et al. 2009; Freeman et al. 2010; Watson et al. 2010). There is aggressive fibroblast proliferation with accumulation of extracellular matrix components (Murakami et al. 1997; Bosch et al. 2001). The reduced extracellular matrix remodeling leads to impaired blood flow and tissue hypoxia (Distler et al. 2007; Freeman et al. 2010). Tissue hypoxia leads to oxidative stress and ROS/RNS production, and the production of ROS/RNS stimulates degranulation of mast cells (Steiner et al. 2003; Freeman et al. 2010). Mast cells release chymase and fibroblast growth factor (FGF) that result in the activation of TGF-β, and TGF-β further stimulates fibroblast proliferation and extracellular matrix accumulation, thus creating additional regions of hypoxia (Shiota et al. 2005; Freeman et al. 2010). The vicious circle in pathogenesis of arthrofibrosis is schematized in Fig. 1 (Freeman et al. 2010). Hypoxia is the key fact that directs the cascade toward arthrofibrosis. Freeman et al. (2010) showed that hypoxia and associated oxidative stress induces metaplastic conversion to fibrocartilage, which, through the process of endochondral ossification, results in heterotopic bone formation (Fig. 1).

Also, in a recent research, Pfitzner et al. (2012) found that bone morphogenetic protein 2 (BMP-2), a low-molecular-weight glycoprotein in the TGF-ß protein superfamily, was overexpressed and its synovial fluid concentrations were higher in patients suffering from arthrofibrosis. They concluded that the synovial BMP-2 concentration might be a potential marker for differentiating between intra- and extra-articular causes of fibrosis and pain.

Histopathology

There are variable reports about histopathologic description of arthrofibrosis (Jackson and Schaefer 1990; Noyes et al. 1991; Gillespie et al. 1993, 1998). It was initially studied in localized forms of arthrofibrosis. In 1987, Paulos et al. (1987) described infrapatellar contracture syndrome (IPCS), and they observed a dense, fibrosclerotic reaction with disorganized collagen in the biopsy specimens. In 1990, Jackson and Schaefer (1990) expressed the "cyclops" nodule histopathologically as peripheral fibrous tissue with a central region of granulation tissue. They also noted bony fragments and cartilaginous tissue in some of their specimens. Thereafter, in 1991, Noyes et al. (1991) reported that in patients

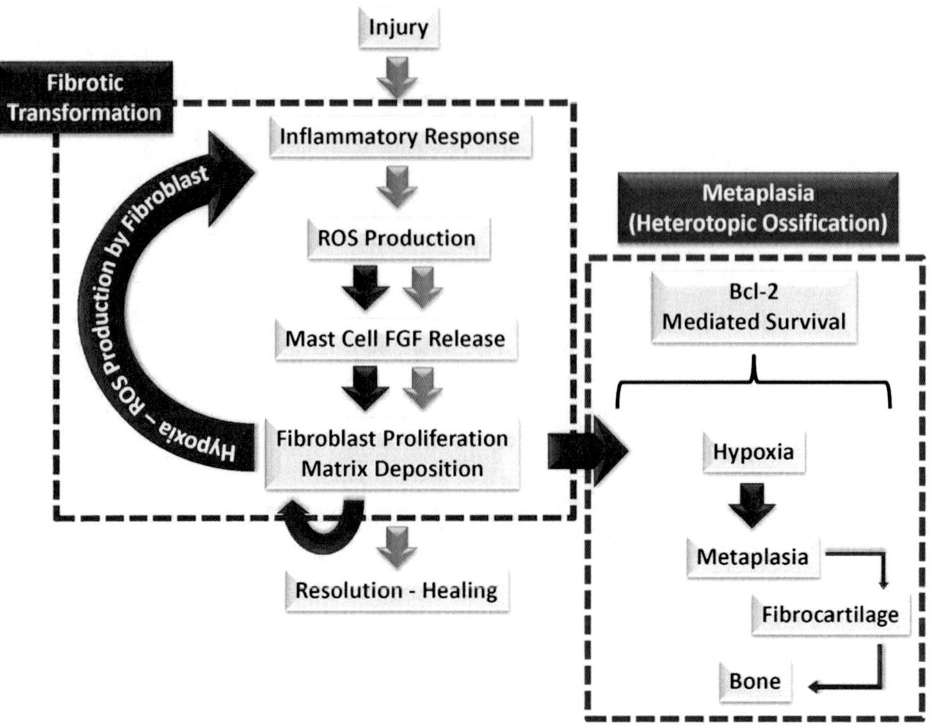

Fig. 1 Arthrofibrotic progression pathway. Normal healing pathway is denoted by *blue arrows*, and disease progression pathway is indicated by *red arrows*. The *red box* indicates the etiology of the oxidative fibrotic transformation process (Freeman et al 2009). The *purple box* indicates the pathology of metaplastic heterotopic ossification (Freeman et al 2010)

with developmental patella infera syndrome, histologically fibroblastic and endothelial proliferation was seen with dense collagen fiber formation in the specimens. In 1993, Gillespie et al. (1993) defined the histopathologic descriptions of arthrofibrosis in 22 surgical specimens: fibrosis, vascular proliferation, and synovial chondrometaplasia. They also found bone formation in two specimens similar to Jackson and Schaefer (1990). The authors proposed that there was a trend toward maturity of synovial chondrometaplasia as the interval between the surgery and resection of arthrofibrosis was lengthened (Gillespie et al. 1993). Murakami et al. (1997) described synovitis in the infrapatellar fat pad following anterior cruciate ligament (ACL) reconstruction that may lead to arthrofibrosis. They found synovial hyperplasia, infiltration of inflammatory cells, vascular proliferation, and PDGF- and TGF-β-positive cells. In 2001, Bosch et al. (2001) took fibrotic tissue samples from 18 patients undergoing open arthrolysis of the knee joint for symptomatic arthrofibrosis and stained the samples for immunohistological analysis. Based on their study, they concluded that arthrofibrosis is the result of a T-cell-mediated immune response resulting in the formation of diffuse scar tissue within the knee joint. In a recent study, Freeman et al. (2010) found that the arthrofibrotic tissues consist of three distinct regions. Two of these regions were fibrotic, one was a highly vascularized area around the periphery of the tissue, and the other area contained disorganized matrix and increased proteoglycan content. Directly contiguous to the fibrotic areas was the third region type, consisting of avascular fibrocartilage, which undergoes endochondral ossification to form bone (Fig. 2).

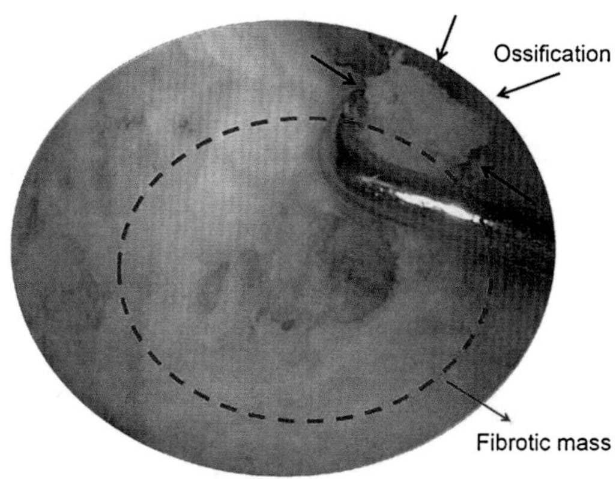

Fig. 2 Arthroscopic view of endochondral ossification adjacent to the fibrotic mass

Symptoms, Clinical Findings, and Classification

Knee motion depends on a smooth articulation between the femur and tibia; a flexible joint capsule; free space in the lateral and medial recesses, intercondylar notch, and suprapatellar pouch; and sufficient meniscal motion. A systematic evaluation of the knee is recommended to ascertain which abnormalities are responsible.

The most common presentation of arthrofibrosis is a patient who has undergone ACL or multiligament reconstructions. The evaluation of patients with arthrofibrosis begins with a patient history for initial trauma or surgery. The clinician should ask about pain, instability, mechanical symptoms, history of knee injuries or surgeries, and the length of immobilization. Arthrofibrosis of the knee is poorly tolerated by patients, and they complain about stiffness, pain, limping, edema around knee, crepitus, and quadriceps weakness.

Physical examination begins with inspection. The skin is inspected for scar formation that gives clues for the etiology of arthrofibrosis. It is also important for the future surgery planning. The signs of CRPS are inspected over the skin. There may be erythema over the skin and sometimes radiance of the skin may be observed. Then, the form of the knee is assessed for fullness due to the fibrotic tissues of hypertrophic synovium, especially on suprapatellar pouch. After the inspection, patellar mobility is evaluated. Typically, the patella exhibits decreased mobility in all directions in patients with arthrofibrosis. Next, ROM is examined both passively and actively and compared to the unaffected knee. The painless end point is pathognomonic clinical sign of arthrofibrosis. A soft block is appropriate for physical therapy, as well as tolerated by the patient. If there is no difference in regard to ROM with physical therapy, arthrofibrosis is suspected even there is no feeling of an end point.

Shelbourne et al. (1996) described a classification system based on the pattern of knee stiffness. Type I patients have normal flexion and $<10°$ extension loss. Type II patients have normal flexion and $>10°$ extension loss. Type III patients have a combined flexion loss of $>25°$ and extension loss of $>10°$ with patellar tightness. Type IV patients have a flexion loss of $\geq 30°$ and extension loss of $>10°$, combined with patella infera and marked patellar tightness.

Arthrofibrosis may be associated with both extension and flexion loss. Scarring can occur from the patella to the intercondylar notch, suprapatellar pouch, and ultimately within the articular surfaces. Capsular and quadriceps contractions further reduce joint mobility. The anatomic site of fibrosis determines the type of motion loss. Adhesions in the suprapatellar pouch, medial gutter, and lateral gutter restrict knee flexion. Causes of extension loss include notch impingement, cyclops lesion, and posterior capsule contracture. Causes of both extension and flexion loss include improper graft position during ACL reconstruction, anterior interval scarring ((IPCS), which causes flexion loss predominantly), soft tissue calcifications, CRPS, and infection (Kim et al. 2004).

Imaging can be very helpful in the evaluation and includes both x-rays and magnetic resonance imaging (MRI) of the knee. X-rays can identify loose bodies and bony blocks within the knee in cases of arthrofibrosis (Fig. 3). The calcification of the infrapatellar fat pad may be seen on lateral x-ray, whereas the calcification of the medial

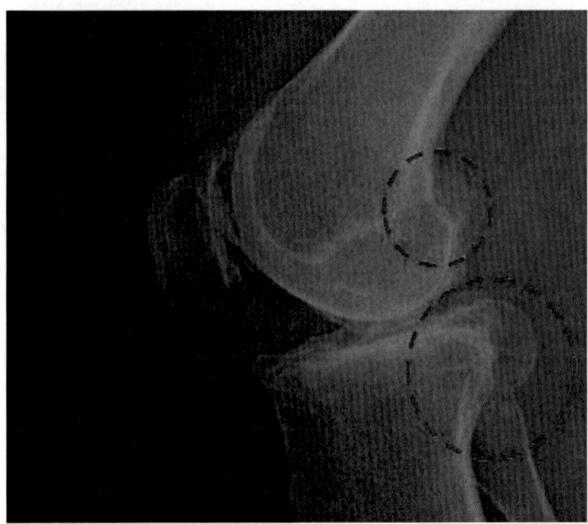

Fig. 3 The radiologic view of bony blocks (*red circles*) in the posterior part of femoral condyles and tibial plateau

collateral ligament (MCL, Pellegrini-Stieda lesion) is best evaluated on AP radiographs. MCL calcification impairs both flexion and extension. MRI can help to both diagnose and determine the extent of the disease.

Cosgarea et al. (1994) further classified arthrofibrosis into two variants: localized intra-articular variants and global arthrofibrosis. The localized variants are described in four groups below.

Cyclops Lesion

In 1990, Jackson and Schaefer (1990) described the cyclops lesion as a nodular and vascular soft tissue mass at the base of the ACL stump that caused isolated loss of extension. This tissue may locate anterior to the ACL body or ACL tibial stump. Similarly, the fibrotic tissues appearing at the roof of the notch can cause isolated loss of extension (Fig. 4). The etiology of a cyclops lesion appears to be multifactorial, and this fibroproliferative tissue originates from drilling debris of the tibial tunnel or from remnants of the native ACL or from the scar tissue occurred by repeated graft impingement of a malpositioned graft (Delincé et al. 1998). After ACL reconstruction, an anteriorly placed femoral tunnel or overtensioned graft can limit knee flexion (Romano et al. 1993; Nabors et al. 1995; Fu et al. 1999). An anteriorly placed ACL graft on the tibia, because of its position, would impinge on the intercondylar notch and limit knee extension. This impingement could lead piling up of the graft fibers anteriorly, causing to the formation of cyclops lesion, which could further limit knee extension (Marzo et al. 1992; Delincé et al. 1998) (Fig. 5a, b).

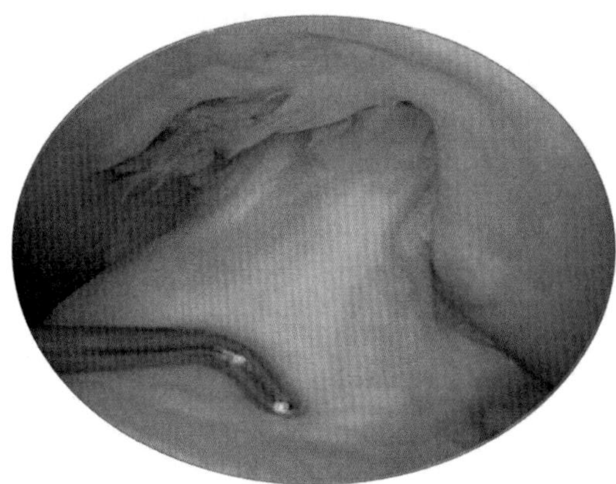

Fig. 4 Variants of cyclops lesion. The tibial roof of the notch is filled with fibrotic tissue

Infrapatellar Contracture Syndrome

The anterior interval is between the infrapatellar fat pad and patellar tendon anteriorly and the anterior border of the tibia and transverse

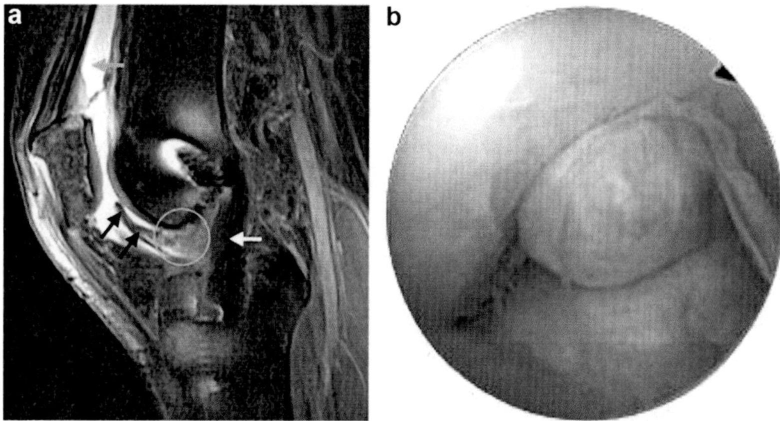

Fig. 5 (**a**) Magnetic resonance image of the fibrotic tissue (*yellow circle*) and piling of graft fibers (*black arrows*) that limit knee extension. (**b**) Arthroscopic view of the cyclops lesion

meniscal ligament posteriorly (Steadman et al. 2008). Trauma or previous surgery may cause hemorrhage or inflammation of the fat pad, which may result in fibrosis. Fibrosis that occurs between the fat pad and the transverse meniscal ligament or the anterior tibia leads to dysfunction of anterior knee structures (e.g., decreased mobility of the patellar tendon) and results in stretching of the surrounding synovial tissue, which may cause pain or loss of knee extension (Steadman et al. 2008).

In 1987, Paulos et al. (1987) described IPCS, which is a severe form of fibrosis of the fat pad with extension loss, flexion loss, and patellar entrapment. A fibrotic band forms between the patella and anterior tibia, which causes patella infera (Fig. 6), thereby resulting in patellar entrapment anterior to the intercondylar notch. Subsequently, the predominant outcome is flexion loss. Sometimes, the fibrotic band appears as a fibrotic nodule, which causes an additional extension loss. Paulos et al. (1987) described three stages of IPCS: the prodromal stage (stage I), the active stage (stage II), and the residual stage (stage III). The prodromal stage (stage I) occurs 2–8 weeks after surgery. Physical examination typically demonstrates swelling and tenderness around the patellar tendon, painful ROM, restricted patellar mobility, and quadriceps muscle weakness and lag. Failure to progress with rehabilitation is an important clue. The active stage (stage II) occurs 6–20 weeks after surgery. In this stage, patients have continued peripatellar swelling, induration of the fat pad, marked quadriceps atrophy,

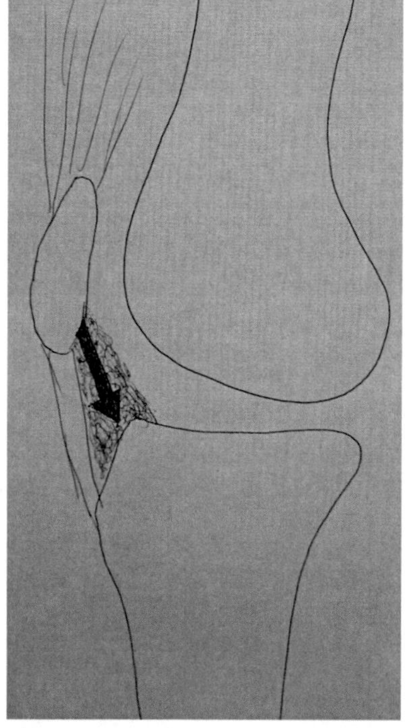

Fig. 6 Infrapatellar contracture syndrome. Fibrosis of the fat pad causing to motion loss and patella infera

worsening knee motion, and severely restricted patellar mobility (especially superior glide). The residual stage (stage III) occurs 8 months to years after surgery and is characterized by marked quadriceps atrophy, fat pad atrophy, patellofemoral crepitus, and in most cases patellofemoral arthrosis. Developmental patella infera is often present.

The clinical diagnosis of IPCS is confirmed with imaging studies. To detect patella infera, preoperative and postoperative lateral radiographs should be compared. The calcification of fat pad may also be observed. The most significant abnormality noted on MRI is pathologic scar formation in the anterior knee. Moreover, the intensity of the fat pad may be abnormal. Also, some accompanying fibrotic adhesions at the medial and lateral gutter and patellofemoral pouch may be seen on MRI. The definitive diagnosis for IPCS is achieved by arthroscopic examination through the superomedial (SM) and superolateral (SL) portals.

Patellar Clunk Syndrome

The term "patellar clunk syndrome" and its pathology were first described by Hozack et al. (1989) in 1989 as a complication in posteriorly stabilized knee prosthesis. This syndrome is described as development of a fibrous nodule just proximal to patella and lodging of the nodule into the intercondylar notch of the femoral component during flexion. Patients experience a painful and audible clunk as their knee was brought from flexion to extension (Hozack et al. 1989; Pollock et al. 2002). It is a well-documented cause of intra-articular mechanical symptoms after total knee arthroplasty (TKA), and its incidence after primary TKA varies from 0 % to 13.3 % (Lonner et al. 2007; Fukunaga et al. 2009).

The exact cause of patellar clunk syndrome had not been identified. Impingement of the anterosuperior edge of the femoral box or the patella component itself into the quadriceps tendon has been theorized to be the cause of the fibrous nodule (Hozack et al. 1989). The etiologic factors are proposed to be the surgical technique, component design, component positioning, extent of surgical trauma, alteration of joint line, patellar height, patellar thickness, and patellar tracking (Hozack et al. 1989; Fukunaga et al. 2009; Frye et al. 2012). For the surgical technique, arthroscopic debridement of the peripatellar synovium, especially at the junction of the rectus femoris tendon and the patella, was advised (Dajani et al. 2010). Also, increased flexion of the femoral component or a proximal position of the patellar component must be avoided during component positioning. Patellar clunk syndrome can occur with posterior cruciate-sparing designs and isolated patellofemoral arthroplasties; however, these complications are predominantly encountered with posterior cruciate-substituting components (Pollock et al. 2002; Sringari and Maheswaran 2005; Lonner et al. 2007; Dajani et al. 2010). Newer prosthesis designs are promising to avoid the syndrome (Clarke et al. 2006; Lonner et al. 2007; Dajani et al. 2010).

Localized Intra-articular Scarring

These fibrotic bands can be classified in two varieties according to anatomic location: the fibrotic bands extending between capsular parts (in suprapatellar pouch, in the medial and lateral gutters) (Fig. 7) and the fibrotic bands extending from capsule to articular cartilage. These two varieties can arise concurrently. The latter fibrotic bands generally extend from the anterior capsule or from fat pad to trochlear cartilage (Fig. 8) and from gutters or from suprapatellar pouch to patellar cartilage (Fig. 9a, b). The most important fibrotic bands that affect prognosis are the bands inserting on the cartilage. If these bands are not debrided in 6 months, the nourishment and homeostasis of the cartilage can be disrupted, which in turn can lead to irreversible damage (Fig. 10).

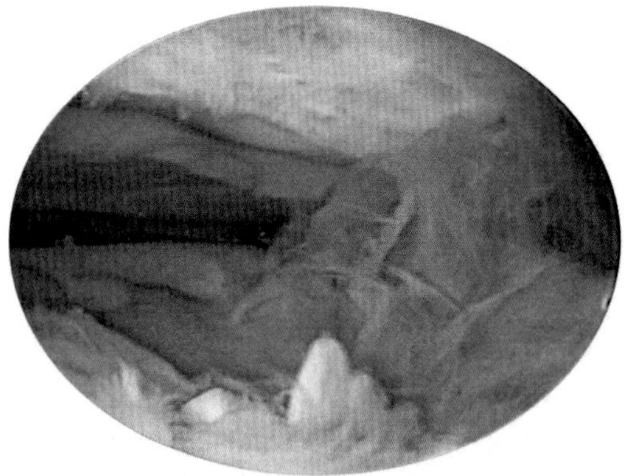

Fig. 7 The superomedial portal view of fibrotic bands extending from patella to suprapatellar pouch

Treatment

A thorough history and physical examination are vital in evaluating a patient with motion loss. It is important to determine whether the patient has a loss of flexion, a loss of extension, or a combination of both. It is also important if the patient has had previous surgery. A thorough study about the previous surgery should be performed. This will aid in understanding the cause of arthrofibrosis (i.e., timing of surgery, multiligament reconstruction, etc.). In the postoperative period, if the expected progress for the ROM cannot be achieved by physical therapy, the surgeon should concern about impending arthrofibrosis.

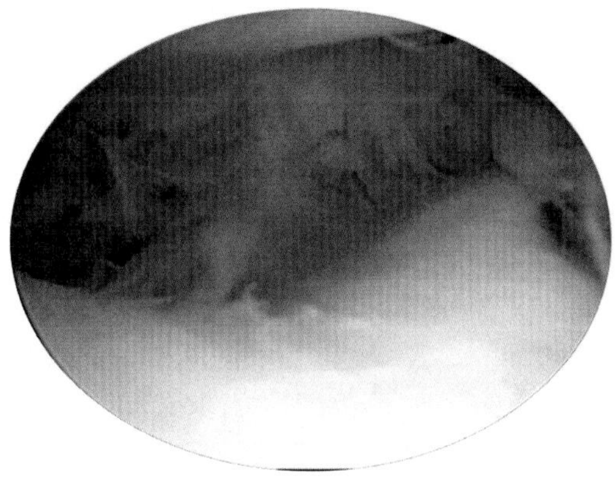

Fig. 8 The superomedial portal view of fibrotic bands extending from anteromedial part of the capsule to trochlea

The initial course of treatment is aggressive physical therapy. Often this requires direct discussion with the physiotherapist involved and patient compliance. Physical therapy should focus on stretching exercises. Nonsteroidal anti-inflammatory medications help to decrease pain and swelling, therefore allowing the patient to tolerate more aggressive physical therapy. For the extension deficits, extension splinting or braces are advised to use while ambulation and sleeping (Shelbourne et al. 1996; Biggs and Shelbourne 2006). Generally, the extension deficits due to posterior capsular tightness relieve well with physical therapy. The physical therapy period is adjusted according to the type and stage of the arthrofibrosis, and the progression of motion is reassessed throughout the therapy (Gillespie et al. 1998).

Additional intervention is indicated in patients who fail initial physical therapy. Manipulation under anesthesia (MUA) has been recommended within 4–12 weeks postoperatively in patients who have not regained full ROM following surgery (Noyes et al. 2000). However, isolated MUA has the risks of intra-articular hemorrhage and recurrence of arthrofibrosis and complications

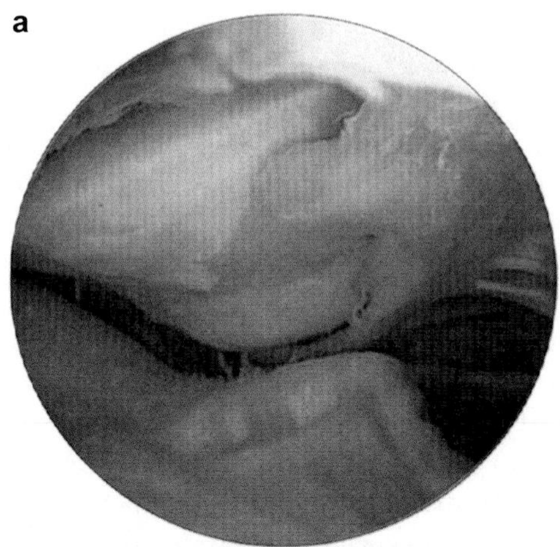

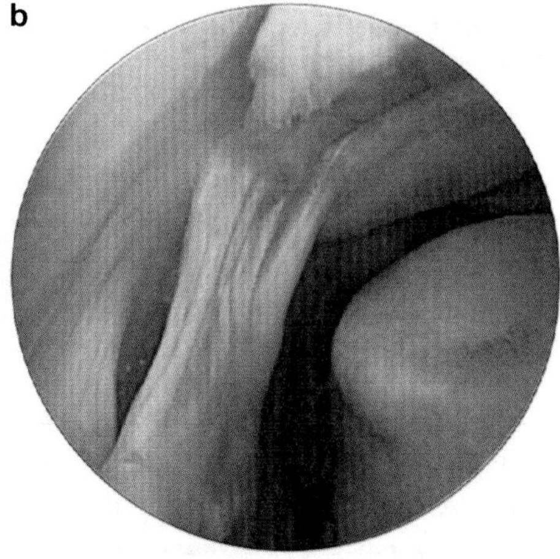

Fig. 9 (**a**) The superomedial portal view of fibrotic bands extending from anterior part of the capsule to medial articular facet of patella. (**b**) The superomedial portal view of fibrotic bands extending from lateral capsule to lateral part of patella, causing to lateral pull of patella

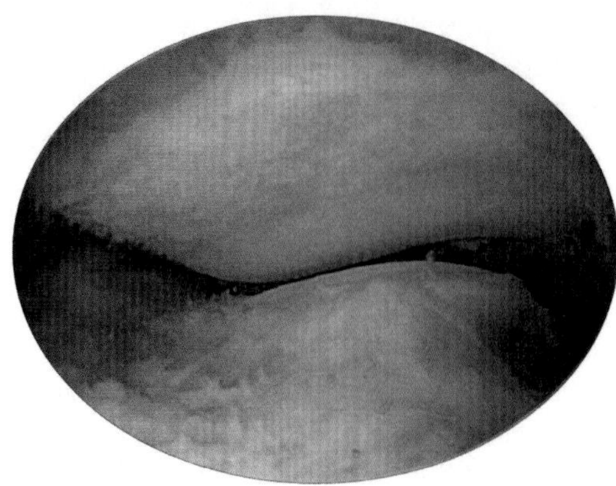

Fig. 10 Arthroscopic view of the overt irreversible damage to patellar cartilage despite debridement of fibrotic bands

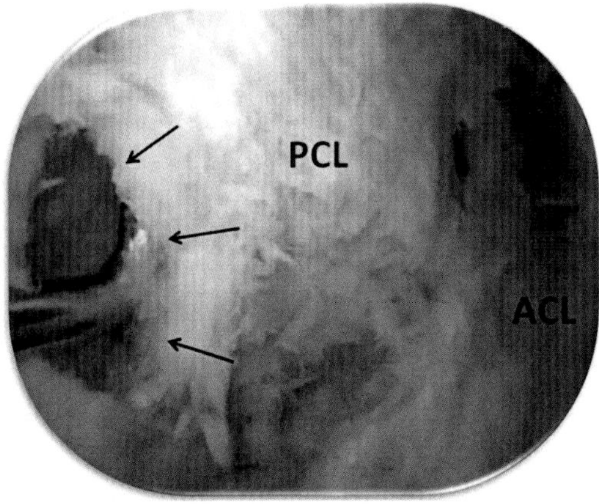

Fig. 11 Posterior cruciate ligament (*PCL*) avulsion fracture is indicated by *black arrows*. It can be seen after isolated manipulation or after arthroscopic arthrolysis and manipulation. ACL, anterior cruciate ligament

such as excessive tibiofemoral and patellofemoral compression with the risk of chondral damage or fracture, rupture of the patellar tendon, distal femoral fracture, posterior cruciate ligament (PCL) avulsion fracture (Fig. 11), and CRPS. Therefore, it is not recommended.

Although it is not logical to determine absolute criteria for surgical intervention, arthroscopic debridement combined with MUA is preferred after 6 weeks of failed conservative treatment. Arthroscopic debridement, open debridement, and combined open and arthroscopic debridement are the surgical treatment modalities for arthrofibrosis. Open procedures are more invasive, extend surgery and postoperative recovery time, increase the risk of postoperative infection, and lead to unpleasant surgical scars. Therefore, arthroscopic debridement gained popularity because of being effective in improving ROM and restoring function with minimal complications. However, arthroscopic treatment is generally most effective when the underlying pathology is predominately intra-articular. When the etiology of the motion loss involves extra-articular structures, often a combined approach involving both arthroscopic and open techniques is indicated (Millett et al. 1999).

Generally, arthroscopic debridement combined with a controlled post-arthroscopic MUA is preferred after the 6 weeks of failed conservative treatment modalities. Sprague et al. (1982) were first to report the results of 24 patients treated with arthroscopic debridement for "fibroarthrosis." They were able to improve ROM 45° at a mean follow-up of 8 months. Many studies reported similar results with knee ROM improvements after arthroscopic debridement with or without knee manipulation (Marzo et al. 1992; Harner et al. 1992; Fisher and Shelbourne 1993; Cosgarea et al. 1994; Shelbourne et al. 1996; Millett et al. 1999; LaPrade et al. 2008; Mariani 2010). Jackson and Schaefer (1990) were the first to describe the cyclops lesion after ACL reconstruction and reported on 13 patients who underwent arthroscopic debridement with knee manipulation and achieved an average improvement of loss of extension from 16° to 3.8°. Similarly, Marzo et al. (1992) reported on 21 patients who improved on an average loss of extension of 11° to an average of 0° at a 1-year follow-up after arthroscopic removal of fibrous nodules in the intercondylar notch. LaPrade et al. (2008) reported the results of 15 patients who underwent isolated arthroscopic posteromedial release. Preoperative knee extension averaged 15° and significantly improved to 0.07° at an average of 24 months' follow-up. Mariani (2010) reported the results of 18 patients with extension deficits that averaged 34° (range, 16–44°) who were treated with posterior capsular release. Extension deficits averaged 3° (range, 0–5°) at a final 1-year follow-up.

Arthroscopic Technique

Regional epidural anesthesia with sedation and the placement of an epidural catheter are preferred. The catheter is necessary for pain control and allows more intensive physical therapy in the immediate postoperative period.

The operative table is set to allow hanging of the operative leg freely, and the nonoperative limb is placed in a leg holder and well padded. A knee holder on the operative leg is not used because this will impede the instruments working in the suprapatellar pouch and restrict MUA. A nonsterile tourniquet is applied as proximal as possible on the thigh to allow easy manipulation of arthroscopic instruments through the superior portals. An arthroscopic pump is routinely used to maintain constant intra-articular pressure between 50 and 60 mmHg.

A four-portal arthroscopy is performed for arthroscopic arthrolysis of the knee. In addition to the universal anterolateral (AL) and anteromedial (AM) portals, a SM portal and a SL portal are prepared. The SM portal is prepared at the most proximal part of the suprapatellar pouch, just medial to quadriceps tendon for the scope. The SL portal is localized 2.5 cm distal to the SM portal and 2.5 cm lateral to the quadriceps tendon. The superior portals are the best portals to view patellofemoral articulation and gutters and also to debride fibrotic adhesions while the knee is in extension (Fig. 12a, b). Moreover, for the treatment of arthrofibrosis, the posteromedial and posterolateral portals are used when needed.

A thorough arthroscopic arthrolysis is the procedure that necessitates a skilled and experienced surgeon. Then, the AL and AM portals are next prepared. At the first look of the arthroscopy, the surgeon may face intensive fibrotic tissue that must be debrided. After that, to evaluate the cause of extension deficit, the anterior portion of intercondylar notch is inspected. Fibrous nodules (cyclops lesion), anterior fibrotic bands, and bony blocks are explored (Fig. 13). In rare overt cases of graft malposition, the ACL or even the PCL grafts might need to be released that can also cause mechanical blocks for full extension. Then, adhesions in the suprapatellar pouch are identified and released with arthroscopic scissors (Fig. 14a, b). The adhesions are released till to the most proximal part of suprapatellar pouch. Once reached to the most proximal part of suprapatellar pouch, SM portal is prepared just medial to quadriceps tendon. Then, the SL portal was localized 2.5 cm distal to the SM portal and 2.5 cm lateral to the quadriceps tendon. Next, the medial and lateral gutters are inspected and releases are performed via the SM and SL portals. The fat pad and peripatellar fibrotic tissues can easily be evaluated by the superior portals. The superior portals are affective especially for arthroscopic arthrolysis of IPCS. Aggressive shavers and arthroscopic scissors are passed through the patellofemoral joint, and the fibrotic tissues are

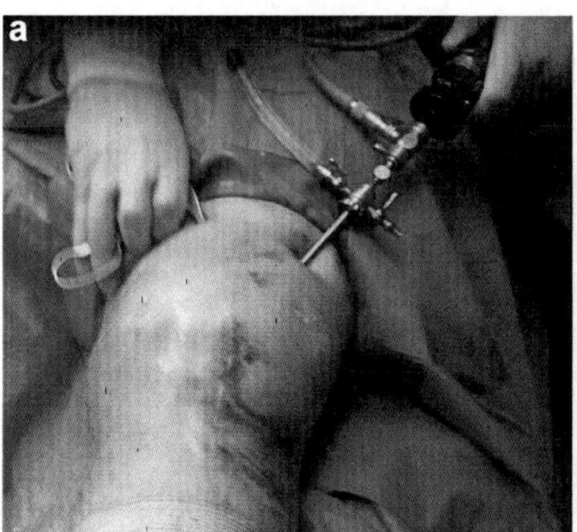

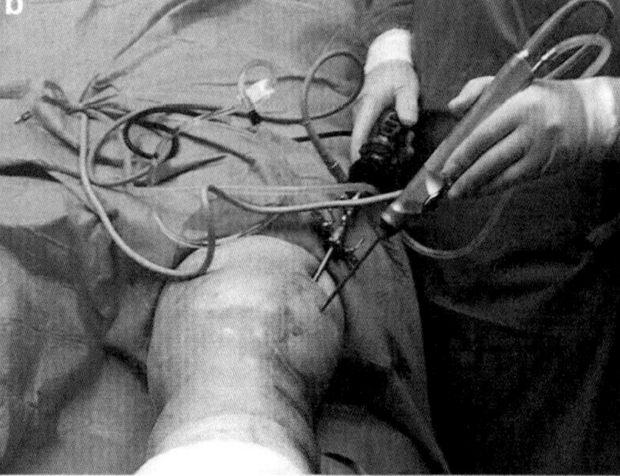

Fig. 12 (**a**, **b**) Arthroscopic arthrolysis of a prosthetic knee by the superior portals to view patellofemoral articulation and gutters

released until the anterior tibial cortex or the normal fat pad is seen. At this step, AM and AL portals can be used when needed. Knee motion is then assessed. If full extension cannot be achieved despite to the removal of anterior scarring, the tibial insertion of the posterior capsule is inspected and the posterior portals are established. To work in the posterior part of the knee, disposable arthroscopic cannulas and sometimes a 70° arthroscope are used. The posterior transseptal portal for arthroscopic surgery of the knee can be used as previously advised (Ahn and Ha 2000). Excision of scar tissue and removal of any loose bodies are performed, paying particular attention not to injure the neurovascular structures. The knee is gently manipulated and ROM is assessed. Postoperative knee motion will not improve from that obtained in surgery. Therefore, if a loss of extension or flexion persists intraoperatively, the maximal range of motion is attempted before leaving the operating room. The whole articular cartilage of three bones is thoroughly evaluated from every portal and chondroplasty is performed, when needed. The chondroplasty is an important issue for arthroscopic arthrolysis of arthrofibrosis. The fibrotic bands which are attached to chondral tissue more than 6 months of duration can cause irreversible chondral damage. Therefore, the fibrotic bands must be debrided thoroughly from the chondral tissue before 6 months. The tourniquet is released and two drains are placed to decrease the occurrence of postoperative hemarthrosis, which can contribute to both pain and adhesions. The drains are left in place for 48 h. An angle adjustable knee brace is locked in full extension.

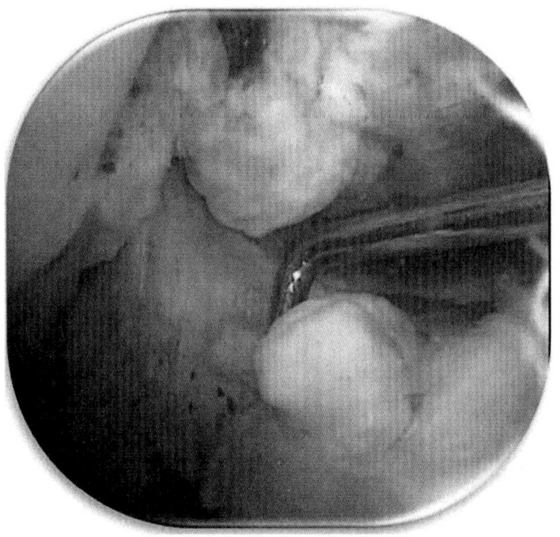

Fig. 13 Bony blocks in the anterior part of tibial plateau

Postoperative Rehabilitation

Patients are hospitalized to take advantage of the analgesic properties provided by the indwelling epidural catheter and postoperatively can have indwelling femoral and sciatic catheters as needed

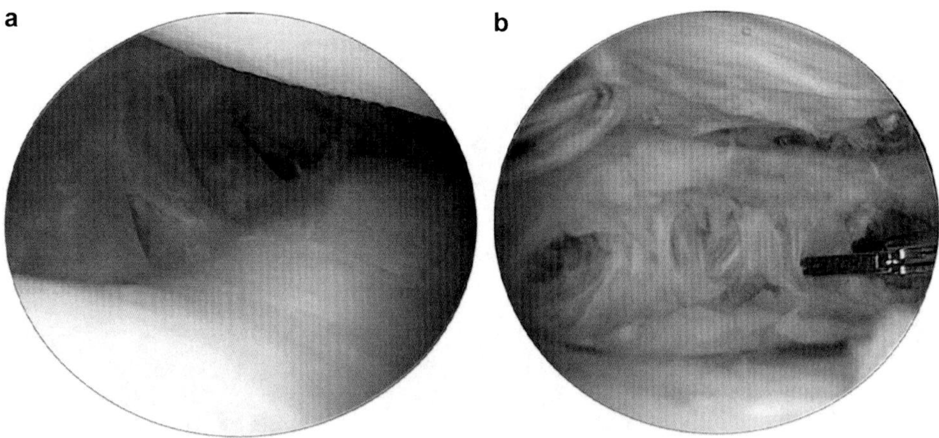

Fig. 14 (**a**) The fibrotic adhesions filling the suprapatellar pouch (anterolateral portal view). (**b**) The adhesions in the suprapatellar pouch are released with arthroscopic scissors via the anteromedial portal

for pain control. But the femoral and sciatic catheters are not comfortable in a mobile extremity. An adjustable knee brace which is locked in full extension is continued until the drains are taken out. Thereafter, physical therapy of the patients is initiated with a continuous passive motion (CPM) machine. Home CPM is continued for 2–6 weeks for 6–8 h a day. Weight bearing is permitted as tolerated. The adjustable angle knee braces are locked in full extension during walking and sleeping. Patellar mobility exercises, extensor mechanism exercises, and full passive and active-assisted ROM exercises are all essential components of therapy.

Prevention

Prevention is the most effective means of avoiding motion loss following knee injury or surgery. Patient selection is the initial key to avoid postoperative motion loss. Before deciding for any knee surgery, associated injuries and the patient's ability to participate postoperative rehabilitation program must be considered.

For ACL reconstruction, timing of the surgery is believed to be very important in preventing the potential development of arthrofibrosis (Beynnon et al. 2005; Magit et al. 2007). In 1990, Strum et al. (1990) reported a significant difference in the incidence of arthrofibrosis between acute (less than 3 weeks after injury) and chronic ACL reconstructions. Subsequently, several studies confirmed this recommendation (Shelbourne et al. 1991; Wasilewski et al. 1993). However, other studies have indicated surgical timing had less of an effect when early motion was instituted (Hunter et al. 1996; Majors and Woodfin 1996). This conclusion was supported in randomized controlled trials and in a recent systematic review (Bottoni et al. 2008; Raviraj et al. 2010; Smith et al. 2010). These authors concluded that there was no difference in clinical outcome between patients who underwent early and those who underwent delayed ACL reconstruction. Finally, in a very recent meta-analysis, Kwok et al. (2013) state that there is no increased risk of postoperative stiffness if an ACL reconstruction is performed as early as the first week after injury, as long as an accelerated rehabilitation protocol is followed postoperatively.

Anatomic placement of the graft is important during ACL or PCL reconstruction. The tunnels should be created at the anatomic native cruciate attachment sites (Ziegler et al. 2011; Anderson et al. 2012). Otherwise, impingement can occur with knee motion, establishing the background for arthrofibrosis. Arthrofibrosis is generally observed with the femoral tunnels that are placed high on the top and anteriorly by a transtibial technique during ACL reconstruction. This causes restriction of knee flexion. If the ACL graft is positioned too anteriorly on the tibial side, impingement of the graft against the roof of the intercondylar notch occurs on extension. Impingement of the graft can be visualized arthroscopically in full extension and flexion before completion of the case. These technical errors may result with cyclops formation.

In the postoperative period, modalities such as ice, compression, elevation, aspiration of a postoperative effusion, physical therapy, nonsteroidal anti-inflammatory drugs, and a short-term course of oral corticosteroids can be used to decrease knee pain and inflammation (Noyes et al. 2000). Postoperative immobilization should be kept to a minimum, and rehabilitation should be started immediately. Because flexion can be achieved more easily than extension, efforts should be directed toward gaining full extension (Chen and Dragoo 2011). Isometric strengthening of the quadriceps helps to restore extension and prevents atrophy. Early patellar mobilization prevents adhesion formation and contracture of the patellar tendon.

The deleterious effects of immobilization on the ligamentous and articular surfaces of joints have been reported in the literature (Enneking and Horowitz 1972; Akeson et al. 1987). Intra-articular changes include fibrotic adhesions between synovial folds and cartilage surfaces, atrophy of cartilage, and cartilage ulceration (Akeson et al. 1987). Also, immobilization may lead to extra-articular changes including disorganization of ligament cellular and fibrillar alignment, weakening of ligament insertion sites, regional osteoporosis, increased force requirements for joint cycling, and increased ligament compliance (Akeson et al. 1987). The beneficial effects of controlled motion and low stress on ligaments with respect to stiffness and strength are the basis of recent postoperative management.

Historically, early postoperative rehabilitation protocols for ACL reconstruction did not permit immediate full ROM and full weight bearing in order to protect the graft. Restricted ROM and limited weight bearing lead to muscle atrophy and may cause to the development of adhesions and soft tissue contractures (Magit et al. 2007; vanGrinsven et al. 2010; Beynnon et al. 2011). Therefore, these rehabilitation regimens were associated with an increased risk of postoperative stiffness. As it was stated in the recent meta-analysis of Kwok et al. (2013), modern rehabilitation protocols declined the risk of arthrofibrosis. The current approach is to encourage the patients for full ROM and full weight bearing as early as possible.

Stiffness After Total Knee Arthroplasty

Stiffness after TKA is a common problem occurring in 8–60 % of patients (Fitzsimmons et al. 2010). For evaluation of a stiff TKA, the surgeon must consider component position in the first glance and take into account the previous factors that contribute to a stiff knee. If motion loss is determined to be caused by malpositioned or loose components, revision TKA is the treatment of choice.

The risk factors for stiffness after TKA can be grouped according to preoperative, intraoperative, and postoperative periods (SchiavonePanni et al. 2009; Ghani et al. 2012). Decreased preoperative ROM is a well-known preoperative risk factor, and also a history of previous surgery and diabetes mellitus are reported to be risk factors for stiffness after TKA (SchiavonePanni et al. 2009). The component positioning is the most important intraoperative risk factor that affects postoperative ROM. Postoperative risk factors leading to decreased ROM include poor patient motivation, lack of compliance with physiotherapy, deep infection, patellar complications, CRPS, and heterotopic ossification (Ghani et al. 2012).

The various treatment options available for arthrofibrosis of the knee are physical therapy, manipulation under anesthesia (MUA), arthroscopic arthrolysis, open arthrolysis, and revision TKA.

If stiffness is encountered within the first 3 months and the patient does not have an infection and has appropriately fixed and positioned components, an aggressive physical therapy and home exercise program are started. However, generally, the results after physical therapy may not be satisfactory. Esler et al. (1999) reported an average increase in knee motion of only 5° in a group of patients with arthrofibrosis after TKA treated with physical therapy alone.

If the physical therapy is not successful within the first 3 months, MUA is often the next step. Manipulations were not performed 3 months after TKA surgery because of decreased effectiveness and the risk of fracture after that time (Seyler et al. 2007). In a recent systematic review, it was proposed that manipulation is more effective during the first few months because there is less adhesive tissue in the knee (Fitzsimmons et al. 2010). Sharma et al. (2008) recommended injection of a local anesthetic and steroid at the time of manipulation to preserve the ROM gained during manipulation.

If manipulation alone is not adequate, the addition of arthroscopic debridement or open arthrolysis is the next step of treatment. In their recent review, Fitzsimmons et al. (2010) concluded that arthroscopy (with manipulation) seems to provide substantial increases in ROM even when performed 1 year after the TKA. They also concluded that the gains in ROM after manipulation and arthroscopy (with manipulation) were similar in patients with arthrofibrosis after TKA, and open arthrolysis provided inferior results. However, in a more recent review, Ghani et al. (2012) reported that open surgical release showed the highest improvement in ROM with a value of 43.4° and manipulation and arthroscopy had a similar mean improvement in ROM being as

38.4° and 36.2°, respectively. Nevertheless, both recent reviews agree that the data are limited to come to a conclusion with a higher quality of evidence. Therefore, well-designed randomized controlled trials with blinded measurement of outcomes are needed to confirm the results found in these systematic reviews.

When a systematic approach is used during arthroscopy, there is no need to open arthrolysis to improve ROM. If the ROM failed to progress to 0–90° in the postoperative 6th week, aggressive physical therapy is enforced for the following 2 weeks. At the end of the 8th week, if the flexion of 90° was not achieved, a MUA is done. If an extension deficit was accompanying to flexion deficit, arthroscopic arthrolysis is added to the procedure. Meanwhile, as a reasonable notion, arthroscopic arthrolysis is performed more aggressively for the native knees than for the prosthetic knees, because of the damage risk on viable chondral tissue of native knees by fibrotic bands. For the prosthetic knees, the surgeon can insist on MUA.

Conclusion

Arthrofibrosis of the knee is not a rare complication. However, because of an unclear and multifactorial etiopathogenesis, to avoid such a complication is sometimes not possible, even following a well-performed surgery and meticulous postoperative physical therapy. Arthrofibrosis may be underdiagnosed, because it usually does not present as a global stiffness of the knee. Therefore, the surgeons must be aware of localized forms of arthrofibrosis. To diagnose and treat arthrofibrosis, a thorough patient history and a systematic evaluation of the knee are vital. The initial treatment must be aggressive physical therapy for the first 6 weeks. If the conservative treatment fails, a comprehensive arthroscopic arthrolysis via multiple arthroscopic portals and MUA must be performed by an experienced surgeon. Finally, a careful and immediate postoperative rehabilitation is mandatory for successful outcomes in the postoperative period.

Cross-References

▸ Rehabilitation of Complex Knee Injuries and Key Points
▸ Special Considerations for Multiple-Ligament Knee Injuries

References

Ahn JH, Ha CW (2000) Posterior trans-septal portal for arthroscopic surgery of the knee joint. Arthroscopy 16:774–779

Akeson WH, Amiel D, Abel MF et al (1987) Effects of immobilization on joints. Clin Orthop Relat Res 219:28–37

Anderson CJ, Ziegler CG, Wijdicks CA et al (2012) Arthroscopically pertinent anatomy of the anterolateral and posteromedial bundles of the posterior cruciate ligament. J Bone Joint Surg Am 94:1936–1945

Baran CP, Zeigler MM, Tridandapani S et al (2004) The role of ROS and RNS in regulating life and death of blood monocytes. Curr Pharm Des 10:855–866, Review

Beynnon BD, Johnson RJ, Abate JA et al (2005) Treatment of anterior cruciate ligament injuries, part I. Am J Sports Med 33:1579–1602, Review

Beynnon BD, Johnson RJ, Naud S et al (2011) Accelerated versus nonaccelerated rehabilitation after anterior cruciate ligament reconstruction: a prospective, randomized, double-blind investigation evaluating knee joint laxity using roentgen stereophotogrammetric analysis. Am J Sports Med 39:2536–2548

Biggs A, Shelbourne KD (2006) Use of knee extension device during rehabilitation of a patient with type 3 arthrofibrosis after ACL reconstruction. N Am J Sports Phys Ther 1:124–131

Bosch U, Zeichen J, Skutek M et al (2001) Arthrofibrosis is the result of a T cell mediated immune response. Knee Surg Sports Traumatol Arthrosc 9:282–289

Bottoni CR, Liddell TR, Trainor TJ et al (2008) Postoperative range of motion following anterior cruciate ligament reconstruction using autograft hamstrings: a prospective, randomized clinical trial of early versus delayed reconstructions. Am J Sports Med 36:656–662

Chen MR, Dragoo JL (2011) Arthroscopic releases for arthrofibrosis of the knee. J Am Acad Orthop Surg 19:709–716, Review

Clarke HD, Fuchs R, Scuderi GR et al (2006) The influence of femoral component design in the elimination of patellar clunk in posterior-stabilized total knee arthroplasty. J Arthroplasty 21:167–171

Cochrane AL, Ricardo SD (2003) Oxidant stress and regulation of chemokines in the development of renal interstitial fibrosis. Contrib Nephrol 139:102–119, Review

Cosgarea AJ, DeHaven KE, Lovelock JE (1994) The surgical treatment of arthrofibrosis of the knee. Am J Sports Med 22:184–191

Dajani KA, Stuart MJ, Dahm DL et al (2010) Arthroscopic treatment of patellar clunk and synovial hyperplasia after total knee arthroplasty. J Arthroplasty 25:97–103

Delincé P, Krallis P, Descamps PY et al (1998) Different aspects of the cyclops lesion following anterior cruciate ligament reconstruction: a multifactorial etiopathogenesis. Arthroscopy 14:869–876

Distler JH, Jüngel A, Pileckyte M et al (2007) Hypoxia-induced increase in the production of extracellular matrix proteins in systemic sclerosis. Arthritis Rheum 56:4203–4215

Enneking WF, Horowitz M (1972) The intra-articular effects of immobilization on the human knee. J Bone Joint Surg Am 54:973–985

Esler CN, Lock K, Harper WM et al (1999) Manipulation of total knee replacements. Is the flexion gained retained? J Bone Joint Surg (Br) 81:27–29

Fisher SE, Shelbourne KD (1993) Arthroscopic treatment of symptomatic extension block complicating anterior cruciate ligament reconstruction. Am J Sports Med 21:558–564

Fitzsimmons SE, Vazquez EA, Bronson MJ (2010) How to treat the stiff total knee arthroplasty?: a systematic review. Clin Orthop Relat Res 468:1096–1106

Freeman TA, Parvizi J, Della Valle CJ et al (2009) Reactive oxygen and nitrogen species induce protein and DNA modifications driving arthrofibrosis following total knee arthroplasty. Fibrogenesis Tissue Repair 2:5

Freeman TA, Parvizi J, Dela Valle CJ et al (2010) Mast cells and hypoxia drive tissue metaplasia and heterotopic ossification in idiopathic arthrofibrosis after total knee arthroplasty. Fibrogenesis Tissue Repair 3:17

Frye BM, Floyd MW, Pham DC et al (2012) Effect of femoral component design on patellofemoral crepitance and patella clunk syndrome after posterior-stabilized total knee arthroplasty. J Arthroplasty 27:1166–1170

Fu FH, Bennett CH, Lattermann C et al (1999) Current trends in anterior cruciate ligament reconstruction. Part 1: biology and biomechanics of reconstruction. Am J Sports Med 27:821–830, Review

Fukunaga K, Kobayashi A, Minoda Y et al (2009) The incidence of the patellar clunk syndrome in a recently designed mobile-bearing posteriorly stabilised total knee replacement. J Bone Joint Surg (Br) 91:463–468

Ghani H, Maffulli N, Khanduja V (2012) Management of stiffness following total knee arthroplasty: a systematic review. Knee 19:751–759

Gillespie MJ, Sebastianelli WJ, Hicks DG et al (1993) The histopathology of arthrofibrosis. Arthroscopy 9:359–360 (abstract)

Gillespie MJ, Friedland J, Dehaven KE (1998) Arthrofibrosis: etiology, classification, histopathology, and treatment. Oper Tech Sports Med 6:102–110

Harner CD, Irrgang JJ, Paul J et al. (1992) Loss of motion after anterior cruciate ligament reconstruction. Am J Sports Med 20:499–506

Hozack WJ, Rothman RH, Booth RE Jr et al (1989) The patellar clunk syndrome. A complication of posterior stabilized total knee arthroplasty. Clin Orthop Relat Res 241:203–208

Hughston JC (1985) Complications of anterior cruciate ligament surgery. Orthop Clin N Am 16:237–240

Hunter RE, Mastrangelo J, Freeman JR et al (1996) The impact of surgical timing on postoperative motion and stability following anterior cruciate ligament reconstruction. Arthroscopy 12:667–674

Ihn H (2002) Pathogenesis of fibrosis: role of TGF-beta and CTGF. Curr Opin Rheumatol 14:681–685, Review

Jackson DW, Schaefer RK (1990) Cyclops syndrome: loss of extension following intra-articular anterior cruciate ligament reconstruction. Arthroscopy 6:171–178

Kim DH, Gill TJ, Millett PJ (2004) Arthroscopic treatment of the arthrofibrotic knee. Arthroscopy 2:187–194

Kwok CS, Harrison T, Servant C (2013) The optimal timing for anterior cruciate ligament reconstruction with respect to the risk of postoperative stiffness. Arthroscopy 29:556–565

LaPrade RF, Pedtke AC, Roethle ST (2008) Arthroscopic posteromedial capsular release for knee flexion contractures. Knee Surg Sports Traumatol Arthrosc 16:469–475

Laubenthal KN, Smidt GL, Kettelkamp DB (1972) A quantitative analysis of knee motion during activities of daily living. Phys Ther 52:34–43

Lonner JH, Jasko JG, Bezwada HP et al (2007) Incidence of patellar clunk with a modern posterior-stabilized knee design. Am J Orthop (Belle Mead NJ) 36:550–553

Magit D, Wolff A, Sutton K et al (2007) Arthrofibrosis of the knee. J Am Acad Orthop Surg 15:682–694, Review

Majors RA, Woodfin B (1996) Achieving full range of motion after anterior cruciate ligament reconstruction. Am J Sports Med 24:350–355

Mariani PP (2010) Arthroscopic release of the posterior compartments in the treatment of extension deficit of knee. Knee Surg Sports Traumatol Arthrosc 18:736–741

Marzo JM, Bowen MK, Warren RF et al (1992) Intraarticular fibrous nodule as a cause of loss of extension following anterior cruciate ligament reconstruction. Arthroscopy 8:10–18

Millett PJ, Williams RJ 3, Wickiewicz TL (1999) Open debridement and soft tissue release as a salvage procedure for the severely arthrofibrotic knee. Am J Sports Med 27:552–561

Murakami S, Muneta T, Ezura Y et al (1997) Quantitative analysis of synovial fibrosis in the infrapatellar fat pad before and after anterior cruciate ligament reconstruction. Am J Sports Med 25:29–34

Nabors ED, Richmond JC, Vannah WM et al (1995) Anterior cruciate ligament graft tensioning in full extension. Am J Sports Med 23:488–492

Noyes FR, Barber-Westin SD (1997) Reconstruction of the anterior and posterior cruciate ligaments after knee dislocation. Use of early protected postoperative motion to decrease arthrofibrosis. Am J Sports Med 25:769–778

Noyes FR, Wojtys EM, Marshall MT (1991) The early diagnosis and treatment of developmental patella infera syndrome. Clin Orthop Relat Res 265:241–252

Noyes FR, Berrios-Torres S, Barber-Westin SD et al (2000) Prevention of permanent arthrofibrosis after anterior cruciate ligament reconstruction alone or combined with associated procedures: a prospective study in 443 knees. Knee Surg Sports Traumatol Arthrosc 8:196–206

O'Brien SJ, Ngeow J, Gibney MA et al (1995) Reflex sympathetic dystrophy of the knee. Causes, diagnosis, and treatment. Am J Sports Med 23:655–659

Paulos LE, Rosenberg TD, Drawbert J et al (1987) Infrapatellar contracture syndrome. An unrecognized cause of knee stiffness with patella entrapment and patella infera. Am J Sports Med 15:331–341

Pfitzner T, Geissler S, Duda G et al (2012) Increased BMP expression in arthrofibrosis after TKA. Knee Surg Sports Traumatol Arthrosc 20:1803–1808

Poli G, Parola M (1997) Oxidative damage and fibrogenesis. Free Radic Biol Med 22:287–305, Review

Pollock DC, Ammeen DJ, Engh GA (2002) Synovial entrapment: a complication of posterior stabilized total knee arthroplasty. J Bone Joint Surg Am 84-A:2174–2178

Raviraj A, Anand A, Kodikal G et al (2010) A comparison of early and delayed arthroscopically-assisted reconstruction of the anterior cruciate ligament using hamstring autograft. J Bone Joint Surg (Br) 92:521–526

Romano VM, Graf BK, Keene JS et al (1993) Anterior cruciate ligament reconstruction. The effect of tibial tunnel placement on range of motion. Am J Sports Med 21:415–418

Sachs RA, Daniel DM, Stone ML et al (1989) Patellofemoral problems after anterior cruciate ligament reconstruction. Am J Sports Med 17:760–765

SchiavonePanni A, Cerciello S, Vasso M et al (2009) Stiffness in total knee arthroplasty. J Orthop Traumatol 10:111–118

Seyler TM, Marker DR, Bhave A et al (2007) Functional problems and arthrofibrosis following total knee arthroplasty. J Bone Joint Surg Am 3:59–69

Sharma V, Maheshwari AV, Tsailas PG et al (2008) The results of knee manipulation for stiffness after total knee arthroplasty with or without an intra-articular steroid injection. Indian J Orthop 42:314–318

Shelbourne KD, Wilckens JH, Mollabashy A et al (1991) Arthrofibrosis in acute anterior cruciate ligament reconstruction. The effect of timing of reconstruction and rehabilitation. Am J Sports Med 19:332–336

Shelbourne KD, Patel DV, Martini DJ (1996) Classification and management of arthrofibrosis of the knee after anterior cruciate ligament reconstruction. Am J Sports Med 24:857–862

Shiota N, Kakizoe E, Shimoura K et al (2005) Effect of mast cell chymase inhibitor on the development of scleroderma in tight-skin mice. Br J Pharmacol 145:424–431

Skutek M, Elsner HA, Slateva K et al (2004) Screening for arthrofibrosis after anterior cruciate ligament reconstruction: analysis of association with human leukocyte antigen. Arthroscopy 20:469–473

Smith TO, Davies L, Hing CB (2010) Early versus delayed surgery for anterior cruciate ligament reconstruction: a systematic review and meta-analysis. Knee Surg Sports Traumatol Arthrosc 18:304–311

Sprague NF 3, O'Connor RL, Fox JM (1982) Arthroscopic treatment of postoperative knee fibroarthrosis. Clin Orthop Relat Res 166:165–172

Sringari T, Maheswaran SS (2005) Patellar clunk syndrome in patellofemoral arthroplasty–a case report. Knee 12:456–457

Steadman JR, Dragoo JL, Hines SL et al (2008) Arthroscopic release for symptomatic scarring of the anterior interval of the knee. Am J Sports Med 36:1763–1769

Steiner DR, Gonzalez NC, Wood JG (2003) Mast cells mediate the microvascular inflammatory response to systemic hypoxia. J Appl Physiol 94:325–334

Strum GM, Friedman MJ, Fox JM et al (1990) Acute anterior cruciate ligament reconstruction. Analysis of complications. Clin Orthop Relat Res 253:184–189

Ushiyama T, Chano T, Inoue K et al (2003) Cytokine production in the infrapatellar fat pad: another source of cytokines in knee synovial fluids. Ann Rheum Dis 62:108–112

vanGrinsven S, van Cingel RE, Holla CJ et al (2010) Evidence-based rehabilitation following anterior cruciate ligament reconstruction. Knee Surg Sports Traumatol Arthrosc 18:1128–1144

Wasilewski SA, Covall DJ, Cohen S (1993) Effect of surgical timing on recovery and associated injuries after anterior cruciate ligament reconstruction. Am J Sports Med 21:338–342

Watson RS, Gouze E, Levings PP et al (2010) Gene delivery of TGF-β1 induces arthrofibrosis and chondrometaplasia of synovium in vivo. Lab Investig 90:1615–1627

Ziegler CG, Pietrini SD, Westerhaus BD et al (2011) Arthroscopically pertinent landmarks for tunnel positioning in single-bundle and double-bundle anterior cruciate ligament reconstructions. Am J Sports Med 39:743–752

Arthroscopic Patellar Instability Surgery

75

Mahmut Nedim Doral, Egemen Turhan, Gazi Huri, Gürhan Dönmez, Mustafa Karahan, Nurzat Elmalı, Onur Bilge, and Defne Kaya

Contents

Abstract

Biomechanically the knee joint has motion complex which includes gliding, rolling, translation, and rotation during their extension to flexion. A significant incidence of knee pain and disability arises from patellofemoral disorders in all ages. Patellar instability is a subjective term that defines pain, blockage, and clinical twisting due to the deterioration of the static and dynamic knee extensor mechanism. An accurate diagnosis relies both on assessing soft tissues and bony tissues together and

M.N. Doral (✉)
Department of Orthopaedics and Traumatology and Department of Sports Medicine, Hacettepe University, Istanbul, Turkey
e-mail: ndoral@hacettepe.edu.tr; mndoral@gmail.com

E. Turhan
Department of Orthopaedics and Traumatology, Hacettepe University School of Medicine, Ankara, Sihhiye, Turkey
e-mail: dregementurhan@yahoo.com

G. Huri
Department of Orthopaedics and Traumatology, Faculty of Medicine, Hacettepe University, Ankara, Turkey

Division of Shoulder Surgery, Department of Orthopaedic Surgery, Johns Hopkins University, Baltimore, MD, USA
e-mail: gazihuri@yahoo.com

G. Dönmez
Faculty of Medicine, Department of Sport Medicine, Hacettepe University School of Medicine, Ankara, Sihhiye, Turkey
e-mail: gurhan@hacettepe.edu.tr; gdonmez_1805@yahoo.com

M. Karahan
Department of Orthopedics and Traumatology, Faculty of Medicine, Acibadem University, Maltepe, Istanbul, Turkey
e-mail: drmustafakarahan@gmail.com; mustafa@karahan.dr.tr

N. Elmalı
Department of Orthopaedics and Traumatology, Dr. Lütfi Kırdar Kartal Education and Research Hospital, İstanbul, Turkey
e-mail: nelmali@hotmail.com

O. Bilge
Department of Orthopaedics and Traumatology, and Department of Sports Medicine, Konya NE University, Meram School of Medicine, Konya, Turkey
e-mail: onurbilgemd@gmail.com

D. Kaya
Department of Physical Therapy and Rehabilitation, Faculty of Health Science, Biruni University, İstanbul, Turkey
e-mail: defne@hacettepe.edu.tr

M.N. Doral, J. Karlsson (eds.), *Sports Injuries*,
DOI 10.1007/978-3-642-36569-0_125

considering pelvic and spinal stabilizers. Under the title of patellar instability, arthroscopic medial plication technique and the importance of the medial patellofemoral ligament in this approach will be discussed.

Introduction

The knee joint is an area of joint pain which is the most frequent reason for seeking medical advice. A significant incidence of the pain arises from patellofemoral (PF) disorders. Patellofemoral pain syndrome term is used to define the clinical cases which cause pain on the anterior part of the knee regarding the pathology in the PF joint.

The PF joint is the part of human muscle–skeleton system on which the joint forces are most loaded (Doral et al. 2009). It has been determined that 3.3 times the body weight is loaded on the PF joint during activities such as climbing or going down the stairs, whereas 7.6 times the body weight is loaded on it during crouching and 20 times increased loads occur during jumping (Panni et al. 2006). The quadriceps muscle power increases by 30 % during full extension. The patella, which is the largest sesamoid bone, has the thickest cartilage in the body with a thickness of 6–7 mm, and it provides the main leverage point of the knee extensor mechanism (White and Sherman 2009). Hyaline cartilage reduces the friction coefficient of the extensor mechanism. The total amount of these joint loads in full extension is balanced at the PF joint level as tensile forces and that is called "patellofemoral joint reaction force." Shortly, it is specified as F1 (quadriceps tendon vector) = F2 (patellar tendon) vector junction. It has a size of 100 + 20 kg (Doral et al. 2009).

Patellofemoral disorders are generally examined in three groups:

1. Pain due to soft tissue disorders
2. Patellar instability
3. Patellofemoral osteoarthritis

Patellar instabilities, namely, "patellar balance disorders," have been the most important of the subjects challenging the knee surgeons. **Patellar instability** is a subjective term defining pain, blockage, and clinical twisting due to the deterioration of the static and dynamic knee extensor mechanism. We can categorize the "patellar instability" title, the main subject of this review, into four subtitles: subluxation (half dislocation), luxation (full dislocation), patella infera (patella below – "patella baja"), and patella supera (patella above – "patella alta") (Boden et al. 1997; Doral et al. 2009).

Patellar laxity or looseness may appear without any subjective symptoms. This finding, which is more prevalent in children, begins to decrease with age. In these cases the individuals can use their extensor mechanisms with a powerful muscle balance and proprioception without any symptoms developing. To sum up, patellar instability, which is used as a subjective term, is formed during dynamic position and patellar laxity and presents itself as an objective finding.

Patellar subluxation and luxation: The incidence of patella dislocation has been reported as 5.8 in 100,000 people. This rate is approximately 5 times more between the ages of 10 and 17 (Fithian et al. 2004; Colvin and West 2008). It is reported that 15–44 % of the acute dislocation cases, which are treated with conservative approaches, have recurrent patellar instability (Hawkins et al. 1986). Acute patella dislocations may occur directly or indirectly. The patella may be forced laterally in direct injuries. Medial dislocations are rare and typically iatrogenic. This results from lateral relaxation due to inadequate technical application and excess medialization or an overaggressive lateral retinacular release. Dislocation develops frequently. Acute patella dislocations are examined in two groups as recurrent (after traumatic dislocation) and habitual, and it is an important condition that causes instability. Habitual dislocations may be related to collagen tissue and the collagen structure of the individual, and it is more commonly seen in cases of Down's syndrome, multiple epiphyseal dysplasia, and Ehlers–Danlos syndrome which have general joint and tissue laxity. In his book, under the title of "continuous patella dislocations," Fulkerson mentions congenital and acquired forms of dislocation and defines the habitual type as recurrent dislocations (Fulkerson 1997). The most important point to note here is that quadriceps fibrosis and soft tissue stiffness around the knee may not be seen in all cases. Quadriceps and vastus medialis obliquus reinforcement is recommended for the traditional conservative approaches of patella dislocations; surgery is preferred in cases of recurrent instabilities and acute osteochondral fractures (Satterfield and Johnson 2005). You should bear in mind that lateral condyle cartilage damage may develop approximately in 30 % of the acute dislocations (Nomura et al. 2003). Many researchers recommend early surgery to prevent recurrent instability from developing because of its high recurrence rate (Ahmad et al. 2000). It is observed that pain complaints continue to exist in most patients even if early surgery corrections reduce the recurrence.

Patella infera and patella supera: Patella height may be evaluated with direct or indirect methods. Indexes such as the "Insall–Salvati," "Blackburne–Peel," and "Caton–Deschamps" ratios are the indirect methods that assess the patella height according to patellar tendon length and tibia proximal. *Blumensaat's line* is drawn on the linear opacity image that the intercondylar notch top forms on lateral knee radiographs. In Blumensaat's method, the distance of the lower patella pole to that line is measured in mm and patella height is assessed. Normally, the lower patella pole needs to be the continuation of Blumensaat's line. Patella supera is at a distance more than 10 mm above the line, whereas patella infera is at a distance more than 10 mm below the line (Seyahi et al. 2006). The Insall–Salvati index is measured by dividing the distance between the lower patella pole and the adherence location of patellar tendon to the tibial tuberosity by the longest diameter between higher back ends and lower front ends of the patella. Greater than 1.2 is considered as patella supera, whereas <0.8 is considered as patella infera for that index which has a normal value of 1 (Seil et al. 2000). The modified Insall–Salvati index is the ratio of the joint surface length of the patella to the distance between the most distal point of the patella joint surface and the attachment point of the patellar tendon to the tibial tuberosity. It is considered in favor of patella infera if this index (normally which should be below 2) has a value of greater than 2. Sometimes this technique may provide erroneous results since the tibia tubercle does not have a sufficient significance. The Blackburne–Peel index is calculated by dividing the straight distance between the lowest point of the patella joint surface and the tangential line passing through the surface of joint surface of the tibia to the length of the patella joint surface. The normal value of the index is 0.8; >1 is considered as patella supera, whereas <0.5 is considered as patella infera. According to some authors, patellar tendon length is another factor that causes instability (Neyret et al. 2002).

The cases that cause the abovementioned situations will result in patellar instability and can be examined in three groups:

1. Local reasons: Trochlear trough failure, undeveloped or small patella, patella being higher or lower, medial patellofemoral ligament (MPFL) damage, vastus medialis obliquus muscle insufficiency, and stretched outer retinaculum and capsule.
2. Sub-morphotype disorders: Increased femoral anteversion and Q angle, genu valgus, genu varus, and genu recurvatum, increased tibial inner rotation as well as tibia varus and valgus deformity, and increased tibial outer rotation and accompanying pronated foot.
3. General reasons: Situations such as Ehlers–Danlos syndrome, multiple epiphyseal dysplasia, nail-patella syndrome, general body joint hyperlaxity, and "short rectus femoris muscle" not relevant to CP carry on from the childhood age, and they may cause PF problems or patellar balance disorders in advancing ages.

Diagnosis

Taking a detailed history and making a careful physical examination is conditional to diagnose these patients accurately so as to successfully treat them. Clinical observation and treatment findings are quite helping in diagnosing patellar instability. Squinting patella which results from the fact two patella turn inward while the patient is standing and shows parallelism with inward torsion of the lower extremities. During walking, foot deformity develops due to skeletal system lower morphotype disorder (pronated feet), Q angle measurement, and grasshopper patella which are the typical symptoms of bilateral subluxated knees and T-sulcus angle. These need to be assessed as major issues.

While assessing the knee joint, the bony tissues (shape of patella, sulcus, and lateral condyle) and soft tissues in active and passive dynamic positions (outer capsule, MPFL, quadriceps, patellar tendon) should be considered together. While examining the biomechanics of the knee joint, it is observed that it makes gliding in flexion movement (patellar rotation with medial and lateral translation), rotation (internal and external rotation), and translocation and some rotation (Post et al. 2002). Patellar tilt, apprehension test, and PF grinding (patellar grinding) test are the treatment methods that are important for the assessment of PF joint. Passive patellar tilt test is a test that shows lateral retinacular tension, and normally the angle of patella lateral edge is parallel to the ground. The patella should be able to be turned 10–15° toward the medial. Otherwise, lateral retinacular tension will occur. The lateral apprehension test is a valuable test for recurrent patella dislocation cases. While the knee is in 30° of flexion, the patella is pushed from the medial to the lateral by applying force. The patient will be afraid during this, and he/she will try to prevent the movement from carrying on by active quadriceps contraction. Patellofemoral grinding (patellar grinding) is a static test. It is desired to reveal the existence of retropatellar pathology by active quadriceps contraction. While examining a patient with patellar instability, a very important point here is that the clinician should not focus only on the knee region and should not ignore the examination of pelvic and spinal stabilizers with the knowledge of the fact that the innervation of the distal alignment starts from the L5–S1 vertebras. Loss of normal torsion of the hip joint and being in retroversion or anteversion positions in the transverse plan will affect the whole alignment of the lower extremity and thus may cause possible patellar instability. Similarly, finding hallux valgus in a person increases the subtalar joint pronation and causes PF joint problems and also patellar instability later on (Menz and Lord 2005; Kaya et al. 2009).

The axis of the PF joint is determined by the Q angle. This angle is the angle between the midpoint of the anterior superior iliac spine and the patella and the lines that connect this point to the tibial tuberosity. Normal values of this angle are 8–14° for men and 11–20° for women, and values exceeding 20° are accepted as abnormal. The reason why this angle has higher values for women is that they have a wider pelvis and there is an increase in knee valgus.

However, it should be borne in mind that the clinical measurement of the Q angle is made in a static environment. It is very difficult to dynamize the Q angle. The question of how much the "walking analysis" will help could not be established. Increasing this angle may cause patellar instability. The risk of dislocation of the patella increases in full extension since Q angle is in full extension. The same angle in a dynamic position will be assessed during 0–30° of flexion. In the case of an increased Q angle, femoral anteversion, external tibial torsion, genu valgus, and tibial tubercle lateralization should be considered (Pınar et al. 1994).

In addition to history and physical evaluation, various monitoring methods are also important for diagnosis. Together with the abovementioned methods, the relation of the patella with the femoral sulcus is observed in tangential radiographs at 30, 45, 60, and 90° flexions in dynamic positions. The Hughston sulcus angle was determined as 118° and Merchant sulcus angle was determined as 138° in defining trochlear dysplasia (Doral et al. 1992). The crossing sign in lateral radiographs, which is the line reaching to the anterior face of the condyle from the deep part of the trochlear trough, shows the supratrochlear protrusion, and the double boundary appearance (trochlear hump) shows hypoplastic condyle and trochlear groove failure (Dejour and Le Coultre 2007). More advanced imaging methods such as computed tomography (CT) and magnetic resonance imaging (MRI) may be used when necessary. Generally MRI is used with X-ray if there is a doubt for osteochondral fracture at medial facet level. Also, in cases of acute traumatic patellar dislocations, the MRI method is superior to the other methods. Direct radiologic methods do not help in most cases since many of these cases occur in a spontaneously reduced manner. Determining the existence of an edema secondary to the contusion in medial patellar facet and in lateral femoral condyle by means of MRI and damaging the integrity of medial patellofemoral ligament not only reinforces the patellar dislocation diagnosis but also helps with planning the treatment.

Arthroscopy is a necessary attempt for dynamic diagnosis and treatment related to PF joint problems, especially patellar instability (Doral et al. 1988). The importance of cine-arthroscopy, under epidural anesthesia, for actively determining all joint movements and revealing the dynamic proximity of the patella with sulcus is unquestionable. Also, the interior joint structure of the cartilage tissue may be monitored with this method. A 70° arthroscope should be used in cine-arthroscopy, and the joint should be entered through the outer edge of the suprapatellar cavity. Other than inflating the joint with liquid, the PF relation may be monitored while the joint is idle. While making the assessment, knee flexion and extension are required from the patient and dynamic position of patella is monitored in 0, 30, 45, and 60° flexions. Following the arthroscopic alignment of the patella, the same images can be rechecked and overcorrection will be prevented and the rate of arthroscopic correction will be increased.

Treatment

To obtain successful results in patellar instability treatment, knee surgery and arthroscopy specialists should work in an absolute harmony with physical therapy and the rehabilitation team. Treatment must be carried out with conservative methods at the beginning, and nonsteroidal anti-inflammatory drugs, devices, physical treatment, and proprioceptive physiotherapy should be applied. The importance of brain–patella coordination should be explained to the patient in detail, and the difficulty of the treatment should be notified both before and after the surgical treatment. Undesired results could be obtained with surgical treatment if this coordination was not restored before surgery. It has been determined that most of the patellar instability patients have weakness on gluteal muscles (Colvin and West 2008). Weakness of the gluteal muscles is due to adduction and inner rotation of femur during load-bearing activities, thereby giving grounds for instability. For this reason, most of the time, strengthening of the gluteal muscles or banding that draw the hip to external rotation should be added to the treatment. While most of the PF diseases respond to the conservative methods, various techniques such as lateral relaxation, medial reinforcement and MPFL reconstruction, proximal and distal alignment procedures, femoral sulcus osteotomy, condyloplasty, patellar osteotomy, autologous chondrocyte transplantation, and patellectomy can be applied as surgical treatment alternatives. That is to say, no treatment method has been defined yet as the golden standard of patellar instability treatment. It is hard to compare them since there are differences between the methods of the studies made on this area and so prospective randomized clinical studies are needed. As the only prospective randomized study in the literature, which compared the nonoperative and operative methods in acute instability treatment, Nikku et al. found no significant differences in terms of recurrent instability with their follow-ups of 2–5 years, and they have recommended to treat the patients with nonoperative conservative methods at the beginning (Nikku et al. 1997).

Under the title of "wrong alignment types" in their CT examinations in chronic cases, Schutzer et al. have specified the surgery principles according to tilt, subluxation, and cartilage damage (Schutzer et al. 1986). However, the clinical experiences of the authors show that patella supera can also cause to some subluxation cases too. Classic "wrong alignment types" which are divided into three main groups are as follows: (1) subluxation without tilt, (2) subluxation with tilt, and (3) tilt without subluxation.

Minor or major surgeries or both of these are applied in subluxation with tilt (where the patella is supera or not). Attempts such as outer retinacular or capsular loosening, medial placation, anteromedial transposition and/or distalization, and proximalization of the tibial tuberosity are made.

In the cases such as increased Q angle, common hyperlaxity, hypermobile patella, genu varus, valgus or recurvatum, excess internal/external tibial torsion, high femoral anteversion, and severely pronated foot patellar alignment should be done with open surgery instead of arthroscopic attempts. However, it should be borne in mind that irrational surgery applications should cause irrecoverable problems in knee extensor mechanism.

Lateral relaxation can be implemented with arthroscopic control. Capsular lateral relaxation may be done for the patients who do not have too much joint laxity and/or with whom subluxation is observed. The capsule should be cut from the surface of patella higher pole to distal by means of a scissors, cautery, or laser. The patella needs to be pushed approximately toward 90° after lateral relaxation (Doral et al. 1992). Lateral relaxation may be applied in combination with methods such as MPFL reconstruction and medial plication if the distance between tibial tubercle and trochlear trough is below 20 mm and there are some PF degenerative changes (Tom and Fulkerson 2007). Even if it is reported in recent publications that isolated lateral relaxation technique provided successful results when it is applied in patellar compression syndrome, it is not recommended in the treatment of patellar instability (Lattermann et al. 2007; Colvin and West 2008). Lateral relaxation should not be done if the patient has distal patellar cartilage lesion, and medial stabilization should be taken care of if there is a medial patellar cartilage lesion. Otherwise these lesions will be triggered and the risk of PF osteoarthritis will be increased.

Arthroscopic medial plication technique is the authors' preferred method in cases of patellar instability. There are some studies which report very good functional results and very low rate of "redislocation" after arthroscopic medial plication in treatment of cases with recurrent patellar instability (Nam and Karzel 2005; Ali and Bhatti 2007). Indications of this technique are extensor mechanism having a normal kinetic, there are no serious changes in terms of patella shape and femoral sulcus angle, Q angle is significant between 20° and 40°, and there is no three-dimensional axis disordered especially in at serious levels. Also, in the cases with severe joint laxity, accelerated proprioceptive physiotherapy should be preferred initially (Fig. 1). Arthroscopy should be considered by the surgeons with patients who have sufficient muscle power and control and especially with recurrent patellar instability or an osteochondral fracture of the patella or at the lateral edge of the trochlear groove. It may also be considered with the first dislocation of a sportsman who has plans to return to sports after a short period of time. Attention must be paid on arthroscopic corrections in case of excess joint looseness, severe cartilage and bone tissue damages, patella infera-supera, and "regional pain syndrome," that is, reflex sympathetic dystrophy cases. In addition to proximodistal and mediolateral corrections in cases of lower extremities with bad alignment, lateral condyloplasty, trochleoplasty, tibial tubercle anteriorization, and/or anteromedialization as Marguet and Fulkerson specified should be done using open surgery techniques (Fulkerson 2002; Dejour and Le Coultre 2007).

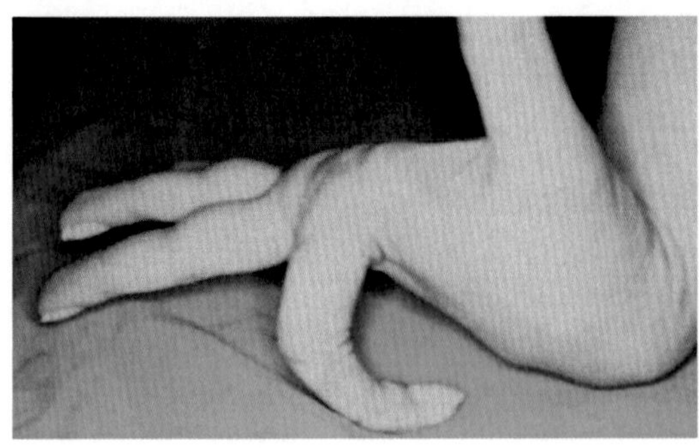

Fig. 1 A patient of with severe joint looseness

Medial facet fractures are more likely in recurrent dislocation cases. Calcifications on radiographic images may be confused with a fracture in the cases where MPFL rupture is from the adherence location to medial facet. Calcifications form in the medial capsule, medial patellotibial ligament, and MPFL as a result of patella dislocation after a trauma. The MPFL is the primary reinforcing ligament of the patella's medial stability (Desio et al. 1998). Anatomically it originates from the region between the adductor tubercle, medial epicondyle, and medial collateral ligament and lies upon 2/3 of the medial patellar edge. MPFL lies down in the second layer of the medial knee and acts as a checkrein for further lateral patellar movement (Warren et al. 1974). Size and power of this extrasynovial ligament which is observed as 90 % in cadaver studies are variant, and it has a shape of an hourglass and its average width is 13 mm (Conlan et al. 1993). In another study, it has been shown that the power required to draw the patella to lateral by 10 mm had decreased by 50 % after cutting the medial structures (Senavongse and Amis 2005). The MPFL is surely damaged by patella dislocations, and it has been determined that it is damaged by adductor tubercle avulsions in 50–80 % of cases (Nomura 1999). Recent approaches mostly recommend its repair or reconstruction.

With the developing techniques, MPFL reconstruction has gained importance. Many authors underline the importance of reinforcing the medial side in the anatomical correction of lateral instability. Anatomical attempts may not be done in the cases where there are no cartilage lesions and severe hemarthrosis. For active sportsmen, MPFL repairs should be done following the arthroscopic joint debridement. However, it should be borne in mind that hemarthrosis exceeding 20 ml may be because of severe cartilage damage. In such cases, lavage, cartilage assessment, and correction of MPFL and medial capsular tears should be done primarily with arthroscopic control especially after first dislocation (Doral et al. 1988). The vastus medialis obliquus muscle integrity should be taken into consideration because of its importance in dynamic medial stabilization (Ahmad et al. 2000).

MPFL reconstruction has an advantage of visualizing the damage to the attachment adjacent to the adductor tubercle. No agreement has been reached in terms of graft selection and graft localization regarding previously described adductor magnus autograft, semitendinosus autograft and allograft, and tibialis anterior allografts (Deie et al. 2005). The surgeon needs to be careful during MPFL reconstruction in terms of possible patella fractures that may develop during graft

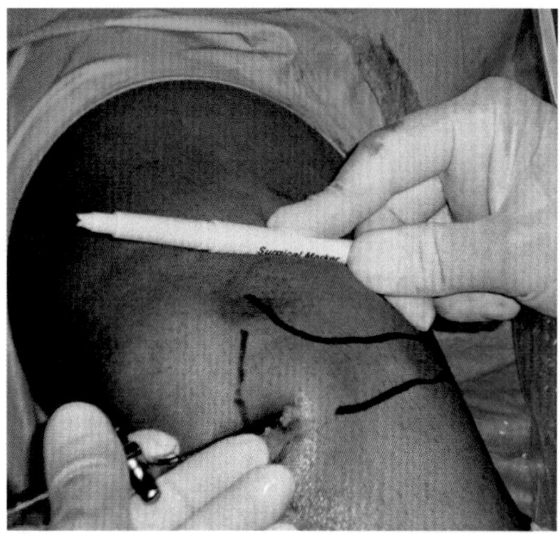

Fig. 2 Drawing of the topographic anatomy of the MPFL

fixation. Dynamic reconstruction of MPFL is preferred to static reconstruction (Ostermeier et al. 2007; Panagopoulos et al. 2008).

The technique can be summarized as follows:

1. Topographic drawing of MPFL is done while the knee is in 30° flexion (Fig. 2).
2. Arthroscopic entrance is made from anterolateral portal. The MPFL is not seen in this location because it is an extracapsular structure. Initially the routine arthroscopic examination of the knee has to be performed in order to search for cartilage damages, particularly the medial facet of patella and lateral femoral condyle (Fig. 3).
3. In the case of small amount of knee flexion, sutures start to be made preferably with #5 PDS (absorbable sutures sometimes anchor, especially absorbable one is preferable), before the adductor tubercle level and by passing them through a position out of the capsule and under the skin (Fig. 4). The intra-articular section is entered by the patella medial side and adductor tubercle which is also the starting point is reached again, and three individual sutures are done at three levels from upside down, and adductor is determined at tubercle level, while knots are tied at 30° of flexion (Fig. 5). No forcing that pushes the patella medially should be implemented. In this

technique, direct procedures are done in case of acute dislocations, whereas same procedure is done with chronic ones by cutting medial capsule with radiofrequency. Lateral capsular relaxation absolutely should not be done if the outer tissues are not tensile.

4. Finally the position of the anchors has to be verified by radiographic measures (Fig. 6a, b).
5. Physiotherapy is started a short time after post-operative compression. No devices are used.

The most important advantages of arthroscopic PF correction are that it has a low morbidity and small amounts of scar tissues because of minimal invasive attempts; it provides a chance for easy revision; it allows early movement; and it has a low cost and a short hospital time (Ali and Bhatti 2007; Doral et al. 2009). The major complications of this method in the early period are hemarthrosis, overcorrection, and cartilage damage, whereas its major complications in the late period are anterior knee pain, reflex sympathetic dystrophy, recurrent dislocations, and PF osteoarthritis. Knowing knee biomechanics well and

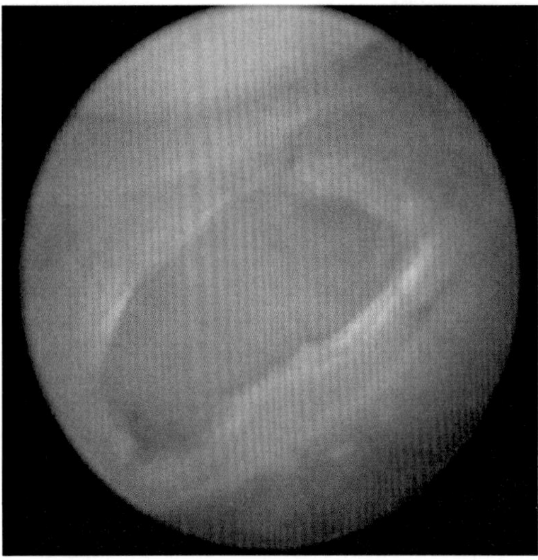

Fig. 3 The demonstration of the cartilage damage over lateral femoral condyle

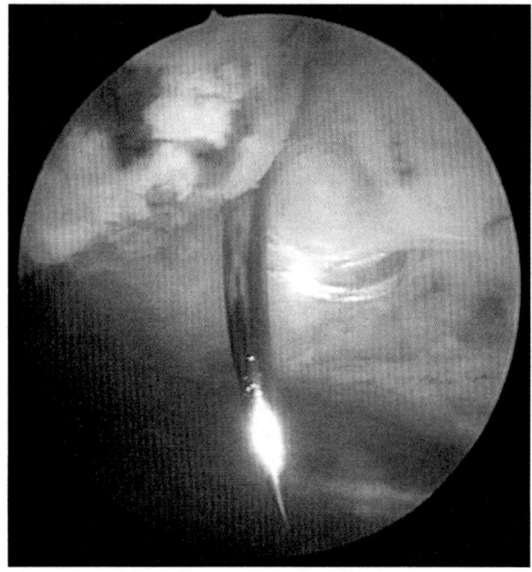

Fig. 4 Determination of anchor suture on adductor tubercle

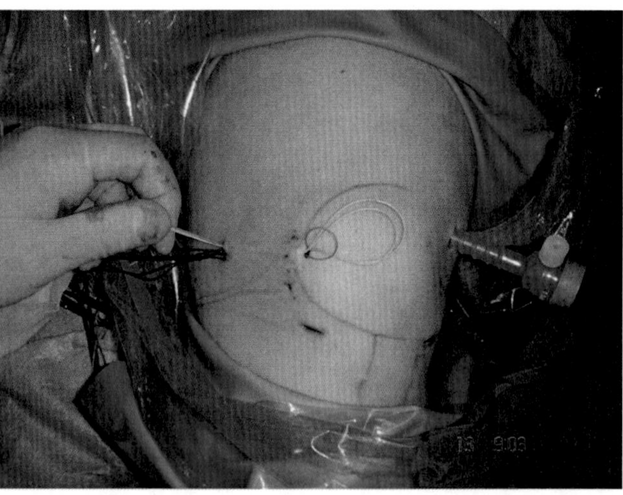

Fig. 5 Passing the suture through the inside of the joint and then passing it between under-skin MPFL with suture passer and ending it at AT

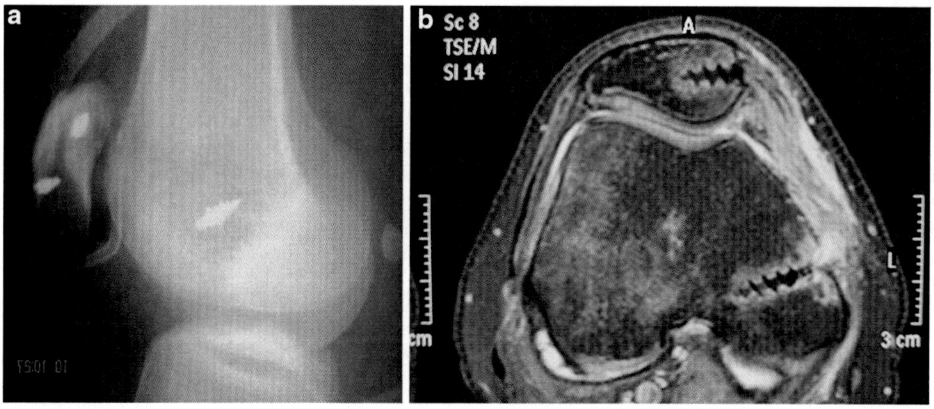

Fig. 6 (**a**) The optimal localization of the suture anchors is seen on the lateral view of the knee. (**b**) The accurate position of the anchors in T2 axial MRI view of knee. *ADT* adductor tubercle, *MF* medial facet, —> suture material (with #5 PDS or Ethibond)

planning before a detailed operation are basic elements required for preventing these complications. Besides, even if MPFL reconstruction provides more stability when compared to a medial tubercle transfer in biomechanical terms, it is insufficient regarding osteosis problems, and it theoretically causes for excess burden to be loaded on medial PF cartilage (Elias and Cosgarea 2006; Ostermeier et al. 2006). Making the knots of sutures without outer capsular relaxation and while the knee is at 30° flexion is the most important stage of the technique in arthroscopic medial approach. Otherwise, medial overcorrection and medial tilt are complications which are hard to rectify.

Conclusion

Patellar instability is an area which is constantly developing. While most of the cases make use of conservative treatment, surgical attempts should obtain successful results if they are implemented by experienced doctors. Planning for underlying pathology should be done in the selection of treatment method. Otherwise, PF osteoarthritis and limitation of movement will be the inevitable long-term results. Besides, it should be borne in mind that irrational surgical treatment implementation will result in some situations on knee extensor mechanism which are impossible to recover from. The most important elements in patella surgery, which is a job similar to fine as tuning a musical instrument, are philosophy and the experience of the surgeon as well as the tissue quality of the patient.

Cross-References

- ▶ Patellar Dislocations: Overview
- ▶ Patellofemoral Problems in Adolescent Athletes
- ▶ Physiotherapy in Patellofemoral Pain Syndrome
- ▶ Radiologic Criteria in Patellar Dislocations
- ▶ Reconstruction of the Medial Patellofemoral Ligament: A Surgical Technique Perspective from an Orthopedic Surgeon
- ▶ Return to Play After Acute Patellar Dislocation
- ▶ Structured Rehabilitation Model for Patients with Patellofemoral Pain Syndrome

References

Ahmad CS, Stein BE, Matuz D et al (2000) Immediate surgical repair of the medial patellar stabilizers for acute patellar dislocation. A review of eight cases. Am J Sports Med 28(6):804–810

Ali S, Bhatti A (2007) Arthroscopic proximal realignment of the patella for recurrent instability: report of a new surgical technique with 1 to 7 years of follow-up. Arthroscopy 23:305–311

Boden BP, Pearsall AW, Garrett WE Jr et al (1997) Patellofemoral instability: evaluation and management. J Am Acad Orthop Surg 5:47–57

Colvin AC, West RV (2008) Patellar instability. J Bone Joint Surg Am 90:2751–2762

Conlan T, Garth WP Jr, Lemons JE (1993) Evaluation of the medial soft-tissue restraints of the extensor mechanism of the knee. J Bone Joint Surg Am 75(5):682–693

Deie M, Ochi M, Sumen Y (2005) A long-term follow-up study after medial patellofemoral ligament reconstruction using the transferred semitendinosus tendon for patellar dislocation. Knee Surg Sports Traumatol Arthrosc 13:522–528

Dejour D, Le Coultre B (2007) Osteotomies in patellofemoral instabilities. Sports Med Arthrosc 15(1):39–46

Desio SM, Burks RT, Bachus KN (1998) Soft tissue restraints to lateral patellar translation in the human knee. Am J Sports Med 26:59–65

Doral MN, Atik OŞ, Şener E (1988) Patellar malalignmentta artroskopik lateral fasyal gevşetme. Acta Orthop Traumatol Turc 22:252–254

Doral MN, Tandoğan R, Acaroğlu E et al (1992) Arthroscopically assisted closed lateral capsular release in the treatment of patellar instability and anterior knee pain syndromes in professional athletes. Proc Int Arthrosc Cong Mapere Med 3(Suppl 3):10

Doral MN, Turhan E, Donmez G (2009) Diz artroskopisi: Artroskopik patellar instabilite cerrahisi. Turkiye Klinikleri J Orthop Traumatol-Spec Top 2(3):80–87

Elias JJ, Cosgarea AJ (2006) Technical errors during medial patellofemoral ligament reconstruction could overload medial patellofemoral cartilage: a computational analysis. Am J Sports Med 34:1478–1485

Fithian DC, Paxton EW, Stone ML et al (2004) Epidemiology and natural history of acute patellar dislocation. Am J Sports Med 32:1114–1121

Fulkerson JP (1997) Disorders of the patellofemoral joint, 3rd edn. William & Wilkins, Philadelphia, pp 211–214

Fulkerson JP (2002) Diagnosis and treatment of patients with patellofemoral pain. Am J Sports Med 30:447–456

Hawkins RJ, Bell RH, Anisette G (1986) Acute patellar dislocations. The natural history. Am J Sports Med 14:117–120

Kaya D, Atay OA, Callaghan M et al (2009) Hallux valgus in patients with patellofemoral pain syndrome. Knee Surg Sports Traumatol Arthrosc 17(11):1364–1367

Lattermann C, Toth J, Bach BR Jr (2007) The role of lateral retinacular release in the treatment of patellar instability. Sports Med Arthrosc 15:57–60

Menz HB, Lord SR (2005) Gait instability in older people with hallux valgus. Foot Ankle Int 26(6):483–489

Nam EK, Karzel RP (2005) Mini-open medial reefing and arthroscopic lateral release for the treatment of recurrent patellar dislocation: a medium-term follow-up. Am J Sports Med 33:220–230

Neyret P, Robinson AH, Le Coultre B (2002) Patellar tendon length–the factor in patellar instability? Knee 9(1):3–6

Nikku R, Nietosvaara Y, Kallio PE et al (1997) Operative versus closed treatment of primary dislocation of the patella. Similar 2-year results in 125 randomized patients. Acta Orthop Scand 68(5):419–423

Nomura E (1999) Classification of lesions of the medial patellofemoral ligament in patellar dislocation. Int Orthop 23(5):260–263

Nomura E, Inoue M, Kurimura M (2003) Chondral and osteochondral injuries associated with acute patellar dislocation. Arthroscopy 19(7):717–721

Ostermeier S, Stukenborg-Colsman C, Hurschler C (2006) In vitro investigation of the effect of medial patellofemoral ligament reconstruction and medial tibial tuberosity transfer on lateral patellar stability. Arthroscopy 22:308–319

Ostermeier S, Holst M, Bohnsack M (2007) In vitro measurement of patellar kinematics following reconstruction of the medial patellofemoral ligament. Knee Surg Sports Traumatol Arthrosc 15:276–285

Panagopoulos A, van Niekerk L, Triantafillopoulos IK (2008) MPFL reconstruction for recurrent patella dislocation: a new surgical technique and review of the literature. Int J Sports Med 29:359–365

Panni AS, Tartarone M, Patricola AA (2006) Patellofemoral problems. In: Volpi P (ed) Football traumatology – current concepts: from prevention to treatment, 1st edn. Springer, Milan, pp 263–274

Pınar H, Akseki D, Karaoğlan O (1994) Kinematic and dynamic axial computed tomography of the patellofemoral joint in patients with anterior knee pain. Knee Surg Sports Traumatol Arthrosc 2(3):170–173

Post WR, Teitge R, Amis A (2002) Patellofemoral malalignment: looking beyond the viewbox. Clin Sports Med 21:521–546

Satterfield WH, Johnson DL (2005) Arthroscopic patellar "Bankart" repair after acute dislocation. Arthroscopy 21(5):627

Schutzer SF, Ramsby GR, Fulkerson JP (1986) Computed tomographic classification of patellofemoral pain patients. Orthop Clin North Am 17:235–248

Seil R, Muller B, Georg T (2000) Reliability and interobserver variability in radiological patellar height ratios. Knee Surg Sports Traumatol Arthrosc 8:231–236

Senavongse W, Amis AA (2005) The effects of articular, retinacular, or muscular deficiencies on patellofemoral joint stability. J Bone Joint Surg Br 87:577–582

Seyahi A, Atalar AC, Koyuncu LÖ (2006) Blumensaat çizgisi ve patella yüksekliği. Acta Orthop Traumatol Turc 40(3):240–247

Tom A, Fulkerson JP (2007) Restoration of native medial patellofemoral ligament support after patella dislocation. Sports Med Arthrosc 15:68–71

Warren LA, Marshall JL, Girgis F (1974) The prime static stabilizer of the medical side of the knee. J Bone Joint Surg Am 56(4):665–674

White BJ, Sherman OH (2009) Patellofemoral instability. Bull NYU Hosp Jt Dis 67(1):22–29

Arthroscopic Repair of Partial Anterior Cruciate Ligament Tears: Perspective from an Orthopedics Surgeon

76

Stephan Lorenz, Stefan Hinterwimmer, and Andreas B. Imhoff

Contents

S. Lorenz (✉) • S. Hinterwimmer
Department of Orthopaedic Sports Medicine, Klinikum rechts der Isar, Technische Universität München, München, Germany
e-mail: Stephan.Lorenz@lrz.tum.de; stephan.lorenz@lrz.tu-muenchen.de; stefan.hinterwimmer@lrz.tu-muenchen.de

A.B. Imhoff
Department of Orthopaedic Sports Medicine, Klinikum rechts der Isar, Technical University of Munich, Munich, Germany
e-mail: Andreas.Imhoff@lrz.tum.de

M.N. Doral, J. Karlsson (eds.), *Sports Injuries*,
DOI 10.1007/978-3-642-36569-0_87

Abstract

The therapy of partial ACL tear is under discussion whether it should be treated conservatively or by operative reconstruction. Instability during stair climbing or direction changes tends to need operative treatment. Exact clinical examination of the knee is mandatory to find minor laxities in translation or rotation. MRI imaging is not highly significant for the diagnosis of the partial tear but can rule out concomitant injuries at the cartilage or meniscus. Meticulous probing of the ACL in a diagnostic arthroscopy under different flexion angles and anterior translation of the tibia seems to be the best test in the diagnosis of a partial tear. If sufficient parts of the ligament remain, an augmentation with a hamstring tendon can be accomplished under preservation of the remaining intact ligament. A further indication for a partial repair is an intact misplaced high-noon ACL reconstruction that can be augmented with a more oblique bundle to gain rotational stability.

This chapter deals with some key points in the diagnosis and therapy of the partial ACL tear. The surgical technique of the augmentation is described in detail.

Introduction

An isolated tear of the AMB or PLB is a rare event. The incidence in a group of patients with pathologic ACL findings lies between

1 % and 13 % (Lorenz et al. 2009; Sonnery-Cottet et al. 2009).

Introduced by Girgis et al. in 1975, the concept of the two functional bundles of the ACL, the anteromedial bundle (AMB) and posterolateral bundle (PLB) , found a broad interest among knee surgeons since the anatomic reconstruction of the ACL with both functional bundles promised a better restoration of the biomechanical behavior of the knee (Girgis et al. 1975). Next to the upcoming popularity of the double-bundle reconstruction, partial augmentation of the ACL also came into the surgeon's mind. The concept of ligament augmentation is appealing, since it may facilitate the positioning and the ingrowth/ligamentization of the graft (Papalia et al. 2014).

The natural course of knees with partial ACL rupture remains uncertain. Patients, who reduced their sport activity level, showed good short- to midterm results. Nevertheless pain and laxity increased in the midterm follow-up (Pujol et al. 2012). The healing rate for meniscal sutures when the ACL was reconstructed at the same time was increased from 57 % to 90 % (Tenuta and Arciero 1994).

There might be a population who takes care of its "instability" also with a partial or complete tear of the ACL. Snyder-Mackler et al. introduced the term of copers and non-copers (Snyder-Mackler et al. 1997).

Clinical Examination

Exact evaluation of the patient's history is essential since most patients with a tear of the AMB or PLB also complain of difficulties descending stairs or giving way while changing directions, respectively (Siebold and Fu 2008). After taking the history, a meticulous clinical examination should follow. Patients with complete tears have a higher-grade pivot-shift test and a bigger side-to-side difference in instrumented measures than patients with partial tears (Dejour et al. 2013). Patients with an isolated tear of the AMB more often have positive anterior drawer and Lachman's tests, while a positive pivot-shift test can be found more often in PLB-deficient patients (Siebold and Fu 2008). In addition, a small (minimal) side-to-side difference (<5 mm) in the anterior drawer and Lachman's test is suspicious for a partial ACL tear during the pivot-shift test. If the standard pivot shift according to MacIntosh and Galway (Galway et al. 1972) is difficult to perform due to high muscle tension, the test described by Losee might be easier to perform (Losee et al. 1978). The collateral ligaments should be examined to rule out combined instability.

It is mandatory to confirm the clinical findings preoperatively under anesthesia.

Radiologic Imaging/MRI

Standard x-rays are obtained to rule out osseous avulsions of either the cruciate or the collateral ligaments. Magnetic resonance imaging (MRI) is the most frequent diagnostic imaging procedure for suspected ACL injuries. It is an accurate, highly sensitive, and specific tool for the diagnosis of ACL tear-associated injuries (Crawford et al. 2007).

Partial ACL tears can heal or progress. Often it is difficult to analyze the rupture pattern in an acute phase since hemorrhage might overemphasize the ruptured part of the ACL. Therefore, MRI may be repeated in these cases after the hemarthrosis resolves. An optimal MRI protocol for ACL tears consists of planes in true axial, sagittal, oblique sagittal (that run parallel to the ACL), and coronal orientation (Araujo et al. 2012). In addition coronal-oblique images are obtained, which run along the long axis of the ACL. The sagittal-oblique planes optimally visualize the functional bundles; the coronal-oblique sequence increases the sensitivity and specificity of diagnosing isolated AM or PL bundle tears (Araujo et al. 2012). The oblique planes are important, since partial tears might be missed with the standard imaging (Dejour et al. 2013). Signs for partial tears in the MRI are signal alterations in the tendon and partially disorganized fibers at the insertions. Overall the MRI is considered as an adjunct for diagnosis of partial ACL tear and to rule out concomitant injuries (Colombet et al. 2010).

Diagnostic Arthroscopy

The diagnostic arthroscopy is a very important tool to evaluate the value of remaining fibers in the ACL. The big advantage of the arthroscopy in contrast to MRI is the chance to check the tension of the functional bundles under different flexion angles and loading conditions (e.g., anterior drawer).

For best visualization of the ACL, the arthroscope should be switched to the anteromedial portal. The anteromedial portal enables the best visualization of the entire medial wall of the lateral condyle and the ACL. Concomitant proximal tears and partial intrasubstance tears of the AM bundle can be ruled out by meticulous probing of the ACL. Nonphysiologic lengthening of the AM bundle can also be detected from this position by probing the AM bundle for laxity while applying a force to translate the tibia anteriorly. Elongated PL bundles are best confirmed by using a probe to test tension in the PLB while internally rotating the tibia (Lorenz et al. 2009). Furthermore, the PLB can be better identified when the patient's knee is placed in the figure-of-four position (Sonnery-Cottet and Chambat 2007).

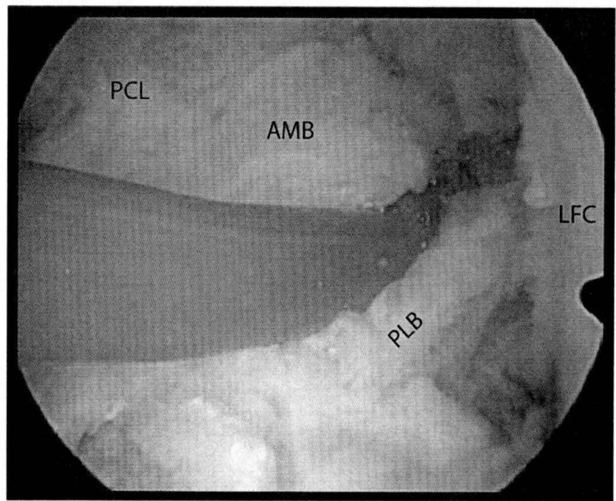

Fig. 1 Preparation of the femoral insertion of the torn anteromedial bundle (*AMB*) with an electrothermal device. The posterolateral bundle (*PLB*) is intact. *PCL* posterior cruciate ligament, *LFC* lateral femoral condyle

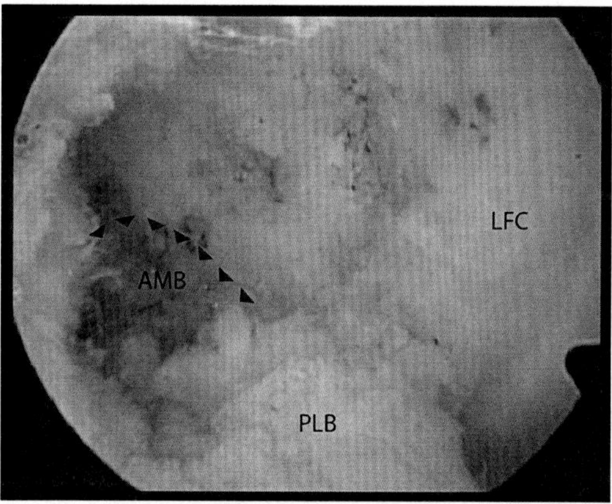

Fig. 2 View from the anteromedial portal. The AMB insertion is marked with *arrowheads*

Surgical Procedure: Partial Augmentation of the Anteromedial and Posterolateral Bundle

The resection of the torn ligament preserving the remaining fibers is of high importance. Insufficient tissue can be removed best by using a low-energy electrocautery device (Fig. 1). Bipolar devices have the advantage of a more superficial tissue penetration. The femoral and tibial insertion sites are prepared and visualized from the anteromedial portal (Fig. 2).

Firstly, the femoral tunnel is created. A 2.4 mm K-wire can be placed under direct view from an accessory anteromedial portal (Fig. 3) (Petersen et al. 2012). For the AMB augmentation, a drill guide with a defined offset can also be used (Fig. 4). Nevertheless the correct position of the K-wire should be controlled from the anteromedial portal before drilling the tunnel with a cannulated drill (Fig. 5).

On the tibial side, a 55-degree angulated tibial drill guide is utilized to place a 2.4 mm K-wire in the center of the AMB footprint (Fig. 6). The tunnel is created with a spiral drill. Due care should be taken not to harm the remaining fibers. Either the drill is forwarded manually at the articular side or a smaller drill is used and the tunnel is enlarged with dilators in 0.5 mm steps (Fig. 7).

Finally, the graft is inserted and fixed by interference screw or suspension sling at the femoral tunnel. Recent fixation devices like the ACL

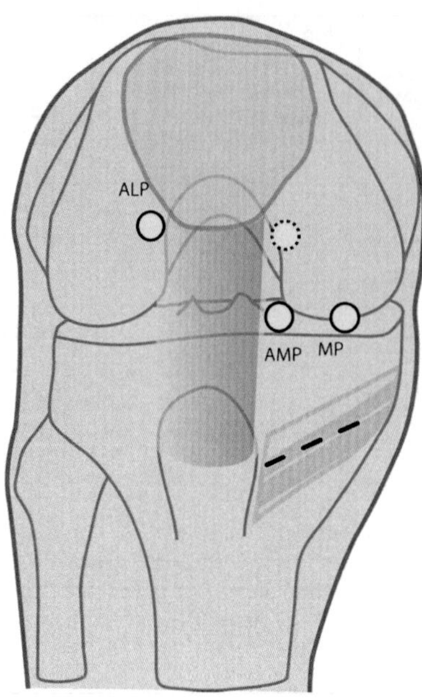

Fig. 3 Standard arthroscopic portals: anterolateral portal (*ALP*), low anteromedial (*AMP*) and medial (*MP*) portal. The *dotted circle* shows the position of an accessory portal that can be utilized for direct visualization of the lateral notch wall according to Petersen et al. (see text)

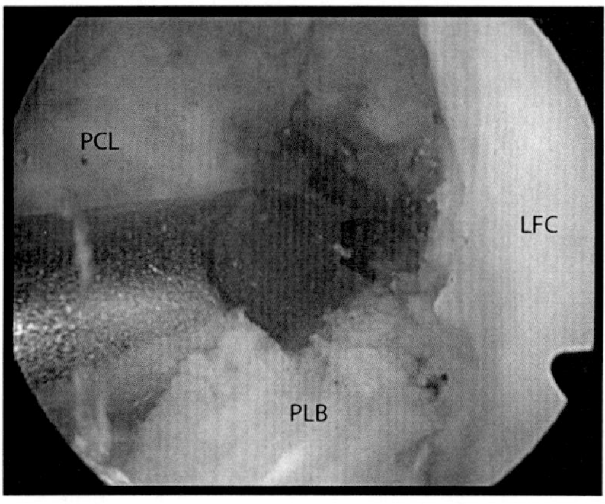

Fig. 4 Position of the drill guide and placement of a K-wire in the center of the AMB insertion. View from the ALP in 100° of flexion

TightRope™ (Arthrex Inc., Naples, FL) seem to have the advantage that the graft can be retightened at the end of the procedure if necessary. On the tibial side, the graft is pretensioned with 60 N by 20-time cycling of the knee joint. The graft fixation with an oversize interference

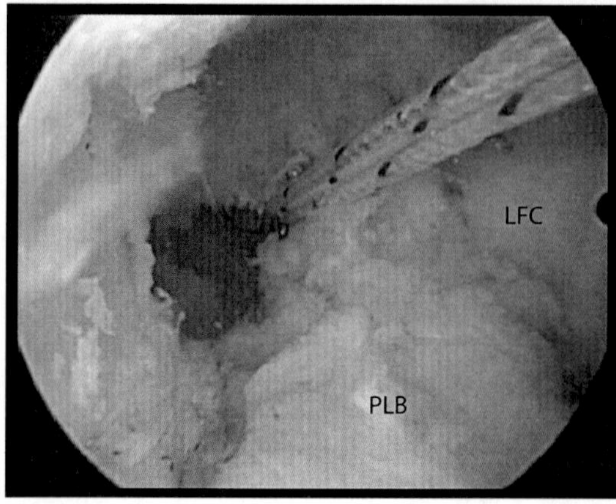

Fig. 5 Femoral tunnel for the AMB with pull-out suture. View from the AMP

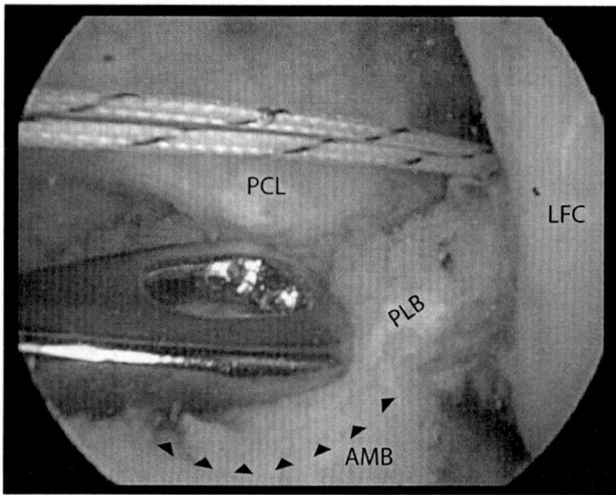

Fig. 6 Placement of a K-wire in front of the intact PLB in the center of the AMB insertion (*arrowheads*). View from the ALP

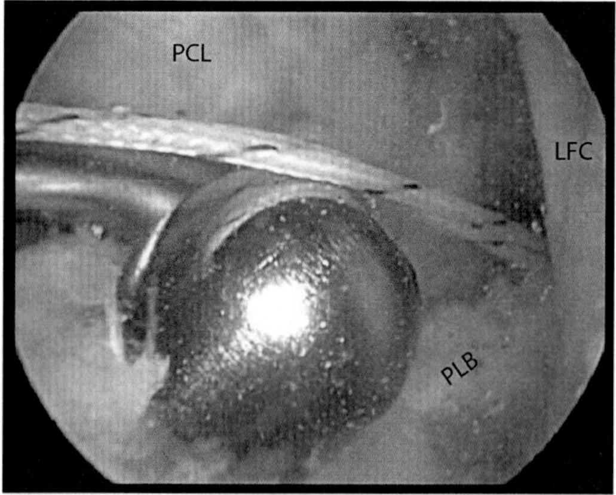

Fig. 7 Step-by-step enlarging of the tibial tunnel with dilators. View from the ALP

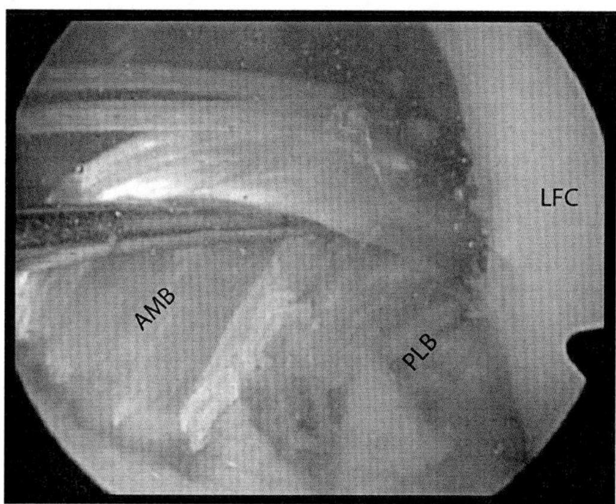

Fig. 8 The AMB graft is pulled in by two strands of the ACL TightRope ™

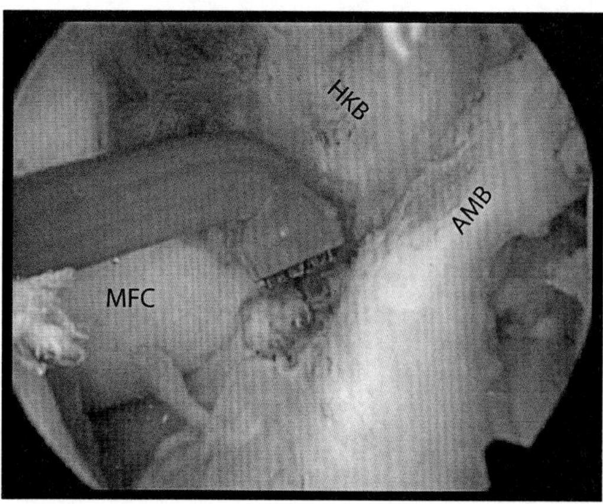

Fig. 10 Cautious preparation of the tibial PL footprint by preserving the AMB

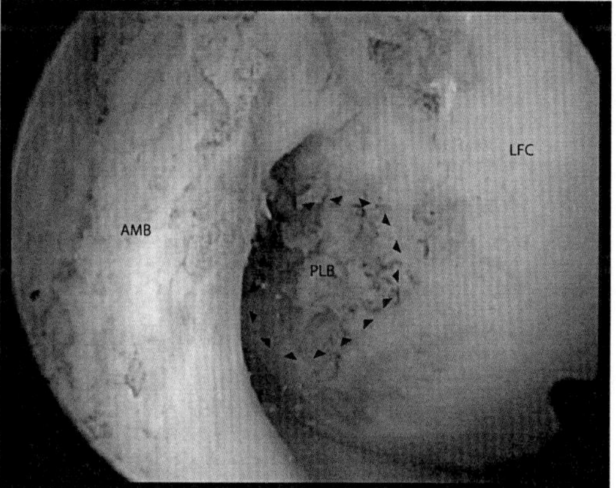

Fig. 9 Preparation of the femoral PLB insertion (*arrowheads*) with an electrothermal device. View from the AMP

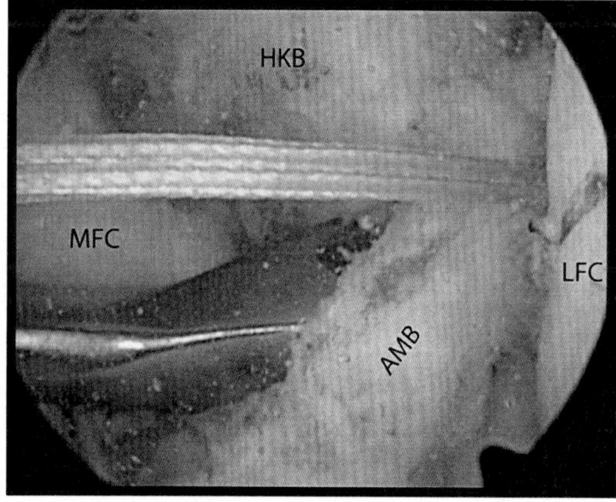

Fig. 11 Placement of a K-wire in the center of the PLB footprint. The suture runs through the previously created femoral PLB tunnel. View from the ALP

screw is accomplished at 15° of flexion. At the end of the procedure, the tension of the graft is checked with a probe (Fig. 8).

The PLB augmentation might be a little more challenging since the position of the tunnel apertures is either covered by the AMB or not clearly defined at the femoral and tibial insertion site, respectively. Therefore, preparation and good visualization are of even more importance than for the AMB augmentation. The insertions are prepared with an electrothermal device. In order to keep the intra-articular water pressure high, the femoral side is prepared first (Fig. 9). If remnants of the PLB fibers are remaining, the K-wire is placed in the center of the insertion. If not, the K-wire should be in line with the AMB in 102° of flexion with a distance of 6 mm of the "shallow" cartilage border (Siebold et al. 2008). The K-wire is overdrilled in more than 90° of flexion in order to preserve the peroneal nerve at the posterolateral aspect of the knee. On the tibial side, the footprint of the PLB is marked with an electrothermal device (Fig. 10). The tibial tunnel is planned and created with a 65° angulated drill guide and overdrilled with a cannulated reamer (Fig. 11). The pull-in suture is pulled through the tibial tunnel (Fig. 12), and the graft (normally a

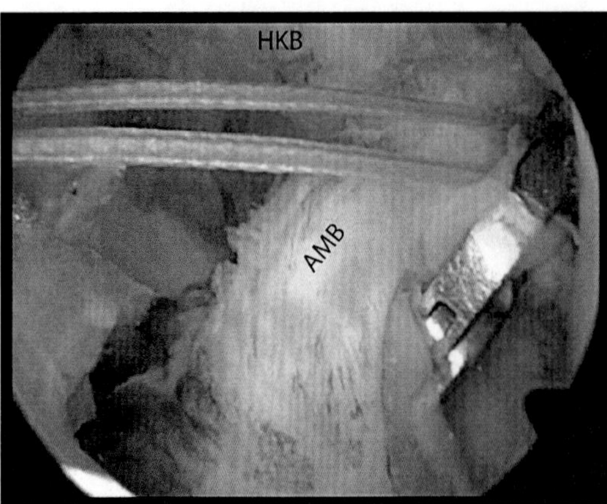

Fig. 12 The pull-in suture is grabbed and pulled through the tibial PLB tunnel

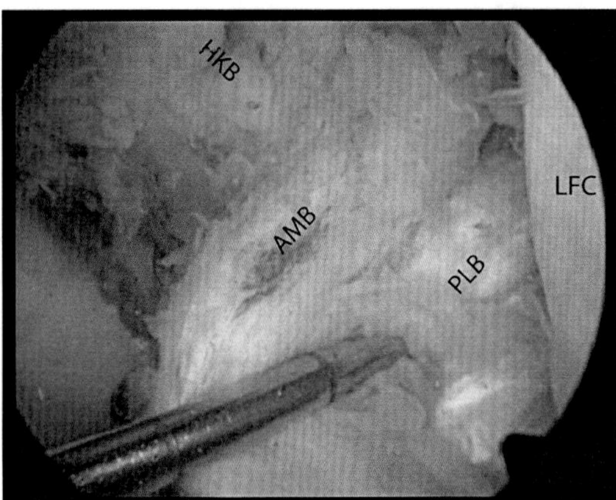

Fig. 13 Final result with the pulled-in PLB graft and the intact AMB

double/triple-looped gracilis tendon) is inserted under direct visualization while the AMB remnants are retracted with a probe (Fig. 13). Femoral fixation is accomplished either by interference screw or suspension sling.

Summary

In summary, a balanced positioning of the tunnels is crucial to perform a successful anatomic partial augmentation of the ACL. In order to prevent unphysiologic tension patterns of the graft that might lead to early graft failure, lack of motion, or persistent instability, grafts should be placed in corresponding insertion sites at femur and tibia (Fig. 14).

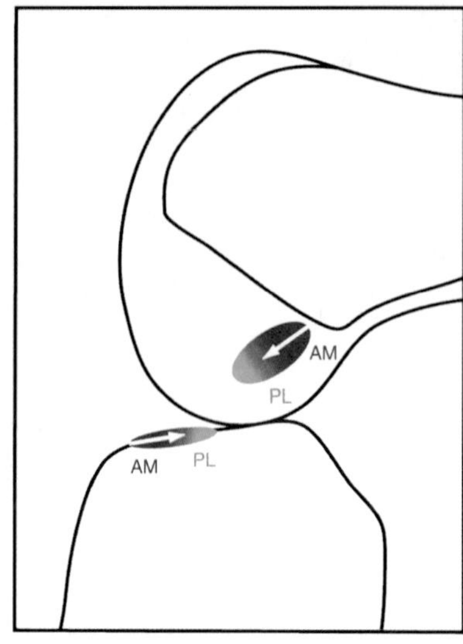

Fig. 14 Schematic drawing of the concept of balanced anatomic placement of tunnels in the femoral and tibial ACL insertion

Cross-References

- ▶ Anterior Cruciate Ligament Augmentation in Partial Ruptures
- ▶ Anterior Cruciate Ligament Injuries and Surgery: Current Evidence and Modern Development
- ▶ Different Techniques of Anterior Cruciate Ligament Reconstruction: Guidelines
- ▶ Double-Tunnel Anatomic Anterior Cruciate Ligament Reconstruction
- ▶ Graft Remodeling and Bony Ingrowth After Anterior Cruciate Ligament Reconstruction
- ▶ Partial Anterior Cruciate Ligament Ruptures: Knee Laxity Measurements and Pivot Shift
- ▶ Perioperative and Postoperative Anterior Cruciate Ligament Rehabilitation Focused on Soft Tissue Grafts
- ▶ Personalized Treatment Algorithms for Anterior Cruciate Ligament Injuries
- ▶ Revision Anterior Cruciate Ligament Reconstruction
- ▶ State of the Art in Anterior Cruciate Ligament Surgery

References

Araujo P, Eck CF, Torabi M, Fu FH (2012) How to optimize the use of MRI in anatomic ACL reconstruction. Knee Surg Sports Traumatol Arthrosc 21:1495–1501

Colombet P, Dejour D, Panisset JC, Siebold R (2010) Current concept of partial anterior cruciate ligament ruptures. Orthop Traumatol Surg Res 96:S109–S118

Crawford R, Walley G, Bridgman S, Maffulli N (2007) Magnetic resonance imaging versus arthroscopy in the diagnosis of knee pathology, concentrating on meniscal lesions and ACL tears: a systematic review. Br Med Bull 84:5–23

Dejour D, Ntagiopoulos P, Saggin PR, Panisset J-C (2013) The diagnostic value of clinical tests, magnetic resonance imaging, and instrumented laxity in the differentiation of complete versus partial anterior cruciate ligament tears. Arthroscopy 29:491–499

Galway H, Beaupre A, MacIntosh D (1972) Pivot shift: a clinical sign of symptomatic anterior cruciate deficiency. J Bone Joint Surg 54-B:763–764

Girgis FG, Marshall JL, Monajem A (1975) The cruciate ligaments of the knee joint. Anatomical, functional and experimental analysis. Clin Orthop Relat Res 106:216–231

Lorenz S, Illingworth KD, Fu FH (2009) Diagnosis of isolated posterolateral bundle tears of the anterior cruciate ligament. Arthroscopy 25:1203–1204, author reply 1204–1205

Losee RE, Johnson TR, Southwick WO (1978) Anterior subluxation of the lateral tibial plateau. A diagnostic test and operative repair. J Bone Joint Surg Am 60 A:1015–1030

Papalia R, Franceschi F, Zampogna B et al (2014) Surgical management of partial tears of the anterior cruciate ligament. Knee Surg Sports Traumatol Arthrosc 22:154–165

Petersen W, Achnich A, Forkel P et al (2012) The high medial portal. Arthroskopie 25:45–46

Pujol N, Colombet P, Cucurulo T et al (2012) Natural history of partial anterior cruciate ligament tears: a systematic literature review. Orthop Traumatol Surg Res 98:S160–S164

Siebold R, Fu FH (2008) Assessment and augmentation of symptomatic anteromedial or posterolateral bundle tears of the anterior cruciate ligament. Arthroscopy 24:1289–1298

Siebold R, Ellert T, Metz S, Metz J (2008) Tibial insertions of the anteromedial and posterolateral bundles of the anterior cruciate ligament: morphometry, arthroscopic landmarks, and orientation model for bone tunnel placement. Arthroscopy 24:154–161

Snyder-Mackler L, Fitzgerald GK, Bartolozzi AR, Ciccotti MG (1997) The relationship between passive joint laxity and functional outcome after anterior cruciate ligament injury. Am J Sports Med 25:191–195

Sonnery-Cottet B, Chambat P (2007) Arthroscopic identification of the anterior cruciate ligament posterolateral bundle: the figure-of-four position. Arthroscopy 23:1128 e1–1128 e3

Sonnery-Cottet B, Barth J, Graveleau N et al (2009) Arthroscopic identification of isolated tear of the posterolateral bundle of the anterior cruciate ligament. Arthroscopy 25:728–732

Tenuta JJ, Arciero RA (1994) Arthroscopic evaluation of meniscal repairs. Factors that effect healing. Am J Sports Med 22:797–802

Arthroscopic Repair of the Meniscus Tears

77

Ugur Haklar, Tekin Kerem Ulku, and Egemen Ayhan

Contents

U. Haklar (✉)
Orthopaedics and Traumatology Department, Bahcesehir University Medical Faculty, Liv Hospital, Istanbul, Turkey
e-mail: dr.haklar@superonline.com

T.K. Ulku
Orthopaedics and Traumatology Department, Camlica Erdem Hospital, Istanbul, Turkey
e-mail: keremulku@gmail.com

E. Ayhan
Orthopaedics and Traumatology Department, Liv Hospital, Istanbul, Turkey
e-mail: egemenay@yahoo.com

M.N. Doral, J. Karlsson (eds.), *Sports Injuries*,
DOI 10.1007/978-3-642-36569-0_72

Abstract

Meniscal tissue is essential for shock absorption, load distribution, joint lubrication, and proprioception. Removal of meniscal tissue usually causes subsequent degeneration of cartilage tissue over time. Therefore, repair rather than removal is essential when possible. Reparability of a tear depends on different factors as does the success of repair. Age, tear configuration, tear location, a patient's activity level, and the presence of additional ACL or chondral injury are among them. During the past three decades, outside-in, inside-out, and all-inside techniques were developed for arthroscopic meniscal repair. In general, the inside-out technique is accepted as the gold standard; however, over the past 10 years, all-inside techniques, with advancement of new designs, have reportedly produced comparable results. Meniscal root tears are also a unique topic deserving of special attention because meniscal extrusion has been proven to have deleterious effects on the articular cartilage.

Introduction

The human meniscus, composed of fibrocartilage tissue, is a very important structure for normal knee function. It acts as a shock absorber, load distributer, lubricator (Fukubayashi and Kurosawa 1980; Ahmed and Burke 1983), and proprioceptor (Baratz et al. 1986) and also assists in joint stability and cartilage nutrition. This vital role in knee stability protects the ACL-deficient knee from arthritic changes (Shoemaker and Markolf 1986). Therefore, a thorough understanding of meniscus anatomy, physiology, biomechanics, and healing properties aids improvements in meniscal repair techniques.

Partial meniscectomy is one of the most common performed surgical procedures of orthopaedic surgery. However, the meniscectomized knee raises concerns about future development of degenerative arthritis (Rupp et al. 2002). For this reason over the past two decades research has focused on retaining as much meniscal tissue as possible. This strategy not only balances contact stress distribution in knee joint but also helps to preserve chondral tissue from arthritic changes. It is this protective effect that makes meniscal repair desirable for tears with a sufficient blood supply to enable healing of a repair.

It has been over a century since the first meniscal repair was reported (Annandale 1885). Initially, open repair techniques were used and popularized by DeHaven et al. in 1978. In 1969, Ikeuchi performed and reported the first arthroscopic meniscal repair (Ikeuchi 1979). Over time, arthroscopic techniques have become more and more popular.

Three main arthroscopic techniques, outside in, inside out, and all inside, are used for meniscal repair. Charles Henning popularized the inside-out technique in 1983 (Henning et al. 1988). Russel Warren used and popularized outside-in technique in 1985 (Warren 1985). The all-inside technique was first used somewhat later around the early 1990s. By advancing technology, newer materials for all-inside repairs were developed. New generation all-inside devices are more stable and stronger biomechanically.

Anatomy

The menisci are semilunar, wedge-shaped specialized chondral tissue that adapts to the round-shaped femoral condyles to the relatively flat tibial plateau surface. They cover approximately 50–55 % of the medial and 60–65 % of the lateral plateau (Bloecker et al. 2012). Lateral meniscus is circular, while medial meniscus is semicircular "C" shaped. Meniscal tissue is thick and pliable at the peripheral part, whereas it tapers to a thin free articular border congruent with respective condylar surface. The medial meniscus is less mobile than the lateral meniscus because of its firm peripheral attachments to the joint capsule (Thompson et al. 1991). The lateral meniscus lacks peripheral attachments at popliteal hiatus and usually has the ligaments of Humphrey and Wrisberg that bind its posterior horn to the medial wall of the intercondylar notch. The anterior intermeniscal ligament attaches anterior horns of the each meniscus.

A microstructural view shows that meniscal tissue is composed of fibrochondrocytes surrounded by an extracellular matrix of collagen (mostly type 1), proteoglycans, glycoproteins, and elastin. Collagen is composed of three different layers. The superficial layer is composed of woven fibrils in a mesh-like pattern. The layer underneath is composed of randomly orientated collagen fibrils, and then there is the deep layer which has circumferential fibrils cross-linked with radial fibers. Circumferential fibrils run from root to root generating hoop stresses.

Another important subject about meniscal anatomy concerning repair is the meniscal blood supply. Capillary vessels penetrate to peripheral 20–30 % of medial and 10–25 % of lateral meniscal tissue (Arnoczky and Warren 1982). This vascular supply pattern has an important role in tear repair. Arnoczky et al. established the vascular zone system where the peripheral 3 mm is a red-red zone that has vascularity, the middle 3–5 mm is a red-white zone with variable vascularity, and the central 3 mm is a white-white zone that has very poor or no blood supply.

The neural supply of meniscal tissue also resembles its blood supply. Peripheral parts receive neural connections which make tears more symptomatic, but the more central parts receive no neural supply (Zimny and Wink 1991).

Suture Materials

There are many different types of suture materials. These materials are generally classified as absorbable versus nonabsorbable and braided versus non-braided.

Absorbable sutures degrade over time. The most commonly used absorbable sutures in orthopaedic surgery are PDS (Ethicon, Somerville, NJ, USA) and Panacryl (Ethicon, Somerville, NJ, USA). Absorbable materials have different absorption lengths. Manufacturers report 180–210 days of absorption time for PDS; however, its strength decreases to 50 % at 4 weeks. A more recent material, Panacryl, has up to 1.5 years of absorption time, and it reportedly retains 60 % of its original strength at 6 months.

Among nonabsorbable sutures, the most commonly used types are Polyblend polyethylene sutures Fiberwire (Arthrex, Naples, FL, USA), Herculine (Linvatec, Largo, FL, USA), and Orthocord (De Puy Mitek, Raynham, MA, USA) and polyester sutures like TiCron (Tyco, Waltham, MA, USA) and Ethibond (Ethicon, Somerville, NJ, USA). Ethibond, Polyblend polyethylene sutures, and TiCron are all braided. Braided and non-braided materials have certain advantages and disadvantages. Braided materials theoretically increase the risk of infection due to their disrupted surfaces; however, they are much easier to handle and knots are much more secure. Braided materials require at least four proper knots for secure fixation. For non-braided materials the most important handicap is their insecurity in knot tying compared to braided which require at least six proper knots to achieve good fixation (Ilahi et al. 2008). They also can cut the tissue because of their less flexible structure. On the other hand, they cause less tissue reaction.

One other important concern is strength of these materials. There are many studies reporting on the failure loads for different suture materials (Barber et al. 2003; Najibi et al. 2010). Among other materials, Polyblend polyethylene sutures have the highest load to failure strengths. When knotted Herculine was strongest (261 ± 44 N), followed by Ultrabraid (244 ± 3 N). Fiberwire is the most resistant against fraying on metallic anchors. Polyblend polyethylene sutures ultimate strength was found to be 2–2.5-fold greater than polyester sutures (Wüst et al. 2006).

Suture Configuration

Suture placement and configuration are another important subject. Many different configurations have been described. Among them are vertical, horizontal, double vertical, vertical mattress, and oblique configurations.

Vertical suturing is generally accepted as the gold standard for meniscal fixation (Henning et al. 1988). Horizontal configurations have the advantage of securing greater meniscal tissue, but it is weaker biomechanically (Karaoğlu et al. 2002).

Many studies report that vertical suture techniques have superior load to failure (Kohn and Siebert 1989; Rimmer et al.1995; Post et al. 1997; Rankin et al. 2002). Song et al. concluded that this superior load may be due to the incorporation of a greater proportion of semicircular-oriented meniscal collagen fibers (Song and Lee 1999). Based on this knowledge Kocabey et al. conducted a study for the pullout strength of oblique suturing and concluded that oblique suturing mixes the advantages of greater meniscal tissue fixation of horizontal sutures and greater proportion of semicircular fiber coverage of vertical sutures. And they advocated that oblique sutures provided better fixation than other techniques.

Suture configuration directly affects the apposition of meniscal tissue. Anatomical reduction is crucial in this step because it is shown that fibrinolysin in synovial fluid directly affects meniscal healing (Andersen et al. 1972). Therefore, configurations that can achieve the best anatomical reduction should be preferred to minimize fluid interposition.

Also, the tear configuration is another subject that determines suture configuration. For radial tears, the double horizontal repair configuration was shown to be effective (Haklar et al. 2008).

Generally, the preferred method is double vertical suturing for longitudinal and bucket handle tears using 5–6 mm intervals (Fig. 1a and b). This is because double vertical system provides better reduction and fixation of meniscal tissue.

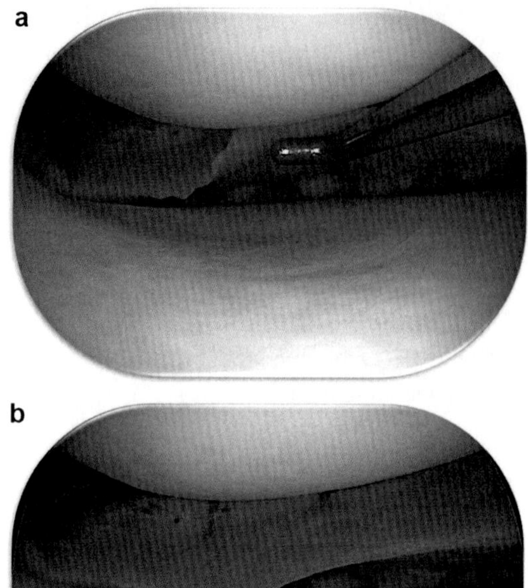

Fig. 1 (**a**) Arthroscopic view of double vertical sutures inferior surface of meniscus. (**b**) Arthroscopic view of double vertical sutures superior surface of meniscus

Meniscal Healing

Meniscal tissue has variable healing capacity. This variability depends on the tear site, tear pattern, and quality of meniscal tissue. Tears within three mm of the meniscosynovial junction have the capacity to heal due to an adequate blood supply, whereas more central tears in the red-white zone have less healing capacity (Arnoczky and Warren 1983). Tears in the white-white zone have a low healing capacity. The judgment to repair or excise a tear should be given by taking many different variables into consideration including the patient's age, tear type, occupation, and activity level and the surgeon's technical preferences. For example, in an elite athlete, the decision also includes the injury timing in season or number of the athlete's expected remaining competitive years.

It is reported that meniscal tissue heals through the normal wound healing pathways of the acute inflammation phase, granulation phase, formation of a fibrovascular scar, and maturation. Experimental tears in a dog model shoved evidences of healing at 10 weeks for peripheral tears (Kambic and McDevitt 2005). Meniscal fibrochondrocytes are also important participants of healing because they synthesize extracellular matrix and proliferate.

It should be kept in mind that healing is not the same with the restoration of biomechanical properties. Therefore, besides radiological studies, biomechanical research should also be emphasized. In some studies (Roeddecker et al. 1993) using rabbit models, it is shown that the energy required to tear a repaired meniscus after 6 weeks is 26 % and after 12 weeks is 23 % of normal meniscus. This increases to 42 % at 12 weeks if fibrin glue is added to repair. This data suggests that even after 12 weeks of repair, the repaired tissue is not as strong as desired. After 4 months of repair usually the healing tissue is visible in second-look arthroscopies (Morgan et al. 1991).

Factors Influencing Meniscal Repair

The indications for meniscal repair, regardless of the chosen repair method, are commonly the same and show some variability among different authors. DeHaven et al. defined factors as the tear location, tear type, configuration, tear size, and stability of meniscal tissue (DeHaven 1999). Peripheral location of tears is key because these tears are in the vascular zone. Cannon and Vittori reported 90 % healing rates for tears less than 2 mm from periphery, 74 % for tears within 3 mm, and 50 % for 4–5 mm from the rim (Cannon and Vittori 1992).

Additional factors can also be listed such as age of the patient, activity level and occupation, presence of concomitant ACL injury, presence of chondral lesions, and time elapsed since the tear happened. Acute tears are more amenable to repair, whereas chronic tears especially the ones in complex configuration are lesser candidates for repair.

Even though there is not a clear age limit, generally less than 30–35 years are considered as to be the best candidates for repair. Stein et al. described improved results for patients less than 30 years of age (Stein et al. 2010). Some authors reported this as 35 years of age. Patients between 35 and 50 years of age have relatively lower healing rates.

For more active patients with high activity level, decreasing the time required to return to full activity should be emphasized. However, this is a debatable subject for elite athletes. At early ages, at the beginning of their career, meniscal repair is the gold standard treatment. Whereas for older athletes or for some elite players at the top of their performance in the middle of the season, meniscectomy can be considered before repair keeping long healing period in mind. Probably the best decision is the one obtained together with the athlete, but the long-term effects of a meniscectomy should not be minimized.

A review of the literature shows many investigators agree that concomitant ACL reconstruction increases the success rates of repairs. Turman and Dudich reported repair success rates as high as 90 % with ACL reconstruction, whereas it was only 60–80 % for isolated tears (Turman and Diduch 2008). A very important point here is to never repair meniscal tissue without planning to reconstruct a torn ACL at the same time or at a planned staged procedure (Haas et al. 2005; Gallacher et al. 2012).

For young patients with concomitant chondral injuries, appropriate tears should be repaired together with the surgeon's selected method of chondral repair. But for older patients with chronic degenerative arthritis especially for patients older than 50 years, meniscal repair should be evaluated carefully.

Application of microfracture to the intercondylar notch or to the medial side of the medial femoral condyle was reported to be effective in meniscal healing after repair (Freedman et al. 2003; Haklar et al. 2013). The technique was described as application of five to eight perforations with a microfracture awl (approximately 3 cm^2) in the medial side of medial femoral condyle or lateral side of lateral femoral condyle depending on repaired meniscal side, after debridement of overlaying synovial tissue. At this level using superior portals for easy viewing and using anteromedial or anterolateral portals for microfracture awl can be appropriate (Fig. 2). Rasping the tear edges to obtain bleeding tissue is also crucial (Ochi et al. 2001). Once the tear is reduced to its original position, both margins of tear tissue should be rasped by using a mechanical rasp. Many types of rasps are commercially available (forward angle, back angle, double sided). By using these rasps and an arthroscopic motorized shaver, the free edges are debrided until establishing a smooth surface free of interposed tissue and tissue with punctate bleeding. A crucial point at this level is not to

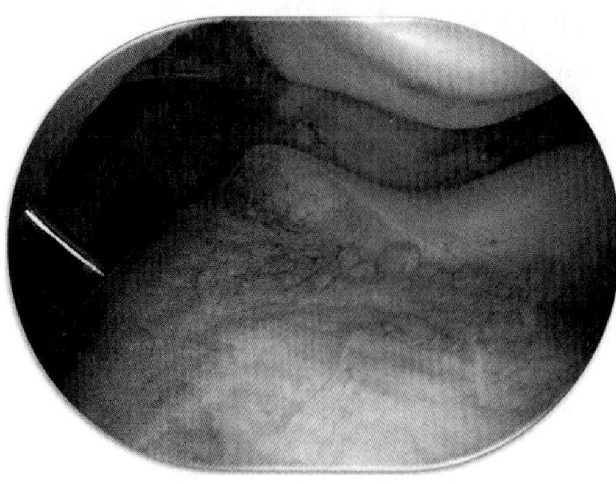

Fig. 2 Microfracture application on medial side of medial femoral condyle. Note the synovial debridement before using microfracture awl in order to prevent subsynovial accumulation of stem cells

debride or rasp any healthy meniscal tissue and decrease meniscal volume.

Originally described by Zhang et al., trephination consists of the use of a trephine which is a special device with a sharp end and connected to a motorized tool or 1 mm k wires to create tunnels in meniscal tissue to provide vascular ingrowth and healing. Different studies advocated superior results when compared with suturing alone (Zhang et al. 1995; Mintzer et al. 1998).

The fibrin clot technique is believed to directly add growth factors to the site of repair. This technique is also somewhat challenging. After a decision to repair is made, 40–60 ml of blood is drawn from the patient. The blood is placed in a glass beaker and stirred with a glass rod. After several minutes of stirring, the blood clot adheres to the rod. Once sufficient clot is formed by using arthroscopic probe, the clot is peeled to a sponge and it is ready to use. Through a plastic cannula it is placed to the joint. The repair site should be prepared so that all the sutures were placed but untied. Once the clot is placed into the repair site, the sutures can be tied.

This topic remains somewhat controversial in our series of medial meniscal tears treated with vertical mattress sutures. Tear length of more than 2 cm was shown to be a significant factor in meniscal healing. However, Kotsovos et al. found no significant differences in healing (Kotsovolos et al. 2006).

Many studies in the literature have described an inverse relation between soft tissue healing and smoking (Hoolinger et al. 2008; Wright et al. 2010). However, not many studies have been reported for smoking and meniscal healing. In a study conducted by Haklar et al., significantly improved results were obtained in meniscal healing for nonsmoking patients (Haklar et al. 2013).

Partial longitudinal tears treated with single vertical sutures have been reported to have a significantly higher healing potential than full thickness tears treated with double vertical sutures.

Biological adjuncts are one of the most studied subjects in meniscal tears currently. Recent studies have evaluated the effects of autologous bone marrow aspirate, CTGF, IL-1, TNF-α, TGF β,1 and VEGF on meniscal healing. Most of which have promising results but deserve further studies (Kopf et al. 2010; Riera et al. 2011). Ishida et al. showed the potent effect of platelet-rich plasma in increasing matrix deposition and proliferation of meniscus cells cultured in monolayer (Ishida et al. 2007).

Outside-In Meniscal Repair Technique

Indications

The outside-in technique is currently a seldom used technique popularized by Russell Warren around the mid-1980s but still deserves mentioning. It is especially useful for anterior horn and body tears (Rodeo and Warren 1996). This technique is generally not recommended for tears of the posterior horn.

Surgical Technique

The technique requires an 18 g needle and a monofilament suture material. Once the tear site is visualized, the first needle is inserted. Transillumination can help to identify the tear site and also can help avoid injuring the cutaneous nerves and vessels. Once the first needle is passed and suture material is sent in through the tear site, either the suture material is retrieved or a "mulberry knot" is tied and used as an internal anchor which can reduce the meniscal tissue. After this step, a second needle is passed through the tear site either in a horizontal or vertical orientation and a subsequent knot is made through a small incision and the two sutures are tied together over the joint capsule (Bloecker et al. 2012).

A modification of this technique is made by placing a metal snare or a monofilament loop from the second needle to retrieve the first one. Then, the suture is tied over the anterior joint capsule. In our practice, we believe that this technique is more suitable because it prevents chondral damage by the knots left inside the joint.

A successful outcome was reported in 87 % of patients repaired by this technique.

Inside-Out Meniscal Repair Technique

Indications

The inside-out technique for meniscal repair is suitable for tears of all parts of the menisci. It is especially very useful for body and posterior horn tears. The technique involves the use of zone-specific cannulas and absorbable or nonabsorbable sutures placed on flexible needles.

The indications for repair are the same as mentioned before. However, certain areas of meniscal tissue are more suitable to be repaired by the inside-out method. Commonly, all medial meniscal tears are best treated with the inside-out technique.

Surgical Technique

The inside-out repair may be performed with different setups. Supine positioning of the patient free leg and a lateral post is our standard setup allowing counter-traction of all compartments of the joint. This positioning allows for a circumferential approach to the knee allowing for an easier approach for suture retrieval.

The basic steps of the surgical technique are diagnostic arthroscopy, prepare ration of the tear site, exposure of the joint capsule, and placement of meniscal sutures.

After anesthesia and appropriate positioning of the patient, standard anterolateral and anteromedial portal incisions are made. A complete diagnostic arthroscopy using a 30° scope is made to correlate the MRI or preoperative findings and to reevaluate the reparability of the tear. Following meniscal evaluation a careful inspection of the cruciate ligaments and chondral tissue is standard.

Preparation of meniscal tissue involves the evaluation of reducibility of the tear (Figs. 3 and 4). Probing the tear combining with appropriate varus-valgus stress usually is the technique most commonly used; however, for significantly displaced bucket handle tears, Yoon et al. proposed outside-in piercing the displaced fragment with a suture

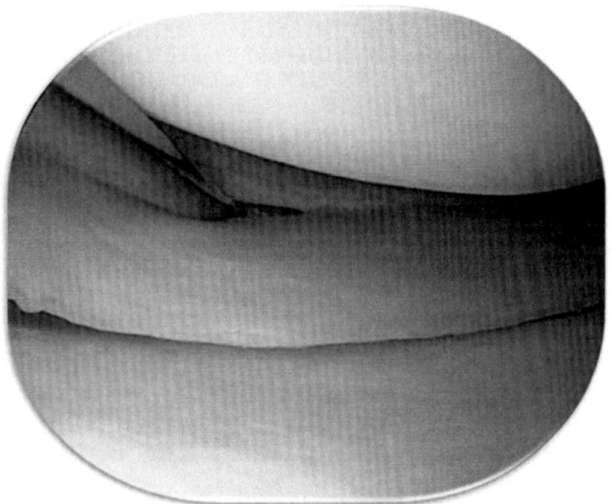

Fig. 3 Arthroscopic view of longitudinal tear in posterior horn of meniscus

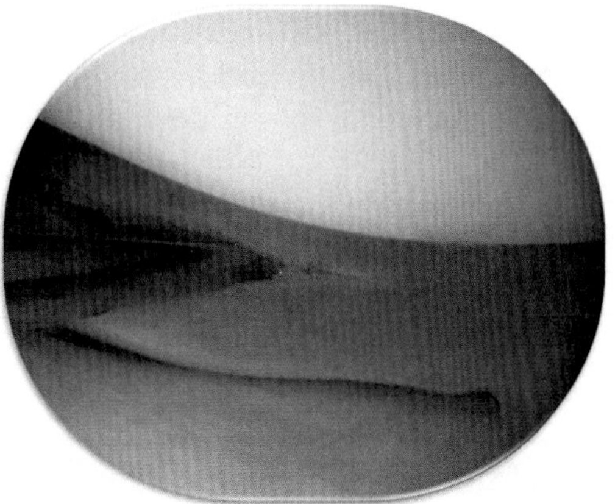

Fig. 4 Probing the tear site

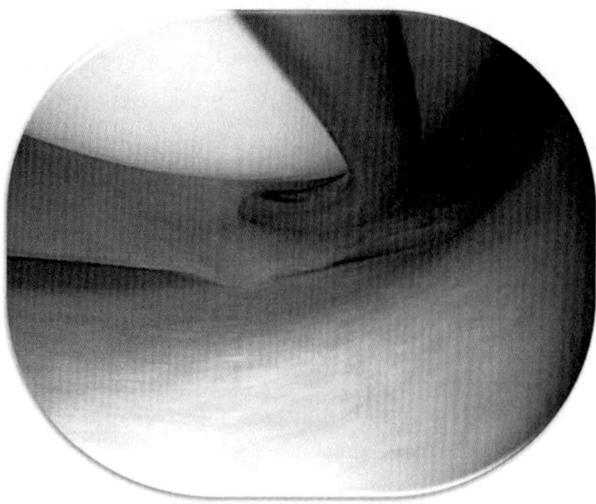

Fig. 5 Arthroscopic view of posterior horn tear with zone-specific cannula inserted, and meniscal tissue is reduced to its anatomical position

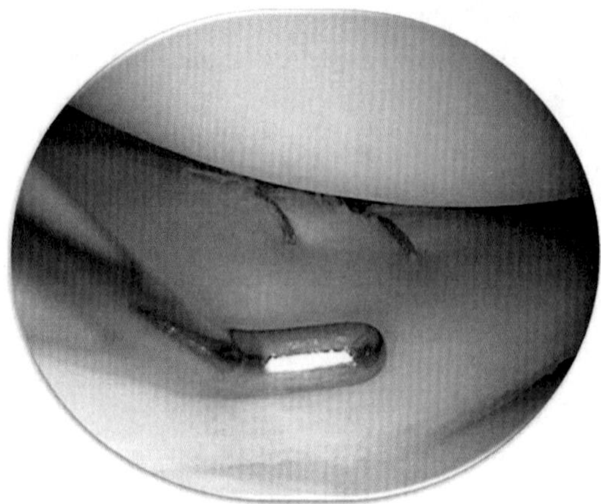

Fig. 6 Arthroscopic view after two all-inside sutures vertically placed using zone-specific cannula system

hook and reducing the displaced fragment (Fig. 5) (Yoon et al. 2009).

Suture placement through the portal is done using zone-specific cannula systems. Variations of this system as single or double barrels are present but we prefer a single barrel system. The double barrel system has the advantage of avoiding repositioning of the cannula after the first needle passage, but because of its large volume, it avoids easy application of vertical suture configuration (Fig. 6). The single barrel system gives the freedom to place the second arm of the stitch. When greater angles of curvature are intended for an anterior horn tear, a far lateral portal can be used to direct cannula.

Anatomical knowledge of the medial and lateral sides of the knee is of vital importance for surgical exposure (Wymenga et al. 2006). Medial exposure starts with the knee in 90° of flexion through a longitudinal or transverse exposure, centered over the joint line and just posterior to the medial collateral ligament. Care should be taken in order to avoid the saphenous nerve which generally lies just posterior to the incision (Wijdicks et al. 2010). Subcutaneous dissection is carried out using Metzenbaum scissors. During dissection, the infrapatellar branches of the saphenous nerve should be protected. This neural tissue lies just posterior to the sartorius muscle in most individuals. Initial flexion positioning of the knee is very important here to keep the nerve posterior. A more extension position moves the nerve anterior and may cause iatrogenic injuries. After subcutaneous dissection, a blunt dissection is carried out to create an interval between the posteromedial joint capsule and the medial head of the gastrocnemius. A popliteal retractor or a spoon is placed here to accept passing needles. The crucial step at this point is to stay anterior to the hamstring tendons. Sutures placed into the posterior horn generally tend to pass inside or posterior to semimembranosus tendon unless directed otherwise. Therefore, the semimembranosus tendon should be identified carefully. A small incision over the semimembranosus can be made to retract the tendon easily. This allows the surgeon to inspect tissues below the tendon clearly. Sutures around the tendon are then retrieved by an arthroscopic probe and tied anteriorly (Fig. 7).

Lateral exposure also involves a straight incision centered just slightly distal to the joint line and just posterior to the fibular collateral ligament. With subcutaneous dissection, the interval between the biceps femoris and the iliotibial band is identified and developed. The common peroneal nerve is at risk here; therefore, posterior retraction of biceps is very important to retract the nerve posteriorly and avoid an iatrogenic injury. The interval between the joint capsule and the

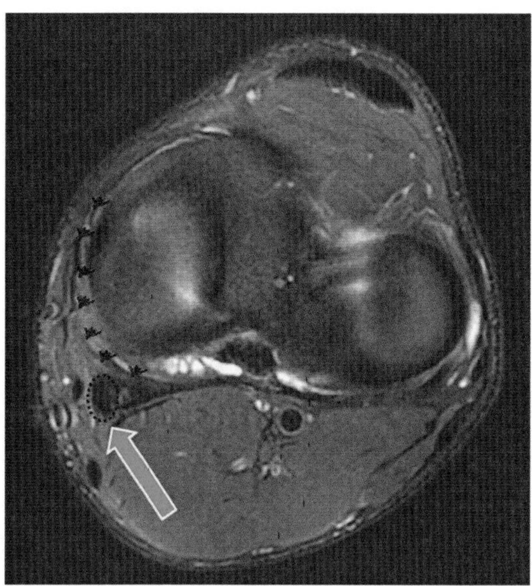

Fig. 7 After meniscal repair using inside-out technique position of knots. All knots are placed anterior to semimembranosus tendon marked with *green arrow*

lateral head of gastrocnemius is the area to position the popliteal retractor.

Suture tying should be done with the knee in 0–20°of flexion for anterior horn tears and at 50–60° of flexion for the posterior horn (Haklar et al. 2013).

All-Inside Meniscal Repair Technique

Indications

The all-inside repair technique has certain advantages compared to the inside-out technique. Elimination of a posterior incision, a potentially shorter operating time, and decreased risk of neurovascular injury are among the advantages. It was believed that inside-out technique allows a better tensioning on meniscal tissue; however, with advances in suture-based fixator systems, even bucket handle tears can often be secured reliably and consistently.

The indications for meniscal repair are mostly the same among all techniques. More posterior tears and tears involving meniscal body are easily approachable by all-inside techniques. However, this depends on the surgeon's preference. Also repair of more posterior tears places neurovascular structures at risk by inside-out technique, skill level, and surgical team. All-inside devices are designed for a more perpendicular approach to tears. Therefore, anterior tears are not very suitable to repair by all-inside techniques.

Specific Devices

Since their introduction to orthopaedic practice in the mid-1990s, there have been gradual changes and improvement in fixation systems. Although there is no consensus which device belongs to which generation, three or four different generations of devices have been introduced.

The first generation devices were similar in their composition of somewhat rigid materials. Mostly they were dart- or arrow-shaped materials They were composed of different proportions of PLLA and polyglactic acid.

The first generation devices had many disadvantages; prominently their rigid structure caused foreign body reaction and chondral damage. Also their biomechanical strength was inferior to traditional suture techniques. These caused the creation of newly designed systems.

Second generation devices, also called hybrid systems, mostly overcame these disadvantages. They had more complex structures combining soft suture materials and somewhat rigid backstops. Different companies introduced many different devices, with some still leaving hard materials, like top hats, onto the meniscus surface which could still cause chondral injury. Over the years of difficulty in the handling and deploying of these devices, larger backstop anchors and weaker suture materials urged the need of newer generation devices.

Devices commonly referred as third generation mostly are modifications of second generation devices. They have smaller backstop anchors, stronger suture materials, easier handles, and easily deployable sliding knots. The most commonly used third generation systems are the FasT-Fix

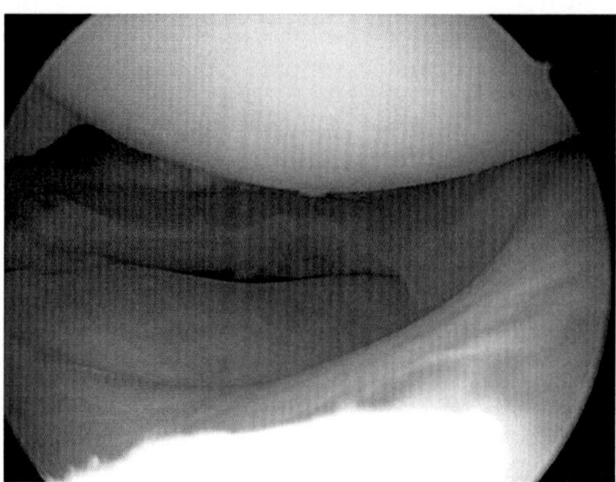

Fig. 8 All-inside meniscal repair using all-inside technique by Meniscal Cinch (Arthrex)

360 for Smith and Nephew (Andover, MA, USA), Crossbow for Linvatec (Largo, FL, USA), Omniscan for Mitek (Westwood, MA, USA), MaxFire and MaxFire MarXmen for Biomet (Warsaw, Indiana, USA), and Cinch for Arthrex (Naples, Florida, USA).

As a commonly used second generation device, the FasT-Fix 360 uses a suture anchor bar as T -Fix did, but it also had another anchor attached to a braided suture which can be deployed by a self-sliding knot. Unlike the FasT-Fix Rapid Lock which used a single backstop anchor behind the capsule and a top-hat anchor brought onto the meniscus, it is tightened until it starts to dimple. For both systems different delivery angles are available.

A third generation Maxfire (Biomet, Warsaw, Indiana, USA) was introduced in March 2007 by Biomet, Cinch, in March 2008 by Arthrex (Arthrex Naples, Florida, USA) (Fig. 8). MaxFire is a suture only system that uses ZipLoop technology. Here a single braided polyethylene is woven through itself two times in opposing directions. The loop is tensioned along the articular side of meniscus so no knots are necessary. After the MaxFire device, Biomet introduced the MaxFire MarXmen which is basically the same as the MaxFire except its special handle design which according to their studies required the least insertion force compared to other all-inside devices. The cinch uses two peek anchors and a sliding pre-tied knot which can be tensioned. Biomet advocates that the ultimate load to failure is approximately 100 N which is highest for all comparable devices. The CrossFix is a suture only device. It deploys two needles at the same time across the tear and a crossing needle passes the polymer to other needle just behind the capsule. The suture is then tightened by a pre-tied sliding knot over the meniscus.

A different design that is commonly described as fourth generation by Linvatec is named the Sequent. It is a special multi-anchor design that allows the surgeon to place four to seven PEEK anchors without removing the device. It creates a continuous running stitch or separate stitches based upon the surgeon's preference. In order to lock the suture, a double rotation is made at each anchor, and once all the sutures are placed and tightened, the suture tail is cut with a cutter device.

Root Repair

Meniscal root tears are unique clinical entities that deserve special interest. As mentioned earlier normal meniscal function depends on circumferally oriented collagen, coronary ligaments, and root attachments that anchor meniscal tissue (Wojtys and Chan 2005). By altering meniscal attachment properties, root tears compromise meniscal kinematics (Lerer et al. 2004; Allaire et al. 2008).

Tears of the lateral meniscal roots commonly accompany ACL injuries (Fu 2010). Recently medial meniscal root tears have been recognized (Brody et al. 2006). Medial meniscal root tears are often the cause of meniscal extrusion, which means a dysfunctional meniscus that causes overloading of the medial femoral condyle and tibial plateau and rapidly progressive arthritis (Habata et al. 2004). Therefore, with the help of this knowledge, new techniques of meniscal root repair have been introduced. Results have been shown to be successful for root tears, and especially meniscal excursion has been reported to decrease significantly (Ahn et al. 2009; Vyas and Harner 2012).

Indications

Indications for meniscal root tear repairs differ between the lateral and medial menisci. Typically lateral meniscal root tears occur as a result of valgus and rotationary loading that causes severe bone bruise in a young active patient (Fu 2010). Therefore, the indication for repair is that of similar to ACL reconstruction. However, for medial root tears, the classical scenario is somewhat different. A common etiology is a 40–50-year-old female with a sudden onset of medial knee pain after a relatively low-energy trauma, such as rising from a chair or stair climbing. For this patient treatment should be tailored according to his/her expectations. Patients who are significantly symptomatic and have a high functional demand deserve a surgical repair to preserve knee kinematics, whereas an overweight or obese patient with lower expectations may be considered for a weight loss consultation, lifestyle modification like avoiding deep squads, rest, or NSAID drugs.

For both meniscus root tears, a common indication and main determinative for root repair is the presence of chondral injury. Therefore, the Rosenberg view is very useful for all patients in preoperative planning.

Surgical Technique

Portals needed include standard AM, AL, and PM portals. After portal establishment, a careful inspection including direct visualization of the posterior root of the medial meniscus is crucial because the meniscus may seem totally normal through a standard arthroscopic approach. This visualization can easily be achieved through a Gillquist view. Using the arthroscope through the AL portal, a motorized shaver is inserted through the AM portal, and the synovial tissue beneath the PM bundle of the PCL is resected. Following this resection, a reverse notchplasty may be done. This should be done sufficient enough to use all the instruments including an aiming guide. The tear site is reevaluated and using a shaver or a rasp, the attachment site should be debrided till a broad bone tissue is visible.

The next step is suture passage in which different suture passer devices can be used according to the surgeon's preference. After passage, loop is retrieved back out from AL portal, and free suture ends are held out to wait for tunnel preparation.

Then using an ACL guide, a tunnel is prepared and a suture passer device is exchanged with the drill, and monofilament is retrieved through this tunnel and the sutures are tied over a button on the tibia.

Complications

The complications of meniscal repair largely depend on the type of repair applied. For the inside-out technique, probably the most important complications are neurovascular complications. The sural and common peroneal nerves for the lateral and saphenous nerve in medial repairs are among the structures at highest risk. Also if a tourniquet is used, deflation prior to wound closure is important for hemostasis because of potential bleeding from the inferior lateral geniculate artery on the lateral side. For all-inside materials, especially for earlier generation devices, chondral injury due to remaining rigid structures in the joint is a common complication.

Arthrofibrosis although not very commonly seen is also a possible complication of meniscal repair surgery together with other knee surgery complications.

Rehabilitation

Rehabilitation protocols after meniscal repair have evolved greatly. But the surgeon's preference is probably still the most important factor. Some surgeons believe in a more conservative approach giving satisfactory results, whereas others support a more accelerated approach.

For a conservative approach 2 weeks of knee immobilization in extension in a brace followed by 10–80° of flexion for two more weeks, and limited weight bearing for two more weeks, a total of 6 weeks is sufficient for most protocols (DeHaven 1999).

Accelerated approach advocates immediate full range of motion followed by weight bearing as tolerated (Barber 1994; Shelbourne et al. 1996). For most tears individualization of physiotherapy is crucial. One of the most important criteria is preinjury activity status. Expectations of an elite athlete, a recreational athlete, and a non-athlete would be different.

Probably the most useful protocol is 0–90° of flexion at first 4 weeks and non-weight bearing or partial weight bearing for the first 3 weeks. After 4 weeks up to 4 months, active max flexion is done as tolerated and, after 4 months terminal flexion, exercises can be started.

Conclusion

Meniscal tissue is a vital tissue for proper knee kinematics. Removal of meniscal tissue usually causes subsequent degeneration of cartilage tissue over time. Reparability of a tear depends on different factors as does the success of repair.

Decision making for meniscal repair is sometimes challenging for most orthopaedic surgeons. However, over the past 10 years, all-inside techniques, especially with advancement of new designs, became easily applicable and have reportedly produced comparable results. Therefore, repair rather than removal is essential when possible.

Cross-References

- ▶ Anatomy and Biomechanics of the Knee
- ▶ Asymptomatic Meniscal Tears
- ▶ Human Meniscus: From Biology to Tissue Engineering Strategies
- ▶ Meniscal Injuries and Discoid Lateral Meniscus in Adolescent Athletes

References

Ahmed AM, Burke DL (1983) In-vitro measurement of static pressure distribution in synovial joints–Part I: tibial surface of the knee. J Biomech Eng 105:216–225

Ahn JH, Lee YS, Chang JY et al (2009) Arthroscopic all inside repair of the lateral meniscus root tear. Knee 16:77–80. Epub

Allaire R, Muriuki M, Gilbertson L et al (2008) Biomechanical consequences of a tear of the posterior root of the medial meniscus. Similar to total meniscectomy. J Bone Joint Surg Am 90:1922–1931

Andersen RB, Gormsen J, Petersen PH (1972) Protease activity in synovial tissue extracts. Scand J Rheumatol 1:75–79

Annandale T (1885) An operation for displaced semilunar cartilage. Br Med J 1:779

Arnoczky SP, Warren RF (1982) Microvasculature of the human meniscus. Am J Sports Med 10:90–95

Arnoczky SP, Warren RF (1983) The microvasculature of the meniscus and its response to injury. An experimental study in the dog. Am J Sports Med 11:131–141

Baratz ME, Fu FH, Mengato R (1986) Meniscal tears: the effect of meniscectomy and of repair on intraarticular contact areas and stress in the human knee. A preliminary report. Am J Sports Med 14:270–275

Barber FA (1994) Accelerated rehabilitation for meniscus repairs. Arthroscopy 10:206–210

Barber FA, Herbert MA, Richards DP (2003) Sutures and suture anchors: update. Arthroscopy 19:985–990

Bloecker K, Wirth W, Hudelmaier M et al (2012) Morphometric differences between the medial and lateral meniscus in healthy men – a three-dimensional analysis using magnetic resonance imaging. Cells Tissues Organs 195:353–364. Epub

Brody JM, Lin HM, Hulstyn MJ et al (2006) Lateral meniscus root tear and meniscus extrusion with anterior cruciate ligament tear. Radiology 239:805–810

Cannon WD Jr, Vittori JM (1992) The incidence of healing in arthroscopic meniscal repairs in anterior cruciate ligament-reconstructed knees versus stable knees. Am J Sports Med 20:176–181

DeHaven KE (1999) Meniscus repair. Am J Sports Med 27:242–250. Review

Freedman KB, Nho SJ, Cole BJ (2003) Marrow stimulating technique to augment meniscus repair. Arthroscopy 19:794–798

Fu F (2010) Master techniques in orthopaedic surgery sports medicine, 1st edn. Lippincott& Williams, Philadelphia, pp 263–271

Fukubayashi T, Kurosawa H (1980) The contact area and pressure distribution pattern of the knee. A study of normal and osteoarthrotic knee joint. Acta Orthop Scand 51:871–879

Gallacher PD, Gilbert RE, Kanes G et al (2012) Outcome of meniscal repair prior compared with concurrent ACL reconstruction. Knee 19:461–463. Epub

Haas AL, Schepsis AA, Hornstein J et al (2005) Meniscal repair using the FasT-Fix all-inside meniscal repair device. Arthroscopy 21:167–175

Habata T, Uematsu K, Hattori K et al (2004) Clinical features of the posterior horn tear in the medial meniscus. Arch Orthop Trauma Surg 124:642–645. Epub

Haklar U, Kocaoglu B, Nalbantoglu U et al (2008) Arthroscopic repair of radial lateral meniscus tear by double horizontal sutures with inside-outside technique. Knee 15:355–359. Epub

Haklar U, Donmez F, Basaran SH et al (2013) Results of arthroscopic repair of partial- or full-thickness longitudinal medial meniscal tears by single or double vertical sutures using the inside-out technique. Am J Sports Med 41:596–602

Henning CE, Clark JR, Lynch MA et al (1988) Arthroscopic meniscus repair with a posterior incision. Instr Course Lect 37:209–221

Hollinger JO, Hart CE, Hirsch SN et al (2008) Recombinant human platelet-derived growth factor: biology and clinical applications. J Bone Joint Surg Am 90(Suppl 1):48–54. Review

Ikeuchi H (1979) Meniscus surgery using the Watanabe arthroscope. Orthop Clin N Am 10:629–642

Ilahi OA, Younas SA, Ho DM et al (2008) Security of knots tied with ethibond, fiberwire, orthocord, or ultrabraid. Am J Sports Med 36:2407–2414. doi:10.1177/0363546508323745. Epub

Ishida K, Kuroda R, Miwa M et al (2007) The regenerative effects of platelet-rich plasma on meniscal cells in vitro and its in vivo application with biodegradable gelatin hydrogel. Tissue Eng 13:1103–1112

Kambic HE, McDevitt CA (2005) Spatial organization of types I and II collagen in the canine meniscus. J Orthop Res 23:142–149

Karaoglu S, Duygulu F, Inan M et al (2002) Improving the biomechanical properties of the T-fix using oblique direction: in vitro study on bovine menisci. Knee Surg Sports Traumatol Arthrosc 10:198–201. Epub

Kohn D, Siebert W (1989) Meniscus suture techniques: a comparative biomechanical cadaver study. Arthroscopy 5:324–327

Kopf S, Birkenfeld F, Becker R et al (2010) Local treatment of meniscal lesions with vascular endothelial growth factor. J Bone Joint Surg Am 92:2682–2691

Kotsovolos ES, Hantes ME, Mastrokalos DS et al (2006) Results of all-inside meniscal repair with the FasT-Fix meniscal repair system. Arthroscopy 22:3–9

Lerer DB, Umans HR, Hu MX et al (2004) The role of meniscal root pathology and radial meniscal tear in medial meniscal extrusion. Skeletal Radiol 33:569–574. Epub

Mintzer CM, Richmond JC, Taylor J et al (1998) Meniscal repair in the young athlete. Am J Sports Med 26:630–633

Morgan CD, Wojtys EM, Casscells CD et al (1991) Arthroscopic meniscal repair evaluated by second-look arthroscopy. Am J Sports Med 19:632–637

Najibi S, Banglmeier R, Matta J et al (2010) Material properties of common suture materials in orthopaedic surgery. Iowa Orthop J 30:84–88

Ochi M, Uchio Y, Okuda K et al (2001) Expression of cytokines after meniscal rasping to promote meniscal healing. Arthroscopy 17:724–731

Post WR, Akers SR, Kish V (1997) Load to failure of common meniscal repair techniques: effects of suture technique and suture material. Arthroscopy 13:731–736

Rankin CC, Lintner DM, Noble PC et al (2002) A biomechanical analysis of meniscal repair techniques. Am J Sports Med 30:492–497

Riera KM, Rothfusz NE, Wilusz RE et al (2011) Interleukin-1, tumor necrosis factor-alpha, and transforming growth factor-beta 1 and integrative meniscal repair: influences on meniscal cell proliferation and migration. Arthritis Res Ther 13:R187. Epub

Rimmer MG, Nawana NS, Keene GC et al (1995) Failure strengths of different meniscal suturing techniques. Arthroscopy 11:146–150

Rodeo SA, Warren RF (1996) Meniscal repair using the outside-to-inside technique. Clin Sports Med 15:469–481

Roeddecker K, Nagelschmidt M, Koebke J et al (1993) Meniscal healing: a histological study in rabbits. Knee Surg Sports Traumatol Arthrosc 1:28–33

Rupp S, Seil R, Kohn D (2002) [Meniscus lesions] [Article in German]. Orthopade 31812-28, 829–831

Shelbourne KD, Patel DV, Adsit WS et al (1996) Rehabilitation after meniscal repair. Clin Sports Med 15:595–612. Review

Shoemaker SC, Markolf KL (1986) The role of the meniscus in the anterior-posterior stability of the loaded anterior cruciate-deficient knee. Effects of partial versus total excision. J Bone Joint Surg Am 68:71–79

Song EK, Lee KB (1999) Biomechanical test comparing the load to failure of the biodegradable meniscus arrow versus meniscal suture. Arthroscopy 15:726–732

Stein T, Mehling AP, Welsch F et al (2010) Long-term outcome after arthroscopic meniscal repair versus arthroscopic partial meniscectomy for traumatic meniscal tears. Am J Sports Med 38:1542–1548

Thompson WO, Thaete FL, Fu FH et al (1991) Tibial meniscal dynamics using three-dimensional reconstruction of magnetic resonance images. Am J Sports Med 19:210–215; discussion 215-6

Turman KA, Diduch DR (2008) Meniscal repair: indications and techniques. J Knee Surg 21:154–162. Review

Vyas D, Harner CD (2012) Meniscus root repair. Sports Med Arthrosc 20:86–94. Review

Warren RF (1985) Arthroscopic meniscus repair. Arthroscopy 1:170–172

Wijdicks CA, Westerhaus BD, Brand EJ et al (2010) Sartorial branch of the saphenous nerve in relation to a medial knee ligament repair or reconstruction. Knee Surg Sports Traumatol Arthrosc 18:1105–1109. Epub

Wojtys EM, Chan DB (2005) Meniscus structure and function. Instr Course Lect 54:323–330. Review

Wright R, Mackey RB, Silva M et al (2010) Smoking and mouse MCL healing. J Knee Surg 23:193–199

Wüst DM, Meyer DC, Favre P et al (2006) Mechanical and handling properties of braided polyblend polyethylene sutures in comparison to braided polyester and monofilament polydioxanone sutures. Arthroscopy 22:1146–1153

Wymenga AB, Kats JJ, Kooloos J et al (2006) Surgical anatomy of the medial collateral ligament and the posteromedial capsule of the knee. Knee Surg Sports Traumatol Arthrosc 14:229–234. Epub

Yoon JR, Muzaffar N, Kang JW et al (2009) A novel technique for arthroscopic reduction and repair of a bucket-handle meniscal tear. Knee Surg Sports Traumatol Arthrosc 17:1332–1335. Epub

Zhang Z, Arnold JA, Williams T et al (1995) Repairs by trephination and suturing of longitudinal injuries in the avascular area of the meniscus in goats. Am J Sports Med 23:35–41

Zimny ML, Wink CS (1991) Neuroreceptors in the tissues of the knee joint. J Electromyogr Kinesiol 1:148–157. doi:10.1016/1050-6411(91)90031-Y

78 Asymptomatic Meniscal Tears

Niv Marom and Gideon Mann

Contents

Abstract

Meniscus tears can occur following a local trauma or spontaneously due to aging and degenerative processes. An asymptomatic meniscal tear finding on MRI scan is common. It ranges from ~5 % in young ages and up to 67 % in older ages. The older the patient is and the more osteoarthritic findings, the higher the prevalence. There is no evidence of a direct link between meniscal tears and knee symptoms in middle-aged and older adults, and it is evident that meniscal tears and knee symptoms are separately connected to osteoarthritis. A diagnosis of an asymptomatic meniscal tear requires careful evaluation and consideration when choosing the appropriate treatment. Once ruling out mechanical complaints and symptoms, the treatment of choice is conservative treatment because there is a lack of evidence of superiority for surgical treatments. Further research is needed for assessing and comparing the efficacy of the various possible treatments.

N. Marom (✉)
Department of Orthopedic Surgery, Meir University Hospital Medical Center, Kfar-Saba, Israel
e-mail: niv.marom@gmail.com

G. Mann
Service of Sports Injuries, Department of Orthopaedic Surgery, Meir Medical Centre, Tel Aviv University, Tel Aviv, Israel
e-mail: gideon.mann.md@gmail.com; gideon.mann@gmail.com

M.N. Doral, J. Karlsson (eds.), *Sports Injuries*,
DOI 10.1007/978-3-642-36569-0_70

Introduction

The knee menisci are two semicircular fibrocartilaginous structures located between the articular cartilage surfaces of the femur and tibia. The main functions of the menisci are for shock absorption and load transmission in the knee, mainly through the distribution of mechanical stress over a large area of the joint cartilage. Loss of meniscal function is recognized as a potential risk factor for both the development of knee osteoarthritis (OA) and cartilage loss in OA (Englund et al. 2007).

Meniscal tears, either traumatic or degenerative, can be symptomatic or asymptomatic. The complex mechanism of knee symptoms production, such as pain and stiffness in cases of meniscal tears, is not yet fully understood. It is conceivable that meniscal lesions that extend to the outer one-third of the meniscus, where neural innervations and nociceptors are present, might directly produce pain. It is also possible that the compromised meniscal function might produce knee pain from other structures within the joint (Mine et al. 2000; Englund et al. 2007).

Magnetic resonance imaging (MRI) is frequently used in the diagnosis of meniscal damage and has high sensitivity and specificity (Crues et al. 1987). The literature has reported that asymptomatic meniscal tears in the general population are a common finding on MRI scans. There is no specific data regarding subgroups of the population, such as: recreational or competitive athletes.

Prevalence in the Young Asymptomatic Population

In the young *asymptomatic* population, the prevalence of MRI finding of a meniscal tear (linear signal within the meniscus that extends to the meniscal surface) was found to be 5.6 % (LaPrade et al. 1994). This study investigated the MRI findings of knees of 54 asymptomatic young subjects with the mean age of 28.5 years old (range, 19–39). Changes of a lesser grade within the meniscus (linear signal that *does not* extend to meniscal surface) were found in up to 24.1 %. There is no other data in literature that focuses on the prevalence of meniscal tears in the young asymptomatic population. It can be assumed that based on current MRI technologies, the prevalence would be higher.

Prevalence in the Asymptomatic Middle-Aged and Elderly Population

When considering an MRI finding of meniscal tear in the *asymptomatic* middle-aged and elderly population, the picture is much more complex.

Englund et al. (2008) showed that the prevalence of an MRI finding of a meniscal tear in an overall sample of 991 subjects with a mean age of 62.3 years (range, 50.1–90.5) was 31 %. The prevalence of meniscal damage increased with increasing age in both sexes, up to 56 % and 51 % among men and women aged 70–90, respectively. A majority of the meniscal tears (61 %) were in subjects who had no knee symptoms.

More evidence of the high prevalence of asymptomatic meniscal tears (based on MRI finding) in the middle-aged and elderly population has been published during the last decade: Bhattacharyya et al. (2003) evaluated a group of 154 patients (age above 45) with clinical symptoms of knee osteoarthritis and a group of 49 age-matched asymptomatic controls. An MRI finding of a medial or lateral meniscal tear was a common finding in the asymptomatic subjects (prevalence=76 %). Zanetti et al. (2005) published their study that prospectively evaluated the clinical course of asymptomatic meniscal lesions diagnosed by MRI. They found 37 % prevalence of asymptomatic meniscal tears in the study group (age range, 18–73 years). Englund et al. (2007) published a study that evaluated the effect of meniscal damage on the development of frequent knee pain, aching, or stiffness in middle-aged and older adults. The authors investigated knees at baseline and at 15 months follow-up. Meniscal damage was common at baseline in both "case knees," who developed knee symptoms during the 15 months follow-up (prevalence=38 %), and "control knees," who remained asymptomatic at 15 months follow-up (prevalence=29 %).

All studies show similar trends; the prevalence of a finding of a meniscal tear rises with increasing age and also increases with more severe

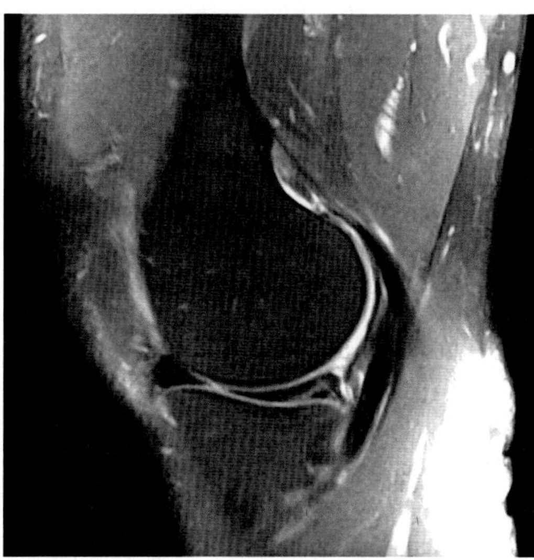

Fig. 1 Sagittal fat-suppressed T2 sequence magnetic resonance image showing a complex medial meniscal tear in an asymptomatic 63-year-old male

radiographic evidence of osteoarthritis. The higher the Kellgren-Lawrence grade, the higher the prevalence of a meniscal tear. Englund et al. (2008) showed a prevalence of more than 80 % of meniscal tears among persons with radiographic evidence of severe osteoarthritis (Kellgren and Lawrence grade of 3 or 4). Figure 1 shows an MRI scan image of a complex degenerative meniscal tear in an asymptomatic 63-year-old male.

Meniscal Tears and Knee Symptoms

In all studies, there was no evidence of a direct link between a meniscal tear finding on MRI scan and knee symptoms. This was evident in all ages and in all grades of osteoarthritis. Healthy knees and osteoarthritic knees with a meniscal tear are not more painful than those without a tear, and the presence of meniscal tears does not necessarily affect functional status. Most studies suggest a linkage between knee symptoms and knee osteoarthritis, irrespective of the presence of meniscal damage (Bhattacharyya et al. 2003; Englund et al. 2007, 2008).

Management

Based on the evidence showed, an MRI finding of an asymptomatic meniscal tear requires careful consideration when choosing the appropriate treatment, especially in the middle-aged and elderly population. Moreover, even when symptomatic knees are concerned, it has been shown above that a meniscal tear is not always the direct cause of symptoms.

As strenuous physical activity and sport-related injuries are more and more common among older ages, as well as the usage of MRI scans for the evaluation of knee injuries, the process of decision making when considering an optimal treatment for a finding of a meniscal tear is more difficult. This process should be based on the history of the patient, proper evaluation of injury mechanism, and presentation and thorough physical examination. A special emphasis should be made on the presence of mechanical complaints or symptoms of the knee, such as: locking, clicking, giving way, sensation of free-floating piece in the knee joint, recurrent episodes of sharp pain, or swelling with no preceded traumatic injury.

The arsenal of treatments for a meniscal tear includes conservative treatment based on an exercise program and surgical treatments: arthroscopic partial meniscus resection, arthroscopic meniscal repair, or meniscus transplant.

As for the asymptomatic meniscal tears with or without evidence of osteoarthritic changes, there is a weak evidence base for the natural history of these tears and the effects and benefits of the various treatment options and their ability to prevent, postpone, or decelerate a potential osteoarthritic process. Since there is no evidence-based data in the literature suggestive of any additional benefit with invasive surgical treatments for these asymptomatic subjects, the mainstay of treatment in these cases should remain the conservative one.

For those with the combination of symptomatic knees, an MRI finding of a meniscal tear, and radiologic evidence of osteoarthritis, the physician must take into consideration the complexity

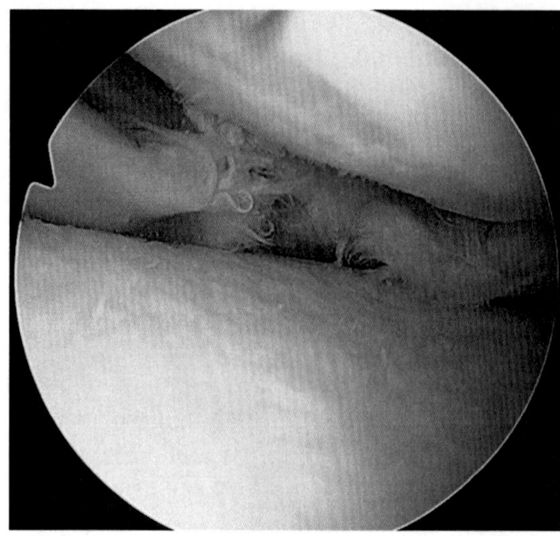

Fig. 2 Arthroscopic image of an asymptomatic degenerative meniscal tear

of the association between meniscal tears, the process of osteoarthritis, and knee symptoms. Because incidental MRI findings of meniscal tears are frequent, with a higher prevalence among those with knee osteoarthritic radiologic changes, it remains difficult to attribute knee symptoms to either the meniscal tear or the osteoarthritic process.

The American Academy of Orthopaedic Surgeons published in 2013 the 2nd edition of the full guideline for treatment of osteoarthritis of the knee and was unable to recommend for or against arthroscopic partial meniscectomy in patients with osteoarthritis of the knee and a torn meniscus (Recommendation number 13). The strength of the recommendation was concluded as inconclusive. Figure 2 shows an arthroscopic image of an asymptomatic degenerative meniscal tear.

Herrlin et al. (2007, 2012) showed that in cases of *symptomatic* nontraumatic degenerative meniscal tear in the middle aged and elderly, arthroscopic partial meniscectomy followed by supervised exercise was not superior to supervised exercise alone in terms of reduced knee pain, improved knee function, and improved quality of life. The exercise program consisted of exercises for improving muscle strength, endurance, and flexibility as well as balance and proprioception. There are no other similar studies or additional relevant data in the literature.

Based on this limited data and until further evidence emerges, an acceptable approach for the treatment of degenerative nontraumatic symptomatic and asymptomatic meniscal tears should be based mainly on conservative modalities, such as a supervised exercise program for improving muscle strength, endurance, and flexibility, as well as balance and proprioception.

Arthroscopic surgical treatments should be considered in cases of traumatic meniscal tears with mechanical complaints and symptoms.

As for the preventive and protective role of meniscal repair or transplant, modern techniques of meniscal repair or transplant aimed at restoring meniscal function have still not been shown to reduce the risk of the development of osteoarthritis, and further research is needed (Englund et al. 2009).

Summary

Meniscal tears in the asymptomatic population are a common finding on MRI scans. The prevalence of asymptomatic meniscal tears ranges from ~5 % in young ages and up to 67 % in older ages. Prevalence is higher the older the patient age is and/or the more radiologic OA findings he has. The published literature shows that there is no direct link between meniscal tears and knee symptoms in middle-aged and older adults; however, meniscal tear and knee symptoms are separately linked to OA findings. Conservative treatment of degenerative meniscal tears in the symptomatic middle aged and elderly includes a training program which was proven to improve knee function and symptoms and quality of life. There are no proven advantages to surgical treatment of middle-aged and elderly degenerative meniscal tears, as long as there are no mechanical complaints of an acute tear. Arthroscopic surgical treatment can be considered in cases of complaints or physical examination findings indicating a mechanical pathology of knee function, such as: locking, clicking, giving way, sensation of free-floating piece in the knee joint, and recurrent episodes of sharp intermittent pain occasionally followed by swelling. Further research is needed in investigating the natural history of asymptomatic meniscal tears, as well as the benefits and outcomes of the various treatments.

Cross-References

- ▶ Arthroscopic Repair of the Meniscus Tears
- ▶ Degenerative Meniscal Tears: Meniscal Cysts
- ▶ Meniscal Allografts: Indications and Results
- ▶ Meniscal Substitutes: Polyurethane Meniscus Implant: Technique and Results
- ▶ Meniscectomy

References

AAOS (2013) The American Academy of Orthopaedic Surgeons. Treatment of osteoarthritis (OA) of the knee, 2nd edn. Full guideline document. Rosemont

Bhattacharyya T, Gale D, Dewire P et al (2003) The clinical importance of meniscal tears demonstrated by magnetic resonance imaging in osteoarthritis of the knee. J Bone Joint Surg Am 85-A(1):4–9

Crues JV 3rd, Mink J, Levy TL et al (1987) Meniscal tears of the knee: accuracy of MR imaging. Radiology 164(2):445–448

Englund M, Niu J, Guermazi A et al (2007) Effect of meniscal damage on the development of frequent knee pain, aching, or stiffness. Arthritis Rheum 56(12):4048

Englund M, Guermazi A, Gale D et al (2008) Incidental meniscal findings on knee MRI in middle-aged and elderly persons. N Engl J Med 359(11):1108–1115

Englund M, Guermazi A, Roemer FW et al (2009) Meniscal tear in knees without surgery and the development of radiographic osteoarthritis among middle-aged and elderly persons: the multicenter osteoarthritis study. Arthritis Rheum 60(3):831–839

Herrlin S, Hållander M, Wang P et al (2007) Arthroscopic or conservative treatment of degenerative medial meniscal tears: a prospective randomized trial. Knee Surg Sports Traumatol Arthrosc 15(4):393–401

Herrlin SV, Wange PO, Lapidus G et al (2012) Is arthroscopic surgery beneficial in treating non-traumatic, degenerative medial meniscal tears? A five year follow-up. Knee Surg Sports Traumatol Arthrosc 21(2):358–364

LaPrade RF, Burnett QM 2nd, Veenstra MA et al (1994) The prevalence of abnormal magnetic resonance imaging findings in asymptomatic knees. Am J Sports Med 22(6):739–745

Mine T, Kimura M, Sakka A et al (2000) Innervation of nociceptors in the menisci of the knee joint: an immunohistochemical study. Arch Orthop Trauma Surg 120(3–4):201–204

Zanetti M, Pfirrmann CW, Schmid MR et al (2005) Clinical course of knees with asymptomatic meniscal abnormalities: findings at 2-year follow-up after MR imaging-based diagnosis. Radiology 237(3):993–997

Combined Anterior and Posterior Cruciate Ligament Injuries

79

Bülent Aksoy, Cem Zeki Esenyel, and F. Erkal Bilen

Contents

B. Aksoy (✉)
Bahçeşehir University, Istanbul, Turkey
e-mail: drbulentaksoy@gmail.com

C.Z. Esenyel
Department of Orthopedics and Traumatology, Vakif Gureba Training and Research Hospital, Fatih, Istanbul, Turkey
e-mail: esenyel@yahoo.com

F.E. Bilen
Head of Shoulder and Elbow Unit, Orthopaedic Surgery, Istanbul Memorial Hospital, Istanbul, Marmara, Turkey
e-mail: bilenfe@me.com; bilenfe@gmail.com

M.N. Doral, J. Karlsson (eds.), *Sports Injuries*,
DOI 10.1007/978-3-642-36569-0_110

Abstract

Combined injuries to the anterior and posterior cruciate ligaments are usually associated with knee dislocations; however, they can also occur with absence of a knee dislocation. Either way, the management of these injuries is fairly demanding. In the presence of a knee dislocation, it is of paramount importance to reduce the knee as soon as possible. Then, the vascular status and the integrity of the cruciate ligaments should be evaluated carefully. Clinical and objective outcomes are closely correlated with the treatment plan. It should be kept in mind that these rare injuries are more encountered in multitrauma patients. The decision of timing for the surgical intervention relies on the stability of the knee joint and accompanying neurovascular injuries. In the absence of ongoing dislocation or subluxation after a closed reduction and neurovascular injury, it is wise to postpone the surgery for at least 2–3 weeks as it will reduce the risk of arthrofibrosis.

Introduction

Multiligament knee injuries are a complex problem which may occur after both sporting injuries and high-velocity injuries (Schenk 1994; Fanelli and Edson 2002; Fanelli 2003; Stannard et al. 2005; Levy et al. 2009). The vascular status of the extremity should be evaluated carefully (Kennedy 1963; Green and Allen 1977; Schenk 1994; Fanelli et al. 2001; Stannard et al. 2005).

The assessment and treatment should be systematically performed in these complex injuries (Fanelli et al. 2001; Stannard et al. 2005; Levy et al. 2009). A complete physical examination and imaging studies are essential to make a correct diagnosis and formulate a correct treatment plan (Wascher et al. 1997; Fanelli and Edson 2002; Stannard et al. 2005; Levy et al. 2009).

Multiligament injuries are often observed after sports injuries and account for less than 2 % of orthopaedic injuries. The male-to-female ratio is 4:1. Incidence of PCL injuries after acute knee injuries is reported to range between 3 % and 40 %. This rate depends on the patient population reported; while it is 3 % in the general population, it is reported as high as 38 % in regional trauma centers (Fanelli and Edson 1995; Fanelli et al. 2001). In patients with multiple trauma, this rate can be as high as 56.5 % (Fanelli et al. 2001; Robertson and Nutton 2006). Combined ACL/PCL tears are present in 45.9 % of these PCL injuries. Posterolateral corner tears accompany up to 41 % of these cases (Fanelli et al. 2001).The accompanying injury together with vascular and neurological damage makes the treatment more complicated in knees with multiple-ligament injuries (Fanelli 2003; Robertson and Nutton 2006; Levy et al. 2009).

Classification

Combined ACL/PCL injuries may or may not present as acute knee dislocations (Fanelli et al. 2001, 2005; Levy et al. 2009). Classification of knee dislocations is based primarily on the direction the tibia dislocates relative to the femur (Kennedy 1963; Schenk 1994; Fanelli et al. 2001, 2005). This results in five different categories:

- Anterior
- Posterior
- Lateral
- Medial
- Rotational

Rotational instability is subdivided as:

- Anteromedial
- Posteromedial
- Anterolateral
- Posterolateral

Anterior and/or posterior dislocations are the most common dislocations. Frassica et al. (Frassica et al. 1991) reported that dislocations in their series consisted of 70 % posterior, 25 % anterior, and 5 % rotational. On the other hand, Green and Allen (Green and Allen 1997) reported that their series constituted 31 % anterior,

25 % posterior, and 3 % rotational dislocations. Rotational dislocations are rare, but posterolateral dislocation is the most common rotational combination. In these cases, the medial femoral condyle dislocates together with a "buttonhole" mechanism piercing the anteromedial capsule which cannot be closed reduced. In addition, the MCL invaginated into the joint and blocks reduction. This buttonhole draws the subcutaneous tissues and the skin attached to the joint capsule into the joint and creates a dimple along the medial joint line (Fanelli et al. 2005).

Although classification according to direction of dislocation is simple, it is not a reliable guide in demonstrating the pattern of the ligament injury (Robertson and Nutton 2006). For this reason, Schenk (Schenk 1994) has defined a different classification for ligament injuries depending on whether there are intra-articular fractures or not, and others have modified this classification.

Other factors to be considered are as follows:

- ***Is it open or closed injury?***

  Open knee dislocations are not uncommon. The reported incidence is between 19 % and 35 % of all dislocations (Fanelli et al. 2001, 2005). An open knee dislocation may be connected to a serious injury related to the soft tissue envelope around the knee and may indicate a bad prognosis. Furthermore, an open injury may require an open ligament reconstruction, or staged reconstruction (Fanelli et al. 2001), since arthroscopically assisted techniques may not always be reliably performed in the acute setting with these open injuries (Fanelli et al. 2001, 2005).
- ***Occurrence as a result of low or high-energy trauma***

  Distinguishing between low- and high-energy injuries is important. Low-energy injuries are usually associated with sports injuries and have a decreased incidence of associated vascular injury. High-energy injuries usually result from motor vehicle accidents or falls from heights. The possibility of a vascular injury in high-velocity injuries is high (Wascher et al. 1997; Fanelli et al. 2001).
- ***Complete dislocation or subluxation of the knee***

  One should be aware of the fact that a complete knee injury may have spontaneously reduced. Any patient who presents with injury to any combination of the three main knee ligaments may have been caused by a knee dislocation.

Mechanisms of Injury

Anterior and posterior knee dislocations are the most common knee dislocations (Fanelli et al. 2001), and their occurrence mechanisms are well described (Fanelli et al. 2001; Fanelli 2003). Hyperextension of the knee resulting in anterior dislocation of the tibia is the most frequent mechanism in regard to the femur (40 %). At 30° of hyperextension of the knee, the posterior capsule is torn (Fanelli et al. 2001, 2005; Fanelli 2003). When extended further to approximately 50°, the ACL, PCL, and popliteal artery can be torn. There is some question whether the ACL or PCL is torn first (Fanelli et al. 2001, 2005). Posterior dislocation (33 %) usually occurs as a result of a posterior stress affecting the proximal tibia when the knee is at 90° of flexion. "Dashboard injuries" are of this type. A varus or valgus stress can cause medial (4 %) or lateral (18 %) dislocations, and these dislocations often occur with tibial plateau fractures (Fanelli 2003).

The most frequent type of concurrent injury is to the posterolateral or medial knee structures depending on the direction of force along with tears of both cruciate ligaments (Robertson and Nutton 2006). The most frequent ACL/PCL posterolateral corner mechanism of injury is forced varus and knee dislocation (Fanelli et al. 2001). The most frequent ACL/PCL medial collateral ligament mechanism of injury is forced valgus and extension (Fanelli et al. 2001).

Initial Evaluation

Evaluation of the acute ACL/PCL-injured knee should include the history of the injury mechanism, physical examination with careful neurovascular examination (arteriogram or CT angiogram), plain and stress radiographs, magnetic resonance imaging studies, examination under anesthesia, and diagnostic arthroscopy (Fanelli et al. 2001; Fanelli 2012).

If the acute ACL/PCL injury has occurred due to the knee dislocation, the vascular and neurological conditions of the injured extremity are evaluated carefully after the first assessment based on the guidelines of Advanced Trauma Life Support in terms of popliteal artery and common peroneal nerve injury, and these evaluations are repeated at certain intervals (Robertson and Nutton 2006). Clinical symptoms are recorded. The clinical diagnosis is supported by plain radiography and the knee is reduced at an earliest possible time under controlled sedation (Robertson and Nutton 2006). In acute ACL/PCL injuries in which a knee dislocation is not documented, the neurovascular status should be carefully assessed, since the knee might have dislocated and spontaneously reduced at the scene of the accident (Fanelli et al. 2001). Wascherand et al. (1997) have reported the incidence of arterial injury in knee dislocations as 14 %. Fanelli et al. (2001) found the incidence of arterial injury as 11 % in the knees in which three ligaments are acutely injured.

Vascular Assessment

The incidence of vascular injury has been reported as 32 % (Fanelli et al. 2005; Remond et al. 2008). When this case is limited only to anterior and posterior injury, then the incidence increases up to 50 %. The popliteal artery is the terminal artery of the leg and has minimal collateral circulation. Furthermore, the popliteal vein is responsible for the majority of the venous outflow from the knee (Fanelli et al. 2005).

The main concern is the injury to the popliteal artery after a knee dislocation and the possibility of losing the extremity. For this reason, it is arguable that in the assessment, not only physical examination should be done but also the ankle-brachial artery index measurement should be included or a CT arteriogram be performed (Levy et al. 2009). However, many studies have been done, and it has been concluded that physical examination is sufficient in the face of normal pedal pulses for the diagnosis of a clinically apparent vascular injury (Levy et al. 2009).

A great majority of arterial injuries occurring after knee dislocations are intimal injures not restricting circulation. Those intimal injuries not blocking circulation changes can turn into an occlusive vein lesion. Observation and follow-up are sufficient for the treatment of intimal damage in patients whose physical examination is normal. Arteriogram is necessary only for the patients whose physical examination is not normal. Most selective arteriography protocols propose serial physical examinations to be performed at least for 48 h (Levy et al. 2009). This will help make a diagnosis without delay for a lesion causing the blockage (Levy et al. 2009).

Physical Examination

Examination in a seriously injured knee starts with a detailed evaluation of neurovascular status and with the inspection of the soft tissue to determine whether there is an open injury. Motor and sensory functions are documented in neurological examination. The peroneal nerve is the most frequently injured nerve in multiple-ligament injuries (Niall et al. 2005; Robertson et al. 2006).

Vascular assessment is also very important. As stated before, repeated physical examination is effective in revealing vascular injury (Stannard et al. 2004; Remond et al. 2008). The distal pulse may be taken in a major arterial injury. Therefore, measurement of the ankle-brachial index (ABI) is preferred, which has excellent sensitivity in a major arterial injury (Mills et al. 2004).If the ABI is greater than 0.9, it is sufficient to examine at intervals. However, if the ABI is less than 0.9, an angiography is required. During the neurovascular examination, compartment syndrome must be ruled out.

Assessment of the anterior cruciate ligament (ACL) can be difficult in the presence of a PCL injury and must be carefully performed. It is important to pay close attention to the position of the tibia in relation to the femur, since increased posterior translation of the tibia on the femur due to a PCL injury may cause a false-positive Lachman test. Stiffness of the endpoint is more important than translation. A distinct endpoint helps ruling out an ACL injury.

In physical examination for combined ACL/PCL injuries when the knee is at 25° and 90° of flexion, there is an abnormal increase in anteroposterior tibiofemoral laxity. The Lachman and pseudo-Lachman tests are positive, the pivot shift test is positive, and tibial step-off is negative (Robertson and Nutton 2006).

The presence of a dimple sign on the anteromedial surface of the knee indicates a posterolateral dislocation and is associated with a high incidence of irreducibility and potential skin necrosis. Thus, an open reduction may be required.

Imaging Studies

Radiographs should include (Fanelli et al. 2001):

- Anteroposterior X-rays of both knees (if possible in standing position)
- Lateral X-rays of both knees
- 30° anteroposterior axial X-rays of both patella
- Intercondylar notch views

These radiographic views will help document reduction of the tibiofemoral and patellofemoral joints, assess bony alignment, and evaluate the cruciate ligaments, the collateral ligaments, and the insertion site of bony avulsions of the cruciates, collateral ligament complexes, and extensor mechanisms (Fanelli et al. 2001).Stress radiographs should also be considered to objectively define the amount of medial or lateral joint line gapping and to assist with determining the site of injury (LaPrade et al. 2008, 2010; Jackman et al. 2008).

Magnetic resonance imagining has a high diagnostic accuracy in acute PLC injuries (Fanelli et al. 2001). It is helpful in specifying the tear location of the cruciate and collateral ligaments and formulating a treatment plan (Fanelli et al. 2001).

In the presence of cyanosis, pallor, weak capillary refill, and decreased peripheral heat, arteriography or CT angiography should be considered (Fanelli et al. 2001).Venography is considered if the clinical picture indicates adequate limb perfusion but obstruction of outflow (Fanelli et al. 2001).

Other Considerations

In acute ACL/PCL injuries, surgical timing depends on the vascular status, reduction stability, skin condition, systemic injuries, open versus closed knee injury, meniscus and articular surface injuries, other orthopaedic injuries, and the collateral or capsular ligaments involved (Fanelli 2003; Fanelli and Harris 2007).

The indications for urgent surgery are (Fanelli et al. 2001; Fanelli 2003):

- Dislocations that cannot be reduced
- Presence of vascular injury
- Open injuries

Surgical Timing

A state of irreducibility or vascular injury necessitates immediate surgical intervention (Fanelli et al. 2001; Fanelli 2003). One should consider four-compartment fasciotomy of the limb when the ischemic time is more than 2.5 h (Fanelli et al. 2001). If the maintenance of reduction cannot be achieved, then the knee should be stabilized to avoid recurrent vascular congestion. In such a case, an early ligament reconstruction or the placement of an external fixator can be necessary (Fanelli et al. 2001).

The main indication for surgery for an isolated ACL/PCL-injured knee is severe functional instability. These knees are at high risk for progressive instability and the development of posttraumatic arthrosis (Fanelli et al. 2001). Surgery should be performed as soon as it is possible, excluding immediate intervention (Fanelli et al. 2001). If possible, a 2–3-week delay in patients who do not have full motion can reduce the risk for arthrofibrosis (Fanelli 2003) because surgery performed 2–3 weeks after injury allows the acute inflammatory phase to subside and the range of motion to be restored (Fanelli et al. 2001). During this period prior to surgery, the knee can be immobilized in a fully extended position (Fanelli et al. 2001; Levy et al. 2009). At 2–3 weeks after injury, enough capsular sealing occurs to allow arthroscopic ACL/PCL reconstruction and to allow for a primary repair or reconstruction of the injured collateral ligament structures with a minimal risk for fluid extravasation into the posterior knee compartments (Fanelli et al. 2001).

Since these injuries are heterogeneous and seen rarely, it is difficult to develop a treatment scheme (Levy et al. 2009).

External Fixation or Hinged Knee Brace Before Surgery?

In cases in which joint reduction cannot be maintained in open dislocations with vascular repair, external fixation may be helpful (Levy et al. 2009).

Open Reconstruction or Closed Reconstruction?

Whether an open or closed reconstruction can be performed depends on the surgical timing and the nature of injury (Levy et al. 2009). There are no randomized controlled studies comparing open reconstruction with arthroscopic reconstruction for knee dislocations (Levy et al. 2009; Dubberley et al. 2001).

In acute knee dislocations, repair or reconstruction may be performed within a week. Because the capsular tissue is torn, open reconstructions may occasionally have to be delayed for 1 week to prevent excessive arthroscopic fluid extravasation, which might theoretically lead to compartment syndrome (Levy et al. 2009). In most cases with knee dislocation, ideally ACL and PCL reconstructions are performed arthroscopically, along with open reconstruction of the LCL/posterolateral corner (PLC) and/or the MCL/posteromedial corner (PMC) (Levy et al. 2009).

Early-Late Ligament Reconstruction

One Step Versus Staged Surgery

There are advantages of performing ACL and PCL reconstructions with concurrent collateral reconstructions at the same time, especially in young patients (Hara et al. 1999). Stability of the knee is achieved; rehabilitation is started early; and an earlier return to activities and work becomes possible. In addition, the risk for developing secondary meniscus tears and cartilage defects due to instability is minimized (Hara et al. 1999). However, the enormity and difficulty of the surgical initiative and risk for developing contracture during the postoperative period for surgeons and surgical teams with inexperience in treating knee dislocations are problems of concurrent reconstruction (Hara et al. 1999). In some series, where reconstructions are performed late or staged in two to three intervals, the incidence of arthrofibrosis has been reported to be low, but there is a concurrent risk of more residual laxity (Levy et al. 2009).

Surgical timing for acute ACL/PCL/lateral side injuries can be based on the lateral side classification defined by Fanelli and Feldman (1997). Type A injuries (e.g., the increase in external rotation only) are concomitant with tears of the popliteofibular ligament and the popliteus tendon (Fanelli and Feldman 1997). Type B injuries (e.g., increase in external rotation and approximately 5 mm increase in varus laxity at 30° of flexion) include the injury to the popliteofibular ligament, popliteus tendon, and lateral (fibular) collateral ligament (Fanelli and Feldman 1997). However, in Type C injuries (e.g., increase in external rotation and subjective increases in varus laxity of about 10 mm at 30° of flexion), the popliteofibular ligament, popliteal tendon, lateral (fibular) collateral ligament, and lateral capsule are injured (Fanelli and Feldman 1997).

In acute ACL/PCL lateral-posterolateral type A and type B injuries within 2–3 weeks together with the arthroscopic reconstruction of ACL and PCL at the same time, primary repair of the posterolateral corner reinforced with allograft or autograft can be performed (Fanelli 2003). In type C injuries with acute combined ACL/PCL tears and combined lateral-posterolateral injures, primary repair of the posterolateral corner reinforced with allograft or autograft is carried out immediately within the first 1–2 weeks. At approximately 4–6 weeks after this approach, an arthroscopic combined ACL/PCL reconstruction is applied (Fanelli 2003; Levy et al. 2009). If the surgeon prefers a one-stage reconstruction, repair and reconstructions of the medial and lateral sides may be performed with a dry or open technique (Levy et al. 2009).

In acute ACL/PCL/medial side injuries, surgical timing can also be determined according to the medial side classification defined by Fanelli and Harris (Fanelli and Harris 2007). There is axial rotation instability (anteromedial or posteromedial) in type A injuries, and there is no valgus laxity (Fanelli and Harris 2007). In type B injuries, there is axial rotation instability and valgus laxity with a distinct endpoint at 30° of flexion (Fanelli and Harris 2007). In type C injuries, there is valgus laxity with an indistinct endpoint at 30° of flexion combined with axial rotation instability (Fanelli and Harris 2007).In acute ACL/PCL medial side injuries, surgical timing is dependent on the degree of injury on the medial side (Fanelli 2003). Low-grade (type A, B) medial collateral tears can be treated successfully with the repair of ACL/PCL arthroscopically after bracing for 4–6 weeks (Fanelli 2003; Levy et al. 2009). Type C medial side injuries combined with ACL/PCL tears are often treated with reconstruction. Medial posteromedial repair/reconstruction is applied within the first week after injury (Fanelli 2003; Levy et al. 2009). And after 3–6 weeks, an arthroscopic combined ACL/PCL reconstruction is performed (Fanelli 2003; Levy et al. 2009). If the surgeon prefers a one-stage reconstruction, the repairs and reconstructions of cruciate ligaments and medial side can be applied in the form of open procedure or dry arthroscopic reconstruction, especially if this procedure is not performed frequently by the surgeon or by his surgical team (Levy et al. 2009).

Indications for surgical reconstruction in chronic ACL/PCL injuries occur when functional instability is present (Fanelli 2003). This can result in early posttraumatic arthrosis in the knee, so the definitions of all structural injuries are important. These injuries may include ligaments, meniscuses, surface of the knee, and tibiofemoral alignment pathologies. Surgical treatment may involve reconstruction of the torn ligaments, osteotomy in the cases of coronal or sagittal plane malalignment, reconstruction of the joint cartilage, and meniscus surgery (resection, repair, transplantation) (Fanelli 2003).

Surgical timing may perhaps be affected by factors beyond the surgeon's control. These factors are the vascular status of the extremity, whether the injury is open or closed, stability of the reduction, and status of the skin, presence of accompanying system injuries, medical comorbidities, other orthopedic injuries, meniscus, and injuries on the joint surface (Levy et al. 2009).

Repair or Reconstruction of the Ligament?

Stannard et al. performed repairs or reconstruction of 57 PLC tears on 56 patients. They reported that while the rate of failure in the group repaired was 37 %, it was 9 % in the reconstructed group, which was significant ($p < 0.05$) (Stannard et al. 2005).

Graft Selection

The ideal graft material should be strong, should provide secure fixation, should be easy to pass through reamed tunnels, should be readily available, and should have a low donor site morbidity (Fanelli et al. 2001). The available options are autograft and allograft sources (Fanelli et al. 2001; Wascher et al. 1999). The sources of graft used more often for ACL and PCL reconstruction are the Achilles tendon allograft, quadriceps tendon, bone-patellar tendon-bone, and hamstring autograft or allograft.

Allograft has some advantages over autograft:

- No donor site morbidity
- Many options with different graft lengths
- Shorter tourniquet time

Additionally, successful results have been reported regarding the use of allograft.

The risk for HIV infection is one in 1.6 million (Levy et al. 2009).

An Achilles tendon allograft is a preferred graft for a reconstruction of the PCL (Fanelli et al. 2001; Fanelli 2003; Levy et al. 2009), because this tendon is strong because of its large cross-sectional area, donor site morbidity does not occur, and provides easy passage with secure fixation (Fanelli 2003; Levy et al. 2009). If a double-bundle PCL reconstruction is to be performed, the Achilles tendon allograft can be used for the anterolateral band and a tibialis anterior allograft can be used for the posteromedial band (Levy et al. 2009; Spiridonov et al. 2011).

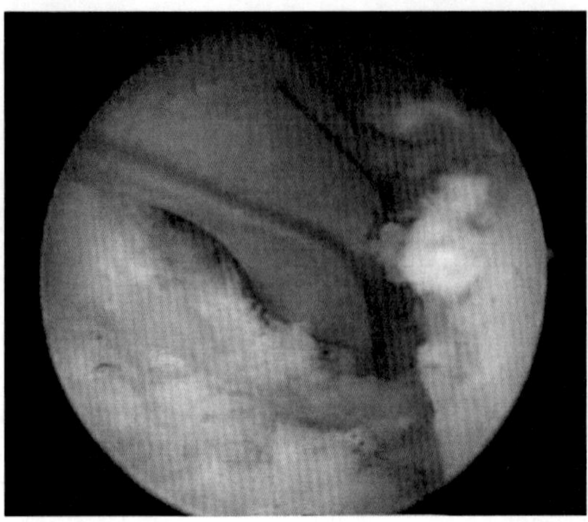

Fig. 1 Specifically curved PCL instrument used to separate the posterior capsule from the tibia

Surgical Technique

The patient is placed in the supine position. The surgical leg is placed to hang down over the edge of the operating table. The healthy extremity is placed on the operating table in full extension or in an abduction leg holder. A lateral support is used for control of the surgical leg. A tourniquet is applied to the thigh. A pump is used to provide fluid outflow.

Concomitant open surgical procedures are performed before arthroscopic surgery for ACL and PCL injuries to prevent fluid leakage.

The arthroscope is first inserted through the anterolateral portal. An accessory extracapsular extra-articular posteromedial safety portal can be created in order to protect the posterior neurovascular structures and control the location of the PCL tibial tunnel to assess whether it is in the correct place. First, intra-articular knee injuries (meniscus tear, cartilage damage) are assessed. If there is a meniscus tear, it is repaired; if it is unrepairable, resection is performed. Then, the ACL and PCL are examined, and locations of detachments are inspected. The inspection of remaining PCL fibers is important to determine the proper direction of the tunnel to be opened. A notchplasty can be performed involving the debridement of the ACL and PCL stumps, the shaping of lateral femoral condyle and intercondylar roof. This is performed to establish the over-the-top position or anatomic position and to prevent the impingement of the ACL graft along the movement arc. Specifically, curved PCL instruments can be used to separate the posterior capsule from the tibia (Fig. 1).

First, the torn ACL is debrided. The tunnels for the ACL are created by using a single-incision technique. An incision is made to the distal medial side of the tibial tubercle. The tibial tunnel begins externally at a point 2–3 cm medial to the tibial tubercle on the anteromedial surface of the proximal tibia. The exit point in the joint should be adjacent to the posterior margin of the anterior horn attachment of the lateral meniscus. This coincides with the center of the tibial footprint or stump of the ACL. The femoral tunnel is placed midway along the lateral intercondylar ridge between the AM and PL bundles on the medial wall of the lateral femoral condyle. The tunnel is left to allow a 1–2 mm posterior cortical wall.

Following the creation of the tibial and femoral tunnels for the ACL, the stump of the PCL remaining in the femur and the synovia surrounding it are debrided. As the adherence place of the PCL to the tibia will not be debrided sufficiently, the shaver to be used for debridement should be inserted through the posteromedial portal. After having created the tibial and femoral tunnels for the ACL, to create the transtibial PCL tunnel, the guide wire is passed starting over the anteromedial surface of the proximal tibia, 6 cm distal to the joint line, and a minimum of 2 cm

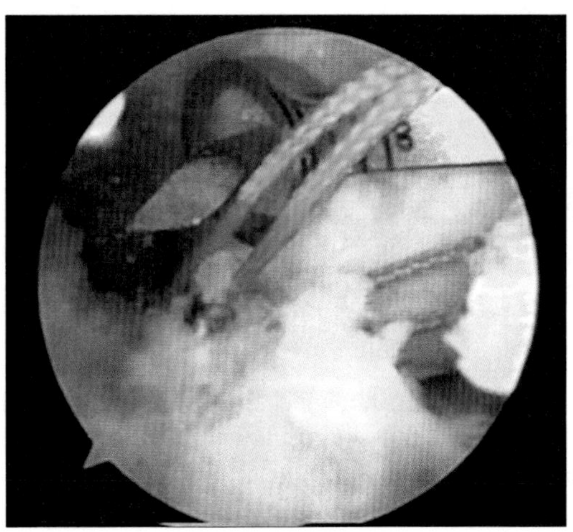

Fig. 2 Photograph showing the femoral tunnel for the PCL

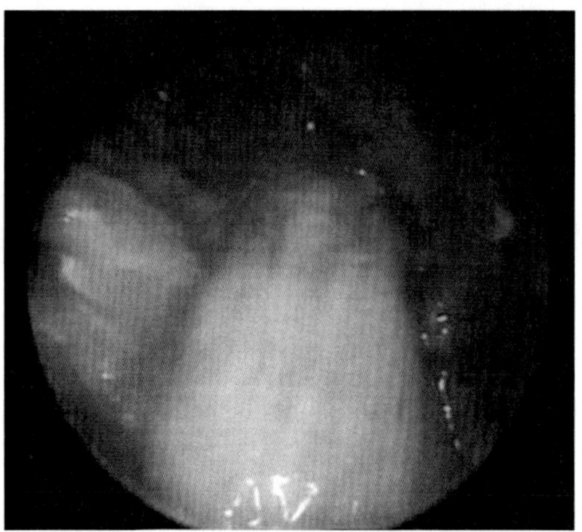

Fig. 3 Photograph showing the PCL after fixation

distal to the tunnel created for the ACL and exiting the inferolateral part of the anatomic adherence area and approximately midway along the PCL facet (Anderson et al. 2012) (Fig. 2). The external position of the femoral tunnel decreases the risk for avascular necrosis or the possibility of the development of subchondral break in the medial femoral condyle. With the construction of the femoral tunnel for the PCL in the specified anatomic region, the distance between the femoral and tibial tunnels in the joint is longer in flexion than in extension. And this provides that the PCL reconstructed at flexion to be tighter. The PCL graft is attached from the femoral side and tibial side is left free at this point in the surgery.

Graft Tensioning and Fixation

The PCL and then ACL are reconstructed once the PLC and the MLC are reconstructed or repaired (Geeslin and LaPrade 2011). Tension is placed on the PCL graft distally and a tension of 20 lb. (9 kg) is applied. This restores the anatomic tibial step-off. Pretensioning is applied to the graft by cycling the knee 25 times, and the graft is adjusted to its place. The knee is placed at 90° of flexion, and the posterior cruciate ligament graft is fixed on the tibial side with a screw, spiked ligament washer and an absorbable interference screw. The knee is bent at 20° of flexion next; valgus force is applied slightly to the knee while the tibia is in neutral rotation, and the fixation of the posterolateral corner is achieved (Geeslin and LaPrade 2011). If a graft tensioning device like Arthrotek is to be used, the anterior cruciate ligament is tensioned to 20 lb. (9 kg).The knee is placed in 0° of flexion, and the final fixation of the anterior cruciate ligament graft is performed. In the medial collateral ligament reconstruction, the graft is tensioned with the knee in 20° of flexion and with the leg in a neutral position. The presence of full range of motion of the joint should be confirmed when the patient is on the operating table (Fanelli 2003; Levy et al. 2009) (Fig. 3).

Technical Tips

The posteromedial safety incision protects the neurovascular structures, confirms subjective tibial tunnel placement in the absence of intraoperative fluoroscopy, and allows the surgical procedure to be performed faster. Attention should be given to the two tibial tunnel directions to have a 1–2 mm bone bridge between the PCL and ACL tibial tunnels. This will reduce the risk of fracture (Fanelli 2003) (Fig. 4).

The order of tensioning: the posterior cruciate ligament is first and then the posterolateral corner, the anterior cruciate ligament, and the medial

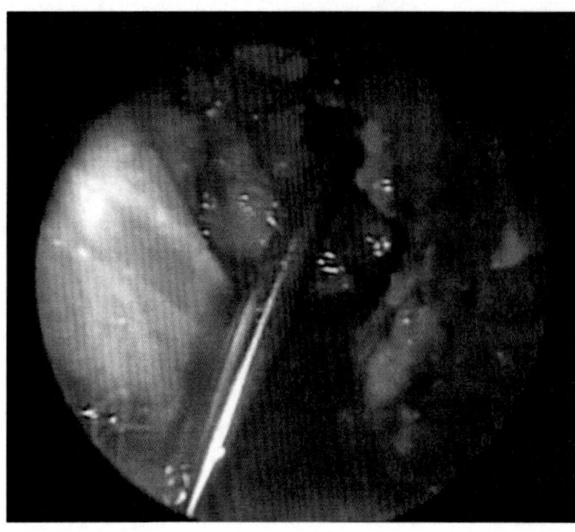

Fig. 4 Note that the two tibial tunnels have an intact bone bridge to prevent fracture

collateral ligament, respectively (Wentorf et al. 2002). The reconstruction of the normal tibial step-off at 90° is a suitable method to create the tibiofemoral relationship.

Postoperative Rehabilitation

The first six postoperative weeks comprises the maximum protection phase. During the first 3 weeks, the knee can be kept at full extension with no weight bearing. In some centers, immediate postoperative motion has been performed with no objective increase in joint laxity and minimal cases of arthrofibrosis. During weeks 4–6, progressive increase of range of motion is achieved. Weight bearing is started at one third of the body weight of the patient and is increased every week at the same rate. In the sixth postoperative week, the patient's full weight bearing is achieved using crutches. During the exercises done to provide joint range of movement, varus or valgus forces are avoided to protect the reconstructed ligaments (Fanelli et al. 2001; Fanelli 2003). Range of motion exercises are progressed using a stationary bike, and closed chain exercises are advanced. During this period, proprioceptive exercises are progressed. Depending on the patient's condition and the progress in the proprioceptive sense, straight-line jogging is initiated between postoperative months of 3 and 4 (Fanelli et al. 2001).

Sports-specific exercises and training are initiated at postoperative months of 4–6. If the following criteria are met, the patient can return to sport after six to nine postoperative months.

- Quadriceps and hamstring strength are 90 % or more than the uninvolved extremity.
- The patient can perform all necessary skills without pain or restriction.

It should be known that a loss of 10–15° of flexion may occur with these complex ligament reconstructions (Fanelli et al. 2001). This reportedly do not cause a functional problem in most patients.

Complications

Potential complications in the treatment of combined ACL/PCL/posterolateral corner injuries are as follows:

- Failure to recognize a vascular injury (arterial or venous)
- Causing an iatrogenic neurovascular injury at the time of reconstruction
- Creating an iatrogenic tibia plateau fracture at the time of reconstruction
- Failure to recognize all components of the instability
- Osteonecrosis of medial femoral condyle
- Loss of knee motion
- Postoperative anterior knee pain
- Recurrent instability

Postoperative adhesions and removal of painful material in the knee are other problems that can be met.

Conclusions

The ACL/PCL and posterolateral corner injuries can be treated successfully at one session with the reconstruction of both cruciate ligaments arthroscopically, together with the repair of the posterolateral corner. The evaluation of the concomitant injuries and surgical strategy are of paramount importance.

References

Anderson CJ, Ziegler CG, Wijdicks CA et al (2012) Arthroscopically pertinent anatomy of the anterolateral and posteromedial bundles of the posterior cruciate ligament. J Bone Joint Surg Am 94(21):1936–1945

Dubberley J, Burnell C, Longstaffe A et al (2001) Irreducible knee dislocation treated by arthroscopic debridement. Arthroscopy 17(3):316–319

Fanelli GC (2003) Evaluation and treatment of the multiligament-injured knee. Arthroscopy 19(10):30–37

Fanelli GC (2012) The multiple ligament injured knee: a practical guide to management, 2nd edn. Springer, Pennsylvania

Fanelli GC, Edson CJ (1995) PCL injuries in trauma patients. Part II. Arthroscopy 11:526–529

Fanelli GC, Edson CJ (2002) Arthroscopically assisted combined anterior and posterior cruciate ligament reconstruction in the multiple ligament injured knee: 2 to 10 years follow-up. Arthroscopy 18:703–714

Fanelli GC, Feldman DD (1997) Management of combined anterior cruciate ligament/posterior cruciate ligament/posterolateral complex injuries of the knee. Oper Tech Sports Med 7:143–149

Fanelli GC, Harris JD (2007) Late MCL (medial collateral ligament) reconstruction. Tech Knee Surg 6:99–105

Fanelli GC, Edson CJ, Maish DR (2001) Combined anterior and posterior cruciate ligament injuries. Tech Orthop 16(2):157–166

Fanelli GC, Orcutt DR, Edson CJ (2005) The multiple-ligament injured knee: evaluation, treatment, and results. Arthroscopy 21(4):471–486

Frassica FJ, Sim FH, Staeheli JW et al (1991) Dislocation of the knee. Clin Orthop Relat Res 263:200–205

Geeslin AG, LaPrade RF (2011) Outcomes of treatment of acute grade-III isolated and combined posterolateral knee injuries: a prospective case series and surgical technique. J Bone Joint Surg Am 93(18):1672–1683

Green NE, Allen BL (1977) Vascular injuries associated with dislocation of the knee. J Bone Joint Surg Am 59:236–239

Hara K, Kubo T, Shimizu C et al (1999) A new arthroscopic method for reconstructing the anterior and posterior cruciate ligaments using a single-incision technique: simultaneous grafting of the autogenous semitendinosus and patellar tendons. Arthroscopy 15(8):871–876

Jackman T, LaPrade RF, Pontinen T et al (2008) Intraobserver and interobserver reliability of the kneeling technique of stress radiography for the evaluation of posterior knee laxity. Am J Sports Med 36(8): 1571–1576

Kennedy JC (1963) Complete dislocation of the knee joint. J Bone Joint Surg Am 45:889–904

LaPrade RF, Heikes C, Bakker AJ et al (2008) The reproducibility and repeatability of varus stress radiographs in the assessment of isolated fibular collateral ligament and grade-III posterolateral knee injuries. An in vitro biomechanical study. J Bone Joint Surg Am 90(10): 2069–2076

LaPrade RF, Bernhardson AS, Griffith CJ et al (2010) Correlation of valgus stress radiographs with medial knee ligament injuries: an in vitro biomechanical study. Am J Sports Med 38(2):330–338

Levy BA, Fanelli GC, Whelan DB et al (2009) Controversies in the treatment of knee dislocations and multiligament reconstruction. J Am Acad Orthop Surg 17(4):197–206

Mills WJ, Barei DP, McNair P (2004) The value of the ankle-brachial index for diagnosing arterial injury after knee dislocation: a prospective study. J Trauma 56(6):1261–1265

Niall DM, Nutton RW, Keating JF (2005) Palsy of the common peroneal nerve after traumatic dislocation of the knee. J Bone Joint Surg Br 87(5):664–667

Remond JM, Levy BA, Dajani KA et al (2008) Detecting vascular injury in lower-extremity orthopedic trauma: the role of CT angiography. Orthopedics 31(8):761–767

Robertson A, Nutton RW (2006) The dislocated knee. Curr Orthop 20:95–102

Robertson A, Nutton RW, Keating JF (2006) Dislocation of the knee. J Bone Joint Surg Br 88(6):706–711

Schenk RC (1994) The dislocated knee. Instr Course Lect 43:127–136

Spiridonov SI, Slinkard NJ, LaPrade RF (2011) Isolated and combined grade-III posterior cruciate ligament tears treated with double-bundle reconstruction with use of endoscopically placed femoral tunnels and grafts: operative technique and clinical outcomes. J Bone Joint Surg Am 93(19):1773–1780

Stannard JP, Sheils TM, Lopez-Ben RR et al (2004) Vascular injuries in knee dislocations: the role of physical examination in determining the need for arteriography. J Bone Joint Surg Am 86-A(5):910–915

Stannard JP, Brown SL, Farris RC et al (2005) The posterolateral corner of the knee: repair versus reconstruction. Am J Sports Med 33:881–888

Wascher DC, Dvirnak PC, Decoster TA (1997) Knee dislocation: initial assessment and implication for treatment. J Orthop Trauma 11:525–529

Wascher DC, Becker JR, Dexter JG et al (1999) Reconstruction of the anterior and posterior cruciate ligaments after knee dislocation. Results using fresh frozen non- irradiated allografts. Am J Sports Med 27:189–196

Wentorf FA, LaPrade RF, Lewis JL et al (2002) The influence of the integrity of posterolateral structures on tibiofemoral orientation when an anterior cruciate ligament graft is tensioned. Am J Sports Med 30(6):796–799

Computer-Assisted Osteotomies for Genu Varum Deformity: Rationale, Surgical Technique, Outcome, and Return to Sports

80

Dominique Saragaglia and René-Christopher Rouchy

Contents

D. Saragaglia (✉) • René-Christopher Rouchy
Department of Orthopaedic Surgery and Sport Traumatology, Grenoble South Teaching Hospital, Grenoble, Échirolles, France
e-mail: DSaragaglia@chu-grenoble.fr; RCRouchy@chu-grenoble.fr

M.N. Doral, J. Karlsson (eds.), *Sports Injuries*,
DOI 10.1007/978-3-642-36569-0_129

Abstract

High tibial osteotomy (HTO) is commonly used for genu varum deformity in young and active patients. Corrective valgus osteotomy may however lead to an oblique joint line in cases of associated femur varum or absence of tibia vara. To avoid this drawback, we use an accurate and reproducible radiological protocol allowing to choose the best indication between HTO, double-level osteotomy (DLO), and distal femoral osteotomy (DFO). Computer navigation of the osteotomies is the best choice to achieve the preoperative goal, above all, to avoid too much overcorrection, which could be detrimental to resume sportive activity. In this chapter, the rationale of this choice will be presented, the operative procedures and their results as well as the possibilities to resume sports.

Introduction

Medial knee osteoarthritis is not uncommon and high tibial osteotomy (HTO) was described for the first time more than 50 years ago (Jackson and Waugh 1961; Merle d'Aubigné and Ramadier 1961; Judet et al. 1964). Nowadays, it remains a good option (Hernigou et al. 1987; Yasuda et al. 1992; Coventry et al. 1993; Lootvoet et al. 1993; Jenny et al. 1998; Rinonapoli et al. 1998; Lerat 2000; Papachristou et al. 2006; Saragaglia et al. 2011; LaPrade et al. 2012) despite the large

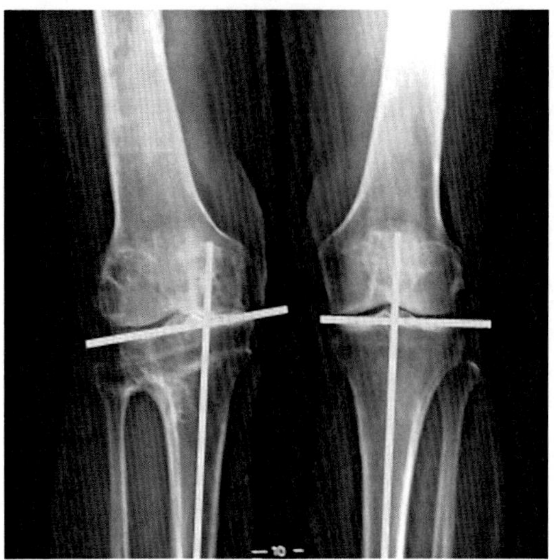

Fig. 1 Severe oblique joint line (*right knee*) after high tibial osteotomy. Notice the extreme tibial valgus

expansion of total knee replacement (TKR) or the revival of unicompartmental knee prosthesis boosted by the less-invasive surgery concept. It is well indicated for "young" and active people (less than 65 years of age) with moderate arthritis (narrowing joint line up to 100 % without any bone wear or instability). Nevertheless, it is a demanding surgery, exposing to excessive over- or undercorrection leading to earlier failure (Saragaglia et al. 2011) or oblique joint line (Fig. 1) being the cause of difficulties when performing later TKR. This oblique joint line corresponds to an excessive valgus of the tibial mechanical axis (Babis et al. 2002). It is all the more frequent when varus is important because of a femoral or a femoral and tibial deformity. The desirable overcorrection (3–6°) to achieve a good clinical result increases even more this oblique joint line.

One can consider combined femoral and tibial osteotomy as a solution to avoid excessive joint line obliquity. However, prior to the advent of computer navigation this was only performed on a limited basis because of the difficulty in obtaining an accurate lower leg axis without any reproducible assistance.

Drawing on our experience with TKR and HTO navigation (Picard et al. 1999; Saragaglia et al. 2001, 2004, 2012; Saragaglia and Roberts 2005), we used the principles of computer-assisted surgery for double-level osteotomy (DLO) hoping to increase the accuracy of this difficult procedure.

The preoperative radiological assessment will be presented as well as the computer-assisted operative procedure, the indications of HTO, DLO, and distal femoral osteotomy (DFO). The rationale behind this way of thinking will be discussed. Moreover, return to sporting activity will be discussed knowing that only a few papers have been published about this topic (Odenbring et al. 1989; Gougoulias et al. 2009; Salzmann et al. 2009; Warme et al. 2011; Bonnin et al. 2013).

Radiological Assessment

Preoperatively standing AP, lateral, and 45° PA weight-bearing views are obtained. In addition, it is essential to obtain AP long-leg standing X-rays to assess the hip-knee-ankle (HKA) angle for preoperative planning. Ramadier's protocol (Ramadier et al. 1982) allows these measurements to be reproducible preoperatively and postoperatively. This protocol can be described as follows: first, to determine accurately the frontal plane by looking for a true lateral view of the knee which is obtained when the posterior margins of the condyles are superimposed; second, to turn 90° around the knee the image intensifier to obtain an accurate long-leg AP standing view, the X-ray being perpendicular to the frontal plane; finally, to draw the footprint on cardboard in order to reproduce the same rotation of the lower leg preoperatively and postoperatively. Using this cardboard by placing the foot in the print, it is easy to do the same view as much as one wants. The long-leg film is critical since the deformity may not be visible on standard knee films (Fig. 2a, b). The HKA angle, the medial distal femoral mechanical angle (MDFMA), and the medial proximal tibial mechanical angle (MPTMA) must be measured (Fig. 3a–c) in order to plan the level of the osteotomy: tibial, femoral, or both.

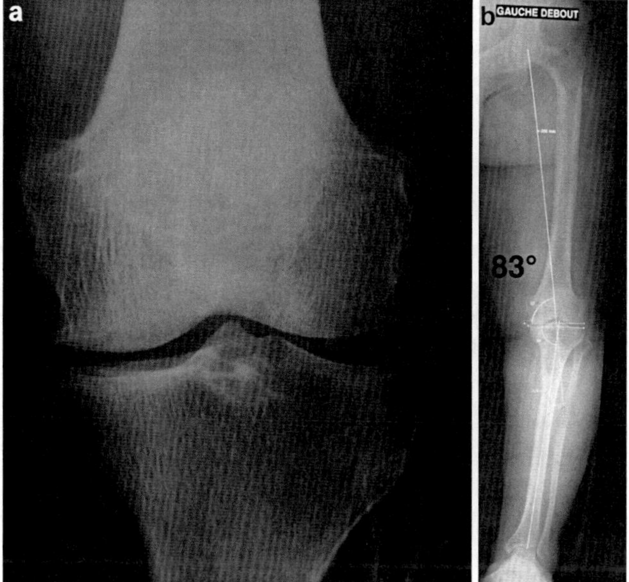

Fig. 2 (**a**) Medial osteoarthritis appearing without severe tibial or femoral deformity. (**b**) Severe genu varum deformity of (**a**) case with medial femoral mechanical angle of 83° which was not predictable on standard X-ray

Grading of osteoarthritis is performed typically using the modified Ahlbäck classification (Saragaglia and Roberts 2005; Table 1).

Surgical Technique

Opening Wedge HTO Computer Navigated

The software is a derivative of the one used for TKA which has been fully described in previous articles (Picard et al. 1999; Saragaglia et al. 2001, 2004) (OrthoPilot® Navigation System, B-Braun-Aesculap, Tuttlingen, Germany). The same principles of real-time acquisition of the rotation center of the hip, knee, and ankle centers and of the anatomical landmarks at the level of the knee joint line and ankle are applied. This allows the mechanical axis of the lower limb to be shown dynamically on the computer screen, i.e., the axis of the lower limb to be seen both pre- and post-osteotomy and to check if the preplanned correction has been established.

A tourniquet is placed at the root of the thigh and the procedure follows in this sequence: The rigid body markers are fixed at the level of the distal femur and proximal tibia allowing acquisition of the centers of the hip, knee, and ankle (Fig. 4). The lower limb mechanical axis then appears on the screen and can be compared with the preoperative radiological goniometry.

A 5–6 cm long incision is made on the proximomedial tibia just at the level of the anterior tuberosity of the tibia. The pes anserinus is incised just above the gracilis tendon and a retractor is placed against the posteromedial corner of the tibia. Then, the superficial medial collateral ligament is released from its tibial insertion to allow an adequate opening of the osteotomy. The HTO is performed 3 cm below the level of the medial joint line, the level confirmed by placing an intra-articular needle. The osteotomy is directed at the fibula head, keeping the saw as horizontal as possible to avoid fracturing the lateral tibial plateau.

With the aid of two osteotomes inserted along the track of the saw cut, the tibia is placed into valgus. These are then replaced by a metal spacer, which is inherently stable and allows the amount of correction to be calmly checked. If there is 8° of varus, one will try a 10–11 mm spacer and make sure that an appropriate hypercorrection is produced real time on the computer screen. If this is

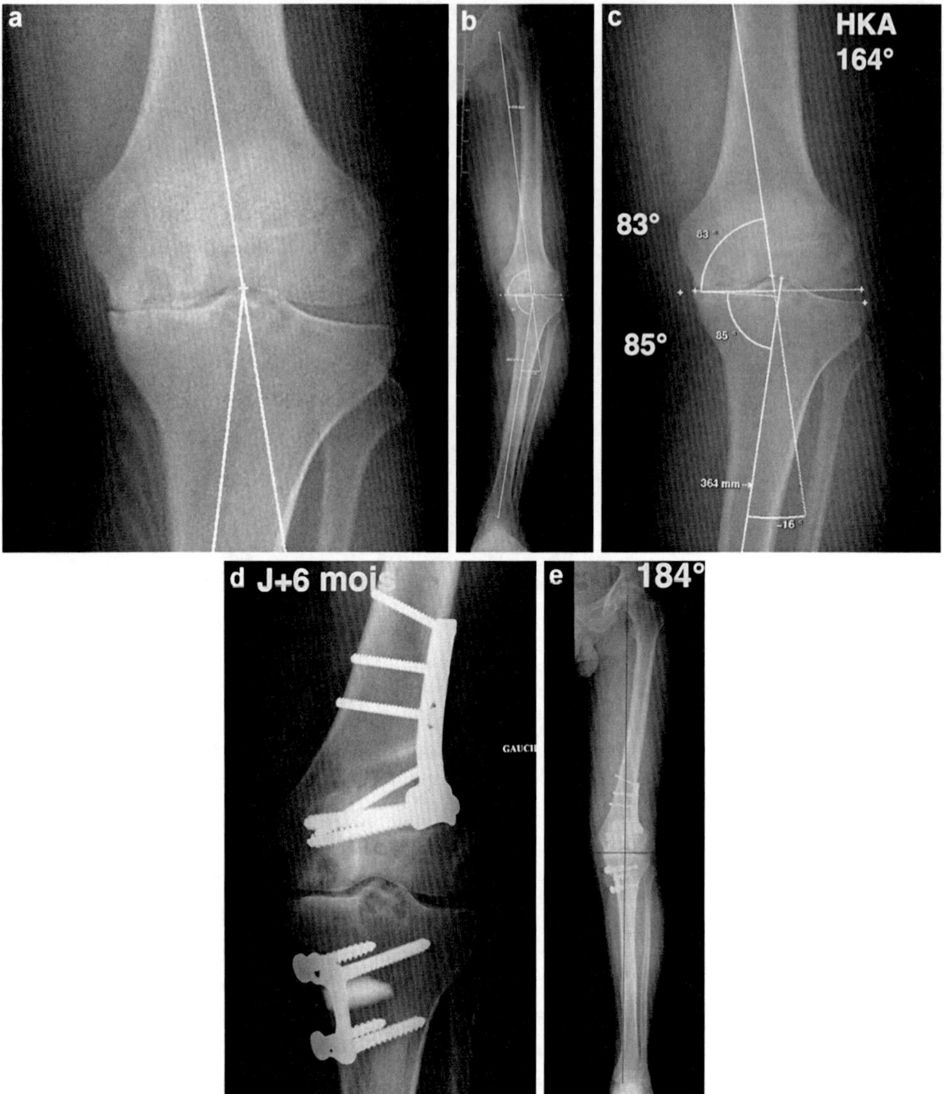

Fig. 3 (**a**) Medial osteoarthritis with necrosis of the medial condyle in a 40-year-old man. (**b**) Severe varus deformity of (**a**) case. (**c**) Centered X-rays of (**a**) case: HKA of 164°, MDFMA of 83°, and MPTMA of 85°. (**d**) Radiological result of (**a**) patient case. Notice after 6 months follow-up, no malunion of the distal femur and proximal tibia and the good healing of the osteotomies as well as the osteonecrosis of the medial condyle. (**e**) Post-operative goniometry of the (**a**) patient case that underwent a DLO. Notice the HKA angle of 184°

Table 1 Modified Ahlbäck criteria according to Saragaglia and Roberts

Grade 1	<50 % joint space narrowing
Grade 2	50–100 % joint space narrowing
Grade 3	100 % narrowing without any bone wear
Grade 4	Bone wear but no lateral instability
Grade 5	Bone wear with lateral compartment decoaptation +/− posterolateral subluxation

insufficient, a thicker spacer may be trialed and the reverse if the correction is too great. The metallic spacer is then replaced with a bioabsorbable tricalcium phosphate wedge (Biosorb®, SBM Company, Lourdes, France) of the desired thickness, and the intervention completed by plating the proximal tibia with a locking screw plate. Then the accuracy of the

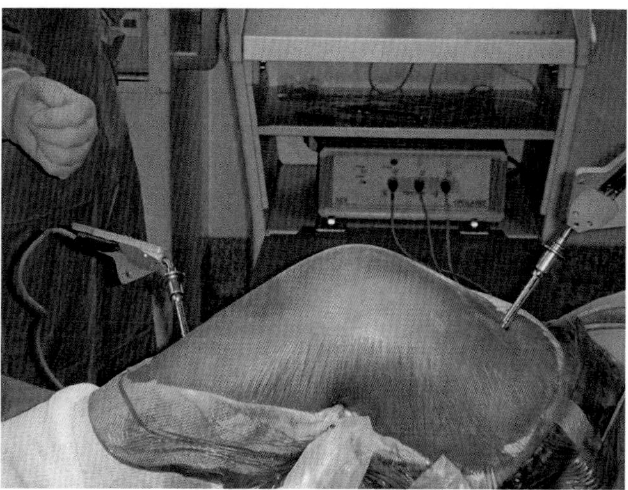

Fig. 4 Left lower leg with rigid bodies at the level of the femur and the tibia

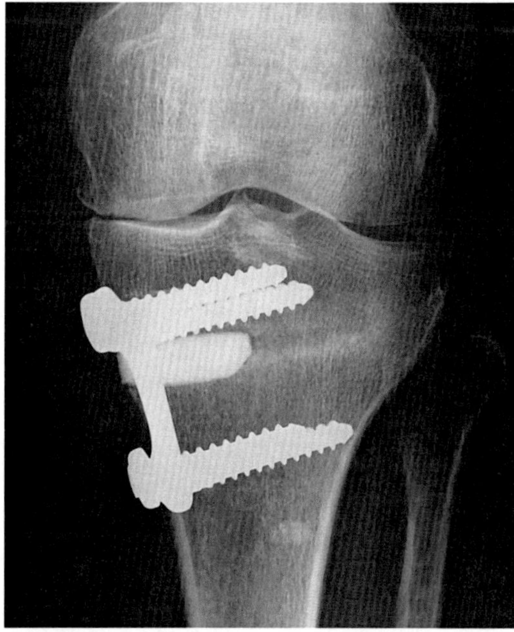

Fig. 5 Radiological result of an HTO (3 months follow-up)

osteosynthesis is checked with the image intensifier (Fig. 5) and the wound is closed.

Computer-Assisted Double-Level Osteotomy

A tourniquet is placed at the proximal aspect of the thigh and the first stage is essentially the same as for that of an HTO: insertion of the rigid body markers (high enough not to hamper the femoral osteotomy and low enough on the other level to avoid interfering with the tibial osteotomy), followed by kinematic acquisition of the hip center, middle of the knee, and tibiotarsal joints in order to find the mechanical axis of the lower limb.

The second stage consists of making the femoral closing osteotomy in the distal femur (in general a 5–6° alteration is made, although sometimes more in congenital femoral varus) and fixing it in position with a locking screw plate. A lateral approach with elevation of the vastus lateralis is chosen, the lateral arthrotomy allowing to locate the tip of the trochlea. The track of the osteotomy lies above the trochlea and is directed obliquely from above laterally to below on the medial femoral cortex. A wedge of bone is then excised from the distal femur with a 4–5 mm lateral base, corresponding to a 5–6° correction. The osteotomy is fixed with the plate after placing the femur into valgus manually. Once this stage is reached, the mechanical axis is rechecked so that the required correction at the level of the tibia can be calculated in order to achieve the preoperative objectives. Then, the wound is closed with a drain.

The last stage is to perform the HTO exactly in the fashion described above. The definitive axis is then displayed on the computer screen and the osteosynthesis is checked with the image intensifier (Fig. 6).

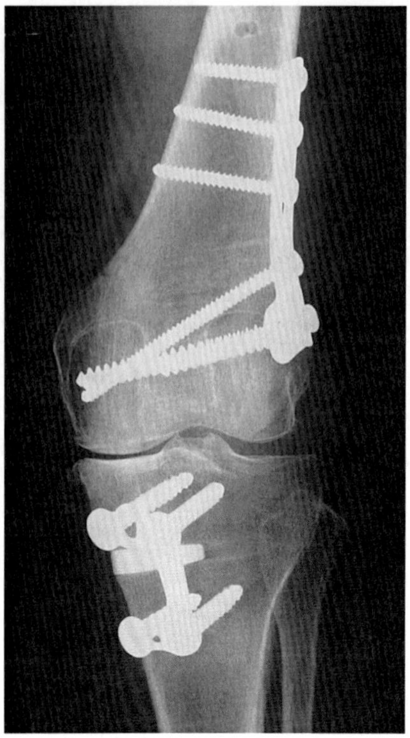

Fig. 6 Radiological result of a DLO (3 months follow-up)

Computer-Assisted Distal Femoral Osteotomy

The procedure is the same as described previously and we prefer to make a closing wedge osteotomy rather than an opening one because of the difficulty to get good stability after plating the distal femur.

Postoperative Management

The patient can stand up the day after the operation and walk with two crutches. Partial weight-bearing is allowed for 30–45 days when performing an HTO and 45–60 days when performing DLO. Full range of motion is regained quickly after HTO (extra-articular procedure) and after 45–60 days for DLO, because of the distal femoral osteotomy, which slows down rehabilitation. It is much more than after HTO but the authors have never seen problems with stiffness in their experience.

Indications

The best indication for osteotomy is a patient with a low arthritis grade (Hernigou et al. 1987; Coventry et al. 1993; Babis et al. 2002) and below 60–65 years. In some cases (very active patients under the age of 50 years), it is possible to perform double-level osteotomy for grade 4 and 5 with a good result (Saragaglia et al. 2012) but this is far from being the rule.

Discussion

The mechanical axis of the lower limb was described by Kapandji (1974) and later taken up by Hungerford and Krackow (1985); it should be 180° with a MDFMA of 93° and a MPTMA of 87° resulting in a joint line perfectly parallel to the ground. However, this assumption is not confirmed in case of osteoarthritis with varus misalignment, because, in a personal unpublished series of 89 TKR, we found a MDFMA of 93° in only 43.8 % of the cases. It was at 90° in 33.7 % of the cases, below 90° in 13.5 %, and above 93° in 9 %.

Thus, before performing high tibial osteotomy, it is crucial to have high-quality and reproducible full-length AP radiographs of the lower limb, according to a specific protocol. The HKA angle, the MDFMA, and the MPTMA should be determined on this goniometry (Fig. 3a–c). Lateral instability testing has become less important than it once was, since the indications for osteotomy in this setting have become rare. In case of femoral valgus (MDFMA >90°), it is illogical to perform a femoral osteotomy because it is better not to create in the femur the error is trying to avoid in the tibia. If the femur is in varus or at 90°, the best is to proceed with a femoral osteotomy to achieve a MDFMA of around 93° (93° +/− 2°) and then complete it with a tibial osteotomy to achieve an HKA angle of 182° +/− 2° in order to avoid too much overcorrection (Fig. 3d, e). Overcorrection, whether femoral or tibial, can distort the anatomy and lead to a much more complicated revision TKR. However, a longer follow-up is needed to prove that overcorrection by +/− 2° is enough for a lasting good result. If the tibia is not in varus (MPTMA over 88°), it is better to perform a femoral osteotomy especially if the femur is at 90° or in varus or contraindicate any osteotomy if it leads to joint line obliquity of more than 5°. Combined distal femoral and proximal tibial osteotomy in the treatment of genu varum is technically difficult. Little has been written about this technique in the literature. Babis et al. 2002 reported on 24 patients (29 knees) operated on with a conventional technique (two closing wedge osteotomies). The mean preoperative HKA angle was 193.3° (i.e., 13.3° of varus); a computer-aided analysis of the mechanical status of the knee for preoperative planning was used. This was limited to preoperative evaluation, and the reliability of the preoperative radiographic evaluation was not assessed. The results showed a mean postoperative HKA angle of 176.9° (169.4–184.9°), a residual varus in two cases (4.6° and 4.9°), and an overcorrection of more than 4° in ten cases and more than 6° in five. It is known that an undercorrection may lead to failure of the operative procedure and a too much overcorrection to cosmetic discomfort and probably to difficulties to return to sport (Warme et al. 2011) especially running-based sports.

The difficulty of the technique comes from the fact that once the first osteotomy is performed, whether femoral or tibial, landmarks change and the ability to achieve a satisfactory alignment with the second osteotomy becomes challenging in the absence of reliable intraoperative landmarks. Martres et al. (2004) suggested performing this operation in two different stages to improve its accuracy and reproducibility. It is also justified to consider that complication occurring at both osteotomy sites could lead to disastrous result. On the other hand, every surgeon operating osteoarthritic knees should be aware of the risk of malunion in the proximal tibia, for a procedure that is often considered temporary, particularly when performing an isolated HTO. In fact, every osteotomy in a young adult is susceptible to lead subsequently to a TKR, and thus it is essential to plan ahead for the iterative surgery called revision.

Computer-assisted surgery allows to assess the femorotibial axis (HKA angle) at every step of the procedure and thus make it more accurate. The first results (Saragaglia et al. 2004) showed in a comparative cohort study of computer-assisted versus conventional HTO a 96 % reproducibility in achieving a mechanical axis of 184° +/− 2° in the computer-navigated group versus 71 % in the conventional osteotomy group ($p < 0.0015$). In another series including 42 cases of DLO (Saragaglia et al. 2012), the authors showed 92.7 % success in reaching the preoperative goal for HKA angle and 88.1 % success in reaching the desired MPTMA (90° +/− 2°), which in terms of performance is remarkable.

Regarding return to sport after osteotomy, little has been published in the literature (Odenbring et al. 1989; Gougoulias et al. 2009; Salzmann et al. 2009; Warme et al. 2011; LaPrade et al. 2012; Bonnin et al. 2013). It is well known that osteotomies allow return to sport, but it is not known if a too much overcorrection or an oblique joint line is compatible with different sporting activities. The best morphotype to play running-based sports (soccer, jogging, tennis, etc.) is neutral or genu varum. When performing an osteotomy getting too much overcorrection, the patient will never be able to play at the same level or will have to change to another sport like golf, cycling, swimming, etc. On the other hand, if few degrees of varus are left, the ability to return to running-based sports may be better but it is riskier regarding pain removal. In other words, the patient must be informed that after surgery he could have pain after strenuous activity (Bonnin et al. 2013). In a personal series of 42 patients (30 HTO and 12 DLO) operated on using navigation, at a mean follow-up of 5.75 +/− 1.3 years (5–8 years), more than 80 % of the patients were always involved in sporting activity which is the same rate as the preoperative one ($p = 0.187$). The frequency of sports sessions per week (2.03 sessions) and duration of activities (5.17 h) did not change significantly after surgery (2.28, $p = 0.214$; 3.83 h, $p = 0.789$, respectively). The mean Lysholm score increased from 64.6 +/−16 to 92.1 +/− 9.3 points ($p < 0{,}001$). The preoperative activity level according to Tegner score and

UCLA score did not decrease significantly after surgery (4.62 and 7.07–4.18 and 6.46, respectively, $p = 0.123$ and 0.117). The mean postoperative KOO Score was 76.17 +/− 20.19. No patient returned to a competitive sport. Many patients were able to do activities such as downhill skiing or mountain biking but very few patients were able to jog or run.

Summary

"Young" patient genu varum deformity can be corrected by high tibial valgus osteotomy, but it is not the sole way to do. The indication is based on an accurate and reproducible radiological protocol including at least standing AP long-leg X-ray. It is useful to measure not only the HKA angle but also the medial distal femoral mechanical angle (MDFMA) and the medial proximal tibial mechanical angle (MPTMA). These measures will guide the surgeon to choose the best indication. When the MDFMA is in valgus (93° or more) and the MPTMA in varus (below 88°), the best option is a HTO. When the MDFMA is in varus (90° or less) and the MPTMA in varus (below 88°), the best indication is DLO. Finally, when the MDFMA is in varus and the MPTMA above 88°, the best indication is DFO. This way of thinking should avoid too much oblique joint line, which is a difficult condition when performing revision to TKA. Regarding return to sport activity, HTO and DLO allows it, but the patient must be informed that residual pain during strenuous sports is not exceptional and return to jogging activities could be a concern.

Cross-References

▶ Arthroscopic Treatment of Knee Osteoarthritis in Athletes
▶ Inlay Joint Resurfacing and High Tibial Osteotomy in Middle-Aged Athletes
▶ Role of Osteotomy for Knee Cartilage, Meniscus, and Ligament Injuries
▶ Sports and High Tibial Osteotomy

References

Babis GC, An KN, Chao EYS et al (2002) Double level osteotomy of the knee: a method to retain joint-line obliquity. J Bone Joint Surg Am 84:1380–1388

Bonnin MP, Laurent JR, Zadegan F et al (2013) Can patients really participate in sport after high tibial osteotomy? Knee Surg Sports Traumatol Arthrosc 21:64–73. doi:10.1007/s00167-011-1461-9

Coventry MB, Ilstrup DM, Wallrichs SL (1993) Proximal tibial osteotomy: a critical long-term study of eighty-seven cases. J Bone Joint Surg Am 75:196–201

Gougoulias N, Khanna A, Maffulli N (2009) Sports activities after lower limb osteotomy. Br Med Bull 91:111–121. doi:10.1093/bmb/ldp023

Hernigou P, Medevielle D, Debeyre J et al (1987) Proximal tibial osteotomy for osteoarthritis with varus deformity: a ten to thirteen-year follow-up study. J Bone Joint Surg Am 69:332–354

Hungerford DS, Krackow KA (1985) Total joint arthroplasty of the knee. Clin Orthop 192:23–30

Jackson JP, Waugh W (1961) Tibial osteotomy for osteoarthritis of the knee. J Bone Joint Surg (Br) 43:746–751

Jenny JY, Tavan A, Jenny G et al (1998) Taux de survie à long terme des ostéotomies tibiales de valgisation pour gonarthrose. Rev Chir Orthop 84:350–357

Judet R, Dupuis JF, Honnard F et al (1964) Désaxations et arthroses du genou. Le genu varum de l'adulte. Indications thérapeutiques, résultats. Rev Chir Orthop 13:1–28

Kapandji IA (1974) Physiologie articulaire. Fascicule II quatrième édition: membre inférieur. Maloine SA (ed), Paris, p 104

LaPrade RF, Spiridonov SI, Nystrom LM et al (2012) Prospective outcomes of young and middle-aged adults with medial compartment osteoarthritis treated with a proximal tibial opening wedge osteotomy. Arthroscopy 28:354–364

Lerat JL (2000) Ostéotomies dans la gonarthrose. Cahiers d'enseignement de la SOFCOT 2000. Elsevier, Paris, pp 165–201

Lootvoet L, Massinon A, Rossillon R et al (1993) Ostéotomie tibiale haute de valgisation pour gonarthrose sur genu varum: à propos d'une série de 193 cas revus après 6 à 10 ans de recul. Rev Chir Orthop 79:375–384

Martres S, Servien E, Aït Si Selmi T et al (2004) Double ostéotomie: indication dans la gonarthrose. Rev Chir Orthop 90(Suppl 6):2S137–2S138

Merle d'Aubigné R, Ramadier JO (1961) Arthrose du genou et surcharge articulaire. Acta Orthop Belg 27:365–375

Odenbring S, Tjornstrand B, Egund N et al (1989) Function after tibial osteotomy for medial gonarthrosis below age 50 years. Acta Orthop Scand 60:527–531

Papachristou G, Plessas S, Sourlas J et al (2006) Deterioration of long-term results following high tibial osteotomy in patients under 60 years of age. Int Orthop 30:406–408

Picard F, Leitner F, Raoult A et al (1999) Computer assisted knee arthroplasty. In: Nichol and Peikenkam (eds). Reschnergestützte Verfahren in Orthopädie und Unfallchirurgie. Steinkopff Darmstadt, Jerosch, Nichol and Peikenkam, pp 461–471

Ramadier JO, Buard JE, Lortat-Jacob A et al (1982) Mesure radiologique des déformations frontales du genou. Procédé du profil vrai radiologique. Rev Chir Orthop 68:75–78

Rinonapoli E, Mancini GB, Corvaglia A et al (1998) Tibial osteotomy for varus gonarthrosis. A 0 to 21-year follow-up study. Clin Orthop 353:185–193

Salzmann GM, Ahrens P, Naal FD et al (2009) Sporting activity after high tibial osteotomy for the treatment of medial compartment knee osteoarthritis. Am J Sports Med 37:312–318. doi:10.1177/0363546508325666

Saragaglia D, Roberts J (2005) Navigated osteotomies around the knee in 170 patients with osteoarthritis secondary to genu varum. Orthopaedics 28(Suppl 10): S1269–S1274

Saragaglia D, Picard F, Chaussard C et al (2001) Mise en place des prothèses totales du genou assistée par ordinateur : comparaison avec la technique conventionnelle. Résultats d'une étude prospective randomisée de 50 cas. Rev Chir Orthop 87:18–28

Saragaglia D, Pradel P, Picard F (2004) L'ostéotomie de valgisation assistée par ordinateur dans le genu varum arthrosique : résultats radiologiques d'une étude cas-témoin de 56 cas. E-mémoires de l'Académie Nationale de Chirurgie 3:21–25, Available at: http://www.bium.univ-paris5.fr/acad-chirurgie

Saragaglia D, Blaysat M, Inman D et al (2011) Outcome of opening-wedge high tibial osteotomy augmented with a Biosorb® wedge and fixed with a plate and screws in 124 patients with a mean of ten years follow-up. Int Orthop 35:1151–1156. doi:10.1007/s00264-010-1102-9

Saragaglia D, Blaysat M, Mercier N et al (2012) Results of forty two computer-assisted double level osteotomies for severe genu varum deformity. Int Orthop 36:999–1003. doi:10.1007/s00264-011-1363-y

Warme BA, Aalderink K, Amendola A (2011) Is there a role for high tibial osteotomies in the athlete? Sports Health 3:59–69. doi:10.1177/1941738109358380

Yasuda K, Majima T, Tsuchida T et al (1992) A ten to 15 year follow-up observation of high tibial osteotomy in medial compartment osteoarthrosis. Clin Orthop Relat Res 282:186–195

81 Costs and Safety of Allografts

Athanasios N. Ververidis and Konstantinos E. Tilkeridis

Contents

A.N. Ververidis (✉) • K.E. Tilkeridis
Department of Orthopaedics, General University Hospital, Democritus University of Thrace, Alexandroupolis, Greece
e-mail: averver@otenet.gr; tilkerorth@yahoo.com

M.N. Doral, J. Karlsson (eds.), *Sports Injuries*,
DOI 10.1007/978-3-642-36569-0_96

Abstract

Allografts are used routinely for sports medicine applications and in a large variety of other non-sports-related surgical procedures. Questions concerning allograft tissue safety remain, such as the actual risk of infection and disease transmission following implantation. Appropriate donor screening, improved donor testing, and adherence to good tissue procurement practices can decrease or eliminate disease transmission from the recipient and infections that are the result of tissue processing. Questions also remain about allograft tissue cost. The main costs represent the efforts that provide the utmost safety in allograft tissue. Concerns about safety, cost, and availability will always limit allograft usage; however, concerns regarding inferior clinical results should not.

Introduction

The use of allograft tissues is becoming increasingly popular, with widespread use among orthopedic surgeons – particularly in knee surgery. In 2005, more than 60,000 allografts were used in knee surgeries by members of the American Orthopaedic Society for Sports Medicine (AOSSM) (McAllister et al. 2007; Vangsness 2007). Allografts have been in vogue in orthopedic medicine for over 20 years; however, questions regarding the safety and cost still remain (Johnson 2004).

Costs of Allografts

First of all, it must be pointed out that it is illegal to buy or sell human organs or tissues. Costs for recovering organs and tissues for donation are never passed on to the donor or the donor family. Many protocols are followed by tissue banks to ensure safety.

Tissue banks insist on *professional expertise* in maintaining uniform and standardized *donor*, *screening*, *testing*, *quality control*, and *state-of-the-art applications* for processing procedures. They also explore advancements in the areas of tissue sterilization and incorporation of bone grafts into the body. Tissue banks must also keep abreast of the development of new products, processing procedures, and Food and Drug Administration (FDA) regulations regarding good manufacturing processes. All these efforts represent the costs of providing the utmost safety in allograft tissue. These expenses are then passed on to the hospital, surgeon, or recipient. Costs are kept at a minimum, but must cover personnel and services in the areas of acquiring, processing, and storage of the allograft (AAOS 2009).

According to Vangsness et al., the average approximate costs of fresh-frozen tissue were $800 for a patellar tendon allograft, $615 for an Achilles tendon, and $640 for menisci (Vangsness et al. 1996). The expenses relating to surgical fees have not been addressed in the literature. There was a study by David W. Cole et al., which presents the cost comparisons between autograft and allograft anterior cruciate ligament (ACL) reconstructive procedures in patients who underwent uncomplicated primary ACL surgical treatment (Cole et al. 2005). The reconstruction of the torn ACL using allograft Achilles tendon was reported to be less expensive than the use of a bone–patellar tendon–bone autograft. The direct surgical fees for the allograft procedure were less than $1,000. The majority of the cost savings for allografts can be attributed to shorter operative time and the lesser likelihood of overnight admission. Nevertheless, this is partially offset by the cost of the allograft itself. Although Cole et al. reported on the cost-effectiveness for the Achilles tendon allograft in ACL reconstruction, a few years later, S. Nagda et al., Barrera Oro et al., and Cooper et al., in their studies, compared the costs associated with anterior cruciate ligament (ACL) reconstruction, with either bone–patellar tendon–bone (BPTB) and hamstring autograft or BPTB, Achilles tendon, and tibialis anterior allograft; they concluded that allograft reconstruction of the ACL was significantly more expensive than autograft reconstruction (Table 1) (Cooper et al. 2010; Nagda et al. 2010; Barrera Oro et al. 2011). It is clear that further analysis is needed to better understand costs and graft selection.

Safety of Allografts

As the use of allograft tissue continues to increase, the safety of allografts will remain an issue of paramount importance (Vangsness 2007).

Disease Transmission from Musculoskeletal Allograft Tissue

The potential for disease transmission is of greatest concern to clinicians and patients.

Table 1 Cost comparison of anterior cruciate ligament reconstruction. Autograft versus allograft

Author/year	Allograft type	Autograft type	Allograft total cost $	Autograft total cost $	p
Cole et al. 2006	Achilles tendon	BPTB[a]	4,622	5,694	$P < 0.0001$
Nagda et al. 2010	BPTB Achilles tendon	BPTB	5,465	4,872	$p = 0.009$
Cooper et al. 2010	Tibialis anterior	Hamstring tendon	5,195	4,072	$P < 0.0001$
Barrera Oro et al. 2011	BPTB	BPTB	4,147	3,154	$P < 0.001$

[a]*BPTB* Bone–patellar tendon–bone

There are several types of infections that can result from the use of these tissues. These include bacterial surface contamination and viral or spore transfer (Johnson 2004).

The most common type of infection is bacterial. This is caused by contamination of the graft or the wound. Viral infection, hepatitis B and C infection, and HIV-1 and HIV-2 infection are also causes for concern. Tuberculosis from allograft use has not been reported in the past 50 years (Johnson 2004).

Disease transmission occurs in two principal ways: either through an infected donor or during tissue procurement, processing, or packaging. Transmission of an infectious agent through an infected donor results from contamination from infectious bacteria in the blood either as the result of prolonged tissue recovery time, occult perimortem infection, or a screening failure (McAllister et al. 2007).

The transmission of disease or infection by the donor to the recipient is always a risk when resorting to the use of allografts, but the prevalence is low, being lower than the risk of transmission by the transplantation of organs (Tomford 1995). Since 1988, only eight cases of bone transplantation-associated HIV infection have been reported, although bacterial allograft infection is more common (Li et al. 2001). Gamma irradiation of allografts is not effective in HIV inactivation at the levels currently used. Therefore, good screening procedures are the most effective means for providing the safest possible allografts (Salzman et al. 1993; Hernigou et al. 1998; Hernigou et al. 2000; Smith et al. 2001). Tomford et al. found an incidence of infection related to the use of allografts of 5 % in patients who had treatment for bone tumors and of 4 % in those who had revision of a hip arthroplasty (Tomford et al. 1990).

Bacterial Infection from Musculoskeletal Allograft Tissue

Historically, the transmission of *bacterial* infection from musculoskeletal tissue has been a rare event. The risk of bacterial infection from allograft tissue is unknown because of several factors: lack of a standardized procurement protocol for tissue harvesting, failure of surgeon to recognize or confirm the allograft as the source of infection (CDC 2002a), and lack of reporting when this complication does occur. However, bacterial infections resulting from allograft contamination may have serious and even fatal consequences (CDC 2002b, 2003).

A case of septic arthritis was reported in 2000, in a 16-year-old girl who had a bone–tendon–bone (BTB) ACL reconstruction. *Pseudomonas aeruginosa*, *Staphylococcus aureus*, and *Enterococcus faecalis* were obtained from cultures. A few days later, a 40-year-old man who received a BTB allograft was diagnosed with septic arthritis. *Pseudomonas aeruginosa* was cultured. Two more cases were reported during the same year: Septic arthritis appeared in a 55-year-old woman who received a BTB allograft. *Citrobacter werkmanii* and group B hemolytic *Streptococci* were cultured. Additionally, septic arthritis developed in a 29-year-old woman from an ACL reconstruction with a BTB allograft. *Klebsiella oxytoca* and *Hafnia alvei* were cultured. Since that cluster of infections, the need for guidelines on screening, disinfecting, sterilizing, and discarding potentially contaminated allografts was recognized. It was clear that a stringent certification mechanism for tissue banks was necessary, with a system for reporting and investigating infections. In addition, safe and effective sterilization methods had to be developed for musculoskeletal tissue (CDC 2000).

In year 2001, the Centers for Disease Control and Prevention (CDC) reported the case of a 23-year-old man who underwent reconstructive knee surgery in Minnesota. He was the recipient of a femoral osteochondral allograft infected with *Clostridium sordellii* and died 3 days after the surgery. Another recipient from the same donor developed a nonfatal septic arthritis (CDC 2001, 2003).

Following these events, the CDC solicited additional reports of allograft-associated infections through electronic list servers, Morbidity and Mortality Weekly Report (MMWR), and by contacting the FDA and state regulatory authorities. Up to March 2002, 26 cases of bacterial infections associated with musculoskeletal allografts had been reported. *Clostridium* species was isolated in 50 % (Kainer et al. 2004). As it is likely that a number of cases were not reported, the number of allograft-acquired infections may actually be higher. The involved allografts included frozen or fresh tendons for ACL reconstruction, fresh femoral condyles with articular cartilage, frozen bone, and menisci. All of these transplanted tissues had been processed aseptically but did not go through terminal sterilization.

In response to these reports, additional steps to reduce the risk of allograft-associated infections have been taken: these include the use and validation of destructive and swab cultures, the elimination of tissues in which bowel flora was isolated, and the review of the time limits for tissue retrieval. Despite these measures, additional infections have been reported (CDC 2002). In September 2003, a 17-year-old patient who had received a cadaver graft for ACL reconstruction was reported to develop septic arthritis. *Streptococcus pyogenes* was isolated. During the following 4 years, there was a single report of a musculoskeletal allograft-associated bacterial infection in year 2006. This infection occurred after a soft-tissue allograft was used for knee ligament reconstruction and was related to *Chryseobacterium meningosepticum* (CDC 2003).

Studies of bacteriologic cultures on preprocessed musculoskeletal allograft tissues have also reported high rates of bacterial contamination in processed musculoskeletal allograft tissue. Malinin et al. reported an 8.1 % incidence of *Clostridium* species contamination, most commonly *Clostridium sordellii*, in musculoskeletal allograft tissue (Malinin et al. 2003). It should be pointed out that the use of terminal sterilization methods such as gamma irradiation (GI) can mainly ensure *bacterial* sterility. This is not the case for viral transmission.

Viral Transmission from Musculoskeletal Allograft Tissue

Viral transmission through allograft tissue is extremely low. Musculoskeletal tissue transplantation has resulted in several reported cases of viral infection, specifically with viral hepatitis, human immunodeficiency virus (HIV), and human T-lymphotropic virus (HTLV). It should be noted that these transmissions occurred before the implementation of guidelines for donor screening for viruses and bacteria and before the availability of currently validated serological tests (Vangsness 2004).

The current risk of contracting HIV from a musculoskeletal allograft has been estimated to be 1 in 1.6 million (Rihn et al. 2003; Caldwell and Shelton 2005; McAllister et al. 2007). The risk of contracting hepatitis B virus (HBV) and hepatitis C virus (HCV) is much higher than the risk of HIV: the current risk of transmitting HCV from unprocessed tissue is 1 in 421,000 (McAllister et al. 2007).

Shutkin, in 1954, was the first to report the transmission of a viral infectious disease with the use of a musculoskeletal tissue. The graft had been obtained from an unprocessed, frozen proximal metaphysis of an above-the-knee amputation. The donor was a 73-year-old man with no previous history of hepatitis or jaundice and had normal liver-function tests (Shutkin 1954).

There are four reports that have documented the transmission of ***hepatitis C*** through transplantation of musculoskeletal allografts. The first documented transmission of hepatitis C was reported in 1992 (Eggen et al. 1992). This was in a patient with no previous risk factors. He had received a frozen unprocessed femoral head from an infected donor who had been transfused 5 years earlier, with no previous history, signs, or symptoms of hepatitis. The second reported case of hepatitis C infection came from a retrospective study in 1992 (Pereira et al. 1992). No clear conclusions could be made in this case because the recipient had also had a previous history of blood transfusions during a coronary-artery bypass and two primary hip replacements. The third case was reported in 1995 (Conrad et al. 1995): a second-generation assay (HCV 2.0) had become available at that time, with the advantage of being more sensitive than the first-generation assay (HCV 1.0). Two donors that had previously been tested negative with the HCV 1.0 were found to be positive with the HCV 2.0. Three patients who had received a nonirradiated frozen proximal femur and two BTB ACL grafts from the second donor were positive. None of these recipients had previous risk factors. The conclusion was that the second donor may have transmitted hepatitis C virus. The fourth case was reported in 2003 (CDC 2003): a patient who had received a BTB allograft developed acute hepatitis C. The donor was a man in his 40s with no history, signs, or symptoms of hepatitis and previous negative tests for hepatitis. The investigation was performed by the CDC by retesting the stored samples of the donor with a third-generation enzyme immuno-analysis. This showed that the donor was negative for anti-HCV but positive for HCV RNA.

HTLV infection after transplantation of frozen allografts was first reported in Sweden in 1993 (Sanzen et al. 1997). A retrospective analysis was performed on 16,000 sera from blood donors. One case was found to be seropositive for HTLV-1. All 16 recipients of this donor were tracked to be tested, and only one was seroconverted. He was a 76-year-old patient who had received a femoral head bone graft to fixate a loose acetabulum during a revision hip arthroplasty. The donor had undergone a total hip arthroplasty, and the femoral head was donated to the bone bank, where it was kept deep-frozen for 1 month before implantation.

HIV transmission through transplantation of musculoskeletal allografts has been documented twice in the USA. The first report was that of a young woman who had received a femoral head allograft from an infected donor, during spinal fusion for idiopathic scoliosis in 1984 (CDC 1988). The donor was tested and found to be positive for HIV *after* the implantation. Both donor and recipient died of complications related to the disease. The donor had not been tested for HIV before donation; he had a history of intravenous drug abuse and had been biopsied for lymphadenopathy a few months before donation. Following this case report, most tissue banks started screening for the virus. This was not, however, sufficient to stop the risk of transmission. The second HIV transmission occurred after transplantation of a bone allograft in 1992 (Simonds et al. 1992). This patient had no previous risk factors and developed HIV after receiving an infected femoral head during revision hip arthroplasty in 1985. The donor had been a 22-year-old man without risk factors and with negative serum tests for HIV. Another four recipients of the kidneys, liver, and heart from the same donor became infected. In addition, three recipients of frozen, unprocessed musculoskeletal allografts contracted the disease (both femoral heads and one BTB graft). However, there was no transmission in 25 recipients of freeze-dried bone chips, freeze-dried segments of fascia lata, tendon, and ligaments.

Proper donor screening and tissue processing are of paramount importance for the prevention of viral disease transmission. However, human error makes disease transmission still possible, and window periods for infection exist when detection may be missed by serological tests (7 days for HIV and HCV, 8 days for HBV) (Tomford et al. 1990).

How to Avoid or Diminish Infection

The best measures that should be taken in order to avoid infection or diminish its incidence, when dealing with bacterial cultures at the extraction, storage, and implantation stages of the allografts, are careful donor selection and application of routine sterile techniques. Routine culturing of allografts tissue in the operating room immediately before implantation is not currently recommended (Caldwell and Shelton 2005; McAllister et al. 2007). For the limitation of infection during allograft procedures, it is important to ensure that the tissue bank that the patient or the hospital is using is certified (Johnson 2004).

Tissue Banking and Regulation

A tissue bank is defined as an organization that provides donor screening, recovery, processing, and storage or distribution of allograft tissue. There are multi-tissue banks that supply musculoskeletal grafts, and there are also dedicated musculoskeletal tissue banks. The American Association of Tissue Banks (AATB) is a private nonprofit peer group organization that was founded in 1976 after the model of the American Association of Blood Banks. It is a scientific, standards-setting organization founded to promote the transplantation of cells and tissue while maintaining quality, minimizing risk to recipients, and maximizing tissue quantities sufficient to meet demand nationally. This association has become a source of information and advice to tissue banking and affiliated organizations in the industry of tissue and cell transplant. The AATB provides certification of personnel and accreditation of organizations that recover and process tissue by publishing standards designed to maintain a safe and adequate supply of transplantable cells and tissues. The AATB standards describe recovery methods, processing, preservation, and distribution of transplantable tissue. These published standards are specific to transmissible disease screening, donor selection criteria, required bacteriological testing, staff training, record-keeping, and maintenance of asepsis, labeling, and storage. These standards meet or exceed the final rule issued by the US FDA CFR 21 1271 (good tissue practices). All donation programs have implemented standardized donor screening protocols as the result of FDA requirements, and all AATB-accredited organizations have additional minimum standards incorporated into their policies. Additional protocols vary and may include age criteria for specific circumstances. As noted previously, the donor age criteria example for sports medicine use is continually being reevaluated and adjusted. It is also important for the surgeon to know the tissue bank from which the tissue came (McGuire et al. 2007; Suarez et al. 2007).

Regulation About Suppliers

In USA the American Association of Tissue Banks requires that its members perform *full screening* that meets US Food and Drug Administration (FDA) requirements; however, secondary sterilization of the grafts is still optional. Surgeons, who use allografts, should know that not all tissue banks are members of AATB and not all tissue banks are inspected (Diaz-de-Rada et al. 2003). The AATB now requires accredited banks to use nucleic acid testing (NAT) for HCV and HIV (American Association of Tissue Banks 2006; McAllister et al. 2007).

The 2004/23/EG guidelines issued by the European Parliament and ratified on 31/3/2004 define the quality and safety standards for the donation, procurement, testing, processing, preservation, storage and distribution of human tissues and cells (Diaz-de-Rada et al. 2003; Pruss et al. 2007). A review by Vangsness et al. in 2003 describes the process of procurement, processing, and storage and is recommended to be read by anyone who is using allograft tissue (Vangsness et al. 2003).

In another article by David McAllister et al., the current concerns of sports medicine surgeons are reviewed, problems associated with allograft usage are identified, the current regulations concerning allograft tissue are cited, and updated information regarding sterilization processes is provided (McAllister et al. 2007).

Screening

The AATB has formulated *guidelines* for its members; these guidelines recommend donor screening.

Screening Steps

The first step in donor screening is to obtain *consent from the donor*. This may be voluntary or may be done by a request made to the family.

Second step: A *history* from the donor's primary caregiver, which should include a listing of any prior infection and risk factors such as male homosexuality, sex for money, illegal drug use, and hemophilia.

Third step: A *physical examination* should be performed to assess the donor for needle wounds or evidence of infection.

Fourth step: *Screening tests* are performed on tissue and blood for hepatitis (B and C) HIV, human T-lymphotropic virus, and syphilis infection. The donor tissue should be obtained aseptically. The tissue should then undergo secondary sterilization. Secondary sterilization would eliminate all possibilities of infection while maintaining all biologic and mechanical properties of the tissue. Nevertheless, no technique currently exists that fulfills these requirements (Johnson 2004; American Association of Tissue Banks 2006).

Procurement

Tissues from donors without risk factors are generally procured in an aseptic environment. Allografts are procured through body donations recovered from donors in the operating room or morgue of hospitals. Most of the banks (89 %) obtain donors through Organ Procurement Organizations (OPOs), which are responsible for identification of potential donors and discussion of donation with the patient's family members (Vangsness et al. 1996). This information is obtained via interview with the patient or next of kin.

Current serological screening involves serologic tests for HIV-I/II antibodies, HIV antigen, polymerase chain reaction-HIV, hepatitis B surface antigen, hepatitis B surface antibodies, hepatitis B core antibodies, HCV antibodies, HTLV-I/II antibodies, and the rapid plasma regain test for syphilis. Most tissue banks accept donors from 15 to 50 years old (Vangsness et al. 1996). The AATB requires that tissue excision shall commence within 15 h of death. If the donor is procured at room temperature, the time limit for most of the banks is 12 h and for refrigerated donors, 24 h (Vangsness et al. 1996; Vangsness 2006). Tissues are kept in quarantine on an average of 5 weeks (range, 14 days to 4 months) until all serologic test results are available (Vangsness et al. 1996). Most banks culture tissues by swab technique and/or by destructive culturing. However, culturing remains under controversy because studies have reported that cultures are only 78–92 % accurate (Veen et al. 1994).

Sterilization–Radiation

Sterilization means inactivation or killing of all forms of life. The ideal method should provide a disease-free graft, without compromising the mechanical characteristics or biologic incorporation. Currently, there is no ideal method to sterilize soft-tissue allografts (King et al. 2004; Branam et al. 2007). In view of this problem, *3 main chemical methods of sterilization have been developed*: *Allowash TM formula* (LifeNet, Virginia Beach, VA), *BioCleanse* Process (Regeneration Technologies, Inc., Alachua, Florida), and *Clearant* Process (Clearant, Inc., Los Angeles, California) (Fideler et al. 1995; King et al. 2004). *The Allowash TM formula* utilizes ultrasonic centrifugation and negative pressure in combination with reagents such as biological detergents, alcohols, and hydrogen peroxide. *BioCleanse* sterilization process is used in the final steps of processing and avoids the use of excessive heat, irradiation, or ethylene oxide. It has been used to effectively clean bone (similar to a dishwasher) and has been reported as resulting in no significant weakness of a BTB graft. *Clearent* is a technique that uses high-dose gamma radiation (5 Mrad) in a proprietary solution of dimethyl sulfoxide (DMSO), ethylene glycol, and a sugar solution (Fideler et al. 1995; King et al. 2004; Branam et al. 2007; Vangsness 2007).

It is important for the surgeon to be aware of the changes in biomechanics that may occur with the use of either chemicals or irradiation. Secondary sterilization with either *ethylene oxide or irradiation* causes biologic and biomechanical damage to the tissue. It should be recognized that allografts may become *weaker* after this sterilization and they may take longer to incorporate into the bony tunnels (Fideler et al. 1995; King et al. 2004). Currently, the average recommended dose of irradiation used in the USA is 1–2.5 Mrad (10–25 kGy) ("low-dose radiation"). This dose is effective in eliminating bacterial surface contamination, but doses more than 3 Mrad are required to kill viruses (Fideler et al. 1995; McAllister et al. 2007). However, there are pressures to tissues banks to develop *chemical techniques that make tissues even safer without degrading either the biologic or biomechanical quality of the tissue*. Therefore, the safety issue must constantly be balanced against efficacy.

Storage

Like sterilization, a perfect storage option does not exist. There are a number of methods and federal guidelines for storing tissue after procurement. These methods are as follows: *fresh allograft, fresh freezing, cryopreservation, and freeze-drying (lyophilization)* (Vangsness et al. 2003; Johnson 2004; Branam et al. 2007). *Fresh grafts* are implanted shortly after harvest. With fresh grafts, a concern for disease transmission exists due to the lack of secondary sterilization and storage processing. Freezing fresh allografts between temperatures −80° and −196° allows for storage of up to 3–5 years; however, *the process kills the cells* (Picture 1). *Cryopreservation* is a process by which the tissue undergoes controlled-rate freezing while cellular water is extracted by glycerol and dimethyl sulfoxide. The graft has a shelf life of 10 years and up to 80 % of cells can remain viable. *Freeze-drying or* lyophilization is an additional storage option. This process results in a residual moisture level of <5 %. An advantage of this process is that the graft can be stored at room temperature for up to 3–5 years (Shelton 2003; Caldwell and Shelton 2005).

Factoring Relative Risk

The relative risks of viral infection following blood transfusion are reported as follows: hepatitis B 1/63,000, hepatitis C 1/100,000, and HIV 1/1,000.000. In comparison, the risk of HIV infection after bone transplantation is 1/1,500.000. The risk of HIV after soft-tissue transplantation with secondary sterilization is 1/1,600.000. To put all this information in the proper perspective, one should remember that the risk of death due to pregnancy is 1/10,000, from administration of penicillin is 1/30,000, and with oral contraceptives is 1/50,000 (Johnson 2004).

Conclusion

In summary, allograft safety has improved greatly over the last 15 years and is a valuable treatment option for today's orthopedic practice. The American Academy believes allografts are safe if used within the guidelines, when they are supplied by an accredited tissue bank, and if the appropriate surgical techniques are employed (Freddie Fu et al. 2008).

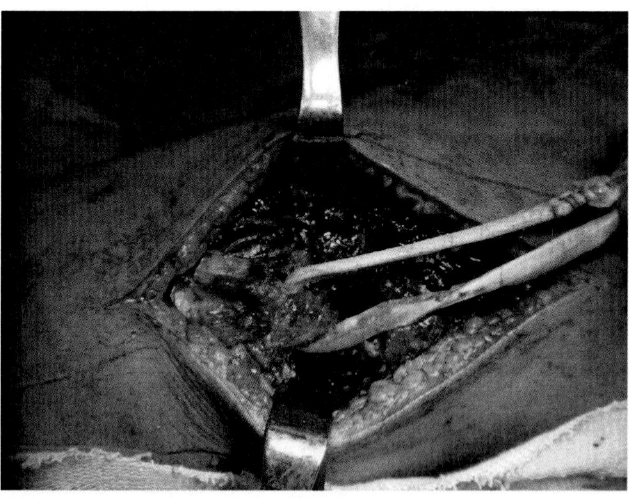

Picture 1 Fresh-frozen tibialis posterior allograft. The allograft has been defrosted and used in a posterolateral corner (*PLC*) of the knee reconstruction

References

American Academy of Orthopaedic Surgeons (2009) Your orthopaedic connection, bone and tissue transplantation, how safe it is? Available at http://orthoinfo.aaos.org/topic.cfm?topic=a00115. Last reviewed and updated: Jan 2009

American Association of Tissue Banks (2006) Standards for tissue banking. American Association of Tissue Banks, MacLean

Barrera Oro F, Sikka RS, Wolters B, Graver R, Boyd JL, Nelson B, Swiontkowski MF (2011) Autograft versus allograft: an economic cost comparison of anterior cruciate ligament reconstruction. Arthroscopy 27 (9):1219–1225

Branam B, Johnson D (2007) Allografts in knee surgery. Orthop Today 30:925

Caldwell PE, Shelton WR (2005) Indications for allografts. Orthop Clin N Am 36(4):459–467

Centers for Disease Control and Prevention (2003) Invasive Streptococcus pyogenes after allograft implantation: Colorado, 2003. MMWR Morb Mortal Wkly Rep 52:1174–1176

Centers for Disease Control and Prevention (2002a) Update: allograft-associated bacterial infections. United States, 2002. MMWR Morb Mortal Wkly Rep 51:207–211

Centers for Disease Control and Prevention (2001a) Septic arthritis following anterior cruciate ligament reconstruction using tendon allografts – Florida and Louisiana, 2000. MMWR 50:1081–1083

Centers for Disease Control and Prevention (2001b) Notice to readers: unexplained deaths following knee surgery – Minnesota. MMWR 50(46):1035–1036

Centers for Disease Control and Prevention (2002b) Update: allograft-associated bacterial infections – United States, 2002. MMWR 51:207–210

Centers for Disease Control and Prevention (CDC) (2003) Hepatitis C virus transmission from an antibody-negative organ and tissue donor – United States 2000–2002. MMWR 52(13):273–276

Centers for Disease Control and Prevention (CDC) (1988) Transmission of HIV through bone transplantation: case report and public health recommendations. MMWR 37:597–599

Cole DW, Ginn AT, Chen GJ, Smith BP, Curl WW, Martin DF, Poehling GG (2005) Cost comparison of anterior cruciate ligament reconstruction: autograft versus allograft. Arthroscopy 21:786–790

Conrad EU, David R, Obermeyer KR et al (1995) Transmission of the hepatitis-C virus by tissue transplantation. J Bone Joint Surg Am 77A:221–224

Cooper MT, Kaeding C (2010) Comparison of the hospital cost of autograft versus allograft soft-tissue anterior cruciate ligament reconstructions. Arthroscopy 26 (11):1478–1482

Diaz-de-Rada P et al (2003) Positive culture in allograft ACL-reconstruction: what to do? Knee Surg Sports Traumatol Arthrosc 11:219–222

Eggen BM, Nordbo SA (1992) Transmission of HCV by organ transplantation. N Engl J Med 326:411–413

Fideler BM, Vangsness CT Jr, Lu B, Orlando C, Moore T (1995) Gamma irradiation: effects on biomechanical properties of human bone-patellar tendon-bone allografts. Am J Sports Med 23:643–646

Fu F (2008) Allografts for orthopedic surgery safer, but still require caution. Orthop Today, Hawaii, 15 Jan 2008. Allograft safety 2008. Presented at Orthopedics Today Hawaii 2008. Lahaina, Maui, Hawaii. http://www.orthosupersite.com/view.asp?rID=25706

Hernigou P, Gras G, Marinello G, Dormont D (2000) Inactivation of HIV by application of heat and radiation: implication in bone banking with irradiated allograft bone. Acta Orthop Scand 71:508–512, 10

Hernigou P, Marinello G, Dormont D (1998) Influence de l'irradiation sur le risque de transmission du virus HIV par allogreffe osseuse. Rev Chir Orthop Reparatrice 84:493–500

Johnson D (2004) All about allografts – select highlights of the 71st annual meeting of the American Academy of Orthopaedic Surgeons, San Francisco

Kainer MA, Linden JV, Whaley DN, Holmes HT, Jarvis WR, Jernigan DB, Archibald LK (2004) Clostridium infections associated with musculoskeletal-tissue allografts. N Engl J Med 350:2564–2571

King WD, Grieb TA, Forng RY (2004) Pathogen inactivation of soft tissue allografts using high dose gamma irradiation with early clinical results. Program and abstracts of the 71st annual meeting of the American Academy of Orthopaedic Surgeons, San Francisco. Paper No 106

Li CM, Ho YR, Liu YC (2001) Transmission of human immunodeficiency virus through bone transplantation: a case report. Formos Med Assoc 100 (5):350–351

Malinin TI, Buck BE, Temple HT, Martinez OV, Fox WP (2003) Incidence of clostridial contamination in donors' musculoskeletal tissue. J Bone Joint Surg (Br) 85:1051–1054

McAllister DR, Joyce MJ, Mann BJ et al (2007) Allograft update. The current status of tissue regulation, procurement, processing, and sterilization. Am J Sport Med 35:2148–2157

McGuire DA, Hendricks SD (2007) Allografts in sports medicine. Oper Tech Sports Med 15:46–52

Nagda SH, Altobelli GG, Bowdry KA, Brewster CE, Lombardo SJ (2010) Cost analysis of outpatient anterior cruciate ligament reconstruction. Autograft versus allograft. Clin Orthop Relat Res 468:1418–1422

Pereira BJ, Milford EL, Kirkman RL et al (1992) Prevalence of hepatitis C virus RNA in organ donors positive for hepatitis C antibody and in the recipients of their organs. N Engl J Med 327:910–915

Pruss A, Von Versen R (2007) Influence of European regulations on quality, safety and availability of cell and tissue allografts in Germany. Handchir Microhir Plast Chir 39(2):81–87

Rihn JA, Harner CD (2003) The use of musculoskeletal allograft tissue in knee surgery. Arthroscopy 19(Suppl 1):51–66

Salzman NP, Psallidopoulos M, Prewett AB, O'Leary R (1993) Detection of HIV in bone allografts prepared from AIDS autopsy tissue. Clin Orthop 292:384–390

Sanzen L, Carlsson A (1997) Transmission of human T-cell lymphotropic virus type 1 by a deep-frozen bone allograft. Acta Orthop 68:70–76

Shelton WR (2003) Arthroscopic allograft surgery of the knee and shoulder: indications, techniques, and risks. Arthroscopy 1(19 Suppl):67–69

Shutkin NM (1954) Homologous serum jaundice transmitted by bank bone: a case report. J Bone Joint Surg Am 36A:160–162

Simonds RJ, Holmberg SD, Hurwitz RL et al (1992) Transmission of human immunodeficiency virus type 1 from a seronegative organ and tissue donor. N Engl J Med 326:726–732

Smith RA, Ingels J, Lochemes JJ, Dutkowsky JP, Pifer LL (2001) Gamma irradiation of HIV-1. J Orthop Res 19:815–819

Suarez LS, Richmond JC (2007) Overview of procurement, processing, and sterilization of soft tissue allografts for sports medicine. Sport Med Arthrosc Rev 15 (3):106–113

Tomford WW (1995) Transmission of disease through transplantation of musculoskeletal allografts. J Bone Joint Surg Am 77(11):1742–1754

Tomford WW, Thongphasuk J, Mankin HJ, Ferraro MJ (1990) Frozen musculoskeletal allografts: a study of the clinical incidence and causes of infection associated with their use. J Bone Joint Surg 72A:1137–1143

Vangsness TC Jr (2007) How safe are soft-tissue allografts? American Academy of Orthopaedic Surgeons/American Association of Orthopaedic Surgeons http://www.aaos.org/news/bulletin/aug07/clinical1.asp

Vangsness TC Jr, Triffon MJ, Joyce MJ, Moore TM (1996) Soft tissue for allograft reconstruction of the human knee: a survey of the American Association of Tissue Banks. Am J Sports Med 24:230–234

Vangsness TC (2004) Overview of allograft soft tissue processing, in-depth look at allograft safety Feb AAOS 2004 Bulletin http://www2.aaos.org/aaos/archives/bulletin/feb04/feature1.htm

Vangsness TC Jr, Garcia IA, Randal M, Kainer MA, Roberts MR, Moore TM (2003) Allograft transplantation in the knee: tissue regulation, procurement, processing, and sterilization. Am J Sports Med 31:474–481

Vangsness CT Jr (2006) Soft-tissue allograft processing controversies. J Knee Surg 19:215–219

Veen MR, Bloem RM, Petit PL (1994) Sensitivity and negative predictive value of swab cultures in musculoskeletal allograft procurement. Clin Orthop 300:259–263

Current Concepts in the Treatment of Posterior Cruciate Ligament Injuries

82

Michael Ellman and Robert F. LaPrade

Contents

M. Ellman (✉)
Department of Orthopedic Surgery, Rush University Medical Center, Chicago, IL, USA
e-mail: mikeellman@gmail.com

R.F. LaPrade
The Steadman Clinic and Steadman Philippon Research Institute, Vail, CO, USA
e-mail: drlaprade@sprivail.org; rlaprade@thesteadmanclinic.com

M.N. Doral, J. Karlsson (eds.), *Sports Injuries*,
DOI 10.1007/978-3-642-36569-0_109

Abstract

Posterior cruciate ligament (PCL) injuries may not be as benign as previously anticipated, yet the literature on PCL injuries is sparse compared to that of the anterior cruciate ligament (ACL). Over the past two decades, however, advances in basic science and clinical research have elucidated a greater understanding of the natural history, anatomy, biomechanics, evaluation, and treatment of PCL injuries. This chapter reviews several principles relating to the diagnosis and treatment of PCL injuries, with a focus on current concepts involving workup, diagnosis, surgical versus nonsurgical management, operative techniques, and rehabilitation strategies following PCL injury.

Introduction

Posterior cruciate ligament (PCL) injuries may be more common than previously anticipated. Historically, PCL tears have been underdiagnosed in clinical practice because isolated injuries are often mildly symptomatic or asymptomatic, and an isolated PCL tear has the potential to heal in many cases. While the incidence of PCL tears has been reported as only 1–3 % of all patients with knee ligament injuries in the general population, PCL tears are diagnosed in almost 40 % of patients with acute knee ligament injuries diagnosed at trauma centers (Miyasaka et al. 1991; Fanelli et al. 1994; Fanelli and Edson 1995).

Further, almost half of PCL injuries diagnosed at trauma centers are combined injuries, with an incidence among these of combined ACL and PCL tears of 46 %, PCL-posterolateral corner (PLC) tears of 41 %, and isolated PCL tears of only 3 % (Fanelli and Edson 1995). Nevertheless, research into treatment of PCL injuries is sparse in comparison to ACL injuries.

Over the past two decades, understanding of the natural history, anatomy, biomechanics, clinical evaluation, indications, and treatment options of both isolated and combined PCL injuries has evolved, elucidating several current concepts in the diagnosis and treatment of PCL tears. Several authors have classically reported good to excellent clinical outcomes following nonoperative treatment of isolated PCL tears (Parolie and Bergfeld 1986; Torg et al. 1989). More recently, however, studies have reported declining clinical outcome scores and early osteoarthritis following severe isolated and combined PCL injuries treated nonoperatively (Strobel et al. 2003; McAllister and Petrigliano 2007; Van de Velde et al. 2009), prompting surgeons to consider operative intervention in these cases. Advances in research have stimulated a better understanding of advantages and disadvantages of nonoperative versus operative treatment options, improvements in surgical techniques, and enhancement of post-injury rehabilitation protocols that help guide the surgeon treating a PCL injury. In this chapter, several principles regarding diagnosis and treatment will be reviewed, with a focus on current concepts involving diagnosis, surgical versus nonsurgical treatment, operative techniques, and rehabilitation strategies following PCL injuries.

Anatomy

The PCL originates from the lateral aspect of the medial femoral condyle at the junction of the medial wall and roof of the intercondylar notch, and passes posteriorly and laterally to attach into a depression on the posterior aspect of the tibia, bordered by a medial and lateral prominence (Fig. 1) (Parolie and Bergfeld 1986). The ligament itself is 32–38 mm long, with an average width of 13 mm (Parolie and Bergfeld 1986). The midsubstance of the ligament is the most compact, approximately one third the diameters of both the femoral and tibial footprints with an average cross-sectional width of 11 mm (Harner et al. 1995). The PCL lies within the joint capsule of the knee, yet it is considered extra-articular because it is enclosed within its own synovial sheath (Matava et al. 2009).

Functionally, the PCL can be divided into three portions based on tensioning patterns. There are two main portions, or bundles: a larger anterolateral (AL) and a smaller posteromedial (PM) bundle (Girgis et al. 1975; Makris et al. 2000;

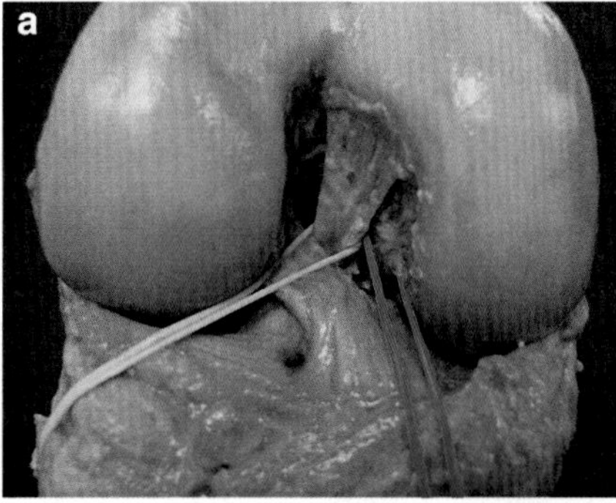

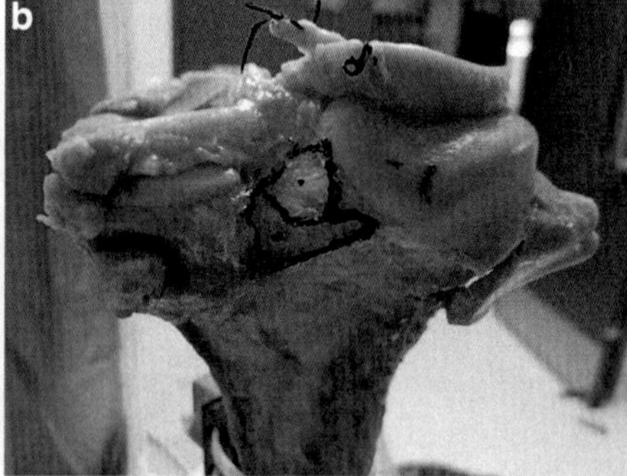

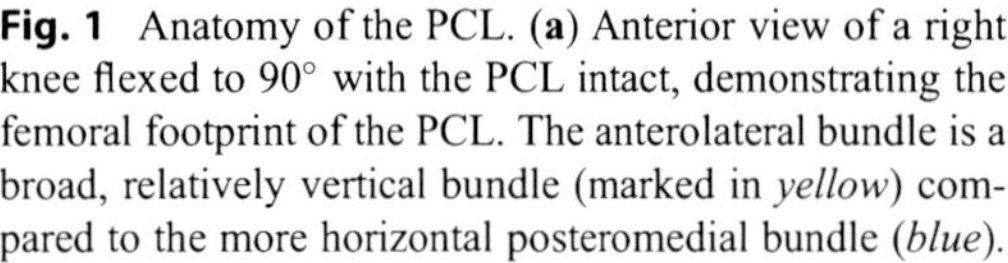

Fig. 1 Anatomy of the PCL. (**a**) Anterior view of a right knee flexed to 90° with the PCL intact, demonstrating the femoral footprint of the PCL. The anterolateral bundle is a broad, relatively vertical bundle (marked in *yellow*) compared to the more horizontal posteromedial bundle (*blue*). (**b**) Posterior view of the tibial footprint of the PCL in a right knee. The posteromedial bundle is distal to the more proximal anterolateral bundle. The average distance between the AL and PM bundle centers on the tibia of 8.9 mm

Lopes et al. 2008), in addition to a third portion, the variable anterior (ligament of Humphrey) and posterior (ligament of Wrisberg) meniscofemoral ligaments (Kennedy et al. 1976; Harner et al. 1995). The terminology of the specific bundles is derived from the relationship of the anatomic location of the femoral origin (anterior or posterior) to the tibial insertion (lateral or medial). The AL bundle serves as the primary restraint to posterior translation of the knee and is under the greatest tension when the knee is at 90° of flexion (Markolf et al. 1997; Covey et al. 2008). It is approximately two times larger in cross-sectional area than the PM bundle (Race and Amis 1994; Harner et al. 1995). The PM bundle, in contrast, provides posterior translation stability as the knee nears full extension (making it the primary stabilizer with knee extension) and has been reported to function as a secondary restraint to external rotation (Markolf et al. 2006; Sekiya et al. 2008). Therefore, tension develops in a reciprocal fashion in each bundle during knee range of motion, with few fibers exhibiting isometric behavior. Interestingly, controversy over the subdivision of the two bundles exists, because the PCL has been previously defined as a continuum of fibers comprising, at a minimum, three or four bundles (Mejia et al. 2002). For the purpose of PCL reconstruction, however, the two-bundle concept has stimulated a movement among surgeons toward double-bundle reconstruction with an attempt to reproduce both bundles of the PCL and achieve a more "anatomic" reconstruction, as opposed to single-bundle reconstruction where the AL bundle alone is reconstructed (Sekiya et al. 2005).

Over the past decade, researchers have placed an increased emphasis on more precisely identifying the osseous landmarks of the PCL in normal knees, in an attempt to allow for anatomic reconstruction of the PCL during either single- or double-bundle reconstruction. On the femoral side, the PCL has a broad, relatively vertical footprint at the anterolateral aspect of the medial femoral condyle, with a midpoint on average 7–8 mm proximal to the articular surface (Fuss 1989; Mejia et al. 2002). The footprint averages 32 mm in diameter (Fig. 1a). In a recent cadaveric study, 75 % of specimens ($n = 20$) demonstrated a semicircular shape of the femoral footprint, while 25 % had an oval shape (Lopes et al. 2008). The authors reported the average area of the femoral footprint to be 209 ± 33.82 mm^2, with the mean area of the AL and PM bundles measuring 118 ± 23.95 mm^2 and 90 ± 16.13 mm^2, respectively, both significantly higher than previously reported values (Harner et al. 1999; Edwards et al. 2007). Two bony prominences were also identified on the femur, the medial intercondylar ridge and the medial bifurcate ridge (Lopes et al. 2008). The medial intercondylar ridge is an osseous prominence 14 mm in length found proximal to the femoral footprint, marking the proximal border of both the AL and PM bundles, running from proximal to distal and anterior to posterior (Lopes et al. 2008; Anderson et al. 2012). The medial bifurcate prominence, shorter in length than the intercondylar ridge, is located between the two fiber bundles (Lopes et al. 2008; Anderson et al. 2012), yet was present in fewer than 50 % of specimens examined in one study (Lopes et al. 2008). The average distance between the AL bundle and the PM bundle centers is approximately 12.1 mm (±1.3). The distal margins of the AL bundle and PM bundle are 1.5 mm (±0.8) and 5.8 mm (±1.7) proximal from the notch articular cartilage, respectively (Anderson et al. 2012).

In contrast to the femoral insertion, the tibial insertion of the PCL is more compact and consistent (Dargel et al. 2006; Edwards et al. 2007; Matava et al. 2009). The two PCL fiber bundles insert onto the tibia without anatomic separation in a centrally located, compact fovea, or facet, on the posterior aspect of the tibia in a depression between the posterior medial and lateral tibial plateaus (Fig. 1b) (Cosgarea and Jay 2001). Recently, Anderson et al. reported that the average distance between the AL and PM bundle centers on the tibia was 8.9 mm (±1.2) (Anderson et al. 2012). The shiny white fibers of the posterior horn of the medial meniscus serve as the anterior border of the tibial PCL footprint, while the bundle ridge consistently defines the posterior margin of the AL bundle and the anterior margin of the PM bundle (Anderson et al. 2012). The center of the two fiber bundles is located ~48 % of the mediolateral width of the tibial plateau from the medial tibial edge (Cosgarea and Jay 2001). Moorman et al. reported that the mean distance from the anterior edge of the PCL tibial insertion to the posterior tibial cortex was 15.6 mm (range, 14–18 mm), while the center of the PCL insertion was, on average, 7 mm anterior to the posterior tibial cortex, with the bulk of the ligament located in the posterior half of the PCL facet (Moorman et al. 2008).

Biomechanics

As previously noted, the PCL provides the primary restraint to posterior tibial translation of the knee (Butler et al. 1980). The mean ultimate load for the AL bundle is 1,120 ± 362 N, which is almost three times more than the mean ultimate load of the PM bundle (419 ± 128 N) (Harner et al. 1995). Similarly, the mean stiffness of the AL component was reported to be 120 ± 37 N/mm, compared with 57 ± 22 N/mm for the PM component. Markolf and colleagues reported near normal knee kinematics when the AL bundle was preserved and the PM bundle was sectioned, and therefore suggested that the AL bundle be the focus of traditional single-bundle reconstruction (Markolf et al. 1997, 2002). Others have reported that the PCL is a nonisometric structure with unequal length and tension throughout knee motion (Jeong et al. 2010), suggesting that neither bundle is dominant in restraining posterior tibial translation throughout the arc of motion.

Natural History

The natural history of isolated PCL injuries is a persistent matter of debate in the literature and has made the subsequent treatment decision-making process difficult. Unlike the ACL, the PCL has an intrinsic ability to heal and often regains continuity following an injury. Several studies have reported that isolated PCL injuries do well with nonoperative treatment (Parolie and Bergfeld 1986; Fowler and Messieh 1987; Torg et al. 1989; Shelbourne et al. 1999a) and chronic PCL injuries are often found during routine preseason sports examinations (Parolie and Bergfeld 1986). Further, several authors have reported no correlation between initial laxity or chronicity of injury and functional status, suggesting that nonoperative treatment may not lead to clinical deterioration over time (Torg et al. 1989; Shelbourne et al. 1999a; Shelbourne and Gray 2002).

More recently, however, clinicians have begun to question the longstanding theory that nonoperative treatment of isolated PCL injuries is the best course of action. Despite its intrinsic ability to heal and potential to regain continuity following a tear, in a PCL-deficient knee, gravity and the forces on the joint from the hamstring muscles can potentially cause the tibia to be positioned in a posteriorly subluxed location relative to the femur (Fowler and Messieh 1987; Shelbourne et al. 1999a, b; Shelbourne and Gray 2002; Shelbourne and Muthukaruppan 2005; Jacobi et al. 2010). This may result in the development of medial compartment and patellofemoral arthritis with chronic PCL deficiency, as well as an increased risk of meniscal tears (Dandy and Pusey 1982; Geissler and Whipple 1993). In a study evaluating the outcome of nonoperative treatment of PCL injury, Keller et al. reported that 65 % of their patients had activity limitations, 90 % reported knee pain during activity, 43 % had problems while walking, and 45 % had persistent knee swelling (Keller et al. 1993). Inouie et al. attempted to identify prognostic factors that can predict outcome and assist in treatment decisions (Inoue et al. 1997). In their study, they reported that gastrocnemius strength and medial and patellofemoral degenerative changes were predictive of functional outcome, while PCL laxity, chronicity of injury, and quadriceps strength were not predictive of outcome (Inoue et al. 1997). Taken together, PCL injuries may not be as benign as originally anticipated, and several factors, many of which remain unidentified at the present time, may influence clinical outcomes following operative or nonoperative treatment.

Treatment

Indications and Contraindications

The approach to treatment of PCL injuries should relate to several patient-specific factors, including the severity of the knee injury (isolated vs. combined), grade of PCL injury (Table 1), timing (acute vs. chronic), clinical presentation (asymptomatic vs. pain/instability), and patient demands or activity level (athletic vs. sedentary). Because of the controversy surrounding the natural history of PCL deficiency and the difficulties in accurately reconstructing the complex function of the PCL operatively, there is no clear consensus regarding the indications for PCL reconstruction. Most authors agree that avulsion fractures of the PCL should be acutely repaired with sutures through drill holes or screw fixation, usually with good results (Espejo-Baena et al. 2000; Kim et al. 2001). In addition, multi-ligamentous injuries involving the PCL should be surgically reconstructed, preferably within 2 weeks of injury to restore knee function (Allen et al. 2004). Outside of these specific scenarios, however, the treatment decision algorithm should be tailored to each patient, taking into account the following factors.

In general, most acute, isolated PCL injuries (grades I and II) are treated nonoperatively. To classify a PCL injury as "isolated," three particular criteria have been reported and may be used in the treatment algorithm (Pierce et al. 2012). These include (1) PCL stress radiographs with <8 mm difference compared to the contralateral knee; (2) <5° of abnormal rotatory laxity at 30° of knee flexion; and (3) no significant collateral injury causing varus/valgus instability. If a PCL injury meets these criteria, it may be considered "isolated," and if given a grade of I or II on physical examination, the patient should undergo a trial of nonoperative treatment. The majority of these patients are able to return to sports within 2–4 weeks after injury.

In contrast, the outcome of isolated, acute grade III PCL injuries is not as predictable and treatment is controversial. Due to the risk of an occult injury to the PLC, it is recommended that the knee either be immobilized in extension for 2–4 weeks or treated in a dynamic PCL brace for 3 months. Healing of the PCL in an elongated (i.e., flexed) position can lead to chronic instability and disability (Shelbourne et al. 1999b), and the use of a cylindrical cast, which applies an anterior drawer force, has demonstrated that placing the PCL in a properly reduced position with less posterior sag allows for improved healing (Jung et al. 2008). Further, immobilization in extension decreases the tension on the anterolateral fibers of the PCL and the PLC, facilitating healing and minimizing posterior tibial translation secondary to hamstring tension and gravity (Harner and Hoher 1998). Following the initial period of immobilization, rehabilitation begins, but not all patients with grade III injuries recover and a large percent have been reported to eventually require PCL reconstruction (Shelbourne and Muthukaruppan 2005; Jung et al. 2008; Pierce et al. 2012). Similarly, acute combined PCL tears (i.e., PCL/PLC) often lead to subjective and objective functional limitations and early arthritis (Shelbourne et al. 1999a; Shelbourne and Gray 2002). Therefore, surgical reconstruction is recommended in these cases.

Table 1 Grading of PCL injury

Grade	Clinical finding	PCL stress radiographs
I	0–5 mm posterior translation	0–7 mm posterior translation
II	5–10 mm posterior translation; flush with MFC	8–11 mm posterior translation
III	>10 mm posterior translation[a]; MTP posterior to MFC; obvious posterior sag	≥12 mm posterior translation $\vec{a}$ suggests combined injury

MFC medial femoral condyle, *MTP* medial tibial plateau
[a]Suggests complete PCL tear

In the setting of a chronic PCL tear, the authors again elect to treat grade I and II injuries nonoperatively, similar to an acute injury of similar severity. Symptomatic patients with recurrent swelling and pain are treated with activity modification and therapy, because at this point in time, surgical reconstruction of acute and chronic grade I or II injuries has not resulted in significant improvement in symptoms or function (Harner and Hoher 1998). Importantly, however, concerns in chronic grade III PCL and combined PCL and PLC injuries include the potential for long-term sequelae of functional limitations and the possible development of early medial and patellofemoral osteoarthritis (Strobel et al. 2003; Van de Velde et al. 2009). Patients often report persistent pain, instability, and loss of function at the time of long-term follow-up with nonoperative treatment of these injuries, and poorer outcomes have also been reported in patients who have increased time between the initial injury and surgical treatment (Jung et al. 2008). Therefore, in cases of chronic grade III PCL injuries with persistent symptoms of pain or instability despite therapy, surgical treatment is recommended.

Surgical Treatment

The primary goal of PCL reconstruction is to restore normal anatomy and reestablish proper laxity. Currently, however, there is no "gold standard" for PCL repair or reconstruction that provides consistently good to excellent results. Although many surgical techniques have been described, the clinical results of PCL reconstruction have not been as reliable as those for reconstruction of the ACL. Controversy exists regarding the optimal location of tibial fixation, number of graft bundles, ideal placement of the femoral tunnel or tunnels, and appropriate graft tension during reconstruction. The current basic science literature is difficult to interpret because most studies differ in several of these variables, making comparisons challenging. Compounding the situation is the fact that only few clinical trials compare one reconstructive method with another and with conflicting results.

Primary Repair

In cases of an acute, displaced PCL bony avulsion, surgical intervention is indicated (Veltri and Warren 1993). Avulsion fractures usually involve the tibial insertion and are typically diagnosed using routine lateral radiographs. If the bone fragment is large, fixation is accomplished with one or two AO screws, with or without washers. Figure 2a, b demonstrates AP and lateral radiographs, respectively, following primary repair of an acute PCL bony avulsion injury using two screws. For smaller fragments, fixation can be achieved using Kirschner wires, tension band wiring, or suture repair through drill holes. The repair should be done in the acute period (less than 3 weeks after injury). In contrast to bony avulsion injuries, results of suture repair of acute or chronic midsubstance tears have generally been unsatisfactory, and reconstruction is typically recommended in this situation (Bianchi 1983). Postoperatively, the knee should be braced in extension, and weight bearing is initially protected. The nature of rehabilitation is based on the quality of fixation. In all cases, once bone healing has occurred (usually 6–8 weeks after surgery), rehabilitation can proceed more aggressively.

PCL Reconstruction

Several different methods of PCL reconstruction have been described. Because of the complexity of tensioning patterns in the two bundles of the PCL, it has been difficult to reproduce the precise function and position of the native ligamentous complex. Current reconstructive techniques include the endoscopic transtibial single-bundle, double-bundle, and tibial inlay techniques.

Graft Selection

Graft types can be divided into autografts, allografts, and synthetic grafts. Autograft sources that are commonly used for PCL reconstruction include the patellar, hamstring, and quadriceps tendons (Allen et al. 2004). Table 2 provides a review of the most commonly used graft sources for PCL reconstruction, with inherent advantages and disadvantages of each. Allografts are an excellent alternative in PCL reconstruction,

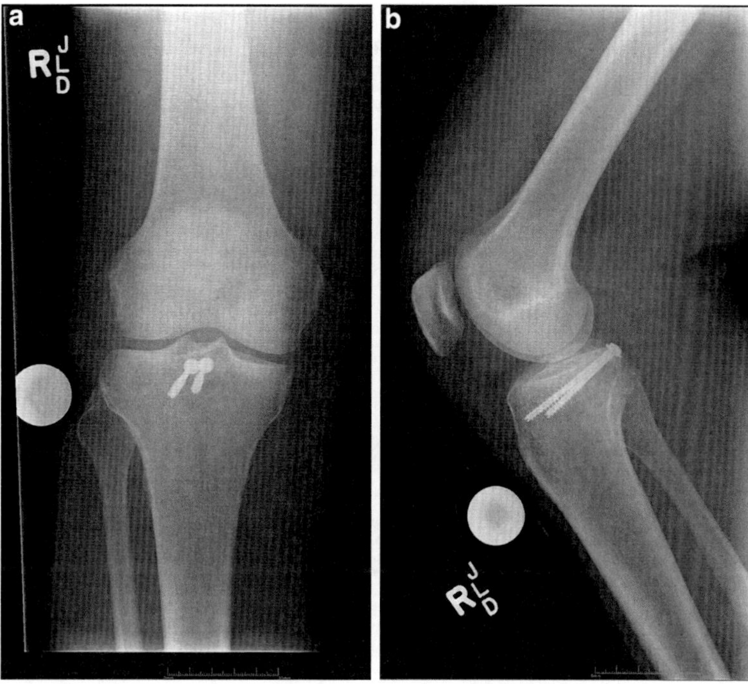

Fig. 2 AP (**a**) and lateral (**b**) postoperative radiographs demonstrating primary repair of a PCL avulsion fracture fixed acutely using screw fixation

Table 2 Graft selection in PCL reconstruction

Graft	Types	Advantages	Disadvantages
Autograft	Patellar tendon	Rigid bony fixation Excellent strength	Donor site morbidity Anterior knee pain Risk patella fracture
	Hamstring tendon	Decreased donor site morbidity Excellent strength	Inferior initial fixation compared to bone
	Quadriceps tendon	Large graft size Generous length Decreased risk graft-tunnel and size mismatch Initial bony tibial fixation	Donor site morbidity Anterior knee pain Risk patella fracture
Allograft	Achilles tendon	Large cross-sectional area Calcaneal bone plug allows rigid initial bony fixation No donor site morbidity	Risk of disease transmission Potential delay in remodeling/ revascularization Cost
	Patellar/quadriceps	Rigid bony fixation Excellent strength No donor site morbidity	See Achilles allograft above
	Hamstring	No donor site morbidity Comparable strength to others	See Achilles allograft above Inferior initial fixation (soft tissue) compared to bone

especially for knee injuries that involve multiple ligaments, for revision surgery, or for patients with general ligamentous laxity (Allen et al. 2004). However, studies have also reported a significant delay in revascularization, cellular repopulation, and maturation of allograft compared to autograft sources (Jackson et al. 1996). The use of synthetic grafts has demonstrated poor results following reconstruction of the ACL, and their use is not currently recommended for PCL reconstruction (Allen et al. 2004).

Transtibial Technique

The transtibial technique utilizes a tibial tunnel for fixation of the PCL within the tibia. It is the most popular of all the PCL reconstruction techniques, allowing the surgeon to perform either a single-bundle or double-bundle reconstruction. However, tibial fixation during transtibial PCL reconstruction is not without controversy. Historically, the transtibial technique involved passing the graft proximally and posteriorly through the tibia and making a 90° turn around the superior edge of the posterior aperture of the tibial tunnel before entering the knee joint (Matava et al. 2009). This 90° bend, or "killer turn," was originally described in patellar tendon grafts and has been shown to create increased internal tendon pressures and potentially lead to graft elongation and failure (Bergfeld et al. 2001). These effects may be attributable to the so-called sawing phenomenon that is elicited when the graft continually abrades the posterior tibia during knee motion (Bergfeld et al. 2001; Matava et al. 2009). Aperture fixation, where the graft is fixed at the posterior aperture of the tunnel, thereby creating the shortest possible graft, is therefore preferable and has been supported by cadaveric testing (Markolf et al. 2003). Markolf and colleagues reported that 15 % of recessed patellar tendon grafts failed at the killer turn after 2,000 loading cycles, while all specimens with flush bone blocks survived testing (Markolf et al. 2003). These findings corroborate the work of Weimann et al. who reported that a rounded posterior edge of the tibial tunnel resulted in less graft damage, with more grafts surviving 2,000 cycles, compared with grafts exposed to sharp tunnel edges that are typically encountered clinically (Weimann et al. 2007).

Despite the aforementioned biomechanical advantages of aperture fixation in the transtibial technique, it is not without difficulty. For example, it requires an interference screw to be placed all the way up the tunnel, which can be technically challenging (Matava et al. 2009). Such screw placement also makes revision reconstruction more difficult if a metallic screw has to be removed. This problem may be avoided through the use of a bioabsorbable screw; however, to date, there has not been a comparison study of metal versus bioabsorbable screws. Further, caution is warranted when drilling the tibial tunnel because of the risk of injury to the adjacent popliteal neurovascular bundle (Matava et al. 2000). All of these factors may contribute to the variable clinical results reported for the transtibial technique.

With regard to tibial fixation, Margheritini et al. studied the kinematic effects and in situ PCL forces of two different types of tibial fixation of Achilles tendon allografts: distal tibial fixation alone using a screw and washer versus combined distal and proximal tibial interference fixation using a bioabsorbable interference screw (Margheritini et al. 2005). Using a cadaveric model with a posterior tibial load applied at various degrees of knee flexion, they reported that combined fixation results in less graft motion in the tibial tunnel, decreased graft deformation, and increased graft stiffness and may eliminate the so-called "windshield wiper" effect that may result in tunnel widening (Margheritini et al. 2005). For these reasons, these authors use combined fixation on the tibia during transtibial reconstruction.

Perhaps the most controversial issue in PCL reconstruction involves the question of whether to reconstruct one or two bundles of the PCL. Compared to the PM bundle, the AL bundle is stiffer, has a higher ultimate load to tensile failure, and is approximately twice the width of the PM bundle (Markolf et al. 2006). Because the PCL is composed of two main bundles, there has recently been renewed interest in restoring both bundles to provide a more "anatomic reconstruction" resulting in a consistent restraint to posterior tibial translation and rotation throughout knee motion.

Single-Bundle Reconstruction

The single-bundle technique is designed to simulate the stronger and stiffer AL bundle of the PCL. The femoral starting point is positioned within the anatomic insertion site of the AL bundle of the intact PCL on the lateral wall of the medial femoral condyle and the roof of the notch. Several studies have reported that the location of the femoral tunnel has more impact on the ability to restore intact knee kinematics than does the location of the tibial tunnel (Sidles et al. 1988; Burns et al. 1995). In addition, the proximal to distal variation of the femoral tunnel has a greater effect on graft performance than does anterior to posterior variation (Sidles et al. 1988; Ogata and McCarthy 1992). Traditionally, the proper placement of the femoral tunnel when reconstructing the AL bundle was 10 mm posterior to the articular cartilage of the medial femoral condyle and 13 mm inferior to the articular cartilage of the medial intercondylar roof (i.e., 2 o'clock position on a right knee) (Morgan et al. 1997). Recently, however, there have been reports indicating poor reliability of the traditional clock-face method for femoral tunnel placement (Apsingi et al. 2009), and a more consistent approach has been introduced by Anderson and colleagues (Anderson et al. 2012), as discussed below in the section on double-bundle reconstruction.

Double-Bundle Reconstruction

The double-bundle technique was initially described by Wirth and Jager in 1984 (Wirth and Jager 1984). It has been hypothesized that double-bundle PCL reconstructions more closely restore normal knee mechanics throughout the entire flexion-extension cycle (Harner et al. 2000). In general, current double-bundle techniques utilize two femoral tunnels in an attempt to recreate the functional anatomy of the AL and PM bundles of the native PCL, with one tibial tunnel. Two separate grafts or a split graft are passed through the tibial tunnel and then fixed in separate, divergent femoral tunnels. The AL femoral tunnel is placed similar to the single-bundle technique, and the PM tunnel (6–7 mm diameter) is placed within the PCL footprint inferior to and slightly deeper in the intercondylar notch than the AL tunnel (3–4 mm off the articular margin, at approximately the 2:30 o'clock position in the right knee or 9:30 in the left knee) (Harner et al. 2000; Allen et al. 2004). In a quantitative analysis of cruciate ligament insertion sites, Harner and Baek identified the PCL femoral insertion area to be approximately 128 mm^2, which is large enough to accommodate both tunnels (Harner et al. 1999).

Recent evidence, however, suggests that the popular clock-face method to identify the femoral PCL attachment site has poor clinical accuracy and reproducibility (Apsingi et al. 2009). Therefore, Anderson et al. recently dissected 20 fresh-frozen human cadaveric knees to better determine arthroscopic landmarks for placement of both tunnels, in an attempt to provide guidelines for femoral and tibial PCL tunnel placement intraoperatively (Anderson et al. 2012). When using an endoscopic double-bundle technique, the center of the femoral AL bundle tunnel should be triangulated on the basis of the trochlear point, the medial arch point, and the medial bifurcate prominence, while the distal edge should be placed adjacent to the articular cartilage. The femoral PM bundle should be placed equidistant from the posterior point and the medial arch point, just distal to the medial intercondylar ridge, with the center an average of 8.6 mm proximal to the articular cartilage margin. With an average distance between the AL and PM bundle of 12.1 mm, utilization of an 11-mm-diameter AL tunnel and a 7-mm PM tunnel would still allow for a 3-mm bone bridge between the two femoral tunnels. Figure 3a demonstrates the use of electrocautery to identify the PCL attachment sites on the femur. As illustrated in Fig. 3b, the anterolateral bundle (larger footprint) is more proximal than the posteromedial footprint (smaller footprint) on the medial femoral condyle.

On the tibia, the center of the more compact single PCL tunnel should be placed just anterosuperior to the bundle ridge, on the medial side of the PCL facet, 9.8 mm from the lateral cartilage point, and 5.0 mm from the medial groove (Fig. 4) (Anderson et al. 2012). An intraoperative lateral radiograph (Fig. 4a) and arthroscopic image (Fig. 4b) demonstrate the proper position of the tibial tunnel guide pin. This corresponds to the center of the tunnel placed one quarter of the total facet length anterior to the posterior tibial cortex (i.e., 7 mm anterior to the posterior cortex) (Moorman et al. 2008). Placement of the tunnel more posteriorly or inferiorly will fail to reproduce

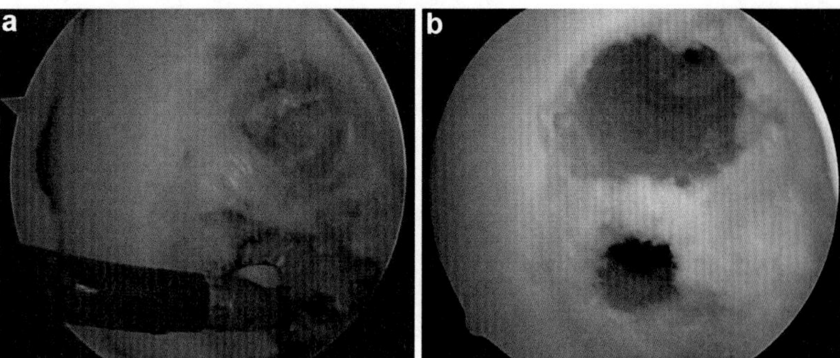

Fig. 3 Anatomic placement of femoral tunnels during endoscopic PCL double-bundle reconstruction. (**a**) Arthroscopic image demonstrating the use of electrocautery to identify the PCL bundle attachment sites on the femur. The anterolateral bundle is more proximal to the posteromedial bundle. (**b**) Arthroscopic image of the anatomic placement of the anterolateral and posteromedial footprints on the medial femoral condyle

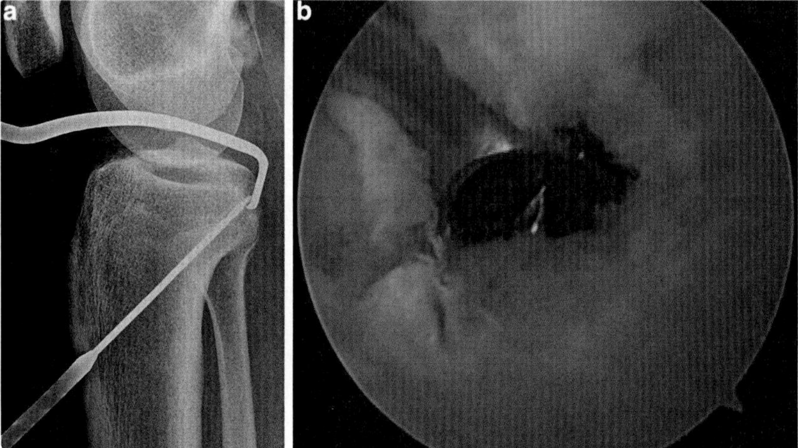

Fig. 4 Anatomic placement of desired tibial tunnel position during endoscopic PCL reconstruction. An intraoperative lateral radiograph (**a**) and arthroscopic image (**b**) demonstrate the proper position for the tibial tunnel guide pin. A large curette protects the soft tissues from posterior over-penetration (**b**)

normal PCL anatomy and risks injury to the popliteal neurovascular bundle, which lies in close proximity to the ligament. In addition, placement of the tunnel more anteriorly could potentially jeopardize the posterior meniscal horns.

To further aid in the movement toward more precise "anatomic reconstruction" of the PCL using the double-bundle technique, Johannsen et al. were the first to quantify radiographic guidelines that may directly assist in PCL reconstruction intraoperatively (Johannsen et al. 2013). Using 20 fresh-frozen cadaver knees labeled with radio-opaque spheres and dye, radiographs were obtained to quantify the femoral and tibial bundle centers and margins using pertinent landmarks. On the AP femur view, the AL and PM bundle centers were 34.1 (±3.0) mm and 29.2 (±3.0) mm lateral to the most medial border of the medial femoral condyle, respectively. The lateral femur images revealed that the AL bundle center was 17.4 (±1.7) mm and PM center was 23.9 (±2.7) mm posteroproximal to a line perpendicular to Blumensaat's line that intersected the anterior margin of the medial femoral condyle cortex. On the tibia, AP images revealed that the AL and PM centers were located 0.2 (±2.1) mm proximal and 4.9 (±2.9) mm distal to the proximal joint line, respectively, while the PCL attachment center was

1.6 (±2.5) mm distal to the proximal joint line. On the lateral view, the ALB center was 8.4 (±1.8) mm, the PCL attachment center was 5.5 (±1.7) mm, and the PMB center was 2.5 (±1.5) mm superior to the champagne glass drop-off of the posterior tibia (Johannsen et al. 2013).

Single-Bundle Versus Double-Bundle Reconstruction

Over the past decade, several studies have been conducted to evaluate the efficacy of single- versus double-bundle reconstructions. To date, however, the literature is inconclusive with regard to superiority of one technique over the other. Harner et al. compared single- and double-bundle PCL reconstructions in a biomechanical study using Achilles and doubled semitendinosus grafts for each respective technique (Harner et al. 2000). The authors reported significant differences in posterior tibial translation following single-bundle reconstruction compared to double-bundle reconstruction and normal knees, and no difference in translation between double-bundle knees and normal knees. The authors concluded that double-bundle reconstruction more closely restores the biomechanics of the intact knee than does single-bundle reconstruction throughout knee range of motion (Harner et al. 2000). In contrast, using a tibial inlay technique, Bergfeld et al. (2005) reported no difference in translation following single- and double-bundle reconstructions at various degrees of flexion, concluding that both single- and double-bundle techniques reproduced posterior laxity of the knee (Bergfeld et al. 2005). Taken together along with other published studies, there are conflicting data and no clear consensus in the literature of one preferred technique over the other (Houe and Jorgensen 2004; Kohen and Sekiya 2009; Kim et al. 2011).

Post-Injury and Postoperative Rehabilitation

Rehabilitation following both nonoperative and operative treatment should focus on progressive weight bearing and emphasize quadriceps strengthening and recovery of proprioception while protecting the healing ligament or graft (Lopez-Vidriero et al. 2010; Pierce et al. 2012). Studies have reported that patients with PCL injuries who regain greater quadriceps strength obtain better functional outcomes (Parolie and Bergfeld 1986). The ultimate goal of rehabilitation protocols should be to reestablish a firm endpoint on the posterior drawer examination with minimal symptomatic, patient-reported instability. Early goals (within 4 weeks of injury/surgery) involve adequate edema/effusion control, limited knee motion exercises, and reactivation of the quadriceps muscle. Any exercise that activates the hamstrings should be avoided in the initial phases of PCL rehabilitation as hamstring contraction can stretch out grafts and cause further injury to the already damaged ligament (Lopez-Vidriero et al. 2010). Further, unlike ACL rehabilitation protocols, initially keeping a patient non-weight bearing immediately following surgery between 2 and 4 weeks is important to prevent strain on the graft, because the PCL is the primary static stabilizer of the knee. Initial phases are followed by a progressive increase in low-impact range of motion and strengthening exercises over time.

Currently, there is a lack of quality studies in the literature investigating the effects of different rehabilitation protocols on PCL treatment outcomes (Watsend et al. 2009; Lopez-Vidriero et al. 2010; Pierce et al. 2012). Pierce et al. were the first to suggest an evidence-based rehabilitation protocol for PCL injuries based on a compilation of previous studies, with stepwise details based on a combination of evidence-based literature and the authors' clinical practice (Pierce et al. 2012). This protocol is summarized in Table 3. Importantly, the authors emphasized several current concepts relating to the use of open kinetic chain (OKC) and closed kinetic chain (CKC) exercises in PCL rehabilitation. While CKC exercises have been the traditional foundation of early rehabilitation protocols, recent evidence demonstrates that OKC rather than CKC exercises may be preferred until the ligament/graft has had adequate time to heal (Mesfar and Shirazi-Adl 2008). OKC exercises are able to isolate single muscle groups for strengthening, which makes them especially important in the early

Table 3 PCL reconstruction rehabilitation protocol

Phase	Precautions	WB status	ROM	Brace	Goals
Phase I	PRICE	NWB (×6 weeks)	Prone passive ROM from 0 to 90° for the first 2 weeks and then progress to full ROM as tolerated	Immobilizer brace (3 days) in extension until patient can transition into PCL-Jack brace	PCL ligament graft protection
0–6 weeks from surgery	Avoid hyperextension and isolated hamstring activation			Jack brace worn at all times (minimum of 24 weeks)	Edema reduction to improve passive ROM and quadriceps activation
	Prevent posterior tibial translation				Address gait mechanics
					Patient education
Phase II	Avoid hyperextension and isolated hamstring activation	Progress to WBAT	Full passive ROM, supine and prone ROM after 6 weeks	Jack brace at all times	PCL ligament protection
6–12 weeks from surgery	Prevent posterior tibial translation				Address gait mechanics during crutch weaning
					Double leg strength through ROM (<70° knee flexion) and single leg static strength exercises
					Reps and set structure to emphasize muscular endurance development
Phase III	Avoid isolated hamstring exercise until week 16	WBAT	Full passive ROM	Jack brace for all activities	Joint protection
13–18 weeks from surgery					Address gait mechanics
					Progressive weight-bearing strength, including progressive hamstring strengthening
					Can progress leg press and knee bends past 70° knee flexion after 16 weeks
Phase IV	None	WBAT	Full active and passive ROM	Jack brace for all activities	Continue to build strength
19–24 weeks from surgery					Single leg endurance to develop power
					Initiate initial sports-specific drills near the end of this phase
					Clinical examination and/or PCL stress radiographs to objectively verify intact PCL
Phase V	None	WBAT	Full active and passive ROM	Wean out of Jack brace	Patient education and return to activity
25–36 weeks from surgery					Sports-specific drills

Adapted and modified from Pierce et al. (2012)
PRICE protect, rest, ice, compress, elevate, *NWB* non-weight bearing, *ROM* range of motion, *WBAT* weight bearing as tolerated

weeks following PCL injury to promote reactivation of the quadriceps muscle (Mesfar and Shirazi-Adl 2008). In contrast, CKC exercises are unable to isolate a single muscle group because they activate antagonistic muscle groups across multiple joints and produce increased shear forces on the healing ligament (Lutz et al. 1993). Therefore, CKC exercises should be initially avoided while OKC exercises are utilized to strengthen the quadriceps during the early stages of rehabilitation (Pierce et al. 2012). Isolated hamstring exercises should be avoided for at least 16 weeks following injury/surgery. Later in the rehabilitation process, squats and leg presses (forms of CKC exercises) are important to increase quadriceps strength, contributing to secondary anteroposterior stability of knee and improving functional outcomes (Pierce et al. 2012).

Return to Sports

Patients are typically allowed to return to sports-related activities once they have painless active range of motion and adequate return of quadriceps strength. Because PCL reconstructions typically yield diminished improvements in objective stability compared with ACL reconstructions, it has been advocated that postoperative rehabilitation should be more conservative and proceed at a slower rate than ACL rehabilitation (Fanelli 2008). Following a standard double-bundle PCL reconstruction, for example, the typical time for return to sports is between 6 and 9 months per the senior author's experience. Nevertheless, a general consensus on return to play fails to exist in the literature for isolated PCL injury.

Role of Bracing

During both nonoperative treatment and postoperative rehabilitation of PCL injuries, it is important to maintain the knee joint in a properly controlled position that allows for healing. If the knee joint is not properly aligned during rehabilitation and healing, posterior dynamic loads from the hamstrings may cause the PCL to heal in an elongated position, resulting in long-term joint instability (Shelbourne et al. 1999a; Jung et al. 2008). A properly controlled joint position, therefore, such as that provided by a brace that applies an anterior force directed to the posterior proximal tibia, may prevent long-term instability and improve outcomes. Theoretical reasons for bracing are numerous and include: (1) protecting the reconstructed PCL and preventing graft elongation postoperatively (rehabilitation), (2) providing external stability to a PCL-deficient knee (functional), and (3) mitigating the development or progression of osteoarthritis in the PCL-deficient knee (prophylactic).

Unfortunately, given that biomechanical studies demonstrate that the PCL is a nonisometric structure with unequal tension throughout knee motion (Covey et al. 1996), it has been difficult to create a knee brace that protects the PCL during the entire arc of knee motion. Most knee braces are "static" in nature, providing the same load throughout the range of knee flexion, and thus fail to provide for the dynamic in vivo load and tension created by the PCL. Only one brace, the PCL-Jack brace (Albrecht, Stephanskirchen, Germany), has been demonstrated to be effective in supporting the tibia with a constant anterior load (Fig. 5) (Jacobi et al. 2010; Spiridonov et al. 2011). This brace, however, is large and bulky, limits the patient from 0° to 90° of knee flexion, and is considered strictly a rehabilitation brace (Jansson et al. 2012). It would not be ideal for a patient seeking long-term use or use during return to athletic activities. Rather, an ideal functional PCL brace would accommodate the larger range of motion necessary for sports participation and be sufficiently low profile enough to allow ease of movement on the athletic field.

A recent study by Jansson et al. reviewed the available literature on the current state of PCL bracing and reported that available PCL braces currently lack evidence validating their biomechanical effectiveness, despite demonstrating beneficial patient outcomes (Jansson et al. 2012). There are few clinical trials or biomechanical studies reporting the effectiveness of PCL bracing to prevent the development of osteoarthritis or post-injury instability. Nevertheless, it is the

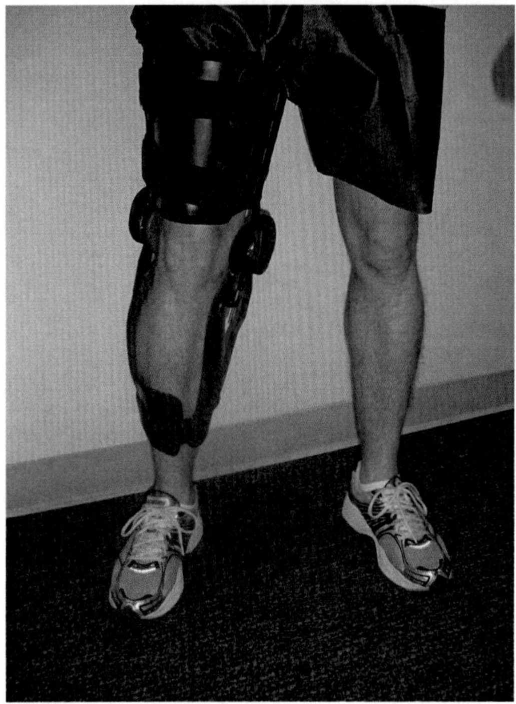

Fig. 5 PCL-Jack brace (Albrecht, Stephanskirchen, Germany)

authors' opinion that nonoperative and postoperative management of PCL injuries should incorporate the use of a brace that supplies a constant anterior tibia force, such as the PCL-Jack brace, for 4–6 months, in order to off-load the forces that would have been applied to the healing PCL.

Further research is warranted to evaluate the efficacy of PCL bracing in preventing long-term instability. There is currently no brace available with biomechanical evidence supporting the capacity to mimic anatomic forces applied by the PCL in the healthy, intact knee. Until this time, the current use of braces in the nonoperative or postoperative setting is likely to remain subject to clinician preference.

Complications

The most serious complication of PCL reconstruction is iatrogenic neurovascular injury. The popliteal artery is especially at risk for injury during tibial tunnel drilling and graft passage. Other early complications following surgery include infection, deep venous thrombosis (DVT), peroneal neuropraxia, and fluid extravasation. Late complications include residual posterior laxity (most common), knee stiffness (loss of flexion greater than extension), medial femoral condyle osteonecrosis, anterior knee pain (following BTB graft), and symptomatic hardware.

Conclusion

PCL injuries are not as benign as once believed. Recent studies examining the biomechanical properties and anatomy of the PCL have led to new surgical techniques in PCL reconstruction that attempt to duplicate the functional behavior of the native PCL throughout the full range of knee motion. Further studies are warranted to more thoroughly evaluate the long-term clinical effectiveness of various surgical techniques, including single-bundle versus double-bundle and tibial inlay PCL reconstruction techniques, in addition to pertinent rehabilitation principles, in an attempt to improve patient outcomes following both operative and nonoperative treatment of PCL injury.

Cross-References

▶ Allografts in Posterior Cruciate Ligament Reconstructions
▶ Combined Anterior and Posterior Cruciate Ligament Injuries
▶ Posterior Cruciate Ligament Reconstruction: New Concepts
▶ Rehabilitation of Complex Knee Injuries and Key Points
▶ Special Considerations for Multiple-Ligament Knee Injuries

References

Allen CR, Rihn J, Harner CD (2004) Posterior cruciate ligament: diagnosis and decision making. In: Miller MD, Cole BJ (eds) Textbook of arthroscopy. Elsevier Health Sciences, Philadelphia

Anderson CJ, Ziegler CG, Wijkicks CA, Engebretsen L et al (2012) Arthroscopically pertinent anatomy of the anterolateral and posteromedial bundles of the posterior cruciate ligament. J Bone Joint Surg Am 94(21):1936–45

Apsingi S, Bull AM, Deehan DJ, Amis AA (2009) Review: femoral tunnel placement for PCL reconstruction in relation to the PCL fibre bundle attachments. Knee Surg Sports Traumatol Arthrosc 17(6):652–659. doi:10.1007/s00167-009-0747-7

Bergfeld JA, McAllister DR, Parker RD, Valdevit AD, Kambic HE (2001) A biomechanical comparison of posterior cruciate ligament reconstruction techniques. Am J Sports Med 29(2):129–136

Bergfeld JA, Graham SM, Parker RD, Valdevit AD, Kambic HE (2005) A biomechanical comparison of posterior cruciate ligament reconstructions using single- and double-bundle tibial inlay techniques. Am J Sports Med 33(7):976–981. doi:10.1177/0363546504273046

Bianchi M (1983) Acute tears of the posterior cruciate ligament: clinical study and results of operative treatment in 27 cases. Am J Sports Med 11(5):308–314

Burns WC 2nd, Draganich LF, Pyevich M, Reider B (1995) The effect of femoral tunnel position and graft tensioning technique on posterior laxity of the posterior cruciate ligament-reconstructed knee. Am J Sports Med 23 (4):424–430

Butler DL, Noyes FR, Grood ES (1980) Ligamentous restraints to anterior-posterior drawer in the human knee. A biomechanical study. J Bone Joint Surg Am 62(2):259–270

Cosgarea AJ, Jay PR (2001) Posterior cruciate ligament injuries: evaluation and management. J Am Acad Orthop Surg 9(5):297–307

Covey DC, Sapega AA, Sherman GM (1996) Testing for isometry during reconstruction of the posterior cruciate ligament. Anatomic and biomechanical considerations. Am J Sports Med 24(6):740–746

Covey DC, Sapega AA, Riffenburgh RH (2008) The effects of sequential sectioning of defined posterior cruciate ligament fiber regions on translational knee motion. Am J Sports Med 36(3):480–486. doi:10.1177/0363546507311097

Dandy DJ, Pusey RJ (1982) The long-term results of unrepaired tears of the posterior cruciate ligament. J Bone Joint Surg Br 64(1):92–94

Dargel J, Pohl P, Tzikaras P, Koebke J (2006) Morphometric side-to-side differences in human cruciate ligament insertions. Surg Radiol Anat SRA 28(4):398–402. doi:10.1007/s00276-006-0107-y

Edwards A, Bull AM, Amis AA (2007) The attachments of the fiber bundles of the posterior cruciate ligament: an anatomic study. Arthrosc J Arthrosc Relat Surg 23 (3):284–290. doi:10.1016/j.arthro.2006.11.005

Espejo-Baena A, Lopez-Arevalo R, Urbano V, Montanez E, Martin F (2000) Arthroscopic repair of the posterior cruciate ligament: two techniques. Arthrosc J Arthrosc Relat Surg 16(6):656–660. doi:10.1053/jars.2000.4626

Fanelli GC (2008) Posterior cruciate ligament rehabilitation: how slow should we go? Arthrosc J Arthrosc Relat Surg 24(2):234–235

Fanelli GC, Edson CJ (1995) Posterior cruciate ligament injuries in trauma patients: part II. Arthrosc J Arthrosc Relat Surg 11(5):526–529

Fanelli GC, Giannotti BF, Edson CJ (1994) The posterior cruciate ligament arthroscopic evaluation and treatment. Arthrosc J Arthrosc Relat Surg 10(6):673–688

Fowler PJ, Messieh SS (1987) Isolated posterior cruciate ligament injuries in athletes. Am J Sports Med 15(6):553–557

Fuss FK (1989) Anatomy of the cruciate ligaments and their function in extension and flexion of the human knee joint. Am J Anat 184(2):165–176. doi:10.1002/aja.1001840208

Geissler WB, Whipple TL (1993) Intraarticular abnormalities in association with posterior cruciate ligament injuries. Am J Sports Med 21(6):846–849

Girgis FG, Marshall JL, Monajem A (1975) The cruciate ligaments of the knee joint. Anatomical, functional and experimental analysis. Clin Orthop Relat Res 106:216–231

Harner CD, Hoher J (1998) Evaluation and treatment of posterior cruciate ligament injuries. Am J Sports Med 26(3):471–482

Harner CD, Xerogeanes JW, Livesay GA, Carlin GJ, Smith BA, Kusayama T, Kashiwaguchi S, Woo SL (1995) The human posterior cruciate ligament complex: an interdisciplinary study. Ligament morphology and biomechanical evaluation. Am J Sports Med 23(6):736–745

Harner CD, Baek GH, Vogrin TM, Carlin GJ, Kashiwaguchi S, Woo SL (1999) Quantitative analysis of human cruciate ligament insertions. Arthrosc J Arthrosc Relat Surg 15(7):741–749

Harner CD, Janaushek MA, Kanamori A, Yagi M, Vogrin TM, Woo SL (2000) Biomechanical analysis of a double-bundle posterior cruciate ligament reconstruction. Am J Sports Med 28(2):144–151

Houe T, Jorgensen U (2004) Arthroscopic posterior cruciate ligament reconstruction: one- vs. two-tunnel technique. Scand J Med Sci Sports 14(2):107–111. doi:10.1111/j.1600-0838.2003.00318.x

Inoue M, Yasuda K, Ohkoshi Y (1997) Factors that affect prognosis of conservatively treated patients with isolated posterior cruciate ligament injury. Paper presented at the 64th annual meeting of the American Academy of Orthopaedic Surgeons, San Francisco

Jackson DW, Corsetti J, Simon TM (1996) Biologic incorporation of allograft anterior cruciate ligament replacements. Clin Orthop Relat Res 324:126–133

Jacobi M, Reischl N, Wahl P, Gautier E, Jakob RP (2010) Acute isolated injury of the posterior cruciate ligament treated by a dynamic anterior drawer brace: a preliminary report. J Bone Joint Surg Br 92(10):1381–1384. doi:10.1302/0301-620X.92B10.24807

Jansson KS, Costello KE, O'Brien L, Wijdicks CA, Laprade RF (2012) A historical perspective of PCL bracing. Knee Surg Sports Traumatol Arthrosc. doi:10.1007/s00167-012-2048-9

Jeong WS, Yoo YS, Kim DY, Shetty NS, Smolinski P, Logishetty K, Ranawat A (2010) An analysis of the posterior cruciate ligament isometric position using an in vivo 3-dimensional computed tomography-based knee joint model. Arthrosc J Arthrosc Relat Surg 26 (10):1333–1339. doi:10.1016/j.arthro.2010.02.016

Johannsen AM, Anderson CJ, Wijdicks CA, Engebretsen L, Laprade RF (2013) Radiographic landmarks for tunnel positioning in PCL reconstructions. J Bone Joint Surg Am 41(1):35–42

Jung YB, Tae SK, Lee YS, Jung HJ, Nam CH, Park SJ (2008) Active non-operative treatment of acute isolated posterior cruciate ligament injury with cylinder cast immobilization. Knee Surg Sports Traumatol Arthrosc 16(8):729–733. doi:10.1007/s00167-008-0531-0

Keller PM, Shelbourne KD, McCarroll JR, Rettig AC (1993) Nonoperatively treated isolated posterior cruciate ligament injuries. Am J Sports Med 21(1):132–136

Kennedy JC, Hawkins RJ, Willis RB, Danylchuck KD (1976) Tension studies of human knee ligaments. Yield point, ultimate failure, and disruption of the cruciate and tibial collateral ligaments. J Bone Joint Surg Am 58(3):350–355

Kim SJ, Shin SJ, Choi NH, Cho SK (2001) Arthroscopically assisted treatment of avulsion fractures of the posterior cruciate ligament from the tibia. J Bone Joint Surg Am 83-A(5):698–708

Kim YM, Lee CA, Matava MJ (2011) Clinical results of arthroscopic single-bundle transtibial posterior cruciate ligament reconstruction: a systematic review. Am J Sports Med 39(2):425–434. doi:10.1177/0363546510374452

Kohen RB, Sekiya JK (2009) Single-bundle versus double-bundle posterior cruciate ligament reconstruction. Arthrosc J Arthrosc Relat Surg 25(12):1470–1477. doi:10.1016/j.arthro.2008.11.006

Lopes OV Jr, Ferretti M, Shen W, Ekdahl M, Smolinski P, Fu FH (2008) Topography of the femoral attachment of the posterior cruciate ligament. J Bone Joint Surg Am 90(2):249–255. doi:10.2106/JBJS.G.00448

Lopez-Vidriero E, Simon DA, Johnson DH (2010) Initial evaluation of posterior cruciate ligament injuries: history, physical examination, imaging studies, surgical and nonsurgical indications. Sports Med Arthrosc Rev 18(4):230–237. doi:10.1097/JSA.0b013e3181fbaf38

Lutz GE, Palmitier RA, An KN, Chao EY (1993) Comparison of tibiofemoral joint forces during open-kinetic-chain and closed-kinetic-chain exercises. J Bone Joint Surg Am 75(5):732–739

Makris CA, Georgoulis AD, Papageorgiou CD, Moebius UG, Soucacos PN (2000) Posterior cruciate ligament architecture: evaluation under microsurgical dissection. Arthrosc J Arthrosc Relat Surg 16(6):627–632. doi:10.1053/jars.2000.9238

Margheritini F, Rihn JA, Mauro CS, Stabile KJ, Woo SL, Harner CD (2005) Biomechanics of initial tibial fixation in posterior cruciate ligament reconstruction. Arthrosc J Arthrosc Relat Surg 21(10):1164–1171. doi:10.1016/j.arthro.2005.06.017

Markolf KL, Slauterbeck JR, Armstrong KL, Shapiro MS, Finerman GA (1997) A biomechanical study of replacement of the posterior cruciate ligament with a graft. Part II: forces in the graft compared with forces in the intact ligament. J Bone Joint Surg Am 79(3):381–386

Markolf KL, Zemanovic JR, McAllister DR (2002) Cyclic loading of posterior cruciate ligament replacements fixed with tibial tunnel and tibial inlay methods. J Bone Joint Surg Am 84-A(4):518–524

Markolf K, Davies M, Zoric B, McAllister D (2003) Effects of bone block position and orientation within the tibial tunnel for posterior cruciate ligament graft reconstructions: a cyclic loading study of bone-patellar tendon-bone allografts. Am J Sports Med 31(5):673–679

Markolf KL, Feeley BT, Tejwani SG, Martin DE, McAllister DR (2006) Changes in knee laxity and ligament force after sectioning the posteromedial bundle of the posterior cruciate ligament. Arthrosc J Arthrosc Relat Surg 22(10):1100–1106. doi:10.1016/j.arthro.2006.05.018

Matava MJ, Sethi NS, Totty WG (2000) Proximity of the posterior cruciate ligament insertion to the popliteal artery as a function of the knee flexion angle: implications for posterior cruciate ligament reconstruction. Arthrosc J Arthrosc Relat Surg 16(8):796–804

Matava MJ, Ellis E, Gruber B (2009) Surgical treatment of posterior cruciate ligament tears: an evolving technique. J Am Acad Orthop Surg 17(7):435–446

McAllister DR, Petrigliano FA (2007) Diagnosis and treatment of posterior cruciate ligament injuries. Curr Sports Med Rep 6(5):293–299

Mejia EA, Noyes FR, Grood ES (2002) Posterior cruciate ligament femoral insertion site characteristics. Importance for reconstructive procedures. Am J Sports Med 30(5):643–651

Mesfar W, Shirazi-Adl A (2008) Knee joint biomechanics in open-kinetic-chain flexion exercises. Clin Biomech (Bristol, Avon) 23(4):477–482. doi:10.1016/j.clinbiomech.2007.11.016

Miyasaka Y, Sakurai M, Yokobori AT Jr, Kuroda S, Ohyama M (1991) Bending and torsion fractures in long bones (a mechanical and radiologic assessment of clinical cases). Biomed Mater Eng 1(1):3–10

Moorman CT 3rd, Murphy Zane MS, Bansai S, Cina SJ, Wickiewicz TL, Warren RF, Kaseta MK (2008) Tibial insertion of the posterior cruciate ligament: a sagittal plane analysis using gross, histologic, and radiographic methods. Arthrosc J Arthrosc Relat Surg 24(3):269–275. doi:10.1016/j.arthro.2007.08.032

Morgan CD, Kalman VR, Grawl DM (1997) The anatomic origin of the posterior cruciate ligament: where is it? Reference landmarks for PCL reconstruction. Arthrosc J Arthrosc Relat Surg 13(3):325–331

Ogata K, McCarthy JA (1992) Measurements of length and tension patterns during reconstruction of the posterior cruciate ligament. Am J Sports Med 20(3):351–355

Parolie JM, Bergfeld JA (1986) Long-term results of nonoperative treatment of isolated posterior cruciate ligament injuries in the athlete. Am J Sports Med 14(1):35–38

Pierce CM, O'Brien L, Griffin LW, Laprade RF (2012) Posterior cruciate ligament tears: functional and post-operative rehabilitation. Knee Surg Sports Traumatol Arthrosc. doi:10.1007/s00167-012-1970-1

Race A, Amis AA (1994) The mechanical properties of the two bundles of the human posterior cruciate ligament. J Biomech 27(1):13–24

Sekiya JK, West RV, Ong BC, Irrgang JJ, Fu FH, Harner CD (2005) Clinical outcomes after isolated arthroscopic single-bundle posterior cruciate ligament reconstruction. Arthrosc J Arthrosc Relat Surg 21(9):1042–1050. doi:10.1016/j.arthro.2005.05.023

Sekiya JK, Whiddon DR, Zehms CT, Miller MD (2008) A clinically relevant assessment of posterior cruciate ligament and posterolateral corner injuries. Evaluation of isolated and combined deficiency. J Bone Joint Surg Am 90(8):1621–1627. doi:10.2106/JBJS.G.01365

Shelbourne KD, Gray T (2002) Natural history of acute posterior cruciate ligament tears. J Knee Surg 15(2):103–107

Shelbourne KD, Muthukaruppan Y (2005) Subjective results of nonoperatively treated, acute, isolated posterior cruciate ligament injuries. Arthrosc J Arthrosc Relat Surg 21(4):457–461. doi:10.1016/j.arthro.2004.11.013

Shelbourne KD, Davis TJ, Patel DV (1999a) The natural history of acute, isolated, nonoperatively treated posterior cruciate ligament injuries. A prospective study. Am J Sports Med 27(3):276–283

Shelbourne KD, Jennings RW, Vahey TN (1999b) Magnetic resonance imaging of posterior cruciate ligament injuries: assessment of healing. Am J Knee Surg 12(4):209–213

Sidles JA, Larson RV, Garbini JL, Downey DJ, Matsen FA 3rd (1988) Ligament length relationships in the moving knee. J Orthop Res 6(4):593–610. doi:10.1002/jor.1100060418

Spiridonov SI, Slinkard NJ, LaPrade RF (2011) Isolated and combined grade-III posterior cruciate ligament tears treated with double-bundle reconstruction with use of endoscopically placed femoral tunnels and grafts: operative technique and clinical outcomes. J Bone Joint Surg Am 93(19):1773–1780. doi:10.2106/JBJS.J.01638

Strobel MJ, Weiler A, Schulz MS, Russe K, Eichhorn HJ (2003) Arthroscopic evaluation of articular cartilage lesions in posterior-cruciate-ligament-deficient knees. Arthrosc J Arthrosc Relat Surg 19(3):262–268. doi:10.1053/jars.2003.50037

Torg JS, Barton TM, Pavlov H, Stine R (1989) Natural history of the posterior cruciate ligament-deficient knee. Clin Orthop Relat Res 246:208–216

Van de Velde SK, Bingham JT, Gill TJ, Li G (2009) Analysis of tibiofemoral cartilage deformation in the posterior cruciate ligament-deficient knee. J Bone Joint Surg Am 91(1):167–175. doi:10.2106/JBJS.H.00177

Veltri DM, Warren RF (1993) Isolated and combined posterior cruciate ligament injuries. J Am Acad Orthop Surg 1(2):67–75

Watsend AM, Osestad TM, Jakobsen RB, Engebretsen L (2009) Clinical studies on posterior cruciate ligament tears have weak design. Knee Surg Sports Traumatol Arthrosc 17(2):140–149. doi:10.1007/s00167-008-0632-9

Weimann A, Wolfert A, Zantop T, Eggers AK, Raschke M, Petersen W (2007) Reducing the "killer turn" in posterior cruciate ligament reconstruction by fixation level and smoothing the tibial aperture. Arthrosc J Arthrosc Relat Surg 23(10):1104–1111. doi:10.1016/j.arthro.2007.04.014

Wirth CJ, Jager M (1984) Dynamic double tendon replacement of the posterior cruciate ligament. Am J Sports Med 12(1):39–43

83 Degenerative Meniscal Tears: Meniscal Cysts

Philippe Beaufils and Nicola Pujol

Contents

P. Beaufils (✉) • N. Pujol
Orthopaedic Department, Versailles Hospital, Le Chesnay, France
e-mail: pbeaufils@ch-versailles.fr; npujol@ch-versailles.fr

M.N. Doral, J. Karlsson (eds.), *Sports Injuries*,
DOI 10.1007/978-3-642-36569-0_69

Abstract

There is not just one but many different types of meniscal tears. Two completely different conditions have to be considered: traumatic lesions and degenerative meniscal lesions. Degenerative meniscal lesions correspond to an aging process and the main question is the relationship between degenerative meniscal lesions and osteoarthritis (OA). Is degenerative meniscal lesions always the early stage of OA or are they true primary DML without OA? The answer is unclear. Practically speaking, when an orthopaedic surgeon is faced with a degenerative meniscal lesion that is assumed to be responsible for the patient's symptoms, one fundamental requirement is to search early signs of macroscopic OA.

The most important guideline in the decision-making process is the principle of meniscal sparing. If there is no OA, leaving the meniscus alone should be the first choice (many DML's are asymptomatic in the general population). If symptoms remain with time, meniscectomy, as partial as possible, could be considered. In the specific group of young athletes presenting a degenerative meniscal lesion (overuse syndrome), meniscus repair must always be considered.

In the case of advanced OA, meniscectomy or arthroscopic debridement may not benefit the patient, and initial treatment should be conservative treatment.

There is not just one but many different types of meniscal tears and consequently not just one, but several potential treatment methods, adapted to the type of lesion and its clinical context. This has led to the concept of meniscal preservation or meniscal sparing, which is based on three pillars: meniscectomy as partial as possible, thanks to arthroscopy, meniscal repair, and benign neglect. In clinical practice, one can be faced with two distinct situations, a traumatic meniscal lesion in a stable or unstable knee or a degenerative meniscal lesion (DML), which is or not associated with macroscopic arthritic changes.

For each of these situations, a specific treatment algorithm is required.

In the degenerate group, leaving the meniscus tear alone should probably be the first choice; meniscectomy could be considered in case of functional treatment failure. Indications for meniscus repair are very selective and non-frequent.

Definition

The definition of a degenerative meniscal lesion (DML) is the conjunction of two criteria:

- Occurrence in the absence of an injury or as a result of decompensation after minor trauma.
- Macroscopic and microscopic alterations which correspond to myxoid degeneration. The meniscal tissue appears yellow. Microscopically, there is an acellular eosinophilic hyaline degeneration, a myxoid degeneration. Myxoid degeneration can be found within the meniscal substance but can also affect the perimeniscal zone which can lead to the formation of perimeniscal cysts (Ferrer-Rocca and Vilalta 1978; Boyer et al. 2010).

Classification

Arthroscopic classification was first proposed in 1983 by Dorfmann and Boyer (Dorfmann et al. 1987; Boyer et al. 2010) (Fig. 1, Table 1).

The classification of Crues et al. (1987) serves as a reference standard for MRI:

- Grade 1 is a high-intensity intrameniscal signal which is round and occupies a variable volume of the meniscus.

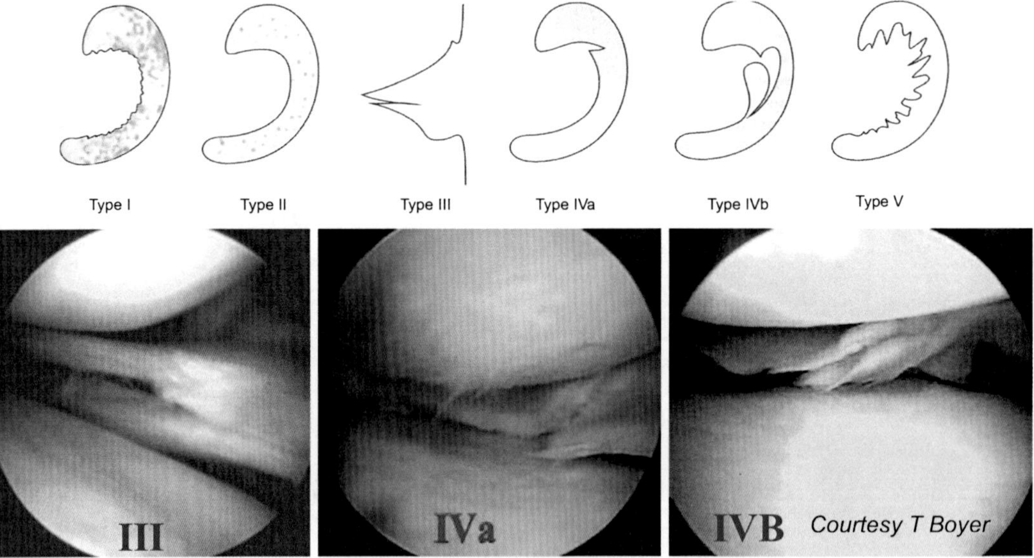

Fig. 1 Arthroscopic classification of degenerative meniscal lesions according to Dorfmann and Boyer (Dorfmann et al. 1987)

- Grade 2 is a high-intensity intrameniscal signal which is linear. It does not involve the surface (Fig. 2a).
- Grade 3 is high-intensity signal extending to the surface of the meniscus. It indicates a true meniscal tear (Fig. 2b).

Pathogenesis

It can be assumed that the aging process of the affected meniscal tissue and its deterioration has advanced to a certain degree. This idea was first introduced by Smillie (Smillie 1978) and Noble (Noble and Erat 1980). Noble, in an analysis of 115 cadaveric or post amputation knee specimens (more than half of which were obtained from subjects aged 65 years or older), documented a lesion of the medial meniscus in 38 %. Their conclusions were subsequently confirmed by arthroscopic and MRI evidence.

Table 1 Classification of degenerative meniscal lesion (Boyer et al. 2010)

Type
Type I: alteration of the meniscus without interruption of its continuity: It is flat and yellow, and its inner edge is frayed
Type II: presence of calcium deposits (meniscocalcinosis)
Type III: horizontal cleavage
Type IV: radial tear (IVa) or a flap (IVb)
Type V: complex lesion

The prevalence of intrameniscal high signal intensity on MRI of asymptomatic subject is high and much more frequent than traumatic lesions. Moreover it increases with age. It is estimated to occur in 5 % of subjects under the age of 30 years, rising progressively to 13–15 % between 30 and 45 years, 25–63 % of subjects above 50 years, and 65 % of subjects above 65 years (Englund et al. 2008; Boyer et al. 2010). Englund et al. (2008) (Fig. 3) observed that MRI meniscus hypersignal intensities were more frequent in the male population than in the female population. Most of these degenerative meniscal tears are actually not causing any symptoms, and they are an incidental finding on MRI.

The relationship between degenerative meniscal lesion and osteoarthritis of the knee is uncertain. Currently, the question whether DML always leads to the development of osteoarthritis or whether the concept of a "primary" lesion is correct remains unanswered.

What is known?

What is the effect of knee OA on the meniscus? It is known that meniscal tears and loss of meniscal function are a strong risk factor for the development of OA (Englund et al. 2009). Englund demonstrated a three times higher risk of OA, in case of minor meniscal lesion, and even

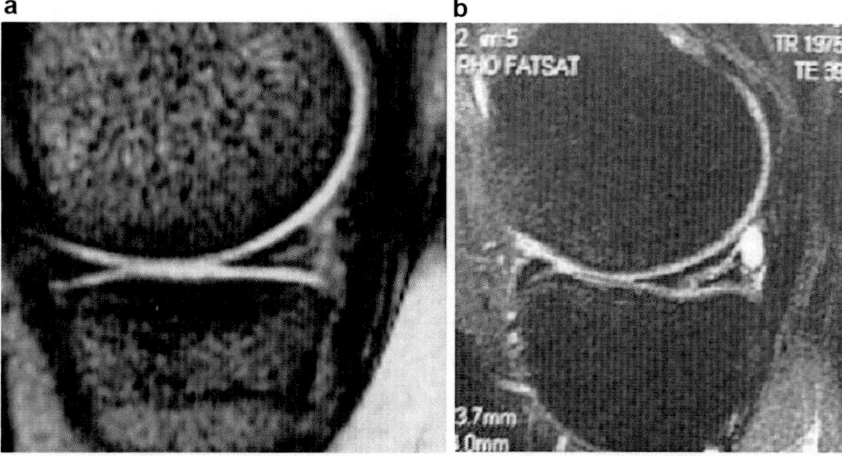

Fig. 2 (**a**) Grade 2 intrameniscal hypersignal. (**b**) Grade 3 hypersignal of the posterior horn (medial meniscus) associated with a parameniscal cyst

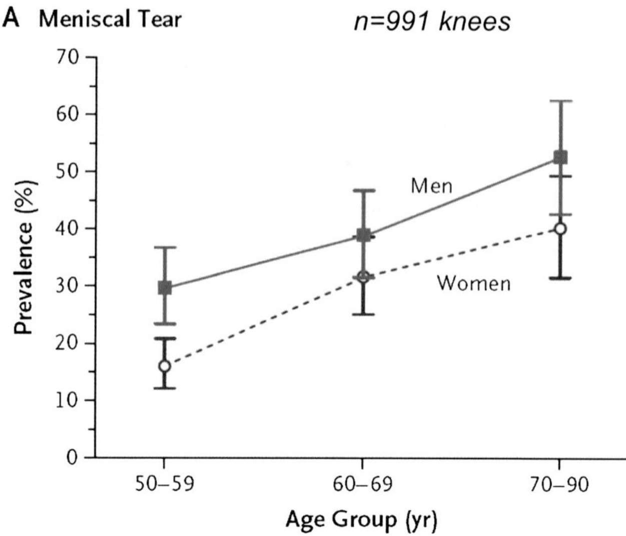

Fig. 3 Prevalence of meniscal lesions according to age and gender (Englund et al. 2008)

seven times, in case of major meniscal tears at 30 months of follow-up compared with normal knees. But it is also known that having the OA puts at increased risk of developing degenerative meniscal tears and meniscal lesions and extrusions. In other words, it is a complex relationship.

What is the relationship between symptoms and MRI abnormalities? Meniscal damage often seems to not be directly causing symptoms, while other features, as a consequence of loss of meniscal function, may do so (Englund et al. 2007).

The questions are:

Is there any continuum between degenerative meniscal lesion and OA? In other words is DML always an early stage of OA?

Are there some "primary" DML without any cartilaginous damage?

These questions have of course major consequences in terms of treatment strategy.

In favor of a strong relationship between DML and osteoarthritis, the prevalence of MRI meniscal abnormalities increases with age, and meniscal tears are systematically associated with osteoarthritic knees (Bhattacharyya et al. 2003; Englund et al. 2007, 2009; Pujol and Boisrenoult 2010a; Zanetti et al. 2003).

In favor of a "primary" lesion, DML are more frequent in men than women (2–1) (Englund et al. 2008), which is exactly the opposite of osteoarthritis. DML may develop earlier, even in young athletes without any chondral degenerative process. Biedert et al. (Biedert 2000; Pujol et al. 2013) recognized a specific group of symptomatic horizontal meniscal cleavage (grade 2 or 3 with or without extra meniscal cyst) which appears in young athletes and can be considered as an overuse syndrome (Fig. 4).

Diagnosis

The key point for a clinician treating a patient presenting with knee pain is therefore to know whether the patient suffers from a DML in a joint with macroscopically intact chondral surfaces or from early-stage osteoarthritis with a coexistent DML.

Surgeons have to ask two questions:

- Is the meniscal lesion responsible for symptoms? It is the concept of painful unstable meniscal lesion.
- Are there signs of osteoarthritis?

In the first case, meniscectomy would be assumed to be a "curative" procedure, while in the second one, it would be purely palliative (the so-called arthroscopic debridement). Because in

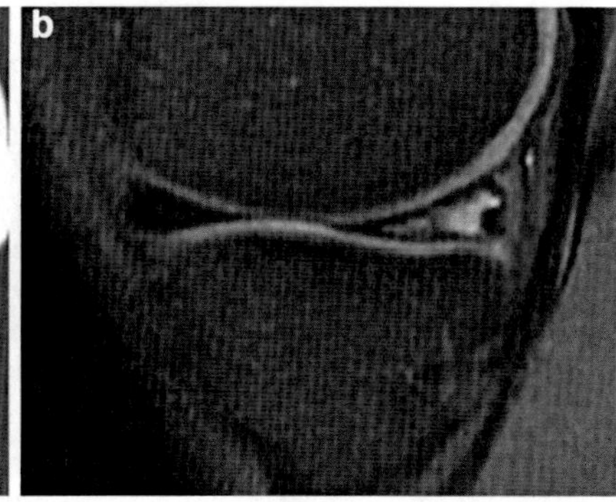

Fig. 4 Seventeen-year-old tennis man with medial complaint. (**a**) Normal arthroCT scan, (**b**) MRI showing a huge intrameniscal hypersignal of the posterior horn

everyday practice, it is impossible to obtain direct information on the microscopic structure of cartilage, its condition is assessed by means of standard radiography and MRI.

The "Painful Unstable Meniscal Tear"

It is well known that meniscal tear itself doesn't cause pain. Pain is due to inflammatory response in the periphery of the meniscus. On the other hand, pain can be due to other causes (i.e., anterior knee pain), and the association of two frequent conditions (knee pain and meniscal hypersignal on MRI) doesn't mean there is a relationship between these two conditions. There is a great difficulty for the clinician: It's quite common to have the patient sent to a MRI scan and they get the report back with the diagnosis of a meniscal tear. Just because the patient has knee pain and a meniscal tear, it's quite easy to draw the conclusion that this tear must be operated upon.

The diagnosis "Painful unstable meniscal lesion" can be established if some of the following criteria are present:

- Sudden onset without significant trauma; for example, during or after sports activities or heavy daily activities (such as squatting, gardening)
- Tenderness on the posterior aspect of the medial or lateral joint line during flexion and corresponding to the spontaneous pain
- Spontaneous clicking knee or during meniscal maneuvers
- MRI demonstrating not only a meniscal hyper signal but signs of a flap (Fig. 5)

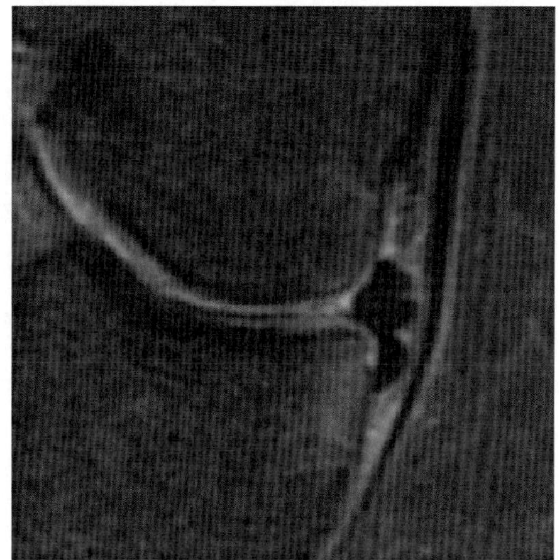

Fig. 5 Displaced flap in the tibial gutter responsible for pain and clicking knee. Note the tibial subchondral bone edema due to the impingement. Typical pattern of "painful unstable meniscus" indicating a meniscectomy

Sign of Osteoarthritis

Clinically speaking, OA can be suspected if there is progressive onset, absence of clicking knee, pain in both knees, or pain at the anterior aspect

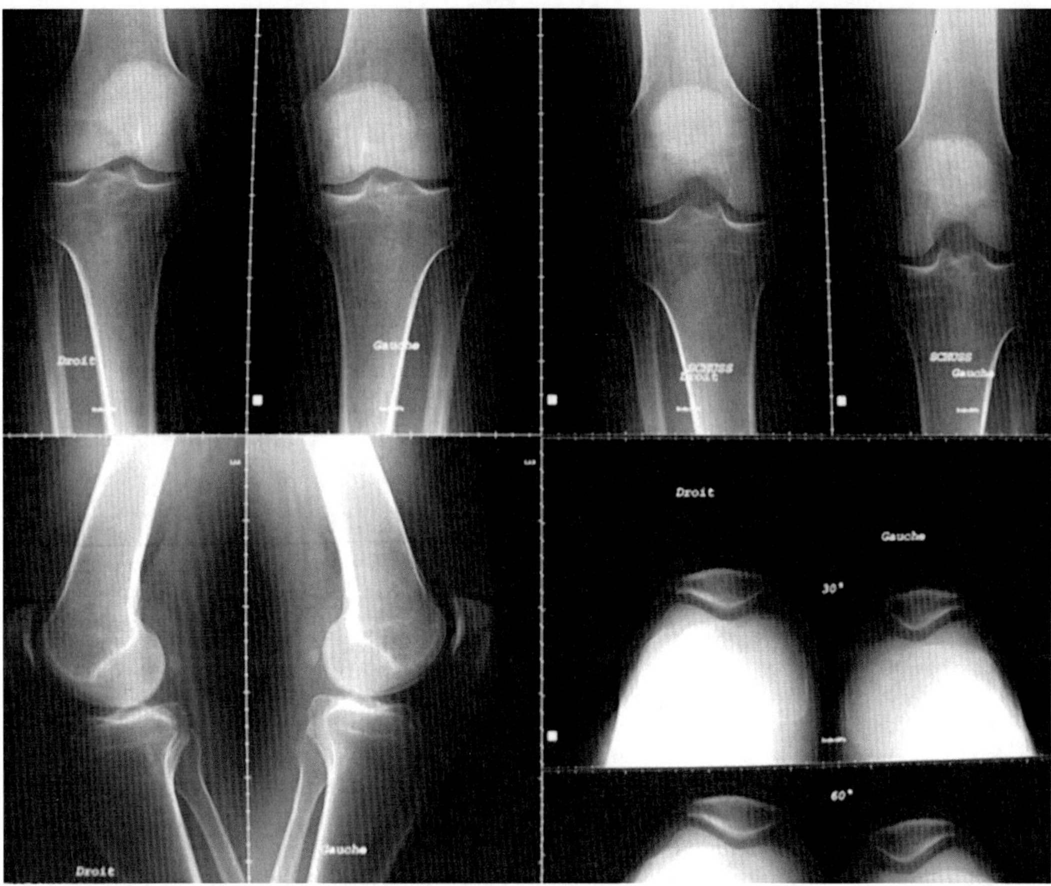

Fig. 6 Standard X-ray protocol: both knees. AP full weight bearing view in extension, schuss view, lateral view, Merchant view

Table 2 Pre- and immediately post meniscectomy joint space measurements according to Prové et al. (2004) coefficient "R" for each appaired serial of measures between both examiners

		Meniscectomized knee	Contralateral knee
Extension	Pre-op	5.8 (±1)	5.8 (±1)
	Post-op	5.6 (±1)	5.8 (±1)
Schuss	Pre-op	5.2 (±1)	5.1 (±1)
	Post-op	5.2 (±1)	5.2 (±1)

of the joint line. But the diagnosis is often provided by imaging techniques.

Radiographs are systematically carried out according to a standardized protocol: comparative X-rays (both knees) including full weight bearing AP view in extension, the so-called schuss view (standing flexed AP view), lateral view, and Merchant view (Fig. 6). The schuss view is very important: it has a good reproducibility. Narrowing of the cartilage space of 2 mm or more is strongly correlated with grade 3 or 4 cartilage degeneration. Meniscectomy itself doesn't modify the joint line width, meaning that joint narrowing is not due to the meniscus itself but is always related to OA (Prove et al. 2004) (Table 2).

MRI shows the meniscus and allows one to characterize the meniscal tear, especially the presence of a flap (Fig. 5). But the cartilage,

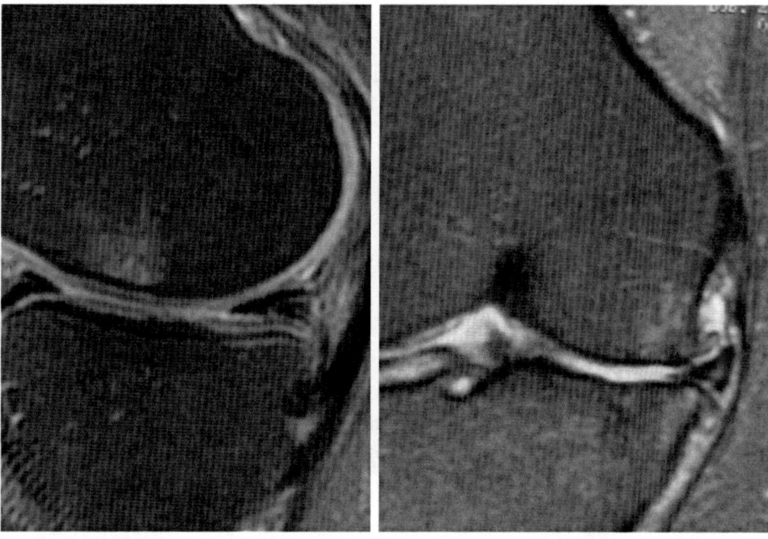

Fig. 7 MRI: early signs of macroscopic osteoarthritis. (**a**) Bone marrow edema in the weight bearing area of the medial condyle, (**b**) medial meniscus extrusion (more than 3 mm)

subchondral bone, and meniscal extrusion must be also assessed in order to detect early signs of osteoarthritis, while standard radiographs may not demonstrate any joint space narrowing.

These early signs consist of meniscal extrusion (Costa et al. 2004) and subchondral abnormalities (Fig. 7). An extrusion more than 3 mm is reported to be strongly related with osteoarthritis and should not be regarded as a meniscal lesion itself, except in particular cases such as root tears (Ahn et al. 2010). The cause of extrusion in the presence of osteoarthritis is not well known. Costa et al. (Costa et al. 2004) found a strong relationship between meniscal extrusion and radial tears, particularly those located within the posterior insertion (root tears) of the meniscus (Ahn et al. 2010).

Whatever the cause, meniscal extrusion is related to a loss of meniscal function and can be interpreted as a functional subtotal meniscectomy. Benefits of arthroscopic meniscectomy of an extruded meniscus is therefore very uncertain (Pujol and Boisrenoult 2010b).

Significance of subchondral hypersignal (bone marrow edema) is not univocal: In the weight bearing area, it could be regarded as an early sign of osteoarthritis, especially if it lies on both sides (femur and tibia: kissing sign). It also can be caused by vascular changes (early stage of osteonecrosis) or subchondral microfractures (Fig. 8), which in these circumstances may be first treated by conservative treatment. The significance of marginal bone marrow edema is more controversial: whether it is due to extrusion (early osteoarthritis) or to impingement with a meniscal displaced flap (Fig. 5).

Meniscal Cyst

Intrameniscal cysts occur in 4–6 % of knees studied with MR imaging (Helms 2002). Meniscal cysts should be considered as a degenerative process. Under pressure, the fluid in the intrameniscal cyst can be squeezed into the adjacent soft tissues, forming a parameniscal cyst. Parameniscal cysts are relatively uncommon (0.27–5 % of meniscal tears) (Hulet et al. 2010). The ratio of lateral to medial meniscal cysts has been reported to be 5–1.

Presenting complaints are usually pain and palpable cyst formation. On the lateral side, the cyst is usually large and disappears in flexion (Pisani's sign). Medial meniscal cysts are usually deeper, more posterior, and smaller, rendering the clinical diagnosis more difficult.

Radiographs are systematically carried out, especially to assess the joint line. One can sometimes find a specific sign of parameniscal cyst, as an erosion of the tibial plateau (Fig. 9a).

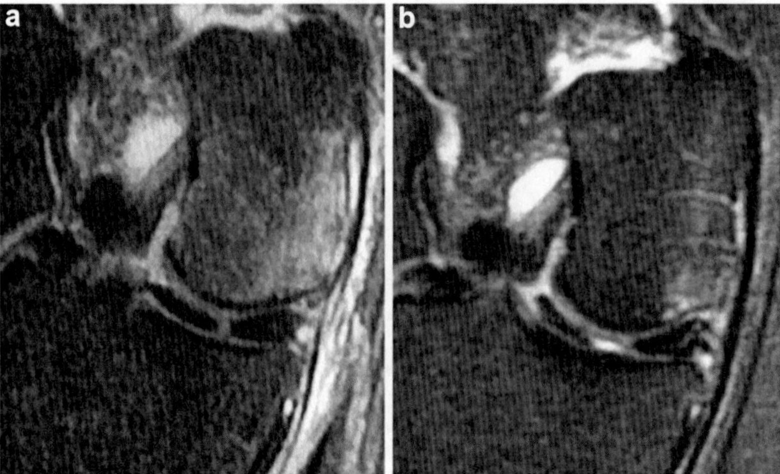

Fig. 8 Sixty-one-year-old patient with medial knee pain. (**a**) MRI shows a meniscal tear of the posterior segment associated with a femoral condylar bone marrow edema. Conservative treatment. (**b**) At 3 months, the patient is asymptomatic with a significant decrease of the condylar hypersignal. Meniscal tear is still there demonstrating that it is not responsible for pain

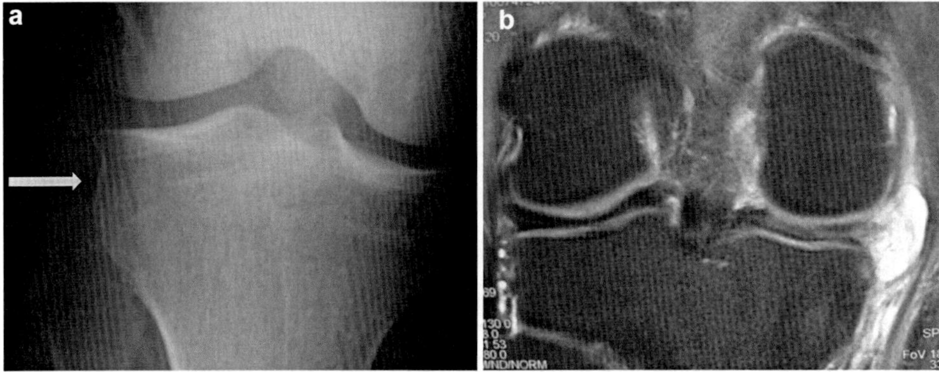

Fig. 9 Meniscal cyst. (**a**) AP standard X-ray demonstrating an erosion of the lateral tibial margin. (**b**) MRI: typical medial meniscal cyst of the mid part

MRI is critical to precisely define the cyst location, the presence of a meniscal tear, and the connection between cyst and meniscus (Fig. 9b). It is important to distinguish between a meniscal cyst associated with a grade 2 intrasubstance meniscal lesion and one with a complete grade 3 tear.

Treatment

It is possible to establish an algorithm for the management of knee pain in these cases (Beaufils et al. 2009; Beaufils 2010) (Fig. 10). Usually, the patient presents with an MRI which shows a meniscal tear. The surgeon must evaluate the patients for signs of early osteoarthritis.

Two different situations must be distinguished:

- There is no macroscopic osteoarthritis on standard radiographs and no early signs of OA on MRI.
- There is evidence of OA

No Evidence of OA

The patient has no joint line pain, the MRI shows a grade 3 meniscal lesion with or without a meniscal cyst, and the subchondral bone signal is unaltered. Treatment in these patients should consist either of benign neglect or arthroscopic meniscectomy because surgical repair is seldom indicated.

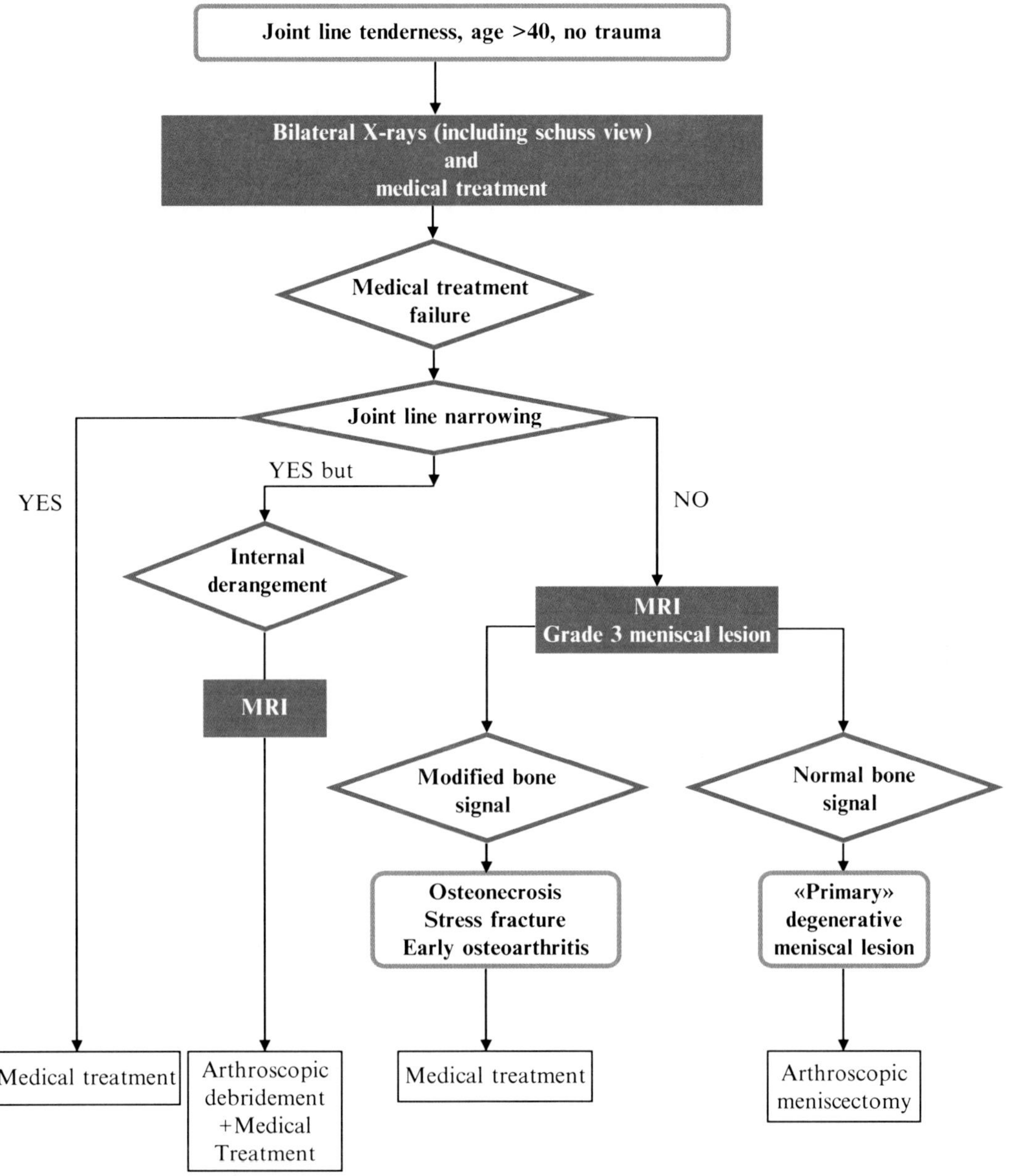

Fig. 10 Algorithm for the management of knee pain in middle-aged patients according to the Haute Autorité de Santé guidelines (Beaufils et al. 2009)

The primary choice is conservative and consists of rest, nonsteroidal anti-inflammatory drugs, and physiotherapy (Weiss et al. 1989; Hede et al. 1990; Baufils et al. 2009; Herrlin et al. 2007; Pujol and Boisrenoult 2010b). Herrlin et al. (2007) compared arthroscopic and conservative treatment in a randomized trial and found that 6 months after treatment, arthroscopic partial medial meniscectomy followed by supervised exercise did not result in less pain and higher knee function compared with supervised exercise alone. A substantial number of degenerative meniscal lesions respond well to conservative treatment, and the symptoms resolve spontaneously even if the lesions do not heal. If improvement fails to occur within a few months (around 6 months), arthroscopic meniscectomy is suggested, especially if the symptoms are made not only of pain but also of clicking or locking suggesting an unstable meniscal tear (i.e., flap) (Figs. 1 and 5).

Which type of meniscectomy should be performed? As partial as possible, resecting the unstable part of the meniscus or more extended to resect the pathological meniscal tissue (meniscal disease)? However, there is no evidence-based answer at this time.

Whatever the type, one can expect a good result. According to Chatain et al. (2001) who reported the results of a large multicenter study conducted by the French Arthroscopy Society, poor results factors are presence of degenerative cartilage lesions (Odd Ratio 2.8), resection of the meniscal wall (Odd Ratio 2.2), and higher age >35 (Odd Ratio 5.0).

In the case of a parameniscal cyst, and when a meniscectomy is indicated, it is very important not only to treat the meniscal tear but also to evacuate the content of the cyst. It is therefore necessary to resect a sufficient amount of the meniscus until the meniscosynovial junction at least at the level of the cyst and to enlarge the opening of the cyst.

To do so, under arthroscopic control, a needle is introduced percutaneously through the cyst to locate the tract junction. Once the meniscus has been resected to the periphery (so-called saucerization), the tract can be enlarged using a forceps punch or a motorized shaver. Mucoid substance appears into the joint indicating the cyst is widely opened. It is then possible to abrade the wall of the cyst with a shaver. Open excision of the cyst, in conjunction with arthroscopic meniscectomy, is only needed in the case of a very large subcutaneous cyst.

Horizontal cleavage, especially grade 2 lesions, with or without parameniscal cyst, in young athletes is a specific group of injuries where meniscus preservation is mandatory.

Biedert (2000) was the first to propose repair in these cases. Rather than an arthroscopic repair, Pujol and Beaufils (2012) use an open technique which allows debriding the intrameniscal lesion, closing the horizontal cleavage, and putting vertical strong bioabsorbable stitches (Fig. 11).

Pujol and Beaufils (Pujol et al. 2013) reviewed 21 patients (24) after 40 months FU. IKDC score was between 87.9 (medial meniscus) and 90.7 (lateral meniscus). There were only four failures (19 %). Functional results deteriorate in patients older than 30 and in grade 3 meniscal lesions.

Root tears have been recently described (Ahn et al. 2010; Vyas and Harner 2012). Degenerate root tears specifically of the medial posterior horn must be differentiated from traumatic root tears which are rare and often associated with an ACL tear and a posterior root tear of the lateral meniscus. Degenerative meniscal root tears are often associated with a meniscal extrusion. In young patients, one should propose meniscal repair rather than meniscectomy: Transtibial root insertion allows to reconstruct the peripheral meniscal rim and insure a functional role to the meniscus (Ahn et al. 2010).

Macroscopic Osteoarthritis

If joint line narrowing is present, especially on the AP 30° flexion view, the diagnosis of osteoarthritis is obvious. Several studies have reported that the outcome of arthroscopic debridement and meniscectomy is roughly similar to the effect of placebo (Moseley et al. 2002; Siparsky et al. 2007). Moseley et al. (2002) randomly assigned 180 patients (mean age 52 years) with OA of the knee to undergo arthroscopic debridement, arthroscopic lavage, or placebo surgery. Patients in the placebo group received skin incisions and underwent a simulated debridement without insertion of the arthroscope. The mean follow-up was 24 months. Subjective results including pain and walking ability were not statistically different between the groups. Siparsky et al. (2007) performed a retrospective, evidence-based review of the current literature on the arthroscopic treatment of osteoarthritis of the knee. Of the 18 relevant studies, one was level I evidence (Moseley et al. 2002), five were level II, six were level III, and six were level IV. They found limited evidence-based research to support the use of arthroscopy as a treatment method for osteoarthritis of the knee. Arthroscopic

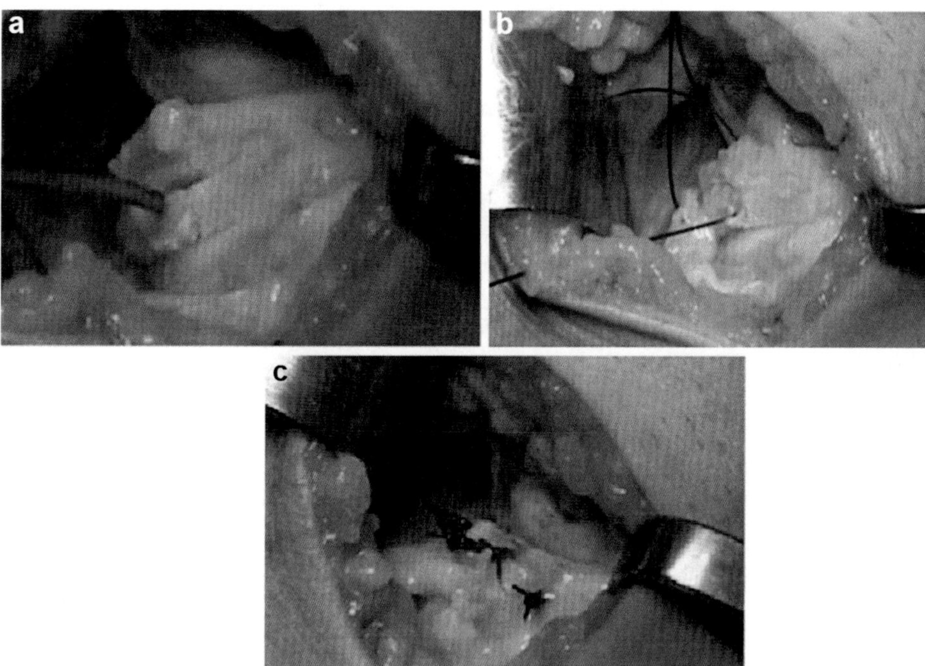

Fig. 11 Open meniscus repair of the medial meniscus (post segment) in young athletes. (**a**) After posterior arthrotomy and meniscosynovial junction release, the horizontal cleavage is clearly visible on the peripheral wall of the meniscus

debridement of meniscus tears and knees with low-grade osteoarthritis may be useful in some patients, but it should not be recommended as a routine treatment for all patients with knee osteoarthritis.

There is no need for arthroscopic debridement in these patients, with the rare exception of acute trauma to the osteoarthritic knee, which can result in an additional traumatic meniscal lesion, or symptoms of internal "derangement" (Pujol and Boisrenoult 2010).

If there is no evidence of joint line narrowing, but the MRI shows a meniscal extrusion or a subchondral bone abnormal signal, treatment should be focused on the cause of the disease, and meniscectomy is not routinely indicated. There is a high risk of postoperative problems such as rapid chondrolysis or subsequent osteonecrosis, especially if a meniscal root tear is debrided rather than repaired. Refraining from surgical treatment should always be considered in such case, except in the rare cases of "internal derangement" with evidence of unstable meniscal tears responsible for bone marrow edema (Fig. 5).

Conclusions

Meniscectomy, one of the most frequent orthopaedic procedures, may be performed too frequently. Meniscus preservation (benign neglect or repair) is probably too rare, even in the case of degenerative meniscal tears. It is not possible to exactly assess the rate of nonsurgical treatment (since many of these patients do not come to the surgeon) so that it is not possible to compare the respective parts of nonsurgical treatment, meniscectomy, or meniscus repair. But it can be assumed that the rate of partial meniscectomies should decrease and the rate of repair or conservative treatment should increase.

Based on a precise diagnosis, treatment principles become clear. And the above-mentioned algorithm can be easily utilized. In these degenerative lesions, waiting before surgical procedure is undertaken never a mistake, except in young athletic patients where early repair is probably necessary to avoid extension of the lesion and allow healing of the tear.

Cross-References

- ▶ Arthroscopic Repair of the Meniscus Tears
- ▶ Arthroscopic Treatment of Knee Osteoarthritis in Athletes
- ▶ Asymptomatic Meniscal Tears
- ▶ Meniscectomy

References

Ahn JH, Lee YS, Yoo JC et al (2010) Results of arthroscopic all-inside repair for lateral meniscus root tear in patients undergoing concomitant anterior cruciate ligament reconstruction. Arthroscopy 26:67–75

Beaufils P (2010) Synthesis -indications. In: Beaufils P, Verdonk R (eds) The meniscus. Springer, Berlin, pp 235–238

Beaufils P, Hulet C, Dhénain M et al (2009) Clinical practice guidelines for the management of meniscal lesions and isolated lesions of the anterior cruciate ligament of the knee in adults. Orthop Traumat Surg Res 95:437–442

Bhattacharyya T, Gale D, Dewire P et al (2003) The clinical importance of meniscal tears demonstrated by magnetic resonance imaging in osteoarthritis of the knee. J Bone Joint Surg Am 85A:4–9

Biedert RM (2000) Treatment of intrasubstance meniscal lesions: a randomized prospective study of four different methods. Knee Surg Sports Traumatol Arthrosc 8:104–108

Boyer T, Dorfmann H, Podgorski A (2010) Degenerative lesions-meniscal cyst. In: Beaufils P, Verdonk R (eds) The meniscus. Springer, Berlin, pp 51–60

Chatain F, Robinson AH, Adeleine P et al (2001) The natural history of the knee following arthroscopic medial meniscectomy. Knee Surg Sports Traumatol Arthrosc 9:15–18

Costa CR, Morrison WB, Carrino JA (2004) Medial meniscus extrusion on knee MRI: is extent associated with severity of degeneration or type of tear? Am J Roentgenol 183:17–23

Crues JV, Mink J, Levy TL et al (1987) Meniscal tears of the knee: accuracy of MR imaging. Radiology 164:445–448

Dorfmann H, Juan LH, Bonvarlet JP et al (1987) Arthroscopy of degenerative lesions of the internal meniscus. Classification and treatment. Rev Rhum Mal osteartic 54:303–310

Englund M, Niu J, Guermazi A et al (2007) Effect of meniscal damage on the development of frequent knee pain, aching, or stiffness. Arthritis Rheum 56:4048–4054

Englund M, Guermazi A, Gale D et al (2008) Incidental meniscal findings on knee MRI in middle-aged and elderly persons. N Engl J Med 359:1108–1115

Englund M, Guermazi A, Roemer FW et al (2009) Meniscal tear in knees without surgery and the development of radiographic osteoarthritis among middle-aged and elderly persons: the Multicenter Osteoarthritis Study. Arthritis Rheum 60:831–839

Ferrer-Rocca O, Vilalta C (1978) Lesions of the meniscus. Part II: horizontal cleavages and lateral cysts. Clin Orthop Rel Res 146:301–307

Hede A, Hempel-Poulsen S, Jensen JS (1990) Symptoms and level of sports activity in patients awaiting arthroscopy for meniscal lesions of the knee. J Bone Joint Surg Am 72A:550–552

Helms CA (2002) The Meniscus: recent advances in MR imaging of the knee. Am J Roentgenol 179:1115–1122

Herrlin S, Hallander M, Wanger P et al (2007) Arthroscopic or conservative treatment of degenerative medial meniscal tears: a prospective randomised trial. Knee Surg Sports Traumatol Arthrosc 15:393–401

Hulet C, Lebel B, Locker B (2010) Meniscal cysts. In: Beaufils P, Verdonk R (eds) The meniscus. Springer, Berlin, pp 137–146

Moseley JB, O'Malley K, Petersen NJ et al (2002) A controlled trial of arthroscopic surgery for osteoarthritis of the knee. N Engl J Med 347:81–88

Noble J, Erat K (1980) In defense of the meniscus. J Bone Joint Surg 62A:7–11

Prove S, Charrois O, Dekeuwer P et al (2004) Comparison of the medial femorotibial joint space before and immediately after meniscectomy. Rev Chir Orthop 90:636–642

Pujol N, Boisrenoult P (2010a) Meniscus and osteoarthritis. In: Beaufils P, Verdonk R (eds) The meniscus. Springe, Berlin, pp 61–66

Pujol N, Boisrenoult P (2010b) Lavage, debridement and osteoarthritis. In: Beaudils P, Verdonk R (eds) The meniscus. Springer, Berlin, pp 229–234

Pujol N, Bohu Y, Boisrenoult P et al (2013) Clinical outcomes of open meniscal repair of horizontal meniscal tears in young patients. Knee Surg Sports Traumatol Arthrosc 21:1530–3

Siparsky P, Ryzewicz M, Peterson B, Bartz R (2007) Arthroscopic treatment of osteoarthritis of the knee: are there any evidence-based indications? Clin Orthop Relat Res 455:107–112

Smillie IS (1978) Injuries of the knee joint, 4th edn. Churchill Livingstone, Edinburgh

Vyas D, Harner CD (2012) Meniscus root repair. Sports Med Arthrosc 20:86–94

Weiss CB, Lundberg M, Hamberg P et al (1989) Non-operative treatment of meniscal tears. J Bone Joint Surg Am 71A:811–822

Zanetti M, Pfirrmann CW, Schmid MR et al (2003) Patients with suspected meniscal tears: prevalence of abnormalities seen on MRI of 100 symptomatic and 100 contralateral asymptomatic knees. Am J Roentgenol 181:635–641

Different Techniques of Anterior Cruciate Ligament Reconstruction: Guidelines

84

Wolf Petersen

Contents

Abstract

Anatomical ACL replacement with medial portal drilling and footprint reconstruction is the technique of choice for patients with symptomatic instability after an ACL rupture (non-coper). The gold standard is the anatomic single-bundle reconstruction with mid-position placement of the tunnel. For patients with a large attachment area, a double-bundle technique could be indicated. Graft options for anatomical ACL reconstruction are the hamstrings, patellar tendon, or the quadriceps tendon with or without bone blocks. Graft choice depends on the individual demands and needs of the patient. A large group of patients can be treated successfully by all three autografts or by nonirradiated allografts. Some subgroups, however, may profit from a specific graft choice. Age, gender, activity, sports, profession, and religious habits should be considered.

Introduction

Personalized or individualized medicine is a new trend in many medical disciplines. Each patient should be treated according to his/her illness and his/her personal characteristics.

In orthopedics and trauma surgery, individual treatment strategies also have become current. An interesting example from sports trauma is anterior cruciate ligament reconstruction surgery (Petersen and Benedetto 2013).

W. Petersen (✉)
Department for Orthopaedic and Trauma Surgery, Martin Luther Hospital, Berlin, Grunewald, Germany
e-mail: w.petersen@mlk-berlin.de

M.N. Doral, J. Karlsson (eds.), *Sports Injuries*,
DOI 10.1007/978-3-642-36569-0_89

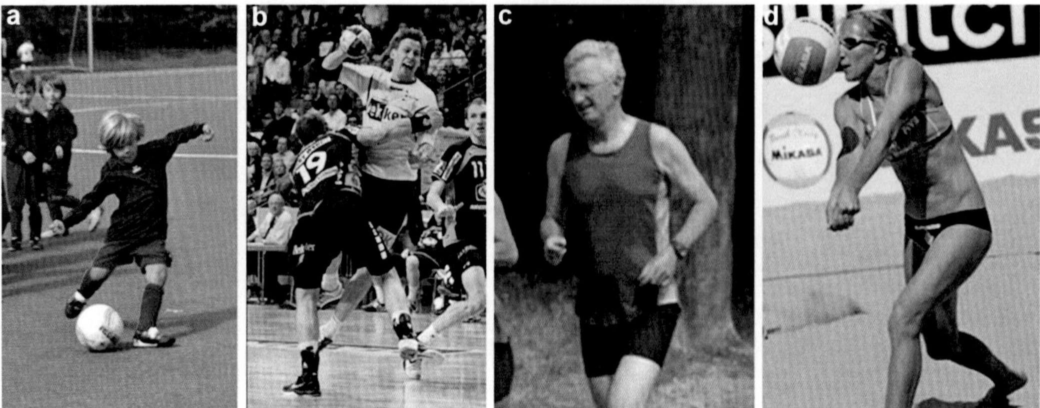

Fig. 1 Different patient groups for ACL reconstruction. (**a**) Young boy, (**b**) professional handball player, (**c**) recreational athlete over 40 years, (**d**) female professional volleyball player

The aim of ACL reconstruction surgery is to treat symptomatic knee instability to prevent subsequent meniscus and cartilage injuries (Petersen 2012; Petersen and Imhoff 2014). A recent meta-analysis has reported that an ACL tear predisposes knees to osteoarthritis, while ACL reconstruction surgery has a role in reducing the risk of developing degenerative changes at 10 years (Ajuied et al. 2013).

For a long time, the different surgical techniques for reconstruction of the anterior cruciate ligament were controversial (e.g., hamstrings vs. patellar tendon grafts, single vs. double-bundle reconstructions). Today, a variety of proven surgical techniques are known. These different techniques, however, face a very heterogeneous patient population (Fig. 1): different concomitant injuries, children, adults, gender, different body sizes, low- or high-level athletes, or senior citizen. It is a challenge for the future to identify the ideal therapy and surgical technique for these different patients.

The Concept of Anatomical ACL Reconstruction

Anatomic techniques for reconstruction of the anterior cruciate ligament have become established in recent years (Zantop and Petersen 2007; Bedi and Altchek 2009; Petersen et al. 2013). Different biomechanical studies have reported that anatomical femoral placement of the graft is more likely to reproduce normal ACL orientation, resulting in a more stable knee (Zantop et al. 2007a; Zantop et al. 2008; Herbort et al. 2010). These authors suggest that achieving anatomical graft placement on the femur is crucial to restoring normal knee function and may theoretically decrease the rate of joint degeneration after ACL reconstruction. Okafor et al. (2014) showed that patients with nonanatomical ACL reconstruction demonstrated a significant decrease in cartilage thickness along the medial intercondylar notch in the operative knee relative to the intact knee. In the anatomic group, no significant changes were observed. These findings suggest that restoring normal knee motion after ACL injury may help to slow the progression of articular cartilage degeneration.

Clinical findings support an anatomical ACL reconstruction concept (Sadoghi et al. 2011). Sadoghi et al. (2011) found significantly superior clinical outcome in anatomical ACL reconstructions in both techniques in terms of higher clinical scores, higher anterior-to-posterior stability, and less pivot shift.

Anatomical ACL reconstruction means that the tunnels must be located within the original insertions of the anterior cruciate ligament (Bedi and Altchek 2009; Achtnich et al. 2013; Petersen et al. 2013) (Fig. 2). For anatomical ACL reconstruction, different grafts can be used as far as they can be inserted in anatomical bone tunnels:

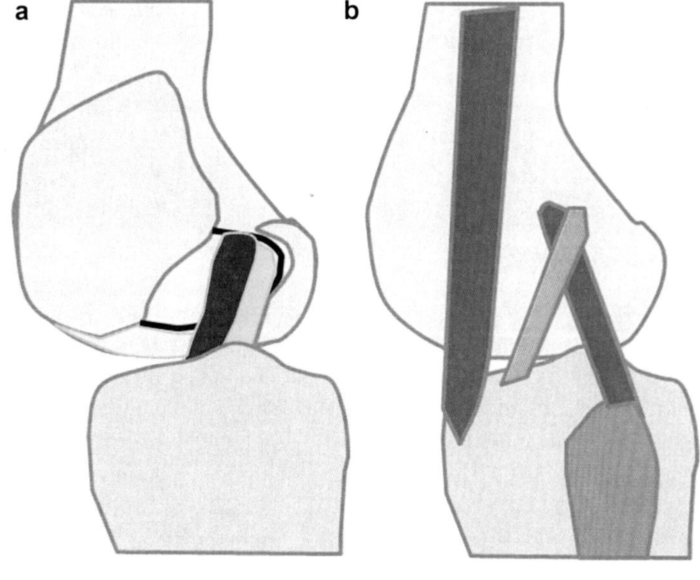

Fig. 2 (**a**) Anatomy of the ACL with the anteromedial and posterolateral bundle, (**b**) the structures of the lateral capsule. The anterolateral ligament is a stabilizer against tibial rotation

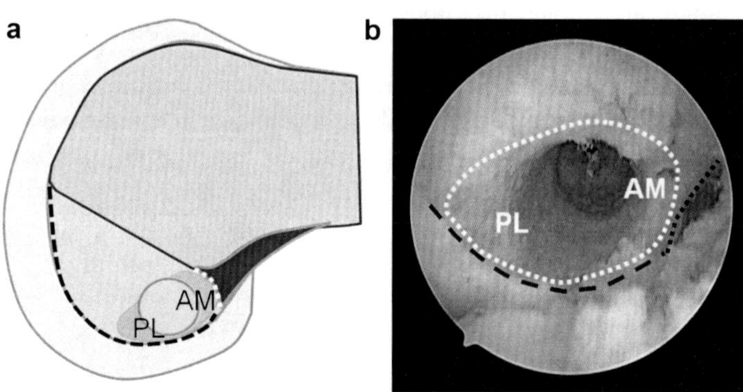

Fig. 3 (**a**) Schematic drawing showing a midportion position of the femoral tunnel, (**b**) femoral tunnel placed in the center of the femoral ACL insertion visualized with the arthroscope in the medial portal

autologous hamstring, quadriceps, and patellar tendon grafts and different allografts (Fig. 3).

The Bundle Concept

With regard to reconstruction of the anterior cruciate ligament, the bundle concept means that only the injured portions are reconstructed. Even remnants of the ACL should be preserved as far as possible to preserve proprioception (Petersen et al. 2013).

In patients with large attachment areas, both bundles of the ACL can be reconstructed separately. This technique is the so-called double-bundle ACL reconstruction (Petersen and Zantop 2007). Two recent meta-analyses showed that the AP and rotational stability are better with a double-bundle reconstruction compared to single-bundle reconstruction (Suomalainen et al. 2012; Tiamklang et al. 2012). Moreover, there is limited evidence for a lower rerupture rate and a lower incidence of meniscal tears after double-bundle reconstruction than after single-bundle reconstruction (Suomalainen et al. 2012; Tiamklang et al. 2012).

A recent study, however, has shown that the personalized use of both techniques (small insertion zones, single bundle; large insertion zones, double bundle) resulted in no difference between the two techniques with regard to stability and clinical scores (Hussein et al. 2012).

Anatomic Single-Bundle Reconstruction

With regard to the higher risk and higher cost of double-bundle reconstruction, single-bundle techniques should be considered as gold standard for ACL reconstruction (Petersen et al. 2013). The correct placement of the bone tunnels is the key to success for ACL reconstruction because nonanatomical tunnel placement is the most frequent factor for failure and revision after ACL surgery (Bedi and Altchek 2009; Herbort et al. 2010; Trojani et al. 2011).

Anatomical ACL reconstruction techniques with round or oval tunnels have been described in the literature (Herbort et al. 2013; Petersen et al. 2013). For a completely torn ACL, the tunnels should be located in the center of the femoral and tibial insertion zone (Achtnich et al. 2013).

An important issue concerning anatomical ACL reconstruction is the drilling technique. Biomechanical and anatomical studies have shown that tunnels created by the anteromedial portal drilling technique match the ACL footprint much closer than tunnels created with the transtibial drilling technique (Bedi et al. 2011). In a biomechanical cadaver study, anteromedial portal ACL reconstruction controlled tibial translation significantly more than the transtibial reconstruction with anterior drawer, Lachman, and pivot-shift examinations (Bedi et al. 2011). In a meta-analysis of clinical studies, Riboh et al. (2013) showed better Lysholm scores for anteromedial drilling techniques. Duffee et al. (2013) showed that transtibial ACL femoral tunnel preparation increases odds of repeat ipsilateral knee surgery.

In a systematic review, some studies found superior rotational stability and clinical outcomes with the anteromedial portal technique, and some found no difference. No studies showed significantly better results with the transtibial technique (Chalmers et al. 2013).

Despite the potential advantages of anteromedial portal reaming, a steep learning curve may exist when transitioning from conventional transtibial ACL reconstruction techniques. Lubowitz (2009) reported several pitfalls which may be associated with anteromedial portal drilling, such as posterior tunnel wall blowout, critically short sockets (less than 20 mm), inferior exit of the guidewire from the lateral thigh approaching critical neurovascular structures, iatrogenic injury to the medial femoral condyle with reamer passage, difficulty with visualization and instrumentation in the requisite hyperflexed position, bending of a rigid guidewire in the hyperflexed position, and difficulty with graft passage and fixation.

According to Behrendt and Richter (2010), the use of a conventional transtibial offset guide might be a pitfall of the anteromedial portal drilling technique, because these guides tend to place the guidewire too far posterior. To overcome this disadvantage, specific offset guides were developed which were designed for use through the anteromedial portal (Anteromedial portal guide, Karl Storz, Tuttlingen, Germany) (Petersen et al. 2013) (Fig. 4).

The anteromedial portal view is essential in anatomical ACL reconstruction. A previous study has reported that the complete femoral ACL footprint can only be visualized with the arthroscope in the anteromedial portal (Petersen and Zantop 2007). From the medial portal, the most important landmarks for femoral tunnel placement can be visualized: the intercondylar line and the cartilage border. The transition between both lines marks the AM bundle insertion.

For anatomical tunnel placement, the tibial stump of the ACL should be left intact (remnant augmentation). In cases with no remnants, the anterior horn of the lateral meniscus is used as landmark (Fig. 5). In single-bundle ACL reconstruction, the K-wire is placed in the center of the tibial ACL footprint. Different autografts (hamstrings, patellar tendon, quadriceps), allografts, and different fixation techniques (interference screws, extracortical buttons, pins, press fit) can be used for this anatomical ACL reconstruction technique.

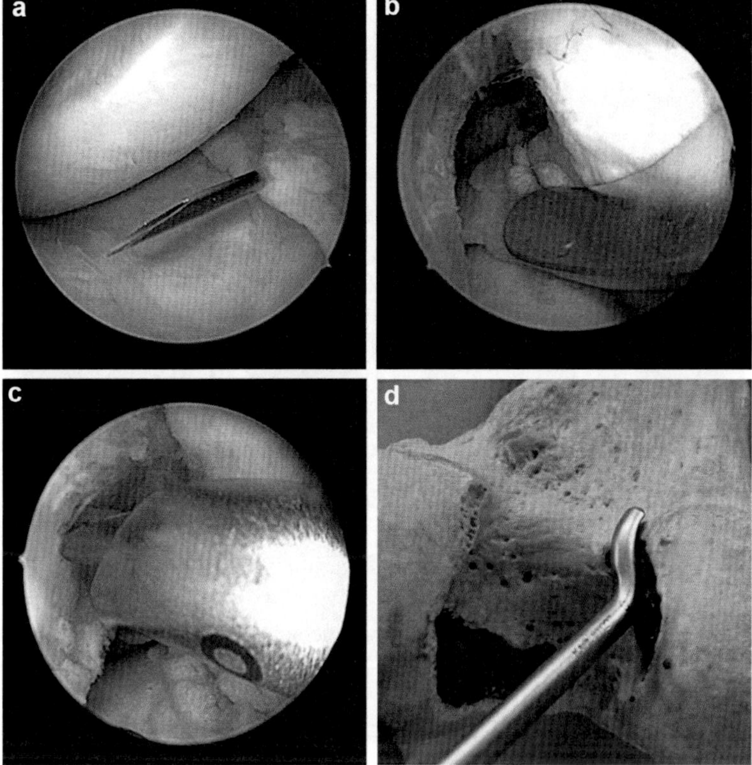

Fig. 4 (**a**) The anteromedial drilling portal is marked by a needle. Care should be taken not to injure the cartilage of the medial femoral condyle by the drill. (**b–d**) The medial portal aimer (Karl Storz, Tuttlingen) is hooked behind the intercondylar line

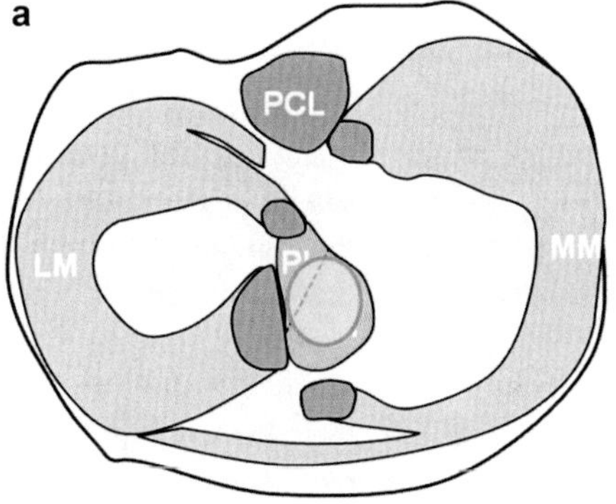

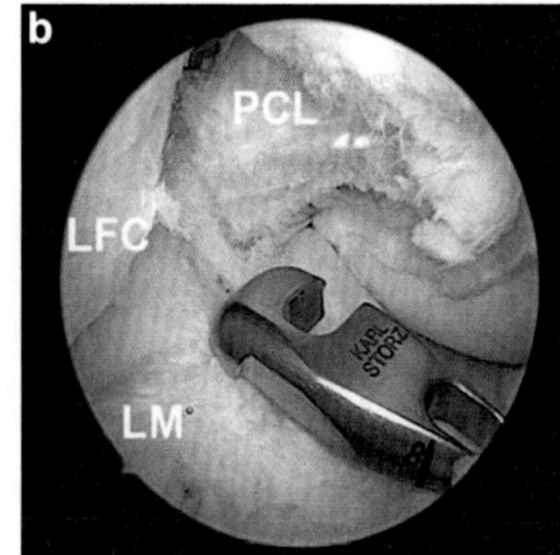

Fig. 5 (**a**) Schematic drawing showing the tibial ACL insertion. (**b**) Tibial aimer (Karl Storz, Tuttlingen) for the guidewire in place

Anatomic Double-Bundle Reconstruction

In patients with large attachment areas, there may be an indication for a double-bundle reconstruction (Siebold and Zantop 2009). That means that the AM and PL bundles are reconstructed separately (Fig. 6).

For the double-bundle technique, the tunnels should be placed within the original AM and PL attachments. At the femur, a bridge of 2–3 mm is left between the two tunnels. At the tibia, confluence of the bone tunnels is frequently observed.

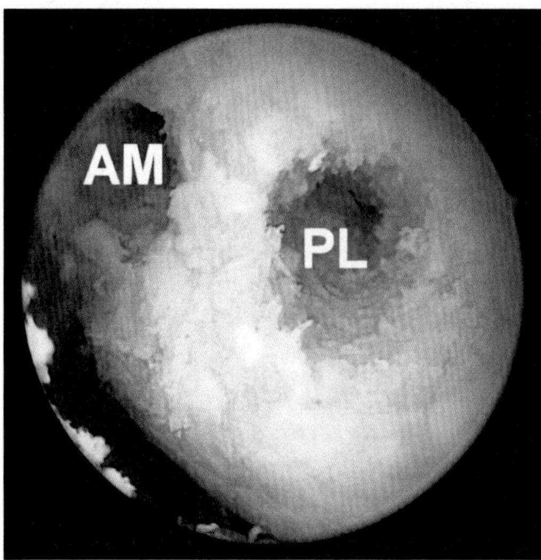

Fig. 6 Double femoral tunnel

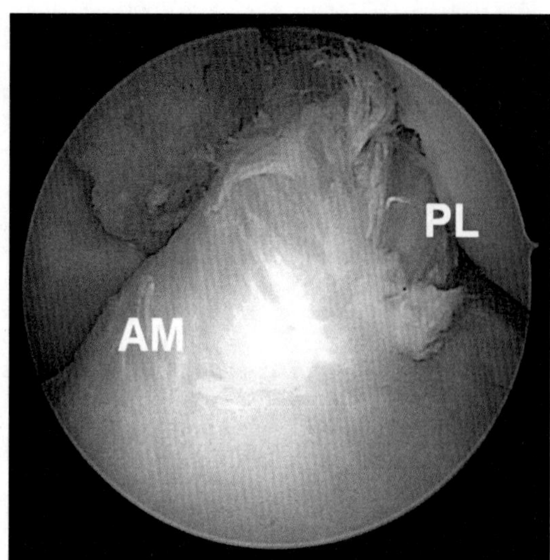

Fig. 7 Reconstruction of a PL bundle

Here the anterior horn of the lateral meniscus serves as a landmark.

Isolated Reconstruction of a Torn Bundle

The so-called double-bundle concept also includes separate reconstructions of the AM and PL bundles in patients with symptomatic partial rupture of the different bundles (Petersen and Zantop 2006) (Fig. 7). The principle of this technique follows that of single-bundle reconstruction with smaller tunnels placed in the center of the AM or PL bundle (Fig. 7).

An advantage of an isolated reconstruction of the AM or PL bundle might be preservation of proprioceptive elements within the remnant (Cha et al. 2012; Kazusa et al. 2013). Moreover, in many cases, a gracilis tendon graft is strong enough to reconstruct one torn bundle. This may be relevant, because the hamstring tendons theoretically act as agonists for the ACL. Furthermore, the medial hamstrings may stabilize against a valgus moment. Therefore, the preservation of the stronger semitendinosus tendon may be advantageous.

However, the clinical evidence for separate bundle augmentation is limited. Comparative clinical studies and long-term results are still missing.

Remnant Augmentation

The preservation of proprioception is also an advantage of the so-called "remnant preservation" technique (Cha et al. 2012). For this technique, as much functional ligament tissue as possible should be preserved. This can be just the tibial stump or the whole elongated ligament. The tendon graft can be pulled into the elongated ligament remnant. Various autografts and allografts can be used for this technique. Most authors prefer the semitendinosus graft for remnant augmentation technique.

This technique seals the tunnels to prevent synovial influx. The vasculature and the cells of the surrounding original ACL tissue promote remodeling. This has been shown by animal studies. Histological studies have also shown that the remnant of the ruptured ACL supports the process of revascularization and remodeling (Nakase et al. 2012; Sun et al. 2013).

The results of the first clinical case series were promising. An increased incidence of cyclops lesions was not observed (Cha et al. 2012). However, long-term results are missing and clinical studies comparing the remnant preservation technique with ACL reconstruction without remnant preservation are lacking.

Remnant preservation techniques can be technically demanding because the remnant tissue might impair the view to the insertion zones. On the other hand, a preserved stump may help to find the correct intra-articular entry point of the femoral and tibial bone tunnel.

Extra-articular Stabilization Techniques

In the recent years, there has been increasing interest in extra-articular procedures because biomechanical studies have shown that additional injury to the lateral capsular structures increases anterior rotational instability significantly (Diermann et al. 2009; Zantop et al. 2007b).

A biomechanical study performed by Engebretsen et al. (1990) reported that the extra-articular reconstruction technique reduces the stress on an intra-articular ACL graft by approximately 43 %. Another biomechanical study using cadaveric knees demonstrated that extra-articular augmentation with a lateral plasty reduces tibial rotation and the displacement of the lateral compartment with less risk of pivoting of the knee (Sydney et al. 1987). Clinical studies could confirm these findings. Several authors found significant improvement in objective knee laxity when adding the extra-articular procedure to a single-bundle ACL reconstruction (Noyes and Barber 1991; Lerat et al. 1998; Marcacci et al. 2009).

However, extra-articular techniques should be used with caution because some authors have reported a greater risk of osteoarthritis in the lateral compartment of the knee (Roth et al. 1987; Strum et al. 1989). The cause might be increased stress on the lateral plateau. A long-term study about a lateral plasty using a semitendinosus graft reconstructing the anterolateral ligament could not demonstrate excessive osteoarthritis in the lateral compartment of the knee (Marcacci et al. 2009).

Today, the exact role of extra-articular augmentation in ACL reconstruction has not been determined. Probably, the majority of ACL reconstruction can be solved by isolated intra-articular reconstruction. However, for patients with an excessive pivot shift or for revision situations, there can be an indication for an extra-articular procedure.

The lateral reconstruction techniques can be divided according to whether a strip of the iliotibial tract is used (Fig. 8) (Müller 1982; Lerat et al. 1998) or if the lateral plasty is performed with an autologous tendon graft Marcacci et al. (2009). Using a semi tendinusus autocraft Noyes and Barber (1991) reported good long-term results after a follow-up of 11 years.

Graft Choice

With regard to a personalized therapy approach, differentiated graft choice is regaining importance (Petersen and Benedetto 2013). Common autologous grafts are the patellar tendon, the hamstring tendons, or the quadriceps tendon. Several different grafts can also be used as allografts (patellar tendon, hamstring tendons, anterior tibialis tendon, and posterior tibialis tendon).

For single-bundle techniques, the hamstring tendons, the patellar tendon, and the quadriceps tendon can be used. For double-bundle reconstruction, mainly hamstring tendons or allografts are most frequently used.

Patellar Versus Hamstring Tendons

Many studies have compared ACL reconstruction with hamstring versus patellar tendon grafts (Biau et al. 2009; Mohtadi et al. 2011; Gifstad et al. 2013; Leys et al. 2012; Mascarenhas et al. 2012). Several well-designed prospective randomized trials do not show a significant difference between the two grafts apart from lesser incidence of anterior knee pain after hamstring tendon ACL reconstruction. In some studies, however, the stability after ACL reconstruction with patellar tendon was higher than after ACL reconstruction with a hamstring graft. Donor-site morbidity such as kneeling pain was also more frequent after ACL reconstruction with a patellar tendon autograft.

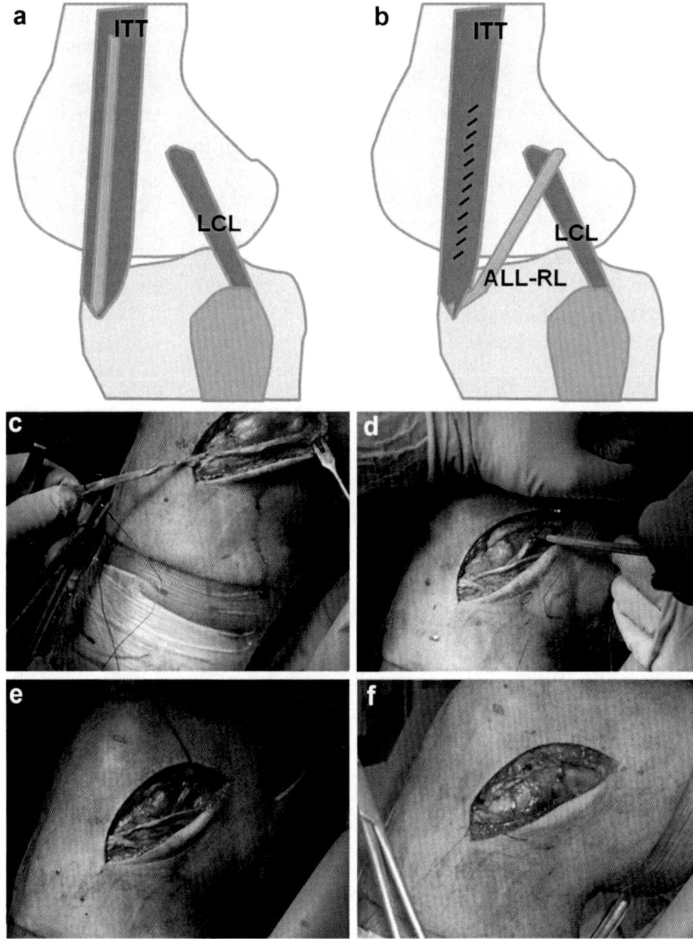

Fig. 8 Extra-articular reconstruction of the ALL with a central stripe from the iliotibial tract

Therefore, in patients with frequent kneeling activities, patellar tendon autografts should be avoided.

A systematic review has shown that the stability in women who were treated with a hamstring tendon graft is less than in female patients who were treated with a patellar tendon autograft (Paterno et al. 2012). Possible explanations involve gender-related differences in bone mineral density or the loss of an active valgus stabilizer. The hamstrings may protect against a valgus moment in patients who are at risk for ACL rupture. Moreover, it is well known that the hamstrings are functional agonists to the ACL, while the quadriceps is an important antagonist.

An indication for use of patellar tendon autografts could exist in young competitive athletes with closed growth plates, because these patients have a high risk for rerupture (Biau et al. 2009; Leys et al. 2012). In this patient group, patellar tendon grafts may be advantageous because the bone blocks may have the advantage that a revision may be easier in case of a rerupture. Mascarenhas et al. (2012) showed that in young athletes, 57 % returned to their preoperative sport after patellar tendon reconstruction and only 44 % after hamstring tendon reconstruction.

The reports regarding the rerupture rates from the literature are contradictory (Barrett et al. 2002; Barrett et al. 2011; Mohtadi et al. 2011; Leys et al. 2012). A recent meta-analysis found no differences between hamstring and patellar tendon ACL reconstruction (Mohtadi et al. 2011). Studies about specific subgroups, however, could demonstrate significant differences in the rerupture rates.

Barrett et al. (2002) compared the clinical results of anterior cruciate ligament reconstruction in female patients using quadruple-looped hamstring autograft versus patellar tendon autograft. The failure rate in the hamstring group was 23 % versus 8 % in the patellar tendon group.

In another study, Barrett et al. (2011) found a significant association between age group and graft failure. Patients 25 years and younger had a significantly higher failure rate than patients older than 25 years. Pairwise comparisons indicated that semitendinosus/gracilis (25.0 %) grafts resulted in significantly higher failure rates than bone-patellar tendon-bone grafts (11.8 %) in the age group of patients 25 years and younger.

For concern, however, is the higher incidence of arthritic changes after ACL replacement with a patellar tendon graft which was reported in some studies (Leys et al. 2012). However, there are also studies that have shown that there is no difference in the incidence of osteoarthritis between hamstring tendon and patellar tendon grafts (Holm et al. 2010).

A theoretical contraindication to the use of the ipsilateral side hamstring grafts could also be a chronic medial instability in the valgus knee. The additional loss of active medial stabilizer may cause a medial collapse.

A specific indication for patellar tendon grafts might be revision surgery. In these cases, the removal of bone blocks may be advantageous to compensate tunnel enlargement.

Several studies have described muscular flexion deficits after harvesting the hamstrings and quadriceps deficits after harvesting (Xergia et al. 2011). In a meta-analysis, these muscular deficits do not appear to affect the clinical results (Mohtadi et al. 2011). Whether the loss of functional ACL agonists might be a reason for the higher rerupture rate after hamstring graft harvesting in young active patients and the increased laxity in women should be the subject of future studies. Further studies also have to find out in which kind of sport the temporary muscular deficits might have relevance.

Quadriceps Tendon

The quadriceps tendon-patellar bone autograft was introduced by Blauth (1984) because it was believed this would minimize donor-site morbidity, including anterior knee pain while providing adequate mechanical strength as a graft. The quadriceps tendon can be used for anatomical ACL reconstruction techniques (Herbort et al. 2013; Forkel and Petersen 2014) and the graft can be harvested with or without bone block. With a bone block graft, a femoral press-fit fixation is possible, and its use may be advantageous in revision situations (Forkel and Petersen 2014).

However, there are few high-quality studies for the quadriceps tendon graft. Recently, Mulford et al. (2012) published a systematic review to identify all clinical studies reporting on the use of the quadriceps tendon autograft in ACL reconstructions. Seventeen articles met the inclusion criteria with a total of 1,580 reconstructions studied. The quadriceps tendon autograft had clinical (Lachman, pivot-shift testing) and functional outcomes (Lysholm and IKDC scores) similar to those reported for the patella tendon and hamstring grafts in the literature. Comparative studies also reported no significant difference between the grafts for any outcome measure. Clinically, there was no difference between central quadriceps tendon autograft with or without bone blocks (Geib et al. 2009).

With regard to the low donor-site morbidity, the quadriceps tendon graft might be an alternative for patellar tendon grafts in cases where a hamstring graft has disadvantages (woman, young athletes). A possible disadvantage of the quadriceps tendon graft is the cosmetically unfavorable scarring above the patella.

Allografts

Allografts are an interesting graft option because allografts are able to eliminate disadvantages associated with donor-site morbidity. Several human tendons such as tibialis anterior, patellar, and Achilles were used. A downside of allograft use is the risk of viral disease transmission (e.g., HIV, hepatitis C). Some sterilization methods (high-dose radiation and ethylene glycol sterilization) are known to affect the collagen structure and the mechanical properties of the graft (Dheerendra 2012). Hence, it is important to know about the graft procurement and sterilization technique when analyzing a research study about allograft ACL reconstruction (Dheerendra et al. 2012). Other disadvantage with using an allograft includes the immunogenic response of the host to the graft and delayed graft incorporation when compared to autografts.

The rate of HIV transmission from a properly screened nonirradiated or non-sterilized allograft is about 1 in 1.5 million (Dheerendra et al. 2012).

A recent meta-analysis could not find significant differences in graft failure rate, postoperative laxity, or patient-reported outcome scores when comparing ACLR with autografts to nonirradiated allografts (Mariscalco et al. 2013). These findings apply to patients in their late 1920s and early 1930s.

Barrett et al. (2010) have reported that the failure rate for allografts in patients younger than 25 years is higher than for autografts (12 % for patellar tendon autografts, 25 % for hamstring tendon autografts, and 29 % for allografts). Therefore, caution is advised when allografts are used in younger, more active cohorts.

Apart from primary ACL reconstruction, the use of allografts is an interesting option in revision surgery when other graft sources are limited.

Children and Adolescents

Conservative treatment of ACL injuries in children and adolescents often leads to poor and unacceptable results with a high rate of meniscal tears (up to 39 %), posttraumatic instabilities, and consecutive degenerative changes (Frosch et al. 2010). After a mean follow-up of 51 months, radiologic evidence of degenerative changes was found in 11 of 18 patients with open growth plates treated conservatively after ACL rupture (Mizuta et al. 1995). Therefore, in children with symptomatic instability due to ACL rupture, reconstruction of the ACL is recommended (Frosch et al. 2010).

Different surgical techniques for children with open growth plates exist: physeal-sparing and extra-anatomic reconstruction methods (over the top) and techniques using transphyseal graft fixation comparable to those used in adults. Surprisingly, a recent meta-analysis has shown that physeal-sparing techniques have a higher risk for postoperative leg-length discrepancies and axis deviations than transphyseal techniques (Frosch et al. 2010). In this study, the overall rate of leg-length differences or axis deviations was 5.8 % with physeal-sparing techniques and 1.9 % with transphyseal techniques (Frosch et al. 2010). An explanation for this unexpected finding might be that with physeal-sparing techniques, there is a higher risk that tangential drilling violates the growth plates.

A downside of transphyseal techniques was the higher rerupture rate (1.4 % vs. 4.2 %).

The relative risk of the occurrence of leg-length discrepancies or axis deviations was also reduced by 45 % when a hamstring transplant was used rather than a patellar tendon (Frosch et al. 2010). Care should be taken not to position bone blocks across open growth plates. The same is true for implants such as interference screws. In the meta-analysis, the rate of leg-length differences or axis deviations was 3.2 % with aperture fixation and 1.4 % when a fixation far from the joint line was used.

In conclusion, transphyseal techniques with bone block-free grafts and extracortical fixation techniques are almost always recommended in children with open physes. There are no reports in the literature about the effect of anteromedial portal drilling on leg axis and length differences. Further studies have to find out if the more horizontal drilling of the femoral tunnel leads to more violation of the growth plate.

Patients Over 40

Surgical treatment for patients older than 40 can be proposed in symptomatic patients who express the need to restore their preinjury activity levels, regardless of their age (Javernick et al. 2006; Legnani et al. 2011). Nonoperative treatment is indicated for older patients who do not perform highly demanding activities, who can cope with instability problems, and for whom quality of life is not affected by knee problems (Legnani et al. 2011).

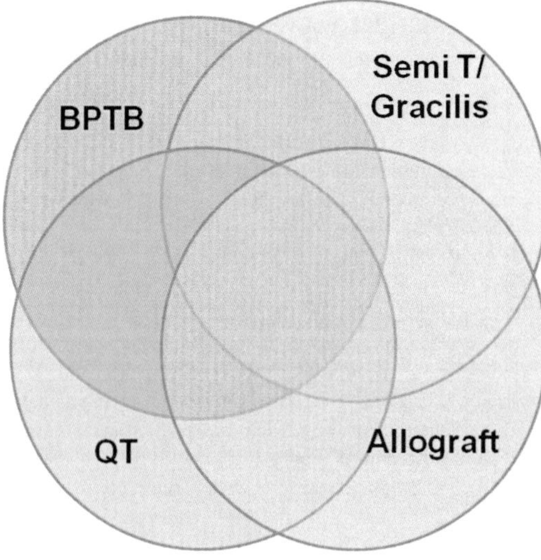

Fig. 9 Schematic drawing showing the overlapping indications for the different auto- and allografts

Results from the Swedish ACL registry have shown that optimal surgical results can be achieved in patients older than 40 years (Desai et al. 2013).

The graft choices in patients older than 40 years are controversial (Legnani et al. 2011). In this age group, the rerupture rate is low. Therefore, hamstring grafts with their low donor-site morbidity are considered to be advantageous in this age group. Moreover, in this population, the incidence is degenerative in the patellofemoral joint and is higher than in younger patients, and a potential osteopenia could increase the risk for patellar fractures (Legnani et al. 2011).

Allografts are also an interesting option for these patients. Barrett et al. (2005) have shown that bone-patellar tendon-bone allograft has advantages such as quicker return to sporting activities but also disadvantages with increased laxity and higher incidence of failure.

Conclusions

Anatomical ACL replacement with medial portal drilling and footprint reconstruction is the technique of choice for patients with symptomatic instability after an ACL rupture (non-coper).

Table 1 Relative indications and relative contraindications for three different autografts, nonirradiated or non-sterilized allografts

Graft	Relative indication	Relative contraindication
Hamstring	Double-bundle technique	Medial instabilities (ipsilateral)
	Large insertion zones	Genu valgum with torsional malalignment
	Partial bundle replacement (Gracilis tendon)	High-risk athletes
	Patients with kneeling activities	Age between growth plate closure and 25 years 16–20
	Patients with patellofemoral problems	
	Athletes who need an intact extensor mechanism	
	Open growth plates	
	Patients older than 40 years	
Patellarsehne	Revisions (bone block)	Kneeling activities
	Patients with a high rerupture risk	Open growth plates (with bone block)
		Femoropatellar pain
Quadrizepssehne	Revisions (bone block)	Femoropatellar pain (bone block)
	Patients with high risk for rerupture	Open growth plates (bone block)
Allografts	Revisions	High-level athletes
	Patients older than 25 years	Patients younger than 25 years

Gold standard is the anatomic single-bundle reconstruction with mid-position placement of the tunnel. For patients with a large insertion zone, a double-bundle technique could be indicated. Graft options for anatomical ACL reconstruction are the hamstrings, patellar tendon, or the quadriceps tendon with or without bone blocks. Several fixation techniques can be chosen. The fixation technique, however, should not interfere with anatomical tunnel placement. Graft choice depends on individual demands and needs of the patient. A large group of patients can be treated successfully by all three autografts or by nonirradiated allografts (Fig. 9). Some subgroups, however, may profit from a specific graft choice.

Table 1 gives an overview of the differential indication and relative contraindications of the various grafts. There is certainly a great deal of overlap in patients in whom all three grafts can be used as an alternative.

Cross-References

- ▶ Anterior Cruciate Ligament Graft Selection and Fixation
- ▶ Anterior Cruciate Ligament Injuries and Surgery: Current Evidence and Modern Development
- ▶ Anterior Cruciate Ligament Injuries Identifiable for Pre-participation Imagiological Analysis: Risk Factors
- ▶ Anterior Cruciate Ligament Injuries in Children
- ▶ Anterior Cruciate Ligament Reconstruction with Autologous Quadriceps Tendon

References

Achtnich A, Stiepani H, Forkel P, Metzlaff S, Hänninen EL, Petersen W (2013) Tunnel widening after anatomic double-bundle and mid-position single-bundle anterior cruciate ligament reconstruction. Arthroscopy 29(9):1514–1524

Ajuied A, Wong F, Smith C, Norris M, Earnshaw P, Back D, Davies A (2013) Anterior cruciate ligament injury and radiologic progression of knee osteoarthritis: a systematic review and meta-analysis. Am J Sports Med 8

Barrett GR, Noojin FK, Hartzog CW, Nash CR (2002) Reconstruction of the anterior cruciate ligament in females: a comparison of hamstring versus patellar tendon autograft. Arthroscopy 18(1):46–54

Barrett G, Stokes D, White M (2005) Anterior cruciate ligament reconstruction in patients older than 40 years: allograft versus autograft patellar tendon. Am J Sports Med 33(10):1505–1512

Barrett GR, Luber K, Replogle WH, Manley JL (2010) Allograft anterior cruciate ligament reconstruction in the young, active patient: tegner activity level and failure rate. Arthroscopy 26(12):1593–1601

Barrett AM, Craft JA, Replogle WH, Hydrick JM, Barrett GR (2011) Anterior cruciate ligament graft failure: a comparison of graft type based on age and Tegner activity level. Am J Sports Med 39(10):2194–2198

Bedi A, Altchek DW (2009) The "footprint" anterior cruciate ligament technique: an anatomic approach to anterior cruciate ligament reconstruction. Arthroscopy 25(10):1128–1138

Bedi A, Musahl V, Steuber V, Kendoff D, Choi D, Allen AA, Pearle AD, Altchek DW (2011) Transtibial versus anteromedial portal reaming in anterior cruciate ligament reconstruction: an anatomic and biomechanical evaluation of surgical technique. Arthroscopy 27(3):380–390

Behrendt S, Richter J (2010) Anterior cruciate ligament reconstruction: drilling a femoral posterolateral tunnel cannot be accomplished using an over-the-top step-off drill guide. Knee Surg Sports Traumatol Arthrosc 18(9):1252–1256

Biau DJ, Katsahian S, Kartus J, Harilainen A, Feller JA, Sajovic M, Ejerhed L, Zaffagnini S, Röpke M, Nizard R (2009) Patellar tendon versus hamstring tendon autografts for reconstructing the anterior cruciate ligament: a meta-analysis based on individual patient data. Am J Sports Med 37(12):2470–2478

Blauth W (1984) 2-strip substitution-plasty of the anterior cruciate ligament with the quadriceps tendon. Unfallheilkunde 87:45–51

Cha J, Choi SH, Kwon JW, Lee SH, Ahn JH (2012) Analysis of cyclops lesions after different anterior cruciate ligament reconstructions: a comparison of the single-bundle and remnant bundle preservation techniques. Skeletal Radiol 41(8):997–1002

Chalmers PN, Mall NA, Cole BJ, Verma NN, Bush-Joseph CA, Bach BR Jr (2013) Anteromedial versus transtibial tunnel drilling in anterior cruciate ligament reconstructions: a systematic review. Arthroscopy 29(7):1235–1242

Desai N, Björnsson H, Samuelsson K, Karlsson J, Forssblad M (2013) Outcomes after ACL reconstruction with focus on older patients: results from The Swedish National Anterior Cruciate Ligament Register. Knee Surg Sports Traumatol Arthrosc 22:379, Dec 10. [Epub ahead of print]PMID: 24318509

Dheerendra A (2012) Anterior cruciate ligament graft choices: a review of current concepts. Open Orthop J 6(Suppl 2: M4):281–286

Diermann N, Schumacher T, Schanz S, Raschke MJ, Petersen W, Zantop (2009) Rotational instability of the knee: internal tibial rotation under a simulated pivot shift test. Arch Orthop Trauma Surg 129(3):340–353

Duffee A, Magnussen RA, Pedroza AD, Flanigan DC, MOON Group, Kaeding CC (2013) Transtibial ACL femoral tunnel preparation increases odds of repeat ipsilateral knee surgery. J Bone Joint Surg Am 95(22):2035–2042

Engebretsen L, Lew WD, Lewis JL, Hunter RE (1990) The effect of an iliotibial tenodesis on intraarticular graft forces and knee joint motion. Am J Sports Med 18:169–176

Forkel P, Petersen W (2014) Anatomic reconstruction of the anterior cruciate ligament with the autologous quadriceps tendon: primary and revision surgery]. Oper Orthop Traumatol 26(1):30–42

Frosch KH, Stengel D, Brodhun T, Stietencron I, Holsten D, Jung C, Reister D, Voigt C, Niemeyer P, Maier M, Hertel P, Jagodzinski M, Lill H (2010) Outcomes and risks of operative treatment of rupture of the anterior cruciate ligament in children and adolescents. Arthroscopy 26(11):1539–1550

Geib TM, Shelton WR, Phelps RA, Clark L (2009) Anterior cruciate ligament reconstruction using quadriceps tendon autograft: intermediate-term outcome. Arthroscopy 25(12):1408–1414

Gifstad T, Sole A, Strand T, Uppheim G, Gr½ntvedt T, Drogset JO (2013) Long-term follow-up of patellar tendon grafts or hamstring tendon grafts in endoscopic ACL reconstructions. nKnee Surg Sports Traumatol Arthrosc. 21(3):576–83. doi: 10.1007/s00167-012-1947-0. Epub 2012 Mar 10

Herbort M, Lenschow S, Fu FH, Petersen W, Zantop T (2010) ACL mismatch reconstructions: influence of different tunnel placement strategies in single-bundle ACL reconstructions on the knee kinematics. Knee Surg Sports Traumatol Arthrosc 18 (11):1551–1558

Herbort M, Tecklenburg K, Zantop T, Raschke MJ, Hoser C, Schulze M, Petersen W, Fink C (2013) Single-bundle anterior cruciate ligament reconstruction: a biomechanical cadaveric study of a rectangular quadriceps and bone-patellar tendon-bone graft configuration versus a round hamstring graft. Arthroscopy 29(12):1981–1990

Holm I, Oiestad BE, Risberg MA, Aune AK (2010) No difference in knee function or prevalence of osteoarthritis after reconstruction of the anterior cruciate ligament with 4-strand hamstring autograft versus patellar tendon-bone autograft: a randomized study with 10-year follow-up. Am J Sports Med 38 (3):448–454

Hussein M, van Eck CF, Cretnik A, Dinevski D, Fu FH (2012) Individualized anterior cruciate ligament surgery: a prospective study comparing anatomic single- and double-bundle reconstruction. Am J Sports Med 40(8):1781–1788

Javernick MA, Potter BK, Mack A, Dekay KB, Murphy KP (2006) Autologous hamstring anterior cruciate ligament reconstruction in patients older than 40. Am J Orthop (Belle Mead NJ) 35(9):430–434

Kazusa H, Nakamae A, Ochi M (2013) Augmentation technique for anterior cruciate ligament injury. Clin Sports Med 32(1):127–140

Legnani C, Terzaghi C, Borgo E, Ventura A (2011) Management of anterior cruciate ligament rupture in patients aged 40 years and older. J Orthop Traumatol 12(4):177–184

Lerat JL, Chotel F, Besse JL (1998) The results after 10–16 years of the treatment of chronic anterior laxity of the knee using reconstruction of the anterior cruciate ligament with a patellar tendon graft combined with an external extra-articular reconstruction [in French]. Rev Chir Orthop Reparatrice Appar Mot 84:712–727

Leys T, Salmon L, Waller A, Linklater J, Pinczewski L (2012) Clinical results and risk 13factors for reinjury 15 years after anterior cruciate ligament reconstruction: a prospective study of hamstring and patellar tendon grafts. Am J Sports Med 40(3):595–605

Lubowitz JH (2009) Anteromedial portal technique for the anterior cruciate ligament femoral socket: pitfalls and solutions. Arthroscopy 25(1):95–101

Marcacci M, Zaffagnini S, Giordano G, Iacono F, Presti ML (2009) Anterior cruciate ligament reconstruction associated with extra-articular tenodesis: a prospective clinical and radiographic evaluation with 10- to 13-year follow-up. Am J Sports Med 37(4):707–714

Mariscalco MW, Magnussen RA, Mehta D, Hewett TE, Flanigan DC, Kaeding CC (2013) Autograft versus nonirradiated allograft tissue for anterior cruciate ligament reconstruction: a systematic review. Am J Sports Med 8:492, [Epub ahead of print] PMID23928319

Mascarenhas R, Tranovich MJ, Kropf EJ, Fu FH, Harner CD (2012) Bone-patellar tendon-bone autograft versus hamstring autograft anterior cruciate ligament reconstruction in the young athlete: a retrospective matched analysis with 2–10 year follow-up. Knee Surg Sports Traumatol Arthrosc 20(8):1520–1527

Mizuta H, Kubota K, Shiraishi M, Otsuka Y, Nagamoto N, Takagi K (1995) The conservative treatment of complete tears of the anterior cruciate ligament in skeletally immature patients. J Bone Joint Surg Br 77:890–894

Mohtadi NG, Chan DS, Dainty KN, Whelan DB (2011) Patellar tendon versus hamstring tendon autograft for anterior cruciate ligament rupture in adults. Cochrane Database Syst Rev 7:9

Mulford JS, Hutchinson SE, Hang JR (2012) Outcomes for primary anterior cruciate reconstruction with the quadriceps autograft: a systematic review. Knee Surg Sports Traumatol Arthrosc 21(8):1882–1888

Müller W (1982) The knee. Springer, New York/ Heidelberg

Nakase J, Toratani T, Kosaka M, Ohashi Y, Tsuchiya H (2012) Roles of ACL remnants in knee stability. Knee Surg Sports Traumatol Arthrosc 21(9):2101–6

Noyes FR, Barber SD (1991) The effect of an extra-articular procedure on allograft reconstructions for chronic ruptures of the anterior cruciate ligament. J Bone Joint Surg Am 73(6):882–892

Okafor EC, Utturkar GM, Widmyer MR, Abebe ES, Collins AT, Taylor DC, Spritzer CE, Moorman CT 3, Garrett WE, Defrate LE (2014) The effects of femoral graft placement on cartilage thickness after anterior cruciate ligament reconstruction. J Biomech 47(1):96–101

Paterno MV, Weed AM, Hewett TE (2012) A between sex comparison of anterior-posterior knee laxity after anterior cruciate ligament reconstruction with patellar tendon or hamstrings autograft: a systematic review. Sports Med 42(2):135–152

Petersen W (2012) Does ACL reconstruction lead to degenerative joint disease or does it prevent osteoarthritis? How to read science. Arthroscopy 28(4):448

Petersen W, Benedetto KP (2013) Personalisierte Medizin in der Orthopädie am Beispiel der Kreuzbandchirurgie. Arthroskopie 26:6–11

Petersen W, Imhoff AB (2014) Reconstruction of the anterior cruciate ligament. Oper Orthop Traumatol 26(1):5–6

Petersen W, Zantop T (2006) Partial rupture of the anterior cruciate ligament. Arthroscopy 22(11):1143–1145

Petersen W, Zantop T (2007) Anatomy of the anterior cruciate ligament with regard to its two bundles. Clin Orthop Relat Res 454:35–47

Petersen W, Forkel P, Achtnich A, Metzlaff S, Zantop T (2013a) Technique of anatomical footprint reconstruction of the ACL with oval tunnels and medial portal aimers. Arch Orthop Trauma Surg 133(6):827–833

Petersen W, Forkel P, Achtnich A, Metzlaff S, Zantop T (2013b) Anatomic reconstruction of the anterior cruciate ligament in single bundle technique. Oper Orthop Traumatol 25(2):185–204

Riboh JC, Hasselblad V, Godin JA, Mather RC 3rd (2013) Transtibial versus independent drilling techniques for anterior cruciate ligament reconstruction: a systematic review, meta-analysis, and meta-regression. Am J Sports Med 41(11):2693–2702

Roth JH, Kennedy JC, Lockstadt H, McCallum CL, Cunning LA (1987) Intraarticular reconstruction of the anterior cruciate ligament with and without extra-articular supplementation by transfer of the biceps femoris tendon. J Bone Joint Surg Am 69:275–278

Sadoghi P, Kröpfl A, Jansson V et al (2011) Impact of tibial and femoral tunnel position on clinical results after anterior cruciate ligament reconstruction. Arthroscopy 27(3):355–359

Siebold R, Zantop T (2009) Anatomic double-bundle ACL reconstruction: a call for indications. Knee Surg Sports Traumatol Arthrosc 17(3):211–212

Strum GM, Fox JM, Ferkel RD (1989) Intraarticular versus intraarticular and extraarticular reconstruction for chronic anterior cruciate ligament instability. Clin Orthop Relat Res 245:188–198

Sun L, Wu B, Tian M, Liu B, Luo Y (2013) Comparison of graft healing in anterior cruciate ligament reconstruction with and without a preserved remnant in rabbits. Knee 20(6):537–544

Suomalainen P, Kannus P, Järvelä T (2012) Double-bundle anterior cruciate ligament reconstruction: a review of literature. Int Orthop 37(2):227–232

Sydney SV, Hayners DW, Hungerford DS (1987) The altered kinematic effect of an iliotibial band tenodesis on the anterior cruciate deficient knee. Orthop Trans 11:340

Tiamklang T, Sumanont S, Foocharoen T, Laopaiboon M (2012) Double-bundle versus single-bundle reconstruction for anterior cruciate ligament rupture in adults. Cochrane Database Syst Rev 14:11

Trojani C, Sbihi A, Djian P, Potel JF, Hulet C, Jouve F, Bussière C, Ehkirch FP, Burdin G, Dubrana F, Beaufils P, Franceschi JP, Chassaing V, Colombet P, Neyret P (2011) Causes for failure of ACL reconstruction and influence of meniscectomies after revision. Knee Surg Sports Traumatol Arthrosc 19 (2):196–201

Xergia SA, McClelland JA, Kvist J, Vasiliadis HS, Georgoulis AD (2011) The influence of graft choice on isokinetic muscle strength 4–24 months after anterior cruciate ligament reconstruction. Knee Surg Sports Traumatol Arthrosc 19(5):768–809

Zantop T, Petersen W (2007) Anatomische Rekonstruktion des vorderen Kreuzbandes. Arthroskopie 20(2):94–104

Zantop T, Herbort M, Raschke MJ, Fu FH, Petersen W (2007a) The role of the anteromedial and posterolateral bundles of the anterior cruciate ligament in anterior tibial translation and internal rotation. Am J Sports Med 35(2):223–227

Zantop T, Schumacher T, Diermann N, Schanz S, Raschke MJ, Petersen W (2007b) Anterolateral rotational knee instability: role of posterolateral structures. Winner of the AGA-DonJoy award 2006. Arch Orthop Trauma Surg 127(9):743–752

Zantop T, Diermann N, Schumacher T, Schanz S, Fu FH, Petersen W (2008) Anatomical and nonanatomical double-bundle anterior cruciate ligament reconstruction: importance of femoral tunnel location on knee kinematics. Am J Sports Med 36(1):65–72

Double-Tunnel Anatomic Anterior Cruciate Ligament Reconstruction

85

Eiji Kondo and Kazunori Yasuda

Contents

E. Kondo (✉)
Department of Advanced Therapeutic Research for Sports Medicine, Hokkaido University, Graduate School of Medicine, Sapporo, Hokkaido, Japan
e-mail: eijik@med.hokudai.ac.jp

K. Yasuda
Department of Sports Medicine and Joint Surgery, Hokkaido University, Graduate School of Medicine, Sapporo, Hokkaido, Japan
e-mail: yasukaz@med.hokudai.ac.jp

M.N. Doral, J. Karlsson (eds.), *Sports Injuries*,
DOI 10.1007/978-3-642-36569-0_92

Abstract

In the early 2000s, a new concept of anatomic reconstruction of the anteromedial and posterolateral bundles of the anterior cruciate ligament (ACL), in which four independent tunnels were created through the center of each anatomic attachment of the two bundles, was proposed. Biomechanical studies have shown that the anatomic double-bundle ACL reconstruction can restore knee stability significantly more closely to the normal level than the conventional single-bundle reconstruction. In clinical evaluations, the anterior and/or rotatory stability of the knee was significantly better with the anatomic double-bundle ACL reconstruction than with the conventional single-bundle reconstruction. To establish the clinical utility of the anatomic double-bundle ACL reconstruction, further clinical studies are needed concerning the effects on rotatory stability, long-term survival of the graft functions, and comparisons with other procedures.

Abbreviations

ACL	Anterior cruciate ligament
AM	Anteromedial bundle
PL	Posterolateral bundles

Introduction

The normal ACL consists of the anteromedial (AM) and posterolateral (PL) bundles, each having different functions (Amis and Dawkins 1991; Sakane et al. 1997). The concept of double-bundle ACL reconstruction was initially described in the 1980s (Mott 1983; Zaricznyj 1987). In 1999, Muneta et al. (1999) described an arthroscopically assisted double-bundle procedure with two tunnels in the femur and the tibia, respectively. In their articles, however, the 10:30-o'clock orientation for the right knee was recommended as the location of the femoral tunnel for the PL bundle. In the early 2000s, only a few clinical articles were published to evaluate the double-bundle procedures (Hamada et al. 2001; Adachi et al. 2004). Concerning these procedures, however, no significant differences were found in the clinical results between single- and double-bundle procedures. No studies have clearly shown a method to identify the location of the femoral attachment of the PL bundle in the arthroscopic visual field. In the early 2000s, Yasuda et al. (2004, 2006) reported a new concept of anatomic reconstruction of the AM and PL bundles of the ACL with 2-year clinical results superior to conventional single-bundle ACL reconstruction (Fig. 1). This procedure has several noteworthy characteristics. First, all four ends of two tendon grafts are grafted at the center of the anatomical attachment of the AM or PL bundle, not only on the femur but also on the tibia. Second, the transtibial tunnel technique is used to create femoral tunnels. In this procedure, the greatest key to success is to create a tibial tunnel with appropriate direction. In other words, a tibial tunnel should be created so that a guidewire for femoral tunnel creation can be easily inserted at a targeted point on the lateral femoral condyle through the tibial tunnel. To create such a tibial tunnel, a specially designed hole-in-one guide was developed. Third, the hamstring tendon "hybrid" graft (Yasuda et al. 1995, 1997), in which the femoral and tibial end is connected with an Endobutton and a polyester tape, was used. Since this report, a number of anatomic, biomechanical, and clinical studies on the anatomic double-bundle reconstruction procedures have been conducted in the field of ACL reconstruction, and several clinical trials have found that postoperative knee stability is superior in the anatomic double-bundle reconstruction compared with conventional single-bundle reconstruction (Aglietti et al. 2007; Yagi et al. 2007; Muneta et al. 2007; Kondo et al. 2008; Jarvela et al. 2008; Siebold et al. 2008). However, the utility of the anatomic double-bundle reconstruction has not yet been established (Streich et al. 2008; Meredick et al. 2008). In this chapter, the surgical procedure and biomechanical and clinical evaluations of anatomic double-bundle ACL reconstruction are explained.

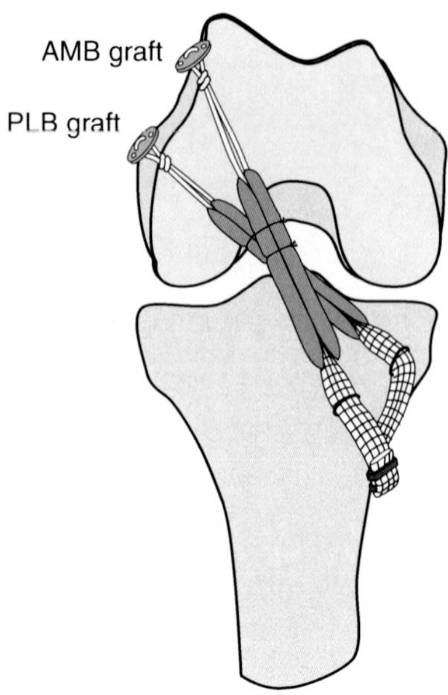

Fig. 1 Anatomic double-bundle ACL reconstruction procedure with hamstring tendon "hybrid" grafts

Operative Procedure

Graft Preparation

Surgery is performed with an air tourniquet in the supine position with the tibia flexed at approximately 90°, in the "Fig. 4 knee position." An approximately 3-cm-long transverse incision is made in the anteromedial portion of the proximal tibia. The semitendinosus and gracilis tendons are harvested using a tendon stripper. When the semitendinosus tendon is thick and long enough, the gracilis tendon is not harvested (Inagaki et al. 2013). The distal half of the semitendinosus tendon (and the gracilis tendon) is doubled and used for AM bundle reconstruction (Kondo et al. 2012b). The remaining proximal half of the semitendinosus tendon is doubled and used for PL bundle reconstruction. During graft preparation, the grafts are pretensioned using a specially designed graft fashioning board. First, the doubled tendons are sutured using a polyester thread. Next, a polyester tape is mechanically connected in series with the end of the doubled tendons, using the original technique. This tape is strong, soft, meshed, 10 mm wide, and 50 cm long. After the length of the femoral tunnel created with the procedure is measured, the selected Endobutton-CL-BTB is attached at the looped end of the tendons according to the manufacturer's guidelines (Fig. 2). The autogenous tendon portion is fashioned so that the 15–20-mm-long autogenous tendon portion can be placed within each bone tunnel. The remaining half of the semitendinosus tendon is also doubled, and the same type of fashioning is performed for the PL bundle graft (Fig. 2). The AM graft diameter ranged from 6 to 7 mm, and the PL graft diameter ranged from 5 to 6 mm. The first advantage of the hybrid graft is that it is stronger and stiffer than the tendon-suture composite (Kondo et al. 2012b). The second advantage is that the tape portions of the two grafts can be simultaneously fixed to the tibia with an initial tension (Yasuda et al. 2008).

Anatomic Double-Bundle Reconstruction Procedure

The procedure is performed in the supine position with the femur horizontal and the tibia flexed at approximately 90°, in the "hanging leg position." This position enables the femoral attachment of the femoral AM and PL bundles to be easily recognized (Kai et al. 2013). The details of this procedure were previously described in the literature (Yasuda et al. 2004, 2006). An arthroscope is inserted through the lateral infrapatellar portal. The ACL remnant is resected, leaving a 1-mm-long ligament tissue at the femoral and tibial insertions to obtain landmarks for inserting guidewire. When an osteophyte was formed at the notch in chronic cases, notchplasty is performed. First, a tibial tunnel for the PL bundle is created. To insert a guidewire, a wire navigator is used as a hole-in-one guide (Fig. 3a, b). The Navi-tip portion of this device is introduced into the joint cavity through the medial infrapatellar portal. The surgeon holds the tibia at 90° of knee flexion, keeping the femur horizontal. The tibial indicator of the Navi-tip is placed at the center of the PL bundle footprint on the tibia (Fig. 4a), which is located at the most posterior aspect of the area between the tibial eminences and 6–7 mm anterior to the posterior cruciate ligament (Fig. 5a). Then, keeping the tibial indicator at this point, the femoral indicator is aimed at the center of the PL bundle footprint on the femur (Fig. 5b). Subsequently, the direction of the extra-articular wire sleeve is automatically decided. The proximal end of the sleeve is fixed on the anteromedial aspect of the tibia through the skin incision made for the

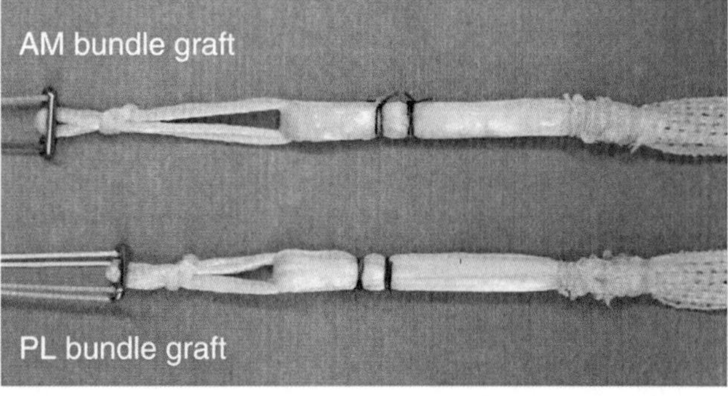

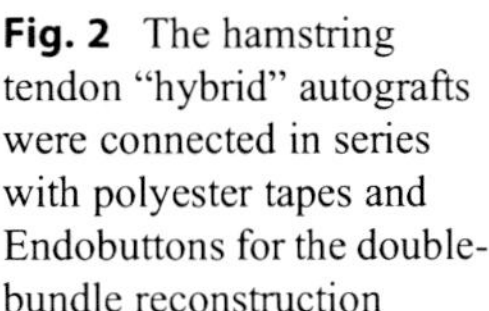

Fig. 2 The hamstring tendon "hybrid" autografts were connected in series with polyester tapes and Endobuttons for the double-bundle reconstruction

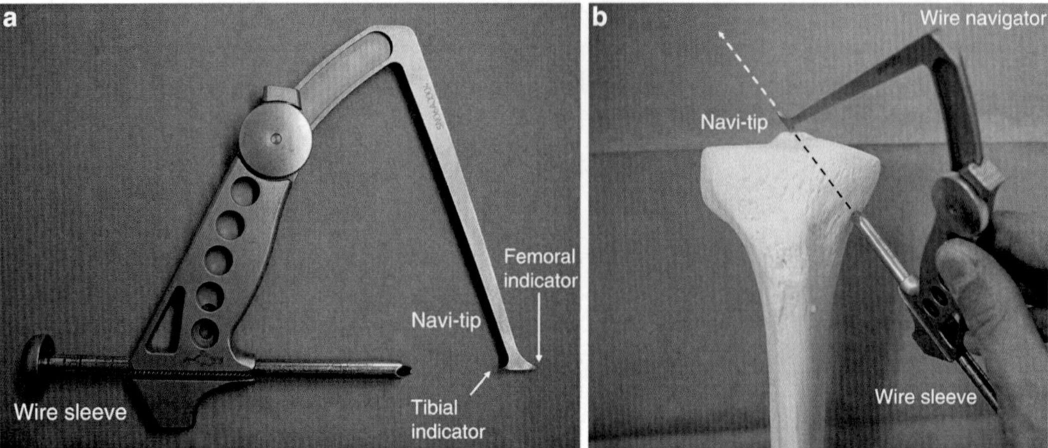

Fig. 3 (**a**) The wire navigator is composed of a Navi-tip and a wire sleeve. The Navi-tip consists of sharp tibial and femoral indicators. (**b**) The axis of the wire sleeve passes through the tip of the tibial indicator. The axis of the wire sleeve is passed through the tip of the tibial indicator. Keeping the tibial indicator at this point, the femoral indicator was aimed at a targeted point on the femur

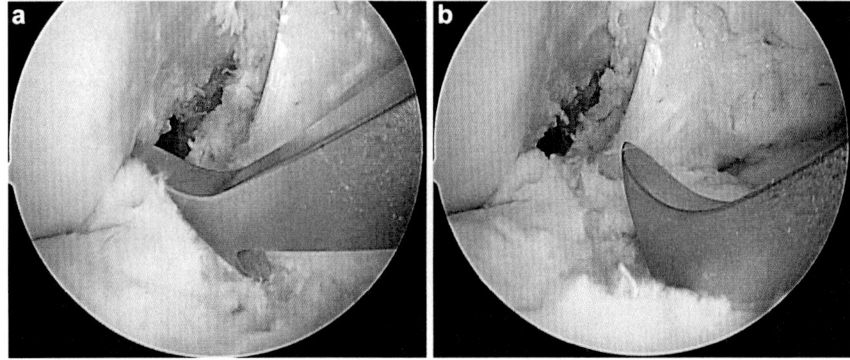

Fig. 4 The Navi-tip of wire navigator for the tibial posterolateral (*PL*) tunnels in arthroscopic surgery. (**a**) The Navi-tip of wire navigator for the tibial anteromedial (*AM*) tunnels in arthroscopic surgery

graft harvest. A guidewire is drilled through the sleeve in the tibia. Then, a tibial tunnel for the AM bundle is drilled. The same wire navigator is used to insert a guidewire. The tibial indicator of the Navi-tip is placed at the center of the tibial footprint of the AM bundle (Fig. 4b). The center is located at a point approximately 8 mm anterior to the guidewire for the PL bundle (Fig. 5a). Keeping the tibial indicator at this point, the femoral indicator is aimed at the center of the femoral footprint of the AM bundle, which is located 5 mm anterior to the most posterior aspect of the notch at the junction of the intercondylar roof and the medial wall of the lateral femoral condyle (Fig. 5b). This point is positioned at the 1:30-o'clock (or 10:30) position (Kai et al. 2013). The wire sleeve is fixed on the anteromedial cortex. At this point, the knee is extended to ensure the tip of the second wire was located at the point 5 mm posterior to the anterior edge of the roof in the intercondylar notch. A guidewire is drilled through the sleeve in the tibia. The two tibial tunnels are made with a cannulated drill corresponding to the measured diameter of the prepared substitute. The AM and PL tibial tunnel angles in anatomic double-bundle ACL reconstruction procedure were clarified. The tibial tunnel angles of the PL bundle averaged 40.7° in the

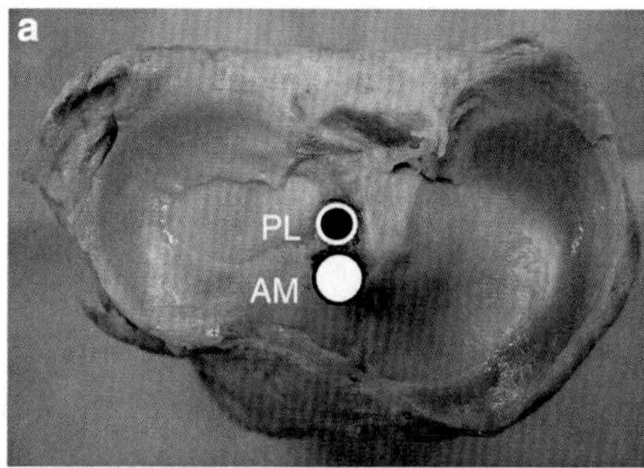

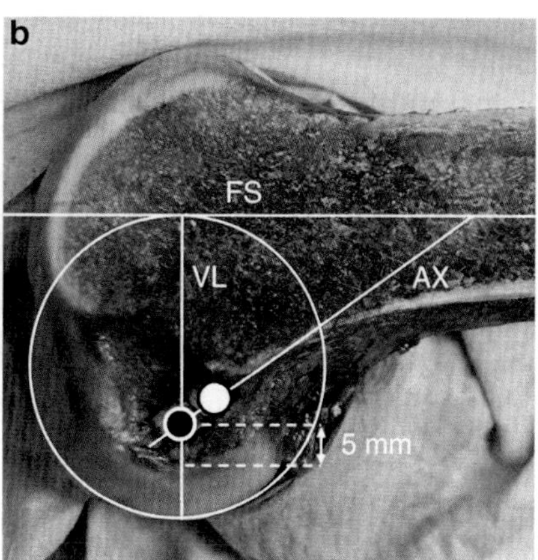

Fig. 5 (**a**) Bone tunnel position in attachment of the ACL on the tibia. AM, tunnel outlet of anteromedial bundle; PL, tunnel outlet of posterolateral bundle. (**b**) Bone tunnel position in attachment of the ACL on the femur. A picture of the lateral condyle was taken with a precise medial view (FS, parallel line of axis of femoral shaft). When a surgeon drew a vertical line (*VL*) through the contact point between the femoral condyle and the tibial plateau on a picture taken at 90° of flexion, this line and the long axis of the ACL attachment (*AX*) crossed at the PL point on the vertical line 5 mm anterior to the edge of the joint cartilage. The center of the attachment of the PL bundle was located approximately at this crossing point

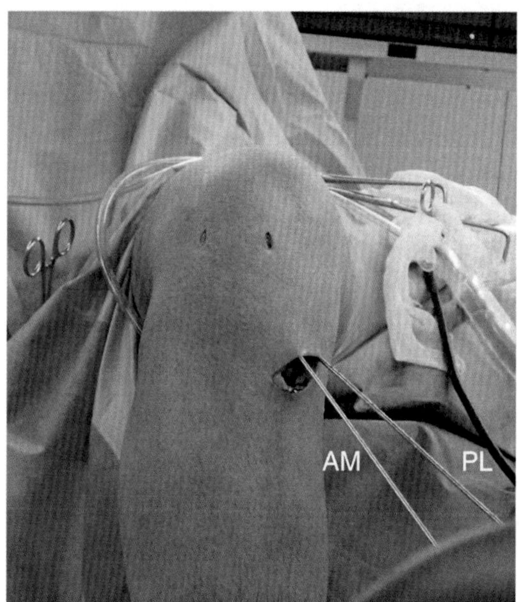

Fig. 6 Two guidewires of the posterolateral (*PL*) and anteromedial (*AM*) tunnels were inserted in the proximal tibia

anteroposterior view (Kondo et al. 2007) (Fig. 6). The given data will be useful for surgeons to evaluate the tunnel positions and standardization postoperatively in anatomic double-bundle reconstruction.

To create two femoral tunnels for the AM and PL bundles in the lateral condyle, first, a guidewire is drilled at the center of the femoral footprint of the AM bundle through the second tibial tunnel, by use of the previously described 5-mm offset guide system (Fig. 7a). With the use of this wire as a guide, a tunnel is made with a 4.5-mm cannulated drill. The length of the tunnel is measured with a scaled probe. The portal for an arthroscope is then changed to the medial infrapatellar portal because it is difficult to precisely identify the attachment of the PL bundle through the lateral infrapatellar portal. The surgeon again holds the tibia at 90° of knee flexion, keeping the femur horizontal. The surgeon manually holds the guidewire and aims it at the center of the PL bundle attachment on the femur through the tibial tunnel. Namely, a surgeon could draw an imaginary vertical line through the contact point between the lateral femoral condyle and the tibial plateau at 90° of knee flexion in the arthroscopic visual field (Fig. 5b). This line and the long axis of the ACL remnant are crossed at the point 5 mm anterior to the edge of the joint cartilage (Fig. 5b). The center of the normal attachment of the PL bundle is located approximately at this crossing point. The surgeon first hammers the wire into the

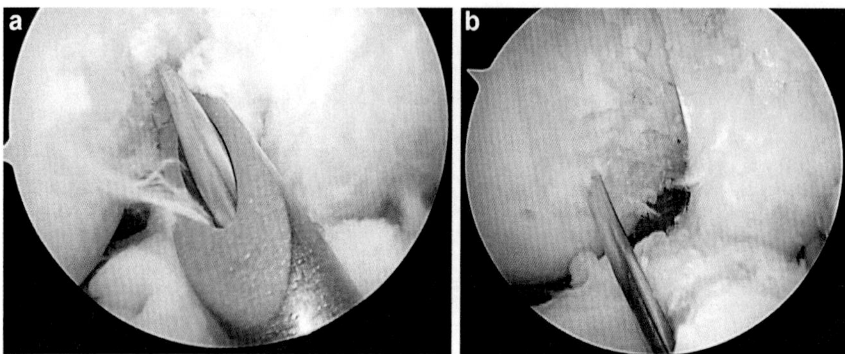

Fig. 7 (**a**) The center of the attachment of the anteromedial (*AM*) bundle was located at the point 5 mm distal from the back of the femur in measurements using the offset guide. (**b**) Insertion of a guidewire for the posterolateral (*PL*) bundle into the femur using the transtibial tunnel technique

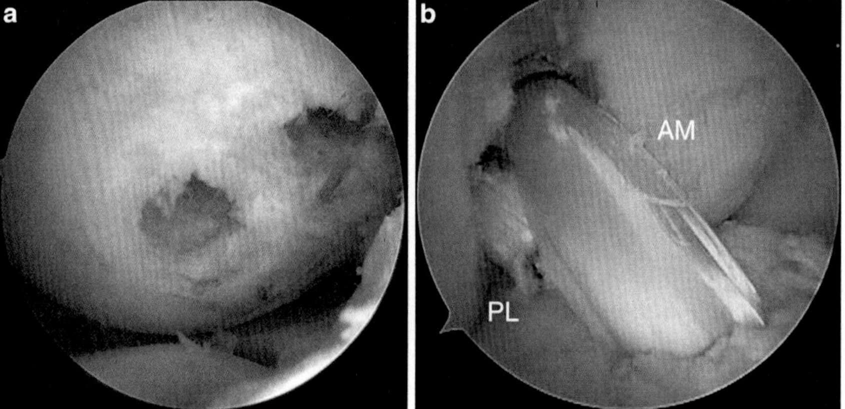

Fig. 8 (**a**) Two tunnels are independently created within the ACL remnant on the femur. (**b**) Two grafts transplanted across the knee joint at the time of surgery at 90° of knee flexion in arthroscopic view by use of the lateral infrapatellar portal. *AM* anteromedial bundle graft, *PL* posterolateral bundle graft

femur and then drills it (Fig. 7b). A 4.5-mm-diameter tunnel is drilled, and its length is measured in the same manner. Finally, two sockets are created for the AM and PL bundles, respectively, with cannulated drills for the Endobutton fixation system, the diameter of which is matched to the two grafts prepared with the technique described below (Fig. 8a).

Graft Tensioning and Fixation

The graft for the PL bundle is introduced through the tibial tunnel to the femoral tunnel using a passing pin. The Endobutton is carefully flipped on the femoral cortical surface. Then, the graft for the AM bundle is placed in the same manner (Fig. 8b). For graft tensioning, the knee is manually flexed to approximately 90° on the operating table. A spring tensiometer is attached at the each end of the polyester tape portion of the graft. An assistant surgeon simultaneously applies tension of 30 N to each graft for 2 min for avoiding graft tension relaxation. In the transtibial tunnel technique, the graft is easily applied an initial tension for avoiding graft impingement to the bone tunnel. Finally, for graft fixation, the knee is flexed to 10° with a sterilized thin pillow placed beneath the thigh, keeping the heel in contact with the operating table (Fig. 9). A surgeon applies tension of 30 N to each graft at 10° of knee flexion and

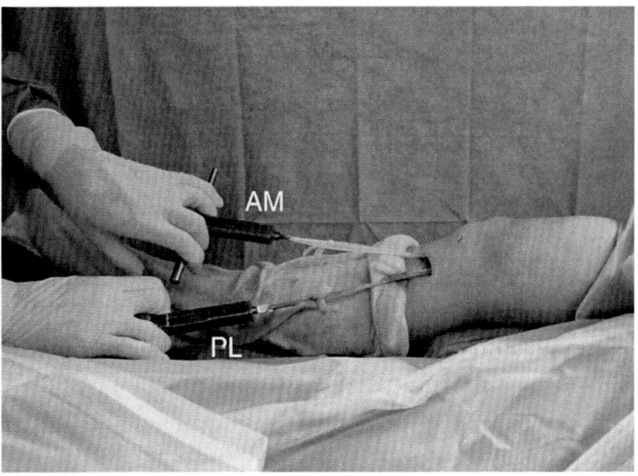

Fig. 9 A surgeon applied tension of 30 N to each graft at 10° of knee flexion and simultaneously secured the two tape portions onto the tibia using two spiked staples in the turnbuckle fashion

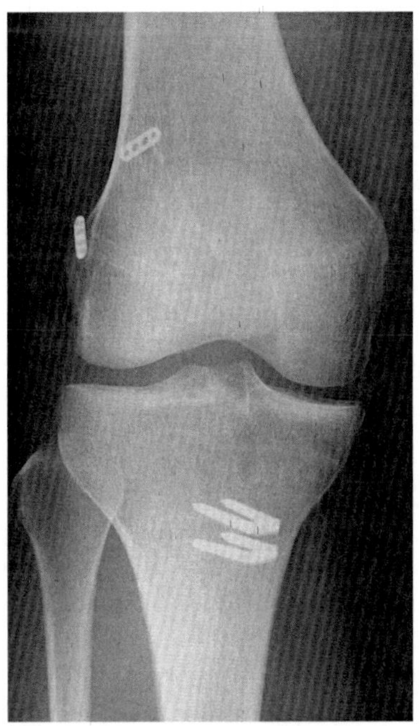

Fig. 10 Postoperative digital radiograph of anatomic double-bundle ACL reconstruction

simultaneously secured the two tape portions onto the tibia using two spiked staples in the turnbuckle fashion.

Postoperative computed digital radiograph (Fig. 10) and three-dimensional computed tomography (Fig. 11) show that each tunnel outlet was created at the center of the anatomical attachment of the AM and PL bundle of the ACL.

Postoperative Management

Postoperative management was performed according to an original rehabilitation protocol (Tohyama et al. 2011). On the basis of previous biomechanical studies, quadriceps and hamstring muscle training are encouraged immediately after surgery. The static squat exercise is started 1 week postoperatively. A postoperative immobilizer is applied for 2 weeks after the operation. Full weight bearing is then allowed with a hinged brace 2 weeks after surgery. Various kinds of athletic training are gradually allowed after 6 weeks, although no running is allowed until 4 months after surgery. Return to full sports activity is generally permitted at 9 months.

Biomechanical Evaluations

During anatomic double-bundle ACL reconstruction, graft tension of the AM and PL grafts was measured using specially designed strain gauge-type tensiometers (Yasuda et al. 2008). The tension-versus-flexion curve pattern of each graft was similar to the normal pattern (Fig. 12). Namely, the curve of the AM suture graft indicated that the tension was highest at full extension and then relaxed with knee flexion between 0 and 30°. The curve then showed a plateau between 30 and 90°, and the tension gradually increased

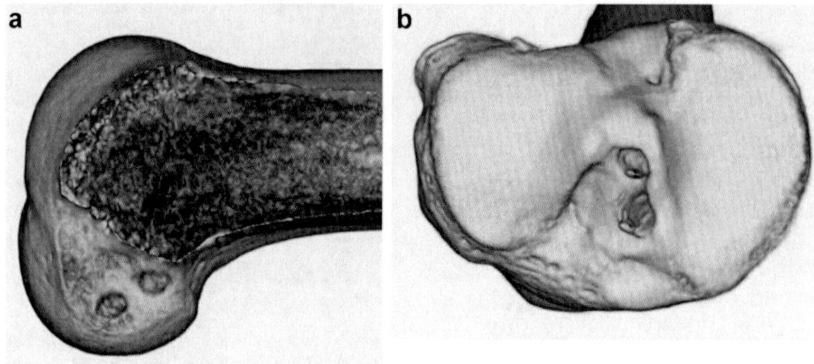

Fig. 11 Postoperative three-dimensional computed tomography showing that each tunnel outlet was created at the center of the anatomical attachment of the anteromedial and posterolateral bundle of the ACL

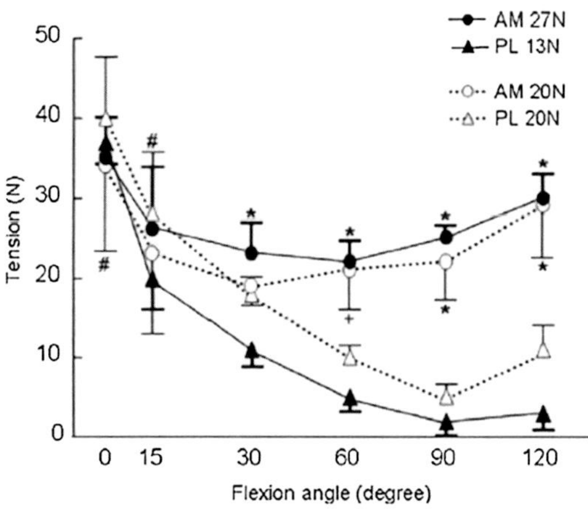

Fig. 12 Mean tension-versus-flexion curves of anteromedial (*AM*) and posterolateral (*PL*) grafts under different initial conditions (with bars showing SDs) (Reprinted with permission from Yasuda et al. 2008)

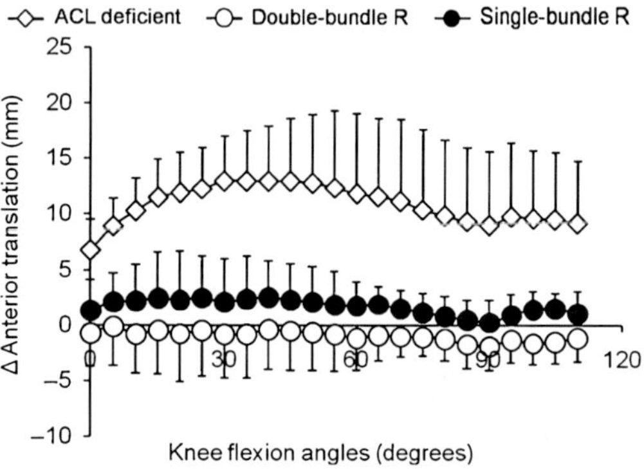

Fig. 13 The difference in anterior translation from the intact knee under 90-N anterior load. The error bars indicate standard deviation (mean and standard deviation). *ACL* anterior cruciate ligament, *R* reconstruction (Reprinted with permission from Kondo et al. 2010)

thereafter. On the other hand, the curve of the PL suture graft showed that the tension was highest at full extension and gradually relaxed with knee flexion between 0 and 90°. The tension increased thereafter. The initial tension significantly affected the absolute graft tension values at each knee flexion angle but did not significantly affect the curve patterns. Thus, these studies suggested that the clinical anatomic double-bundle procedures can reconstruct the knee having biomechanical functions closer to the normal range than single-bundle reconstruction if surgeons have sufficient surgical skills to precisely perform the appropriate anatomic double-bundle procedures.

Next, the anatomic double-bundle reconstruction procedure was compared with the conventional single-bundle procedure using cadaveric knees (Kondo et al. 2010). The knees were mounted in a 6 degree-of-freedom rig using the various loading conditions. Tibiofemoral kinematics was recorded with an optical tracking system for intact, ACL-deficient knee, anatomic double-bundle reconstruction, and conventional single-bundle reconstruction. Anterior laxity with anterior tibial load, rotational laxity with internal tibial torque, and anterior laxity in the simulated pivot-shift test were significantly less in the double-bundle reconstruction compared with the conventional single-bundle reconstruction (Fig. 13). This work suggests that the postoperative anterior translation and internal rotation stability after anatomic double-bundle ACL reconstruction were significantly better than after single-bundle reconstruction, in both static tests and the pivot shift.

Clinical Evaluations

In 2006 Yasuda et al. reported the first prospective comparative study to compare anatomic double-bundle procedure with conventional single-bundle and nonanatomic double-bundle (Rosenberg's) procedures in 72 patients (Yasuda et al. 2006). The side-to-side anterior laxity was significantly lower in the anatomic double-bundle group than in the single-bundle group, although there was no significant difference between the nonanatomic double-bundle and single-bundle groups. Concerning the pivot-shift test, the anatomic double-bundle group was significantly superior to the single-bundle group. There were no significant differences in the IKDC evaluation, the range of knee motion, and the quadriceps and hamstring muscle torque. In addition, the grafted tendons in 136 patients were morphologically evaluated using postoperative second-look arthroscopy (Kondo and Yasuda 2007). After anatomic double-bundle ACL reconstruction, the AM bundle was evaluated as excellent in 79.5 % of the cases, fair in 16.7 %, and poor in 3.8 %, and the PL bundle was evaluated as excellent in 75.8 %, fair in 21.2 %, and poor in 3.0 %. Both the AM and PL bundles were clearly visible after the anatomic double-bundle anterior cruciate ligament reconstruction at 1–2 years after surgery (Fig. 14). In 2008 Kondo et al. reported on a large prospective comparative study of 328 patients, in which the anatomic double-bundle group was significantly superior to the single-bundle group in terms of anterior laxity and pivot-shift testing (Kondo et al. 2008). There were no significant differences in the other clinical evaluations or the rate of complications (Table 1).

Discussion

Biomechanical studies have found that the anatomic double-bundle ACL reconstruction can restore knee stability significantly more closely to the normal level than the conventional single-bundle reconstruction (Kondo et al. 2010). Intraoperative measurement studies showed that the clinically available anatomic double-bundle procedures can reconstruct knee stability significantly better and improve knee function close to the normal level at the time immediately after surgery compared with the conventional single-bundle procedures (Yasuda et al. 2008). However, surgeon should note that the grafted tendon tissues are necrotized at first in any type of ACL reconstruction and then revascularized with mechanical deterioration (Kondo et al. 2012a). Therefore, short- and long-term follow-up studies are essential to evaluate the clinical utility of the anatomic double-bundle reconstruction. In previously published original trials using hamstring tendons, the anterior and/or rotatory stability of the knee was significantly better after the anatomic double-bundle ACL reconstruction than the conventional single-bundle reconstruction (Yasuda et al. 2006; Aglietti et al. 2007; Yagi et al. 2007; Muneta et al. 2007; Kondo et al. 2008;

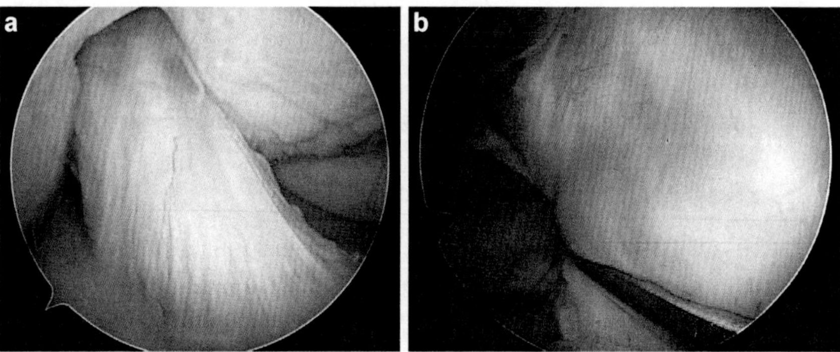

Fig. 14 (**a**) Arthroscopic view of transplanted anteromedial bundle graft. (**b**) Arthroscopic view of transplanted posterolateral bundle graft (Reprinted with permission from Kondo and Yasuda 2007)

Table 1 Comparisons in the clinical outcome between single-bundle and double-bundle groups (Reprinted with permission from Kondo et al. 2008)

	Single-bundle group (n = 157)	Double-bundle group (n = 171)
The loss of knee motion		
Loss of extension (>5°)	3 patients	7 patients
Loss of flexion (>15°)	9 patients	2 patients
The mean Lysholm knee score	96.5 (5.8) points	97.3 (3.3) points
The IKDC evaluation		
A (normal)	97 patients	110 patients
B (nearly normal)	48 patients	58 patients
C (nearly abnormal)	10 patients	3 patients
D (abnormal)	2 patients	0 patient
The mean isokinetic peak torque[a]		
Quadriceps muscle	88.9 (16.7) %	89.4 (14.4) %
Hamstring muscles	90.9 (20.4) %	94.3 (19.5) %

[a]The ratio (%) of the treated knee to the uninjured knee

Jarvela et al. 2008; Siebold et al. 2008). However, one original trial (Streich et al. 2008) and one meta-analysis study (Meredick et al. 2008) reported that there were no differences in the results between the two types of reconstructions. Thus, controversies on this issue still remain. In the actual clinical field, one of the most significant factors affecting the clinical outcome is the surgical skill of the surgeon who performs the anatomic double-bundle ACL reconstruction. It is most essential in anatomic double-bundle ACL reconstruction to create four independent tunnels at the center of the four anatomic attachments of the AM and PL bundles, respectively (Yasuda et al. 2004). Therefore, orthopedic surgeons who intend to perform the anatomic double-bundle ACL reconstruction should have sufficient training and surgical skills to perform the essence of the procedure. In previous reports, tunnel creation techniques for the anatomic AM and PL bundle reconstruction have been classified into a few different types: the transtibial tunnel technique, the transportal technique, and the double-incision outside-in technique. With each technique, it is possible for surgeons to create four independent tunnels at the center of the four anatomic attachments of the AM and PL bundles, respectively. However, the three techniques have both advantages and disadvantages. Therefore, orthopedic surgeons are required to master these techniques and should use the most suitable technique for each surgery.

In addition, an advanced system should have been established to more precisely measure the anterior and rotatory laxity after ACL reconstruction in the near future. There are clinically available devices to measure in vivo kinematics during athletic activities, and clinical evaluation criteria concerning the secondary injuries of the meniscus and the cartilage that occur during the long-term follow-up examination after ACL reconstruction. Efforts to establish a better evaluation system will advance ACL reconstruction surgery in the near future. At present time, many controversies remain in the field of anatomic double-bundle ACL reconstruction. Therefore, orthopedic surgeons should not discard any method of single- and anatomic double-bundle reconstruction. Further clinical studies are needed to establish the utility of each procedure. However, the anatomic double-bundle reconstruction will provide patients with ACL insufficiency at least an option when considering ACL reconstruction procedures, particularly when the hamstring tendons are used as a graft tissue.

Cross-References

- ▶ Anatomic Double-Tunnel Anterior Cruciate Ligament Reconstruction: Evolution and Principles
- ▶ Anterior Cruciate Ligament Graft Selection and Fixation
- ▶ Anterior Cruciate Ligament Injuries and Surgery: Current Evidence and Modern Development
- ▶ Alternative Techniques for Double-Tunnel Anatomic Anterior Cruciate Ligament Reconstruction
- ▶ Different Techniques of Anterior Cruciate Ligament Reconstruction: Guidelines

- ▶ Graft Remodeling and Bony Ingrowth After Anterior Cruciate Ligament Reconstruction
- ▶ Perioperative and Postoperative Anterior Cruciate Ligament Rehabilitation Focused on Soft Tissue Grafts
- ▶ Personalized Treatment Algorithms for Anterior Cruciate Ligament Injuries
- ▶ Single Versus Double Anterior Cruciate Ligament Reconstruction in Athletes
- ▶ State of the Art in Anterior Cruciate Ligament Surgery
- ▶ Structured Rehabilitation Model with Clinical Outcomes After Anterior Cruciate Ligament Reconstruction

References

Adachi N, Ochi M, Uchio Y et al (2004) Reconstruction of the anterior cruciate ligament. Single- versus double-bundle multistranded hamstring tendons. J Bone Joint Surg (Br) 86:515–520

Aglietti P, Giron F, Cuomo P et al (2007) Single- and double-incision double-bundle ACL reconstruction. Clin Orthop Relat Res 454:108–113

Amis A, Dawkins GPC (1991) Functional anatomy of the anterior cruciate ligament: fiber bundle actions related to ligament replacement and injuries. J Bone Joint Surg (Br) 73:260–267

Hamada M, Shino K, Horibe S et al (2001) Single- versus bisocket anterior cruciate ligament reconstruction using autogenous multiple-stranded hamstring tendons with Endobutton femoral fixation: a prospective study. Arthroscopy 17:801–807

Inagaki Y, Kondo E, Kitamura N et al (2013) Prospective clinical comparisons of semitendinosus versus semitendinosus and gracilis tendon autografts for anatomic double-bundle anterior cruciate ligament reconstruction. J Orthop Sci 18:754–761

Jarvela T, Moisala AS, Sihvonen R et al (2008) Double-bundle anterior cruciate ligament reconstruction using hamstring autografts and bioabsorbable interference screw fixation: prospective, randomized clinical study with two-year results. Am J Sports Med 36:290–297

Kai S, Kondo E, Kitamura N et al (2013) A quantitative technique to create a femoral tunnel at the averaged center of the anteromedial bundle attachment in anatomic double-bundle anterior cruciate ligament reconstruction. BMC Musculoskelet Disord 14:189

Kondo E, Yasuda K (2007) Second-look arthroscopic evaluations of anatomic double-bundle anterior cruciate ligament reconstruction: relation with postoperative knee stability. Arthroscopy 23:1198–1209

Kondo E, Yasuda K, Ichiyama H et al (2007) Radiologic evaluation of femoral and tibial tunnels created with the transtibial tunnel technique for anatomic double-bundle anterior cruciate ligament reconstruction. Arthroscopy 23:869–876

Kondo E, Yasuda K, Azuma H et al (2008) Prospective clinical comparisons of anatomic double-bundle versus single-bundle anterior cruciate ligament reconstruction procedures in 328 consecutive patients. Am J Sports Med 36:1675–1687

Kondo E, Merican AM, Yasuda K et al (2010) Biomechanical comparisons of knee stability after anterior cruciate ligament reconstruction between 2 clinically available transtibial procedures: anatomic double bundle versus single bundle. Am J Sports Med 38:1349–1358

Kondo E, Yasuda K, Katsura T et al (2012a) Biomechanical and histological evaluations of the doubled semitendinosus tendon autograft after anterior cruciate ligament reconstruction in sheep. Am J Sports Med 40:315–324

Kondo E, Yasuda K, Miyatake S et al (2012b) Clinical comparison of two suspensory fixation devices for anatomic double-bundle anterior cruciate ligament reconstruction. Knee Surg Sports Traumatol Arthrosc 20:1261–1267

Meredick RB, Vance KJ, Appleby D et al (2008) Outcome of single-bundle versus double-bundle reconstruction of the anterior cruciate ligament: a meta-analysis. Am J Sports Med 36:1414–1421

Mott HW (1983) Semitendinosus anatomic reconstruction for cruciate ligament insufficiency. Clin Orthop Relat Res 172:90–92

Muneta T, Sekiya I, Yagishita K et al (1999) Two-bundle reconstruction of the anterior cruciate ligament using semitendinosus tendon with Endobuttons: operative technique and preliminary results. Arthroscopy 15:618–624

Muneta T, Koga H, Mochizuki T et al (2007) A prospective randomized study of 4-strand semitendinosus tendon anterior cruciate ligament reconstruction comparing single-bundle and double-bundle techniques. Arthroscopy 23:618–628

Sakane M, Fox RJ, Woo SL et al (1997) In situ forces in the anterior cruciate ligament and its bundles in response to anterior tibial loads. J Orthop Res 15:285–293

Siebold R, Dehler C, Ellert T (2008) Prospective randomized comparison of double-bundle versus single-bundle anterior cruciate ligament reconstruction. Arthroscopy 24:137–145

Streich NA, Friedrich K, Gotterbarm T et al (2008) Reconstruction of the ACL with a semitendinosus tendon graft: a prospective randomized single blinded comparison of double bundle versus single-bundle technique in male athletes. Knee Surg Sports Traumatol Arthrosc 16:232–238

Tohyama H, Kondo E, Hayashi R et al (2011) Gender-based differences in outcome after anatomic double-bundle anterior cruciate ligament reconstruction with hamstring tendon autografts. Am J Sports Med 39:1849–1857

Yagi M, Kuroda R, Nagamune K et al (2007) Double bundle ACL reconstruction can improve rotational stability. Clin Orthop Relat Res 454:100–107

Yasuda K, Tsujino J, Ohkoshi Y et al (1995) Graft site morbidity with autogenous semitendinosus and gracilis tendons. Am J Sports Med 23:706–714

Yasuda K, Tsujino J, Tanabe Y et al (1997) Effects of initial graft tension on clinical outcome after anterior cruciate ligament reconstruction: autogenous doubled hamstring tendons connected in series with polyester tapes. Am J Sports Med 25:99–106

Yasuda K, Kondo E, Ichiyama H et al (2004) Anatomical reconstruction of the anteromedial and posterolateral bundles of the anterior cruciate ligament using hamstring tendon grafts. Arthroscopy 20:1015–1025

Yasuda K, Kondo E, Ichiyama H et al (2006) Clinical evaluation of anatomic double-bundle anterior cruciate ligament reconstruction procedure using hamstring tendon grafts: comparisons among 3 different procedures. Arthroscopy 22:240–251

Yasuda K, Ichiyama H, Kondo E et al (2008) An in vivo biomechanical study on the tension-versus-knee flexion angle curves of 2 grafts in anatomic double-bundle anterior cruciate ligament reconstruction: effects of initial tension and internal tibial rotation. Arthroscopy 24:276–284

Zaricznyj B (1987) Reconstruction of the anterior cruciate ligament of the knee using a doubled tendon graft. Clin Orthop Relat Res 220:162–175

Factors Affecting Return to Sport After Anterior Cruciate Ligament Reconstruction

86

Alberto Gobbi, Georgios Karnatzikos, and Dnyanesh G. Lad

Contents

A. Gobbi (✉) • G. Karnatzikos • D.G. Lad
Orthopaedic Arthroscopic Surgery International (O.A.S.I.)
Bioresearch Foundation, Gobbi Onlus, Milan, Italy
e-mail: gobbi@cartilagedoctor.it;
info@oasibioresearchfoundation.org; giokarnes@gmail.com; dnyaneshlad@gmail.com; fellow@oasiortopedia.it

M.N. Doral, J. Karlsson (eds.), *Sports Injuries*,
DOI 10.1007/978-3-642-36569-0_264

Abstract

Athletes with an ACL injury commonly ask when they will be able to return to sport. The answer has always been ambiguous, ranging from a few weeks to a few months. Some athletes, even after ACL reconstruction and completion of the prescribed rehabilitation, are unable to resume their pre-injury activities. It is important to identify factors which will determine the athletes' ability to return to sport. Standard knee scales are a valuable tool for evaluating the progression of knee recovery following ACL reconstruction. However, the psychological profile and motivation of the patient are also important.

Introduction

The risk of anterior cruciate ligament (ACL) injury is significantly greater in individuals who participate in pivoting sport. At present, ACL reconstruction is the gold standard after its injury in the young athletic population (Dye et al. 1998). The most widely used techniques for reconstruction include patellar tendon and hamstring autograft or allografts (Jarvinen et al. 1995; Aglietti et al. 1997; Frank and Jackson 1997; Gobbi et al. 2003a, b). The combined use of a strong graft and good fixation with an appropriate rehabilitation program should restore the knee function and allow the return to sport. However, there are those who even after ACL reconstruction and completion of the prescribed rehabilitation are unable to resume their pre-injury activities (Gobbi and Francisco 2006). This problem is most pronounced in the athletic population where expectations and demands are higher when compared to sedentary or even normal individuals (Daniel et al. 1994; Nakayama et al. 2000; Jerre et al. 2001; Pantano et al. 2001). Few studies have assessed the effectiveness of specific rehabilitation protocols with regard to restoring normal muscle strength, balance, proprioception, and other neuromuscular indices required for high-risk activities such as cutting, twisting, and pivoting. Outcome assessment after ACL reconstruction has commonly used knee scoring systems like the Lysholm, Noyes, International Knee Documentation Committee (IKDC), and Tegner scores with success usually equated with acceptable restoration of measurable parameters such as strength, stability, and functional level (Lysholm et al. 1982, 1984; Tegner and Lysholm 1985; Noyes et al. 1989; Hefti et al. 1993; Sgaglione et al. 1995; Senert et al. 1999). Additional evaluation schemes like the Marx scale (knee activity rating scale) can also be used; this scale enables the measurement of activity rather than the health status of the patient by assessing the frequency of specific physical tasks that normally are difficult for someone who has a pathologic knee condition (Marx et al. 2001). Furthermore, attention should be placed on the patient's psychological profile because this also can contribute to the treatment outcome (Goh and Boyle 1997; Morrey 1999). Kinesiophobia (fear of movement) stems from an athlete associating certain activities with a repeated ACL injury. Although a certain element of fear is natural, increased levels of kinesiophobia may well correlate with a lack of return to sport (Flanigan et al. 2013).

Assessment of Factors

One hundred athlete patients who met the inclusion criteria were evaluated (Gobbi and Francisco 2006).

Inclusion Criteria:

1. Nonprofessional athletes playing in competitive sport at regional or national level or participating in recreational sport at least three times per week
2. Patients with a normal contralateral knee
3. Patients who have had partial meniscectomies
4. Those willing to follow-up at 3, 6, 12, and 24 months
5. Those that were willing to follow a standard postoperative rehabilitation program

Exclusion criteria:

1. Previous open knee surgery
2. Injury to the contralateral knee
3. Grade III–IV chondral damage and significant associated ligament injury requiring reconstruction

Through a simple random sampling technique, the 100 athletes [67 males, 33 females, mean age of 28 years (17–50 years)] were assigned with the specific type of reconstruction technique to be used – patellar tendon (PT) reconstruction and hamstring tendon (HT) reconstruction. All the athletes reported ACL injury during participation in sport activities (Table 1). The mean interval from injury to knee reconstruction was 8.9 months. Eight patients had minor previous surgery on the involved knee consisting of diagnostic arthroscopy with partial meniscectomy. All surgeries were performed by the same surgeon, while

Table 1 Sport activity in patients who had ACL reconstruction

Sport activity (PT)	No. of patients	Sport activity (HT)	No. of patients
Soccer	16	Skiing	21
Skiing	9	Soccer	14
Motocross	8	Motocross	6
Basketball	5	Trekking	2
Volleyball	4	Tennis	2
Cycling	3	Volleyball	1
Tennis	2	Karate	1
Running	1	Swimming	1
Gymnastics	1	Aerobics	1
Horseback riding	1	Basketball	1
Total	50		50

PT patellar tendon, *HT* hamstring tendon

Table 2 Psychological data questionnaire

	Not important	Slightly important	Very important
How important is it for you to be involved in competitive sport?	1	2	3
How fast do you expect to return to your sport after surgery?	1 year (1)	6 months (2)	3 months (3)
How much time are you willing to spend for rehabilitation after surgery?	Once a week (1)	3 times a week (2)	Every day (3)
Do you have any doubts in your ability to return to your previous sport?	Yes (0)		No (3)
Would you be content if after your surgery you can only manage to go back to an activity level that is less than your pre-injury sporting level?	Yes (0)		No (3)
After your surgery, would you be willing to settle for a less strenuous sporting activity than you were previously engaged in?	Yes (0)		No (3)

rehabilitation was conducted for 6 months in the same rehabilitation center.

To document the progression of the patients' recovery, clinical evaluations were conducted by the surgeon and a physical therapist preoperatively and then at 3, 6, and 12 months following the ACL reconstruction. Final follow-up was performed at a minimum of 24 months by an independent examiner. Subjective and objective assessment was conducted using the IKDC evaluation scales. Further evaluations were carried out using the Lysholm, Noyes, and Tegner scales. In addition, the single assessment numeric evaluation (SANE) was used to subjectively assess their knee function and symptoms; computerized analysis of anterior knee laxity was performed using the OSI CA 4000 arthrometer (Orthopedic System Inc., Hayward, CA, USA) preoperatively and then at 6 and 12 months (Neuschwander et al. 1996).

Isokinetic testing for analysis of muscle strength was performed with Biodex multijoint system (Biodex, Shirley, NY, USA) at 3, 6, and 12 months after surgery. The maximum peak torque in flexion and extension was determined at speeds of 60, 180, and 300°/s, and the total work ratio and the hamstring/quadriceps ratio were calculated. A knee activity rating scale (Marx scale) was also used preoperatively and at final follow-up to measure the patients' activities and the frequency by which they are able to perform specific physical tasks that would be difficult for someone who has a pathologic knee condition. The scores range from 0 to 16; a higher score indicates a better functional capacity on the part of the patient to resume pre-injury activity levels. To determine the patients' psychological profile, a specific questionnaire (psychovitality) was administered prior to surgery (Table 2).

Patient Evaluation

Knee Scores

Objective IKDC knee scores of normal or nearly normal, obtained of the 100 patients treated, demonstrated a significant improvement ($P < 0.05$) from preoperative values. Eighty-eight percent of PT- and 90 % of HT-reconstructed knees attained normal or nearly normal knees (IKDC A or B) on final evaluation which was not significant.

The mean Tegner activity score demonstrated no significant difference ($P > 0.05$) from 7.6 points pre-injury to 6 points on final follow-up.

The mean Noyes and Lysholm scores, on the other hand, showed statistical improvement (Fig. 1). The mean subjective knee score of 47 points preoperatively improved to 85 points at final follow-up among the 100 patients treated using the IKDC evaluation form which compared the injured knee to the patient's uninjured contralateral knee.

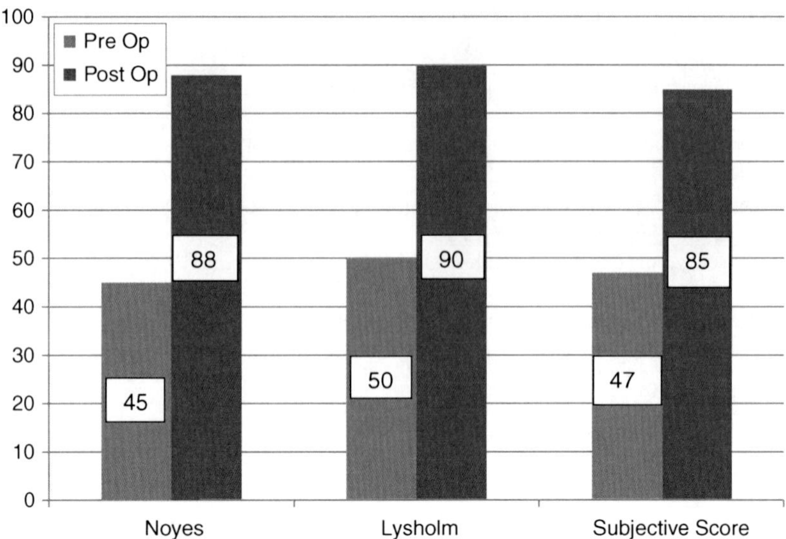

Fig. 1 Preop and post-op knee scores

Analyzing the scores obtained in terms of the type of graft used revealed no significant difference ($P < 0.05$).

Comparing the scores obtained by those who "returned to sport" against those who "did not return at the same level of sport activity" revealed no significant differences. In the same way, patients who completely ceased participation in sport activity demonstrated no significant differences from those who "returned to sport at a lower level."

Isokinetic tests and computed analysis conducted at 60°/s 3 months following surgery demonstrated decreased quadriceps strength in the PT group and decreased hamstring strength in the HT group. Tests conducted at 60, 180, and 300°/s in extension 1 year postoperatively demonstrated no statistically significant difference between the PT and HT groups. One-year evaluation in flexion revealed significant difference ($P = 0.0164$) in HT group at 60 and 180°/s, while at 300°/s no difference was detected.

Anterior laxity tests performed with computed analysis (OSI) carried out at 3 months and 1 and 2 years from knee reconstruction demonstrated 90 % of the 100 patients treated to have less than 3 mm side-to-side difference, 8 % with 3–5 mm difference, and 2 % to have more than 5 mm difference; no statistically significant difference was noted among the two grafts.

Knee Activity Rating Scale (Marx Scale)

Scores obtained from 26 of the 35 patients who "did not return to sport" had a mean of 7.5 points (0–16) with only 17.1 % obtaining a score $\geq$15 points. This group of patients reported some difficulty in resuming running, cutting, decelerating, and pivoting activities. On the other hand, a mean score of 15 points (9–16) was documented among 26 of the 65 patients who "returned to sport." In this group, 53.3 % scored $\geq$15 points because they did not encounter any difficulty doing the same activities. Statistical analysis demonstrated a significant difference ($P < 0.001$) between patients who "returned" and those who "did not return" to their previous sport.

Psychovitality Questionnaire (Table 2)

Data from the psychological questionnaire administered before surgery demonstrated that 28.6 % of the athletes that "did not return to sport" scored $\geq$15 points. On the other hand, 67 % of the athletes that "returned to sport" scored $\geq$15 points. Statistical analysis using the Mann–Whitney *U* test revealed a significant difference ($P < 0.001$) between these two groups. Athletes who were able to return to previous sport had a mean score of 16.5, while those

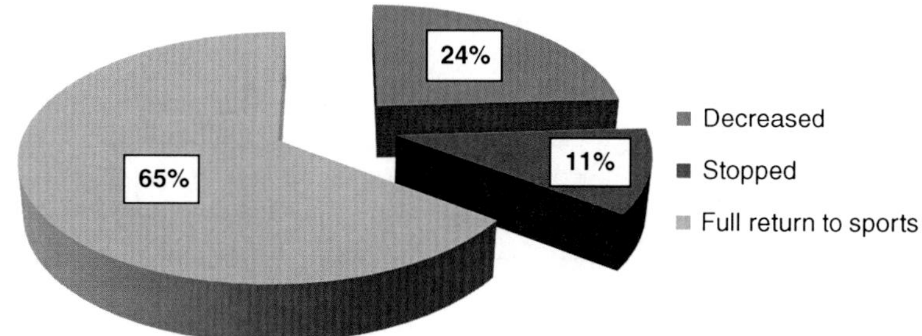

Fig. 2 Outcomes following ACL reconstruction

Table 3 Factors related to patients' inability to return to sport

Graft type	Reason for inability to return to sport	No. of patients
	Fear of new injury	2
Patellar tendon	Pain due to chondropathy	2
	Extensor deficit	1
	Reasons unrelated to surgery	1
Hamstring tendon	Strength deficit	2
	Pain related to chondropathy	1
	Pain at tibial fixation site	1
	Reasons unrelated to surgery	1

who changed or completely stopped any sport activity had an average score of 9 points.

Return to Sport

The reason for inability to return to sport is described in Fig. 2 and Table 3.

Discussion

ACL reconstruction in athletes is carried out to achieve a stable knee that will enable them to return to their desired activities. For athletes with an ACL tear, the outcome of reconstruction becomes more important because expectations of returning to pre-injury activity levels are usually higher. Unfortunately, even with the present techniques in knee reconstruction, a successful return to sport cannot be guaranteed. Restoration of mechanical restraints is the initial step in achieving knee functional recovery, but factors including the patient's motivation and willingness to complete the prescribed rehabilitation program may also play a role in influencing outcome.

Commonly utilized knee evaluation scales remain good indicators in evaluating the results of ACL reconstructions. In those cases, where return to the same level of previous sport after ACL reconstruction is not achieved, two additional scales can be utilized: the knee activity rating scale (Marx scale) and the psychovitality questionnaire (Noyes et al. 1983, 1989; Sgaglione et al. 1995; Senert et al. 1999). The Marx scale questions the components of physical function common to different sporting activities, putting more focus on measuring activity rather than health status.

The psychological questionnaire, on the other hand, focuses on factors like the patient's commitment, willingness, and interest in resuming pre-injury activity levels. Information extracted from these additional scales can provide the data necessary to go beyond the objective measures available with standard knee scales. The importance of using these two questionnaires cannot be undermined especially in cases where good results with IKDC, Lysholm, Tegner, and Noyes scales are obtained, and yet the athlete remains unable to resume previous activity levels.

This study demonstrated that only 65 % of athletes were able to resume the same sport activity at the same level following ACL reconstruction, while the remaining 35 % for various reasons decreased their level of activity (24 %) or completely ceased sport participation (11 %) (Table 3).

Aglietti et al. (1997) and Jarvinen et al. (1995) demonstrated similar results in their studies with

53 % and 40 % patients, respectively, "returned to sport" following knee reconstruction. On the other hand, Nakayama et al. (2000) reported a 92 % incidence of return to sport among 50 young athletes reviewed. However, in all these studies mentioned, the main focus was on the technique utilized for reconstruction (PT vs. HT) followed by analysis of outcome using standard knee rating scales. In cases where less satisfactory results were obtained, possible contributory factors were enumerated but not thoroughly discussed.

Restoration of ligament stability is just one of several factors required to facilitate return of athletes to sport. Patient selection, type of sport, and factors which include pain, patellofemoral dysfunction, change in lifestyle, rehabilitation, and concomitant injuries to the joint may lead to a less than desired result in an ACL-reconstructed knee (Noyes et al. 1983; Macdonald et al. 1996). In a recently published article, Flanigan et al. have reported that teen and young adults who are less likely to be affected by life-related events like marriage, childbirth, and increased job demands (commonly cited by non-returners) have a greater potential to return to sport than an older athlete (Flanigan et al. 2013).

Some studies emphasized the importance of early recovery of knee function as a significant determinant of the long-term outcome of reconstructed knees (Noyes et al. 1989; Neuschwander et al. 1996; Senert et al. 1999). Furthermore, other factors such as proprioception and neuromuscular control have also been cited to influence the outcome (Solomonow et al. 1987; Wojtys and Huston 1994, 2000; Adachi et al. 2002; Ochi et al. 2002). In general, a progressive neuromuscular control rehabilitation program should be made to minimize the risk of injury and to promote a greater chance of successful return to competition (Lephart et al. 1997; Friden et al. 2001; Georgoulis et al. 2001; Risberg et al. 2001; Beynnon et al. 2002).

Psychological profile of patients has been found to exert a certain degree of influence in the final outcome of treatment. Morrey et al. (1999) demonstrated that significant mood changes throughout rehabilitation may be a contributing factor to poor psychological and physical outcomes. Furthermore, Pantano et al. (2001) emphasized that a variety of psychosocial factors including motivation influence the level of activity following surgical procedures. It is important for the surgeon to also understand the etiology of kinesiophobia. Although a lot is not yet known of this entity, Picavet et al. have reported that kinesiophobia and pain catastrophizing (an exaggerated psychological response in anticipation of pain) were definitely associated with lower activity levels (Picavet et al. 2002). The recognition of the variety of factors influencing the outcome following an ACL reconstruction is important, especially when developing a sport-specific postoperative rehabilitation program focused on facilitating the full return of athletes to previous levels of activity.

In a systematic review published in 2011, Arden et al. concluded that only about half of patients return to competitive sport after ACL reconstruction surgery. Also, approximately 90 % of patients achieved successful outcomes in terms of impairment-based measures of knee function after ACL reconstruction surgery, which suggests that factors other than knee function could be contributing to the lack of return to sport (Arden et al. 2011).

Conclusions

The most common question asked after an ACL reconstruction is "Doctor, when will I be able to play again?" This question may be asked not only by the athlete, but by parents, teammates, coaches, and sometimes even the media. The answer has always been ambiguous, ranging from a few weeks to a few months. It is important hence to identify factors which will determine the athletes' ability to return to sport. Standard knee scales like IKDC, Lysholm, Noyes, and Tegner are valuable tools for evaluating the progression of knee recovery following ACL reconstruction. However, the psychological profile and motivation of the patient are also important. The additional use of the Marx knee activity rating scale and the psychovitality evaluation can provide additional data on the patient's functional capabilities and psychological profile which could be useful in determining the capacity of athletes to resume pre-injury activity levels.

Cross-References

- Perioperative and Postoperative Anterior Cruciate Ligament Rehabilitation Focused on Soft Tissue Grafts
- Return to the Field for Football (Soccer) After Anterior Cruciate Ligament Reconstruction: Guidelines
- Structured Rehabilitation Model with Clinical Outcomes After Anterior Cruciate Ligament Reconstruction

References

Adachi N, Ochi M, Uchio Y et al (2002) Mechanoreceptors in the anterior cruciate ligament contribute to the joint position sense. Acta Orthop Scand 73:330–334

Aglietti P, Buzzi R, Zaccherotti G et al (1997) A comparison between patellar tendon versus doubled semitendinosus/gracilis tendon for anterior cruciate ligament reconstruction. A minimum five year follow-up. J Sports Traumatol Relat Res 19:57–68

Arden CL, Webster KE, Taylor NF, Feller JA (2011) Return to sport following anterior cruciate reconstruction surgery: a systematic review and meta-analysis of the state of play. Br J Sports Med 45:596–606

Beynnon BD, Johnson RJ, Fleming BC (2002) The science of anterior cruciate ligament rehabilitation. Clin Orthop 402:9–20

Daniel D, Stone M, Dobson B et al (1994) Fate of the ACL-injured patient. A prospective outcome study. Am J Sports Med 22(5):632–644

Dye S, Wojtys E, Fu F et al (1998) Factors contributing to function of the knee joint after injury of reconstruction of the anterior cruciate ligament. J Bone Joint Surg 80A:1380–1393

Flanigan D, Everhart J, Pedroza A, Smith T, Kaeding C (2013) Fear of reinjury (kinesiophobia) and persistent knee symptoms Are common factors for lack of return to sport after anterior cruciate ligament reconstruction. Arthrosc: J Arthrosc Relat Surg 29(8):1322–1329

Frank CB, Jackson DW (1997) The science of reconstruction of the anterior cruciate ligament. J Bone Joint Surg 79A:1556–1576

Friden T, Roberts D, Ageberg E et al (2001) Review of knee proprioception and the relation to extremity function after an anterior cruciate ligament rupture. J Orthop Sports Phys Ther 31:567–576

Georgoulis AD, Pappa L, Moebius U et al (2001) The presence of proprioceptive mechanoreceptors in the remnants of the ruptured ACL as a possible source of re-innervation of the ACL autograft. Knee Surg Sports Traumatol Arthrosc 9:364–368

Gobbi A, Francisco R (2006) Factors affecting return to sports after anterior cruciate ligament reconstruction with patellar tendon and hamstring graft: a prospective clinical investigation. Knee Surg Sports Traumatol Arthrosc 14:1021–1028

Gobbi A, Tuy B, Mahajan S et al (2003a) Quadrupled bone-semitendinosus anterior cruciate ligament reconstruction: a clinical investigation in a group of athletes. Arthroscopy 19(7):691–699

Gobbi A, Tuy B, Mahajan S et al (2003b) Patellar tendon versus quadrupled bone-semitendinosus anterior cruciate ligament reconstruction: a prospective clinical investigation in athletes. Arthroscopy 19(6): 592–601

Goh S, Boyle J (1997) Self-evaluation and functional testing two to four years post ACL reconstruction. Aust J Physiother 43:255–262

Hefti F, Muller W, Jakob R et al (1993) Evaluation of knee ligament injuries with the IKDC form. Knee Surg Sports Traumatol Arthrosc 1:226–234

Jarvinen M, Natri A, Lehto M et al (1995) Reconstruction of chronic anterior cruciate ligament insufficiency in athletes using a bone-patellar tendon bone autograft. Int Orthop 19:1–6

Jerre R, Ejerhed L, Wallmon A et al (2001) Functional outcome of anterior cruciate ligament reconstruction in recreational and competitive athletes. Scand J Med Sci Sports 11(6):342–346

Lephart SM, Pincivero DM, Giraldo JL et al (1997) Current concepts: the role of proprioception in the management and rehabilitation of athletic injuries. J Bone Joint Surg 25B:130–137

Lysholm J, Gilquist J (1982) Evaluation of knee ligament surgery results with special emphasis on use of a scoring scale. Am J Sports Med 10:150–154

Lysholm J, Tegner Y, Gilquist J (1984) Functional importance of different clinical findings in the unstable knee. Acta Orthop Scand 55:472

Macdonald PB, Hedden D, Pacin O et al (1996) Proprioception in anterior cruciate ligament-deficient and reconstructed knees. Am J Sports Med 24:774–778

Marx R, Stump T, Jones E et al (2001) Development and evaluation of an activity rating scale for disorders of the knee. Am J Sports Med 29(2):213–218

Morrey MA, Stuart MJ, Smith AM et al (1999) A longitudinal examination of athletes' emotional and cognitive responses to anterior cruciate ligament. Clin J Sport Med 9:63–69

Nakayama Y, Shirai Y, Narita T et al (2000) Knee functions and a return to sports activity in competitive athletes following anterior cruciate ligament reconstruction. J Nippon Med Sch 67:172–176

Neuschwander D, Drez D Jr, Heck S (1996) Pain dysfunction syndrome of the knee. Orthopaedics 19(1):27–32

Noyes FR, Matthews DS, Mooar PA et al (1983) The symptomatic anterior cruciate deficient knee. Part II: the results of rehabilitation, activity modification and counseling on functional disability. J Bone Joint Surg 65A:163–174

Noyes FR, Barber SD, Mooar LA (1989) A rationale for assessing sports activity levels and limitations in knee disorders. Clin Orthop 246:238–249

Ochi M, Iwasa J, Uchio Y et al (2002) Induction of somatosensory evoked potentials by mechanical stimulation in reconstructed anterior cruciate ligaments. J Bone Joint Surg 84B:761–766

Pantano KJ, Irrgang JJ, Burdett R et al (2001) A pilot study on the relationship between physical impairment and activity restriction in persons with anterior cruciate ligament reconstruction at long-term follow-up. Knee Surg Sports Traumatol Arthrosc 9:369–378

Picavet HS, Vlaeyen JW, Schouten JS (2002) Pain catastrophizing and kinesiophobia: predictors of chronic low back pain. Am J Epidemiol 156:1028–1034

Risberg MA, Mork M, Jenssen HK et al (2001) Design and implementation of a neuromuscular training program following anterior cruciate ligament reconstruction. J Orthop Sports Phys Ther 31:620–631

Senert N, Kartus J, Kohler K et al (1999) Analysis of subjective, objective and functional examination tests after anterior cruciate ligament reconstruction. A follow-up of 527 patients. Knee Surg Sports Traumatol Arthrosc 7:160–165

Sgaglione N, Del Pizzo W, Fox J et al (1995) Critical analysis of knee ligament rating systems. Am J Sports Med 23:660–667

Solomonow M, Baratta R, Zhou BH et al (1987) The synergistic action of the anterior cruciate ligament and thigh muscles in maintaining joint stability. Am J Sports Med 15:207–213

Tegner Y, Lysholm J (1985) Rating systems in the evaluation of knee ligament injuries. Clin Orthop 1958:43–49

Wojtys WM, Huston LJ (1994) Neuromuscular performance in normal and anterior cruciate ligament-deficient lower extremities. Am J Sports Med 22:89–104

Wojtys WM, Huston LJ (2000) Longitudinal effects of anterior cruciate ligament injury and patellar tendon autograft reconstruction on neuromuscular performance. Am J Sports Med 28:336–344

Knee Ligament Surgery: Future Perspectives

87

Megan Wolf, Christopher D. Murawski, Bart Muller, Marcus Hofbauer, James Ward, and Freddie H. Fu

Contents

Abstract

Ligament injuries are commonly encountered in sports medicine. Current research is focused upon the augmentation of healing after ligament injury and reconstruction (an emphasis placed on anterior cruciate ligament (ACL) reconstruction) with the use of biological substances or biomechanical techniques. The evolution of surgical techniques to more anatomical reconstructions and rehabilitation focused upon graft healing can possibly decrease the rate of failure. An objective assessment of graft healing with tools such as magnetic resonance imaging may provide valuable insight as to when a person should be cleared to return to athletic participation. Ultimately, the goal of ligament repair and reconstruction is to individualize both the surgery and the recovery to meet each patient's anatomy and lifestyle.

M. Wolf (✉) • C.D. Murawski • F.H. Fu
Department of Orthopaedic Surgery, University of Pittsburgh School of Medicine, Pittsburgh, PA, USA
e-mail: orthowolf15@gmail.com; cdmurawski@gmail.com; ffu@upmc.edu

B. Muller
Department of Orthopaedic Surgery, University of Pittsburgh, Pittsburgh, PA, USA

Department of Orthopaedic Surgery, Academic Medical Center, University of Amsterdam, Amsterdam, NH, Netherlands
e-mail: bart.muller@live.nl

M. Hofbauer
Department of Trauma Surgery, Medical University of Vienna, Vienna, Austria
e-mail: marcus.hofbauer@meduniwien.ac.at

J. Ward
Department of Orthopaedic Surgery, University of Pittsburgh Medical Center, Pittsburgh, PA, USA
e-mail: jamespward@gmail.com

M.N. Doral, J. Karlsson (eds.), *Sports Injuries*,
DOI 10.1007/978-3-642-36569-0_119

ACL Reconstruction

An estimated 200,000 Anterior cruciate ligament (ACL) reconstruction are performed each year in the United States alone (Kim et al. 2011). The incidence of graft failure after anatomical *ACL reconstruction* has been reported to be as high as 29.9 % (Salmon et al. 2006). In order to decrease this rate of failure, advancements in the field of biologics and biomechanical augmentation of healing after *ACL reconstruction* remain topics of intense research. Furthermore, the individualization of *ACL reconstruction* and assessment of healing before return to sports may provide methods for decreasing the rates of failure after surgery.

Augmentation of Healing

Biologics: PRP

Platelet-rich plasma (PRP), 1-2 has gained popularity in the popular media since the recent advertisement of its use and reported success with professional athletes. However, evidence for its use in *ACL reconstruction* within the basic science and clinical literature remains controversial.

Animal studies have reported that the addition of *PRP* can promote wound healing after ACL transection and suture repair via recruitment of fibroblasts and endothelial cells and collagen production. However, the relationship between increased cellular and molecular content does not necessarily translate to improved tensile properties. While some animal models of ACL suture repair and reconstruction with *PRP* report improved mechanical characteristics compared with controls (Murray et al. 2007; Joshi et al. 2009), others report no significant effect (Murray et al. 2009; Spindler et al. 2009). Joshi et al. (2009) studied the effect of a collagen-platelet composite (CPC) on porcine ACL transection and repair and found a temporal effect on the mechanical properties of the ligament. *PRP* may cause an earlier inflammatory response in a healing ACL or graft, leading to increased cellularity and vascularity, but this in turn may lead to earlier decreases in mechanical strength.

While animal studies have shown some benefits for the addition of *PRP* in ACL repair and reconstruction, clinical studies have failed to either confirm or disprove a clinical advantage. The addition of *PRP* into femoral and tibial tunnels reported no difference versus control at either 3 months (Mirzatolooci et al. 2013), 6 months (de Almeida et al. 2012), or 24 months (Nin et al. 2009) postoperatively in terms of pain, stability, or range of motion. Researchers have also evaluated graft maturation analyzed by magnetic resonance imaging (MRI). Orrego et al. (2008) reported that while no difference in graft maturation was seen at 3 months postoperatively, at 6 months follow-up, patients who underwent *ACL reconstruction* with hamstring autograft augmented with platelet concentrate and bone plug showed significantly higher low-intensity signal than controls. Another group (Radice et al. 2010) studied *ACL reconstruction* with bone-patellar tendon-bone autograft supplemented with *PRP* gel and found that the study group needed 48 % of the time to achieve graft maturation compared with control. However, other studies have failed to show similar significant results (Nin et al. 2009; Figueroa et al. 2010).

Currently, the clinical research regarding the use of *PRP* in *ACL reconstruction* is conflicted. The addition of *PRP* has the theoretical potential to hasten *graft healing* and subsequent return to sports. However, *platelet-rich plasma* as an entity must be defined in terms of percentage of components and mechanism of preparation before study results can be adequately incorporated into clinical practice.

Biomechanical Augmentation

ACL reconstruction creates an inherently different insertion type than the native enthesis. The native insertion site is termed "direct," meaning that it is composed of four zones: the ligament, unmineralized fibrocartilage, mineralized fibrocartilage, and bone. In contrast, graft-tunnel healing is affected by multiple surgical and postsurgical factors and becomes an "indirect" insertion (similar to the *medial collateral ligament*), composed mainly of specialized collagen fibers, termed Sharpey's fibers. In order to strengthen and accelerate the healing of this new enthesis, researchers are studying low-intensity pulsed ultrasound (LIPUS) and extracorporeal shockwave therapy (ESWT), which have previously been shown to accelerate healing in the bone, cartilage, and tendon defects (Cook et al. 2001; Ko et al. 2001; Wang et al. 2001).

Low-intensity pulsed ultrasound treatment is a daily treatment lasting about 20–30 min, administered in bursts of 200 ms at a frequency of 1.5 MHz (Walsh et al. 2007). Early research of LIPUS on *ACL reconstruction* has reported promising results. In a study of *ACL reconstruction* in adult sheep, LIPUS-exposed subjects demonstrated more mature organization at the tendon-bone interface, resulting in greater peak loads and stiffer constructs than control (Walsh et al. 2007). However, LIPUS treatment may prove to be too time-intensive for practical use. Extracorporal shockwave therapy may prove a favorable option because only two to three treatments are required. Wang et al. (2005) demonstrated, in a rabbit model of *ACL reconstruction*, that ESWT increased bone formation in tunnels, improved tensile strength, and resisted pullout at the tendon-bone junction versus control. While ESWT appears advantageous, controversies still exist concerning the number of pulses and sessions. Moreover, heavy activity must be avoided after initial therapy due to decreased ability of the tissue to bear load (Bosch et al. 2007). While these modalities offer promise in ACL *graft healing*, further studies are needed to elucidate their place in clinical use.

Individualization of ACL Reconstruction

The authors believe that the future of knee ligament surgery rests with individualization. While multiple surgical techniques, graft options, and rehabilitation protocols have been studied with regard to *ACL reconstruction*, decisions regarding these options must be determined by the patient anatomy and their performance requirements.

Determination of Single-Bundle Versus Double-Bundle ACL Reconstruction

Recently, studies have shown that conventional *ACL reconstruction* fails to restore the ligament to its anatomical position (Kopf et al. 2010), which has provided inadequate outcomes (Lewis et al. 2008). Thus, a move toward understanding the anatomy of the anterior cruciate ligament in order to anatomically restore the ACL size and location has been undertaken.

The size and shape of the ACL and its surrounding structures vary between patients (Kopf et al. 2011; Ziegler et al. 2011). In order to restore maximum biomechanical stability and function, the percentage of reconstructed area of the insertion site should be optimized. Size, measured preoperatively on magnetic resonance imaging (MRI) as described by Schreiber et al. (2010) or intraoperatively, may assist in the determination of the feasibility of double-bundle (DB) reconstruction. Hussein et al. (2012) reported in a prospective cohort study on single-bundle versus double-bundle *ACL reconstruction* that patients with tibial insertion sites less than 16 mm in length should undergo SB reconstruction, whereas those with larger tibial insertion sites (greater than or equal to 16 mm) should be considered to undergo DB reconstruction in order to adequately restore the native insertion site (Fig. 1). With this understanding, recent studies have looked at using oval dilators as opposed to standard circular drills in order to more closely match the shape and orientation of the native ACL insertion site (Petersen et al. 2013).

Understanding the anatomy of the intercondylar notch may also assist in the determination of SB versus DB anatomical *ACL reconstruction*. Smaller notches have been reported to have a higher risk for initial ACL injury (LaPrade and Burnett 1994; Sonnery-Cottet et al. 2011). Furthermore, non-anatomical tunnel placement may lead to graft failure and loss of extension (Howell and Taylor 1993). Therefore, intraoperative measurement of the intercondylar notch width may provide a guide as to the use of the SB or DB technique (Fig. 2). Van Eck et al (2010) propose that, to decrease the incidence of "overstuffing" the notch and because of technical difficulties with a narrow

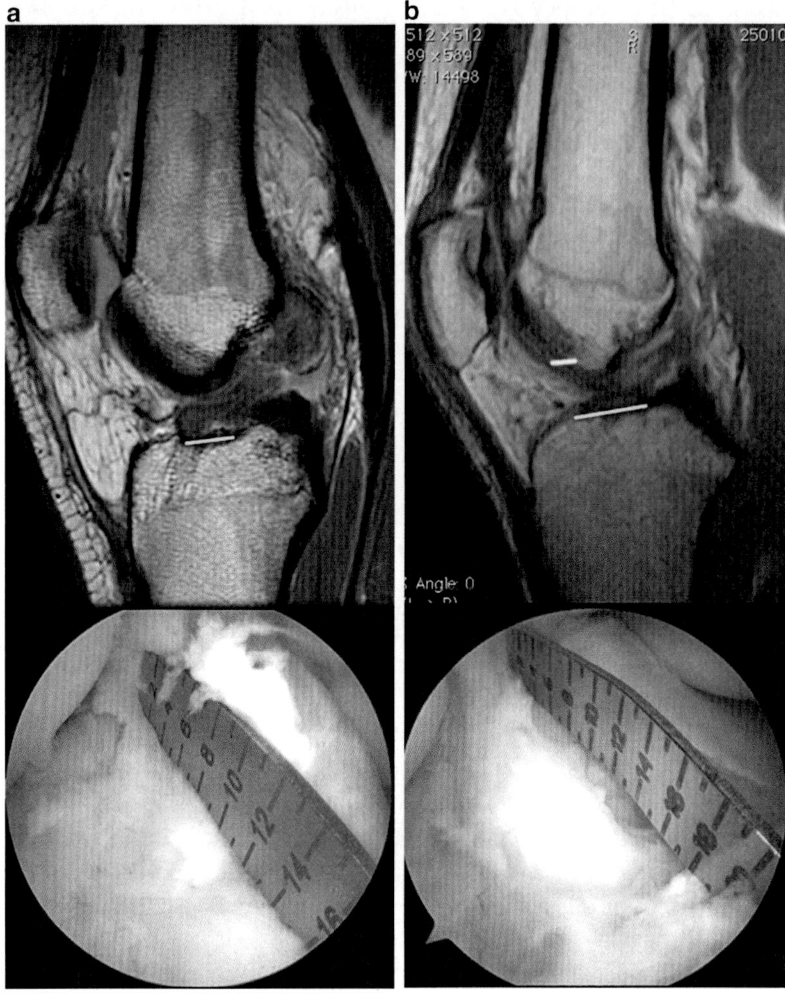

Fig. 1 ACL tibial insertion site width preoperative measurement using MRI and intraoperative measurement using an arthroscopic ruler. (**a**) Patients with tibial insertion site measurements less than 16 mm should undergo single-bundle ACL reconstruction, whereas (**b**) patients with tibial insertion site measurements greater than 16 mm can be considered for double-bundle ACL reconstruction

notch, SB reconstruction should be considered for intercondylar notches with a width less than 12 mm.

Finally, decisions regarding graft options should also account for individual age, activity level, concomitant injuries, previous surgeries, and patient and surgeon preferences. Individualization of *ACL reconstruction* should be based upon individual anatomy, preferences, and lifestyle. Further research is needed in order to characterize these decisions completely.

MRI Assessment of Graft Healing

The push for earlier return to sports from athletes and coaches contrasts significantly with the surgeon's desire for complete healing and recovery in order to decrease the risk of reinjury. However, a reliable, noninvasive method for the assessment of *graft healing* must be developed and characterized in order to determine when a patient can return to sports with a lower chance of graft failure. MRI has recently been studied as such a method.

Contrast medium enhancement MRI reflects remodeling and vascular composition within the graft. Animal studies have looked into the structure and biomechanical properties of ACL grafts and their relation to MRI appearance. Weiler et al (2001) studied the correlation of graft biomechanical properties in a sheep model of *ACL reconstruction* with Achilles tendon autograft

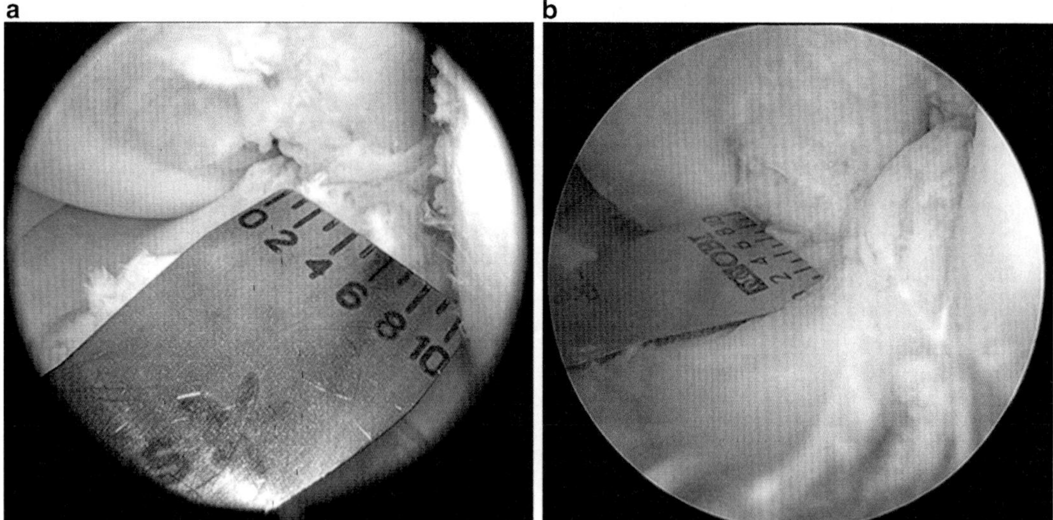

Fig. 2 Intraoperative measurement of intercondylar notch width using an arthroscopic ruler. (**a**) Single-bundle ACL reconstruction should be considered for narrow notch widths (defined as <12 mm). (**b**) Double-bundle ACL reconstruction can be considered for notch widths >12 mm

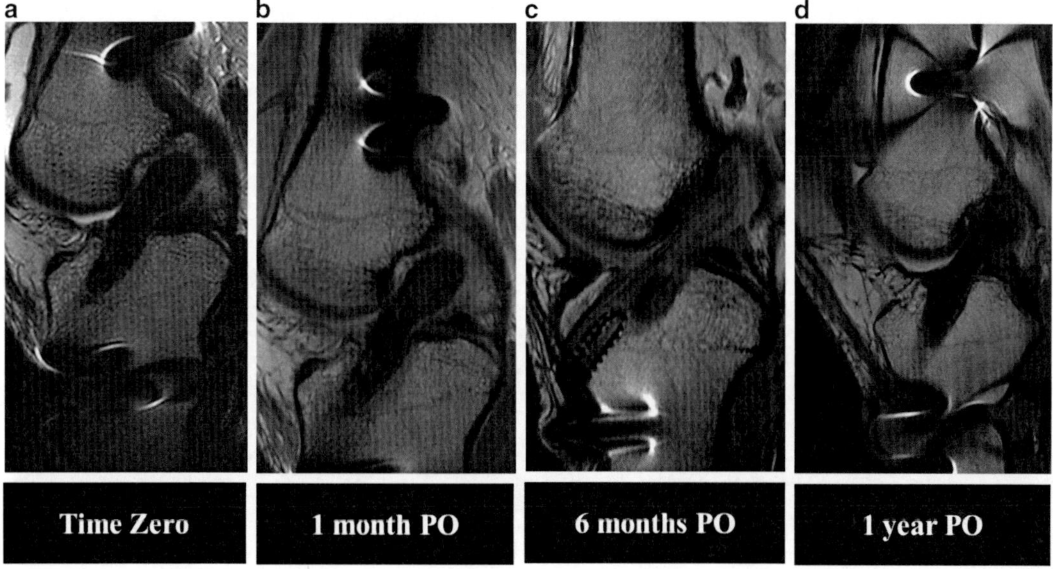

Fig. 3 MRI of ACL reconstruction using a quadriceps graft at (**a**) time zero, (**b**) 1 month post-op, (**c**) 6 months post-op, and (**d**) 1 year post-op. In the early postoperative period, the graft becomes hyperintense with increasing vascularity, with a peak around 6 months post-op. The graft then becomes hypointense, which may reflect healing and thus increase tensile strength

and found a significant negative correlation between graft signal intensity and load to failure, stiffness, and tensile strength. Therefore, a graft will first become hyperintense with increased vascularity and poor biomechanical properties and then hypointense with increasing tensile strength (Fig. 3). Furthermore, Ntoulia et al. (2011) showed in the clinical setting that graft located in the tunnel revascularized to a greater degree than the intra-articular graft portion. This correlates with the findings that early graft failure tends to occur within the bone tunnel. Another study (Muramatsu et al. 2008) looked at the difference in signal intensity between autograft and allograft and found that autograft signal intensity peaked between 4 and 6 months, whereas allograft signal intensity peaked at 12–24 months. This may show that the autograft may undergo peak revascularization and thus diminished tensile properties, at a significantly earlier time than allograft.

Return to sports criteria should therefore be considered when viewing postoperative MRI imaging and choice of graft. Using this tool to assess *graft healing* may be the future for understanding the safest time for a patient to return to full activity.

MCL: Double-Bundle Versus Single-Bundle Reconstruction

The *medial collateral ligament* is the most commonly injured knee ligament. The extra-articular location of the *MCL* allows for healing due to the abundant blood supply. Traditionally, isolated *MCL* injuries have been treated conservatively with an emphasis on early rehabilitation and range of motion because immobilization has been shown to significantly decrease load to failure (Thornton et al. 2005). Although healing occurs, 13 % of patients develop signs of early radiographic osteoarthritis (Lundberg and Messner 1996). Therefore, recent studies on isolated *MCL* injuries have focused on decreasing healing time and efficacy through the use of supplemental biological and physical therapies. For multiple-ligament injuries, controversy exists for the repair or reconstruction of the *MCL* in order to provide supplemental stability to the knee.

The *medial collateral ligament* is composed of the superficial fibers (superficial *MCL*), deep meniscocapsular structures (deep *MCL*), and the posterior oblique ligament (POL) (LaPrade et al. 2007). The superficial *MCL* is the primary static medial stabilizer of the knee (Warren and Marshall 1979), whereas the POL stabilizes the knee against valgus stress in 45–90° of flexion (Borden et al. 2002). Because of the dynamics of both ligaments, a double-bundle reconstruction technique has been reported to better resist valgus and external rotations than a single-bundle reconstruction in cadaver models (Feeley et al. 2009). Two techniques for double-bundle reconstruction have been described, utilizing four tunnels or three tunnels in order to reconstruct both the superficial *MCL* and the POL (Fig. 4). Cadaveric studies have shown near-normal stability without overconstraint using four tunnels (Coobs et al. 2010), and clinical studies have shown improved overall patient function and stability and return to previous activity utilizing both techniques (Kim et al. 2008; Lind et al. 2009; Laprade and Wijdicks 2012). Studies comparing double-bundle and single-bundle reconstruction techniques and conservative treatment are needed in order to determine the efficacy and the appropriate population.

Posterolateral Corner

The *posterolateral corner* is composed of multiple structures that provide both static and dynamic stability to resist varus rotation, external tibial rotation, and posterior tibial translation (Fig. 5). These structures include the static stabilizers (lateral collateral ligament, fabellofibular ligament, popliteofibular ligament, joint capsule, and coronary ligaments) and the dynamic stabilizers (biceps femoris and popliteus muscle-tendon units) (LaPrade et al. 2003). The identification of a *posterolateral corner* injury, especially in combination with cruciate ligament injury, is important because cruciate ligament grafts will see increased forces if not treated (Harner et al. 2000; LaPrade et al. 2002). Furthermore, O'Brien and colleagues (1991) found that 15 % of *ACL reconstructions* failed due to untreated *posterolateral corner* injuries. A high suspicion of injury should be maintained for patients with high-energy trauma; however, noncontact hyperextension-twisting injury is also common. Special tests, such as varus testing and the dial test, may be used to identify isolated *posterolateral corner* and concomitant PCL injury. MRI may be useful to identify, but cannot exclude, acute *posterolateral corner* injuries (LaPrade et al. 2000). In a

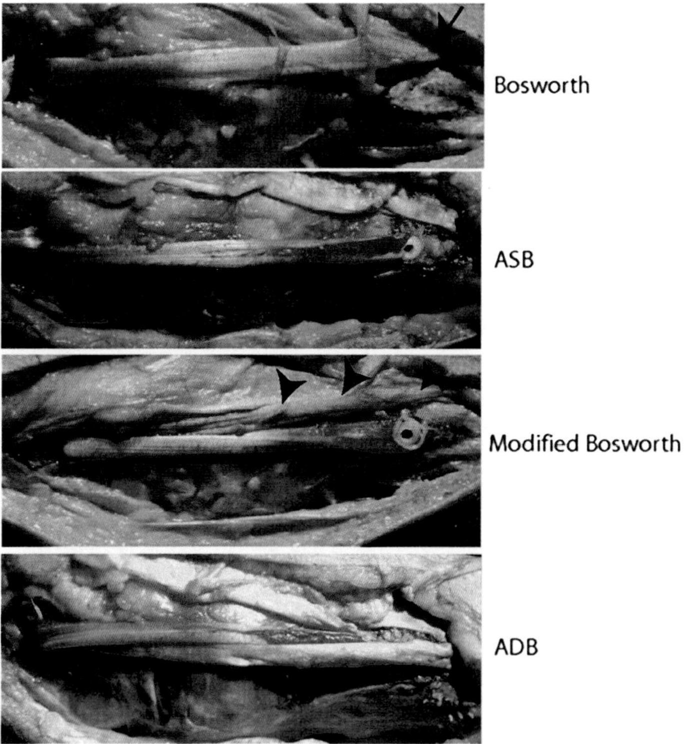

Fig. 4 Reconstruction techniques of the MCL on cadaveric knees. See citation for details of the technique. "The Bosworth technique was performed with the semitendinosus tendon taken from its origin (*arrow*) to the insertion of the MCL on the femur. The anatomical single-bundle (*ASB*) reconstruction was performed with the semitendinosus graft secured at the superficial MCL origin and the distal attachment of the distal MCL. The modified Bosworth was performed with the semitendinosus tendon looped proximally (*arrowheads*) from its insertion around a proximal staple and attached distally with an Intrafix screw. The anatomical double-bundle (*ADB*) reconstruction had one loop of semitendinosus tendon around a staple in the anatomical origin of the MCL" (Feeley et al., Am J Sports Med 37 (6):1123–30, copyright © The Author(s). Reprinted with Permission of SAGE Publications)

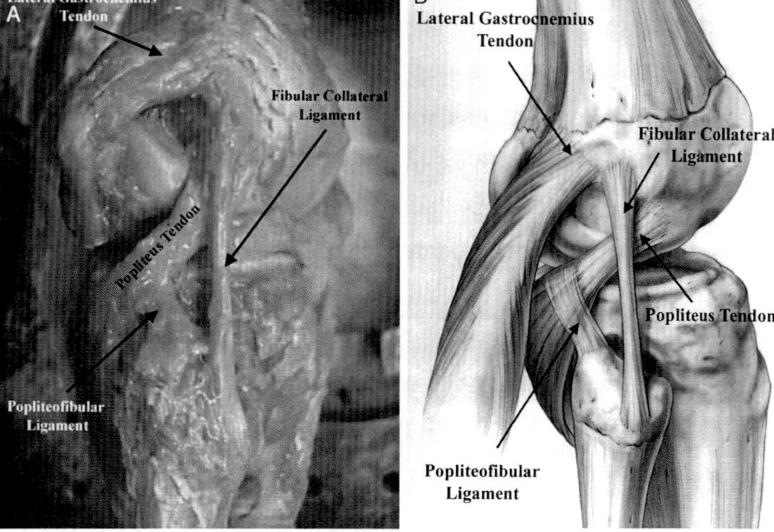

Fig. 5 Anatomy of the posterolateral corner, cadaveric dissection (**a**), and illustration (**b**). Lateral view, right knee (LaPrade et al., Am J Sports Med 31 (6):854–60, copyright © 2003 American Orthopaedic Society for Sports Medicine. Reprinted by Permission of SAGE Publications)

retrospective study by Pacheco et al. (2011), the authors found that only 4/15 (27 %) of *posterolateral corner* injuries could be identified on MRI greater than 12 weeks after injury.

The management of *posterolateral corner* injuries is controversial. Most authors advocate nonsurgical treatment with early immobilization and progressive range of motion for grade I and some grade II *posterolateral corner* injuries (Kannus 1989; Krukhaug et al. 1998); conversely, for grade III and some grade II injuries, surgical management is required. Recent studies have shown that repairs performed early (within 3 weeks after injury) provide superior results compared to reconstruction, especially for bony avulsion injuries (Geeslin and LaPrade 2011). However, because *posterolateral corner* injuries are often missed, the presentation (greater than 3 weeks after injury) of chronic injury requires reconstruction due to the inability to localize structures. Furthermore, the reconstruction of chronic injury has been shown to have better outcomes, especially in multi-ligamentous injury (Stannard et al. 2005; LaPrade et al. 2010; Levy et al. 2010). *Posterolateral corner* injury is a frequently missed diagnosis, which can affect the outcome of concomitant ligament reconstruction. Efforts must be taken in order to identify this injury early, so anatomical repair and precautions may be taken in order for the patient to have the best possible outcome (Laprade et al. 2014).

Conclusion

Innovations for knee ligament surgery, and specifically *anterior cruciate ligament reconstruction*, are continually improving and changing in order to decrease the rates of failure and improve outcomes. Anatomical reconstruction, individualization, augmentation, and assessment of *graft healing* are at the forefront of research. Although some smaller studies have shown promise for these methods, more research and better clinical studies are needed in order to provide proper guidelines for the utilization of materials such as *PRP*, LIPUS, and ESWT. Furthermore, with improvements in imaging, healing may be assessed in order to allow physicians to have objective data as to when a patient may return to their pre-injury levels of activity.

Cross-References

- ▶ Allografts in Anterior Cruciate Ligament Reconstruction
- ▶ Alternative Techniques for Double-Tunnel Anatomic Anterior Cruciate Ligament Reconstruction
- ▶ Anatomic Double-Tunnel Anterior Cruciate Ligament Reconstruction: Evolution and Principles
- ▶ Anterior Cruciate Ligament Graft Selection and Fixation
- ▶ Anterior Cruciate Ligament Injuries and Surgery: Current Evidence and Modern Development
- ▶ Anterior Cruciate Ligament Reconstruction with Autologous Quadriceps Tendon
- ▶ Different Techniques of Anterior Cruciate Ligament Reconstruction: Guidelines
- ▶ Double-Tunnel Anatomic Anterior Cruciate Ligament Reconstruction
- ▶ Graft Remodeling and Bony Ingrowth After Anterior Cruciate Ligament Reconstruction
- ▶ Platelet-Rich Plasma: From Laboratory to the Clinic
- ▶ Reconstruction of the Posterolateral Corner of the Knee
- ▶ Role of Growth Factors in Anterior Cruciate Ligament Surgery
- ▶ Single Versus Double Anterior Cruciate Ligament Reconstruction in Athletes
- ▶ State of the Art in Anterior Cruciate Ligament Surgery

References

Borden PS, Kantaras AT, Caborn DNM (2002) Medial collateral ligament reconstruction with allograft using a double-bundle technique. Arthroscopy 18(4): 1–6

Bosch G, Lin YL, van Schie HT, van De Lest CH et al (2007) Effect of extracorporeal shock wave therapy on the biochemical composition and metabolic activity of tenocytes in normal tendinous structures in ponies. Equine Vet J 39(3):226–231

Coobs BR, Wijdicks CA, Armitage BM et al (2010) An in vitro analysis of an anatomical medial knee reconstruction. Am J Sports Med 38(2):339–347

Cook SD, Salkeld SL, Popich-Patron LS et al (2001) Improved cartilage repair after treatment with low-intensity pulsed ultrasound. Clin Orthop Relat Res 391:S231–S243

de Almeida AM, Demange MK, Sobrado MF et al (2012) Patellar tendon healing with platelet-rich plasma: a prospective randomized controlled trial. Am J Sports Med 40(6):1282–1288

Feeley BT, Muller MS, Allen AA et al (2009) Biomechanical comparison of medial collateral ligament reconstructions using computer-assisted navigation. Am J Sports Med 37(6):1123–1130

Figueroa D, Melean P, Calvo R et al (2010) Magnetic resonance imaging evaluation of the integration and maturation of semitendinosus-gracilis graft in anterior cruciate ligament reconstruction using autologous platelet concentrate. Arthroscopy 26(10):1318–1325

Geeslin AG, LaPrade RF (2011) Outcomes of treatment of acute grade-III isolated and combined posterolateral knee injuries: a prospective case series and surgical technique. J Bone Joint Surg Am 93(18):1672–1683

Harner CD, Vogrin TM, Hoher J et al (2000) Biomechanical analysis of a posterior cruciate ligament reconstruction. Deficiency of the posterolateral structures as a cause of graft failure. Am J Sports Med 28(1):32–39

Howell SM, Taylor MA (1993) Failure of reconstruction of the anterior cruciate ligament due to impingement by the intercondylar roof. J Bone Joint Surg Am 75(7): 1044–1055

Hussein M, van Eck CF, Cretnik A et al (2012) Individualized anterior cruciate ligament surgery: a prospective study comparing anatomic single- and double-bundle reconstruction. Am J Sports Med 40(8):1781–1788

Joshi SM, Mastrangelo AN, Magarian EM et al (2009) Collagen-platelet composite enhances biomechanical and histologic healing of the porcine anterior cruciate ligament. Am J Sports Med 37(12):2401–2410

Kannus P (1989) Nonoperative treatment of grade II and III sprains of the lateral ligament compartment of the knee. Am J Sports Med 17(1):83–88

Kim SJ, Lee DH, Kim TE et al (2008) Concomitant reconstruction of the medial collateral and posterior oblique ligaments for medial instability of the knee. J Bone Joint Surg (Br) 90(10):1323–1327

Kim S, Bosque J, Meehan JP et al (2011) Increase in outpatient knee arthroscopy in the United States: a comparison of National Surveys of Ambulatory Surgery, 1996 and 2006. J Bone Joint Surg Am 93(11):994–1000

Ko JY, Chen HS, Chen LM (2001) Treatment of lateral epicondylitis of the elbow with shock waves. Clin Orthop Relat Res 387:60–67

Kopf S, Forsythe B, Wong AK et al (2010) Nonanatomic tunnel position in traditional transtibial single-bundle anterior cruciate ligament reconstruction evaluated by three-dimensional computed tomography. J Bone Joint Surg Am 92(6):1427–1431

Kopf S, Pombo MW, Szczodry M et al (2011) Size variability of the human anterior cruciate ligament insertion sites. Am J Sports Med 39(1):108–113

Krukhaug Y, Molster A, Rodt A et al (1998) Lateral ligament injuries of the knee. Knee Surg Sports Traumatol Arthrosc 6(1):21–25

LaPrade RF, Burnett QM (1994) Femoral intercondylar notch stenosis and correlation to anterior cruciate ligament injuries. A prospective study. Am J Sports Med 22(2):198–202

Laprade RF, Wijdicks CA (2012) Surgical technique: development of an anatomic medial knee reconstruction. Clin Orthop Relat Res 470(3):806–814

LaPrade RF, Gilbert TJ, Bollom TS et al (2000) The magnetic resonance imaging appearance of individual structures of the posterolateral knee. A prospective study of normal knees and knees with surgically verified grade III injuries. Am J Sports Med 28(2):191–199

LaPrade RF, Muench C, Wentorf F et al (2002) The effect of injury to the posterolateral structures of the knee on force in a posterior cruciate ligament graft: a biomechanical study. Am J Sports Med 30(2): 233–238

LaPrade RF, Ly TV, Wentorf FA et al (2003) The posterolateral attachments of the knee: a qualitative and quantitative morphologic analysis of the fibular collateral ligament, popliteus tendon, popliteofibular ligament, and lateral gastrocnemius tendon. Am J Sports Med 31(6):854–860

LaPrade RF, Engebretsen AH, Ly TV et al (2007) The anatomy of the medial part of the knee. J Bone Joint Surg Am 89(9):2000–2010

LaPrade RF, Johansen S, Agel J et al (2010) Outcomes of an anatomic posterolateral knee reconstruction. J Bone Joint Surg Am 92(1):16–22

Laprade RF, Griffith CJ, Coobs BR et al (2014) Improving outcomes for posterolateral knee injuries. J Orthop Res 32(4):485–491

Levy BA, Dajani KA, Morgan JA et al (2010) Repair versus reconstruction of the fibular collateral ligament and posterolateral corner in the multiligament-injured knee. Am J Sports Med 38(4):804–809

Lewis PB, Parameswaran AD, Rue JP et al (2008) Systematic review of single-bundle anterior cruciate ligament reconstruction outcomes: a baseline assessment for consideration of double-bundle techniques. Am J Sports Med 36(10):2028–2036

Lind M, Jakobsen BW, Lund B et al (2009) Anatomical reconstruction of the medial collateral ligament and posteromedial corner of the knee in patients with chronic medial collateral ligament instability. Am J Sports Med 37(6):1116–1122

Lundberg M, Messner K (1996) Long-term prognosis of isolated partial medial collateral ligament ruptures. A ten-year clinical and radiographic evaluation of a prospectively observed group of patients. Am J Sports Med 24(2):160–163

Mirzatolooci F, Alamdari MT, Khalkhali HR (2013) The impact of platelet-rich plasma on the prevention of tunnel widening in anterior cruciate ligament reconstruction using quadrupled autologous hamstring tendon: a randomized clinical trial. Bone Joint J 95B:65–69

Muramatsu K, Hachiya Y, Izawa H (2008) Serial evaluation of human anterior cruciate ligament grafts by contrast-enhanced magnetic resonance imaging: comparison of allografts and autografts. Arthroscopy 24(9): 1038–1044

Murray MM, Spindler KP, Ballard P et al (2007) Enhanced histologic repair in a central wound in the anterior cruciate ligament with a collagen-platelet-rich plasma scaffold. J Orthop Res 25(8):1007–1017

Murray MM, Palmer M, Abreu E et al (2009) Platelet-rich plasma alone is not sufficient to enhance suture repair of the ACL in skeletally immature animals: an in vivo study. J Orthop Res 27(5):639–645

Nin JR, Gasque GM, Azcarate AV et al (2009) Has platelet-rich plasma any role in anterior cruciate ligament allograft healing? Arthroscopy 25(11):1206–1213

Ntoulia A, Papadopoulou F, Ristanis S et al (2011) Revascularization process of the bone–patellar tendon–bone autograft evaluated by contrast-enhanced magnetic resonance imaging 6 and 12 months after anterior cruciate ligament reconstruction. Am J Sports Med 39(7):1478–1486

O'Brien SJ, Warren RF, Pavlov H et al (1991) Reconstruction of the chronically insufficient anterior cruciate ligament with the central third of the patellar ligament. J Bone Joint Surg Am 73(2):278–286

Orrego M, Larrain C, Rosales J et al (2008) Effects of platelet concentrate and a bone plug on the healing of hamstring tendons in a bone tunnel. Arthroscopy 24(12):1373–1380

Pacheco RJ, Ayre CA, Bollen SR (2011) Posterolateral corner injuries of the knee: a serious injury commonly missed. J Bone Joint Surg (Br) 93(2):194–197

Petersen W, Forkel P, Achtnich A et al (2013) Technique of anatomical footprint reconstruction of the ACL with oval tunnels and medial portal aimers. Arch Orthop Trauma Surg 133(6):827–833

Radice F, Yanez R, Gutierrez V et al (2010) Comparison of magnetic resonance imaging findings in anterior cruciate ligament grafts with and without autologous platelet-derived growth factors. Arthroscopy 26(1):50–57

Salmon LJ, Russell VJ, Refshauge K et al (2006) Long-term outcome of endoscopic anterior cruciate ligament reconstruction with patellar tendon autograft: minimum 13-year review. Am J Sports Med 34(5):721–732

Schreiber VM, van Eck CF, Fu FH (2010) Anatomic double-bundle ACL reconstruction. Sports Med Arthrosc 18(1):27–32

Sonnery-Cottet B, Archbold P, Cucurulo T et al (2011) The influence of the tibial slope and the size of the intercondylar notch on rupture of the anterior cruciate ligament. J Bone Joint Surg (Br) 93(11): 1475–1478

Spindler KP, Murray MM, Carey JL et al (2009) The use of platelets to affect functional healing of an anterior cruciate ligament (ACL) autograft in a caprine ACL reconstruction model. J Orthop Res 27(5):631–638

Stannard JP, Brown SL, Farris RC et al (2005) The posterolateral corner of the knee: repair versus reconstruction. Am J Sports Med 33(6):881–888

Thornton GM, Johnson JC, Maser RV et al (2005) Strength of medial structures of the knee joint are decreased by isolated injury to the medial collateral ligament and subsequent joint immobilization. J Orthop Res 23(5): 1191–1198

van Eck CF, Lesniak BP, Schreiber VM et al (2010) Anatomic single- and double-bundle anterior cruciate ligament reconstruction flowchart. Arthroscopy 26(2): 258–268

Walsh WR, Stephens P, Vizesi F et al (2007) Effects of low-intensity pulsed ultrasound on tendon-bone healing in an intra-articular sheep knee model. Arthroscopy 23(2):197–204

Wang CJ, Chen HS, Chen CE et al (2001) Treatment of nonunions of long bone fractures with shock waves. Clin Orthop Relat Res 387:95–101

Wang CJ, Wang FS, Yang KD et al (2005) The effect of shock wave treatment at the tendon-bone interface-an histomorphological and biomechanical study in rabbits. J Orthop Res 23(2):274–280

Warren LF, Marshall JL (1979) The supporting structures and layers on the medial side of the knee: an anatomical analysis. J Bone Joint Surg Am 61(1):56–62

Weiler A, Peters G, Maurer J et al (2001) Biomechanical properties and vascularity of an anterior cruciate ligament graft can be predicted by contrast-enhanced magnetic resonance imaging. A two-year study in sheep. Am J Sports Med 29(6):751–761

Ziegler CG, Pietrini SD, Westerhaus BD et al (2011) Arthroscopically pertinent landmarks for tunnel positioning in single-bundle and double-bundle anterior cruciate ligament reconstructions. Am J Sports Med 39(4):743–752

Graft Remodeling and Bony Ingrowth After Anterior Cruciate Ligament Reconstruction

88

Sven Scheffler and Roland Becker

Contents

Abstract

The following chapter will provide a concise overview about the biological changes of an autologous graft following reconstruction of the anterior cruciate ligament. Detailed attention is paid to the healing processes that occur at the intra-articular and at the intra-tunnel graft regions. The specific biological changes leading to adaptation of the intra-articular graft region towards an ACL-like structure and the formation of a neoinsertion of the ACL graft are outlined. Time-specific phases are defined, which show distinct differences in remodeling activity. Overall information of this chapter will help to understand when *graft remodeling and incorporation* will be completed and full functional recovery can be expected.

Introduction

A successful reconstruction of the anterior cruciate ligament (ACL) requires an understanding of several factors that influence long-term function of the knee joint. At time of reconstruction, the structural and mechanical properties of the selected graft tissue and the mechanical behavior and fixation strength of its fixation materials will determine time-zero knee stability. However, the ensuing biological remodeling of the intra-articular graft and the incorporation of its intra-tunnel region will change the overall mechanical stability of the reconstructed knee joint over time.

S. Scheffler (✉)
Sporthopaedicum, Charite Universitatsmedizin, Berlin, Germany
e-mail: scheffler@sporthopaedicum.de

R. Becker
Klinik für Orthopädie und Unfallchirurgie, Städtische Klinikum Brandenburg, Hochstrasse, Brandenburg an der Havel, Germany
e-mail: roland_becker@yahoo.de

M.N. Doral, J. Karlsson (eds.), *Sports Injuries*,
DOI 10.1007/978-3-642-36569-0_98

Several studies have analyzed the various changes that occur during graft healing and osseous incorporation (Amiel et al. 1986; Ballock et al. 1989; Kleiner et al. 1989; Rodeo et al. 1993; Rougraff et al. 1993; Grana et al. 1994; Howell et al. 1995; Liu et al. 1997; Kuroda et al. 2000; Goradia et al. 2000a; Papageorgiou et al. 2001; Tomita et al. 2001; Weiler et al. 2001, 2002; Yamakado et al. 2002; Kobayashi et al. 2005; Scheffler et al. 2008a). Most of our current knowledge on intra-articular graft remodeling and bony graft incorporation stems from in vivo animal studies (Ballock et al. 1989; Kleiner et al. 1989; Grana et al. 1994; Ng et al. 1996; Goradia et al. 2000a, b; Kuroda et al. 2000; Ishibashi et al. 2001; Papageorgiou et al. 2001; Tomita et al. 2001; Weiler et al. 2002; Nebelung et al. 2003; Kawakami et al. 2004; Kobayashi et al. 2005; Rodeo et al. 2006; Arai et al. 2008; Scheffler et al. 2008a). Few human biopsy studies exist (Rougraff et al. 1993; Falconiero et al. 1998; Rougraff and Shelbourne 1999; Zaffagnini et al. 2007; Claes et al. 2011; Janssen et al. 2011). Both animal and human in vitro and in vivo studies have demonstrated three characteristic stages of graft healing after ACL reconstruction:

1. ***Phase of early graft healing***: It is the central part of the graft necroses and there is hypocellularity and no detectable revascularization of the graft tissue. The peripheral part shows more vital tissue, which is supplied by synovial fluid. There is a significant impairment of the biomechanical properties of the graft.
2. ***Phase of proliferation***: It is the most intensive phase of remodeling activity and revascularization, which starts from the periphery to the central part of the tendon. Metabolically highly active cells move into the tendon.
3. ***Phase of ligamentization***: The phase is characterized by restructuring of the graft towards the properties of the intact ACL and by development of a new mature neoinsertion (Scheffler et al. 2008b; Claes et al. 2011).

Early Graft Healing Phase

Immediately after ACL reconstruction, the characteristic organization of the extracellular matrix and cellular structure of the avascular graft starts to slowly dissolve (Liu et al. 1997; Goradia et al. 2000b; Dustmann et al. 2008). During the first four postoperative weeks, graft necrosis and hypocellularity are mainly found in the graft's center (Fig. 1) (Amiel et al. 1986; Kleiner et al. 1989; Kuroda et al. 2000; Dustmann et al. 2008; Scheffler et al. 2008a). Ultrastructural cell changes, such as mitochondrial swelling, dilatation of the endoplasmic reticulum and

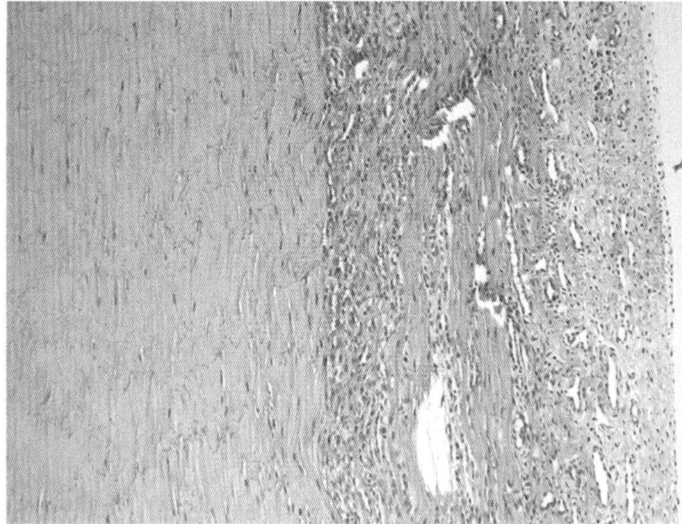

Fig. 1 Histomorphological appearance of the intra-articular graft substance during the first 4 weeks of healing (H&E, cross section of sheep flexor tendon ACL graft, magnification 10×, *S*, Surface of the graft, *C*, Center of the graft)

intracytoplasmic deposition of lipids, and macroscopic swelling and increased cross-sectional area, illustrate the progression of graft necrosis and degradation (Goradia et al. 2000b). At the same time, an influx of host cells can be observed into the graft's periphery (Kleiner et al. 1986, 1989; Yoshikawa et al. 2004; Kobayashi et al. 2005) (Fig. 1). Yoshikawa et al. (2004; Kobayashi et al. 2005) were able to demonstrate that all original graft cells were completely replaced by 2–4 weeks in an animal model of ACL reconstruction. The exact source of these cells was unclear, but it has been speculated that the stump of the native ACL and bone marrow elements originating from drilling maneuvers might play an important role this repopulation (Kleiner et al. 1986). It is therefore believed that preservation of the ACL stump and Hoffa's fat pad might be beneficial. During this time, no graft revascularization can be seen (Kleiner et al. 1989; Yoshikawa et al. 2006; Scheffler et al. 2008a). Due to the slow progression of graft remodeling during the first 4 weeks, overall graft integrity is maintained and only a slow decrease of the graft's mechanical properties was shown (Shino and Horibe 1991; Papageorgiou et al. 2001).

During the first 4 weeks, no bony integration or mechanical bridging occurs between the graft and the surrounding bone (Rodeo et al. 1993; Grana et al. 1994; Goradia et al. 2000a; Papageorgiou et al. 2001; Weiler et al. 2002; Rodeo et al. 2006). Only a poorly organized vascular and highly cellular fibrous tissue is formed between the graft and the adjacent bony wall without any structural linking (Rodeo et al. 1993). An increasing number of host cells invade the graft from the surrounding bone (Rodeo et al. 2006). The mechanical strength of the overall reconstruction is therefore relying on the graft's fixation devices, which have been shown to provide fixation strength far below the graft's structural properties (Goradia et al. 2000a; Weiler et al. 2001; Scheffler et al. 2008a). However, recent studies suggested that activities of daily living, full-weight bearing, biking, or continuous knee motion without significant acceleration or deceleration resulted into loading of the ACL <400 N (Shelburne and Pandy 1998; Fujiya et al. 2011). All current fixation devices are designed to safely withstand such loads, allowing for safe early rehabilitation. The importance of immediate loading for graft healing has been analyzed in several studies (Ohno et al. 1993; Majima et al. 2003). Ohno et al. (1993) reported that stress deprivation of a patellar tendon in vivo resulted into significant loss of tensile strength at 1 week with further deterioration until 6 weeks of healing. Similar findings were reported by Majima et al. (2003), who detected a significantly higher loss in tensile strength of an ACL graft between the first and third week of healing after complete stress shielding. They explained this observation with ultrastructural changes in the collagen composition that shifted to small diameter fibrils, which were reported to provide less mechanical strength than the large diameter fibrils typically found in the intact ACL (Majima et al. 2003). Contrary, overloading of the graft has also been shown to impair graft healing. Tohyama et al. found in their model of an in situ frozen patellar tendon that a reduction of the cross-sectional area of the tendon by half (thereby doubling the tendon stress during loading) resulted in substantially reduced tensile strength after only 3 weeks, whereas only a slight increase in tendon stress (reduction of cross-sectional area by only a third) did not significantly impair the mechanical strength of the ACL graft (Kuroda et al. 2000; Tohyama and Yasuda 2002; Yoshikawa et al. 2006; Scheffler et al. 2008a; Dustmann et al. 2008).

Proliferation Phase

The early healing phase is followed by a time period of maximum remodeling activity of the intra-articular graft. In animal studies, this phase has been described to occur between the 4th and 12th postoperative week and is termed the proliferation phase of ACL healing (Amiel et al. 1986; Scheffler et al. 2008a, b). During this phase, the increasing graft necrosis triggers the release of growth factors that stimulate cell migration and proliferation and extracellular matrix degradation and restoration as well as revascularization (Kuroda et al. 2000; Yoshikawa et al. 2006;

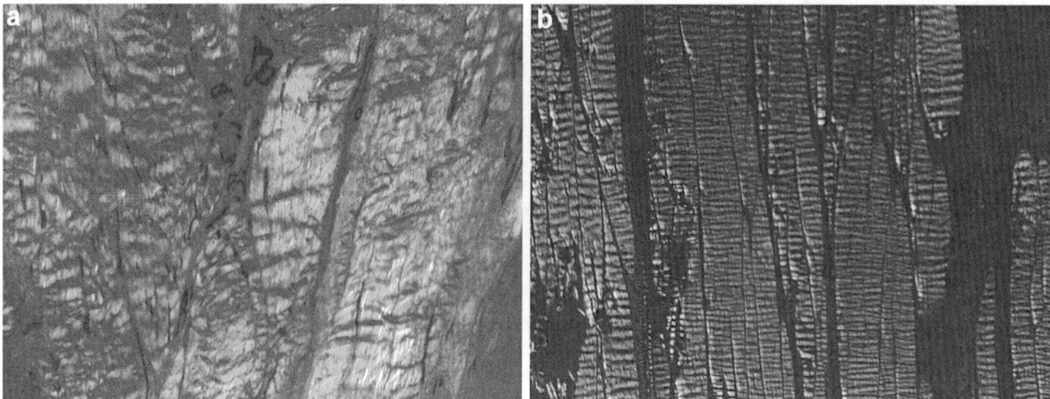

Fig. 2 Crimp pattern, polarization microscopy, 5× magnification; (**a**) sheep ACL autograft 12 weeks, (**b**) sheep intact ACL

Dustmann et al. 2008; Scheffler et al. 2008a). The typical collagen fiber distribution and organization is completely lost and replaced by an irregular crimp pattern and a decrease of collagen fibril density (Fig. 2). This is followed by increased collagen synthesis and a shift from large diameter collagen fibrils to small diameter fibrils and an increased collagen III synthesis (with lower mechanical strength than type I collagen) (Ng et al. 1996).

At the same time, graft cellularity constantly increases (Ballock et al. 1989; Kleiner et al. 1989; Papageorgiou et al. 2001; Scheffler et al. 2008a) and substantially surpasses that of the intact ACL. Revascularization (Weiler et al. 2001; Unterhauser et al. 2003; Yoshikawa et al. 2006; Scheffler et al. 2008a) progresses from the periphery to the entire graft diameter at 12 weeks (Weiler et al. 2001; Scheffler et al. 2005, 2008a). Specific fibroblasts appear in the healing graft, so-called myofibroblasts, which play an important role in the reorganization of the collagen matrix. Due to their contractile cell properties, restoration of the in situ graft tension is achieved (Dustmann et al. 2008). The maximum remodeling activity results into significant reduction of the mechanical properties of the intra-articular graft region. All animal studies showed the lowest structural and mechanical properties of the healing ACL graft at this time point, with consistent failure at the intra-articular graft region (Rodeo et al. 1993; Goradia et al. 2000a; Papageorgiou et al. 2001; Weiler et al. 2001; Nebelung et al. 2003; Scheffler et al. 2008a). As a result of the impairment of the graft's biomechanical properties, significantly increased anterior-posterior knee laxity was measured (Scheffler et al. 2008a). Kondo et al. studied the failure loads and stiffness of an ACL reconstruction in sheep using a doubled free tendon graft. They reported failure loads of less than 30 % and 50 % after 12 and 52 weeks respectively. However, no difference in stiffness was observed after 52 weeks in comparison to the intact ACL (Kondo et al. 2012). Other studies suggest that the initial graft's synovialization might have an impact on the restoration of the structural properties of the intact ACL. Mayr et al. found that a synovialized transplant such as the flexor digitorum superficial tendon graft showed significantly lower failure loads than a non-synovialized patella tendon-bone graft during early healing (12 weeks). However, these differences disappeared during the ensuing remodeling phase until 6 months postoperatively (Mayr et al. 2012).

These reduced biomechanical properties of healing grafts in animal models seem to contradict the successful clinical outcomes after ACL reconstruction in humans, especially with the proposition of immediate aggressive rehabilitation and no reports of increased ACL reconstruction failures during this time. The few available biopsy studies (Rougraff et al. 1993; Falconiero et al. 1998; Rougraff and Shelbourne 1999; Zaffagnini et al. 2007; Sánchez et al. 2010; Claes et al. 2011; Janssen et al. 2011) describe substantial differences between the remodeling activity of human and animal ACL grafts during the first 3 months of healing. Remodeling activity was less pronounced, and complete loss and replacement of all intrinsic graft cells were not observed in human biopsy studies. Graft necrosis or degeneration never involved more than 30 % of the graft's biopsies (Rougraff and Shelbourne 1999), while neovascularization was also not as excessive as in animal model. Large areas of human healing grafts stayed unchanged, displaying normal collagen alignment and crimp pattern.

On the other hand, analyses of biopsies from human ACL grafts also revealed similar findings as in animal studies with loss of collagen organization mainly occurring in areas of neovascularization (Scheffler et al. 2008b; Janssen et al. 2011). The remodeling cascade of (limited) graft necrosis, recellularization, revascularization, and restoration of collagen crimp and three-dimensional structural reorganization followed similar time patterns of the early healing and proliferation phases found in animal studies, suggesting that also the human ACL graft might have its lowest mechanical strength around 6–8 weeks postoperatively (Rougraff and Shelbourne 1999; Zaffagnini et al. 2007).

It is valid to conclude that loading of the graft must be high enough to stimulate graft cell activity, as a prerequisite of cellular and extracellular remodeling, leading to preservation of graft stability, but without compromising graft integrity, which could possibly result into an early stretching of the ACL reconstruction (Rodeo et al. 1993; Grana et al. 1994; Liu et al. 1997; Weiler et al. 2002Scheffler et al. 2008b).

At the beginning of the fourth postoperative week, a neoinsertion of the intra-tunnel graft region starts to develop (Rodeo et al. 1993, 2006). The timeline of intra-tunnel graft incorporation strongly depends on the type of graft tissue. Bone-patellar tendon-bone grafts undergo bone-to-bone healing, while soft-tissue grafts, such as hamstring tendons, require tendon-bone incorporation. It has been shown that bone-to-bone incorporation occurs faster than tendon-to-bone healing (Ishibashi et al. 2001; Kawakami et al. 2004).

Rodeo et al. (2006) found that the interface between the graft and tunnel wall becomes more organized and less vascular and cellular after the fourth week of healing. Special collagen fibers can be identified, so-called Sharpey fibers that connect the graft to the tunnel wall. The intra-tunnel region of the graft becomes recellularized with fibroblast-like cells. Increased osteoclast activity along the tunnel wall is seen as early as 2 weeks postoperatively. By 8 weeks, a continuous line of lamellar bone can be found between the graft and osseous tunnel wall. The development of Sharpey-like fibers has been viewed to be the earliest sign of osseous to soft-tissue graft incorporation (Rodeo et al. 1993; Grana et al. 1994; Liu et al. 1997; Weiler et al. 2002). However, it is unclear what density of Sharpey-like fibers is required to provide a solid graft incorporation, since several authors described a very sparse occurrence in their animal models and in human tissue harvested during second look arthroscopies. Rodeo et al., Goradia et al., and Grana et al. all found an increasing density of Sharpey-like fibers, with ongoing time, which they described as a solid indirect tendon insertion (Rodeo et al. 1993; Grana et al. 1994; Goradia et al. 2000a). It is known that an indirect type of ligament insertion is mechanically inferior compared to a direct type of insertion (Weiler et al. 2002). Several studies investigating tendon-to-bone healing reported identical findings with the development of an indirect graft insertion within the tunnel (Rodeo et al. 1993; Grana et al. 1994; Goradia et al. 2000a; Rodeo et al. 2006). A direct type of insertion, which is characteristic for the native ACL, could not be identified within the tunnel. However, a new formation of cartilage and fibrocartilage was discovered around the 6th–12th postoperative week at the tunnel apertures, especially at locations where compression of the graft against the bony walls was found rather than shear stress as it typically occurs between the graft and tunnel walls (Weiler et al. 2002; Rodeo et al. 2006; Scheffler et al. 2008a). The transition zone at the tunnel apertures was still poorly organized and did not fully resemble the typical direct insertion of the native ACL, which shows a distinct zone of mineralized cartilage and non-mineralized cartilage, connecting the femoral and tibial bones to the graft (Rodeo et al. 2006; Scheffler et al. 2008a).

Ligamentization Phase

The time beyond 3 months of healing is usually called the "ligamentization or maturation phase." It is characterized by the ongoing process of continuous remodeling of the ACL graft towards the morphology and restoration of the mechanical strength of the intact ACL. A clear endpoint of this phase, when no further changes in histological appearance can be observed, cannot be defined since certain changes still occur even years after ACL reconstruction. Rougraff et al. found areas of degeneration, neovascularization, and hypercellularity even 3 years after ACL reconstruction (Rougraff et al. 1993; Rougraff and Shelbourne 1999). It is still a matter of debate whether a full restoration of the biological and mechanical properties of the intact ACL is possible or whether it is more a transformation of graft tissue that resembles but not fully replicates the properties of the intact ACL.

Cellularity of the healing graft slowly returns to levels of the native ACL by 6 months (Shino et al. 1984; Jones et al. 1987; Ballock et al. 1989; Scheffler et al. 2005, 2008a; Dustmann et al. 2008). Revascularization continues to the center of the graft, while the increased vascular density of the graft's periphery slowly subsides with overall graft vascularity returning to values of the intact ACL by 6–12 months after surgery (Goradia et al. 2000b; Weiler et al. 2001; Scheffler et al. 2008a). In animal models, it could be observed that a homogenous vessel distribution of the complete graft does not occur until the end of 12 months of healing (Scheffler et al. 2008a). The loss of structural organization of the extracellular matrix as a result of the high remodeling activity of the proliferation phase is repaired. Restoration of collagen fiber alignment is observed, which microscopically starts to resemble the appearance of the intact ACL around 6–12 months after reconstruction (Ng et al. 1996; Dustmann et al. 2008). However, collagen crimp and the strict parallel alignment of the collagen fibers are only partially restored (Ng et al. 1996; Dustmann et al. 2008). Also, the typical composition of collagen fibers of varying diameter of the intact ACL is never fully restored (Ballock et al. 1989; Dustmann et al. 2008; Scheffler et al. 2008a). The increased synthesis of collagen type III of the proliferation phase decreases during the ligamentization phase, but the overall collagen type III content continues to be significantly higher than in the intact ACL even at 2 years (Liu et al. 1997). Therefore, the healing ACL graft rather resembles than shows full restoration of the morphology of the intact ACL, which explains the term "ligamentization."

The continuous presence of small diameter collagen fibrils and increased type III collagen content in animal models have been used to explain the significantly lower mechanical and structural properties of the healing graft compared to the intact ACL, even after long-term healing of up to 2 years (Liu et al. 1997; Weiler et al. 2001). However, all published studies observed a substantial improvement of the mechanical properties of the ACL-reconstructed knee joints during the phase of ligamentization with maximum values discovered at around 1 year. Some studies were able to show that the compromised mechanical properties of the ACL graft still allowed for restoration of anterior-posterior (AP) stability of the knee joint to the laxity of the healthy contralateral side (Falconiero et al. 1998; Scheffler et al. 2008a), while others observed significantly lower AP stability even 3 years after reconstruction (Ng et al. 1995).

In summary, animal in vivo studies revealed that overall restoration of graft integrity and histological appearance was completed between 6 and 12 months of healing, acquiring similar morphology as the intact ACL. This is also substantiated by the mechanical properties that reach their maximum strength around 12 months without any significant improvements thereafter. However, characteristic differences, especially in extracellular matrix composition, remain and do not reach the initial mechanical strength of the intact ACL.

Human biopsy studies showed a similar biological progression during the ligamentization phase as it was shown in animal models. However, the timeline of these biological changes was different: studies in humans were shown to undergo a prolonged remodeling process compared to animal models (Rougraff et al. 1993; Falconiero et al. 1998; Marumo et al. 2005; Sánchez et al. 2010; Claes et al. 2011; Janssen et al. 2011). In a recent study by Janssen et al., cellularity and myofibroblast expression was increased until 2 years after ACL reconstruction (Janssen et al. 2011). Collagen orientation did not return to normal in their study period up to 117 months after ACL reconstruction (Janssen et al. 2011). Rougraff et al. (1993) found the highest remodeling activity between 3 and 10 months and concluded that the proliferation phase seemed to be delayed compared to animal models. Similar findings were made by Falconiero et al. (1998) analyzing biopsies of patellar tendon and hamstring tendon ACL reconstructions. They found that hypercellularity and hypervascularity had not returned to native ACL values before 6–12 months, although collagen fiber alignment was restored around 6 months. Full histological maturity was not found before 12 months of healing. Other human biopsy studies (Rougraff et al. 1993; Falconiero et al. 1998; Janssen et al. 2011) even found increased cell counts and differing fiber alignment beyond 1 year with grafts showing continuous remodeling activity up to 3 years before becoming indistinguishable from the intact ACL. Remodeling of the extracellular matrix also seems to continue beyond 1 year of healing. Marumo et al. found that the collagen crosslink ratio of hamstring tendon autografts slowly changed to values of the native ACL at 1 year, while still being substantially different at 6 months postoperatively (Marumo et al. 2005). Zaffagnini et al. confirmed the observations in animal models (Ng et al. 1996; Goradia et al. 2000a) that human hamstring ACL grafts showed a replacement of large by small diameter fibrils, which did not change even after more than 2 years (Zaffagnini et al. 2007).

The neovascularization of human ACL grafts was analyzed using MRI technology. Howell et al. did not demonstrate any discernible blood supply in an unimpinged 4-strand hamstring ACL graft during the 2 years after (Howell et al. 1995). The graft retained the same hypovascular appearance as it is typically seen in the intact ACL. Revascularization was only seen in the periligamentous soft tissues as early as 1 month, postulating that diffusion rather than revascularization of the graft itself might be of relevance for biological graft remodeling. Other human biopsy studies demonstrated neovascularization of the healing graft, such as for hamstring tendons (Falconiero et al. 1998; Rodeo et al. 2006; Scheffler et al. 2008a; Janssen et al. 2011). Gohil et al. found in their MRI analysis of human hamstring ACL grafts that revascularization could be seen as early as 2 months within the graft's midsubstance (Gohil et al. 2007). In another study by Vogrin et al. (2010), looking at the effect of autologous platelet concentrate on ACL healing, revascularization started at 4–6 weeks after ACL reconstruction. Janssen et al. (2011) examined the biopsies of their 67 patients with clinically successful 4-strand hamstring autograft ACL reconstruction and found an increase in vessel density over 24 months.

As the intra-articular graft remodels towards an ACL-like structure, the bony graft incorporation matures simultaneously. Beyond the 12th week of healing, several studies observed that the organization of the transition zone between the graft and its tunnel wall becomes more organized, the density of Sharpey-like fibers increases, and upregulated osteoclast activity is seen, with small lamellar bone formations appearing in the bone-graft interface (Rodeo et al. 2006). More importantly, a mature neoinsertion develops at the tunnel aperture. Weiler et al. (2002) found in their thorough analysis of tendon-bone healing a clear distinction of the four transition zones from the graft via a zone of non-mineralized cartilage – mineralized cartilage and bone at around 6 months postoperatively in their sheep model of ACL

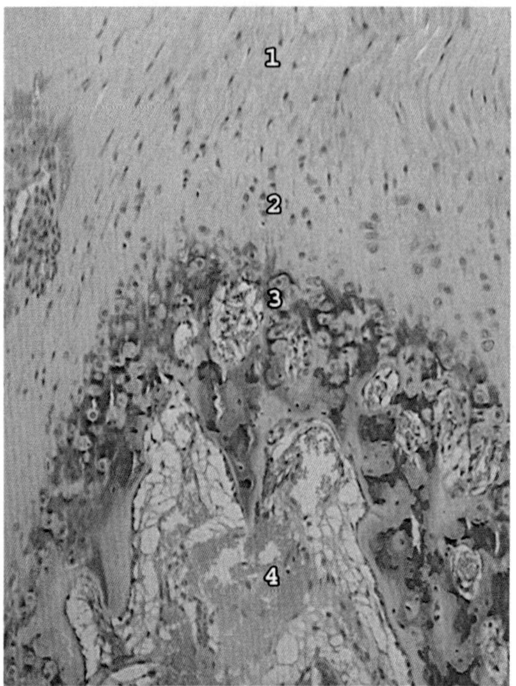

Fig. 3 Neoinsertion of healing ACL at the tunnel aperture. Direkte Bandinsertion Grad IV mit klassischem Vierzonenaufbau (1-Band, 2-Faserknorpel, 3-Kalkknorpel, 4-Knochen) in der Alcian-Blau-Färbung, Tibia, AB, 100×

reconstruction using interference screw fixation (Fig. 3). Full maturity was observed at 1 year postoperatively, with no visible histological changes thereafter at 2 years. Identical findings were made by Scheffler et al. (2008a) using the identical animal model, but no joint-line fixation. The only difference they found was a delay in the development of a mature direct tendon-bone insertion, which also completed at 1 year, but showed a lesser degree of maturity at 6 months compared to the study by Weiler et al. (2002).

The importance of the establishment of a neoinsertion is underlined by changing failure modes of ACL-reconstructed knee joints as shown in several in vivo animal studies (Rodeo et al. 2006; Scheffler et al. 2008a). Tendon pullout from the osseous tunnel is observed during the first 6 weeks of healing (Rodeo et al. 1993; Scheffler et al. 2008a), which is due to the lack of a biological insertion of the graft to the bone. The failure mode changes to intra-articular graft failure around 8–12 weeks at the lowest failure loads during the postoperative time. This can be explained by the establishment of an immature biological graft incorporation, primarily in the bone tunnel, and the substantial deterioration of the intra-articular graft structure due to intensive remodeling activity. With ongoing time at 6–12 months postoperatively, failure mode remains mainly at the intra-articular graft region or by bony peel off of the graft at the joint line. Now failure loads and stiffness of the healing graft increase and reach maximum values at around 1 year (Rodeo et al. 2006; Scheffler et al. 2008a). This is a result of the formation of a mature neoinsertion and restoration of structural graft integrity.

Summary

In summary, all studies, whether animal or human biopsy studies, have confirmed characteristic changes of an ACL graft during the course of healing. While it has become clear that the remodeling intensity of human ACL grafts seems to be less pronounced than in animal models and that therefore the impairment of the graft's biomechanical properties during the early healing period is reduced, it has also been shown that a human ACL graft continues to remodel far beyond 1 year after reconstruction. The actual relevance of these findings for the *graft's mechanical function* is unknown. No information has been published until today on the bony graft incorporation in humans. Today's knowledge is therefore based on animal in vivo studies, which showed the development of a mature neoinsertion between 6 and 12 months for soft-tissue grafts. All this information should be implemented into rehabilitation protocols that must be aimed to support and optimize the biological remodeling of an ACL graft by supplying necessary mechanical stimulus without compromising the graft's integrity early on and then returning to full loading of the reconstructed knee joint as early as bony graft incorporation is completed and intra-articular graft remodeling has restored a fully functional ACL replacement.

Cross-References

- ▶ Anterior Cruciate Ligament Graft Selection and Fixation
- ▶ Different Techniques of Anterior Cruciate Ligament Reconstruction: Guidelines
- ▶ Perioperative and Postoperative Anterior Cruciate Ligament Rehabilitation Focused on Soft Tissue Grafts
- ▶ Return to Play Decision-Making Following Anterior Cruciate Ligament Reconstruction: Multi-factor Considerations
- ▶ Role of Growth Factors in Anterior Cruciate Ligament Surgery
- ▶ Structured Rehabilitation Model with Clinical Outcomes After Anterior Cruciate Ligament Reconstruction

References

Amiel D, Kleiner JB, Roux RD et al (1986) The phenomenon of "ligamentization": anterior cruciate ligament reconstruction with autogenous patellar tendon. J Orthop Res 4:162–172

Arai Y, Hara K, Takahashi T et al (2008) Evaluation of the vascular status of autogenous hamstring tendon grafts after anterior cruciate ligament reconstruction in humans using magnetic resonance angiography. Knee Surg Sports Traumatol Arthrosc 16:342–347. doi:10.1007/s00167-007-0478-6

Ballock RT, Woo SL, Lyon RM et al (1989) Use of patellar tendon autograft for anterior cruciate ligament reconstruction in the rabbit: a long-term histologic and biomechanical study. J Orthop Res 7:474–485

Claes S, Verdonk P, Forsyth R, Bellemans J (2011) The "ligamentization" process in anterior cruciate ligament reconstruction: what happens to the human graft? A systematic review of the literature. Am J Sports Med 39:2476–2483. doi:10.1177/0363546511402662

Dustmann M, Schmidt T, Gangey I et al (2008) The extracellular remodeling of free-soft-tissue autografts and allografts for reconstruction of the anterior cruciate ligament: a comparison study in a sheep model. Knee Surg Sports Traumatol Arthrosc 16:360–369. doi:10.1007/s00167-007-0471-0

Falconiero RP, DiStefano VJ, Cook TM (1998) Revascularization and ligamentization of autogenous anterior cruciate ligament grafts in humans. Arthroscopy 14:197–205

Fujiya H, Kousa P, Fleming BC et al (2011) Effect of muscle loads and torque applied to the tibia on the strain behavior of the anterior cruciate ligament: an in vitro investigation. Clin Biomech (Bristol, Avon) 26:1005–1011. doi:10.1016/j.clinbiomech.2011.06.006

Gohil S, Annear PO, Breidahl W (2007) Anterior cruciate ligament reconstruction using autologous double hamstrings: a comparison of standard versus minimal debridement techniques using MRI to assess revascularisation. A randomised prospective study with a one-year follow-up. J Bone Joint Surg Br 89:1165–1171. doi:10.1302/0301-620X.89B9.19339

Goradia VK, Rochat MC, Grana WA et al (2000a) Tendon-to-bone healing of a semitendinosus tendon autograft used for ACL reconstruction in a sheep model. Am J Knee Surg 13:143–151

Goradia VK, Rochat MC, Kida M, Grana WA (2000b) Natural history of a hamstring tendon autograft used for anterior cruciate ligament reconstruction in a sheep model. Am J Sports Med 28:40–46

Grana WA, Egle DM, Mahnken R, Goodhart CW (1994) An analysis of autograft fixation after anterior cruciate ligament reconstruction in a rabbit model. Am J Sports Med 22:344–351

Howell SM, Knox KE, Farley TE, Taylor MA (1995) Revascularization of a human anterior cruciate ligament graft during the first two years of implantation. Am J Sports Med 23:42–49

Ishibashi Y, Toh S, Okamura Y et al (2001) Graft incorporation within the tibial bone tunnel after anterior cruciate ligament reconstruction with bone-patellar tendon-bone autograft. Am J Sports Med 29:473–479

Janssen RPA, van der Wijk J, Fiedler A et al (2011) Remodelling of human hamstring autografts after anterior cruciate ligament reconstruction. Knee Surg Sports Traumatol Arthrosc 19:1299–1306. doi:10.1007/s00167-011-1419-y

Jones JR, Smibert JG, McCullough CJ et al (1987) Tendon implantation into bone: an experimental study. J Hand Surg Br 12:306–312

Kawakami H, Shino K, Hamada M et al (2004) Graft healing in a bone tunnel: bone-attached graft with screw fixation versus bone-free graft with extra-articular suture fixation. Knee Surg Sports Traumatol Arthrosc. doi:10.1007/s00167-003-0484-2

Kleiner JB, Amiel D, Roux RD, Akeson WH (1986) Origin of replacement cells for the anterior cruciate ligament autograft. J Orthop Res 4:466–474

Kleiner JB, Amiel D, Harwood FL, Akeson WH (1989) Early histologic, metabolic, and vascular assessment of anterior cruciate ligament autografts. J Orthop Res 7:235–242

Kobayashi M, Watanabe N, Oshima Y et al (2005) The fate of host and graft cells in early healing of bone tunnel after tendon graft. Am J Sports Med 33:1892–1897

Kondo E, Yasuda K, Katsura T et al (2012) Biomechanical and histological evaluations of the doubled semitendinosus tendon autograft after anterior cruciate ligament reconstruction in sheep. Am J Sports Med 40:315–324. doi:10.1177/0363546511426417

Kuroda R, Kurosaka M, Yoshiya S, Mizuno K (2000) Localization of growth factors in the reconstructed anterior cruciate ligament: immunohistological study in dogs. Knee Surg Sports Traumatol Arthrosc 8:120–126

Liu SH, Panossian V, al-Shaikh R et al (1997) Morphology and matrix composition during early tendon to bone healing. Clin Orthop Relat Res 339:253–260

Majima T, Yasuda K, Tsuchida T et al (2003) Stress shielding of patellar tendon: effect on small-diameter collagen fibrils in a rabbit model. J Orthop Sci 8:836–841. doi:10.1007/s00776-003-0707-x

Marumo K, Saito M, Yamagishi T, Fujii K (2005) The "ligamentization" process in human anterior cruciate ligament reconstruction with autogenous patellar and hamstring tendons: a biochemical study. Am J Sports Med 33:1166–1173. doi:10.1177/0363546504271973

Mayr HO, Stoehr A, Dietrich M et al (2012) Graft-dependent differences in the ligamentization process of anterior cruciate ligament grafts in a sheep trial. Knee Surg Sports Traumatol Arthrosc 20:947–956. doi:10.1007/s00167-011-1678-7

Nebelung W, Becker R, Urbach D et al (2003) Histological findings of tendon-bone healing following anterior cruciate ligament reconstruction with hamstring grafts. Arch Orthop Trauma Surg 123:158–163. doi:10.1007/s00402-002-0463-y

Ng GY, Oakes BW, Deacon OW et al (1995) Biomechanics of patellar tendon autograft for reconstruction of the anterior cruciate ligament in the goat: three-year study. J Orthop Res 13:602–608

Ng GY, Oakes BW, Deacon OW et al (1996) Long-term study of the biochemistry and biomechanics of anterior cruciate ligament-patellar tendon autografts in goats. J Orthop Res 14:851–856

Ohno K, Yasuda K, Yamamoto N et al (1993) Effects of complete stress-shielding on the mechanical properties and histology of in situ frozen patellar tendon. J Orthop Res 11:592–602

Papageorgiou CD, Ma CB, Abramowitch SD et al (2001) A multidisciplinary study of the healing of an intraarticular anterior cruciate ligament graft in a goat model. Am J Sports Med 29:620–626

Rodeo SA, Arnoczky SP, Torzilli PA et al (1993) Tendon-healing in a bone tunnel. A biomechanical and histological study in the dog. J Bone Joint Surg Am 75:1795–1803

Rodeo SA, Kawamura S, Kim HJ et al (2006) Tendon healing in a bone tunnel differs at the tunnel entrance versus the tunnel exit: an effect of graft-tunnel motion? Am J Sports Med 34:1790–1800. doi:10.1177/0363546506290059

Rougraff BT, Shelbourne KD (1999) Early histologic appearance of human patellar tendon autografts used for anterior cruciate ligament reconstruction. Knee Surg Sports Traumatol Arthrosc 7:9–14

Rougraff B, Shelbourne KD, Gerth PK, Warner J (1993) Arthroscopic and histologic analysis of human patellar tendon autografts used for anterior cruciate ligament reconstruction. Am J Sports Med 21:277–284

Sánchez M, Anitua E, Azofra J et al (2010) Ligamentization of tendon grafts treated with an endogenous preparation rich in growth factors: gross morphology and histology. Arthroscopy 26:470–480. doi:10.1016/j.arthro.2009.08.019

Scheffler SU, Dustmann M, Gangey I, et al. (2005) The biological healing and restoration of the mechanical properties of free soft-tissue allografts lag behind autologous ACL reconstruction in the sheep model. In: Washington, D.C., USA, p abstract no.0236

Scheffler SU, Schmidt T, Gangéy I et al (2008a) Fresh-frozen free-tendon allografts versus autografts in anterior cruciate ligament reconstruction: delayed remodeling and inferior mechanical function during long-term healing in sheep. Arthroscopy 24:448–458. doi:10.1016/j.arthro.2007.10.011

Scheffler SU, Unterhauser FN, Weiler A (2008b) Graft remodeling and ligamentization after cruciate ligament reconstruction. Knee Surg Sports Traumatol Arthrosc 16:834–842. doi:10.1007/s00167-008-0560-8

Shelburne KB, Pandy MG (1998) Determinants of cruciate-ligament loading during rehabilitation exercise. Clin Biomech (Bristol, Avon) 13:403–413

Shino K, Horibe S (1991) Experimental ligament reconstruction by allogeneic tendon graft in a canine model. Acta Orthop Belg 57(Suppl 2):44–53

Shino K, Kawasaki T, Hirose H et al (1984) Replacement of the anterior cruciate ligament by an allogeneic tendon graft. An experimental study in the dog. J Bone Joint Surg Br 66:672–681

Tohyama H, Yasuda K (2002) The effect of increased stress on the patellar tendon. J Bone Joint Surg Br 84:440–446

Tomita F, Yasuda K, Mikami S et al (2001) Comparisons of intraosseous graft healing between the doubled flexor tendon graft and the bone-patellar tendon-bone graft in anterior cruciate ligament reconstruction. Arthroscopy 17:461–476

Unterhauser FN, Bail HJ, Höher J et al (2003) Endoligamentous revascularization of an anterior cruciate ligament graft. Clin Orthop Relat Res 414:276–288

Vogrin M, Rupreht M, Dinevski D et al (2010) Effects of a platelet gel on early graft revascularization after anterior cruciate ligament reconstruction: a prospective, randomized, double-blind, clinical trial. Eur Surg Res 45:77–85. doi:10.1159/000318597

Weiler A, Peters G, Maurer J et al (2001) Biomechanical properties and vascularity of an anterior cruciate ligament graft can be predicted by contrast-enhanced magnetic resonance imaging. A two-year study in sheep. Am J Sports Med 29:751–761

Weiler A, Hoffmann RFG, Bail HJ et al (2002) Tendon healing in a bone tunnel. Part II: histologic analysis after biodegradable interference fit fixation in a model of anterior cruciate ligament reconstruction in sheep. Arthroscopy 18:124–135

Yamakado K, Kitaoka K, Yamada H et al (2002) The influence of mechanical stress on graft healing in a bone tunnel. Arthrosc J Arthrosc Relat Surg 18:82–90. doi:10.1053/jars.2002.25966

Yoshikawa T, Tohyama H, Enomoto H, et al. (2004) Temporal changes in relationships between fibroblast repopulation, VEGF expression and angiogenesis in the patellar tendon graft after anterior cruciate ligament reconstruction. In: San Francisco, USA, p Paper 0236

Yoshikawa T, Tohyama H, Enomoto H et al (2006) Expression of vascular endothelial growth factor and angiogenesis in patellar tendon grafts in the early phase after anterior cruciate ligament reconstruction. Knee Surg Sports Traumatol Arthrosc 14:804–810. doi:10.1007/s00167-006-0051-8

Zaffagnini S, De Pasquale V, Marchesini Reggiani L et al (2007) Neoligamentization process of BTPB used for ACL graft: histological evaluation from 6 months to 10 years. Knee 14:87–93. doi:10.1016/j.knee.2006.11.006

Human Meniscus: From Biology to Tissue Engineering Strategies

89

Hélder Pereira, Ibrahim Fatih Cengiz, Joana Silva-Correia, Joaquim Miguel Oliveira, Rui Luís Reis, and João Espregueira-Mendes

Contents

Abstract

Once meniscus is damaged, a cascade of events occurs leading to degenerative joint changes of the knee. The morbidity of patients can significantly increase overtime and degeneration of the cartilage can progress, resulting in arthritis. Possibilities for treatment of meniscus lesions are primordially focused in repair and replacement (e.g., acellular scaffolds and meniscus allograft transplantation). Tissue Engineering and Regenerative Medicine have been providing new options in medical practice. However, these disciplines require deep understanding of the target tissue and physiopathology of the implicated disorder. In order to overcome the

H. Pereira (✉)
3B's Research Group – Biomaterials, Biodegradables and Biomimetics, Headquarters of the European Institute of Excellence on Tissue Engineering and Regenerative Medicine, University of Minho, Taipas, Guimarães, Portugal

ICVS/3B's – PT Government Associated Laboratory, Guimarães, Portugal

Clínica Espregueira–Mendes F.C. Porto Stadium – FIFA Medical Centre of Excellence, Porto, Portugal

Orthopedic Department, Centro Hospitalar Póvoa de Varzim, Vila do Conde, Portugal
e-mail: heldermdpereira@gmail.com

I.F. Cengiz • J. Silva-Correia
3B's Research Group – Biomaterials, Biodegradables and Biomimetics, Headquarters of the European Institute of Excellence on Tissue Engineering and Regenerative Medicine, University of Minho, Taipas, Guimarães, Portugal

ICVS/3B's – PT Government Associated Laboratory, Guimarães, Portugal
e-mail: fatih.cengiz@dep.uminho.pt; joana.correia@dep.uminho.pt

J.M. Oliveira
3B's Research Group – Biomaterials, Biodegradables and Biomimetics, Headquarters of the European Institute of Excellence on Tissue Engineering and Regenerative Medicine, University of Minho, Taipas, Guimarães, Portugal

ICVS/3B's – PT Government Associated Laboratory, Braga/Guimarães, Portugal

FIFA Medical Centre of Excellence, Clínica Espregueira–Mendes F.C. Porto Stadium, Porto, Portugal
e-mail: miguel.oliveira@dep.uminho.pt

M.N. Doral, J. Karlsson (eds.), *Sports Injuries*,
DOI 10.1007/978-3-642-36569-0_73

current limitations, fundamental studies have been made for developing reliable strategies aiming to obtain superior tissue healing. Herein, it is presented the most relevant insights and research directions on the fundamental biology and biomechanics of meniscus. The principles of tissue engineering (triad) and the significant in vitro and in vivo reports addressing meniscus regeneration are included, once these will provide the basements for future clinical directions.

Introduction

Meniscus is a complex tissue with an autonomous repair capability that is mostly restricted to the vascularized region, in the stable knee (Pereira et al. 2013c). Also for this fact, it still subsists as one of the most frequent injuries leading to orthopedic surgery (Garrett et al. 2006), thus causing work absenteeism and, in some cases, sports invalidity.

In the last few years, meniscal replacement/repair and regeneration are gaining increased attention (Lubowitz and Poehling 2011) as an alternative to meniscectomy. This is mainly due to the long-term functional instability of the knee and appearing of early osteoarthritis (Fayard et al. 2010) as a consequence of meniscus removal (Fig. 1).

Meniscus lesions treatment possibilities are still limited and quite often not very effective. This is not only due to the recent interest in its preservation but more importantly due to the fact that meniscus is poorly studied as compared to other tissues, in respect to: biomechanics, vascularity, innervation, cellularity, and extracellular matrix (ECM) composition.

Replacement of meniscus can be both total and partial (Monllau et al. 2010) and comprehends the use of cadaveric tissue. Repair strategies are almost restricted to suturing techniques, and its application greatly dependent on healing prognosis of meniscus which by its turn is dictated by location of the lesion, i.e., if it is limited to the vascular or extends to central and avascular zone (Kohn and Siebert 1989).

In the last few years, tissue engineering (TE) regeneration has emerged as a new world of treatment possibilities. This recent field of knowledge demands deep comprehension of tissue biology, architecture, and natural mechanisms of repair. Furthermore, several tissue-engineered products are still being tested preclinically and will undoubtedly require prior clinical validation until reaching the clinics (Pereira et al. 2011). Thus, the process of product development will require many years as most of biomaterials, scaffolds, and formulations need to be optimized in vitro and in vivo using different processing routes, cell types, and animal models.

R.L. Reis
Clínica Espregueira–Mendes F.C. Porto Stadium, FIFA Medical Centre of Excellence, Porto, Portugal

Orthopaedic Department, Hospital de S. Sebastião, Feira, Portugal

ICVS/3B's – PT Government Associated Laboratory, Braga/Guimarães, Portugal

3B's Research Group – Biomaterials, Biodegradables and Biomimetics, Head- quarters of the European Institute of Excellence on Tissue Engineering and Regenerative Medicine, University of Minho, Taipas, Guimarães, Portugal
e-mail: rgreis@dep.uminho.pt

J. Espregueira-Mendes
3B's Research Group – Biomaterials, Biodegradables and Biomimetics, Headquarters of the European Institute of Excellence on Tissue Engineering and Regenerative Medicine, University of Minho, Taipas, Guimarães, Portugal

Clínica Espregueira–Mendes F.C. Porto Stadium – FIFA Medical Centre of Excellence, Porto, Portugal

Orthopedic Department, Centro Hospitalar Póvoa de Varzim, Vila do Conde, Portugal

ICVS/3B's – PT Government Associated Laboratory, Braga/Guimarães, Portugal

Orthopaedic Department, Hospital S. Sebastião, Feira, Portugal
e-mail: jem@espregueira.com; joaoespregueira@netcabo.pt

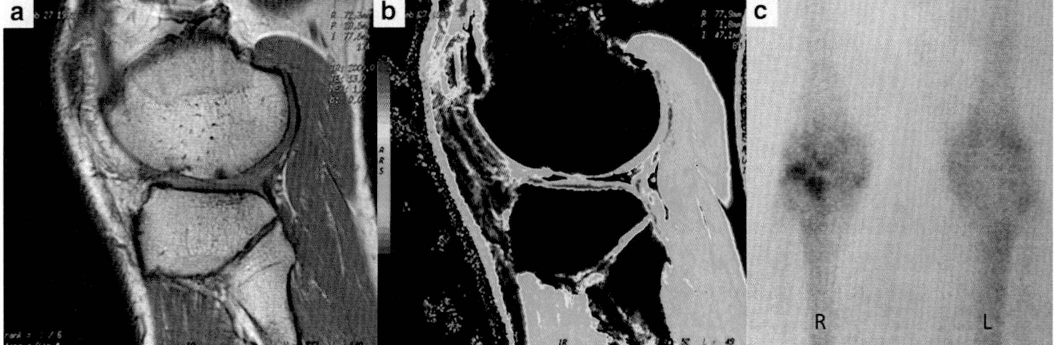

Fig. 1 Clinical case concerning 27 years old patient, 2 years after lateral meniscectomy. T2 MRI sagittal view of lateral compartment where absence of lateral meniscus can be noticed besides osteochondral lesion of femoral condyle (**a**); correspondent T2-mapping MRI image demonstrating cartilage and subchondral bone changes (**b**); Corresponding delayed phase bone scan demonstrates increased signal in the affected compartment related to stress overload after meniscectomy (**c**)

Fundamental Aspects on Meniscus Tissue

Biology

The fundamental knowledge on meniscus biology has evolved significantly in recent years (Verdonk et al. 2005). It has been reported that meniscus fibrocartilage tissue composition greatly varies with age and gender and upon injury/disease (Sweigart and Athanasiou 2001). In addition, lateral and medial menisci also present significant differences in respect to shape (Fig. 2), vascular network, and composition. From gross morphology, it is possible to observe the C-shape of medial meniscus, whereas lateral meniscus is more sharply curved. In respect to vasculature, meniscus has three distinct zones: vascularized (r-r), central or intermediate (r-w), and avascular (w-w) (Fig. 3). From histological images, there can be observed a higher blood vessels network at the r-r zone, and these are mainly limited to the meniscus periphery with a variable penetration in medial (10–30 %) and lateral menisci (10–25 %). A network of nerves is accompanying the blood vessels. Smaller nerves and axons run radially in convoluted patterns, and mostly nerves can be found in the interstitial tissue of the peripheral zone of the meniscus and in the anterior and posterior horns, while the inner menisci core has no nerves (Brian et al. 1985).

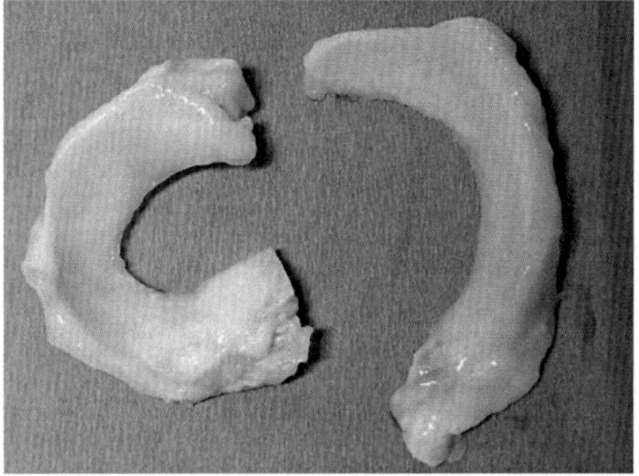

Fig. 2 Photography of lateral (*left*) and medial (*right*) menisci harvested from human donor

Meniscus composition studies have been shown that it possess a water content of about 72 %, and the remnant portion consists of an organic component, where an asymmetric distribution of cells are embedded (2 % DNA of total organic component) (Herwig et al. 1984; Makris et al. 2011).

In respect to cellularity, chondrocyte-like, fibroblast-like, and intermediate cells have been observed in the meniscus (Ghadially et al. 1978), though classification of meniscus cells has no consensus (Nakata et al. 2001). The outer zone cells have an oval, fusiform shape, i.e., fibroblast-like cells. The cells in the inner portion have round morphology and are embedded in an ECM, thus called fibrochondrocytes or chondrocyte-like cells

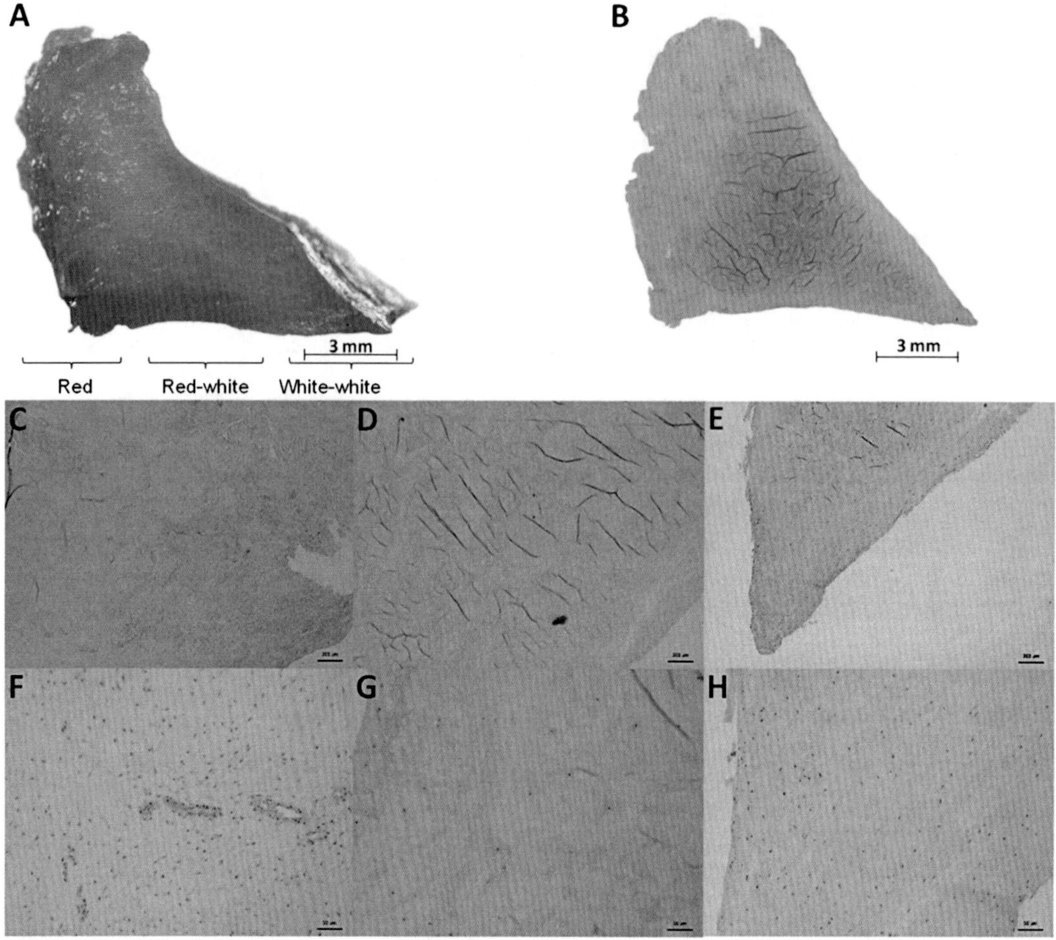

Fig. 3 A stereomicroscopy image of a part of a human meniscus (**a**), a hematoxylin and eosin-stained histological micrograph showing the complete cross section of a human meniscus (**b**), hematoxylin-eosin-stained micrographs of meniscus obtained from vascular region (**c**, **f**), from intermediate region (**d**, **g**) and from avascular region (**e**, **h**) at two different magnifications. The scale bar indicates 3 mm in (**a**, **b**), 200 μm in (**c**–**e**), and 50 μm in (**f**–**h**)

(Verdonk et al. 2005). Another type of flattened and fusiform cells can be found at the superficial zone of the meniscus. It has been advanced with the possibility of being specific progenitor cells (Van der Bracht et al. 2007). The outer zone cells presents a higher migration capability and seems to exhibit lower adhesion strengths as compared to the ones present in the inner portion (Gunja et al. 2012). Furthermore, it has also been recognized that paracrine signaling by these MSCs might play a decisive role in stimulating repair responses (Pasa and Visna 2005).

Pereira et al. has recently investigated the cell phenotypes and distribution within the different segments and zones of meniscus tissue in 44 patients (Pereira et al. 2014). The histomorphometry revealed a gradual decrease of cell density from vascular (outer) to avascular (inner) zones, in all segments (anterior, middle, and posterior) of both lateral and medial menisci. Complementarily, a lower cell density in anterior segments of both (lateral or medial) menisci as compared to middle or posterior segments was observed. Isolated cells presented both rounded and fusiform-like morphology. Cell sorting analysis revealed that CD44, CD73, CD90, and CD105 surface markers were being expressed by more than 97 % of cells. CD31 (2.3 % ± 0.8 %)

and CD34 (3.2 % ± 1.0 %) were also expressed by a cell population. The CD45 marker for hematopoietic stem cells was present in 0.2 % ± 0.1 %, but this small population might play a role on chondrogenic differentiation of mesenchymal stem cells (MSCs), as previously suggested (Pasa and Visna 2005).

The ECM surrounding the meniscus cells contains different types of collagen (75 % of total organic component) and glycosaminoglycans (GAGs, 17 % of total organic component) (Melrose et al. 2005), with small percentages of glycoproteins. Collagen type I is the major of ECM fibrils, but types III and V are also present. Chondoitin-6-sulfate, dermatan sulfate, chondroitin-4-sulfate, and keratin sulfate are the main types of GAGs (Herwig et al. 1984). Aggrecan constitutes the major large proteoglycan of the meniscus (Scott et al. 1997), and its main function is to enable the meniscus to absorb water (Makris et al. 2011). Adhesion glycoproteins and elastin (<1 % of total organic component) can be also found in meniscus, but the role of the latter is not yet fully understood (Ghosh and Taylor 1987; McDevitt and Webber 1992). The adhesion glycoproteins present in the human meniscus are fibronectin, thrombospondin, and collagen VI (Miller and McDevitt 1991) and act as anchor sites between ECM and cells.

Biomechanics

Lateral and medial menisci are located in each knee and are attached between the tibial and femoral surfaces, thus covering two-thirds of the tibia plateau. Meniscus has a unique role on preserving knee joint stability, and total contact area is reduced by a third to a half in the fully extended knee, upon its removal (Kurosawa et al. 1980). Fukubayashi and Kurosawa (1980) reported that meniscectomy induces deleterious consequences in articular cartilage, subchondral bone, and proximal tibia's trabecular bone and cortex.

Due to its anatomical features and attachment to medial collateral ligament, the medial meniscus has limited mobility as compared to the lateral one. In the stable knee (with functioning central pivot ligaments), the medial meniscus has smaller contribution on anterior tibial displacement constraint. The anterior cruciate ligament impairs anterior knee motion prior to significant contact of femoral condyle with posterior horn of medial meniscus and tibial plateau (Levy et al. 1982). There are significant differences between both femorotibial compartments on the knee joint to be considered. Lateral tibial plateau is prone to have a more convex shape opposing to a more concave shape on the medial compartment (Levy et al. 1982; McDermott et al. 2008). This fact helps us to recognize that the loss of the lateral meniscus leads to significant decrease on femorotibial congruence as shown in Fig. 1.

The lateral meniscus carries most of the load transfer on the lateral compartment (70 % opposing to 50 % in the medial) (Walker and Hajek 1972), while in the medial compartment force transmission is distributed between the articular cartilage and meniscus (Bourne et al. 1984).

The biomechanical response of the menisci to forces acting on tibiofemoral joints results from their macro-geometry, fine architecture, and insertional ligaments (McDermott et al. 2008). The collagen bundles of the superficial layer are randomly orientated somewhat similarly to articular hyaline cartilage (Beaupre et al. 1986). This way it provides lower friction between articular surfaces during joint motion. Beneath these surface layers, the bulk of meniscal tissue presents two different regions concerning collagen fibers: the inner one-third bundles display a radial pattern, whereas the outer two-thirds are oriented circumferentially.

Accordingly, it has been suggested that the inner third may function mainly in compression, while the outer two-thirds will function mostly in tension. Furthermore, some radially orientated collagen fibers can also be found within the bulk of the meniscal tissue, resisting longitudinal splitting of the circumferential collagen bundles. These are known as "tie fibers" (Bullough et al. 1970).

Viscoelastic behavior of the meniscus correlates with ECM composition (Makris et al. 2011). It presents a rubber-like pattern at high loading frequencies, while at lower frequencies viscous dissipation occurs (Makris et al. 2011; Pereira et al. 2014). These biomechanical features are not much dependent of collagen content but mainly correlate with GAGs and water content: higher with increasing GAGs and lower with increasing water (Bursac et al. 2009).

Killian et al. (2010) has reported segmental and zonal variation in GAGs content, size, and cellular density in animal meniscus. Similarly to the asymmetric distribution of cells and blood vessels within the different meniscus, mechanical properties (Bursac et al. 2009) also vary. Recently our group (Pereira et al. 2014) evaluated the mechanical properties in each segment of fresh lateral and medial human menisci, at physiological-like conditions (37 °C and pH 7.4). Mean age of all evaluated patients ($n = 44$) was 59 (SD = 3.0), mean height was 161 cm (SD = 10), mean weight was 74 kg (SD = 11), and mean body mass index (BMI) was 28.7 (SD = 3.53). Significant differences between the measurement of E' and $tan\ \delta$ between the medial and lateral menisci were found. Medial meniscus presented higher E' and $tan\ \delta$ as compared to lateral. The analysis of data revealed a significant difference between the measurements of E' and $tan\ \delta$ for anterior, middle, and posterior segments of lateral and medial menisci. When considering combined analysis of both menisci (medial and lateral together), posterior segments are stiffer as compared to the middle ones, and these are significantly stiffer than anterior. Anterior segments presented a significant lower E' but higher $tan\ \delta$ as compared to middle or posterior ones, in both types of menisci.

Regeneration of Meniscus: Principle of Tissue Engineering

Tissue engineering (TE) advances promise to create a revolution in clinical medicine by means of employing life sciences and engineering principles toward restoring or even improving tissue functioning. TE takes place in the domain of regenerative medicine, which covers also other fields including cellular and gene therapies. The objective of TE is to regenerate the damaged tissues by using three main components (Fig. 4)

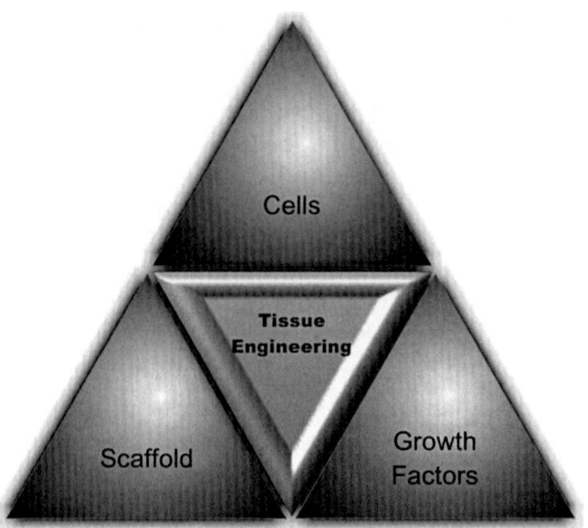

Fig. 4 Three main components of tissue engineering. A scaffold is a 3D structure that is manufactured from biodegradable biomaterials and in which cells are seeded; cells are the basic constituent of a tissue by synthesizing the matrix of the tissue; and growth factors are polypeptides that regulate the activities of cells

that are scaffolds, cells, and growth factors (GFs) or bioactive agents, which are used alone or preferably in combination to mimic the native tissue.

Scaffolds are three-dimensional (3D) porous structures that are manufactured from biodegradable biomaterials in which cells are seeded. Since cells need to survive and grow inside the scaffolds, it should serve more than a physical construct that has the right size and shape. Cells interact with scaffold and the outcome of the interaction is linked with the success of biomimicry of the ECM of the damaged/diseased tissue. The scaffold acts preferably as a temporary matrix, and its degradation products should not elicit the toxic effect or acute inflammation. Ideally, a TE scaffold has high porosity with adequate pore size and high interconnectivity to facilitate cell migration, ingrowth, and scaffold-cell interactions (Freyman et al. 2001; Noeth et al. 2010; Puppi et al. 2010). Moreover, the surface of an ideal scaffold promotes adhesion and proliferation of cells.

Cells are the basic constituent of a tissue by synthesizing the ECM of the tissue. Both stem cells and differentiated cell have been employed in TE strategies. A mature differentiated cell (e.g., fibrochondrocyte) has a certain function in the tissue. Stem cells are undifferentiated cells, and they have the ability of self-renewal and differentiation into a certain type of specialized cells. A possible classification of stem cells is based on the tissue from which they are isolated: adult or embryonic stem cells. Adult stem cells (Young and Black 2004) are relatively more specialized and partially differentiated. Embryonic stem cells (Rippon and Bishop 2004) have a greater natural potential since they are isolated during the embryonic stages of development. Stem cells can be classified by their potential as totipotent, pluripotent, multipotent, and unipotent. Totipotent and pluripotent stem cells are embryonic stem cells, and totipotent stem cells possess the greatest potential with their ability to differentiate into all body cell types. However, multipotent and unipotent stem cells are adult stem cells which able to differentiate into only a certain type of cells (Alison et al. 2002).

The principle of TE involves the expansion of the patient's own cells in vitro and the consequent seeding into an appropriate scaffold. Then, either directly or after in vitro conditioning, the cell-scaffold construct is implanted into the corresponding site of the body. The tissue regeneration occur by the ECM synthesis of the cells, while the scaffold biodegrades over time. Even though TE is a developing and promising research field, effective clinical applications have not yet achieved (Pereira et al. 2011).

TE strategies have been considered for the treatment of partial meniscus defects that cannot heal by themselves (Pereira et al. 2011; Verdonk et al. 2012). So far, only acellular scaffolds alone (polyurethane- or collagen-based) are employed in clinical studies. However, there is a possibility to develop strategies where all main components of the TE are used. With such kind of strategy, the native meniscus tissue could be mimicked and in this way failure rates can be minimized, and better clinical results could be achieved (Pereira et al. 2011).

Scaffolds Alone

So far only acellular scaffolds are employed in TE strategies for clinical meniscus partial replacement (Pereira et al. 2011; Verdonk et al. 2012). The use of collagen-based constructs (CMI, at present known as Menaflex®, ReGen Biologics, USA) were reported, mostly for the treatment of medial meniscus defects of hundreds of patients (Linke et al. 2006; Genovese et al. 2007; Zaffagnini et al. 2007; Rodkey et al. 2008; Bulgheroni et al. 2010; Monllau et al. 2011; Zaffagnini et al. 2011; Hirschmann et al. 2012), and more recently for the treatment of lateral meniscus defects as well (Zaffagnini et al. 2012).

In the evaluations of the biopsy specimens, no severe inflammation or immune response of clinical relevance was observed (Pereira et al. 2011). Assessments by second look arthroscopy or MRI revealed that shrinkage of the implants might occur over time. However, this phenomenon is not yet accurately elucidated to determine the extent of this decrease and to evaluate how the outcome is affected. It was reported also that the mechanical properties of implant material were not adequate (Zaffagnini et al. 2011). Moreover, the obtained neo-tissue showed some dissimilarity in characteristics with the native fibrocartilaginous meniscus tissue (Pereira et al. 2011). Polyurethane-based (Actifit®, Orteq Ltd, London, United Kingdom) is the other clinically evaluated implant. It was reported that it could be used for the clinical treatment of pain associated to irreparable partial meniscus lesions (Efe et al. 2012; Verdonk et al. 2012). In addition, it also allows tissue ingrowth (Verdonk et al. 2011). Nevertheless, histologically the neo-tissue was different from the native meniscus tissue, and the pattern of re-cellularization thus should be further investigated in a near future (Pereira et al. 2011). These drawbacks accentuate the need for developing a new generation of products/scaffolds and more advanced TE strategies to regenerate meniscus tissue.

Additionally, a number of other scaffolding biomaterials are being developed and studied with or without cells, but they are not yet employed in clinical studies. These biomaterials include: silk fibroin (Yan et al. 2012), polycaprolactone-polyurethane (Welsing et al. 2008), hyaluronic acid-polycaprolactone (Kon et al. 2008), and polyglycolic acid (Kang et al. 2006).

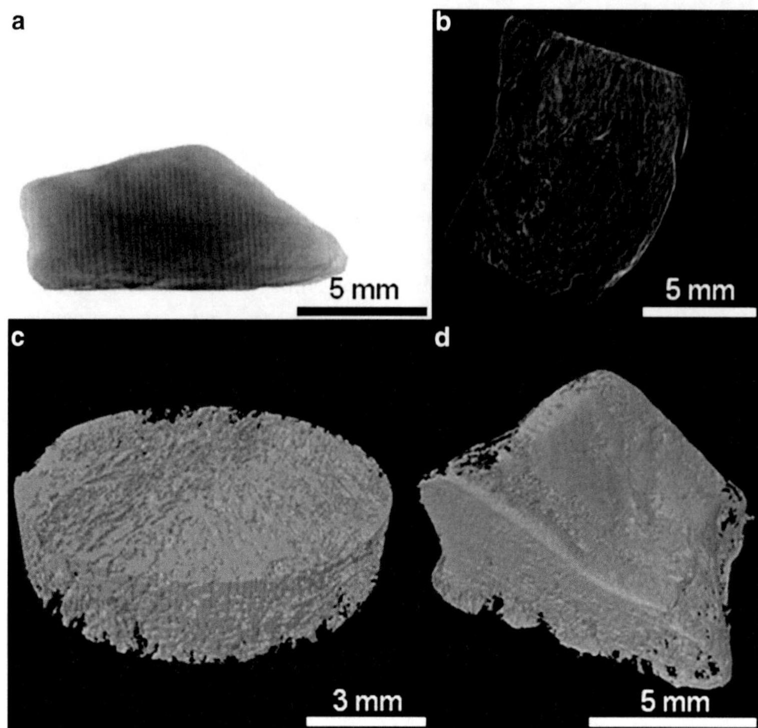

Fig. 5 An X-ray image of a freeze-dried portion of a human medial meniscus acquired with a high-resolution microcomputed tomography equipment, SkyScan 1072 scanner, (SkyScan, Kontich, Belgium) (**a**), and respective 2D (**b**) and 3D reconstructions of the images showing the internal (**c**) and entire (**d**) architectures of the tissue. Images were obtained by using CT Analyzer and CTvox, image-processing softwares from SkyScan

One of the requirements for TE scaffolds is that they should present an adequate structural architecture. Besides, their size and shape should be correct. The conventional scaffold manufacturing methods lack the ability of precise controlling of size and geometry single pores and the interconnectivity and anatomically correct size of the whole construct. Rapid prototyping (RP) techniques are relatively new methods by which a physical construct can be created layer by layer using a computer-aided design developed from computer-based medical imaging modalities (e.g., computed tomography, CT or magnetic resonance imaging, MRI). Using a RP technique, manufacture-customized scaffolds in correct anatomical shape can be manufactured (Moroni et al. 2006).

Knowledge on the internal architecture of meniscus is one of the requirements to develop advanced TE constructs which mimic the native tissue. Quantitative data on internal architectural features can be obtained by μ-CT characterization. These data include the values of pore size, porosity, and trabeculae thickness and their distribution across the sample, as well as the value of interconnectivity. Figure 5 presents images obtained from μ-CT characterization of a portion of freeze-dried healthy human medial meniscus. Notwithstanding the recent advances, biological characterization of human meniscus is not yet completed (Verdonk et al. 2005; Pereira et al. 2011), for example, recognition of different cell populations, its ultrastructure (Verdonk et al. 2005), determination of segmental distributions of cells, and ECM. Once the information on these topics is revealed, it will be exploited by the TE. Thus, RP is very advantageous since it does not only provide the possibility of manufacturing patient-specific scaffolds with the right architecture, namely, layer-specific desired pore size, porosity, and interconnectivity, but also the right distribution of different cell populations within the meniscus (Pereira et al. 2013). In this way, the biomechanical properties and microstructure of the TE constructs can be optimized to mimic the native meniscus tissue.

Delivery of Growth Factors

Growth factors (GFs) represent many polypeptides that transmit signals and have a specific effect on the cell activity (Babensee et al. 2000). GFs can bind to the specific receptors of the target cells. The effect could be stimulation or inhibition of adhesion, proliferation, migration, differentiation, and gene expression of the cells. Therefore, incorporating GFs into TE strategies for meniscus repair has a great potential to provide better results. One of the important GFs in chondrogenesis is insulin-like growth factor-1 (IGF-1) (Patil et al. 2012). Thus, it might be expected for IGF-1 to have a role in the regeneration of meniscus (Zhang et al. 2009). Zhang et al. (2009) followed an approach where growth factor gene therapy and TE are combined and performed a preclinical study with IGF-1 transfected cells that were incorporated into injectable gels. The results showed that the repaired meniscal defects were similar to native meniscus (Zhang et al. 2009).

Huey and Athanasiou (2011) demonstrated with a scaffold-free approach that two bioactive agents – chondroitinase-ABC (C-ABC) and transforming growth factor-β1 (TGF-β1) – can be used for maturational growth of meniscus neo-tissue both biochemically and biomechanically similar to native meniscus tissue. In another study, MacBarb et al. (2012) developed fibrocartilage tissue with a range of functional properties close to that of native tissues by means of treating a range of co-cultures of meniscus cells and articular cartilage cells in different ratios with C-ABC and TGF-β1. In another study (Gu et al. 2012), in vitro chondrogenic differentiation of myoblasts was achieved with cartilage-derived morphogenetic protein-2 (CDMP-2) alone or together with TGF-β1 where using these two bioactive agents together improved the outcome. It was reported that myoblasts could be convenient cell source for meniscus TE (Gu et al. 2012).

In the study of Ionescu et al. (2012), it was shown that in vivo short-term delivery of basic fibroblast growth factor (bFGF) and in vivo sustained delivery of transforming growth factor-β3 (TGF-β3) stimulated meniscus repair owing to their promitotic and pro-matrix formative effects, respectively. Hoben et al. (2009) investigated a large number of strategies for the differentiation of human embryonic stem cells to fibrochondrocyte-like cells by using a variety of GFs, including TGF-β3, bone morphogenetic protein (BMP)-2, -4, and -6 that were combined with different co-cultures. It was reported that the combination of BMP-4 and TGF-β3 resulted in the most effective combination for collagen and GAG synthesis (Hoben et al. 2009).

Additionally, platelet-rich plasma and exogenous fibrin clots contain growth factors. Ishida et al. (2007) showed that platelet-rich plasma that was introduced into gelatin hydrogel improved the healing of meniscal defects. Kamimura and Kimura (2011) reported that the exogenous fibrin clots serve as a scaffold to enhance the healing process of meniscus by its GFs.

Cell-Based Strategies

Recently, Pereira et al. (2011) reported a systematic review on TE strategies aimed at regeneration of meniscus lesions. It was shown that there is a mismatch between the strategies employed in clinical trials and preclinical studies. Most clinical trials applications pursue acellular strategies, while most preclinical studies exploit cells and/or GFs to achieve better results. The strategy of using cell-laden scaffolds (Kang et al. 2006; Martinek et al. 2006; Weinand et al. 2006a, b; Angele et al. 2008; Kon et al. 2008; Yamasaki et al. 2008; Scotti et al. 2009; Weinand et al. 2009) has been reported in several preclinical studies.

Zellner et al. (2010) studied the role of MSCs in meniscus tissue engineering. It was reported that stem cells provide a good healing, i.e., the TE constructs that were implanted into the avascular region of rabbit meniscus resulted in meniscus-like repair tissue. Stapleton et al. assessed (2011) the in vivo immunocompatibility and the capacity for cellular attachment of de-cellularized porcine meniscus scaffold which could be re-cellularized in vitro before implantation if desired.

Weinand et al. (2006a, b) studied vicryl mesh scaffolds seeded with autologous (Weinand et al. 2006a) or allogenic (Weinand et al. 2006b) chondrocytes from different types of cartilage tissues. It was reported that inclusion of cells into the scaffold improves the healing of avascular meniscus (Weinand et al. 2006a). In the study of Martinek et al. (2006), it was shown that collagen-based meniscus implant that is seeded with autologous fibrochondrocytes performs better than the acellular implant for partial meniscus replacement. Besides, it was also reported that stem cell-seeded hyaluronan/gelatin composite scaffold has higher ability to repair meniscus defects as compared to the acellular scaffold (Angele et al. 2008).

Bioreactors

Bioreactors are devices that are used to mimic the in vivo conditions for cell culturing in TE applications. Bioreactors can control the conditions in the culture media, for example, the oxygen ratio, pH, temperature, nutrients, and osmolality (Griffith and Naughton 2002; Martin and Vermette 2005; Pörtner et al. 2005). With a bioreactor, uniform cell seeding and improved mass transfer between the culture and the cells can be achieved. In this way, the tissue regeneration could be enhanced in vitro. In TE, depending on the application different types of bioreactors can be used, for example, spinner flasks, flow perfusion bioreactors, rotating wall vessels, and mechanical stimulation bioreactor (Griffith and Naughton 2002; Martin and Vermette 2005; Pörtner et al. 2005).

Petri et al. studied (Petri et al. 2012) the effects of continuous perfusion and mechanical stimulation of cyclic compression on human bone marrow stromal cell-laden collagen meniscus implants. The results showed that differentiation of cells was improved by mechanical stimulation, whereas proliferation of the cells was promoted by continuous perfusion (Petri et al. 2012). In another study with the aim of developing a meniscus implant, Martínez et al. (2012) showed that fibroblast-laded micro-channeled cellulose scaffolds that were cultivated in a dynamic compression bioreactor had aligned cells and collagen fibers and increased collagen synthesis. Moreover, Fox et al. (2010) cultivated the TE constructs that were fibroblast-like synoviocytes-laden synthetic scaffolds with incorporation of bFGF alone/with TGF-β3, in a rotating bioreactor, and showed their potential for avascular meniscus regeneration (Fox et al. 2010). Ideally, a "complete" bioreactor for meniscus TE research would be capable to mimic the complexity of compressive, strain, and shear forces acting on medial and lateral menisci, once they play different roles within knee kinematics (McDermott et al. 2008). This remains a non-accomplished target and subject of ongoing research (Pereira et al. 2013). However, it is very important to understand its relevance in the development of a tissue/implant within the laboratory, capable to combine the key features of the native meniscus and suitable for human transplantation (Pereira et al. 2013). Such implant would probably be capable to overcome some currently recognized pitfalls attributed to cadaveric allograft transplantation (Monllau et al. 2010).

Summary

Meniscus is a complex and challenging tissue, and once damaged it possesses limited repair ability. Current meniscus replacement with a matched size donor allograft meniscus is used to treat the symptoms of early arthritis, such as pain and swelling of the knee, but not all patients are eligible. Only those who are young and active and have minimal degenerative joint changes are considered good candidates for the replacement procedure. Future tissue-engineered strategies might broaden these indications in future. By its turn, repair of meniscus ruptures (vertical tears) using suturing technique via arthroscopy can be used alone or in combination with bioactive agents in order to enhance fibrovascular scar proliferation. The type of rupture, time elapsed after injury, joint stability, and overall biomechanical degeneration of the joint should also be borne in mind and included in the equation prior to treatment. Healing ability is also decreased in complex or degenerative tears, central tears, and tears in unstable knees. Tissue engineering meniscus is most advantageous as it envisions a total regeneration of the damaged tissue. Combination of adequate scaffolds (patient-customized) with cells (differentiated or undifferentiated or even genetically modified cells) may be advantageous in those patients where repair/replacement approaches fail such as elderly and patients with pathological conditions associated. Despite being promising from the technological and clinical point of views, tissue-engineered products might require many years before reaching the full range of its clinical use, once its application is highly regulated and dependent on country-specific legislations. These barriers might even hinder its widespread application. Furthermore, TE technologies and solutions are still considered as expensive and difficult to reach for most patients. For these reasons, the clinical exploitation of tissue-engineered products is greatly dependent and dictated not only by the future technological developments but more importantly on correct research protocols. Correct selection of cases and adequate follow-up are mandatory in the early clinical application of any promising therapy. Controlled application of therapies still under research will impair unnecessary costs and losses and will have determinant impact if it can be supported by insurance companies and national health systems.

Cross-References

- ▶ Anterior Cruciate Ligament Injuries with Concomittant Meniscal Pathologies
- ▶ Anatomy and Biomechanics of the Knee
- ▶ Arthroscopic Repair of the Meniscus Tears
- ▶ Meniscal Allografts: Indications and Results
- ▶ Meniscal Injuries and Discoid Lateral Meniscus in Adolescent Athletes
- ▶ Meniscal Substitutes: Polyurethane Meniscus Implant: Technique and Results
- ▶ Meniscectomy
- ▶ Meniscus Reconstruction Using a New Collagen Meniscus Implant
- ▶ Meniscus Variations

References

Alison MR, Poulsom R, Forbes S, Wright NA (2002) An introduction to stem cells. J Pathol 197:419–423

Angele P, Johnstone B, Kujat R, Zellner J, Nerlich M, Goldberg V et al (2008) Stem cell based tissue engineering for meniscus repair. J Biomed Mater Res A 85:445–455

Babensee JE, McIntire LV, Mikos AG (2000) Growth factor delivery for tissue engineering. Pharm Res 17:497–504

Beaupre A, Choukroun R, Guidouin R, Garneau R, Gerardin H, Cardou A (1986) Knee menisci. Correlation between microstructure and biomechanics. Clin Orthop Relat Res 208:72–75

Bourne RB, Finlay JB, Papadopoulos P, Andreae P (1984) The effect of medial meniscectomy on strain distribution in the proximal part of the tibia. J Bone Joint Surg Am 66:1431–1437

Brian D, Mackenzie WG, Shim SS, Leung G (1985) The vascular and nerve supply of the human meniscus. Arthrosc J Arthrosc Relat Surg 1:58–62

Bulgheroni P, Murena L, Ratti C, Bulgheroni E, Ronga M, Cherubino P (2010) Follow-up of collagen meniscus implant patients: clinical, radiological, and magnetic resonance imaging results at 5 years. Knee 17:224–229

Bullough PG, Munuera L, Murphy J, Weinstein AM (1970) The strength of the menisci of the knee as it relates to their fine structure. J Bone Joint Surg (Br) 52:564–567

Bursac P, Arnoczky S, York A (2009) Dynamic compressive behavior of human meniscus correlates with its extracellular matrix composition. Biorheology 46:227–237

Efe T, Getgood A, Schofer MD, Fuchs-Winkelmann S, Mann D, Paletta JR et al (2012) The safety and short-term efficacy of a novel polyurethane meniscal scaffold for the treatment of segmental medial meniscus deficiency. Knee Surg Sports Traumatol Arthrosc 20:1822–1830

Fayard JM, Pereira H, Servien E, Lustig S, Neyret P (2010) Meniscectomy global results-complications. Springer, Berlin/Heidelberg, pp 177–190

Fox DB, Warnock JJ, Stoker AM, Luther JK, Cockrell M (2010) Effects of growth factors on equine synovial fibroblasts seeded on synthetic scaffolds for avascular meniscal tissue engineering. Res Vet Sci 88:326–332

Freyman TM, Yannas IV, Gibson LJ (2001) Cellular materials as porous scaffolds for tissue engineering. Prog Mater Sci 46:273–282

Fukubayashi T, Kurosawa H (1980) The contact area and pressure distribution pattern of the knee. A study of normal and osteoarthrotic knee joints. Acta Orthop Scand 51:871–879

Garrett WE Jr, Swiontkowski MF, Weinstein JN, Callaghan J, Rosier RN, Berry DJ et al (2006) American board of orthopaedic surgery practice of the orthopaedic surgeon: part-II, certification examination case mix. J Bone Joint Surg Am 88:660–667

Genovese E, Angeretti MG, Ronga M, Leonardi A, Novario R, Callegari L et al (2007) Follow-up of collagen meniscus implants by MRI. Radiol Med 112:1036–1048

Ghadially FN, Thomas I, Yong N, Lalonde JM (1978) Ultrastructure of rabbit semilunar cartilages. J Anat 125:499–517

Ghosh P, Taylor TK (1987) The knee joint meniscus. A fibrocartilage of some distinction. Clin Orthop Relat Res 224:52–63

Griffith LG, Naughton G (2002) Tissue engineering–current challenges and expanding opportunities. Science 295:1009–1014

Gu Y, Wang Y, Dai H, Lu L, Cheng Y, Zhu W (2012) Chondrogenic differentiation of canine myoblasts induced by cartilage-derived morphogenetic protein-2 and transforming growth factor-β1 in vitro. Mol Med Rep 5:767–772

Gunja NJ, Dujari D, Chen A, Luengo A, Fong JV, Hung CT (2012) Migration responses of outer and inner meniscus cells to applied direct current electric fields. J Orthop Res 30:103–111

Herwig J, Egner E, Buddecke E (1984) Chemical changes of human knee joint menisci in various stages of degeneration. Ann Rheum Dis 43:635–640

Hirschmann MT, Keller L, Hirschmann A, Schenk L, Berbig R, Lüthi U et al (2012) One-year clinical and MR imaging outcome after partial meniscal replacement in stabilized knees using a collagen meniscus implant. Knee Surg Sports Traumatol Arthrosc 21 (3):740–747

Hoben GM, Willard VP, Athanasiou KA (2009) Fibrochondrogenesis of hESCs: growth factor combinations and cocultures. Stem Cells Dev 18:283–292

Huey DJ, Athanasiou KA (2011) Maturational growth of self-assembled, functional menisci as a result of TGF-β1 and enzymatic chondroitinase-ABC stimulation. Biomaterials 32:2052–2058

Ionescu LC, Lee GC, Huang KL, Mauck RL (2012) Growth factor supplementation improves native and engineered meniscus repair in vitro. Acta Biomater 8:3687–3694

Ishida K, Kuroda R, Miwa M, Tabata Y, Hokugo A, Kawamoto T et al (2007) The regenerative effects of platelet-rich plasma on meniscal cells in vitro and its in vivo application with biodegradable gelatin hydrogel. Tissue Eng 13:1103–1112

Kamimura T, Kimura M (2011) Repair of horizontal meniscal cleavage tears with exogenous fibrin clots. Knee Surg Sports Traumatol Arthrosc 19:1154–1157

Kang SW, Son SM, Lee JS, Lee ES, Lee KY, Park SG et al (2006) Regeneration of whole meniscus using meniscal cells and polymer scaffolds in a rabbit total meniscectomy model. J Biomed Mater Res A 78:659–671

Killian ML, Lepinski NM, Haut RC, Haut Donahue TL (2010) Regional and zonal histo-morphological characteristics of the lapine menisci. Anat Rec (Hoboken) 293:1991–2000

Kohn D, Siebert W (1989) Meniscus suture techniques: a comparative biomechanical cadaver study. Arthrosc J Arthrosc Relat Surg 5:324–327

Kon E, Chiari C, Marcacci M, Delcogliano M, Salter DM, Martin I et al (2008) Tissue engineering for total meniscal substitution: animal study in sheep model. Tissue Eng Part A 14:1067–1080

Kurosawa H, Fukubayashi T, Nakajima H (1980) Load-bearing mode of the knee joint: physical behavior of the knee joint with or without menisci. Clin Orthop Relat Res 149:283–290

Levy IM, Torzilli PA, Warren RF (1982) The effect of medial meniscectomy on anterior-posterior motion of the knee. J Bone Joint Surg Am 64:883–888

Linke RD, Ulmer M, Imhoff AB (2006) Replacement of the meniscus with a collagen implant (CMI). Oper Orthop Traumatol 18:453–462

Lubowitz JH, Poehling GG (2011) Save the meniscus. Arthroscopy 27:301–302

MacBarb RF, Makris EA, Hu JC, and Athanasiou KA (2012) A chondroitinase-ABC and TGF-β1 treatment regimen for enhancing the mechanical properties of tissue engineered fibrocartilage. Acta Biomater

Makris EA, Hadidi P, Athanasiou KA (2011) The knee meniscus: structure-function, pathophysiology, current repair techniques, and prospects for regeneration. Biomaterials 32:7411–7431

Martin Y, Vermette P (2005) Bioreactors for tissue mass culture: design, characterization, and recent advances. Biomaterials 26:7481–7503

Martinek V, Ueblacker P, Braun K, Nitschke S, Mannhardt R, Specht K et al (2006) Second generation of meniscus transplantation: in-vivo study with tissue engineered meniscus replacement. Arch Orthop Trauma Surg 126:228–234

Martínez H, Brackmann C, Enejder A, Gatenholm P (2012) Mechanical stimulation of fibroblasts in micro-channeled bacterial cellulose scaffolds enhances production of oriented collagen fibers. J Biomed Mater Res A 100:948–957

McDermott ID, Masouros SD, Amis AA (2008) Biomechanics of the menisci of the knee. Curr Orthop 22:193–201

McDevitt CA, Webber RJ (1992) The ultrastructure and biochemistry of meniscal cartilage. Clin Orthop Relat Res 252:8–18

Melrose J, Smith S, Cake M, Read R, Whitelock J (2005) Comparative spatial and temporal localisation of perlecan, aggrecan and type I, II and IV collagen in the ovine meniscus: an ageing study. Histochem Cell Biol 124:225–235

Miller RR, McDevitt CA (1991) Thrombospondin in ligament, meniscus and intervertebral disc. Biochim Biophys Acta 1115:85–88

Monllau JC, González-Lucena G, Gelber PE, Pelfort X (2010) Allograft meniscus transplantation: a current review. Tech Knee Surg 9:107–113

Monllau JC, Gelber PE, Abat F, Pelfort X, Abad R, Hinarejos P et al (2011) Outcome after partial medial meniscus substitution with the collagen meniscal implant at a minimum of 10 years' follow-up. Arthroscopy 27:933–943

Moroni L, de Wijn JR, van Blitterswijk CA (2006) 3D fiber-deposited scaffolds for tissue engineering: influence of pores geometry and architecture on dynamic mechanical properties. Biomaterials 27:974–985

Nakata K, Shino K, Hamada M, Mae T, Miyama T, Shinjo H et al (2001) Human meniscus cell: characterization of the primary culture and use for tissue engineering. Clin Orthop Relat Res 391:S208–S218

Noeth U, Rackwitz L, Steinert AF, Tuan RS (2010) Cell delivery therapeutics for musculoskeletal regeneration. Adv Drug Deliv Rev 62:765–783

Pasa L and Visna P (2005) Suture of meniscus. SCRIPTA MEDICA (BRNO) 78(3):135–150

Patil AS, Sable RB, Kothari RM (2012) Role of insulin-like growth factors (IGFs), their receptors and genetic regulation in the chondrogenesis and growth of the mandibular condylar cartilage. J Cell Physiol 227:1796–1804

Pereira H, Frias AM, Oliveira JM, Espregueira-Mendes J, Reis RL (2011) Tissue engineering and regenerative medicine strategies in meniscus lesions. Arthroscopy 27:1706–1719

Pereira H, Caridade SG, Frias AM, Silva-Correia J, Pereira DR, Cengiz IF et al (2014) Biomechanical and cellular segmental characterization of human meniscus: building the basis for tissue engineering therapies. Osteoarthritis and Cartilage (submitted)

Pereira H, Silva-Correia J, Oliveira JM, Reis RL, Espregueira-Mendes J (2013) Future trends in the treatment of meniscus lesions: from repair to regeneration. In: Verdonk R, Espregueira-Mendes J, Monllau JC (eds) Meniscal transplantation. Springer, Heidelberg/New York/Dordrecht/London, pp 103–114

Pereira H, Silva-Correia J, Oliveira JM, Reis RL, Espregueira-Mendes J (2013c) The meniscus: basic science. In: Verdonk R, Espregueira-Mendes J, Monllau JC (eds) Meniscal transplantation. Springer, Heidelberg/New York/Dordrecht/London, pp 7–14

Petri M, Ufer K, Toma I, Becher C, Liodakis E, Brand S et al (2012) Effects of perfusion and cyclic compression on in vitro tissue engineered meniscus implants. Knee Surg Sports Traumatol Arthrosc 20:223–231

Pörtner R, Nagel-Heyer S, Goepfert C, Adamietz P, Meenen NM (2005) Bioreactor design for tissue engineering. J Biosci Bioeng 100:235–245

Puppi D, Chiellini F, Piras AM, Chiellini E (2010) Polymeric materials for bone and cartilage repair. Prog Polym Sci 35:403–440

Rippon HJ, Bishop AE (2004) Embryonic stem cells. Cell Prolif 37:23–34

Rodkey WG, DeHaven KE, Montgomery WH 3rd, Baker CL Jr, Beck CL Jr, Hormel SE et al (2008) Comparison of the collagen meniscus implant with partial meniscectomy. A prospective randomized trial. J Bone Joint Surg Am 90:1413–1426

Scott PG, Nakano T, Dodd CM (1997) Isolation and characterization of small proteoglycans from different zones of the porcine knee meniscus. Biochim Biophys Acta 1336:254–262

Scotti C, Pozzi A, Mangiavini L, Vitari F, Boschetti F, Domeneghini C et al (2009) Healing of meniscal tissue by cellular fibrin glue: an in vivo study. Knee Surg Sports Traumatol Arthrosc 17:645–651

Stapleton TW, Ingram J, Fisher J, Ingham E (2011) Investigation of the regenerative capacity of an acellular porcine medial meniscus for tissue engineering applications. Tissue Eng Part A 17:231–242

Sweigart MA, Athanasiou KA (2001) Toward tissue engineering of the knee meniscus. Tissue Eng 7:111–129

Van der Bracht H, Verdonk R, Verbruggen G, Elewaut D, Verdonk P (2007) Cell based meniscus tissue engineering. In: Ashammakhi N, Reis R, Chiellini E (eds) Topics in tissue engineering, 508 vol 3. Expertissues, Guimarães, Portugal, pp 6756–6763

Verdonk PC, Forsyth RG, Wang J, Almqvist KF, Verdonk R, Veys EM et al (2005) Characterisation of human knee meniscus cell phenotype. Osteoarthritis Cartilage 13:548–560

Verdonk R, Verdonk P, Huysse W, Forsyth R, Heinrichs EL (2011) Tissue ingrowth after implantation of a novel, biodegradable polyurethane scaffold for treatment of partial meniscal lesions. Am J Sports Med 39:774–782

Verdonk P, Beaufils P, Bellemans J, Djian P, Heinrichs EL, Huysse W et al (2012) Successful treatment of painful irreparable partial meniscal defects with a polyurethane scaffold: two-year safety and clinical outcomes. Am J Sports Med 40:844–853

Walker PS, Hajek JV (1972) The load-bearing area in the knee joint. J Biomech 5:581–589

Weinand C, Peretti GM, Adams SB Jr, Bonassar LJ, Randolph MA, Gill TJ (2006a) An allogenic cell-based implant for meniscal lesions. Am J Sports Med 34:1779–1789

Weinand C, Peretti GM, Adams SB Jr, Randolph MA, Savvidis E, Gill TJ (2006b) Healing potential of transplanted allogeneic chondrocytes of three different sources in lesions of the avascular zone of the meniscus: a pilot study. Arch Orthop Trauma Surg 126:599–605

Weinand C, Xu JW, Peretti GM, Bonassar LJ, Gill TJ (2009) Conditions affecting cell seeding onto three-dimensional scaffolds for cellular-based biodegradable implants. J Biomed Mater Res B Appl Biomater 91:80–87

Welsing RT, van Tienen TG, Ramrattan N, Heijkants R, Schouten AJ, Veth RP et al (2008) Effect on tissue differentiation and articular cartilage degradation of a polymer meniscus implant: a 2-year follow-up study in dogs. Am J Sports Med 36:1978–1989

Yamasaki T, Deie M, Shinomiya R, Yasunaga Y, Yanada S, Ochi M (2008) Transplantation of meniscus regenerated by tissue engineering with a scaffold derived from a rat meniscus and mesenchymal stromal cells derived from rat bone marrow. Artif Organs 32:519–524

Yan LP, Oliveira JM, Oliveira AL, Caridade SG, Mano JF, Reis RL (2012) Macro/microporous silk fibroin scaffolds with potential for articular cartilage and meniscus tissue engineering applications. Acta Biomater 8:289–301

Young HE, Black AC (2004) Adult stem cells. Anat Rec A Discov Mol Cell Evol Biol 276A:75–102

Zaffagnini S, Giordano G, Vascellari A, Bruni D, Neri MP, Iacono F et al (2007) Arthroscopic collagen meniscus implant results at 6 to 8 years follow up. Knee Surg Sports Traumatol Arthrosc 15:175–183

Zaffagnini S, Marcheggiani Muccioli GM, Lopomo N, Bruni D, Giordano G, Ravazzolo G et al (2011) Prospective long-term outcomes of the medial collagen meniscus implant versus partial medial meniscectomy: a minimum 10-year follow-up study. Am J Sports Med 39:977–985

Zaffagnini S, Marcheggiani Muccioli GM, Bulgheroni P, Bulgheroni E, Grassi A, Bonanzinga T et al (2012) Arthroscopic collagen meniscus implantation for partial lateral meniscal defects: a 2-year minimum follow-up study. Am J Sports Med 40:2281–2288

Zellner J, Mueller M, Berner A, Dienstknecht T, Kujat R, Nerlich M et al (2010) Role of mesenchymal stem cells in tissue engineering of meniscus. J Biomed Mater Res A 94:1150–1161

Zhang H, Leng P, Zhang J (2009) Enhanced meniscal repair by overexpression of hIGF-1 in a full-thickness model. Clin Orthop Relat Res 467:3165–3174

Knee Dislocations

90

Mark A. Bergin, James Ward, Bruno Ohashi, and Volker Musahl

Contents

M.A. Bergin (✉)
University of Pittsburgh, Pittsburgh, PA, USA
e-mail: mbergin.md@gmail.com

J. Ward
Department of Orthopaedic Surgery, University of Pittsburgh Medical Center, Pittsburgh, PA, USA
e-mail: wardjp@upmc.edu

B. Ohashi
Center for Orthopaedics and Traumatology of Brasilia, Brasilia, DF, Brazil
e-mail: brunohashi@yahoo.com

V. Musahl
Department of Orthopaedic Surgery, University of Pittsburgh Medical Center, Pittsburgh, PA, USA

Division of Sports Medicine, Orthopaedic Surgery, University of Pittsburgh, Pittsburgh, PA, USA
e-mail: musahlv@upmc.edu

M.N. Doral, J. Karlsson (eds.), *Sports Injuries*,
DOI 10.1007/978-3-642-36569-0_123

Abstract

A knee dislocation is a potentially devastating injury that must be managed appropriately from initial presentation through potentially several interventions and surgeries. A high suspicion for neurovascular injuries should be maintained at all times, and just because it is not obvious at initial presentation does not mean that one has not occurred. Surgical management should be well thought out and planned because complications such as wound problems, compartment syndrome, neurovascular injury, and stiffness are more common than in less severe extremity injuries.

Introduction

Knee dislocations can be among the most devastating injuries to the lower extremity and are true orthopedic emergencies. A knee dislocation is defined as a disruption of the normal anatomic relationship of the distal femur and proximal tibia, and it necessarily involves injury to two or more of the ligamentous supporting structures about the knee (Kennedy 1963; Brautigan and Johnson 2000; Klimkiewicz et al. 2001; Rihn et al. 2004). A knee dislocation may present as an occult dislocation or "subluxation" that has occurred and spontaneously reduced, or as a gross deformity and persistent dislocation of the tibiofemoral joint. In addition to ligamentous injury, neurovascular injuries are frequent with knee dislocations, occurring in anywhere from 15 % to 50 % of these injuries, and they are associated with poor outcome (Green and Allen 1977; Shelbourne and Klootwyk 2000; Wascher 2000; Stannard et al. 2004). A knee dislocation may also involve significant meniscal and capsular injury and may or may not have an associated fracture. Dislocations are frequently caused by high-velocity trauma, but can result from seemingly minimal trauma such as a misstep from a curb with a low-velocity knee dislocation due to morbid obesity; so one must maintain a high index of suspicion when evaluating patients (Azar et al. 2011). Treatment options have evolved from initial nonoperative treatment to continually evolving surgical and arthroscopic techniques with increasing awareness of procedure timing after injury.

Anatomy

There is minimal stability conferred by the bony anatomy of the knee, as most of the stability is due to the ligamentous structures, including the two bundles of the anterior cruciate ligament (ACL), the anteromedial (AM) and posterolateral (PL) bundles, the two bundles of the posterior cruciate ligament (PCL), and the anterolateral (AL) and posteromedial (PM) bundles, along with the anterior and posterior meniscofemoral ligaments, the medial collateral ligament (MCL), and fibular (lateral) collateral ligament (FCL) including the posterolateral corner structures (PLC). The posterolateral corner generally refers to the iliotibial band (ITB), the biceps femoris, the FCL, the popliteus muscle and tendon, the popliteofibular ligament, the fabellofibular ligament, and the lateral joint capsule.

Several neurovascular structures run in close proximity to the knee joint and have a high potential for injury at the time of knee dislocation. Structures within the popliteal fossa, including the popliteal artery, popliteal vein, and tibial nerve, are immediately adjacent to the posterior capsule just to the lateral of midline and can all be subject to injury (Kim et al. 2010). They are particularly vulnerable because they are tethered above and below the knee by the adductor hiatus and the gastrocnemius-soleus arch, respectively. The common peroneal nerve, which courses deep to the biceps femoris and then runs superficial to the fibular head as it courses anteriorly and distally in the leg, is also at high risk for being injured as it courses over the lateral aspect of the fibular head.

Classification

Many classification systems exist for knee dislocations. The most common description of knee dislocations is directional and refers to the tibial

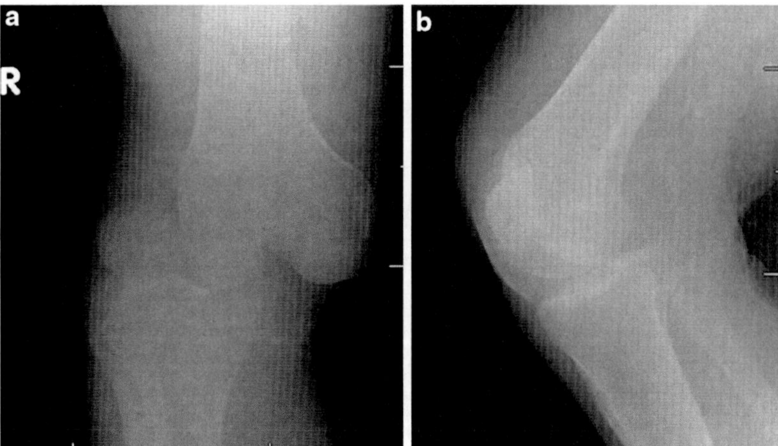

Fig. 1 (**a**) AP X-ray of a lateral knee dislocation. (**b**) Lateral X-ray of a lateral knee dislocation

displacement relative to the femur (Kennedy 1963). In decreasing order of incidence, these are described as anterior, posterior, lateral, medial, and rotatory, with rotatory being subdivided into anteromedial, anterolateral, posteromedial, and posterolateral (Kennedy 1963; Green and Allen 1977; Fig. 1a, b). This type of classification however fails to take into account occult or spontaneously reduced knee dislocations.

Several other methods of classification have also been developed including those based on mechanism of injury and perceived "high"- and "low"-energy mechanisms (Shelbourne et al. 1991a, Hagino et al. 1998). Anatomic classification of knee dislocations has been described by Schenk and ranges from disruption of one cruciate ligament (KD-I) to disruption of all four knee ligaments (KD-IV) (Eastlack et al. 1997). In this classification system, a concomitant fracture is indicated by (KD V) and associated neurologic and arterial vascular injury represented by (N) and (C), respectively (Eastlack et al. 1997).

Due to the severe, unique, and complicated nature of knee dislocations, most of these injuries are not accurately represented by these classification systems. Therefore, it is preferred to describe knee dislocations based on timing of presentation, acute versus chronic; based on specific anatomic structure injured, along with grade of injury; and based on specific description of concomitant neurologic or vascular injury (Harner et al. 2004). An example of the above is a patient whose radiographs can be seen in Fig. 2a, b. This patient sustained an acute, occult knee dislocation, involving a grade three injury to the proximal MCL, a grade three ACL midsubstance injury, a fibular head avulsion fracture, and a bony avulsion of the tibial PCL and was neurovascular intact (Fig. 2a, b).

Evaluation

History and Clinical Presentation

Knee dislocations can present in many different circumstances ranging from an obese patient limping into the physician's office after a slip and fall having sustained a knee dislocation or "subluxation" with spontaneous reduction, to a person in a high-speed motor vehicle collision brought to the emergency room with obvious gross deformity to the knee joint and to anywhere in between including during sports participation. Despite knee dislocation being a rare event, a high index of suspicion for this injury must be maintained. Knee dislocations may be missed if the evaluating physician underestimates the severity of knee injury based on injury mechanism alone or if the treating physician is distracted by other life-threatening injuries after a severe trauma. Regardless of presentation, a detailed and systematic workup must be initiated immediately in order to diagnose and treat any potentially limb-threatening neurovascular injuries.

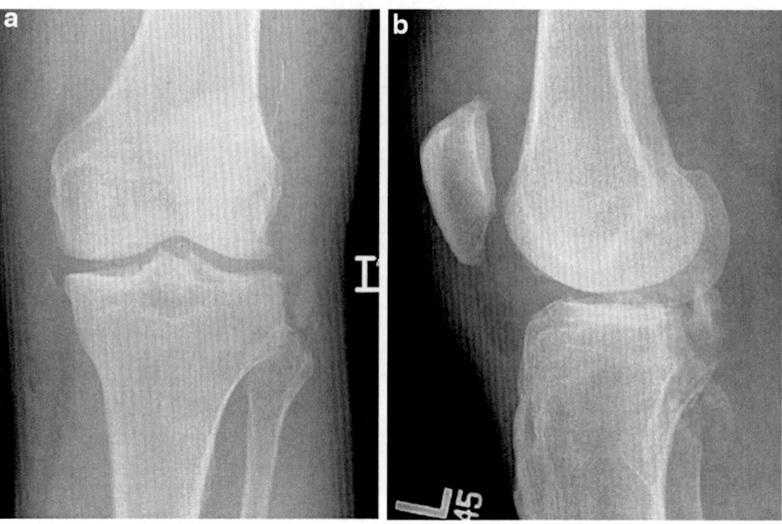

Fig. 2 (**a**) AP X-ray of an occult knee dislocation with fibular head fracture and PCL avulsion fracture. (**b**) Lateral X-ray of occult knee dislocation with fibular head fracture and PCL avulsion fracture

The direction of force at the time of injury will dictate the structures that are injured and the position of dislocation. Anterior dislocations most frequently result from a hyperextension mechanism (Kennedy 1963; Green and Allen 1977; Gustilo and Cabatan 1993). At approximately 30° of hyperextension, injury to the posterior capsule is initiated. This is followed by injury to the ACL and PCL as the severity of hyperextension increases, with injury to the popliteal artery occurring after 50° of hyperextension (Kennedy 1963).

Posterior dislocations are the result of a posteriorly directed force to the anterior tibia (Green and Allen 1977). These injuries can frequently occur due to a blow to the anterior tibia while playing sport or due to a dashboard injury in a motor vehicle collision (Taylor et al. 1972; Gustilo and Cabatan 1993). The PCL is the main restraint to posterior forces and is necessarily disrupted in posterior knee dislocations. The patella and/or the extensor mechanism and the ACL are also frequently injured (Kennedy 1963).

Medial, lateral, and rotatory dislocations are typically due to varus, valgus, and combined forces, respectively (Gustilo and Cabatan 1993). These types of knee dislocations are frequently occult and usually present with a slightly subluxed knee rather than a grossly dislocated knee. Medial dislocations more commonly present with an associated fracture and, as such, must always be concerned for a knee dislocation with evidence of a medial tibial plateau fracture on imaging (Brautigan and Johnson 2000). Lateral knee dislocations are frequently complicated by injury to the common peroneal nerve and have the potential to be unable to be reduced due to the medial femoral condyle "buttonholing" through the medial capsule (Taylor et al. 1972). In this scenario, the patient will likely present with gross deformity about the knee joint and with a "dimple sign," indicative of the medial capsular tissues being trapped in the joint (Taylor et al. 1972).

Lastly, the patient with a knee dislocation may present with a cold leg without pulses, a warm leg without palpable pulses, or a dusky appearance to the skin below the injury level at the knee. They may also present complaining of numbness on the dorsum of the foot and/or inability to dorsiflex or plantar flex the ipsilateral foot. Whatever the clinical presentation may be, the clinician must have a high suspicion for neurovascular insult and must immediately evaluate these structures with the physical exam and further diagnostic studies as indicated.

Physical Examination

A complete and systematic examination is mandatory when there is a clinically apparent knee dislocation, or concern for occult knee dislocation, so that injuries are not missed. Initial management will depend on the overall condition of the patient and the clinical setting at the time of primary evaluation. Whether treating an athlete at a sporting event with a dislocated knee, or seeing a patient in the emergency room with the same injury, the patient should be managed according to Advanced Trauma Life Support (ATLS) protocol, and once airway, breathing, and circulation are confirmed, an attempt to reduce the dislocated knee should be made.

The initial musculoskeletal examination begins with inspection. The skin should be examined for any lacerations or traumatic arthrotomies. The color of the skin should also be closely examined distally to the injury for any evidence of vascular insufficiency. Any dimpling of the anteromedial knee should be noted as mentioned above, this could represent an irreducible dislocation (Taylor et al. 1972). The condition of the soft tissues of the entire lower extremity should also be noted with a high degree of suspicion for an associated compartment syndrome.

Neurovascular Examination

A complete neurovascular examination must be carried out. Any active bleeding or expanding hematoma is indicative of a possible popliteal artery injury. Two mechanisms of arterial injury have been described. With an anterior dislocation and hyperextension deformity to the knee joint, the popliteal artery is stretched and this traction can cause intimal tears to the vessel. This patient may have intact pulses initially with apparent distal perfusion; however, late thrombosis can occur placing the entire limb in jeopardy. With a posterior dislocation, there is a greater likelihood of popliteal artery transection or tearing (Green and Allen 1977). A vascular surgeon should be consulted immediately to evaluate this injury.

Distal pulses, including posterior tibial and dorsalis pedis pulses, should be checked; however, palpable pulses alone cannot rule out an arterial injury. These pulses should be compared to the contralateral limb. Serial ankle–brachial index (ABI) exams should be checked for both lower extremities and compared as well. Any side-to-side difference, or absolute value of less than 0.9, should be treated as a likely vascular injury, and further workup should be initiated. If there is no difference, then the ABI exams should be frequently repeated to ensure that late signs of vascular compromise do not develop.

In place of serial exams, some authors now recommend angiographic studies, for example, CT angiogram, regardless of physical exam findings (Seroyer et al. 2008; Fig. 3). This is controversial because many surgeons argue that these invasive vascular studies are not warranted in patients without clear signs of vascular injury on physical exam. In a recent study by Mills et al., ABI exams demonstrated 100 % sensitivity, specificity, and positive predictive value in that all patients with an ABI of greater than 0.9 had no vascular injury and all patients with an ABI of less than 0.9 had a vascular injury (Mills et al. 2004). Nevertheless, if there is any question about potential vascular injury, a CT angiogram should be obtained.

After the evaluation of the patient's vascular status, attention should be turned to the neurologic examination and, more specifically, evaluation of the common peroneal nerve. Common peroneal nerve injuries are reported to occur in between 14 % and 35 % of knee dislocations (Hegyes et al. 2000). Nerve injury ranges from stretch injury, to complete disruption of the nerve. Whether evaluating a patient immediately after injury on the field of play, in the emergency department, or several days later in the clinic, the timing of nerve dysfunction is critical to evaluate and consider. Examination consists of sensory and motor evaluation distal to the knee injury, specifically assessing at the sensation distribution over the dorsum of the foot and ankle and great toe dorsiflexion. If the patient states that sensation and motor function were intact immediately after the injury and have deteriorated since that time, concern for expanding hematoma is warranted and emergent decompression should be considered. Documentation of nerve function is also important preoperatively so that there is no question about the status of the nerve prior to surgical

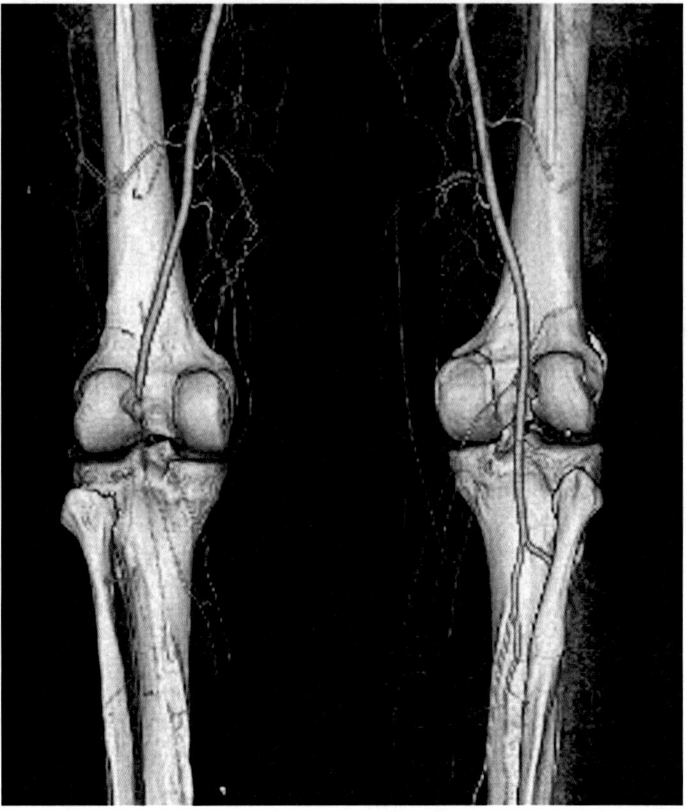

Fig. 3 Three-dimensional reconstruction of CT angiogram to evaluate for arterial injury after knee dislocation. The knee on the left has discontinuity of the popliteal artery in the posterior knee indicating injury at that level

intervention. Many of these nerve injuries have a poor prognosis despite maintaining nerve continuity, with less than 50 % of patients regaining any useful nerve function (Niall et al. 2005).

Knee Examination

Lastly, examination of the knee should be carried out, but may be difficult due to the acute and devastating nature of the injury. Alignment should be assessed and the knee should be confirmed to be reduced. Comparison to the contralateral, uninjured knee should be performed and may give important information when considering surgical intervention with regard to the patient's native coronal plane alignment. One must always consider that the contralateral knee may be injured also an attempt at a straight leg raise may be performed and gives important information about the extensor mechanism. The knee may only have a limited range of motion, but any crepitus should alert the examiner to possible fracture. A large effusion may be present, but may also be reduced due to significant capsular injury. The ligamentous examination can be performed with a pillow under the injured knee for the patient's comfort, and in this position, varus, valgus, and a Lachman examination can be performed with reasonable accuracy. The knee can generally be flexed to 50° or 60°, and the normal 1 cm anterior "step-off" of the medial tibial plateau relative to the medial femoral condyle should be felt for. If this "step-off" is reduced or absent, then injury to the PCL is likely. Varus and valgus stress tests can be performed at both full extension, evaluating cruciate and capsular integrity, and 30° of flexion, where the collateral ligaments are isolated. Rotational evaluation may be very difficult with an acute injury especially at 90° of flexion; however, increased tibial external rotation at 30° of flexion should raise concerns for a posterolateral corner (PLC) injury or a severe medial knee injury.

Imaging

Initial imaging of the dislocated knee should consist of plain radiographs, at least anteroposterior and lateral views of the knee in question. Except in cases of vascular compromise, an attempt at a closed reduction should not be delayed until radiographs are obtained. Initial radiographs should be closely inspected for any small changes in coronal or sagittal plane alignment. Fractures, including fracture of the fibular head or tibial plateau, are common and should raise concern for the severity of injury. Reduction of the knee must be confirmed on X-ray examination, and if reduction is not possible, then the patient should be taken to the operating room where reduction may be fluoroscopically confirmed and reduction maintained with external fixation as necessary. A CT scan may also give added information about fractures and reduction of the tibiofemoral joint, and if a CT angiogram is obtained for vascular evaluation, then this information is readily available.

After initial evaluation including neurovascular examination and confirmation of reduction on radiographs or CT, an MRI should be obtained to further detail the injury to the involved extremity. MRI allows for detailed evaluation of ligamentous structures about the knee including both cruciate and collateral ligaments. MRI can also give further information about meniscal injury, cartilage damage, and capsular injury.

Initial Management and Treatment Options

Initial Management

Management of the dislocated knee should proceed according to a stepwise algorithm to maximize patient outcome and avoid potential complications. The first priority is that reduction of the knee is emergently attempted and reduction immediately confirmed. If reduction is unable to be maintained by closed means, then operative management is warranted in the form of surgical reduction and placement of external fixation. The use of initial external fixation is indicated for more complex injuries as in cases with associated vascular injury, compartment syndrome, or open dislocations for wound management.

Nonoperative Treatment

Historically, nonoperative treatment was the standard of care for knee dislocations (Kennedy 1963; Taylor et al. 1972); however, more recently, studies have reported improved outcomes with surgical management (Dedmond and Almekinders 2001; Richter et al. 2002). Nonoperative treatment may still be the treatment of choice for some patients with severe injuries to vital organ systems that require attention prior to extremity injuries. A recent meta-analysis by Dedmond et al. showed improved postoperative Lysholm scores in the operatively treated group by almost 20 points when compared to nonoperative treatment (Dedmond and Almekinders 2001). Richter et al. showed similar improvement in outcome scores at 8-year follow-up (Richter et al. 2002). Nonoperative treatment in the literature usually consists of immobilization of the effected extremity in full extension using either a cast or external fixator for 3–6 weeks followed by progressive range of motion.

Operative Management

Preoperative Considerations

After initial treatment and stabilization of a patient with a knee dislocation, further operative treatment is generally warranted, and if any subsequent surgical procedure is to be considered, a venous ultrasound 1 day prior to each procedure can rule out a potentially fatal deep venous thrombosis (DVT) and subsequent pulmonary embolism (PE). Acute treatment of knee dislocations usually involves a combination of direct ligament repair and ligament reconstruction. Graft choices should be considered including ipsilateral quadriceps tendon or patellar tendon autografts or

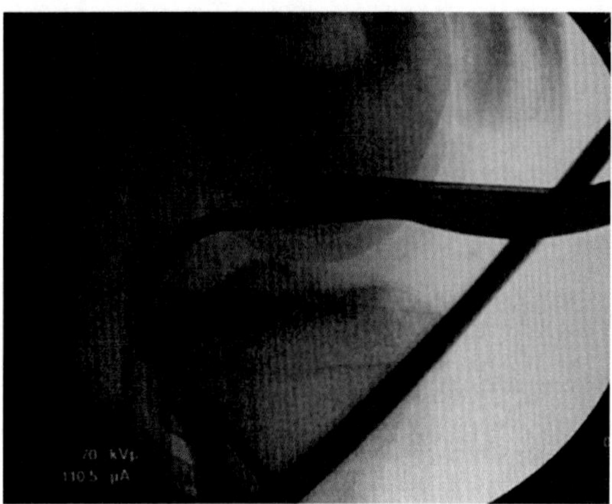

Fig. 4 Intraoperative fluoroscopy for placement of PCL tibial tunnel

contralateral knee grafts. Allografts are generally the preferred graft choice with the advantage of no donor site morbidity, more options for graft sizes, and potentially less operative time during the procedure (Fanelli and Feldmann 1998; Harner et al. 2004; Levy et al. 2009). The use of a tourniquet is contraindicated if vascular injury is present or vascular repair has been performed. Intraoperative fluoroscopy can be an invaluable asset for the assessment of tunnel placement and correction of subluxation during the procedure (Fig. 4).

Surgical Timing: The Staged Approach

The spectrum and variable combination of injuries when dealing with knee dislocations makes it very difficult to follow a rigid algorithm for repair and/or reconstruction of the knee's stabilizing structures. However, when dealing with these injures, one must consider them in terms of four main stabilizing structures of the knee, ACL, PCL, MCL, and posterolateral side.

Due to the complexity of these injuries, a multidisciplinary team approach is necessary. Experienced teams, including surgeons and surgical technicians, are better prepared to deal with the difficult decisions involved in this type of trauma.

An individualized approach to each patient needs to be performed, taking into account the complex and multiple ligament injuries to the knee. The surgeon needs to choose between a single-stage or two-stage procedure considering the benefits of an early surgery and the risks of postoperative stiffness and infection due to external fixation or soft tissue injury (Mohtadi et al. 1991; Shelbourne et al. 1991b; Levy et al. 2010).

As previously mentioned, if external fixation is initially indicated, a definitive approach should be performed from 3 to 6 weeks post-injury. Reconstruction/repair of all ligaments needs to be performed, after soft tissue recovery and the inflammatory response from trauma have decreased (Levy et al. 2010).

Many knee dislocations involve injury to the medial or lateral structures and variable injury to the ACL and/or PCL. When any of the posterolateral corner structures are injured, and the injury is acute (less than 3 weeks), acute direct repair of the biceps femoris, iliotibial band, and lateral capsule is preferred, while reconstruction of the FCL, popliteofibular ligament, and popliteus tendon is recommended (Fig. 5). Reconstruction of the cruciate ligaments can also be concurrently performed.

If the medial side of the knee is acutely injured, then nonoperative management can be initially attempted as long as the MCL remains in close approximation to the femur and tibia. If there is tissue interposed and healing is unlikely (Fig. 6), similar to the Stener lesion in the thumb, in which the distal MCL is flipped over the pes anserinus tendons, then the MCL is acutely repaired or reconstructed and torn cruciate ligaments are concurrently reconstructed to allow for early knee motion. Range of motion and stability are assessed at postoperative visits as for the lateral repairs, and manipulation and/or cruciate ligament reconstruction is undertaken as indicated , if initially delayed. Using this treatment algorithm with medial sided injuries, arthrofibrosis due to early cruciate ligament reconstruction can be avoided.

The patient's range of motion and stability are carefully examined at postoperative visits and serial radiographs are obtained. If postoperative range of motion is poor, manipulation is generally carried out at 10–12 weeks after the initial procedure as indicated.

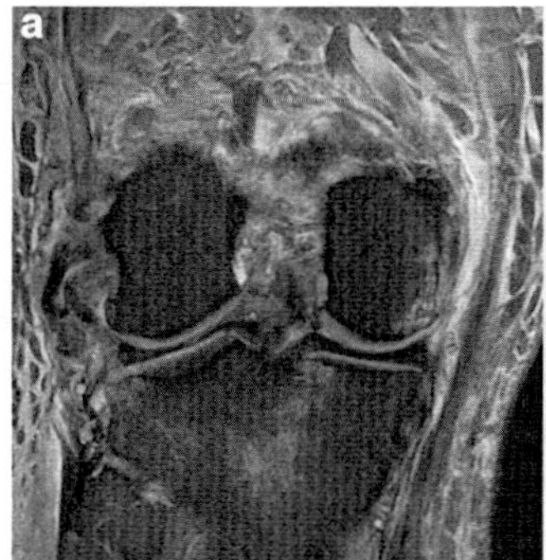

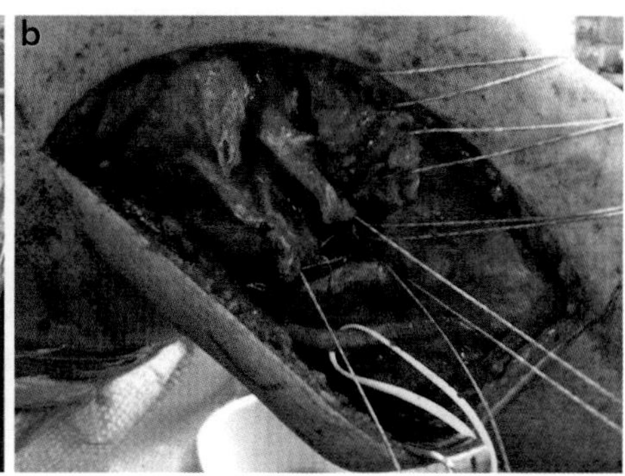

Fig. 5 (a) MRI of posterolateral corner injury with injury to the biceps, LCL, popliteus, and ITB. (b) Direct repair of the posterolateral corner structures with a yellow vessel loop around the peroneal nerve

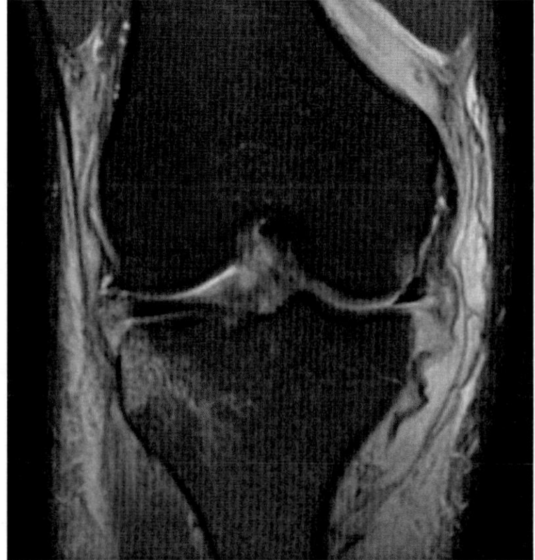

Fig. 6 Tibial avulsion of MCL with proximal retraction

Surgical Timing: Immediate Reconstruction

Most recent studies have shown improved postoperative outcomes with acute reconstructions of the medial and/or lateral sides and of the cruciate ligaments (Noyes and Barber-Westin 1997; Wascher et al. 1999; Harner et al. 2004). Both Noyes et al. and Wascher et al. showed improved patient outcomes in those patients who were treated acutely (Noyes and Barber-Westin 1997; Wascher et al. 1999). Harner et al. showed similar findings with no difference in postoperative range of motion and consistently improved laxity tests in both groups (Harner et al. 2004). Immediate reconstruction can be undertaken, but a high degree of awareness and suspicion for both intraoperative and postoperative complications and swelling must be maintained at all times.

Surgical Technique

Surgical Setup

An examination under anesthesia (EUA) is performed to correlate prior MRI and physical exam findings and to assess for any potential healing of the medial structures or PCL depending on surgical timing. A bump for the foot and lateral post is used so that the knee may be positioned at 90° of flexion (Fig. 7).

Medial Structures

Based on preoperative MRI and EUA, the medial structures of the knee, the MCL, the posterior oblique ligament (POL), and the posteromedial capsule can be assessed. When medial injuries are combined with cruciate injuries, the cruciate ligaments are generally reconstructed first. If the MCL is avulsed off the tibial insertion, it can be repaired (Fig. 8a, b) after the insertion site has been debrided and prepared. For the more common, proximal MCL injuries, repair is often difficult due to poor tissue quality of the proximal MCL (POL) and posteromedial capsule (Potter et al. 2002). In rare cases, these tissues may be advanced and reattached to the femur using suture anchors; however, due to the severity of injury of knee dislocations, a reconstruction is often required.

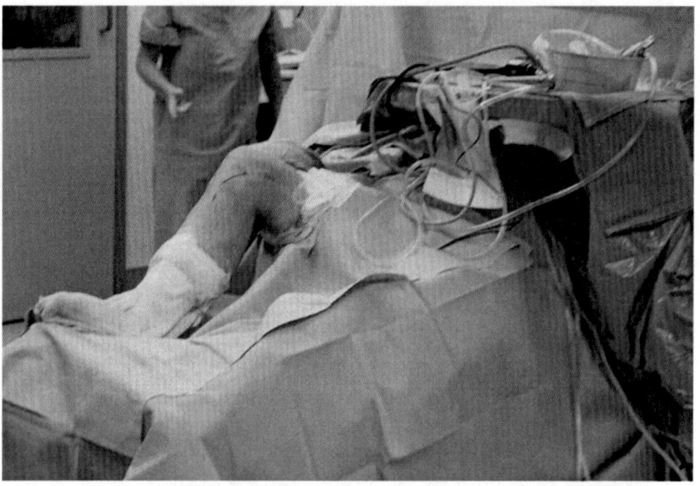

Fig. 7 Operating room set up for surgical management of knee dislocation

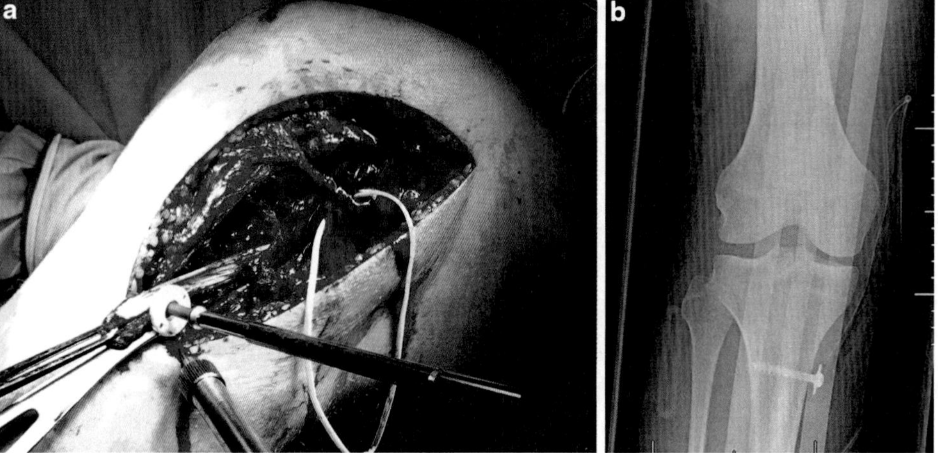

Fig. 8 (**a**) Repair of grade 3 tibial-sided injury using a screw and spiked washer. (**b**) Post-op AP X-ray after MCL tibial-sided repair

The MCL may be reconstructed as described by Bosworth et al. by using the semitendinosus tendon attached at the pes anserinus and dissecting it out proximally. The free end may then be attached to the medial epicondyle of the femur at the isometric point by screw and washer (Bosworth 1952). Despite good historical results with this technique, generally a more anatomical double-bundle MCL reconstruction is preferred (Feeley et al. 2009; Coobs et al. 2010; Lind et al. 2010). The graft is fixed with a staple on the femur and interference screw on the tibia and tensioned with a varus force applied to the knee at 30° of flexion (Fig. 9a, b).

Lateral Structures

A standard lateral hockey stick incision is used to address injuries to the lateral side extending from 5 cm distal to Gerdy's tubercle to 5 cm proximal and posterior to the lateral epicondyle (Terry and LaPrade 1996). Dissection is carried out down to fascia and the peroneal nerve is exposed proximally, outside of the zone of injury, and then carried out from proximal to distal. When intraneural hematoma is found to be compromising nerve function, the epineurium is incised and the hematoma is evacuated.

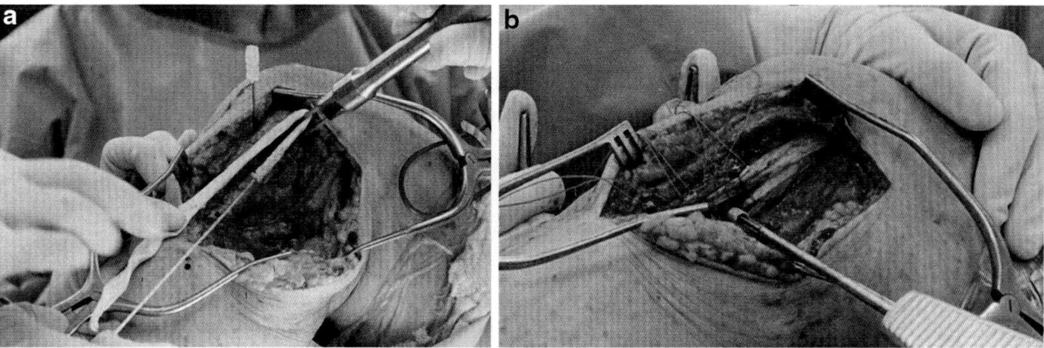

Fig. 9 (**a**) Femoral fixation with stable for double-bundle MCL reconstruction with allograft. (**b**) Tibial-sided fixation for double-bundle MCL reconstruction with allograft

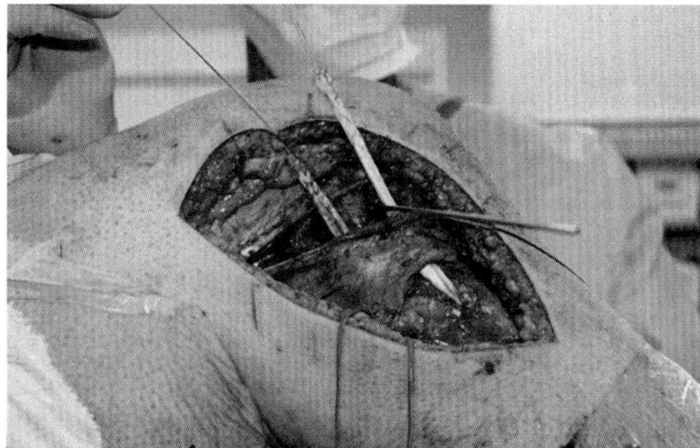

Fig. 10 Fibular-based PLC reconstruction

With direct repair, which is rarely possible, the popliteus is usually addressed first and may be injured at the femoral attachment site or at the musculotendinous junction. If it is injured at the femoral insertion site, it can frequently be advanced and reattached by docking it in a short tunnel or by suture post-fixation. If the popliteus is injured at the musculotendinous junction, it can be tenodesed to the posterolateral corner of the tibia or at the insertion site of the popliteofibular ligament (PFL) on the fibular head, which is just medial and posterior to the insertion of the FCL and biceps tendon (Lunden et al. 2010).

When the posterolateral corner must be reconstructed due to insufficient tissue for repair or time from injury greater than 1 month, a fibular-based technique may be employed (Fig. 10). There are several variations on technique, but the first step is to locate the peroneal nerve posterior and medial to the long head of the biceps tendon. Neurolysis is performed and the nerve is exposed throughout the incision to make sure it is tension-free and that its location is known throughout the case. An allograft tendon may be used to ensure enough length for reconstruction. One 7 mm tunnel is drilled in the fibular head from the FCL attachment on the lateral side to the popliteofibular ligament attachment site on the posteromedial aspect. The graft is passed through the tunnel and the more posterior and medial limb is brought up to the popliteus attachment site on the femur, and the more anterior and lateral limb is brought up to the LCL attachment site on the femur. The two limbs are then docked into short tunnels and may be fixed over the medial side of the distal femur. A two-limbed fibula and tibia-based reconstruction may also be employed as described by LaPrade et al. (2004).

Bi-Cruciate Reconstruction

Arthroscopy is begun in standard fashion with special attention paid to fluid extravasation throughout the procedure. Anatomic single-bundle PCL and ACL reconstructions are performed using an allograft. The PCL is addressed first, and a posterior–medial (PM) portal is created with the use of a spinal needle and the scope may be placed in the anterolateral (AL) or (PM) portals and debridement carried out through the other. A 70° arthroscope is very helpful. The PCL tibial footprint is carefully debrided under direct visualization with care taken to avoid the neurovascular structures; a c-arm may also be utilized. The footprint is visualized in a medial to lateral direction arthroscopically and may be confirmed on the sagittal view with intraoperative fluoroscopy. A tibial PCL guide is placed in the knee and the guide pin advanced carefully under fluoroscopic and arthroscopic visualization towards the tibial attachment site of the PCL, approximately 1.6 mm distal to the proximal joint line (Johannsen et al. 2012; Fig. 11). It is advanced through the posterior cortex by hand and the position is again confirmed with fluoroscopy. The guide pin is over-reamed to the size of the allograft and again advanced through the posterior cortex by hand. The femoral PCL tunnel is then drilled through the low (AL) portal and the scope in the anteromedial (AM) portal (Fig. 12). A double-bundle PCL reconstruction can also be performed using the same AL portal from inside out (Spiridonov et al. 2010). The tibial tunnel for the ACL is then drilled in standard fashion with care taken to avoid the PCL tunnel. The femoral ACL tunnel is drilled using a flexible guide through the (AM) portal at 100° of knee flexion (Fig. 13). The PCL graft is passed through the tibia and pulled up into the femur, followed by passage of the ACL graft. The PCL graft is secured on the femoral side and then secured on the tibial side with the knee at 90° of knee flexion with an anterior drawer applied to the leg. The ACL graft is secured on the femoral side and lastly on the tibial

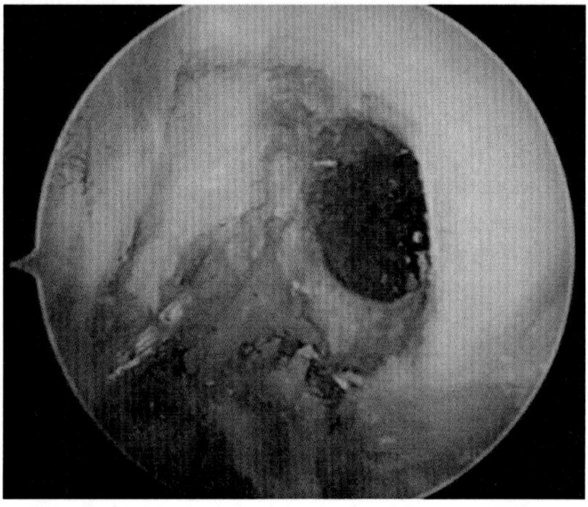

Fig. 12 Femoral PCL tunnel of a right knee viewed from AM portal and drilled through AL portal

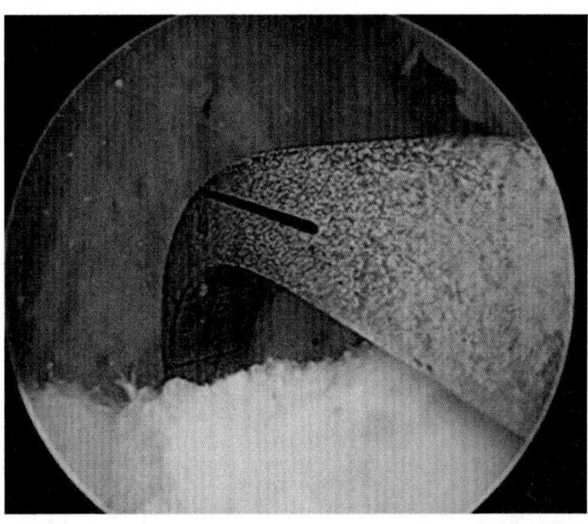

Fig. 11 Tibial PCL guide viewed arthroscopically from the front of the knee

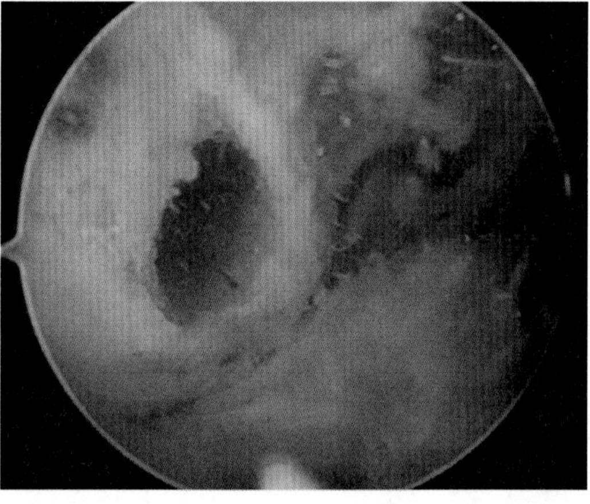

Fig. 13 Femoral ACL tunnel of a right knee drilled with flexible reamer through AM portal, viewed through AL portal

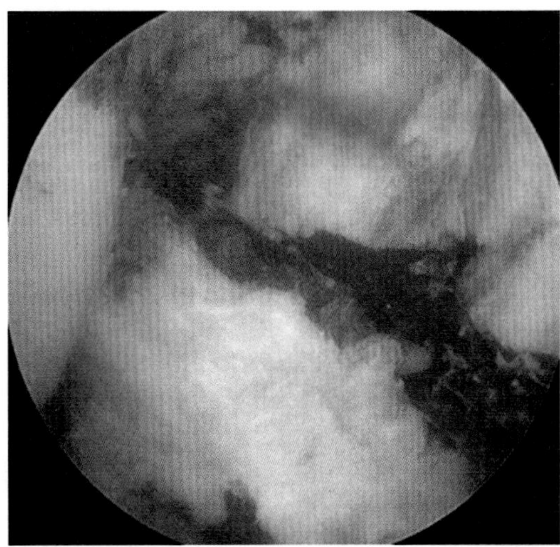

Fig. 14 Arthroscopic picture after right knee bi-cruciate reconstruction

side with the leg in full extension (Fig. 14). The graft may be fixed with graft sutures tied over a screw and washer post. Cortical bone graft can be used in a press-fit fashion to enhance aperture fixation of the grafts. Cortical grafts may be harvested by using core reamers when drilling tunnels or from allograft bone. Examination is immediately performed to assess tension and correction of laxity.

Postoperative

Initial postoperative protocol consists of 6 weeks of non-weight-bearing immobilization with the knee locked in full extension in a knee immobilizer when not undergoing motion in PT. In addition, if available, the use of a PCL jack brace may be initiated at postoperative days 2–3 to allow for early knee motion which protects the PCL reconstruction. The patient is mobilized with physical therapy and quadriceps strengthening is begun immediately. At 6 weeks postoperative, weight bearing is allowed with crutches initially, and the crutches are weaned away over the next few weeks. Active and passive motion exercises are continued during this time. At 6 weeks, extension should be full and flexion should be greater than 90°. From 4 to 6 months, closed-chain strengthening exercises are done progressing to open-chain and straight-line jogging around 6 months. After 6 months the focus is continued strengthening and initiation of functional rehab and activities. Return to play or strenuous work may be considered as early as the seventh month if swelling is absent and strength is 90 % of the contralateral leg. A functional brace may be used for return to sport based on injury.

Conclusions

A knee dislocation is a potentially devastating injury that must be managed appropriately from initial presentation through potentially several interventions and surgeries. A high suspicion for neurovascular injuries should be maintained at all times, and just because one is not obvious at initial presentation does not mean that one has not occurred. Surgical management should be well thought out and planned because complications such as wound problems, compartment syndrome, neurovascular injury, and stiffness are more common than in less severe extremity injuries.

Cross-References

- ▶ Acute Posterior Dislocations and Posterior Fracture–Dislocations of the Shoulder
- ▶ Allografts in Anterior Cruciate Ligament Reconstruction
- ▶ Allografts in Posterior Cruciate Ligament Reconstructions
- ▶ Anterior Cruciate Ligament Injuries and Surgery: Current Evidence and Modern Development
- ▶ Combined Anterior and Posterior Cruciate Ligament Injuries
- ▶ Different Techniques of Anterior Cruciate Ligament Reconstruction: Guidelines
- ▶ On-the-Field Management of American Football Injuries
- ▶ Personalized Treatment Algorithms for Anterior Cruciate Ligament Injuries
- ▶ Rehabilitation of Complex Knee Injuries and Key Points

References

Azar FM, Brandt JC, Miller RH 3rd, Phillips BB (2011) Ultra-low-velocity knee dislocations. Am J Sports Med 39(10):2170–2174

Bosworth DM (1952) Transplantation of the semitendinosus for repair of laceration of medial collateral ligament of the knee. J Bone Joint Surg Am 34-A(1):196–202

Brautigan B, Johnson DL (2000) The epidemiology of knee dislocations. Clin Sports Med 19(3):387–397

Dedmond BT, Almekinders LC (2001) Operative versus nonoperative treatment of knee dislocations: a meta-analysis. Am J Knee Surg 14(1):33–38

Eastlack RK, Schenck RC Jr, Guarducci C (1997) The dislocated knee: classification, treatment, and outcome. U S Army Med Dept J 12:1–9

Fanelli GC, Feldmann DD (1998) The use of allograft tissue in knee ligament reconstruction. In: Serge Parisien J (ed) Current techniques in arthroscopy. Thieme, New York, pp 47–55

Fanelli GC, Giannotti BF, Edson CJ (1996) Arthroscopically assisted combined posterior cruciate ligament/posterior lateral complex reconstruction. Arthroscopy 12(5):521–530

Feeley BT, Muller MS, Allen AA, Granchi CC, Pearle AD (2009) Biomechanical comparison of medial collateral ligament reconstructions using computer-assisted navigation. Am J Sports Med 37:1123

Green NE, Allen BL (1977) Vascular injuries associated with dislocation of the knee. J Bone Joint Surg Am 59(2):236–239

Gustilo RB, Cabatan DM (1993) Traumatic dislocation of the knee. In: Kyle RF, Gustilo RB, Templeman D (eds) Fractures and dislocations, vol 2. Mosby, St. Louis, pp 885–895

Hagino RT, DeCaprio JD, Valentine RJ, Clagett GP (1998) Spontaneous popliteal vascular injury in the morbidly obese. J Vasc Surg 28(3):458–462, discussion 462–453

Harner CD, Waltrip RL, Bennett CH, Francis KA, Cole B, Irrgang JJ (2004) Surgical management of knee dislocations. J Bone Joint Surg Am 86-A(2):262–273

Hegyes MS, Richardson MW, Miller MD (2000) Knee dislocation. Complications of nonoperative and operative management. Clin Sports Med 19(3):519–543

Kennedy JC (1963) Complete dislocation of the knee joint. J Bone Joint Surg Am 45:889–904

Khanna G, Herrera DA, Wolters BW, Dajani KA, Levy BA (2008) Staged protocol for high energy knee dislocation: initial spanning external fixation versus hinged knee brace. Annual meeting of the Arthroscopy Association of North America. Washington, DC

Kim J, Allaire R, Harner CD (2010) Vascular safety during high tibial osteotomy: a cadaveric angiographic study. Am J Sports Med 38(4):810–815

Klimkiewicz J, Petrie R, Harner CD (2001) The dislocated knee. In: Scott WN, Insall JN (eds) Surgery of the knee, vol 1. Churchill Livingstone, Edinburgh, pp 892–905

LaPrade RF, Johansen S, Wentorf FA, Engebretsen L, Esterberg JL, Tso A (2004) An analysis of an anatomical posterolateral knee reconstruction: an in vitro biomechanical study and development of a surgical technique. Am J Sports Med 32(6):1405–1414

Levy BA, Fanelli GC, Whelan DB, Stannard JP, Macdonald PA, Boyd JL, Marx RG, Stuart MJ (2009) Controversies in the treatment of knee dislocations and multiligament reconstruction. J Am Acad Orthop Surg 17(4):197–206

Levy BA, Krych AJ, Shah JP, Morgan JA, Stuart MJ (2010) Staged protocol for initial management of the dislocated knee. Knee Surg Sports Traumatol Arthrosc 18:1630–1637

Lunden JB, Bzdusek PJ, Monson JK, Malcomson KW, LaPrade RF (2010) Current concepts in the recognition and treatment of posterolateral corner injuries of the knee. J Orthop Sports Phys Ther 40(8):502–516

Mills WJ, Barei DP, McNair P (2004) The value of the ankle-brachial index for diagnosing arterial injury after knee dislocation: a prospective study. J Trauma 56(6):1261–1265

Mohtadi NG, Webster-Bogaert S, Fowler PJ (1991) Limitation of motion following anterior cruciate ligament reconstruction. A case-control study. Am J Sports Med 19(6):620–624, discussion 624–625

Niall DM, Nutton RW, Keating JF (2005) Palsy of the common peroneal nerve after traumatic dislocation of the knee. J Bone Joint Surg (Br) 87(5):664–667

Noyes FR, Barber-Westin SD (1997) Reconstruction of the anterior and posterior cruciate ligaments after knee dislocation. Use of early protected postoperative motion to decrease arthrofibrosis. Am J Sports Med 25(6):769–778

Potter HG, Weinstein M, Allen AA, Wickiewicz TL, Helfet DL (2002) Magnetic resonance imaging of the multiple-ligament injured knee. J Orthop Trauma 16(5):330–339

Richter M, Bosch U, Wippermann B, Hofmann A, Krettek C (2002) Comparison of surgical repair or reconstruction of the cruciate ligaments versus nonsurgical treatment in patients with traumatic knee dislocations. Am J Sports Med 30(5):718–727

Rihn JA, Groff YJ, Harner CD, Cha PS (2004) The acutely dislocated knee: evaluation and management. J Am Acad Orthop Surg 12(5):334–346

Seroyer ST, Musahl V, Harner CD (2008) Management of the acute knee dislocation: the Pittsburgh experience. Injury 39(7):710–718

Shelbourne KD, Klootwyk TE (2000) Low-velocity knee dislocation with sports injuries. Treatment principles. Clin Sports Med 19(3):443–456

Shelbourne KD, Porter DA, Clingman JA, McCarroll JR, Rettig AC (1991a) Low-velocity knee dislocation. Orthop Rev 20(11):995–1004

Shelbourne KD, Wilckens JH, Mollabashy A, DeCarlo M (1991b) Arthrofibrosis in acute anterior cruciate ligament reconstruction. The effect of timing of reconstruction and rehabilitation. Am J Sports Med 19(4):332–336

Spiridonov SI, Slinkard NJ, LaPrade RF (2010) Isolated and combined grade-III posterior cruciate ligament tears treated with double-bundle reconstruction with use of endoscopically placed femoral tunnels and grafts. J Bone Joint Surg Am 93:1773–1780

Stannard JP, Sheils TM, Lopez-Ben RR, McGwin G Jr, Robinson JT, Volgas DA (2004) Vascular injuries in knee dislocations: the role of physical examination in determining the need for arteriography. J Bone Joint Surg Am 86-A(5):910–915

Taylor AR, Arden GP, Rainey HA (1972) Traumatic dislocation of the knee. A report of forty-three cases with special reference to conservative treatment. J Bone Joint Surg (Br) 54(1):96–102

Terry GC, LaPrade RF (1996) The posterolateral aspect of the knee. Anatomy and surgical approach. Am J Sports Med 24(6):732–739

Wascher DC (2000) High-velocity knee dislocation with vascular injury. Treatment principles. Clin Sports Med 19(3):457–477

Wascher DC, Becker JR, Dexter JG, Blevins FT (1999) Reconstruction of the anterior and posterior cruciate ligaments after knee dislocation. Results using fresh-frozen nonirradiated allografts. Am J Sports Med 27(2):189–196

Lateral Knee Pain

91

Murat Bozkurt and Metin Dogan

Contents

M. Bozkurt (✉)
Department of Orthopaedics and Traumatology, Yildirium Beyazit University, Faculty of Medicine, Ankara, Turkey

Department of Orthopedics and Traumatology, Ankara Atatürk Training and Research Hospital, Ankara, Turkey
e-mail: nmbozkurt@yahoo.com; nmbozkurt@gmail.com

M. Dogan
Department of Orthopedics and Traumatology, Ankara Atatürk Training and Research Hospital, Ankara, Turkey
e-mail: drmetindogan@gmail.com

M.N. Doral, J. Karlsson (eds.), *Sports Injuries*,
DOI 10.1007/978-3-642-36569-0_278

Abstract
Lateral knee pain is a type of pain occurring on the outer side of the knee. Its onset may either be gradual over time or sudden following an injury. It may have a wide variety of symptoms. This type of pain may lead to suffering in the nature of a general ache or a sharp pain as well as to restricted mobility.

Introduction

Lateral knee pain is a type of pain occurring on the outer side of the knee. Its onset may either be gradual over time or sudden following an injury. It may have a wide variety of symptoms. This type of pain may lead to suffering in the nature of a general ache or a sharp pain as well as to restricted mobility. A number of different causes may result in the development of lateral knee pain. The most common causes are iliotibial band friction syndrome and lateral cartilage injuries.

Iliotibial Band Syndrome

İliotibial band syndrome is a common cause of lateral knee pain, especially in runners (Ellis et al. 2007; Hamill et al. 2008). It may be classified as an overuse syndrome, and conservative approaches are proven quite successful in its treatment. Biomechanical factors have a significant role in its development, but still the etiology behind it is far away from being clear.

Anatomy

The iliotibial band (ITB) originates from the outer lip of the anterior iliac crest, anterior border of the ilium, and outer surface of anterior superior iliac spine. The tensor fascia lata originates here also, and its fascia blends with the ITB at the lateroanterior thigh one-third of the way distally. The intermuscular septum connects the ITB to the linea aspera femoris until inserting just proximal to the lateral femoral condyle (Fig. 1).

At this point, the ITB expands up to Gerdy's tubercle of the lateral tibial plateau into which it inserts. It also helps the lateral collateral ligament and the posterolateral joint capsule for the purpose of knee stabilization.

The primary synergistic muscles are the hip abductors. These muscles are the gluteus medius, gluteus minimus, and upper fibers of the gluteus maximus. Their nerve supply comes from the superior gluteal nerve, which is a branch off of the L4, L5, and S1 nerve roots (Fairclough et al. 2006).

Typically, iliotibial band syndrome affects people with heavy exercise programs. Such an overuse results into a soft tissue damage beyond the extent that could be self-repaired by the body. When knee is brought into flexion, the iliotibial band moves towards posterior along the lateral femoral condyle. Its contact with the condyle is maximum when knee is between 20° and 30° of flexion. In patients with iliotibial band syndrome, magnetic resonance imaging (MRI) studies have shown that the distal iliotibial band becomes thickened.

Incidence of iliotibial band syndrome varies around 1.6–52 % depending on the activity level of the study population. The same has been shown in a study to be 12 % among the runners as a running-related complaint (Linenger and Christensen 1992).

Iliotibial band syndrome is of multifactorial etiology, involving overuse and misexercise as most commonly associated factors. Sudden changes in surface, speed, distance, shoes, and exercise frequency may cause injury. Etiology also includes other factors: genu varum, overpronation, poor hip adductor muscle, and leg length discrepancy.

It has been claimed that leg length discrepancy gives rise to ITB syndrome as it changes hip adduction in the walking cycle which in turn deteriorates the pelvic tilt and the sacral balance increasing the stress applied on the iliotibial band and the tensor fascia lata. Similarly genu varum acts to increase the stress.

Clinics

The diagnosis is usually made based on a characteristic history and physical examination.

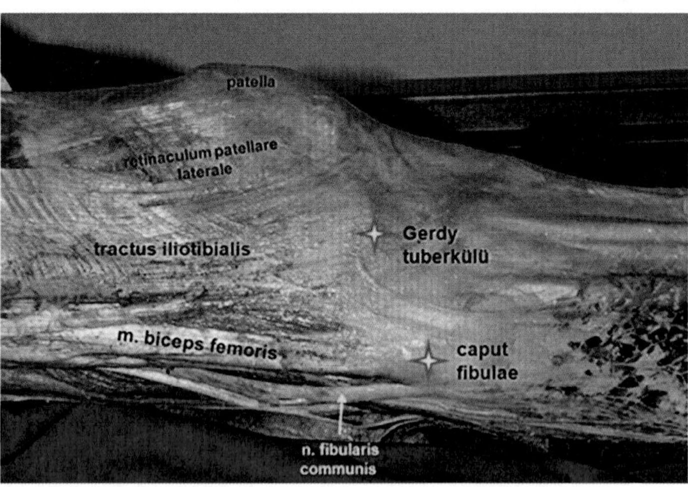

Fig. 1 Tractus of iliotibial band

Pain although is mainly localized along the lateral side of the knee may show up in hip as well. Pain worsens with the activity. While pain is generally felt during the exercise, it may be felt depending on the progression of the syndrome even during walking. Tenderness is noted particularly at about 1–2 cm proximal to the knee joint. Pain could be induced by pressing on the epicondyle and the iliotibial band during the first 30° of an active joint movement. Crepitation might be recognized. Provocative tests such as Noble test, Ober test, Renee Creak test, and Thomas test might be used for diagnosis.

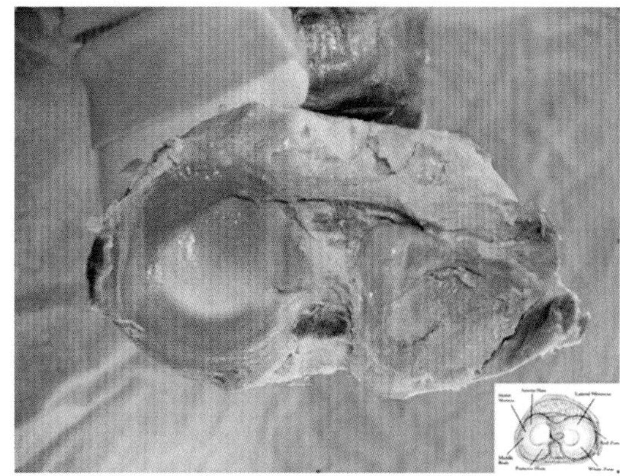

Fig. 2 Anatomy of menisci

Treatment

Failure with the conservative therapy shall stand for a surgical indication. Conservative therapy includes rest, stretching and strengthening exercises, anti-inflammatory medication, other therapy modalities, and biomechanical correction of limb length discrepancies and pes planus. A minimum time period of 3 months should be allowed before any surgery is scheduled. When conservative therapy ends up as unsuccessful, surgery might be considered for patient with greater expectations. Most common approach is the resection of posterior edge of the iliotibial band and the bursa, if necessary.

Lateral Meniscus Abnormality

Menisci enable load transfer and absorbance of shock to the knee joint in addition to contributing to joint stability and ensuring lubrication. Menisci rank at top among the most frequently injured structures at the knee joint (Solomon et al. 2005).

Medial meniscus is in "C" shape whereas the lateral one is featuring as an incomplete circle and having more mobility (Fig. 2). Medial meniscus tears occur more often. Superior and inferior branches of the medial and lateral geniculate arteries supply the peripheral third of the menisci via the perimeniscal capillary plexus (Arnoczky et al. 1998).

Tears at the lateral meniscus generally lead to a localized pain at the joint line. Meniscal pain occurs during torsional, weight-bearing knee movements (classically pivoting on the knee while walking) as a sharp stab lasting several seconds, often followed by a dull ache for several hours. Pain is not observed at rest. It may cause the knee to lock up.

Diagnosis

It may manifest itself with joint effusion, tenderness along the joint line, and pain during flexion. In general, McMurray and Apley test results are positive. Although they are specific, these tests are not sensitive. While specificity reaches up to 57–98 % and 80–99 % in various studies, sensitivity, on the other hand, is limited to 10–66 % and 16–58 % (Jarit and Bosco 2010). Thessaly test, having a sensitivity of 90 % and specificity of 98 % in detecting meniscal injury, comes up as the most beneficial test for meniscus injuries (Harison et al. 2009).

Magnetic resonance imaging is the gold standard, first choice for investigation of suspected meniscal tears (Crawford et al. 2007; Vincken et al. 2007; Liodakis et al. 2009; Bernstein 2010). An MRI is 70–90 % accurate in identifying whether the meniscus has been torn and how badly. However, meniscus tears do not always appear on MRIs. An arthroscope is close to 100 % accurate in diagnosing these tears (Fig. 3).

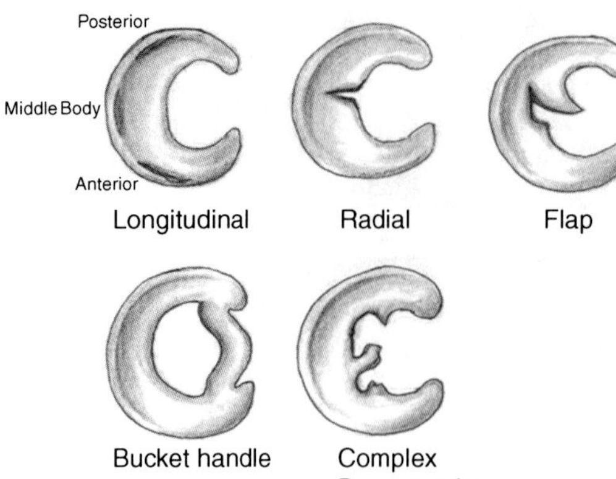

Fig. 3 Types of meniscal tear

Treatment

Nonsurgical approaches constitute an essential part of the treatment. The rapid conservative approach includes the RICE regimen:

- Rest (with weight bearing as tolerated or with crutches)
- Ice
- Compression bandaging
- Elevation of the affected limb to minimize acute swelling and inflammation

Long-term approaches are made up of activity modification, nonsteroidal anti-inflammatory drugs (NSAIDs), and physiotherapy (Rimington et al. 2009; De Carlo and Armstrong 2010; Lim et al. 2010).

Intense physiotherapy composed of range of motion, proprioceptive work, and muscle strengthening exercise is of utmost importance. Nonsurgical approaches are promising for certain types of meniscal tears in patients without joint function loss, who suffer minimal pain with no swelling.

Surgical approach is remarkably successful for young patients who suffer vertical tears at the vascularized one-third peripheral section of the meniscus called "red-red zone" (Jarit 2010). Repair of meniscus tears at sites with poor vascularization is controversial (Krych et al. 2008). Meniscal tears at such a site need to be resected. However, menisectomy is a risk factor for the development of osteoarthritis in the long term (Papalia et al. 2011). Meniscal allografts and scaffolds have given quite good results in young patient with a menisectomy history (Verdonk et al. 2005; Cole et al. 2006; Sekiya et al. 2006).

Lateral Compartment Arthritis

Introduction

Degenerative joint diseases may affect any or all of the knee compartments. Degenerative changes are most commonly found in medial compartment of the knee joint, followed successively by the patellofemoral and lateral compartments (Gresham and Rathey 1975; Johnson and Bodell 1981; Altman et al. 1987). When one conducts a regular gait pattern, force is predominantly exerted on the medial compartment of the knee (Harrington 1983; Goh et al. 1993; Andriacchi 1994). That weight shifted to lateral plateau requires development of valgus deformity. In their study with early-stage symptomatic knee osteoarthritis patients, Khan et al. determined that each degree of increase in alignment change creates a risk contributing to further development of osteoarthritis (Khan et al. 2008).

Genu Valgum Deformity

In most cases, genu valgum deformity is a result of dysplastic lateral femoral condyle which creates a pathologic loading at the lateral compartment of knee followed by bone and cartilage destruction. This condition has been evidenced by experimental models (Goodman et al. 1991; Cooke et al. 1994; Poilvache et al. 1996).

Discoid Lateral Meniscus

Discoid meniscus has been reported to affect 1.4–15.5 % of the population. In children, the total arthroscopic excision of a discoid meniscus accelerates the occurrence of degenerative changes in the following years. Impact of lateral menisectomy on subsequent arthrosis development has also been shown on animal models (Root and Liener 1995).

Osteonecrosis

Lateral compartment arthrosis may be the major complication of a spontaneous osteonecrosis at the lateral femoral compartment (Lotke and Ecker 1988; Ecker and Lotke 1994). Typically, this clinic condition is presented with an acute onset of pain in women older than 55 years.

Trauma

Lateral compartment arthritis may also arise from a trauma such as a lateral tibial plateau fracture.

Patients suffering arthritis at the lateral compartment of knee joint typically have pain at the outer side of the knee. There may or may not be concurrent patellofemoral complaints depending on the degree of degeneration. Lateral compartment arthritis may manifest with an apparent genu valgum deformity. An apparent deformity is defined as a deformity which exceeds 7–10° of femoral tibial valgus angulation (Whiteside 1993; Miyasaka et al. 1997). As a result of an advanced valgus deformity, the lateral structures, i.e., lateral collateral ligament, iliotibial band, and lateral capsule, might become contracted. This kind of deformity may become fixed over time.

Diagnosis

Evaluation of a knee with lateral arthritis needs radiographs of the involved knee primarily from anteroposterior projection and secondarily from lateral and patellofemoral projections. Typical findings to be inferred from the graphs include narrowing of the lateral joint space, subchondral cyst formation, sclerosis, and osteophytic formation. Cases which have a joint space narrowing due to the erosion of the posterior femoral condyle that may not be visible on a routine anteroposterior film might be made visible on a weight-bearing posteroanterior radiograph keeping knee at a flexion of 45°, useful for the diagnosis of joint findings (Dervin et al. 2001) (Fig. 4).

For the purpose of preoperative planning of a lateral unicompartmental knee arthroplasty, an anteroposterior radiograph taken with applied varus stress might be useful. Provided that normal alignment is achieved with applied stress, performance of unicompartmental knee arthroplasty is justified.

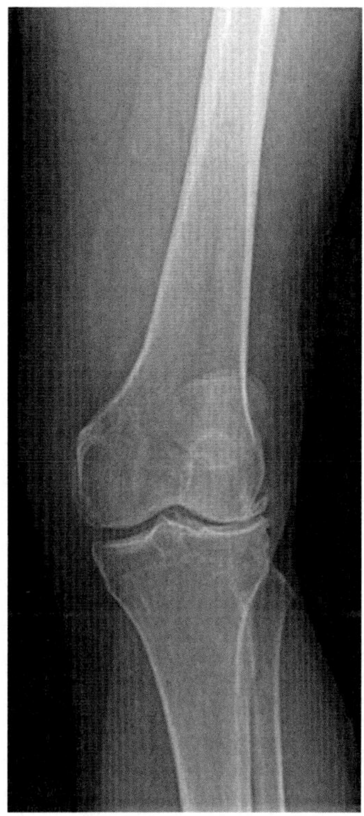

Fig. 4 Radiography of lateral arthrosis

Nonoperative Treatment

Compared to the varus deformities, valgus deformities are better tolerated, and arthritic changes occur in the lateral compartment over a longer time period than in the medial compartment. There is a lack of controlled studies in this field, but still nonoperative approaches may be effective in relieving the complaints of early-stage patients. Nonoperative treatment modalities include:

- Activity modification
- Weight reduction
- Oral analgesics
- Aerobic conditioning of the lower extremity muscles
- Unloader bracing
- Shoe modification
- Use of a cane during ambulation

Even if a surgery has already been scheduled for a patient, management of nonoperative approaches is favorable in order to elaborate the patient's needs, to understand the patient's complaints, and to educate the patient. The fact that unloader braces are able to relieve pain in knees with flexible valgus indicates that corrective osteotomy or unicompartmental knee arthroplasty would be effective.

Surgical Options

Corrective osteotomy, hemiarthroplasty of the knee, and total knee replacement are options for surgical approach to lateral arthritis.

A thorough evaluation of patient's preoperative history, physical examination, and radiographs is crucial when drawing the surgical strategy. If a patient has a history of a lateral tibial plateau fracture, the possibility of a defect in the lateral plateau should be considered and choices such as augmentation or allograft application shall be taken into account when applying arthroplasty. The need of augmentation to femoral component may arise during the total knee arthroplasty, in case a hypoplastic femoral condyle is present.

Corrective Osteotomy

Corrective osteotomy is the act of correcting pathologic misalignment at the lower extremity aiming load reduction on the lateral compartment. Previous studies have arthroscopically demonstrated regeneration of articular cartilage and proliferation of fibrocartilage at the concerned compartment following the osteotomy (Coventry 1973; Insall 1993).

The following criteria are applicable for corrective osteotomy: age younger than 65 years, isolated Ahlback grade I or II lateral compartmental arthrosis, minimum ligamentous laxity, 90° or greater arc of motion of the knee, and a flexion contracture of less than 15–20° (Hanssen 2001).

In literature, osteotomies with a medial closing wedge or lateral opening wedge supported by a tricortical autograft have been described. Tibial osteotomies are rarely used for valgus deformities.

Osteotomy might be correlated with simultaneous joint debridement and arthroscopy directed to solve meniscus pathologies, despite the clinical outcomes fail to suggest a significant improvement.

Unicompartmental Knee Arthroplasty

Unicompartmental knee arthroplasty may be a favorable alternative to eliminate the complaints in selected patients (Marmor 1984; Ohdera et al. 2001). In comparison to corrective osteotomy, unicompartmental knee arthroplasty has a quicker success rate and less early complications. In comparison to total knee arthroplasty, likewise, it is advantageous as it has an almost normal knee biomechanics owing to preserving both cruciate ligaments, in addition to yielding a lower morbidity, smaller incision, and decreased bone and blood loss (Scott and Santore 1981).

Contraindications to unicompartmental arthroplasty are symptomatic arthrosis in other compartments of knee, instability, fixed valgus knee, and a notable inflammatory arthritis. Total knee arthroplasty might be preferred in these cases.

Lateral Collateral Ligament Injury

Introduction

Collateral ligament injuries are common knee pathologies, the medial type being more frequent. Lateral collateral ligament (LCL) is a part of ligaments complex referred to as posterolateral corner. Posterolateral corner includes the LCL, the popliteofibular ligament, the popliteus ligament, the arcuate ligament, the short lateral ligament, and the posterolateral joint capsule. LCL is separated from the lateral meniscus by a fat pad (Fu et al. 1994).

An injury to the LCL is primarily caused by varus forces applied to the knee. Excessive lateral rotation of the knee might be another cause. In multiple injuries which involve LCL, disruption with a concurrent peroneal nerve injury and posterolateral corner structures may occur concomitantly with arterial injuries. A history of varus force applied to the knee is usual among patients.

Pain and stiffness are localized to the lateral knee. Long-term erythema may happen. Often there is swelling. Instability may occur depending on the severity of the trauma, though it is not very common. Injury is usually sports related in young people while it is an outcome of falling down in elderly.

During physical examination LCL injury is palpable with the knee in 20° of flexion. Tenderness might be noted at any point along the LCL. Isolated tenderness, if present, at the proximal or distal insertion points, suggests injuries of avulsion type. Varus stress test is performed when the knee is in flexion of 20–25° and repeated when the knee is extended. Laxity and pain observed during the varus test in flexion points out an injury at the LCL. If the same findings persist in the test with the knee extended, an additional injury to the posterior capsule might be spoken.

Classification by severity of injury:

- Grade I – less than 5 cm laxity (partial tear)
- Grade II – 5–10 cm laxity
- Grade III – more than 10 cm laxity (complete tear)

A lateral collateral ligament injury is mostly diagnosed clinically (Pimentel 2006; Strayer and Lang 2006). Avulsion fractures might be identified through plain radiographs. MRI is used to figure out any soft tissue injuries such as ACL, PCL, or meniscus that are likely to coexist. MRI is very sensitive in determining LCL injury but is not reliable for differentiating and grading the same (Crotty et al. 1996; Beall et al. 2007). Best visualization of LCL is through coronal sections. It tends to be of low signal intensity and have uniform thickness. Partial tears are characterized by edema. A complete LCL tear may be associated with a small avulsion of the styloid process of the fibular head and with marked edema.

Treatment

LCL injury, due to the difference of collagen density in its composition, has a poorer recovery when compared to MCL injury. Grade I and II LCL injuries shall be followed for 4–6 weeks while patient is using a hinged brace, thus the approach is similar to that of a MCL injury. Surgical treatment is widely performed on grade III injuries since there is a rotational instability arising from concurrent injuries of other structures of posterolateral corner. In order to avoid patients to develop instability in the long term, brace use and physiotherapy can be continued as long as 3 months (Bin and Nam 2007; Wahl and Nicandri 2008).

Proximal Tibiofibular Joint Injury

Proximal tibiofibular joint, a cause of lateral knee pain, tends to be neglected most of the time as it has a limited reference in literature. There are only a few reports about this joint. The proximal tibiofibular joint is a synovial type of joint acting as a mode to dissipate any torsional stresses and lateral tibial bending moments exerted on the lower leg and to transmit axial loads in weight bearing (Bozkurt et al. 2003, 2004).

The patient presenting with PTFJ dysfunction experienced a dull ache located on the lateral aspect of the knee and the pain can radiate distally or proximally, and hamstring tightness was present. Knee and ankle movements may exacerbate the pain, while rest relieves it. Examination reveals a painful fibular head. Full knee extension may be lacking due to hamstring tightness or pain in the PTFJ, and the manipulation of this joint results in immediate and dramatic relief of symptoms in this type of patients (De Franca 1992).

There are numerous proximal tibiofibular joint disorders which may give rise to lateral knee pain. Moreover, many adjacent structures can affect the proximal tibiofibular joint and hence cause pain. Pathologies pertaining to the proximal tibiofibular joint include osteoarthritis, neoplasms, ganglion cysts, pigmented villonodular synovitis, and trauma.

Anatomy

The proximal tibiofibular articulation (connecting the head of fibula and lateral condyle of tibia) is an "arthrodial" or "plane-type" joint which allows only slight gliding movement between the two surfaces. The contiguous surfaces of the bones are covered with cartilage and are connected with an articular capsule. This is reinforced by two or three broad, flat bands of ligament (anterosuperior ligament) in front and a single thick band of ligament (posterosuperior ligament) behind. Posterolateral knee stability is highly dependent on the tendon of popliteus which lies quite close to the posterosuperior ligament. Therefore, an injury at this site has a potential to affect all these structures.

The proximal tibiofibular joint has been shown to be in relation to knee joint in 105 of the adult population, MR arthrography demonstrating a ratio of up to 64 %. Due to this relation and its functional connection with the knee joint, the proximal tibiofibular joint has been interpreted as 4th compartment of the knee (Bozkurt et al. 2003).

The common peroneal nerve lies in vicinity to the lower edge of the joint. An injury at this site may result in drop foot and partial loss of feeling at concerned foot.

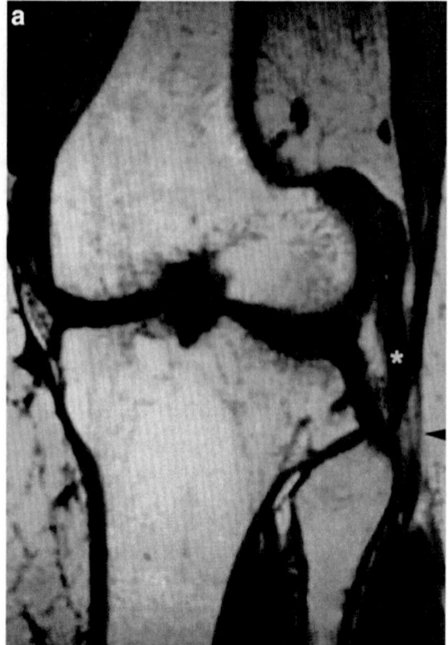

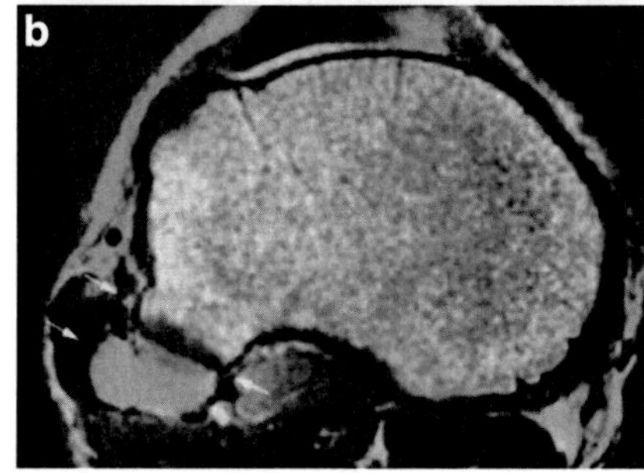

Fig. 5 (**a**) Partial rupture of biceps femoris tendon by the black arrowhead and hypertrophy of LCL (*) on paracoronal T1-weighted MR image. (**b**) Partial rupture of ATiFL and PTiFL by the white arrows on axial T1-weighted MR image

Pathologies of Proximal Tibiofibular Joint

Arthrosis: may accompany an arthrosis at the knee joint but it may also be found in isolated form. Therefore, it may be the reason of a lateral knee pain that persists after a total knee arthroplasty. In a similar manner with the other joints, radiological imaging may show subchondral cysts, osteophyte formation, joint space narrowing, and subchondral sclerosis.

Neoplasm: a diverse range of neoplasm types such as osteochondroma, osteoblastoma, osteosarcoma, and nerve sheath tumors (schwannomas and neurofibromas) may affect the proximal tibiofibular joint.

Trauma: the proximal tibiofibular joint is generally affected by direct traumas, but it may also be affected indirectly by varus, hyperflexion, or hyperextension injuries. As a result, fracture, dislocation, ligament strain, or tear may develop. Since the tendon of the popliteus muscle and the proximal tibiofibular joint are closely related, they need to be carefully evaluated in isolated injuries and complex posterolateral corner injuries. The posterolateral corner is a complex structure composed of the lateral collateral ligament, the popliteus muscle and tendon, and the arcuate complex. Please note that a diagnosis pertaining to the posterolateral corner may involve more than one structure (Recondo et al. 2000). An avulsion fracture of the fibular head to which the arcuate ligament, also known as "arcuate sign," inserts

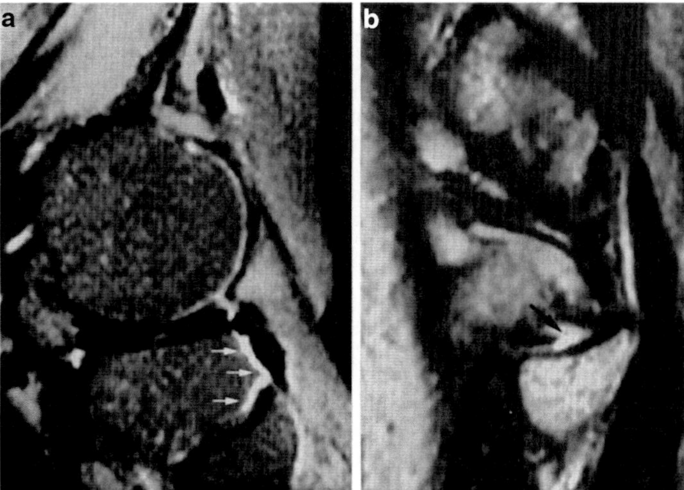

Fig. 6 Effusion in the PTFJ by the arrows of two different cases on sagittal T2-weighted MR images

may be an indicator of posterolateral instability (Huang et al. 2003). Mechanism of injury is mostly through a direct trauma applied on anteromedial tibia when the knee is in extension. PCL and ACL injuries usually accompany to this instability in extension. Unrepaired cases develop chronic knee instability (Hughston and Jacobson 1985) (Figs. 5 and 6).

Ganglion: a tumorlike, joint-involving structure with a tendon capsule or muscle origin. This rare structure might be associated with compression of the common peroneal nerve (Miskovsky et al. 2004).

Pigmented Villonodular Synovitis (PVNS): characterized by synovial hypertrophy. Most often it affects the knee and has a monoarticular involvement with an onset in individuals in their 30s or 40s. Imaging reveals large, globular areas of low T1 and T2 signal outlining the hypertrophied synovium.

Conclusion

Lateral knee pain is a type of pain occurring on the outer side of the knee. A number of different causes may result in the development of the lateral knee pain. Understanding the causes of the lateral knee pain is very important for determining a better treatment approach.

Cross-References

▸ Anatomy and Biomechanics of the Knee
▸ Lateral Knee Pain
▸ Meniscal Injuries and Discoid Lateral Meniscus in Adolescent Athletes
▸ Proximal Tibiofibular Syndesmotic Disruptions in Sport

References

Altman RD, Fries JF, Bloch DA et al (1987) Radiographic assessment of progression in osteoarthritis. Arthritis Rheum 30(11):1214–1225

Andriacchi TP (1994) Dynamics of knee malalignment. Orthop Clin North Am 25(3):395–403

Arnoczky SP, Warren RF, Spivak JM (1998) Meniscal repair using an exogenous fibrin clot. An experimental study in dogs. J Bone Joint Surg Am 70:1209–1217

Beall DP, Googe JD, Moss JT et al (2007) Magnetic resonance imaging of the collateral ligaments and the anatomic quadrants of the knee. Radiol Clin North Am 45(6):983–1002, vi

Bernstein J (2010) In brief: meniscal tears. Clin Orthop Related Res 468:1190–1192

Bin SI, Nam TS (2007) Surgical outcome of 2-stage management of multiple knee ligament injuries after knee dislocation. Arthroscopy 23(10):1066–1072

Bozkurt M, Yilmaz E, Atlihan D et al (2003) The proximal tibiofibular joint: an anatomic study. Clin Orthop Relat Res 406:136–140

Bozkurt M, Yilmaz E, Akseki D et al (2004) The evaluation of proximal tibiofibular joint for patients with lateral knee pain. Knee 11:307–312

Cole BJ, Dennis MG, Lee SJ et al (2006) Prospective evaluation of allograft meniscus transplantation: a minimum 2-year follow-up. Am J Sports Med 34:919–927

Cooke TDV, Bryant JT, Scudamore RA (1994) Biomechanical factors in alignment and arthritic disorders of the knee. In: Fu FH, Harner CD, Vince KG (eds) Knee surgery. Lippincott Williams & Wilkins, Baltimore, p 1061

Coventry MB (1973) Osteotomy about the knee for degenerative and rheumatoid arthritis. J Bone Joint Surg Am 55(1):23–48

Crawford R, Walley G, Bridgman S, Maffulli N (2007) Magnetic resonance imaging versus arthroscopy in the diagnosis of knee pathology, concentrating on meniscal lesions and ACL tears: a systematic review. Br Med Bull 84:5–23

Crotty JM, Monu JU, Pope TL Jr (1996) Magnetic resonance imaging of the musculoskeletal system. Part 4. The knee. Clin Orthop Relat Res 330:288–303

De Carlo M, Armstrong B (2010) Rehabilitation of the knee following sports injury. Clin Sports Med 29:81–106

De Franca GG (1992) Proximal tibiofibular joint dysfunction and chronic knee and low back pain. J Manip Physiol Ther 15(6):382–387

Dervin GF, Feibel RJ, Rody K, Grabowski J (2001) 3-Foot standing AP versus 45 degrees PA radiograph for osteoarthritis of the knee. Clin J Sport Med 11(1):10–16

Ecker ML, Lotke PA (1994) Spontaneous osteonecrosis of the knee. J Am Acad Orthop Surg 2(3):173–178

Ellis R, Hing W, Reid D (2007) Iliotibial band friction syndrome–a systematic review. Man Ther 12(3):200–208

Fairclough J, Hayashi K, Toumi H et al (2006) The functional anatomy of the iliotibial band during flexion and extension of the knee: implications for understanding iliotibial band syndrome. J Anat 208(3):309–316

Fu FH, Harner CD, Johnson DL et al (1994) Biomechanics of knee ligaments: basic concepts and clinical application. Instr Course Lect 43:137–148

Goh JC, Bose K, Khoo BC (1993) Gait analysis study on patients with varus osteoarthrosis of the knee. Clin Orthop Relat Res 294:223–231

Goodman SB, Lee J, Smith RL et al (1991) Mechanical overload of a single compartment induces early degenerative changes in the rabbit knee: a preliminary study. J Invest Surg 4(2):161–170

Gresham GE, Rathey UK (1975) Osteoarthritis in knees of aged persons. Relationship between roentgenographic and clinical manifestations. JAMA 233(2):168–170

Hamill J, Miller R, Noehren B, Davis I (2008) A prospective study of iliotibial band strain in runners. Clin Biomech 23:1018–1025

Hanssen AD (2001) Osteotomy about the knee: American perspective. In: Surgery of the knee. Churchill Livingstone, New York, pp 1461–1462

Harrington IJ (1983) Static and dynamic loading patterns in knee joints with deformities. J Bone Joint Surg Am 65(2):247–259

Harrison BK, Abell BE, Gibson TW (2009) The Thessaly test for detection of meniscal tears: validation of a new physical examination technique for primary care medicine. Clin J Sport Med 19:9–12

Huang GS, Yu JS, Munshi M et al (2003) Avulsion fracture of the head of the fibula ("arcuate" sign): MR imaging findings predictive of injuries to the posterolateral ligaments and posterior cruciate ligament. Am J Roentgenol 180:381–387

Hughston JC, Jacobson KE (1985) Chronic posterolateral rotatory instability of the knee. J Bone Joint Surg Am 67:351–359

Insall JN (1993) Osteotomy. In: Surgery of the knee, 2nd edn. Churchill Livingstone, New York, p 635

Jarit G, Bosco J (2010) Meniscal repair and reconstruction. Bull NYU Hosp Jt Dis 68:84–90

Johnson EW Jr, Bodell LS (1981) Corrective supracondylar osteotomy for painful genu valgum. Mayo Clin Proc 56(2):87–92

Khan FA, Koff MF, Noiseux NO et al (2008) Effect of local alignment on compartmental patterns of knee osteoarthritis. J Bone Joint Surg Am 90(9):1961–1969

Krych AJ, McIntosh AL, Voll AE et al (2008) Arthroscopic repair of isolated meniscal tears in patients 18 years and younger. Am J Sports Med 36:1283–1289

Lim HC, Bae JH, Wang JH et al (2010) Non-operative treatment of degenerative posterior root tear of the medial meniscus. Knee Surg Sports Traumatol Arthrosc 18:535–539

Linenger JM, Christensen CP (1992) Is iliotibial band syndrome overlooked? Phys Sports Med 20:98–108

Liodakis E, Hankemeier S, Jagodzinski M et al (2009) The role of preoperative MRI in knee arthroscopy: a retrospective analysis of 2,000 patients. Knee Surg Sports Traumatol Arthrosc 17:1102–1106

Lotke PA, Ecker ML (1988) Osteonecrosis of the knee. J Bone Joint Surg Am 70(3):470–473

Marmor L (1984) Lateral compartment arthroplasty of the knee. Clin Orthop Relat Res 115–21

Miskovsky S, Kaeding C, Weis L (2004) Proximal tibiofibular joint ganglion cysts: excision, recurrence, and joint arthrodesis. Am J Sports Med 32:1022–1028

Miyasaka KC, Ranawat CS, Mullaji A (1997) 10- to 20-year followup of total knee arthroplasty for valgus deformities. Clin Orthop Relat Res 345:29–37

Ohdera T, Tokunaga J, Kobayashi A (2001) Unicompartmental knee arthroplasty for lateral gonarthrosis: midterm results. J Arthroplasty 16(2):196–200

Papalia R, Del Buono A, Osti L et al (2011) Meniscectomy as a risk factor for knee osteoarthritis: a systematic review. Br Med Bull 2011:89–106

Pimentel L (2006) Orthopedic trauma: office management of major joint injury. Med Clin North Am 90(2):355–382

Poilvache PL, Insall JN, Scuderi GR, et al (1996) Rotational landmarks and sizing of the distal femur in total knee arthroplasty. Clin Orthop Relat Res 331:35–46

Recondo JA, Salvador E, Villanua JA et al (2000) Lateral stabilizing structures of the knee: functional anatomy and injuries assessed with MR imaging. RadioGraphics 20(spec no):S91–S102

Rimington T, Mallik K, Evans D et al (2009) A prospective study of the nonoperative treatment of degenerative meniscus tears. Orthopedics 32:8

Root L, Liener UC (1995) Discoid lateral meniscus in children. Long-term follow-up after excision. J Bone Joint Surg Am 77(9):1357–1361

Scott RD, Santore RF (1981) Unicondylar unicompartmental replacement for osteoarthritis of the knee. J Bone Joint Surg Am 63(4):536–544

Sekiya JK, West RV, Groff YJ et al (2006) Clinical outcomes following isolated lateral meniscal allograft transplantation. Arthroscopy 22:771–780

Solomon L, Warwick D, Nayagam S (2005) Apley's concise system of orthopaedics and fractures, 3rd edn. Hodder Arnold, London

Strayer RJ, Lang ES (2006) Evidence-based emergency medicine/systematic review abstract. Does this patient have a torn meniscus or ligament of the knee? Ann Emerg Med 47(5):499–501

Verdonk PC, Demurie A, Almqvist KF et al (2005) Transplantation of viable meniscal allograft. Survivorship analysis and clinical outcome of one hundred cases. J Bone Joint Surg Am 87:715–724

Vincken PW, ter Braak AP, van Erkel AR et al (2007) MR imaging: effectiveness and costs at triage of patients with nonacute knee symptoms. Radiology 242:85–93

Wahl CJ, Nicandri G (2008) Single-Achilles allograft posterior cruciate ligament and medial collateral ligament reconstruction: a technique to avoid osseous tunnel intersection, improve construct stiffness, and save on allograft utilization. Arthroscopy 24(4):486–489

Whiteside LA (1993) Correction of ligament and bone defects in total arthroplasty of the severely valgus knee. Clin Orthop Relat Res 288:234–245

Medial Collateral Ligament and Anterior Cruciate Ligament Synergy: Functional Interdependence

92

John Nyland, Mahmut Nedim Doral, Yee Han Dave Lee, Jefferson Brand, Matthias Jacobi, Sukeshrao Sankineni, Alberto Gobbi, and Roland Jakob

Contents

J. Nyland (✉)
Kosair Charities College of Health and Natural Sciences, Spalding University, Louisville, USA
e-mail: jnyland@spalding.edu

M.N. Doral
Department of Orthopaedics and Traumatology and Department of Sports Medicine, Hacettepe University, Istanbul, Turkey
e-mail: ndoral@haceteppe.edu.tr; mndoral@gmail.com

Y.H.D. Lee
Department of Orthopedic Surgery, Changi General Hospital, Singapore, Singapore
e-mail: davelyh@singnet.com.sg

J. Brand
Fellowship-Trained Sports Medicine Specialist, Heartland Orthopedic Specialists, Alexandria, MN, USA
e-mail: jbrand@heartlandorthopedics.com

M. Jacobi
Orthopadie am Rosenberg, St. Gallen, SG, Switzerland
e-mail: m.s.jacobi@gmx.ch

S. Sankineni
Sports Medicine, OASI Bioresearch Foundation Gobbi NPO, Orthopaedic Arthroscopic Surgery International, Milan, Italy
e-mail: sukeshrao.sankineni@gmail.com

A. Gobbi
Orthopaedic Arthroscopic Surgery International (O.A.S.I.) Bioresearch Foundation, Gobbi Onlus, Milan, Italy
e-mail: gobbi@cartilagedoc.it; sportmd@tin.it

R. Jakob
Department of Orthopaedic Surgery, Hopital Cantonal, Fribourg, Switzerland
e-mail: jakobroland@gmx.ch

M.N. Doral, J. Karlsson (eds.), *Sports Injuries*,
DOI 10.1007/978-3-642-36569-0_113

Abstract

The ACL functions in synergy with adjacent structures. This chapter discusses how medial capsuloligamentous dysfunction changes knee biomechanics, which might compromise ACL health or reconstruction integrity and potentially lead to failure. The MCL-ACL functional relationship and its influence on meniscus and articular cartilage health should be considered when planning knee rehabilitation and conditioning programs. Early intervention to attenuate the pathomechanics of faulty frontal plane alignment during single leg jump landings and the use of protective functional knee bracing should be considered prior to rehabilitation program advancement to sports-specific training.

Introduction

The MCL is the most frequently injured knee ligament (Miyasaka et al. 1991). It provides important frontal plane valgus knee stability and rotational translatory stability during single leg stance. Injury to the MCL is typically of noncontact athletic etiology when frontal plane alignment during single leg stance is disturbed, the hip is adducted-internally rotated, and the knee is abducted (Griffith et al. 2009; Powers 2010; Hewett and Myer 2011). This combination of events tends to excessively load the deep and superficial MCL leading to increased pain and laxity in minor cases and a frank capsuloligamentous tear in more severe cases. What has been long believed an inconsequential injury when occurring in isolation, a minor MCL sprain takes on greater importance with consideration of its synergistic role with the ACL and direct attachment to the medial meniscus. The noncontractile stabilization function provided by the deep and superficial MCL, the medial meniscus, and the ACL contributes significantly to knee motion control. The displacement magnitude and/or frequency of repetitive frontal plane loading may contribute to dysfunction among these stabilizers promoting frank ACL injury and functional impairment. These same mechanisms may likewise contribute to ACL graft failure particularly when soft tissue grafts are used, and these problems become magnified when foot-subtalar joint motion is poorly controlled in the presence of excessive, repetitive, and/or high displacement foot pronation and tibial rotation (Joseph et al. 2008).

Hughston and Eilers (1973) have been credited as being the first to report the synergism between the ACL and the MCL. Anterior tibia displacement is restricted not only by the ACL but also by the conformity of the meniscus and its attachment to the posterior oblique ligament. Similarly, both the ACL and medial capsuloligamentous complex check valgus instability (Hughston and Eilers 1973). The MCL and posteromedial capsule (PMC) are restraints to not only external rotation but internal rotation with the PMC serving a greater role in extension and the superficial MCL a greater role in flexion (Robinson et al. 2006; Griffith et al. 2009; Wijdicks et al. 2009). With these crucial functional roles considered, combined ACL and MCL injuries (Figs. 1 and 2) result in altered knee kinematics, of which we have an imperfect understanding. If these knee kinematics are not restored to pre-injury status, further joint laxity (Tapper et al. 2009) and knee osteoarthritis (Frank et al. 2012) are more likely to occur. In knees with multiple ligament injuries, 71 % involve combined ACL and MCL injury (Kaeding et al. 2005).

ACL, MCL, and Meniscus Synergy for Articular Cartilage Protection

The meniscus is a crucial load-bearing structure, optimizing contact area and minimizing contact stress. Peak contact stresses have been shown to increase proportionally with the amount of meniscus removed; therefore, the strategy in meniscus surgery is to preserve the greatest amount of meniscus possible (Lee et al. 2006). With an isolated ACL injury, the greatest increase in anterior-posterior translational knee laxity occurs between 20 and 30° flexion (Levy et al. 1982; Shoemaker and Markolf 1986; Levy et al. 1989). Levy

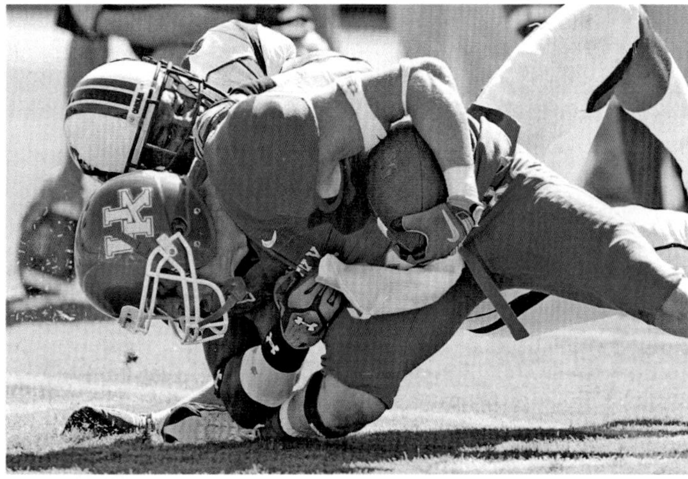

Fig. 1 A football player injuring the MCL a combined knee valgus, flexion, and external rotation injury mechanism (Photo courtesy of Dr. Darren L. Johnson)

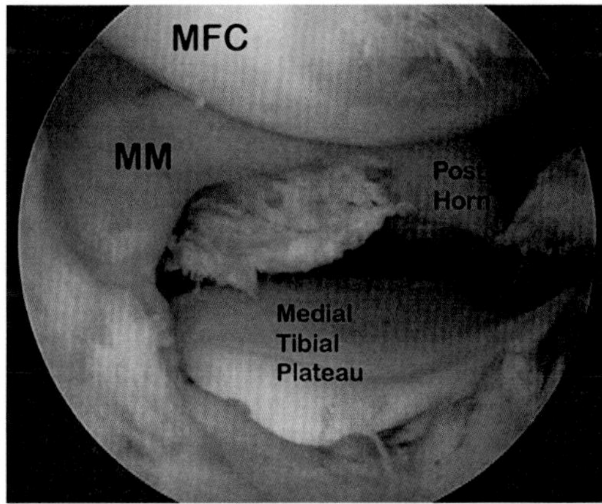

Fig. 2 Arthroscopic picture of the left knee with tibial side medial injury viewed through the anterolateral portal. The medial meniscus is elevated relative to the medial tibial plateau and a portion of the deep medial collateral ligament protruding under the medial meniscus. The medial femoral condyle (*MFC*), medial meniscus (*MM*), and the posterior horn of the medial meniscus (*post horn*) are marked for orientation. The ACL sustained a complete mid-substance tear (Photo courtesy of Dr. Darren L. Johnson)

et al. (1982) reported that in an ACL-deficient knee, the medial meniscus restricts anterior tibial displacement, and a meniscectomy further compromises knee stability by allowing additional anterior displacement. In the ACL-deficient knee, the menisci help maintain a balanced position of the tibia on the femur. The menisci resist the tendency for the tibia to translate and sublux anteriorly when joint load is applied. The posterior horn of the medial meniscus has been reported to be the most effective portion of the meniscus in resisting anterior tibial translatory forces (Shoemaker and Markolf 1986).

The interdependence of the ACL and menisci has been elegantly demonstrated by the work of Papageorgiou et al. (2001) who reported that the relationship between the ACL and the meniscus is substantial, such that injury or impairment of either one of these structures predisposes the other to injury or impairment. Papageorgiou et al. (2001) reported that anterior tibial translation increased following ACL transection, consequently doubling the forces applied to the medial meniscus. Following ACL reconstruction, the anterior tibial translations and forces acting on the medial meniscus were restored to the levels of an intact knee. Several reports have demonstrated how ACL deficiency substantially increases medial meniscus forces generating an increased meniscal tear risk (Warren and Levy 1983; Allen et al. 2000). Hollis et al. (2000) identified statistically significant increases in meniscal strain in ACL-deficient knees compared to intact specimens. Following ACL reconstruction, this strain was reduced to the level of ACL-intact knees. These results support the potential benefit of ACL reconstruction in preventing meniscal injuries.

Papageorgiou et al. (2001) showed the direct effect of a meniscectomy on the reconstructed ACL graft reporting that the in situ forces in the ACL graft increased up to 50 % following medial meniscectomy. In a biomechanical study of combined medial meniscus transplantation and ACL reconstruction, Spang et al. (2010) reported that medial meniscectomy produced a significant increase in tibial displacement relative to the femur and increased ACL strain. They also reported that meniscal allograft transplantation restored displacement and ACL strain values to normal. This implies that performing a subtotal meniscectomy during an ACL reconstruction may increase the chance of ACL graft failure. The medial meniscus contributes directly to ACL stability. In contrast, it has long been believed that the lateral meniscus provides a lesser contribution.

Levy et al. (1989) confirmed that the lateral meniscus was not an efficient posterior wedge to resist anterior tibial translation on the femur, and lateral meniscectomy in an ACL-deficient knee resulted in insignificant increases in anterior tibial translation. The prevailing consensus was that the medial meniscus, but not the lateral meniscus, acted as an important secondary passive restraint to anterior tibial translation. These studies however assessed knee stability only under uniplanar anterior loading forces (Levy et al. 1982, 1989).

Despite the importance of the medial meniscus in ACL stabilization (and vice versa), interestingly, the lateral meniscus is more commonly injured concomitantly with ACL injury (Shelbourne and Gray 2000). With this understanding in mind, Musahl et al. (2010) designed a biomechanical study to investigate the role of the lateral meniscus as a restraint to anterior tibial translation during pivoting. They concluded that the lateral meniscus is a more important anterior tibial translation restraint when the knee is subjected to combined valgus and rotatory loads such as those that occur during a quick, pivoting maneuver.

The movement of the knee is a result of dynamic and static interactions between its various ligaments, other contractile and noncontractile soft tissue structures, and the geometric constraints of the articular surfaces. Among these structures, the ACL and MCL serve crucial roles in maintaining valgus knee stability. Studies have confirmed the synergism between these structures and a possible role in articular cartilage protection (Inoue et al. 1987; Sakane et al. 1999). Injury to either of these important structures may lead to the development of early onset knee osteoarthritis. This is believed to occur as a result of increased tibiofemoral contact stress in conjunction with increased valgus knee instability and/or increased anterior tibial translation. Inoue et al. (1987) reported that valgus knee instability following MCL injury was partly alleviated by the compensatory effects of the ACL. Sakane et al. (1999) reported that knees with combined ACL and MCL deficiency displayed greater anterior tibial translation relative to isolated ACL deficiency at 60° flexion. Matsumoto et al. (2001) postulated that the MCL prevents valgus instability by restraining medial joint space opening while the ACL prevents tibial internal rotation and decreases the valgus rotation angle. The combined effect of these ligaments reduces the valgus knee instability and potential damage to the articular cartilage.

Wu et al. (2002) reported that patients who had undergone any amount of meniscal resection concomitantly with ACL reconstruction had significantly more subjective complaints and activity limitations as measured by the subjective IKDC survey and Lysholm score, respectively. In their long-term follow-up study of patients who underwent ACL reconstruction, Shelbourne and Gray (2000) concluded that the long-term subjective and objective results of a successful ACL reconstruction were directly affected by the status of the menisci and articular surfaces at a mean 8.6 years post-ACL reconstruction. Among a group of 482 patients with objective follow-up and 928 patients with subjective follow-up, they reported that individuals with intact menisci and healthy articular cartilage had a mean subjective IKDC of 94, 97 % had normal or near normal radiographic ratings, and 87 % had normal (A) or nearly normal (B) objective IKDC scores. In contrast, only 70 % of patients who had undergone concomitant partial or total lateral meniscectomy had normal or nearly normal objective IKDC scores, 63 % of patients had normal or nearly normal objective IKDC scores, and only 60 % of patients who had both menisci removed had normal or nearly normal objective IKDC scores. Meniscus and articular cartilage health status was directly related to ACL reconstruction success.

Although the direct relationship between abnormal tibiofemoral contact stress and altered knee kinematics following a combined ACL-MCL injury is poorly understood, related damage to the articular cartilage and resultant knee osteoarthritis is likely (Inaba et al. 1990; Imhauser et al. 2013). Imhauser et al. (2013) reported that ACL deficiency created increased mean tibiofemoral contact stress in the posterior knee regions which were partly alleviated with ACL reconstruction. They emphasized that current ACL reconstruction procedures do not precisely simulate the multi-planar constraint provided by the native ACL, suggesting that this could partly explain the reason for the development of knee osteoarthritis despite seemingly successful ACL reconstruction. Subtle increases in tibial translation in combination with the complex knee joint geometry may create the altered contact patterns that lead to osteoarthritic changes following combined ACL and MCL injury. Increased medial tibial translation may shift the center of peak tibiofemoral contact pressure laterally, increasing compression between the medial femoral condyle and the medial tibial eminence, creating patterns of articular cartilage degeneration. The possibility of this mechanism is supported by in vivo studies (Defrate et al. 2006; Li et al. 2007) of ACL-deficient patients, in which an increase in medial tibial translation and a lateral shift in the location of peak articular cartilage contact (toward the medial tibial eminence in the medial compartment) were observed. Impaired MCL function, which normally helps restrain this motion, could lead to an increased predisposition to medial femoral condyle articular cartilage damage. This belief was corroborated by Frank et al. (2012) who evaluated the role of knee instability in development of knee osteoarthritis using an ovine model. They reported that animals with combined transection of the ACL and MCL had significant kinematic abnormalities, onset of knee osteoarthritis by 20 weeks post-injury, and associated changes in medial-lateral tibial translation.

Natural and Enhanced Healing of an Injured MCL

In young, athletically active individuals, up to 90 % of all knee injuries involve the MCL, ACL, or some combination of both (Miyasaka et al. 1991; Halinen et al. 2009). Healing of MCL injuries with laxity exceeding 5 mm is more likely to develop a less-organized collagen alignment, has increased residual laxity, and provides reduced valgus knee loading resistance post-healing. Biomechanical deficits from reduced MCL tissue integrity in combination with soft tissue graft ACL reconstruction may necessitate a delay in or restriction of patient participation in sports that require sudden running directional changes and single leg jump landings (Anoka et al. 2012). This reinforces the importance of restoring an effective MCL checkrein function, especially if the patient has genetically hyperelastic knee tissues or decreased dynamic neuromuscular stiffness. Since the primary reason for weakness in a healing MCL relates to histologic flaws including smaller than normal collagen fibril size and abnormal collagen cross-linking (Amiel et al. 1995; Lee et al. 1998), interest has increased regarding methods to improve tissue quality. Use of growth factors and bioscaffolds may create mechanically stronger MCL tissue that can better withstand valgus knee stress than natural healing. Others have proposed use of MCL lesion site puncturing or "lancing" to promote growth factor acquisition from local bleeding (Jones et al. 2009) with and without the addition of cross-fiber massage methods (Loghmani and Warden 2009). Cross-fiber massage refers to the manual application of forces transverse to the direction of the underlying collagen substructure in order to induce physiological and/or structural tissue changes (Loghmani and Warden 2009).

"Minor" MCL Laxity and Pathomechanical Single Leg Jump Landings

Genetically excessive connective tissue extensibility in association with poor neuromuscular control of the trunk, hip, and knee during single leg jump landings with coxa vara-genu valgum postural alignment may predispose an athlete to knee injury (Powers 2010; Hewett and Myer 2011). If excessive capsuloligamentous knee tissue laxity (Smith et al. 2005; Konopinski et al. 2012) coincides with the single leg frontal plane loading predisposition (Ford et al. 2010), capsuloligamentous knee injury is more likely, particularly among female athletes. When a seemingly minor MCL injury occurs in association with a noncontact single leg loading mechanism such as jump landings or running direction changes, clinicians should be cognizant of the likelihood for this seemingly minor injury to progress to a more traumatic ACL injury mechanism in combination with more severe MCL injury, medial meniscus tearing, and articular cartilage injury. While a seemingly minor MCL injury may represent a relatively unremarkable event given the continuum of possible knee injuries, its onset has the potential to be the first step toward sustaining a more devastating major knee injury whose effects may negatively impact the athletes for the rest of their life, particularly if athletic performance technique and neuromuscular control impairments exist (Ford et al. 2010; Powers 2010; Hewett and Myer 2011).

A Simple Surgical Technique for Combined Partial ACL Injury and MCL Injury

Having a fully functional ACL is crucial for knee stability; however, other structures that are often injured simultaneously also warrant attention. For example, the MCL reinforces the medial joint capsule, serving as the primary restraint to valgus knee stress. Combined ACL and MCL function prevents anteromedial knee displacement and restrains knee valgus opening (Ma et al. 2000; Shin et al. 2009). For these reasons, it may be necessary to repair the injured MCL simultaneously when a partial ACL injury is observed to restore stability, decrease the likelihood of future knee osteoarthritis, and return patients to their previous activity level (Doral et al. 2013).

Prior to surgery, a complete ligamentous knee examination (pivot shift test, Lachman test, anterior drawer test, dial test, anteromedial drawer test, varus/valgus stress tests) is performed with the patient in a supine position. To be accurate, the patient must be completely relaxed or under anesthesia. Although valgus stress radiographs accurately and reliability measure medial compartment gapping, they cannot definitively differentiate between meniscofemoral- and meniscotibial-based injuries (Laprade et al. 2010). A grade III MCL injury should be suspected when greater than 3.2 mm of medial compartment gapping is observed, compared to the contralateral knee at 20° flexion (Laprade et al. 2010).

A coauthor (MND) has designed a new technique for managing combined partial ACL and MCL injury. Arthroscopy is performed through standard portals. Both anteromedial and posterolateral ACL bundles are evaluated thoroughly. Shrinkage using radiofrequency current is applied if one of these bundles is partially torn or elongated to reestablish natural length. After identifying the midpoint of the medial joint line, a 1 mm incision is made at the proximal MCL attachment at the adductor tubercle. Percutaneous MCL reefing is then performed and the MCL is augmented using bioabsorbable #2 PDS (Ethicon, Johnson and Johnson, New Brunswick, NJ, USA) suture from the distal femur over the adductor tubercle to the proximal tibia (Fig. 3). The suture is passed through the loop twice at the distal aspect of the MCL. Knee stability is then evaluated using valgus stress testing with the knee in full extension and at 30° degree flexion. After further reefing, the suture needle is passed in a distal-proximal-distal sequence through the MCL fibers. Lastly, the free suture ends are tied together at the distal MCL insertion. Prior to closure, platelet-rich plasma (PRP) is injected into the

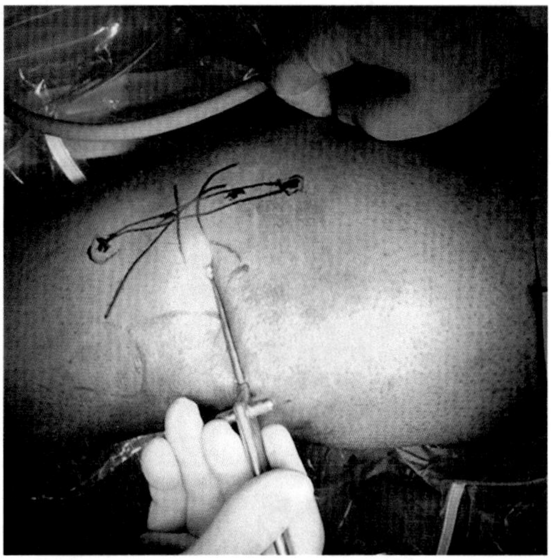

Fig. 3 Identification and demarcation of key surgical landmarks at the medial knee for percutaneous MCL repair

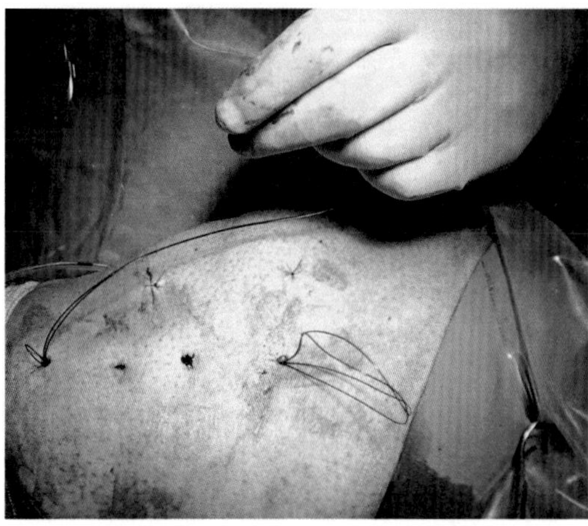

Fig. 4 Percutaneous sutures are initiated from proximal anterior aspect of the MCL and continued distally to the tibial insertion in a double-loop fashion using PDS #2 suture material (Ethicon, Johnson and Johnson, Somerville, NJ, USA)

injured region of the ACL and MCL to facilitate a growth factor-induced healing response (Fig. 4) (Doral et al. 2013). Early patient outcomes at 6 months post-surgery have revealed comparable isokinetic knee extensor and flexor strength and single leg hop test performance between the surgical and healthy, contralateral lower extremity. Two-year follow-up has revealed that many patients returned successfully to recreational soccer and tennis without need for a functional knee brace.

Anatomical ACL Reconstruction

At this time, we remain unsure that anatomical or "footprint" simulated ACL reconstruction provides improved rotational knee control kinematics and clinical outcomes compared to conventional transtibial surgical approaches. Anatomical or footprint ACL reconstructions, particularly double-bundle reconstructions, have been shown to more closely restore normal knee kinematics using in vitro biomechanical study models (Yagi et al. 2007; Seon et al. 2010; Tsai et al. 2010) and with clinical trials (van Eck et al. 2012). Based on these studies, one would expect significantly reduced evidence of knee osteoarthritis since normalized knee kinematics better replicate the pre-injury state. Unfortunately, to date, the clinical advantages have been quite limited compared with conventional transtibial tunnel drilling techniques, largely due to limitations in clinical research study designs and measurement methods (van Eck et al. 2012). Current clinical knowledge, limited as it is, suggests that knee kinematics are not restored to their normal state with ACL reconstruction alone for management of a combined ACL and MCL injury.

In the sheep model, residual knee laxity from combined ACL and MCL transection leads to knee osteoarthritis (Frank et al. 2012). Zaffagnini et al. (2011) evaluated patients at 3 years following double-bundle ACL reconstructions for the treatment of either isolated ACL injury or combined ACL and grade II MCL injury. The MCL injuries were managed conservatively. With Telos-assisted knee valgus stress testing, these patients displayed significantly greater laxity (1.7 mm versus 0.9 mm) compared to patients with isolated ACL injury. Anterior knee laxity evaluated using a KT-2000 arthrometer (Medmetric Corp., San Diego, CA, USA) and other clinical parameters did not display significant group differences. Animal model research evidence, as reported by Frank et al. (2012), and clinical experience, as reported by Kaeding et al. (2005), suggest that the residual laxity with valgus loading may lead to earlier onset of knee osteoarthritis and impaired function.

Although "footprint" ACL reconstruction, particularly with a double-bundle graft configuration, may restore normal knee kinematics at time zero, evidence that this leads to improved clinical outcomes and decreased knee osteoarthritis is minimal. Lacking long-term clinical patient outcome results at this time, we cannot conclude that "footprint" ACL reconstructions will be sufficient to improve the health longevity for the combined ACL- and MCL-injured knee any better than conventional transtibial drilling approaches. In addition to the need for longer clinical follow-up, future studies should include more accurate and precise means of evaluating multi-planar knee stability and comparative trials of different MCL treatment methods in combination with single- and double-bundle "footprint" ACL reconstruction methods.

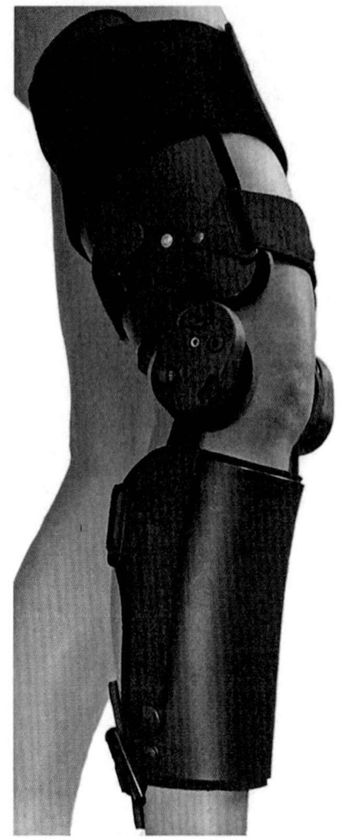

Fig. 5 The "ACL-Jack Brace" (Albrecht GmbH, Germany), a lower extremity brace with a padded anterior tibial cuff designed to provide a posterior translatory force to the healing ACL avoiding quadriceps femoris-induced anterior drawer

Primary ACL Repair

The acutely injured ACL has poor healing capacity that generally results in persisting knee instability. Therefore, surgical reconstruction has become the treatment of choice to restore ACL function in the younger, more active patient. The question remains however if fresh ACL tears can be treated conservatively in athletically active adult patients resulting in a healthy, stable knee. The potential for restoring non-impaired ACL function through primary repair that maintains native anatomy, insertions, neurosensory receptors, and biomechanical characteristics warrants consideration. Jakob et al. (2006) described their primary ACL repair experiences with the "ACL-Jack Brace" (Albrecht GmbH, Stephanskirchen, Germany), a lower extremity brace with a padded anterior tibial cuff designed to provide a posterior translatory force to the healing ACL avoiding the quadriceps femoris-induced anterior drawer (Fig. 5). A total of 86 patients including skiers, soccer players, judokas, and other recreational athletes participated in this study. Eight patients underwent concurrent suture-based meniscus repair. Twenty-four patients underwent arthroscopic realignment and fixation of anteriorly displaced ACL fibers using either Tissucol fibrin glue (Baxter, Deerfield, IL, USA) or Ultra FAST-FIX (Smith and Nephew, Andover, MA, USA) suture devices. Clinical knee examination including bilateral comparison of knee laxity (Rolimeter, Aircast, DJO, Vista, CA, USA) was performed at the time of injury prior to intervention and at 6, 12, and 24 months post-injury. Magnetic resonance imaging was also performed at the time of injury and at 6 months post-injury. Of the 86 patients, two were lost to follow-up. Of the 84 remaining patients, 18 (21 %) required a secondary ACL reconstruction because of persisting instability or repeat tear of the healed ligament within 2 years follow-up. The survivors ($n = 66$) showed respectable longitudinal

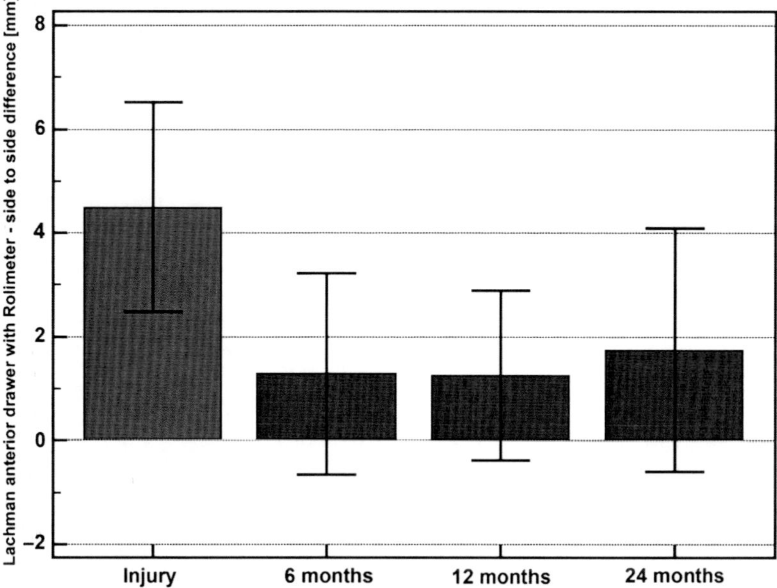

Fig. 6 Side-to-side anterior knee laxity differences between the injured and contralateral, non-injured knee following ACL-Jack Brace use

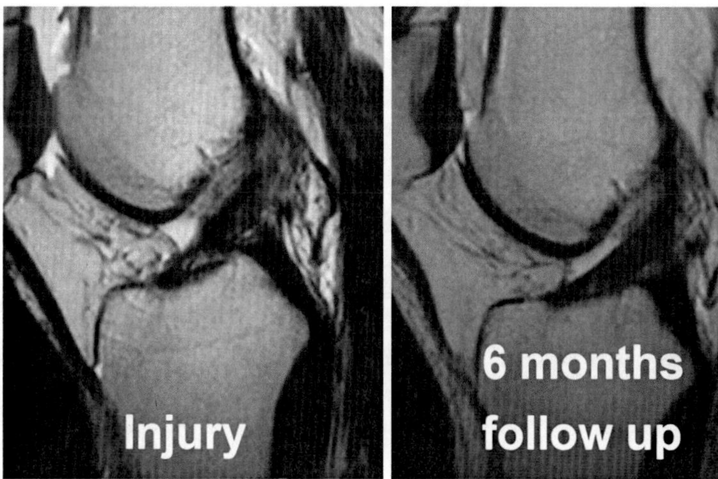

Fig. 7 MRI of healing ACL at 6 months post-intervention

findings for side-to-side anterior knee laxity comparisons (Fig. 6). Longitudinal findings for patient self-reported IKDC-perceived knee function survey revealed a pre-injury baseline score of 97 ± 5.2 (mean ± standard deviation) and a score of 90 ± 8.7 at 2-year follow-up. The mean pre-injury Tegner score was 7. At 2-year follow-up, it was 6. Of the 66 patients who completed the study, 39 (59 %) reached their pre-injury Tegner activity level. Patients that did best and appeared to be most pleased with the procedure were 30–40-year-old women. The highest failure rate was observed among young men with higher-level sport activity interests. Ligament healing was documented on MRI at 6 months (Fig. 7). Patient satisfaction at 2-year follow-up based on a 100 point scale with end range descriptors of 0 = not satisfied and 100 = completely satisfied was generally high (89 % ± 15). The main complications encountered in the survivor group were skin problems over the anterior tibial rim due to the posteriorly directed force of the tibial brace pad ($n = 10$, 15.2 %). One case of knee arthrofibrosis was observed. The results of this study show that healing of the freshly injured ACL is, under optimal conditions, better than generally assumed. Avoidance of the anterior tibial drawer force of the quadriceps femoris muscle during the healing period seems to be a key factor. However, the biomechanical integrity of the healed ACL was not investigated. Based on these findings, future studies need to consider the use of biochemical mediators such as platelet-rich plasma, stem cells, or other repair-enhancing factors, in addition to brace design and use modifications to enhance patient compliance. These findings also support the need for further research regarding stump remnant-sparing ACL reconstruction and internal bracing of the freshly injured ACL with bioscaffolds.

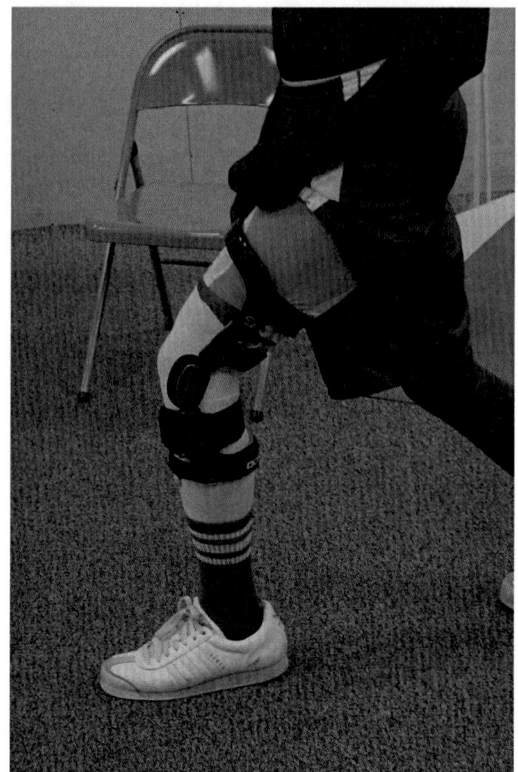

Fig. 8 Strap-based, functional de-rotation ACL brace

Functional Knee Bracing, Orthotics, Neuromuscular and Sensorimotor Control Training

The greatest priority with functional knee bracing for ACL deficiency or graft protection rests in its ability to control frontal plane knee motion and medial femoral condyle lift-off (Anoka et al. 2012). The current state of functional brace technology may also help restrain excessive transverse plane internal-external knee rotation. However, these smaller magnitude rotations are best managed as secondary concerns related to frontal plane knee movement control. Early use of more rigid, strap-based functional knee braces can protect the healing MCL as well as the ACL graft during the first year post-surgery which is when most of the remodeling phase occurs (Claes et al. 2011) (Fig. 8). Following the first year post-ACL reconstruction, simple collateral hinges affixed to sleeve-based braces can provide good frontal plane knee control in a less restrictive brace when the athlete is deemed ready for less restraint (Fig. 9). During brace use, the athlete should be encouraged to perform some range of motion and neuromuscular and strength training exercises outside of the brace as prolonged brace use may tend to impair knee joint kinematics and otherwise contribute to altered neuromuscular responsiveness (Fig. 10). Supervised time spent

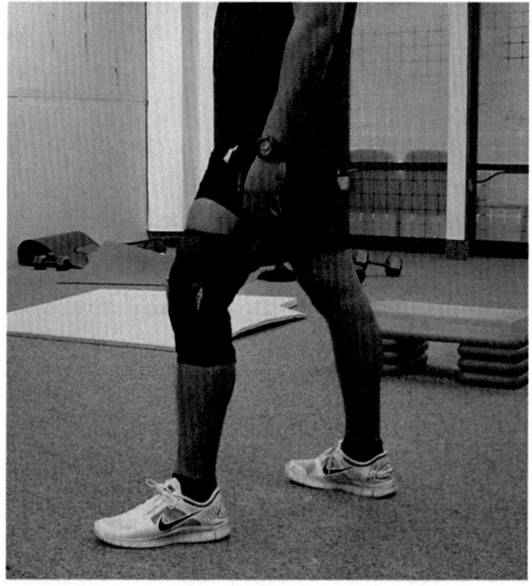

Fig. 9 Simple sleeve-based knee brace with collateral hinges

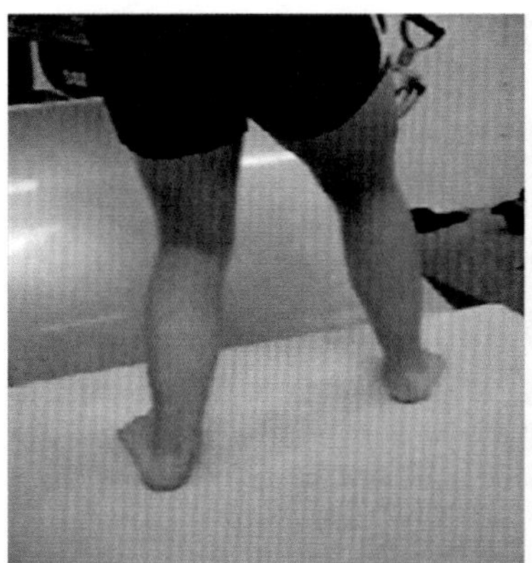

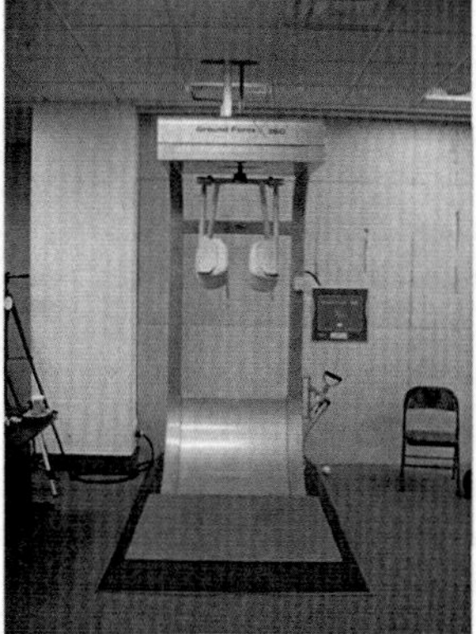

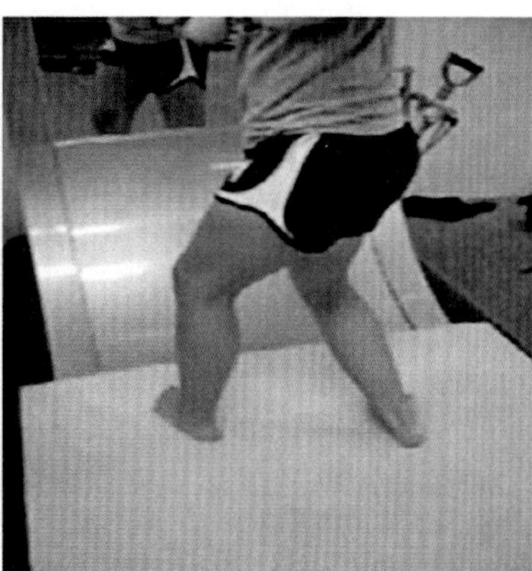

Fig. 10 Ground Force 360 device (Center of Rotational Exercise, Clearwater, FL, USA) center figure; left foot pronation, leg and thigh internal rotation, and knee valgus during resisted right trunk rotation (*left figure*); right foot pronation, leg and thigh internal rotation, and knee valgus during resisted left trunk rotation (*right figure*). Device provides a unique, safe evaluation and training environment to increase awareness of potentially injurious lower extremity postural alignment during loading and to improve trunk and lower extremity neuromuscular control and coordination

training appropriate sports movement postures and neuromuscular control responses outside of the knee brace during rehabilitation, sports-specific training, and following return to sports is essential (Nyland et al. 2010).

Summary

The functional integrity of the MCL is directly linked to ACL, meniscus, and articular cartilage health. Previous notions of minor MCL injuries from noncontact mechanisms being inconsequential requiring a few weeks for healing to take place prior to return to play may be a terrible assumption if poor lower extremity neuromuscular control and faulty postural alignment coexist. At the time of index ACL repair or reconstruction, attention must be paid to MCL functional status to insure successful surgery, particularly when soft tissue grafts are used. Developments in less invasive ACL and MCL repair methods show promise. However, at this time, success with these procedures is greatest for recreational athletes with lower performance expectations. Future well-designed studies of surgical repair of these tissues with biologically mediated healing factors warrant attention, particularly those that include long-term biomechanical tissue integrity and objective patient clinical outcome assessments.

Cross-References

- ▶ Anterior Cruciate Ligament Injuries: Prevention Strategies
- ▶ Perioperative and Postoperative Anterior Cruciate Ligament Rehabilitation Focused on Soft Tissue Grafts
- ▶ Prevention of Knee Injuries in Soccer Players
- ▶ Role of Biologicals in Meniscus Surgery
- ▶ Role of Growth Factors in Anterior Cruciate Ligament Surgery
- ▶ Structured Rehabilitation Model with Clinical Outcomes After Anterior Cruciate Ligament Reconstruction

References

Allen CR, Wong EK, Livesay GA et al (2000) Importance of the medial meniscus in the anterior cruciate ligament-deficient knee. J Orthop Res 18:109–115

Amiel D, Nagineni CN, Choi SH et al (1995) Intrinsic properties of ACL and MCL cells and their responses to growth factors. Med Sci Sports Exerc 27:844–851

Anoka N, Nyland J, McGinnis M et al (2012) Consideration of growth factors and bio-scaffolds for treatment of combined grade II MCL and ACL injury. Knee Surg Sports Traumatol Arthrosc 20(5):878–888

Claes S, Verdonk P, Forsyth R et al (2011) The "ligamentization" process in anterior cruciate ligament reconstruction: what happens to the human graft? a systematic review of the literature. Am J Sports Med 39(11):2476–2483

DeFrate LE, Papannagari R, Gill TJ et al (2006) The 6 degrees of freedom kinematics of the knee after anterior cruciate ligament deficiency: an in vivo imaging analysis. Am J Sports Med 34(8):1240–1246

Doral MN, Kaya D, Huri G et al (2013) Minimal invasive acute medial collateral ligament stabilization with partial anterior cruciate ligament deficiency: preliminary results of 16-patients case series and review of the literature. Clin Exp Med Sci 1(2):69–81

Ford KR, Shapiro R, Myer GD et al (2010) Longitudinal sex differences during landing in knee abduction in young athletes. Med Sci Sports Exerc 42(10): 1923–1931

Frank CB, Beveridge JE, Huebner KD et al (2012) Complete ACL/MCL deficiency induces variable degrees of instability in sheep with specific kinematic abnormalities correlating with degrees of early osteoarthritis. J Orthop Res 30(3):384–392

Griffith CJ, LaPrade RF, Johansen S, Armitage B, Wijdicks C, Engebretsen L (2009) Medial knee injury: part 1, static function of the individual components of the main medial knee structures. Am J Sports Med 37(9):1762–1770

Halinen J, Lindahl J, Hirvensalo E (2009) Range of motion and quadriceps muscle power after early surgical treatment of acute combined anterior cruciate and grade-III medial collateral ligament injuries. J Bone Joint Surg 91A(6):1305–1312

Hewett TE, Myer GD (2011) The mechanistic connection between the trunk, hip, knee and anterior cruciate ligament injury. Exerc Sport Sci Rev 39(4):161–166

Hollis JM, Pearsall AW IV, Niciforos PG (2000) Change in meniscal strain with anterior cruciate ligament injury and after reconstruction. Am J Sports Med 28:700–704

Hughston J, Eilers A (1973) The role of the posterior oblique ligament in repairs of the acute medial (collateral) ligament tears of the knee. J Bone Joint Surg 55A(5):923–940

Imhauser C, Mauro C, Choi D et al (2013) Abnormal tibiofemoral contact stress and its association with altered kinematics after center-center anterior cruciate ligament reconstruction: an in vitro study. Am J Sports Med 41(4):815–825

Inaba HI, Arai MA, Watanabe WW (1990) Influence of the varus-valgus instability on the contact of the femoro-tibial joint. Proc Inst Mech Eng H 204(1):61–64

Inoue M, McGurk-Burleson E, Hollis JM et al (1987) Treatment of the medial collateral ligament injury. I: the importance of anterior cruciate ligament on the varus-valgus knee laxity. Am J Sports Med 15(1): 15–21

Jakob R, Jacobi M, Gautier E (2006) Successful treatment of fresh ACL injuries with the Reverse Jack Brace. Annual meeting of the Swiss Society of Orthopedics, 21 Sept 2006, Luzern

Jones L, Bismil Q, Alyas F et al (2009) Persistent symptoms following non operative management in low grade MCL injury of the knee – the role of the deep MCL. Knee 16:64–68

Joseph M, Tiberio D, Baird JL et al (2008) Knee valgus during drop jumps in National Collegiate Athletic Association Division I female athletes: the effect of a medial post. Am J Sports Med 36(2):285–289

Kaeding C, Pedroza A, Parker R et al (2005) Intra-articular findings in the reconstructed multiligament-injured knee. Arthroscopy 21(4):424–430

Konopinski MD, Jones GJ, Johnson MI (2012) The effect of hypermobility on the incidence of injuries in elite-level professional soccer players: a cohort study. Am J Sports Med 40(4):763–769

Laprade RF, Bernhardson AS, Griffith CJ, Macalena JA, Wijdicks CA (2010) Correlation of valgus stress radiographs with medial knee ligament injuries: An in vitro biomechanical study. Am J Sports Med 38(2):330–338

Lee J, Harwood FL, Akeson WH et al (1998) Growth factor expression in healing rabbit medial collateral and anterior cruciate ligaments. Iowa Orthop 18:19–25

Lee SJ, Aadalen KJ, Malaviya P et al (2006) Tibiofemoral contact mechanics after serial medial meniscectomies in the human cadaveric knee. Am J Sports Med 34:1334–1344

Levy IM, Torzilli PA, Gould JD et al (1989) The effect of lateral meniscectomy on motion of the knee. J Bone Joint Surg 71A(3):401–406

Levy IM, Torzilli PA, Warren RF (1982) The effect of medial meniscectomy on anterior-posterior motion of the knee. J Bone Joint Surg 64A(6):883–888

Li G, Papannagari R, DeFrate LE et al (2007) The effects of ACL deficiency on mediolateral translation and varus-valgus rotation. Acta Orthop 78(3):355–360

Loghmani MT, Warden SJ (2009) Instrument-assisted cross-fiber massage accelerates knee ligament healing. J Orthop Sports Phys Ther 39:506–514

Ma CB, Papageorgiou CD, Debski RE et al (2000) Interaction between the ACL graft and MCL in a combined ACL + MCL knee injury using a goat model. Acta Orthop Scand 71(4):387–393

Matsumoto H, Suda Y, Otani T et al (2001) Roles of the anterior cruciate ligament and the medial collateral ligament in preventing valgus instability. J Orthop Sci 6(1):28–32

Miyasaka KC, Daniel DM, Stone ML et al (1991) The incidence of knee ligament injuries in the general population. Am J Knee Surg 4:3–8

Musahl V, Citak M, O'Loughlin PF et al (2010) The effect of medial versus lateral meniscectomy on the stability of the anterior cruciate ligament deficient knee. Am J Sports Med 38:1591–1597

Nyland J, Brand E, Fisher B (2010) Update on rehabilitation following ACL reconstruction. Open Access Journal of Sports Medicine. http://www.dovepress.com/update-on-rehabilitation-following-acl-reconstruction-peer-reviewed-article-OAJSM

Papageorgiou CD, Gil JE, Kanamori A et al (2001) The biomechanical interdependence between the anterior cruciate ligament replacement graft and the medial meniscus. Am J Sports Med 29:226–231

Powers CM (2010) The influence of abnormal hip mechanics on knee injury: a biomechanical perspective. J Orthop Sports Phys Ther 40(2):42–51

Robinson J, Bull A, Thomas RR et al (2006) The role of medial collateral ligament and posteromedial capsule in controlling knee laxity. Am J Sports Med 34(11): 1815–1823

Sakane M, Livesay GA, Fox RJ et al (1999) Relative contribution of the ACL, MCL, and bony contact to the anterior stability of the knee. Knee Surg Sports Traumatol Arthrosc 7(2):93–97

Seon JK, Gadikota HR, Wu JL et al (2010) Comparison of single- and double-bundle anterior cruciate ligament reconstructions in restoration of knee kinematics and anterior cruciate ligament forces. Am J Sports Med 38(7):1359–1367

Shelbourne KD, Gray T (2000) Results of anterior cruciate ligament reconstruction based on meniscus and articular cartilage status at the time of surgery: five- to fifteen-year evaluations. Am J Sports Med 28(4):446–452

Shin CS, Chaudhari AM, Andriacchi TP (2009) The effect of isolated valgus moments on ACL strain during single-leg landing: a simulation study. J Biomech 42(3):280–285

Shoemaker SC, Markolf KL (1986) The role of the meniscus in the anterior-posterior stability of the loaded anterior cruciate-deficient knee. Effects of partial versus total excision. J Bone Joint Surg 68A:71–79

Smith R, Damodaran AK, Swaminathan S et al (2005) Hypermobility and sports injuries in junior netball players. Br J Sports Med 39(9):628–631

Spang JT, Dang ABC, Mazzocca A et al (2010) The effect of medial meniscectomy and meniscal allograft transplantation on knee and anterior cruciate ligament biomechanics. Arthroscopy 26:192–201

Tapper J, Funakoshi Y, Hariu M et al (2009) ACL/MCL transection affects knee ligament insertion distance of healing and intact ligaments during gait in the ovine model. J Biomech 42(12):1825–1833

Tsai AG, Wijdicks CA, Walsh MP et al (2010) Comparative kinematic evaluation of all-inside single-bundle and double-bundle anterior cruciate ligament reconstruction: a biomechanical study. Am J Sports Med 38(2):263–272

van Eck CF, Kopf S, Irrgang JJ et al (2012) Single-bundle versus double-bundle reconstruction for anterior cruciate ligament rupture: a meta-analysis – does anatomy matter? Arthroscopy 28(3):405–424

Warren RF, Levy IM (1983) Meniscal lesions associated with anterior cruciate ligament injury. Clin Orthop Relat Res 172:32–37

Wijdicks CA, Griffith CJ, LaPrade RF, Spiridonov SI, Johansen S, Armitage BM, Engebretsen L (2009) Medial knee injury: part 2, load sharing between the posterior oblique ligament and superficial medial collateral ligament. Am J Sports Med 37(9):1771–1776

Wu HW, Hackett T, Richmond JC (2002) Effect of meniscal and articular surface status on knee stability, function and symptoms after anterior cruciate ligament reconstruction. A long-term prospective study. Am J Sports Med 30:845–850

Yagi M, Kuroda R, Nagamune K et al (2007) Double-bundle ACL reconstruction can improve rotational stability. Clin Orthop Relat Res 454:100–107

Zaffagnini S, Bonanzinga T, Marcheggiani M et al (2011) Does chronic medial collateral ligament laxity influence the outcome of anterior cruciate ligament reconstruction?: a prospective evaluation with a minimum three-year follow-up. J Bone Joint Surg Br 93(8):1060–1064

Medial Side Instability and Reconstruction

93

Iftach Hetsroni, Robert G. Marx, and Gideon Mann

Contents

I. Hetsroni (✉)
Department of Orthopedic Surgery, Meir Medical Centre, Kfar Saba, Israel

Service of Sports Injuries, Department of Orthopaedic Surgery, Meir Medical Centre, Tel Aviv University, Tel Aviv, Israel
e-mail: iftachhetsroni@gmail.com

R.G. Marx
Foster Center for Clinical Outcome Research, Hospital for Special Surgery, New York, NY, USA

Weill Medical College of Cornell University, New York, NY, USA
e-mail: MarxR@hss.edu

G. Mann
Service of Sports Injuries, Department of Orthopaedic Surgery, Meir Medical Centre, Tel Aviv University, Tel Aviv, Israel
e-mail: Gideon.mann.md@gmail.com

M.N. Doral, J. Karlsson (eds.), *Sports Injuries*,
DOI 10.1007/978-3-642-36569-0_114

Abstract

The primary structure that provides stability to the medial side of the knee during valgus loads is the medial collateral ligament (MCL) complex. In this chapter key anatomy of this ligament is reviewed, a stepwise clinical assessment to recognize medial side instability is suggested, and surgical techniques to address medial instability are discussed.

Function and Anatomy of the MCL Complex

The medial collateral ligament (MCL) is the primary restraint to valgus stability of the knee. At 20–30° flexion, it provides approximately 80 % of the restraining force, whereas at full extension, it provides approximately 60 % of the restraining force with the posteromedial capsule, posterior oblique ligament (POL), and ACL providing the remaining restraint (Grood et al. 1981). The MCL has three major components: (1) the superficial MCL, which is the largest; (2) the deep MCL; and (3) the posterior oblique ligament (La Prade et al. 2007). The superficial MCL originates on an average of 3.2 mm proximal and 4.8 mm posterior to the medial epicondyle and inserts on the proximal tibia, just anterior to the posteromedial crest of the tibia and posterior to the pes anserinus insertion (La Prade et al. 2007). The deep portion of the MCL is a thickened part of the medial joint capsule, lying deep to the superficial part of the

MCL, and has meniscotibial and meniscofemoral components. The femoral attachment is 12.6 mm distal and deep to the femoral attachment of the superficial MCL, and the tibial attachment lies just distal to the edge of the articular cartilage of the medial tibial plateau, 3.2 mm distal to the medial joint line (La Prade et al. 2007). The POL, primarily functioning as an additional medial knee restraint when the knee is extended, is a fibrous extension of the distal aspect of the semimembranosus that blends with the posteromedial joint capsule. Its major and central portion attaches on the femur 7.7 mm distal and 2.9 mm anterior to the gastrocnemius tubercle (La Prade et al. 2007), which is just proximal and posterior to the femoral insertion of the superficial MCL.

Clinical Assessment of Medial Side Instability

History

Patients with MCL dysfunction are likely to complain of a sense of instability during activities that involve planting with pivoting or cutting maneuvers. While this presentation is typical to patients with ACL deficiency as well, MCL dysfunction, either with or without ACL dysfunction, may result also in a sense of instability during activities that overload the knee valgus restraints in particular. This may specifically occur, for example, when passing a soccer ball with the injured limb. In rare chronic cases of MCL attenuation in patients with valgus malalignment, valgus thrust gait may develop, resulting in a sense of the injured knee becoming more knocked-kneed during the stance phase of the gait cycle (Hetsroni et al. 2014). This is analogous to varus thrust gait that may develop in chronic cases of lateral constraints attenuation.

Physical Examination

Physical examination should begin with assessment of alignment and gait. Specific attention should be paid to valgus malalignment with or without noticeable valgus thrust gait. When excessive valgus is confirmed with hip-to-ankle AP x-rays in a patient with increased medial side laxity, it is theorized that valgus moments applied to the medial ligaments play a role in the instability. Therefore, a varus-directed osteotomy to correct the alignment should be thought of as a first step before addressing surgically any attenuation of the medial collateral ligament complex (Phisitkul et al. 2006). This may result in decreasing valgus moments and consequently may lead to improvement in the sense of instability (Hetsroni et al. 2014). Following assessment of alignment and gait, the knee is examined for intra-articular fluid, patellofemoral joint pain, patellofemoral tracking and stability, range of knee flexion and extension, and cruciate and collateral ligament laxities. The uninjured contralateral knee is used as a baseline for comparison. MCL laxity should be tested and graded with valgus stress applied at 0° and at 20–30° of knee flexion. MCL laxity differences graded as 0 corresponds to a 0–2 mm side-to-side medial opening difference, Grade 1+ corresponds to 3–5 mm difference, Grade 2+ corresponds to 6–10 mm difference, and Grade 3+ corresponds to more than 10 mm difference (Hughston and Eilers 1973; Fanelli and Harris 2007; Wijdicks et al. 2010).

Imaging

Stress x-rays can be used to ascertain that the medial rather than the lateral restraints are the source for the increased collateral laxity observed. It can also provide further quantification of medial laxity. However, the amount of medial gapping on stress x-rays that correlates with a specific grade of MCL laxity has not been well documented in vivo. Recently, reference values were provided, but this was tested in a cadaveric model using elderly subjects, which may not apply to young or middle-aged living humans (LaPrade et al. 2010).

When operative management is considered, the following examinations conclude the clinical assessment and grading of medial collateral laxity:

1. *Examination under anesthesia*: The operated knee should be examined under anesthesia and compared with the nonoperated side for range of motion and ligament laxity prior to arthroscopic surgery. Physical examination of the MCL relies both on the patient's ability to relax and the clinician's skill to detect the amount of medial opening and the presence or absence of an end point. In the anesthetized patient, ligament evaluation is facilitated, in the absence of muscle guarding.
2. *Arthroscopic evaluation*: Following arthroscopic examination of the knee, a quantitative assessment of medial compartment gapping can be performed using the tip of the arthroscopic probe as a scale after its length is measured and confirmed outside the knee. Medial compartment gapping of above 5 mm between the articular surfaces of the medial femoral condyle and medial tibial plateau is suggestive of Grade 2+ MCL laxity (Canata et al. 2012), whereas 10 mm or above of medial gapping is suggestive of Grade 3+ MCL laxity (Marx and Hetsroni 2012, Fig. 1).

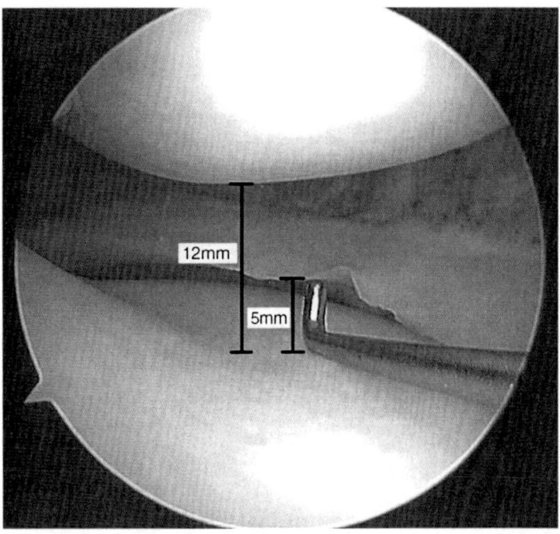

Fig. 1 Arthroscopic view of a right knee, suggesting Grade 3+ MCL laxity (Reprinted from Hetsroni I, Canata GL, Marx RG (2014) Medial Collateral ligament laxity in revision ACL reconstruction. In: Marx, Robert G (ed) Revision ACL Reconstruction: Indications and Technique, with permission from Springer)

Management of Medial Side Instability

The majority of MCL complex lesions involve midsubstance and femoral-sided soft tissue tears (Fig. 2). These lesions can be treated nonoperatively with bracing for 6–8 weeks, resulting in excellent outcomes (Indelicato 1983). Nevertheless, indications for acute direct repair of the MCL complex do exist and include: (1) displaced bony avulsion of the femoral insertion, (2) open MCL disruption, and (3) MCL avulsion of the tibial insertion (Fig. 3) and particularly when a Stener-like lesion is observed (i.e., the superficial MCL fibers flip over and superficial to the pes anserinus tendons) (Corten et al. 2010). In rare cases, chronic medial side instability may persist and require surgical intervention. Such interventions involve either medial complex plication or MCL reconstruction.

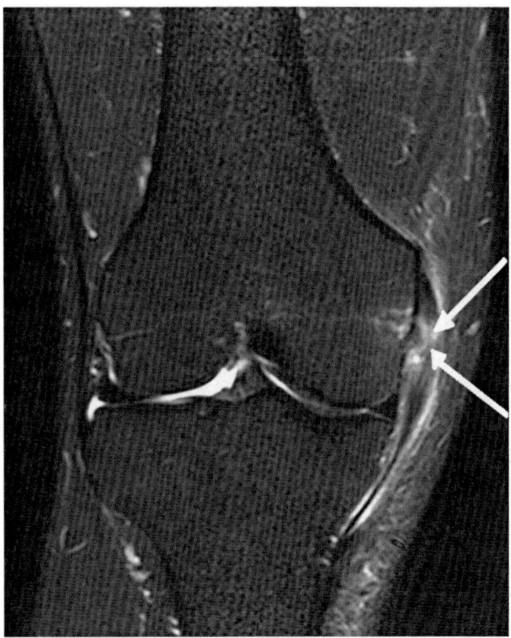

Fig. 2 Coronal MRI image of a right knee, showing midsubstance, femoral-sided MCL rupture. This injury has excellent nonoperative healing potential (*white arrows*)

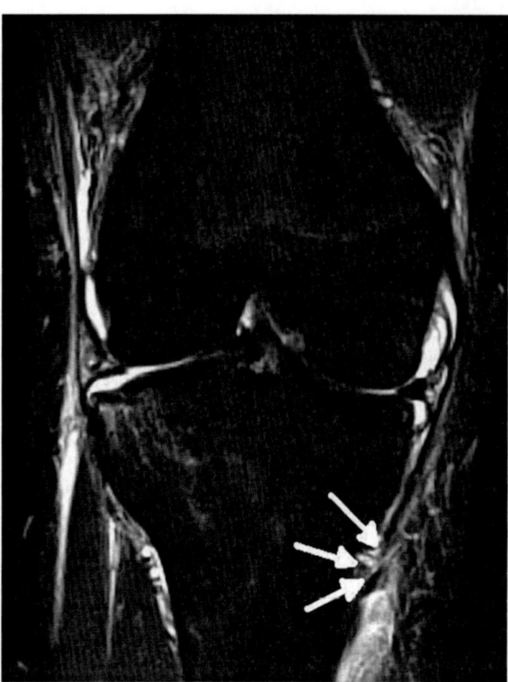

Fig. 3 Coronal MRI image of a right knee, showing distal MCL avulsion of the tibial insertion (*white arrows*)

Medial Complex Plication

Direct MCL repair with medial plication has been described in the setting of primary ACL reconstruction (Robins et al. 1993) and in revision ACL reconstructions where persistent Grade 2+ medial instability was demonstrated after fixing the ACL graft (Canata et al. 2012).

Surgical technique (Canata et al. 2012): In case the procedure is performed alongside ACL reconstruction, repair and plication is performed after the ACL graft is fixed. A 3–5 cm longitudinal incision is made over the medial epicondyle. The sartorial fascia is incised, revealing the MCL-POL layer. Three figure-of-eight Number 2 Ethibond® sutures are then placed. Each suture starts at the medial epicondyle area and extends about 1 cm distally, pulling subsequently the distal portion of the MCL-POL layer towards the medial epicondyle. One suture extends distally and slightly posterior, one extends directly distally, and one extends distally and slightly anterior. Additional sutures can then be added as needed in order to decrease any remaining medial laxity. Postoperative rehabilitation guidelines include keeping crutch-protected gait for 4 weeks with weight-bearing as tolerated and using a knee brace for 6 weeks to prevent excessive valgus loads but without restriction of flexion-extension range of motion. Recently, minimum 2-year outcomes were reported using this technique in a group of 36 patients with a mean age of 37 years (range, 15–70 years) (Canata et al. 2012). Mean International Knee Documentation Committee (IKDC)-subjective score improved from 36 preoperatively to 94, mean Knee Osteoarthritis Outcome Score (KOOS) improved from 45 to 93, and mean Lysholm score improved from 40 to 93 at latest follow-up. At latest follow-up, valgus and external rotation laxities were normal in all cases. It should be noticed that this technique relies on pulling the MCL complex in a distal-to-proximal direction towards the medial epicondyle. Thus, tibial-sided disruption of the MCL complex is a contraindication to performing this technique. In this case (i.e., tibial-sided chronic MCL disruption), MCL reconstruction should be preferred.

MCL Reconstruction

In cases involving chronic Grade 3+ medial side laxity, MCL reconstruction should be considered. One of the earliest techniques developed to reconstruct the MCL was described by Bosworth in the early 1950s (Bosworth 1952). In this technique the tibial insertion of the semitendinosus tendon is left intact at the pes anserinus, and the tendon is fixed proximally on the femur, recreating an isometric MCL graft. Later on, several modifications have been suggested. After the tendon is fixed on the femur, the remaining graft tissue can be looped back in a distal-posterior direction and then fixed to the proximal posteromedial tibia (Lind et al. 2009) or looped around the direct head of the semimembranosus (Kim et al. 2008) in order to recreate the function of the POL. Double-bundle constructs have also been described to optimize medial knee restraint (Borden et al. 2002; Feeley et al. 2009a; Wijdicks et al. 2010). Allograft tissue can be used for this purpose as well (Borden et al. 2002; Fanelli and Tomaszewski 2007; Wijdicks et al. 2010). While good outcomes have been generally reported after using these MCL reconstruction techniques, up to 20° loss of knee flexion or extension has been reported in 20 % of some of these patients (Lind et al. 2009). Also, leaving the semitendinosus attachment intact at the pes anserinus and using it as an MCL graft (Azar 2006; Bosworth 1952; Kim et al. 2008; Lind et al. 2009) could result in a "too-anterior" tibial attachment of the graft since the tibial insertion of the native MCL is posterior to the pes anserinus (Feeley et al. 2009; La Prade et al. 2007). This may result in suboptimal restraint of medial laxity in full extension unless a posteromedial limb is added in order to recreate the POL function of the medial complex. Harvesting a dynamic medial stabilizer (i.e., semitendinosus) that normally applies adduction moments during gait in an already MCL-deficient knee is another theoretical concern. And lastly, few technical considerations that relate to these techniques might pose some concerns as well. Double-bundle MCL reconstructions are more complex to perform compared to single-bundle reconstructions, corresponding to their need for more graft tissue, multiple attachment sites or an increased number of tunnels on the femur and on the tibia, and number of fixation devices (i.e., screws, washers, staples, etc.) (Borden et al. 2002; Fanelli and Tomaszewski 2007; Feeley et al. 2009; Kim et al. 2008; Wijdicks et al. 2010). With the addition of tunnels on the femur or on the tibia, there is also added risk of tunnel convergence, particularly when concomitant ACL or PCL reconstruction is performed in a combined or multiple ligament-injured knee scenario. Moreover, medial to lateral side-to-side tunnels on the tibia, and particularly when two tunnels are needed, increase the risk of iatrogenic injury to the common peroneal nerve on the lateral side. Recently, a technique that uses an Achilles tendon allograft to reconstruct the MCL has been reported (Marx and Hetsroni 2012). Advantages related to this technique include avoiding donor site morbidity, sparing the semitendinosus tendon which is a potential contributor for dynamic medial stability, secure fixation with bone-to-bone healing on the femur, avoiding the need for side-to-side tunnels on the femur or on the tibia which practically eliminates the risk of tunnel convergence in a combined or multiple ligament knee reconstruction, and limited skin incisions that do not cross the knee joint.

Surgical technique (Marx and Hetsroni 2012): In case the procedure is performed alongside an ACL reconstruction, reconstructing the MCL is performed after the ACL graft is fixed on the femur, as follows: (1) The Achilles allograft is prepared on a side table with a 9 mm diameter by 18 mm length bone plug. (2) A 3 cm longitudinal skin incision is made over the medial epicondyle area. (3) A guide pin is inserted 3–5 mm proximal and posterior to the apex of the medial epicondyle, parallel to the joint line on the AP view, and in a 15° anterior direction to avoid the intercondylar notch. The location of the guide pin can be confirmed with fluoroscopy. (4) The skin is undermined from the femoral insertion area of the guide pin to the MCL insertion area on the tibia, creating a subcutaneous tunnel for future graft passage. (5) A suture loop is placed around the guide pin and brought distally under the skin through the subcutaneous tunnel just created. (6) The distal suture ends are held against the tibia at the estimated anatomic MCL graft distal attachment, just posterior to the pes anserinus insertion. Isometricity of the suture loop is tested through knee motion from 0 to 90°. The tibial insertion point against which the suture ends are held is modified, if needed, until the suture loop is isometric. (7) The isometric point is marked on the tibia with a Bovey. (8) Soft tissue around the femoral guide pin is debrided to expose the area of future femoral socket aperture and allow for an easy insertion of the Achilles-bone plug into the socket. (9) A 9 mm diameter by 20 mm depth femoral socket is created around the guide pin. (10) The Achilles-bone plug is docked in the femoral socket and fixed with a 7 mm diameter by 20 mm length interference screw. (11) The Achilles tendon tissue is then passed through the subcutaneous tunnel in a distal direction towards the marked distal tibial insertion area for the graft (Fig. 4). (12) After the ACL graft, when performed, is fixed on the tibia, the MCL

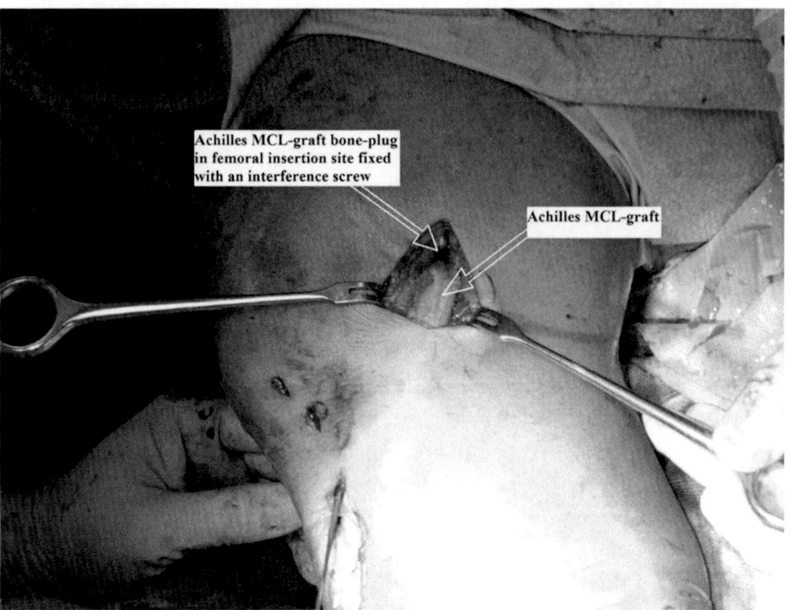

Fig. 4 The Achilles MCL graft bone plug is fixed on the femur of a right knee with an interference screw. The tendon is then passed under the skin to its isometric tibial insertion area

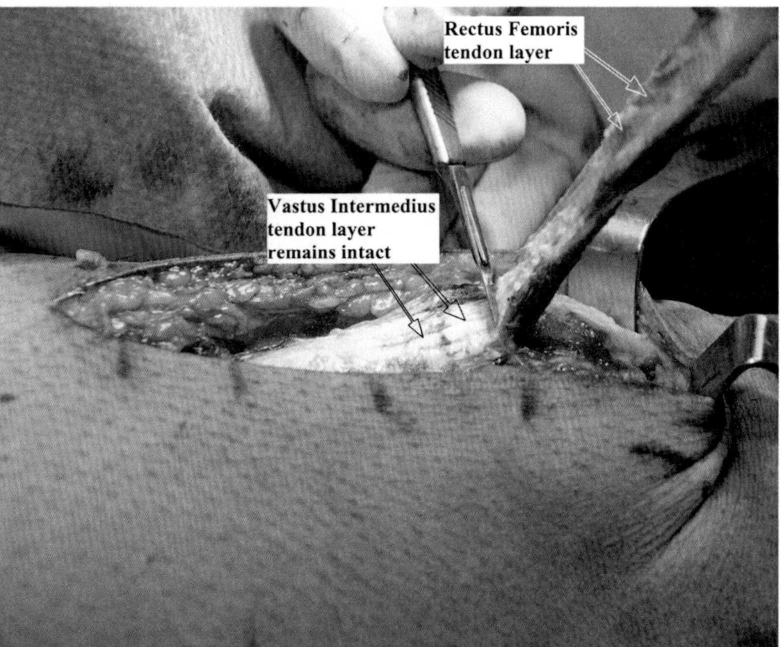

Fig. 5 The rectus femoris layer of the quadriceps tendon is harvested, and the vastus intermedius tendon layer is left intact

graft is tensioned with the knee at 20° flexion and under gentle varus stress and fixed over the isometric point on the tibia with a 4.5 mm diameter cortical screw and 17 mm spiked washer. (13) The subcutaneous tissue and skin are closed. Postoperative rehabilitation guidelines include keeping crutch-protected gait for 4 weeks with weight-bearing as tolerated and using a knee brace for 6 weeks to protect the graft against excessive valgus loads. Recently, minimum 2-year outcomes were reported after using this technique either with primary ACL reconstruction or

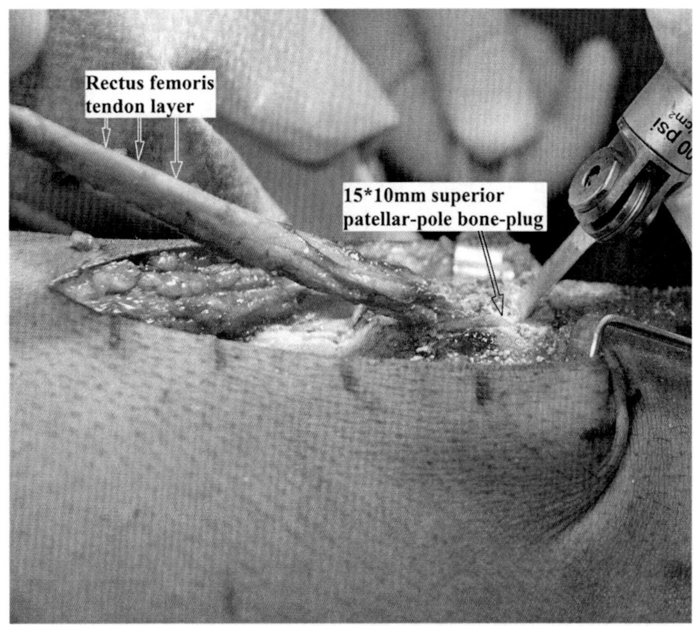

Fig. 6 More than 10 cm long of the tendon is harvested with a 15 mm long by 10 mm wide superior patellar-pole bone plug

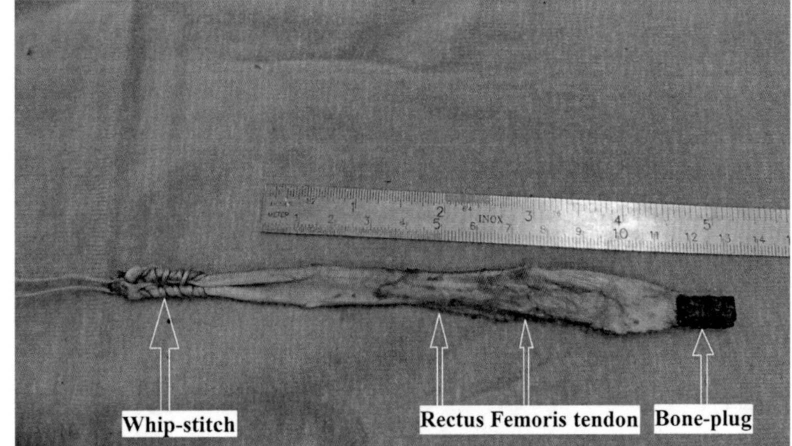

Fig. 7 The graft is prepared in a similar manner to the Achilles-bone allograft, creating a 9 mm diameter bone plug, whipstitched at the tendon end

revision ACL reconstruction in a group of patients with a mean age of 34 years (range, 19–60 years) (Marx and Hetsroni 2012). Latest follow-up examinations revealed that all patients had no or minimal side-to-side medial laxity (Grade 0–1+) with a firm end point. In those patients that had MCL reconstruction with a primary ACL reconstruction, latest follow-up scores were as follows: Mean IKDC-subjective score was 91, mean KOOS-sports subset was 92, and mean Lysholm score was 93. These patients also reported that they have returned to their pre-injury activity levels. In patients that had MCL reconstruction with a revision ACL reconstruction, despite restoring Grade 0–1+ medial knee laxity with this MCL reconstruction technique, functional scores were inferior, and patients did not return to their pre-injury activity levels. Another report recently described the outcome of MCL reconstruction using the Achilles allograft technique in the setting of multiligament-injured knees in a group of patients who had mean age of 37 years (range, 19–53 years) and minimum 2 years follow-up (Liu et al. 2013). At latest follow-up, valgus stress radiographs at 20° flexion showed that medial side-to-side laxity difference was effectively restored to normal, mean IKDC-subjective score improved from 49 before the operation to 84, and mean Lysholm score improved from 69 before the operation to 88. When nonirradiated, high-quality, Achilles tendon-bone allograft is not available, we have found quadriceps tendon-bone autograft can offer a good alternative. In this case, only the rectus femoris layer of the quadriceps tendon is harvested, leaving the vastus intermedius tendon layer and the knee joint capsule intact (Fig. 5). More than 10 cm long of the tendon is harvested with a 15 mm long by 10 mm wide superior patellar-pole bone plug (Fig. 6). The graft is then prepared in a similar manner to the Achilles-bone allograft described before, creating a 9 mm diameter bone plug, and whipstitched at the tendon end (Fig. 7). The resemblance between the Achilles-bone allograft and the rectus femoris-bone autograft enables to follow similar surgical steps to reconstruct the MCL (Figs. 8 and 9).

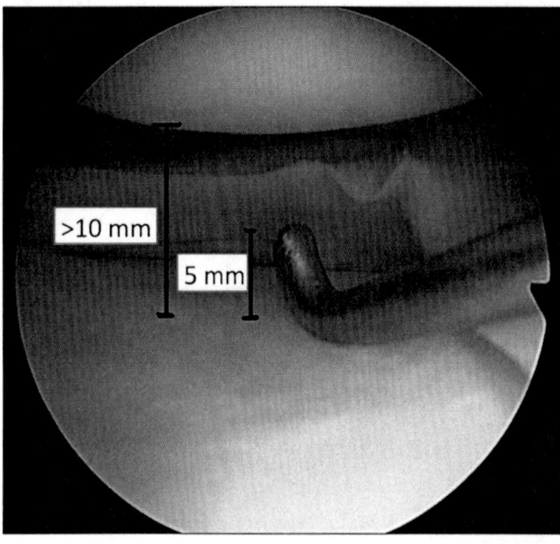

Fig. 8 Intraoperative left knee arthroscopic view of a 19-year-old female that presented chronic tibial-sided Grade 3+ MCL instability

Summary

The MCL complex is the primary structure that provides stability to the medial side of the knee during valgus loads. While the majority of MCL lesions heal without surgery, some injuries remain symptomatic and may require surgical intervention. These cases most commonly involve tibial-sided MCL ruptures which do not heal satisfactorily, combined or multiple ligament-injured knees, or cases that require revision ACL reconstruction and demonstrate concomitant chronic collateral instability. In order to consider the need for surgery and plan the most suitable intervention, a thorough evaluation should include a complete physical examination of the knee in the awake patient as well as under anesthesia, stress radiographs in selected cases, and arthroscopic

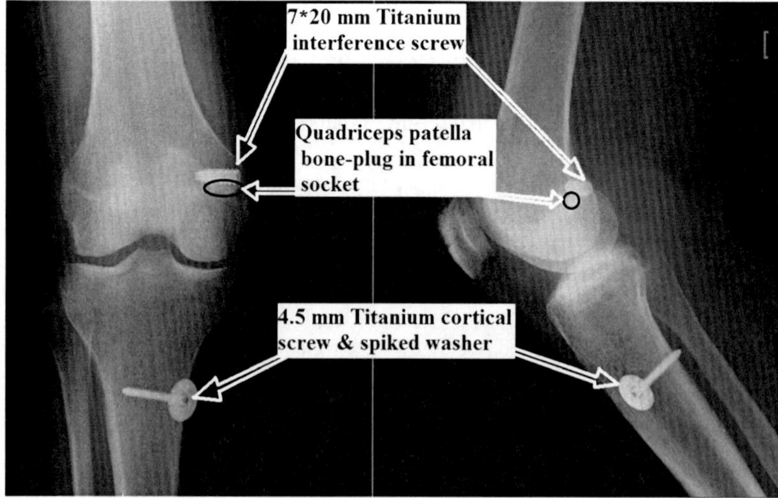

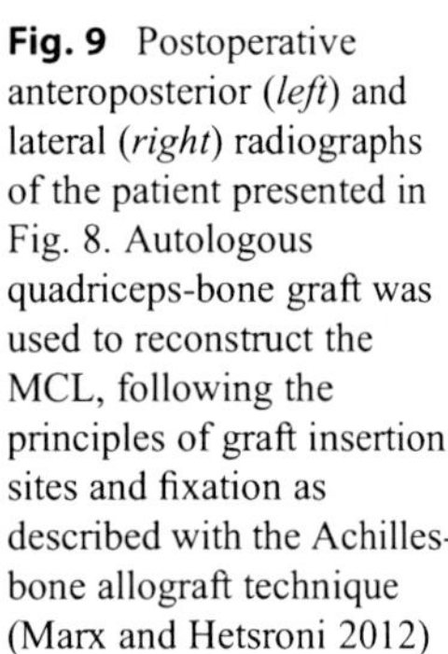

Fig. 9 Postoperative anteroposterior (*left*) and lateral (*right*) radiographs of the patient presented in Fig. 8. Autologous quadriceps-bone graft was used to reconstruct the MCL, following the principles of graft insertion sites and fixation as described with the Achilles-bone allograft technique (Marx and Hetsroni 2012)

assessment of the amount of medial compartment gapping. Good outcomes and restoration of normal medial laxity have been generally reported after MCL repair or reconstruction performed by multiple techniques, but return to pre-injury activity levels in athletes may not be predictable in cases that involve MCL reconstruction in the setting of concomitant revision ACL reconstruction or multiple ligament knee reconstruction.

References

Azar FM (2006) Evaluation and treatment of chronic medial collateral ligament injuries of the knee. Sports Med Arthrosc Rev 14:84–90

Borden PS, Kantaras AT, Caborn DNM (2002) Medial collateral ligament reconstruction with allograft using a double-bundle technique. Arthroscopy 18:E19

Bosworth DM (1952) Transplantation of the semitendinosus for repair of laceration of medial collateral ligament of the knee. J Bone Joint Surg Am 34:196–202

Canata GL, Chiey A, Leoni T (2012) Surgical technique: does mini-invasive medial collateral ligament and posterior oblique ligament repair restore knee stability in combined chronic medial and ACL injuries? Clin Orthop Relat Res 470:791–797

Corten K, Hoser C, Fink C et al (2010) Case reports: a Stener-like lesion of the medial collateral ligament of the knee. Clin Orthop Relat Res 468:289–293

Fanelli GC, Harris JD (2007) Late medial collateral ligament reconstruction. Tech Knee Surg 6:99–105

Fanelli GC, Tomaszewski DJ (2007) Allograft use in the treatment of the multiple ligament injured knee. Sports Med Arthrosc Rev 15:139–148

Feeley BT, Muller MS, Allen AA et al (2009a) Biomechanical comparison of medial collateral ligament reconstructions using computer-assisted navigation. Am J Sports Med 37:1123–1130

Feeley BT, Muller MS, Allen AA et al (2009b) Isometry of medial collateral ligament reconstruction. Knee Surg Sports Traumatol Arthrosc 17:1078–1082

Grood ES, Noyes FR, Butler DL et al (1981) Ligamentous and capsular restraints preventing straight medial and lateral laxity in intact human cadaver knees. J Bone Joint Surg Am 63:1257–1269

Hetsroni I, Lyman S, Pearle AD et al (2014) The effect of lateral opening wedge distal femoral osteotomy on medial knee opening. Knee Surg Sports Traumatol Arthrosc 22:1659–1665

Hughston JC, Eilers AF (1973) The role of the posterior oblique ligament in repairs of acute medial (collateral) ligament tears of the knee. J Bone Joint Surg Am 55:923–940

Indelicato PA (1983) Non-operative treatment of complete tears of the medial collateral ligament of the knee. J Bone Joint Surg Am 65:323–329

Kim SJ, Lee DH, Kim TE et al (2008) Concomitant reconstruction of the medial collateral and posterior oblique ligaments for medial instability of the knee. J Bone Joint Surg Br 90:1323–1327

La Prade RF, Engebretsen AH, Ly TV et al (2007) The anatomy of the medial part of the knee. J Bone Joint Surg Am 89:2000–2010

LaPrade RF, Bernhardson AS, Griffith CJ et al (2010) Correlation of valgus stress radiographs with medial knee ligament injuries: an in vitro biomechanical study. Am J Sports Med 38:330–338

Lind M, Jakobsen BW, Lund B et al (2009) Anatomical reconstruction of the medial collateral ligament and posteromedial corner of the knee in patients with chronic medial collateral ligament instability. Am J Sports Med 37:1116–1122

Liu X, Feng H, Zhang H et al (2013) Surgical treatment of subacute and chronic valgus instability in multiligament-injured knees with superficial medial collateral ligament reconstruction using Achilles allografts: a quantitative analysis with a minimum 2-year follow-up. Am J Sports Med 41:1044–1050

Marx RG, Hetsroni I (2012) Surgical technique: medial collateral ligament reconstruction using Achilles allograft for combined knee ligament injury. Clin Orthop Relat Res 470:798–805

Phisitkul P, Wolf BR, Amendola A (2006) Role of high tibial and distal femoral osteotomies in the treatment of lateral-posterolateral and medial instabilities of the knee. Sports Med Arthrosc Rev 14:96–104

Robins AJ, Newman AP, Burks RT (1993) Postoperative return of motion in anterior cruciate ligament and medial collateral ligament injuries: the effect of medial collateral ligament rupture locations. Am J Sports Med 21:20–25

Wijdicks CA, Griffith CJ, Johansen S et al (2010) Injuries to the medial collateral ligament and associated medial structures of the knee. J Bone Joint Surg Am 92:1266–1280

Anatomic Anterior Cruciate Ligament Reconstruction: Surgical Techniques

94

Anne L. Versteeg, Bas A. C. M. Pijnenburg, and Charles H. Brown Jr.

Contents

A.L. Versteeg (✉)
Department of Orthopaedics Surgery, University Medical Center Utrecht, Utrecht, The Netherlands
e-mail: annelversteeg@gmail.com

B.A.C.M. Pijnenburg
Department of Orthopaedic Surgery, Ziekenhuis Amstelland, Amstelveen, AM, The Netherlands
e-mail: bpijnenburg@gmail.com; bpijnenburg@gmail.com

C.H. Brown Jr.
International Knee and Joint Centre, Abu Dhabi, United Arab Emirates
e-mail: charliebrowngoestosa@yahoo.com

M.N. Doral, J. Karlsson (eds.), *Sports Injuries*,
DOI 10.1007/978-3-642-36569-0_260

Abstract

Rupture of the anterior cruciate ligament (ACL) is a common sports injury. In order to return to their pre-injury level, many patients elect to undergo an ACL reconstruction. Over the past decade, the concept of ACL reconstruction has evolved from a surgical technique that emphasized placement of the ACL femoral tunnel at a location that minimized the change in length of the ACL graft with flexion/extension of the knee (isometry) and placement of the tibial tunnel at a location that minimized the potential for roof impingement to a surgical technique in which the bone tunnels are placed within the native ACL attachment sites (anatomic ACL reconstruction). This chapter will review the anatomy and biomechanics of the ACL, define what an anatomic ACL reconstruction is and where to place the bone tunnels, and compare the location and ACL graft orientation achieved by the transtibial, anteromedial portal, and outside–in surgical techniques.

Introduction

Rupture of the anterior cruciate ligament (ACL) is common in sports involving cutting, pivoting, deceleration or sudden stops, and landing from a jump (Olsen et al. 2004; Hewett et al. 2005; Krosshaug et al. 2007; Silvers and Mandelbaum 2007; Zantop and Petersen 2008; Koga et al. 2010). The incidence of ACL rupture has been reported to be 1 in 3,000 people in the general population in the United States (Miyasaka et al. 1991). In order to return to their pre-injury status, many patients elect to undergo ACL reconstruction. The incidence of ACL reconstruction has been reported to be 29.6–52 per 100,000 in the general population (Csintalan et al. 2008; Janssen et al. 2012). ACL reconstruction is the fourth most commonly performed procedure by the American Board of Orthopaedic Surgery applicants in their first 2 years of practice (Harner et al. 2003). In the United States alone, it is estimated that approximately 300,000 ACL reconstructions are performed annually (Chang et al. 2013). Most isolated ACL ruptures occur as a result of a noncontact, deceleration, valgus-external rotation injury (Olsen et al. 2004; Hewett et al. 2005; Krosshaug et al 2007; Silvers and Mandelbaum 2007; Zantop and Petersen 2008; Koga et al. 2010). Other mechanisms for noncontact ACL injuries include hyperextension and hyperflexion of the knee (Olsen et al. 2004; Krosshaug et al 2007; Silvers and Mandelbaum 2007; Zantop and Petersen 2008; Koga et al. 2010). A complete rupture of the ACL may result in chronic instability of the knee, which can lead to meniscal tears, secondary damage to the articular cartilage, and an early onset of osteoarthritis (Jonsson et al. 2004; Andriacchi et al. 2006; Stergiou et al. 2007; Andriacchi et al. 2009; Yasada et al. 2011). Restoring stability to the knee is therefore an important goal when treating patients with a torn ACL. This chapter will review the anatomy and biomechanics of the ACL, define what an anatomic ACL reconstruction is and where to place the bone tunnels, and compare the location and ACL graft orientation achieved by the transtibial, anteromedial portal, and outside–in surgical techniques.

Anatomy and Biomechanics of the ACL

Differing terms are often used to describe locations and directions in the knee. The use of differing terms is often a source of confusion when reading anatomical studies and surgical technique papers related to the ACL. Anatomical terms, such as proximal, distal, anterior, and posterior, are used to describe positions and directions in the extended knee. Arthroscopic terminology, high (superior), low (inferior), shallow, and deep, is used to describe the knee at 90° flexion, as viewed by the arthroscopic surgeon (Amis and Jakob 1998; Edward et al. 2008; Karlsson et al. 2011). To avoid confusion, in this chapter locations and directions in the knee will be described according to the above convention (Fig. 1).

The femoral attachment of the ACL has an oval- or elliptical-shaped attachment site on the lower third of the inner wall of the lateral femoral condyle (Girgis et al. 1975; Bach 1989; Bernard et al. 1997; Harner et al. 2003; Columbet et al. 2006; Heming et al. 2007; Edward et al. 2008; Purnell et al. 2008; Tsukada et al. 2008; Feretti et al. 2012; Fig. 2). There are no ACL fibers which attach directly to the roof of the intercondylar notch (Purnell et al. 2008; Fig. 3). There is a great deal of variation in the size of the ACL femoral attachment site (Harner et al. 2003; Edward et al. 2008; Kopf et al. 2009, 2011). The length of the ACL femoral attachment site has been reported to range from 14 to 23 mm, and the width from 7.8 to 11.2 mm (Columbet et al. 2006; Heming et al. 2007; Baer et al. 2008; Edward et al. 2008; Purnell et al. 2008; Kopf et al. 2009; Sasaki et al 2012). Arthroscopic measurements using a malleable ACL ruler in 137 patients undergoing primary ACL reconstruction found the length of the ACL femoral attachment site to vary from 12 to 20 mm, with a mean length of 16.5 mm (Kopf et al. 2012). In two-thirds of the patients, the ACL femoral attachment site length was between 16 and 18 mm; 25 % had an attachment site length less than 16 mm, and 11 % had an attachment site length greater than 18 mm (Kopf et al. 2012). The ACL femoral attachment site is defined by two bony ridges located on the lower third of the inner side of the lateral femoral condyle, the lateral intercondylar and the lateral bifurcate ridges (Fu and Jordan 2007; Baer et al. 2008; Purnell et al. 2008; Shino et al. 2010; van Eck et al. 2010; Ziegler et al. 2011; Feretti et al. 2012; Sasaki et al. 2012; Fig. 4). The lateral intercondylar

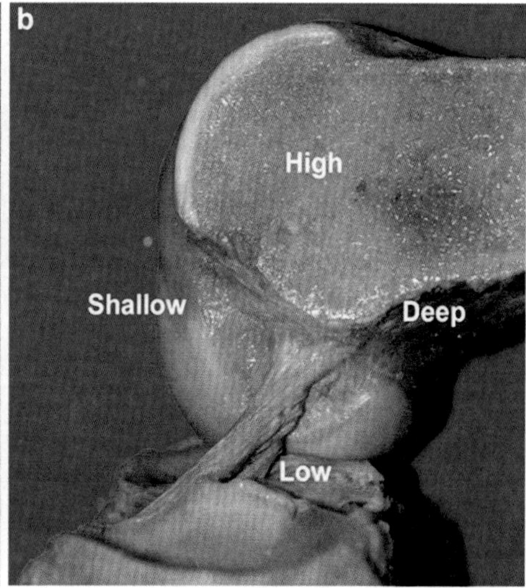

Fig. 1 This figure illustrates the anatomic terminology versus the arthroscopic terminology as demonstrated in a right knee cadaveric specimen. (**a**), the knee is in full extension and the anatomic nomenclature is shown. (**b**), the knee is in 90° of flexion and the arthroscopic terminology is shown

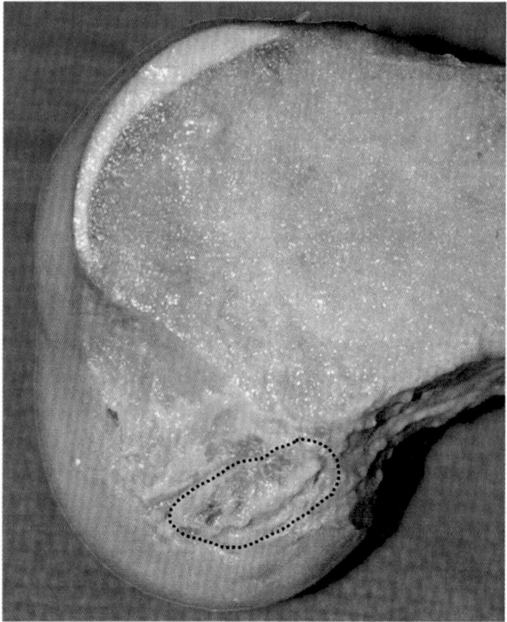

Fig. 2 Right knee. The fibers of the ACL attach to lower third of the medial wall of the lateral femoral condyle in the shape of an ellipse

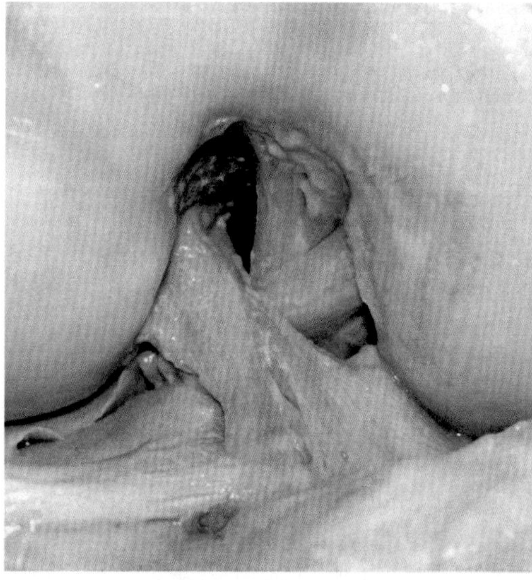

Fig. 3 Right knee. The femoral attachment of the ACL is entirely along the lateral wall of the intercondylar notch. There are no ACL fibers which directly insert onto the roof of the intercondylar notch

ridge, also called "the resident's ridge," was first described by Dr. William Clancy Jr. (Hutchinson and Ash 2003; Purnell et al. 2008). With the knee at 90° of flexion (arthroscopic position), the lateral intercondylar ridge runs from a deep to shallow position in the notch at a 35° angle with respect to the long axis of the femoral shaft (Purnell et al. 2008; Fig. 5). The lateral intercondylar ridge is an important bony landmark for the placement of the ACL femoral tunnel since it has been

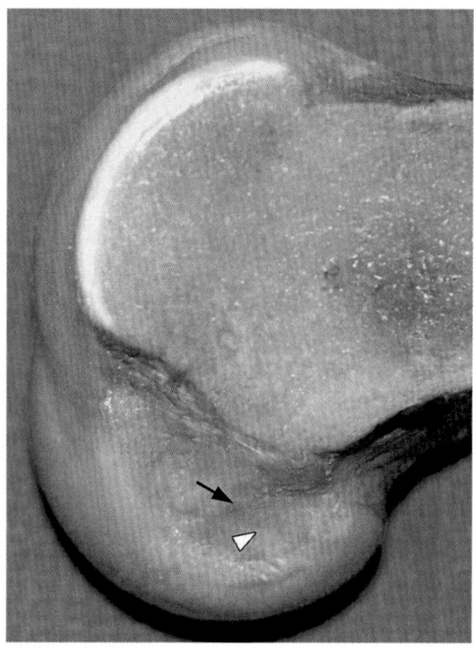

Fig. 4 Right knee. The ACL femoral attachment site is located on the lower third of the inner side of the lateral femoral condyle. The ACL femoral attachment site is defined by the lateral intercondylar ridge (*black arrow*) and the lateral bifurcate ridge (*white arrow head*)

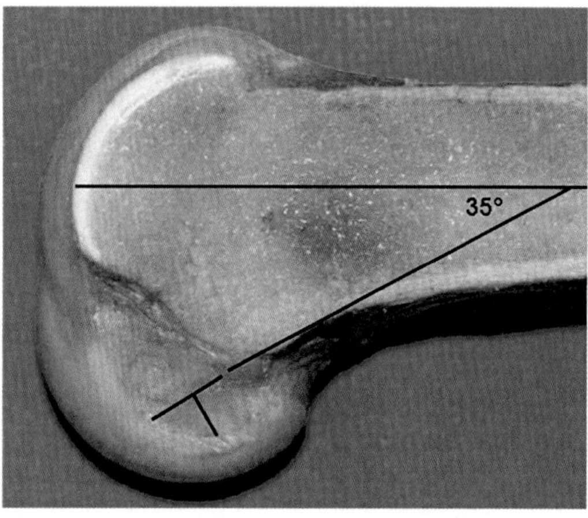

Fig. 5 The lateral intercondylar ridge runs from a deep to shallow position along the inner side of the lateral femoral condyle at a 35° angle with respect to the long axis of the femoral shaft

shown that the native ACL always attaches inferior (posterior) to this ridge (Baer et al. 2008; Purnell et al. 2008; Shino et al. 2010; Feretti et al. 2012; Sasaki et al. 2012). The lateral intercondylar ridge can be identified arthroscopically in 88 % of subacute and chronic ACL-deficient knees and is therefore a consistent anatomic landmark to assist the knee surgeon with anatomic placement of the ACL femoral tunnel (van Eck et al. 2010). The lateral bifurcate ridge runs perpendicular to the lateral intercondylar ridge and divides the ACL femoral attachment site into the attachment site areas for the anteromedial (AM) and posterolateral (PL) bundles (Feretti et al. 2012). The lateral bifurcate ridge was indentified arthroscopically in only 48 % of subacute and chronic knees (van Eck et al. 2010).

The ACL inserts onto the tibia in a depression or fovea in the anterior intercondylar area between the medial and lateral tibial plateaus (condyles) (Purnell et al. 2008; Ziegler et al. 2011). Confusion exists in the terminology used to describe bony landmarks in the anterior intercondylar area. Using anatomic terminology the bony landmarks are the intercondylar eminence (tibial spine), which lies between the medial and lateral tibial condyles; the medial and lateral intercondylar tubercles, which lie at the ends of the intercondylar eminence and are often incorrectly called the medial and lateral tibial spines; and the medial intercondylar ridge of the tibia, which is an anterior extension of the medial intercondylar tubercle (Purnell et al. 2008; Ziegler et al. 2011; Fig. 6). The posterior fibers of the ACL insert onto the tibia just anterior to a curved ridge (the ACL ridge) that runs between the medial and lateral intercondylar tubercles (Purnell et al. 2008). There are no ACL fibers which insert directly on the intercondylar eminence. Medially, the ACL inserts just lateral to and not onto the tip of the medial intercondylar tubercle (Edward et al. 2008; Purnell et al. 2008; Feretti et al. 2012). The medial border of the ACL tibial attachment site is defined by a distinct bony ridge, the medial intercondylar ridge of the tibia (Purnell et al. 2008). The medial intercondylar ridge of the tibia extends anteriorly from the medial intercondylar tubercle. Medially, the ACL fibers insert directly onto this ridge. There are no ACL fibers that insert medial to this ridge. There is no distinct lateral border of the ACL; the fibers blend

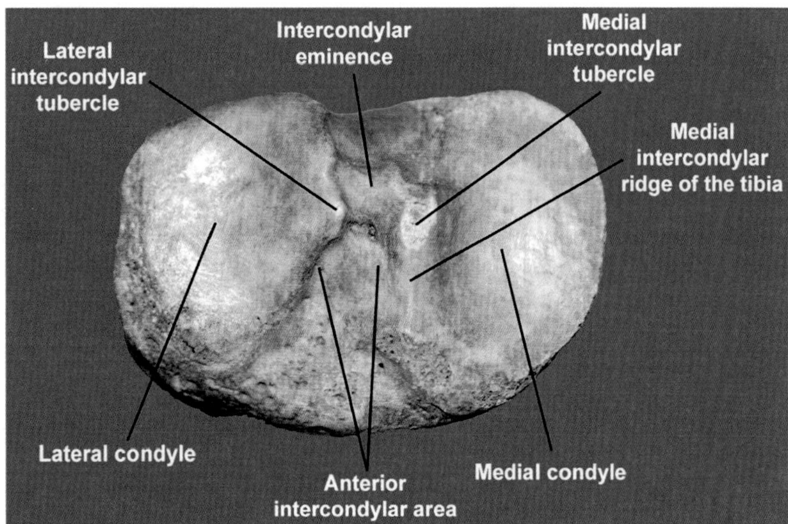

Fig. 6 Right knee. Bony topography of the proximal tibia

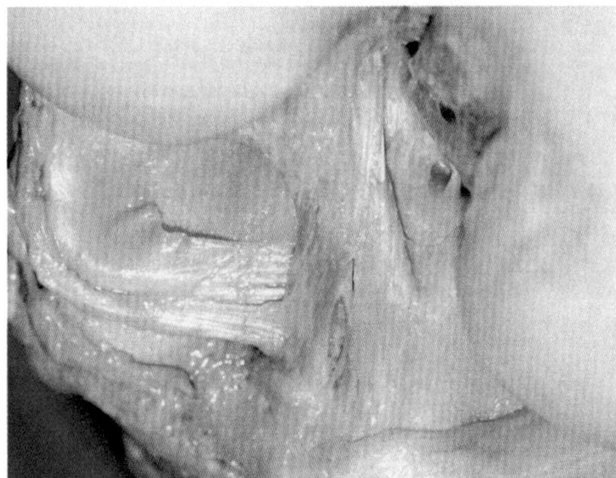

Fig. 7 Right knee. The majority of the ACL fibers insert onto the tibia anterior to posterior edge of the anterior horn of the lateral meniscus

into the anterior horn of the lateral meniscus. The majority of the ACL fibers insert onto the tibia anterior to the posterior edge of the anterior horn of the lateral meniscus (Fig. 7). The anterior border of the ACL tibial attachment site is marked by the intermeniscal or transverse ligament (Kongcharoensombat et al. 2011).

The ACL tibial attachment site has been reported to be wider and longer than the ACL femoral attachment site and the shape to vary from oval to triangular (Harner et al. 1999; Edwards et al. 2007; Kongcharoensombat et al. 2011). Similar to the ACL femoral attachment site, there is great variation in the length and width of the ACL tibial attachment site (Edwards et al. 2007; Heming et al. 2007; Purnell et al 2008; Kopf et al. 2009, 2011; Hwang et al 2012). In human cadaveric knees, the length of the ACL tibial attachment site has been reported to range from 14 to 29 mm, and the width from 9 to 12.7 mm (Edwards et al. 2007; Heming et al. 2007; Purnell et al 2008; Kopf et al. 2009, 2011; Hwang et al. 2012). Arthroscopic measurements with a malleable ACL ruler in 137 patients undergoing ACL reconstruction found the length of the ACL tibial attachment site to range from 12 to 22 mm with a mean value of 17 mm (Kopf et al. 2011). In two-thirds of the patients, the length of the ACL tibial attachment site was between 16 and 18 mm; in approximately half of the remaining patients, the tibial attachment site length was less than 16 mm, and in the other remaining half greater than 18 mm.

It is generally accepted that the ACL consists of two functional bundles, the anteromedial (AM) and the posterolateral (PL) bundles (Girgis et al. 1975; Harner et al. 1999; Columbet et al. 2006; Edwards et al. 2007; Petersen and Zantop 2007; Baer et al. 2008; Edwards et al. 2008; Tsukada et al. 2008; Yasada et al. 2011; Ziegler et al. 2011). The two bundles are named according to their insertion onto the tibia (Fig. 8). Although there is debate as to

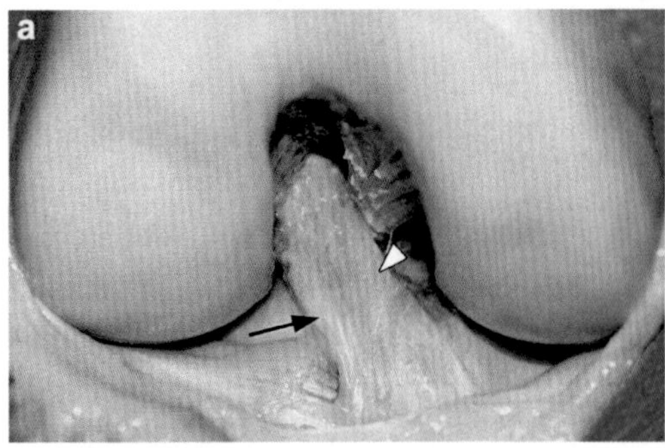

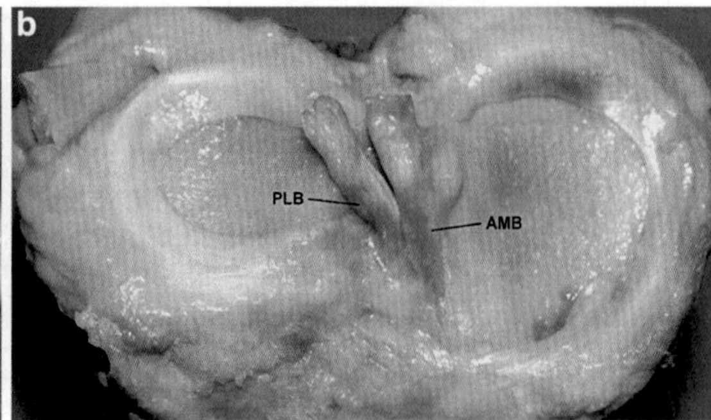

Fig. 8 Right knee. (**a**), the anteromedial (*AM*) bundle fibers are shown by the *white arrow head* and the postero-lateral (*PL*) bundle fibers by the *black arrow*. (**b**), the bundles are named according to their insertion onto the tibia. The AM bundle fibers attach anterior and medial and the PL bundle fibers posterior and lateral

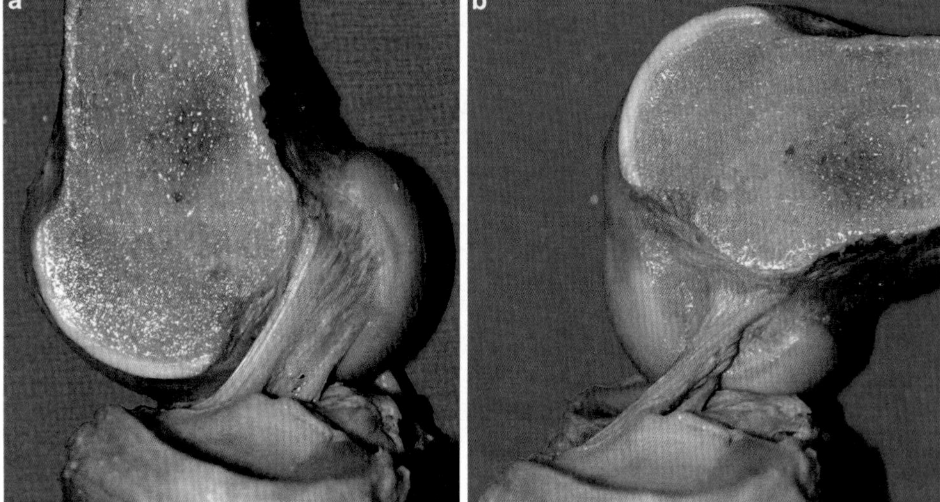

Fig. 9 Right knee. (**a**), in extension the PL bundle is tight and the AM bundle slightly relaxed. (**b**), in flexion the PL bundle is slack and the AM bundle is tight

whether there is a true anatomic division of the ACL into two bundles, it is generally agreed that two separate bundles can be distinguished by the tension that varies in the ligament fibers with flexion/extension of the knee (Girgis et al. 1975; Petersen and Zantop 2007; Baer et al. 2008; Noyes 2009; Yasada et al. 2011; Amis 2012). With the knee in extension, the ACL femoral attachment site is vertically oriented and the PL bundle is tight and the AM bundle is slightly relaxed (Amis and Dawkins 1991; Petersen and Zantop 2007; Baer et al. 2008; Yasada et al. 2011; Amis 2012) With flexion of the knee, the ACL femoral attachment site rotates and becomes more horizontal, the PL bundle fibers shorten and slacken, and the AM bundle fibers lengthen and tighten (Girgis et al. 1975; Amis and Dawkins 1991; Petersen and Zantop 2007; Baer et al. 2008; Yasada et al. 2011; Amis 2012; Fig. 9).

The ACL is the primary restraint against anterior tibial translation, providing 87 % of the total restraining force at 30° of flexion and 85 % at 90° of flexion (Butler et al. 1980). The ACL is a secondary restraint against valgus and varus rotation (Grood 1992). The ACL may act as restraint to internal tibial rotation, but there are conflicting data and opinions on this point (Zantop et al. 2007; Jones and Grimshaw 2011; Amis

2012). Some studies have shown that sectioning of the entire ACL leads to a small increase in internal tibial rotation (Zantop et al. 2007; Jones and Grimshaw 2011; Amis 2012). However, this small increase (2–4°) may be difficult to detect clinically and therefore may not be clinically relevant (Jones and Grimshaw 2011; Amis 2012). Other studies have shown that the ACL has no effect on resisting internal tibial rotation. Internal tibial rotation is resisted primarily by the lateral extra-articular structures (Nakamura et al. 2009). At the present time, the role of the ACL in resisting internal tibial rotation is unclear. One of the primary functions of the ACL is to resist the combined motions of anterior tibial translation and internal tibial rotation and the resulting anterior subluxation of the lateral and medial compartments that represent the pivot-shift phenomenon (Zantop et al. 2007; Nakamura et al. 2009; Jones and Grimshaw 2011; Amis 2012). As a result of their changing tensioning patterns during flexion/extension of the knee, the two ACL bundles play different roles in restoring the stability of the knee. The AM bundle is dominant in resisting anterior tibial translation in the flexed knee, whereas the PL bundle is more important in resisting anterior tibial translation in the extended knee (Amis 2012). It has been hypothesized that the two ACL bundles have different roles with respect to controlling rotational motion of the knee. It has been postulated that the AM bundle which is more vertically oriented in the coronal plane and more closely aligned with the axis of rotation plays a much smaller role in controlling tibial rotation compared to the PL bundle (Amis 2012). Due to the fact that the PL bundle is oriented more horizontally in the coronal plane and better aligned to mechanically resist tibial rotation, it has been postulated that the PL bundle plays a more important role in controlling tibial rotation compared to the AM bundle (Amis 2012). However, biomechanical studies have found conflicting results with respect to the role that the two ACL bundles play in controlling rotation. Most studies have shown only small increases in tibial rotation after sectioning the PL bundle alone (Zantop et al. 2007; Jones and Grimshaw 2011; Amis 2012).

Evolution of Intra-articular ACL Reconstruction

Over the last decade, the concept of ACL reconstruction has evolved from a surgical technique in which the objectives were placement of the ACL femoral tunnel at a location that minimized the change in length of the ACL graft with flexion/extension of the knee (isometry) and placement of the tibial tunnel at a location that minimized the potential for roof and PCL Posterior Cruciate Ligament impingement toward an "anatomic" surgical technique which attempts to reproduce the anatomy of the native ACL (Karlsson et al. 2011; van Eck et al. 2011; Schindler 2012; Brown et al. 2013; Chambat et al. 2013; Fig. 10). This change was prompted by the recognition that positioning the ACL femoral tunnel at the most isometric location on the lateral femoral condyle and positioning the ACL tibial tunnel in a location that avoided roof and PCL impingement of the ACL graft would often result in the bone tunnels of the ACL reconstruction lying outside of the native ACL attachment sites (Yaru et al. 1992; Arnold et al. 2001; Kopf et al. 2010; Marchant et al. 2010; Kopf et al. 2012; Chambat et al. 2013; Iriuchishima et al. 2013).

It was understood early on that in order to meet the simultaneous requirements of maintaining knee joint stability and allowing a full range of motion, an intra-articular ACL replacement graft could not be placed at liberty within the knee joint (Graf 1987; Sapega et al. 1990; Grood 1992; Bylski-Austrow et al. 1993). Placement of the ACL graft in a position where it would undergo excessive lengthening (tightening) would lead to graft failure or loss of motion, and placement of the graft in a location where it would undergo excessive slackening or loosening would cause pathologic laxity of the knee (Sapega et al. 1990; Grood 1992). The concept of "isometry" was developed as a solution to minimize excessive tightening and slackening of the ACL graft (Graf 1987; Schindler 2012). The goal of "isometric" ACL graft placement was to place the ACL graft in a location that would allow full range of motion of the knee while minimizing elongation of the

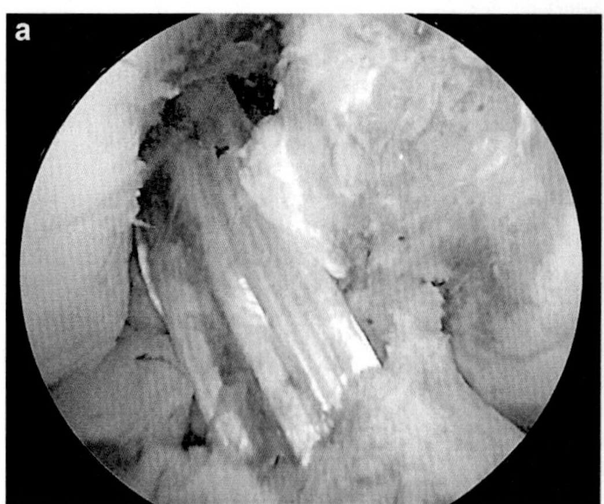
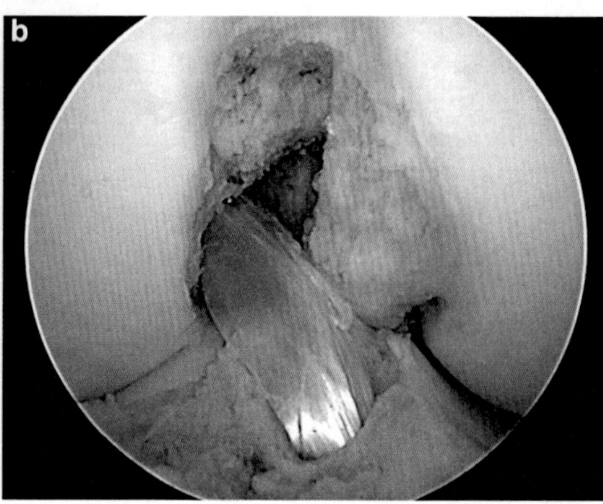
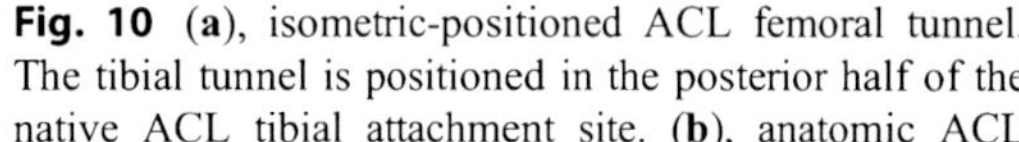

Fig. 10 (**a**), isometric-positioned ACL femoral tunnel. The tibial tunnel is positioned in the posterior half of the native ACL tibial attachment site. (**b**), anatomic ACL reconstruction. The tibial and femoral tunnels are positioned at the center of the native ACL attachment sites

graft (Graf 1987; Sapega et al. 1990; Schindler 2012). Experimental studies demonstrated that the most "isometric" location required the ACL femoral tunnel to be placed higher and deeper in the notch than the native ACL femoral attachment site (Graf 1987; Siddles et al. 1988; Hefzy et al. 1989; Sapega et al. 1990; Schindler 2012). In order to reach this "isometric" femoral tunnel position with a transtibial technique and to simultaneously avoid roof impingement of the ACL graft, it was necessary to position the ACL tibial tunnel in the posterior part of the native ACL tibial attachment site (Yaru et al. 1992; Noyes 2009; Kopf et al. 2010; Marchant et al. 2010; Kopf et al. 2012; Iriuchishima et al. 2013). The combination of a high-deep ACL femoral tunnel and a posterior ACL tibial tunnel produced a nonanatomic ACL graft which was vertically oriented in the sagittal and coronal planes (Heming et al. 2007; Hantes et al. 2009; Noyes 2009; Kopf et al. 2010; Marchant et al. 2010; Bowers et al. 2011; Kopf et al. 2012; Iriuchishima et al. 2013). Biomechanical and clinical studies have demonstrated that a vertical ACL graft may control anterior tibial translation but often fails to control the combined motions of anterior tibial translation and internal tibial rotation which occur during the pivot-shift phenomenon (Yagi et al. 2002; Loh et al. 2003; SCopp et al. 2004; Yamamoto et al. 2004; Musahl et al. 2005; Heming et al. 2007; Lee et al. 2007; Moisala et al. 2007; Noyes 2009; Ristanis et al. 2009; Steiner et al. 2009; Herbort et al. 2010; Kato et al. 2010; Marchant et al. 2010; Bedi et al. 2011; Kondo et al. 2011; Sadoghi et al. 2011; Driscoll et al. 2012; Park et al. 2012; Inderhaug et al. 2013; Kato et al. 2013). The inability of a vertical ACL graft to control the pivot-shift phenomenon may result in the patient continuing to complain of instability symptoms and experiencing giving-way episodes despite having an intact ACL graft and normal or near-normal anterior tibial translation (Lee et al. 2007; Marchant et al. 2010; Inderhaug et al. 2013). It has been proven biomechanically and clinically that placing the bone tunnels of the ACL graft within the native ACL attachment sites better restores anterior tibial translation, rotational stability, and normal knee kinematics compared to an "isometric," nonanatomic ACL reconstruction (Yagi et al. 2002; Scopp et al. 2004; Yamamoto et al. 2004; Musahl et al. 2005; Moisala et al. 2007; Steiner et al. 2009; Alentorn-Geli et al. 2010; Herbort et al. 2010; Kato et al. 2010; Bedi et al. 2011; Kondo et al. 2011; Sadoghi et al. 2011; Driscoll et al. 2012; Hussein et al. 2012a; Kato et al. 2013; Wang et al. 2013). In an attempt to improve knee kinematics and rotational stability after ACL reconstruction, the concept of anatomic ACL reconstruction has emerged.

What Is Anatomic ACL Reconstruction?

According to van Eck et al. (2011), "Anatomic ACL reconstruction is defined as the functional restoration of the ACL to its native dimensions, collagen orientation, and insertion sites." Operationally, an "anatomic" ACL reconstruction refers to a single-bundle (SB) or double-bundle (DB) reconstruction, an ACL augmentation or remnant preservation procedure, or a revision ACL reconstruction in which the femoral and tibial bone tunnels are placed within the native ACL attachment sites. According to Karlsson et al. (2011), there are four principles of anatomic ACL reconstruction. The first principle of anatomic ACL reconstruction is to reproduce as closely as possible the size, shape, and location of the native ACL attachment sites (Karlsson et al. 2011; Siebold 2011; van Eck et al. 2011). The second principle is to restore the two functional bundles of the ACL (Karlsson et al. 2011; van Eck et al. 2011). In order to create an ACL graft that mimics the functional behavior of the two ACL bundles, it is necessary to reproduce the size, shape, and location of the native ACL attachment sites. The third principle is that the ACL graft should reproduce the tensioning pattern of the native ACL (Karlsson et al. 2011; van Eck et al. 2011). The AM bundle fibers of the native ACL are taut throughout the range of motion, while the PL bundle fibers tighten rapidly during the last 30° of extension (Amis and Dawkins 1991; Amis 2012). The reconstructed ACL graft should mimic this tensioning pattern. The final principle of anatomic ACL reconstruction is to individualize the surgical procedure for each patient. Every patient and every knee is different, so the same surgical procedure may not necessarily be performed in each case (Karlsson et al. 2011; van Eck et al. 2011; Hussein et al. 2012b). A commonly held misconception is that anatomic ACL reconstruction implies that the surgeon must perform a DB ACL reconstruction. It is important to recognize that anatomic ACL reconstruction is a concept and not a specific surgical procedure, and reproducing the two functional bundles of the ACL does not always require the surgeon to perform a DB ACL reconstruction. The concept of anatomic ACL reconstruction can be applied to a SB reconstruction, a DB reconstruction, an augmentation procedure for a partial ACL tear, an ACL remnant preservation procedure, and a revision ACL reconstruction with an intact ACL graft (Fig. 11). The specific surgical procedure should be based on the ACL injury pattern (complete ACL tear, partial ACL tear, ACL injury with intact ACL remnants), the size of the native ACL attachment sites, and the degree of rotational laxity (Hussein et al. 2012b; Hofbauer et al. 2013). Hussein et al. (2012b) have shown that when anatomic ACL reconstructions are individualized to the size, shape, and orientation of the patient's native ACL, SB and DB ACL reconstructions yield similar subjective and objective results.

One of the major objectives of anatomic ACL reconstruction is to reproduce as closely as possible the size, shape, and location of the native ACL attachment sites (Karlsson et al. 2011; Siebold 2011; van Eck et al. 2011). During surgery, a malleable ACL ruler can be used to measure the length and width of the ACL attachment sites (Kopf et al. 2011; Siebold 2011; Brown et al. 2013; Fig. 12). These measurements can be helpful to the surgeon when selecting the type of ACL replacement graft and the surgical procedure (Siebold 2011). Four-strand hamstring tendon grafts may adequately restore 12–14 mm-long ACL attachment sites, whereas attachment sites that are 16 mm or longer may be better restored with larger-diameter ACL grafts such as 5- and 6-strand hamstring tendon grafts, a bone–patellar tendon–bone graft, or a quadriceps tendon graft (Siebold 2011; van Eck et al. 2011). Restoring the maximum percentage of the ACL attachment sites requires performing a DB ACL reconstruction (Siebold 2011; van Eck et al. 2011). This concept is supported by recent clinical studies that have demonstrated a higher failure rate for hamstring

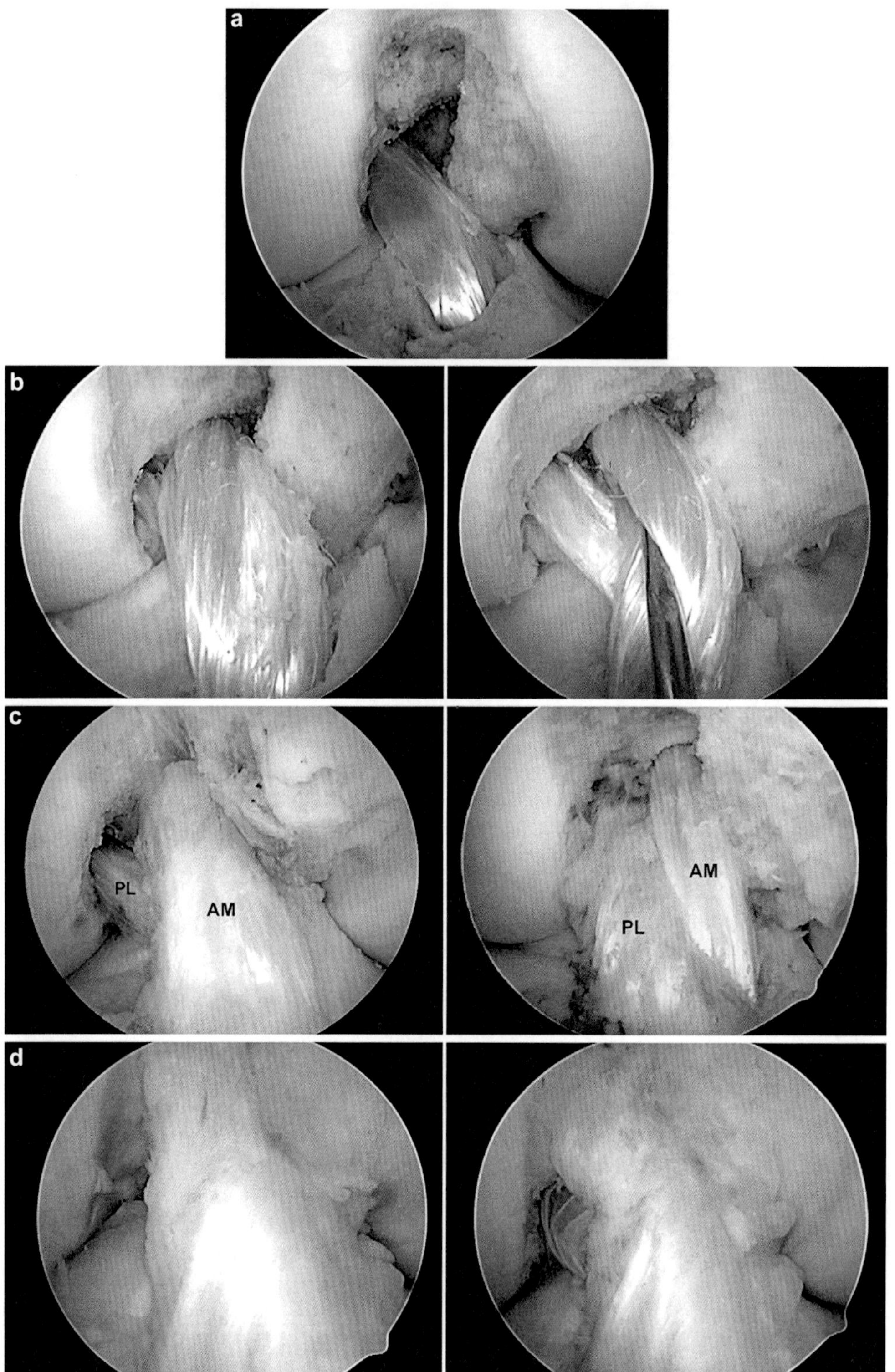

Fig. 11 (continued)

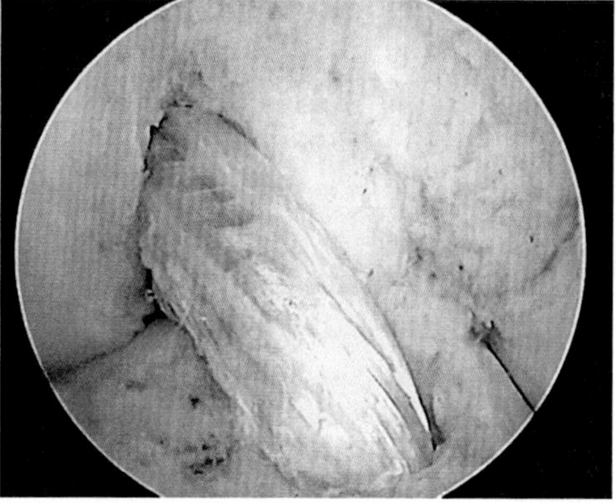

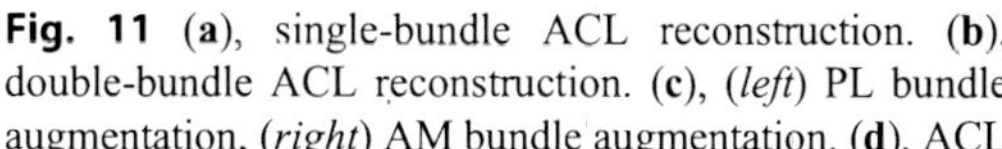

Fig. 11 (**a**), single-bundle ACL reconstruction. (**b**), double-bundle ACL reconstruction. (**c**), (*left*) PL bundle augmentation, (*right*) AM bundle augmentation. (**d**), ACL remnant preservation. (**e**), revision ACL reconstruction with intact ACL graft

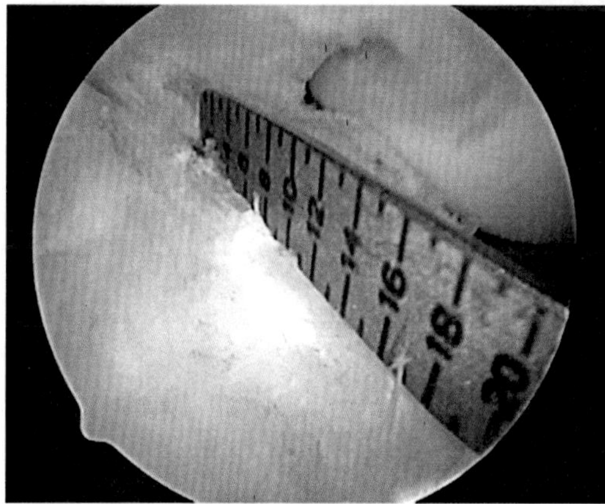

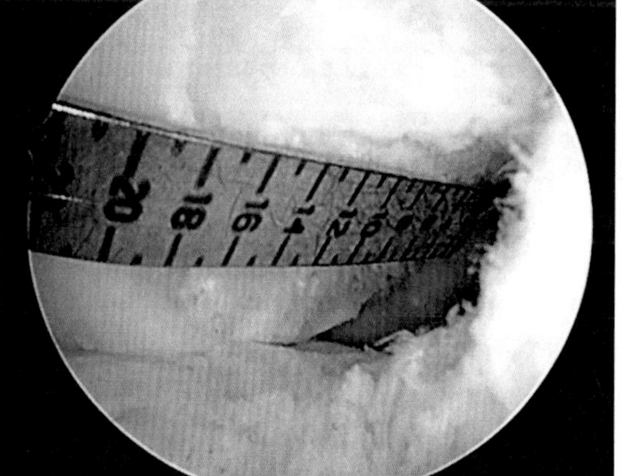

Fig. 12 Malleable ACL ruler is used to measure the length of the ACL tibial (*left*) and femoral attachment sites

tendon ACL reconstructions when the diameter of the hamstring tendon ACL graft is less than 8 mm (Magnussen et al. 2012; Park et al. 2012).

ACL Graft Placement

Proper placement of the ACL graft is critical to the success and clinical outcome of ACL reconstruction (Grood 1992; Wetzler et al. 1998; Getelman and Friedman 1999; Sommer et al. 2000; Loh et al. 2003; Jonsson et al. 2004; Musahl et al. 2005; Moisala et al. 2007; Ristanis et al. 2009; Marchant et al. 2010; Wright et al. 2010; Sadoghi et al. 2011; Trojani et al. 2011; Lind et al. 2012; Whitehead 2013). Malposition of the ACL bone tunnels is the most common technical error leading to recurrent instability and a failed ACL reconstruction (Wetzler et al. 1998; Getelman and Friedman 1999; Sommer et al. 2000; Marchant et al. 2010; Wright et al. 2010; Kamath et al. 2011; Trojani et al. 2011; Lind et al. 2012; Whitehead 2013). Proper placement of the ACL femoral tunnel is especially important because the length and tension of the ACL graft are most influenced by the position of the ACL femoral tunnel (Hefzy and Grood 1986; Hefzy et al. 1989; Grood 1992; Bylski-Austrow et al. 1993). Malposition of the ACL femoral tunnel can cause the ACL graft to undergo

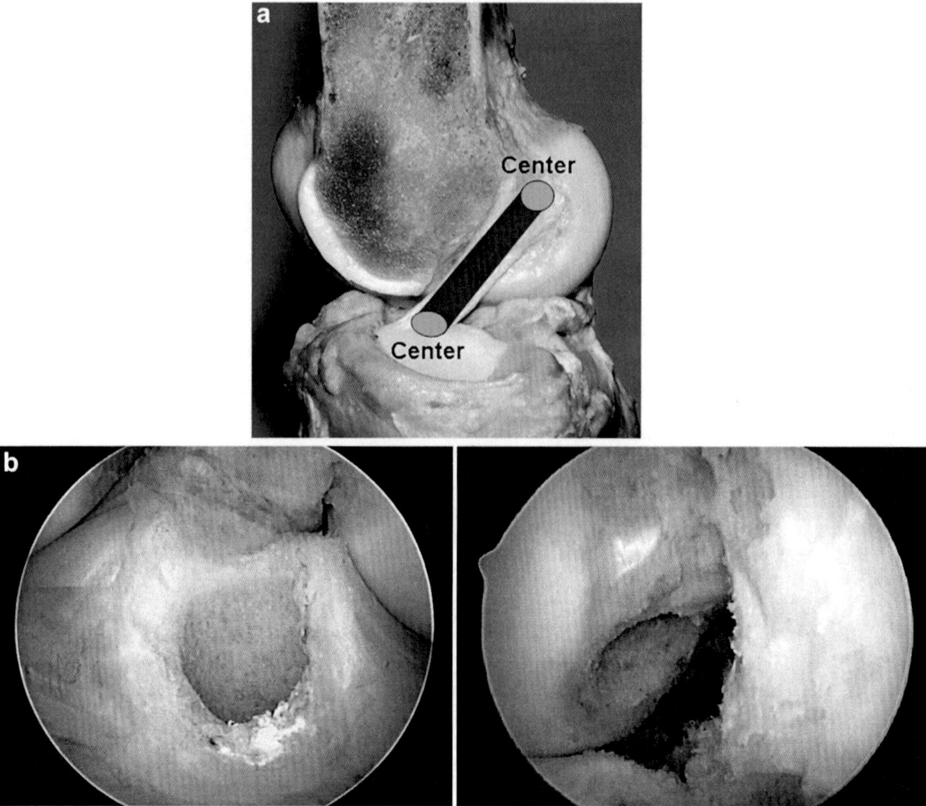

Fig. 13 (**a**), Center-to-center placement for single-bundle ACL reconstruction. (**b**), tibial (*left*) and femoral (*right*) bone tunnels for single-bundle ACL reconstruction are placed at the center of the native ACL attachment sites

excessive tightening or loosening with range of motion of the knee. Excessive loosening of the ACL graft can result in pathologic laxity of the knee, whereas excessive tightening may result in graft failure or loss of motion of the knee. Biomechanical and clinical studies have also shown that proper placement of the ACL femoral tunnel plays an important role in controlling tibial rotation (the pivot-shift phenomenon) and anterior translation of the tibia (Lachman and anterior drawer test) (Yagi et al. 2002; Loh et al. 2003; Scopp et al. 2004; Yamamoto et al. 2004; Musahl et al. 2005; Lee et al. 2007; Moisala et al. 2007; Ristanis et al. 2009; Steiner et al. 2009; Kato et al. 2010; Marchant et al. 2010; Bedi et al. 2011; Kondo et al. 2011; Sadoghi et al. 2011; Driscoll et al. 2012; Kato et al. 2013). It has been hypothesized that abnormal tibial rotation following ACL reconstruction, as well as in the ACL-deficient knee, plays an important role in the development of osteoarthritis (Jonsson et al. 2004; Andriacchi et al. 2006; Stergiou et al. 2007; Andriacchi et al. 2009; Wang et al. 2013). Proper placement of the ACL femoral tunnel is therefore critical to achieving a full range of motion and restoring stability to the knee and ultimately trying to prevent the long-term development of osteoarthritis.

This chapter will focus on recommendations for SB ACL reconstruction, as globally it is the most common surgical technique used to perform an ACL reconstruction (Chechik et al. 2013). For SB ACL reconstruction, it has been recommended that the bone tunnels be placed at the center of the native ACL femoral and tibial attachment sites (Karlsson et al. 2011; Kondo et al. 2011; van Eck et al. 2011; Hussein et al. 2012a, b; Brown et al. 2013; Fig. 13). This recommendation is based on biomechanical and clinical studies which demonstrate that compared to PL, high AM graft placement, or other matched ACL tunnel positions located within the native ACL attachment sites, a SB ACL graft placed at the center of the native ACL attachment sites is more effective at controlling anterior tibial translation and the pivot-shift phenomenon and more closely reproduces normal knee kinematics (Herbort et al. 2010; Kato et al. 2010; Kondo et al. 2011; Hussein et al. 2012a; Kato et al. 2013). Although, not all surgeons agree with the concept of center-to-center placement for anatomic SB ACL reconstructions, it is widely accepted that the bone tunnels for an anatomic ACL reconstruction should be placed within the native ACL attachment sites. Using the center of the ACL femoral attachment site as a defined anatomic reference point, surgeons may choose to place their ACL bone tunnels in the native ACL femoral attachment site according to different philosophies. Moving the center of the ACL femoral tunnel toward the center of the AM bundle will result in a more isometric, vertical ACL graft that experiences lower in situ graft forces. ACL grafts which experience lower in situ graft forces may be less likely to rupture. However, the lower rupture rate may come at the expense of inferior rotational control and increased shear forces on the articular cartilage which may predispose the development of early osteoarthritis. Moving the center of the ACL femoral tunnel toward the central region of the native ACL attachment site and the region of the PL bundle fibers will result in an anisometric ACL graft that undergoes larger length changes with flexion/extension of the knee. ACL grafts placed in this region will demonstrate rapid tightening in the last 20° of extension. Although placing the ACL graft in central and shallow region of the native ACL attachment site will result in greater length changes with flexion/extension of the knee, the resulting ACL graft will be more horizontally oriented and thus better aligned to control rotational laxity. However, the better rotational control of this graft placement may come at the expense of higher in situ ACL graft forces and possibly a higher graft rupture rate.

ACL Reconstruction Surgical Techniques

The two-incision, arthroscopically assisted intra-articular ACL reconstruction surgical technique was first introduced in the mid-1980s (Bach 1989; Schindler 2012; Chambat et al. 2013). In the two-incision surgical technique, the ACL femoral tunnel is drilled independent of the tibial tunnel from an outside–in direction through a small distal femoral incision. With independent drilling of the ACL femoral tunnel, it is possible to consistently position the ACL femoral tunnel within the native ACL femoral attachment site (Abebe et al. 2009; Chang et al. 2013; Kim et al. 2013; Robert et al. 2013; Shin et al. 2013). The only disadvantage to drilling the ACL femoral tunnel using an outside–in drilling technique is the need to make a second distal femoral incision. However, with the development of new drill guides and retro reaming drills, outside–in drilling of the ACL femoral tunnel can now be accomplished through a small stab incision. Long-term clinical studies of ACL reconstructions performed using the two-incision approach with outside–in drilling of the ACL femoral tunnel have demonstrated excellent subjective and objective clinical outcomes with a low percentage of knees having a positive pivot-shift test (Bach et al. 1998).

The transtibial surgical technique was developed in the early 1990s (Hardin et al. 1992; McCulloch et al. 2007; Schindler 2012; Chambat et al. 2013). In the transtibial surgical technique, the ACL femoral tunnel is drilled through the ACL tibial tunnel. For the past 20 years, this has been the most popular surgical technique for ACL reconstruction. There were many reasons for the popularity of the transtibial technique. It eliminated the need to make a second incision, thus decreasing operating time and surgical morbidity. The technique also allowed reliable and reproducible isometric femoral tunnel placement. Since only one skin incision was required, the procedure was more cosmetically acceptable to patients. Another reason for the popularity of the technique was that it utilized an offset ACL femoral aimer which made the surgical procedure reproducible in the hands of the average knee surgeon. Other reasons for the popularity of the transtibial technique were that there was no need to hyperflex the knee. During surgery the ACL femoral tunnel could be drilled with the knee at the more familiar 90° of flexion, and in fact the technique was capable of producing longer femoral tunnel lengths which was advantageous when using suspensory ACL femoral fixation devices. The major disadvantage and limitation of the transtibial technique is that the position of the ACL femoral tunnel is dependent on the position of the ACL tibial tunnel. Drilling the ACL femoral tunnel through a posteriorly positioned ACL tibial tunnel often resulted in the ACL femoral tunnel being located high and deep ("high AM" position), outside of the native ACL femoral attachment site. The combination of a posterior tibial tunnel position and a high, deep ACL femoral tunnel position often produced a vertical ACL graft which controlled anterior tibial translation but often failed to control the pivot-shift phenomenon (Yagi et al. 2002; Loh et al. 2003; Scopp et al. 2004; Yamamoto et al. 2004; Musahl et al. 2005; Heming et al. 2007; Lee et al. 2007; Moisala et al. 2007; Noyes 2009; Ristanis et al. 2009; Steiner et al. 2009; Herbort et al. 2010; Kato et al. 2010; Marchant et al. 2010; Bedi et al. 2011; Kondo et al. 2011; Sadoghi et al. 2011; Driscoll et al. 2012; Park et al. 2012; Inderhaug et al. 2013; Kato et al. 2013). A 10-year follow-up study of hamstring ACL reconstructions performed using the transtibial technique found that although 86 % of the patients had normal or near-normal anterior tibial translation, 20 % had a positive pivot-shift test and 42 % had a pivot glide (Inderhaug et al. 2013).

Advocates of the transtibial technique have claimed that it is possible to position the ACL femoral tunnel in the center of the ACL femoral attachment site (Piasecki et al. 2011). However, it has been shown that in order to position the ACL femoral tunnel in the center of the ACL femoral attachment site, a very medial and proximal starting position for the ACL tibial tunnel must be chosen (Heming et al. 2007; Piasecki et al. 2011). This starting position may result in a very short tibial tunnel which limits the length of the ACL graft available for healing in the tibial tunnel. A short tibial tunnel may also result in a graft–tunnel mismatch which can compromise fixation of bone–patellar tendon–bone grafts. In the transtibial technique, anatomic ACL femoral tunnel placement is facilitated by drilling a 10–11 mm diameter tibial tunnel (Piasecki et al. 2011). A large-diameter tibial tunnel may allow the offset femoral tunnel to be rotated down the lateral wall of the intercondylar notch, thus achieving a more anatomic placement of the ACL femoral tunnel. However, due to the smaller tibial tunnels used for hamstring tendon ACL reconstructions, the transtibial drilling technique does not allow the surgeon to position the ACL femoral tunnel for a hamstring tendon ACL reconstruction within the native ACL femoral attachment site (Strauss et al. 2011).

The medial portal surgical technique for ACL reconstruction was first developed to address the issues of ACL graft laceration, violation of the posterior wall of the ACL femoral tunnel, divergence of ACL femoral interference screws, and graft–tunnel length mismatch associated with bone–patellar tendon–bone autograft ACL reconstructions performed using a transtibial technique (Schindler 2012; Brown et al. 2013). In the medial portal surgical technique, the ACL femoral tunnel is drilled through an anteromedial (AM) or accessory anteromedial (AAM) portal with the knee flexed to 120° or higher. Hyperflexion of the knee is necessary to avoid having the femoral guide pin exit the lateral soft tissues too posteriorly. The peroneal nerve and posterior neurovascular structures are at risk for injury when the femoral guide pin exits the lateral soft tissues in a too posterior position (Hall et al. 2008; Lubowitz 2009; Nakamura et al. 2009; Otani et al. 2011; Brown et al. 2013). Drilling the ACL femoral tunnel through a medial portal provides several advantages compared to the traditional transtibial technique (Brown et al. 2013). First, the ACL femoral tunnel is drilled independently of the tibial tunnel which allows the femoral tunnel to be consistently placed within the native

ACL femoral attachment site (Bowers et al. 2011; Chang et al. 2013; Kim et al. 2013; Robert et al. 2013; Shin et al. 2013). Secondly, the intra-articular and the external starting positions for the tibial tunnel and the angle of the tibial tunnel do not have to be chosen to accommodate drilling of the ACL femoral tunnel. Therefore, the surgeon can position the tibial tunnel in the center of the tibial attachment site and is free to drill a steeper and thus longer tibial tunnel. A longer tibial tunnel minimizes the potential for graft–tunnel length mismatch. Thirdly, in the medial portal technique, femoral interference fixation screws are inserted through the same medial portal which was used to drill the ACL femoral tunnel, thus minimizing screw–tunnel divergence. Finally, the medial portal technique provides improved arthroscopic visualization during ACL femoral tunnel drilling since the ACL femoral tunnel can be drilled under ideal arthroscopic conditions without the loss of joint distention due to fluid extravasation out of the tibial tunnel. Disadvantages of drilling the ACL femoral tunnel through a medial portal include the need to hyperflex the knee and the potential for short femoral tunnels (Lubowitz 2009). Hyperflexion can potentially compromise arthroscopic visualization and lead to spatial disorientation in the notch compared to drilling at the more familiar 90° of knee flexion (Lubowitz 2009). The introduction of flexible drills allows the ACL femoral tunnel to be drilled at 90° of flexion, so this disadvantage no longer necessarily exists. Unless special attention is paid to proper portal placement, drilling the ACL femoral tunnel through a medial portal can result in short femoral tunnel lengths (Lubowitz 2009; Bedi et al. 2010; Chang et al. 2011; Brown et al. 2013). A short femoral tunnel can potentially compromise ACL graft fixation when using suspensory femoral fixation methods. However, with attention to detail, these potential issues can usually be overcome (Brown et al. 2013). The fact that this technique allows independent drilling of the ACL femoral tunnel and allows for consistent anatomic ACL femoral tunnel placement is viewed by most surgeons as outweighing the disadvantages or technical challenges of the technique. As a result, the medial portal technique has become the preferred surgical technique for performing ACL reconstruction (Chechik et al. 2013).

Comparison of the Transtibial, Medial Portal, and Outside–In Drilling Techniques

The different surgical techniques for drilling the ACL femoral tunnel primarily affect the following parameters: ACL femoral tunnel length, angulation of the ACL femoral tunnel in the coronal and sagittal planes, the ability of the ACL femoral tunnel to cover the native ACL femoral attachment site, and the ability to accurately place the ACL femoral tunnel within the native ACL femoral attachment site. Bedi et al. (2010) investigated the effect of transtibial versus AM portal drilling on ACL femoral tunnel length and coronal plane obliquity of the ACL femoral tunnel in human cadaveric knees. AM portal drilling was found to achieve slightly greater ACL femoral tunnel obliquity compared to transtibial drilling. However, there was a much higher risk of short femoral tunnel lengths (<25 mm) and posterior tunnel wall blowout with AM portal drilling. The authors concluded that AM portal drilling achieved slightly greater ACL femoral tunnel obliquity but cautioned that there was a substantially greater risk of obtaining a short (<25 mm) femoral tunnel length and posterior wall blowout.

Chang et al. (2011) compared modified transtibial and AM portal drilling techniques with respect to ACL femoral tunnel obliquity and femoral length in 105 patients who underwent ACL reconstruction with a four-strand hamstring tendon autograft. Obliquity of the ACL femoral tunnel was measured on postoperative tunnel-view radiographs, and femoral tunnel length was directly measured at the time of surgery using a depth probe. The mean coronal obliquity of the ACL femoral tunnel in the transtibial group was 61.7° compared to 55.9° for the AM portal group, and the mean femoral tunnel length was 43.3 mm in the transtibial group and 34.2 mm in the AM portal group. Both of these differences were statistically significant. Twenty-six percent of the knees in the AM portal group had a femoral tunnel length less than 30 mm versus 1.8 % in the transtibial group. Similar to Bedi et al. (2010), the authors concluded that AM portal drilling can achieve a more oblique ACL femoral tunnel position, but the resulting femoral tunnels can be substantially shorter than tunnels obtained using the transtibial technique.

Larson et al. (2012) compared four different femoral tunnel drilling techniques in human cadaveric knees. In group 1, the ACL femoral tunnel was drilled using a transtibial technique. In group 2, the femoral tunnel was drilling through the AM portal with a rigid drill. In group 3, the femoral tunnel was drilled through the AM portal with a flexible reamer. In group 4, the femoral tunnel was drilled using an outside–in technique. Measurements of the ACL femoral tunnel length, tunnel aperture, and tunnel placement were made from 3-D CT scans. Although there was no significant difference between the groups regarding the length or width of the resulting ACL femoral tunnel, there was a trend toward femoral tunnels in group 3 having a longer length and cross-sectional area. Mean femoral tunnel length was as follows: transtibial = 42 mm, AM portal-rigid drill = 38 mm, AM portal-flexible drill = 29 mm, and outside–in = 32 mm. Transtibial tunnels were significantly longer than AM portal-flexible reamer tunnels. The AM portal-flexible drill group was closest to the length obtained with transtibial drilling. Mean coronal obliquity for transtibial drilling was 63°, AM portal-rigid drill was 61°, AM portal-flexible drill was 52°, and outside–in was 45°. The difference in coronal obliquity between outside–in and transtibial and outside–in and AM portal-rigid drill was statistically significant. This study demonstrates that outside–in drilling produces the most oblique femoral tunnels and transtibial drilling the most vertical.

Chang et al. (2013) compared AM portal drilling in 63 knees versus outside–in drilling in 54 knees that had undergone primary ACL reconstruction with a four-strand hamstring tendon autograft. Femoral tunnel positions were compared on a postoperative tunnel-view radiograph. There was no significant difference in the femoral tunnel obliquity or femoral tunnel length between the AM portal and outside–in groups. However, the AM portal group had a greater percentage of knees (14 % versus 0 %) with a femoral tunnel length of less than 30 mm. The authors concluded that outside–in drilling of the ACL femoral tunnel can achieve similar ACL femoral tunnel obliquity in the coronal plane as AM portal drilling with a smaller risk of the femoral tunnel being less than 30 mm.

Hantes et al. (2009) evaluated differences in ACL graft orientation between four-strand hamstring tendon autograft ACL reconstructions performed using transtibial and AM portal drilling techniques. Postoperative MRI scans were used to measure ACL graft orientation in the coronal and sagittal planes. The mean coronal plane ACL graft obliquity was 71° in the transtibial group compared to 52° for the AM group. There was no difference in the sagittal plane obliquity of the ACL graft between the two techniques. However, neither group was able to reproduce the sagittal inclination angle of the normal ACL. The ability of AM portal drilling to achieve a more oblique orientation of the ACL graft in the coronal plane was attributed to the fact that the ACL femoral tunnel was drilled independent of the tibial tunnel, thus giving the surgeon the freedom to place the ACL graft in a more anatomical position.

These studies demonstrate that AM portal and outside–in femoral tunnel drilling techniques achieve greater obliquity in the coronal plane but shorter femoral tunnels compared to transtibial drilling. The issue of short femoral tunnels can be addressed by drilling the ACL femoral tunnel through a low accessory anteromedial (AAM) portal (Tompkins et al. 2012; Brown et al. 2013; Tompkins et al. 2013). The medial-lateral placement of the AAM portal determines both the length and aperture shape of the ACL femoral tunnel (Hensler et al. 2011; Brown et al. 2013). Positioning the AAM portal more medially results in a more perpendicular orientation of the drill bit with respect to the lateral wall of the notch and produces a shorter ACL femoral tunnel length and a more circular-shaped tunnel aperture (Hensler et al. 2011; Brown et al. 2013). Positioning the

AAM portal more laterally, toward the medial border of the patellar ligament, orients the drill bit more obliquely with respect to the lateral wall of the notch and produces a longer ACL femoral tunnel length and a more elliptically shaped ACL femoral tunnel aperture (Hensler et al. 2011; Brown et al. 2013).

The ability to achieve acceptable (longer) ACL femoral tunnel length by drilling the femoral tunnel through an AAM portal has been confirmed by Tompkins et al. (2013). In this study the authors measured the ACL femoral tunnel length in 106 consecutive patients undergoing primary ACL reconstruction with drilling of the femoral tunnel through an AAM portal with the knee in maximum hyperflexion. During surgery, the ACL femoral tunnel length was measured directly using a depth probe. The average femoral tunnel length was 37 mm (range 26–45 mm) with all but one tunnel longer than 30 mm. The authors concluded that the use of an AAM portal for independent drilling of the femoral tunnel with the knee in maximum hyperflexion was capable of consistently producing ACL femoral tunnel lengths greater than 30 mm without posterior tunnel wall fractures.

The ability of different ACL femoral drilling techniques to accurately place the femoral tunnel within the native ACL attachment site and the ability of the different techniques to restore the geometry of the ACL femoral attachment site has also been investigated. Kaseta et al. (2008) compared the ability of two different ACL reconstruction techniques to place a femoral guide pin near the center of the ACL femoral attachment site in a human cadaver knee model. Two different methods of femoral guide pin placement were compared, a transtibial technique in which the femoral guide pin was placed through a tibial tunnel and a two-incision technique in which the femoral guide pin was placed from an outside–in direction, independent of the tibial tunnel. The bony and cartilage geometry and the ACL femoral attachment site were recorded using a 3-D digitizing stylus and this data was used to generate a 3-D surface model of each knee. The 3-D models were used to establish anatomic coordinate systems to measure the position of the guide pins relative to the center of the native ACL. The independent (outside–in) technique allowed the guide pin to be placed closer to the center of the native ACL femoral attachment site compared with the transtibial technique. The transtibial technique placed the guide pin at a mean distance of 7.9 mm from the center of the ACL, whereas the guide pins placed using the independent outside–in technique were at a mean distance of 1.9 mm from the center of the ACL. The guide pins placed using the transtibial technique were 5.1 mm anterior (high) and 3.6 mm proximal (deep) from the center of the ACL compared to 0.3 mm anterior (high) and 1.0 mm distal (shallow) for the outside–in technique. This study demonstrated that independent drilling is able to position guide pins closer to the center of the native ACL femoral attachment site compared to the transtibial technique.

Abebe et al. (2009) performed an in vivo imaging analysis comparing transtibial and outside–in ACL femoral tunnel drilling in 16 patients following primary ACL reconstruction. There were eight patients in the transtibial group and eight patients in the outside–in group. 3-T MRI and 3-D modeling techniques were used to measure femoral tunnel placement of the ACL reconstructions relative to the native ACL femoral attachment site. The transtibial technique placed the center of the ACL femoral tunnel at a mean distance of 8.5 mm from the center of the ACL femoral attachment site compared to 3.2 mm for the outside–in drilling technique. The transtibial technique placed the tunnels anterior (high) and proximal (deep) in the notch compared to the outside–in technique. The center of the ACL femoral tunnel in the transtibial group was at a mean distance of 5 mm in the anterior (high) direction and 5.7 mm in the proximal (deep) direction from the center of the ACL femoral attachment site. The center of the ACL femoral tunnel in the outside–in drilling technique was at a mean distance of 0.9 mm in the posterior (low) direction and 1.7 mm in the proximal (deep) direction from the center of the ACL femoral attachment site (Fig. 14). The authors concluded that the outside–in drilling technique allowed for more anatomic femoral tunnel placement compared with the transtibial technique.

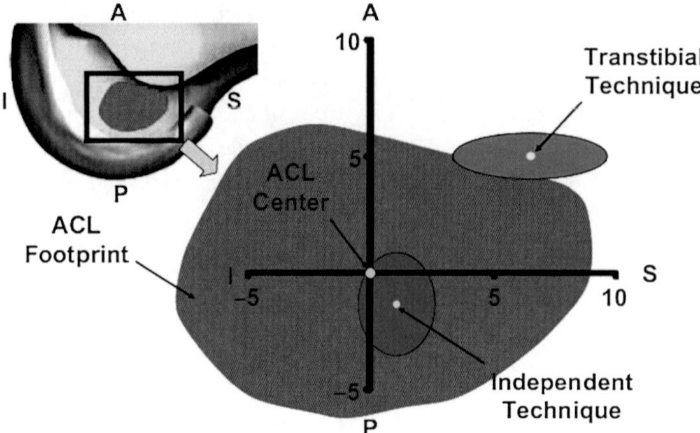

Fig. 14 The average position of the center of the tunnels using the transtibial and tibial tunnel-independent techniques relative to the center of the ACL in mm, mean ± standard deviation. Tunnel placement using the transtibial technique resulted in tunnels which were high and deep compared to the tibial tunnel-independent technique (with permission from the American Journal of Sports Medicine)

Silva et al. (2012) compared 20 patients that had a four-strand hamstring tendon autograft ACL reconstruction performed using a transtibial technique with 20 patients in which the ACL reconstruction was performed using AM portal drilling. The goal of the surgery was to place the femoral and tibial tunnels within the boundaries defined by the centers of the AM and PL bundle attachment sites. Postoperative CT scans were used to determine the position of the center of the ACL femoral and tibial tunnels in the sagittal plane. The position of the center of the ACL femoral tunnel was measured using the Bernard-Hertel (Bernard and Hertel 1996; Bernard et al. 1997) radiographic grid method, and the center of the tibial tunnel was measured using the method of Staubli and Rauschning (1994). There was no difference in the shallow–deep position of the ACL femoral tunnel between the two techniques. However, the center of the ACL femoral tunnel was significantly higher in the transtibial group. The center of the ACL tibial tunnel in the transtibial group was more posterior compared to the AM portal technique. Thirteen (65 %) of the tunnels in the transtibial group were posterior to the center of the PL bundle. In the AM portal group, 3 tunnels (15 %) were located anterior to the center of the AM bundle. This study demonstrated that the transtibial technique placed the femoral and tibial bone tunnels further away from the center of the ACL attachment sites, higher (anterior) on the femoral side, and more posterior on the tibial side compared to the AM portal technique.

Bowers et al. (2011) compared ACL tunnel position and ACL graft obliquity achieved with transtibial and AM portal drilling techniques. Thirty patients were prospectively studied after undergoing primary ACL reconstruction using a bone–patellar tendon–bone autograft. There were 15 patients in the transtibial group and 15 patients in the AM portal group. The ACL reconstructions were performed by 1 of 8 high-volume, fellowship-trained sports medicine surgeons who attempted to optimize femoral tunnel position and reproduce the graft obliquity of the native ACL. Tunnel location and ACL graft obliquity were accessed using 3-D knee models created with high-resolution MRI and imaging analysis software. No significant differences in the femoral centroid position were observed between the two groups. However, on the tibial side, the position of the tibial tunnel centroid in the transtibial group was significantly more posterior than the AM portal group and the native ACL. There was no significant difference in the medial-lateral tibial tunnel centroid position between the two groups. Sagittal plane obliquity in the AM group (52.2°) was closely restored to that of the native ACL

(53.5°), but the transtibial group was significantly more vertical (66.9°) than the native ACL. Coronal plane obliquity of both groups was significantly greater than that of the native ACL. There was 66.3 % overlap of the ACL graft with respect to the native ACL tibial attachment site in the AM portal group. The part of the ACL graft that did not overlap fell mostly medial to the native ACL tibial attachment site. The overlap for the transtibial group was 38 %, with 62 % of the tunnels positioned predominantly posterior and slightly medial to the native ACL tibial attachment site. The authors concluded that although both techniques could reproduce the native ACL femoral attachment site with similar accuracy, the transtibial technique required significantly greater posterior placement of the tibial tunnel which resulted in decreased ACL graft obliquity in the sagittal plane. One factor not accounted for in this study was the fact that the ACL reconstructions were performed using bone–patellar tendon–bone autografts. Piasecki et al. (2011) have shown that it is possible to position the ACL femoral tunnel near the center of the ACL femoral attachment site using a transtibial technique with a 10–11 mm diameter tibial tunnel and a proximal and medial external starting position for the tibial tunnel. However, using this same external starting position, it is not possible to position the ACL femoral tunnel near the center of the ACL femoral attachment site with a transtibial technique using smaller tibial tunnels necessary for hamstring tendon ACL grafts (Strauss et al. 2011). Therefore, the findings of this study apply only to the situation where the ACL reconstruction is performed with a bone–patellar tendon–bone ACL graft. For a hamstring ACL reconstruction, an alternative to the transtibial approach must be used to place the ACL femoral tunnel near the center of the ACL femoral attachment site (Strauss et al. 2011).

Tompkins et al. (2012) compared the ability of traditional transtibial and AAM portal drilling to place the ACL femoral tunnel within the native ACL femoral attachment site in ten matched paired cadaveric human knee specimens. Tunnel placement was documented by dual-energy CT scanning with a technique optimized for ligament evaluation. The AAM portal technique placed significantly more of the ACL femoral tunnel aperture within the native ACL femoral attachment site (98 %) compared to 61 % for the transtibial technique. The AAM portal technique also placed the center of the ACL femoral tunnel significantly closer to the center of the native ACL femoral attachment site (3.6 mm) than the transtibial technique (6 mm). Average femoral tunnel lengths were shorter for the AAM portal technique (37.8 mm) compared to the transtibial technique (41.1 mm). However, this difference was not statistically significant. The authors concluded that drilling the ACL femoral tunnel through an AAM placed more of the ACL femoral tunnel aperture within the native ACL femoral attachment site and placed the femoral tunnel closer to the center of the ACL femoral attachment site than the traditional transtibial technique.

Gadikota et al. (2012) investigated the relationship between femoral tunnels created by the transtibial, AM portal, and outside–in techniques in a controlled laboratory study using human cadaveric knees. The femoral tunnels for each technique were created using an 8 mm reamer. No significant difference was observed between the three groups in the total coverage of the ACL femoral footprint (AM = 55.0 %, outside–in = 56.8 %, transtibial = 51.0 %). Coverage of the PL bundle area of the ACL femoral footprint by the transtibial technique (26.4 %) was significantly lower than the AM portal (42.2 %) and outside–in (61.5 %) techniques. No significant differences were observed between the three groups in terms of coverage of the AM bundle area of the femoral footprint. On average, 72.9 % the transtibial tunnel was inside of the native ACL femoral attachment site. This was significantly less than the AM portal (86.4 %) and outside–in (89.2 %) tunnels. There was no significant difference in the percentage of the ACL femoral tunnel inside of the ACL femoral attachment site between the AM portal and outside–in techniques (Fig. 15). In summary, the study found that similar coverage of the ACL femoral attachment site can be achieved by tunnels created by the transtibial, AM portal, and outside–in techniques. However, tibial tunnel-independent techniques were able to cover a

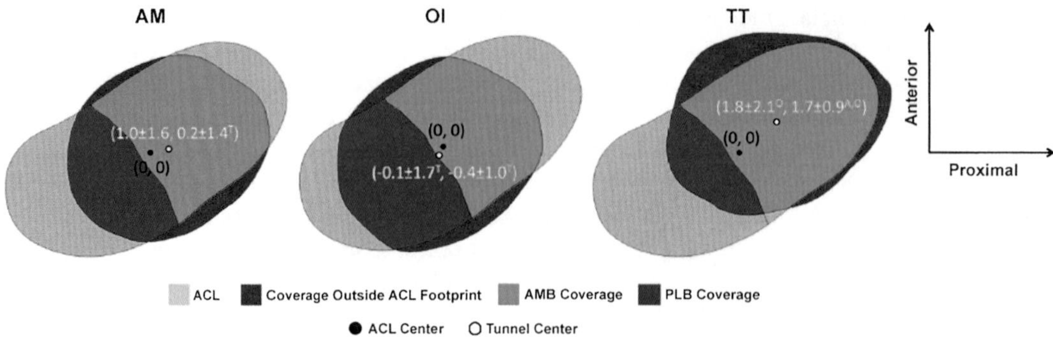

Fig. 15 Average native ACL and femoral tunnel footprints. The *white circles* represent the location of the femoral tunnel for the different surgical techniques. *AM* anteromedial portal technique, *OI* outside–in technique, *TT* transtibial technique (with permission from the American Journal of Sports Medicine)

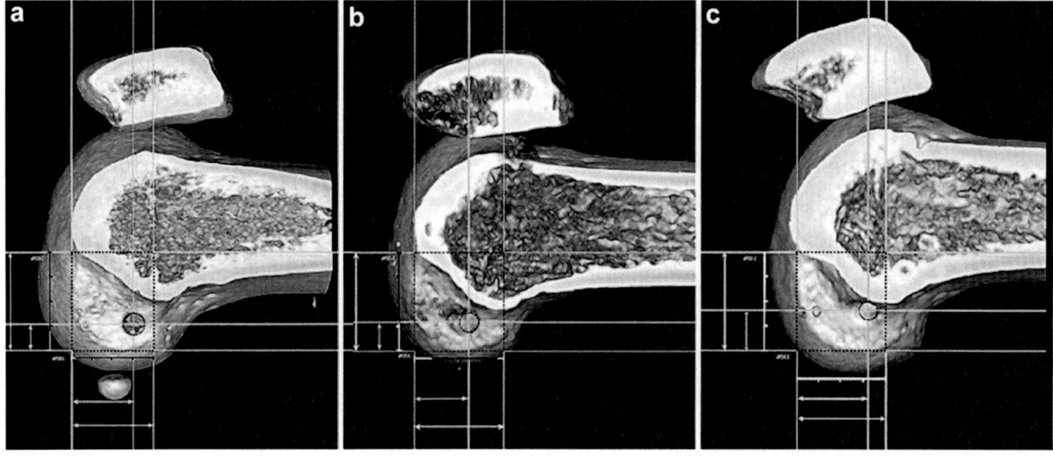

Fig. 16 Illustrations of the (**a**) outside–in, (**b**) anteromedial portal, and (**c**) transtibial surgical techniques. The transtibial technique resulted in a higher femoral tunnel placement than either the anteromedial or outside–in techniques (with permission from the American Journal of Sports Medicine)

larger portion of the PL bundle area of the ACL femoral attachment site.

Shin et al. (2013) prospectively evaluated 153 patients who underwent four-strand hamstring tendon graft ACL reconstruction using the AM portal ($n = 73$), outside–in ($n = 38$), and transtibial ($n = 42$) techniques. The ACL femoral tunnel position for each patient was determined using a 3-D CT scan. There was no significant difference in the shallow-to-deep ACL femoral tunnel position among the three groups. However, the ACL femoral tunnel for the transtibial group was significantly higher than the AM portal or outside–in techniques in the high–low direction (Fig. 16). There was no significant difference in the high–low position between the AM portal and outside–in groups. The authors concluded that the transtibial technique positioned the ACL femoral tunnel higher (more anterior) than the AM portal and outside–in techniques.

In vivo video motion analysis has recently been used to investigate the effects of ACL reconstruction surgical technique on knee joint kinematics. Zampeli et al. (2012) evaluated the effect of coronal and sagittal plane ACL graft obliquity on tibial rotation range of motion during dynamic pivoting activities after bone–patellar tendon–bone autograft ACL reconstruction. The study population involved 19 ACL-reconstructed patients (mean age, 29 years; mean time interval postoperatively, 19.9 months) and 19 matched control subjects (mean age, 30.6 years). Both groups were evaluated using motion analysis during descending a stairway and pivoting and landing from a jump and pivoting. MRI was used to measure the coronal and sagittal ACL graft angles. Although the ACL reconstruction group was unable to restore tibial rotation range of motion back to that of the normal contralateral knee or the healthy control knees, there was a highly significant positive correlation between ACL graft obliquity in the coronal plane and tibial rotation range of motion. No correlation was found between tibial rotation range of motion and sagittal ACL graft angle. The findings of this study show that tibial rotation range of motion was better restored in ACL-reconstructed patients with a more oblique ACL graft orientation in the coronal plane.

Wang et al. (2013) compared the effectiveness of the transtibial and AM portal ACL reconstruction techniques in restoring knee joint kinematics during normal gait. There were 12 patients in the transtibial group and 12 patients in the AM portal group. The control group consisted of 20 healthy participants with no history of lower extremity injuries. The ACL reconstructions were performed by a single surgeon using 4-strand hamstring tendon autografts. When the diameter of the 4-strand hamstring autograft was less than 8 mm, the graft construct was augmented with a single semitendinosus allograft to increase the size of the combined graft to 9 or 10 mm. A video motion capture system was used to record the motion data. The peak femoral external rotations during level walking were greater for both the reconstructed groups (transtibial = 5.7°, AM portal = 4.9°) compared with the controls (3.2°), but the differences were statistically significant for only the transtibial group. The transtibial group had significantly greater average femoral anterior–posterior translation on the tibial plateau during the stance phase compared to the AM portal and control groups (transtibial = 23.8 mm, AM portal = 16.2 mm, controls = 16.9 mm). The transtibial group was also found to have significantly greater average femoral anterior–posterior translation after toe off compared to the AM portal and control groups (TT = 22.2 mm, AM portal = 12.3 mm, control = 13.2 mm). This study demonstrated that surgical technique has an effect on knee kinematics. The AM portal technique improved anterior–posterior stability of the knee during the swing phase as well as axial rotational stability at midstance compared with the transtibial technique.

There are few published clinical studies comparing the results of the transtibial and AM portal techniques. Alentorn-Geli et al. (2010) compared the outcomes of ACL reconstruction performed with bone–patellar tendon–bone autograft using transtibial or AM portal drilling of the femoral tunnel in a homogeneous group of soccer players. All operations were performed by the senior surgeon and differed only in the drilling technique of the femoral tunnel. There were 21 patients in the transtibial group and 26 in the AM portal group. All patients were evaluated 2–5 years after the index surgical procedure. The patients were evaluated with standard outcome measures. Compared with the transtibial group, there was a significant reduction in recovery time in the AM portal group. Manual maximum anterior tibial translation as measured by a KT-1000 arthrometer was significantly reduced in the AM portal group (transtibial = 1.9 mm, AM portal = 0.2 mm). The objective IKDC score, Lachman test, and pivot-shift test were significantly better in the AM portal group. Seventy-nine percent of the patients in the AM portal group had a negative pivot shift compared to 41 % in the transtibial group. The authors concluded, "the AM portal technique significantly improved the anterior–posterior and rotational knee stability, and overall IKDC scores compared to the transtibial technique."

Kim et al. (2011) compared the clinical results of 33 patients who underwent SB ACL reconstruction with an autograft or allograft bone–patellar tendon–bone graft using a 3-portal technique with a control group of 33 patients that had undergone a similar procedure using a transtibial technique. Both groups were evaluated with standard clinical outcome measures. Femoral tunnel obliquity was measured on a postoperative knee view x-ray. There was no significant difference in the Lachman test or KT-1000 arthrometer measurements between the two groups. However, there was a significant difference in the results of the pivot-shift test between the two groups, with 90 % of the patients in the AM portal group having a negative pivot-shift test compared to 79 % in the transtibial group. Although the Lysholm and IKDC scores were higher for the AM portal groups, this difference did not reach statistical significance. Femoral tunnel obliquity was significantly greater in the transtibial group (59°) compared to the AM portal group (31°). The authors concluded that ACL reconstruction using two anteromedial portals was effective in restoring the anatomy of the ACL and obtaining good clinical results, because the technique allowed for a better field of view and lower ACL graft obliquity compared to the transtibial technique.

Recently, Chalmers et al. (2013) performed a systematic review of the literature for biomechanical and clinical studies directly comparing the ability of the transtibial and AM portal ACL reconstruction techniques to achieve rotational stability of the knee. They identified five clinical (Level II or III studies) and four cadaveric studies that directly compared the transtibial and AM portal techniques. Two clinical studies and two cadaveric studies demonstrated superior rotational stability with the AM portal group, whereas one clinical and two cadaveric studies showed no difference. Clinical outcomes were similarly mixed with some studies showing a significantly quicker return to play and better IKDC and Lysholm scores with the AM portal technique, whereas other studies showed no difference. However, no study showed significantly better results with the transtibial technique. According to the authors, "This study shows that the AM portal technique of ACLR may be more likely to produce improved clinical and biomechanical outcomes but that the TT technique is capable of producing similar outcomes."

To summarize the AM portal and outside–in ACL reconstruction techniques can be expected to achieve similar femoral tunnel lengths, while the transtibial technique can be expected to achieve femoral tunnel lengths significantly longer than either the AM portal or outside–in techniques. There are significant differences in the ACL femoral and tibial tunnel positions achieved with the AM portal, outside–in, and transtibial techniques. Transtibial drilling is more likely to position the ACL femoral tunnel significantly higher and deeper along the lateral wall of the notch, and the tibial tunnel more posteriorly in the native ACL tibial attachment site. Biomechanical and clinical studies have demonstrated that positioning an ACL graft in a high-deep femoral tunnel and a posterior tibial tunnel results in a vertical ACL graft in both the coronal and sagittal planes. Vertical ACL grafts may control anterior tibial translation but often fail to control the pivot-shift phenomenon. There does not seem to be a significant difference in the femoral or tibial tunnel positions achieved using the AM portal and outside–in techniques, and both of these techniques can consistently place the ACL femoral and tibial tunnels near the center of the native ACL attachment sites. As a result, vertical ACL grafts are less likely to be achieved using these techniques. There are also differences in the ability of the ACL femoral tunnel created by the three techniques to achieve coverage of the ACL femoral attachment site. Coverage of the PL part of the ACL femoral attachment site is lowest with femoral tunnels drilled using the transtibial technique. There does not appear to be any differences in coverage of the PL area of the ACL femoral attachment site between the AM and outside–in techniques. The three techniques have equal ability to produce a femoral tunnel which covers the AM part of the ACL femoral attachment site. The transtibial technique has the largest percentage of the femoral tunnel outside of the ACL femoral attachment site.

Obliquity of the ACL graft is an important issue since biomechanical and clinical studies have demonstrated that greater coronal obliquity of the ACL graft is associated with better rotational stability, better clinical outcomes, and better restoration of normal knee kinematics. The AM portal and outside–in techniques have been shown to achieve greater femoral tunnel and ACL graft coronal plane obliquity compared to the transtibial technique. Kinematic studies have shown that greater coronal plane obliquity of the ACL graft better restores tibial rotation and knee kinematics (Zampeli et al. 2012; Wang et al. 2013). One of the objectives of anatomic ACL reconstruction is to prevent the development of osteoarthritis. Abnormal tibial rotation in the ACL-deficient and ACL-reconstructed knee has been related to inferior functional outcomes and patient satisfaction and a lower rate of return to sports and has also been considered a predominant etiologic factor for the development of osteoarthritis (Jonsson et al. 2004; Kocher et al. 2004; Andriacchi et al. 2006; Stergiou et al. 2007; Andriacchi et al. 2009). The ability of the AM portal and outside–in techniques to achieve greater coronal plane obliquity of the ACL graft is a significant advantage over the transtibial technique.

Based on the best available biomechanical, clinical, and kinematic studies, there appears to be little advantage to the transtibial technique. Although that it is possible to position a bone–patellar tendon–bone ACL graft near the center of the native ACL femoral and tibial attachment sites using a transtibial technique, numerous modifications including the use of an accessory transpatellar tendon portal for placement of the tibial aimer, use of a external tibial tunnel starting position at the junction of the pes anserinus and medial collateral ligament fibers, adequate rotation of the 7 mm offset femoral aiming device to improve lateralization of the tunnel, and adjustment of the tibial aimer to achieve 55–60° of angulation of the tibial tunnel in the coronal plane are necessary (Piasecki et al. 2011; Chalmers et al. 2013). Even with these modifications it is impossible to position a hamstring tendon ACL graft within the native ACL femoral attachment site (Strauss et al. 2011). Given these limitations, transtibial drilling of the ACL femoral tunnel has a limited role when performing anatomic ACL reconstruction.

Summary

Anatomic ACL reconstruction is defined as "the functional restoration of the ACL to its native dimensions, collagen orientation and insertion sites" (van Eck et al. 2011). Biomechanical and clinical studies have demonstrated that an anatomic ACL reconstruction with the bone tunnels placed at the center of the native femoral and tibial attachment sites is more effective at controlling anterior tibial translation and anterolateral tibial rotation compared to a nonanatomic ACL reconstruction. Anatomic ACL graft placement has been demonstrated to improve rotational stability and produce better clinical outcomes and better restore normal knee kinematics. Different surgical techniques such as the transtibial, anteromedial portal, and outside–in technique are used to perform an ACL reconstruction. The anteromedial portal and outside–in techniques can be used to consistently place the ACL femoral tunnel within the native ACL femoral attachment site and have become the preferred surgical techniques when performing an ACL reconstruction.

Cross-References

- ▸ Anatomic Double-Tunnel Anterior Cruciate Ligament Reconstruction: Evolution and Principles
- ▸ Anterior Cruciate Ligament Graft Selection and Fixation
- ▸ Different Techniques of Anterior Cruciate Ligament Reconstruction: Guidelines
- ▸ Personalized Treatment Algorithms for Anterior Cruciate Ligament Injuries
- ▸ Revision Anterior Cruciate Ligament Reconstruction
- ▸ Single Versus Double Anterior Cruciate Ligament Reconstruction in Athletes

References

Abebe CS, Moorman CT, Dziedzic C et al (2009) Femoral tunnel placement during anterior cruciate ligament reconstruction: an in vivo imaging analysis comparing transtibial and 2-incision tibial tunnel-independent techniques. Am J Sports Med 37(10):1904–1911

Alentorn-Geli E, Samitier G, Alvarez P, Steinbacher G, Cugat R (2010) Anteromedial portal versus transtibial drilling techniques in ACL reconstruction: a blinded cross-sectional study at two- to five-year follow-up. Int Orthop 34(5):747–754

Amis AA (2012) The functions of the fibre bundles of the anterior cruciate ligament in anterior drawer, rotational laxity and the pivot shift. Knee Surg Sports Traumatol Arthrosc 20(4):613–620

Amis AA, Dawkins GP (1991) Functional anatomy of the anterior cruciate ligament: fiber bundle actions related to ligament replacements and injuries. J Bone Joint Surg Br 73:260–267

Amis A, Jakob R (1998) Anterior cruciate ligament graft positioning, tensioning and twisting. Knee Surg Sports Traumatol Arthrosc 6(S1):S2–S12

Andriacchi TP, Briant PL, Bevill SL, Koo S (2006) Rotational changes at the knee after ACL injury cause cartilage thinning. Clin Orthop Relat Res 442:39–44

Andriacchi TP, Seungbum K, Scanlan SF (2009) Gait mechanics influence healthy cartilage morphology and osteoarthritis of the knee. J Bone Joint Surg 91-A (supplement):95–101

Arnold MP, Kooloos J, van Kampen A (2001) Single-incision technique misses the anatomical femoral anterior cruciate ligament insertion: a cadaver study. Knee Surg Sports Traumatol Arthrosc 9(4):194–199

Bach BR (1989) Arthroscopy-assisted patellar tendon substitution for anterior cruciate ligament insufficiency. Surgical technique. Am J Knee Surg 2:3–20

Bach BR, Tradonsky S, Bojchuk J et al (1998) Arthroscopically assisted anterior cruciate ligament reconstruction using patellar tendon autograft. Five- to nine-year follow-up evaluation. Am J Sports Med 26:20–29

Baer GS, Feretti M, Fu FH (2008) Anatomy of the ACL. In: Fu FH, Cohen SB (eds) Current concepts in ACL reconstruction, 1st edn. Slack, Thorofare, pp 27–32

Bedi A, Raphael B, Maderazo A, Pavlov H, Williams RJ (2010) Transtibial versus anteromedial portal drilling for anterior cruciate ligament reconstruction: a cadaveric study of femoral tunnel length and obliquity. Arthroscopy 26(3):342–350

Bedi A, Musahl V, Steuber V et al (2011) Transtibial versus anteromedial portal reaming in anterior cruciate ligament reconstruction: an anatomic and biomechanical evaluation of surgical technique. Arthroscopy 27(3):380–390

Bernard M, Hertel P (1996) Intraoperative and postoperative insertion control of anterior cruciate ligamentplasty. A radiologic measuring method (quadrant method). Unfallchirurg 99:332–340

Bernard M, Hertel P, Hornung H et al (1997) Femoral insertion of the ACL. Radiographic quadrant method. Am J Knee Surg 10:14–22

Bowers AL, Bedi A, Lipman JD et al (2011) Comparison of anterior cruciate ligament tunnel position and graft obliquity with transtibial and anteromedial portal femoral tunnel reaming technique using high-resolution magnetic resonance imaging. Arthroscopy 27(11):1511–1522

Brown CH, Spalding T, Robb C (2013) Medial portal technique for single-bundle anatomical anterior cruciate (ACL) reconstruction. Int Orthop 37:253–269

Butler DL, Noyes FR, Grood ES (1980) Ligamentous restraints to anterior-posterior drawer in the human knee. A biomechanical study. J Bone Joint Surg Am 62:259–270

Bylski-Austrow DL, Grood ES, Hefsy MS (1993) Anterior cruciate ligament replacements: a mechanical study of femoral attachment location, flexion angle of tensioning, and initial tensioning. J Orthop Res 8:522–531

Chalmers PN, Mall NA, Cole BJ et al (2013) Anteromedial versus transtibial tunnel drilling in anterior cruciate ligament reconstructions: a systematic review. Arthroscopy 29:1235–1242

Chambat P, Guier C, Sonnery-Cottet B et al (2013) The evolution of ACL reconstruction over the last fifty years. Int Orthop 37:181–186

Chang CB, Choi J-Y, Koh IJ, Lee KJ et al (2011) Comparisons of femoral tunnel position and length in anterior cruciate ligament reconstruction: modified transtibial versus anteromedial portal techniques. Arthroscopy 27(10):1389–1394

Chang MJ, Chang CB, Won HH, Je MS, Kim TK (2013) Anteromedial portal versus outside–in technique for creating femoral tunnels in anatomic anterior cruciate ligament reconstructions. Arthroscopy 29(9):1533–1539

Chechik O, Amar E, Khashan M et al (2013) An international survey on anterior cruciate ligament reconstruction practices. Int Orthop 37:201–206

Columbet P, Robinson J, Christel P et al (2006) Morphology of anterior cruciate ligament attachments for anatomic reconstruction: a cadaveric dissection and radiographic study. Arthroscopy 22(9):984–992

Csintalan RP, Inacio MCS, Funahashi TT (2008) Incidence rate of anterior cruciate ligament reconstruction. Perm J 12(3):17–21

Driscoll MD, Isabell GP, Conditt MA et al (2012) Comparison of 2 femoral tunnel locations in anatomic single-bundle anterior cruciate ligament reconstruction: a biomechanical study. Arthroscopy 28:1481–1489

Edward A, Bull AM, Amis AA (2008) The attachment of the anteromedial and posterolateral fibre bundles of the anterior cruciate ligament: part II: femoral attachment. Knee Surg Sports Traumatol Arthrosc 16:29–36

Edwards A, Bull AMJ, Amis AA (2007) The attachments of the anteromedial and posterolateral fibre bundles of the anterior cruciate ligament. Part 1: tibial attachment. Knee Surg Sports Traumatol Arthrosc 15:1414–1421

Feretti M, Doca D, Ingham SM, Cohen M, Fu FH (2012) Bony and soft tissue landmarks of the ACL tibial insertion site: an anatomical study. Knee Surg Sports Traumatol Arthrosc 20:62–68

Fu FH, Jordan SS (2007) The lateral intercondylar ridge – a key to anatomic anterior cruciate ligament reconstruction. J Bone Joint Surg Am 89A:2103–2104

Gadikota HR, Sim JA, Hosseini A, Gill TJ, Li G (2012) The relationship between femoral tunnel created by the transtibial, anteromedial portal, and outside–in techniques and the anterior cruciate ligament footprint. Am J Sports Med 40(4):882–888

Getelman MH, Friedman MJ (1999) Revision anterior cruciate ligament reconstruction surgery. J Am Acad Orthop Surg 7:189–198

Girgis FG, Marshall JL, Al-Monajem A (1975) The cruciate ligaments of the knee joint. Anatomical, functional and experimental analysis. Clin Orthop 106:216–231

Graf B (1987) Isometric placement of substitutes for the anterior cruciate ligament. In: Wgackson D, David Orer, YR. The anterior cruciate deficient knee. New concepts in ligament repair. C.V. Mosby, St Louis, pp 102–113

Grood ES (1992) Placement of knee ligament grafts. In: Finerman GA, Noyes FR (eds) Biology and biomechanics of the traumatized synovial joint: the knee as a model. American Academy of Orthopaedic Surgeons, Rosemont

Hall MP, Ryzewicz M, Walsh PJ et al (2008) Risk of iatrogenic injury to the peroneal nerve during posterolateral femoral tunnel placement in double-bundle anterior cruciate ligament reconstruction. Am J Sports Med 37(1):109–113

Hantes ME, Zachos VC, Liantsis A (2009) Differences in graft orientation using the transtibial and anteromedial portal technique in anterior cruciate ligament reconstructions: a magnetic resonance imaging study. Knee Surg Sports Traumatol Arthrosc 17:880–886

Hardin GT, Bach BR, Bush-Joseph CA (1992) Endoscopic single-incision anterior cruciate ligament reconstruction using patellar tendon autograft. Am J Knee Surg 5:144–155

Harner CD, Baek GH, Vogrin TM et al (1999) Quantitative analysis of human cruciate ligament insertions. Arthroscopy 15:741–749

Harner CD, Rihn JA, Vogrin TM (2003) Specialty update: what's new in sports medicine. JBJS(Am) 85(6):1173–1181

Hefzy MS, Grood ES (1986) Sensitivity of insertion locations on the length patterns of anterior cruciate ligament fibers. J Biomech Eng 108:73–82

Hefzy MS, Grood ES, Noyes FR (1989) Factors affecting the region of most isometric femoral attachments. Part II: anterior cruciate ligament. Am J Sports Med 17:208–216

Heming JF, Rand J, Steiner ME (2007) Anatomical limitations of transtibial drilling in anterior cruciate ligament reconstruction. Am J Sports Med 35(10):1708–1715

Hensler D, Working Z, Illingworth K, Thorhauer E, Tashman S, Fu F (2011) Medial portal drilling: effects on the femoral tunnel aperture morphology during anterior cruciate ligament reconstruction. J Bone Joint Surg Am 93:2063–2071

Herbort M, Lenschow S, Fu FH, Petersen W, Zantop T (2010) ACL mismatch reconstructions: influence of different tunnel placement strategies in single-bundle ACL reconstruction. Knee Surg Sports Traumatol Arthrosc 18:1551–1558

Hewett TE, Myer GD, Ford KR et al (2005) Biomechanical measures of neuromuscular control and valgus loading of the knee predict anterior cruciate ligament injury risk in female athletes: a prospective study. Am J Sports Med 33(4):492–501

Hofbauer M, Muller B, Murawski CD et al (2013) The concept of individualized anatomic anterior cruciate ligament (ACL) reconstruction. Knee Surg Sports Traumatol Arthrosc. Published online 6 June 2013 22:979–986

Hussein M, Van Eck CF, Cretnik A et al (2012a) Prospective randomized clinical evaluation of conventional single-bundle, anatomic single-bundle, and anatomic double-bundle anterior cruciate ligament reconstruction: 281 cases with 3- to 5-year follow-up. Am J Sports Med 40(3):512–520

Hussein M, Van Eck CF, Cretnik A et al (2012b) Individualized anterior cruciate ligament surgery: a prospective study comparing anatomic single- and double-bundle reconstruction. Am J Sports Med 40(8):1781–1788

Hutchinson MR, Ash SA (2003) Resident's ridge: assessing the cortical thickness of the lateral wall and roof of the intercondylar notch. Arthroscopy 19(9):931–935

Hwang MD, Piefer JW, Lubowitz JH (2012) Anterior cruciate ligament tibial footprint anatomy: systematic review of the 21st century literature. Arthroscopy 28(5):728–734

Inderhaug E, Strand T, Fisher-Bredenbeck C, Solheim E (2013) Long-term results after reconstruction of the ACL with hamstring autograft and transtibial drilling. Knee Surg Sports Traumatol Arthrosc 21:2004–2010

Iriuchishima T, Shirakura K, Fu FH (2013) Graft impingement in anterior cruciate ligament reconstruction. Knee Surg Sports Traumatol Arthrosc 21(3):664–670

Janssen KW, Orchard JW, Driscoll R, van Mechelen W (2012) High incidence and costs for anterior cruciate ligament reconstructions performed in Australia from 2003–2004 to 2007–2008: time for an anterior cruciate ligament register by Scandinavian model? Scand J Med Sci Sports 22(4):495–501

Jones CDS, Grimshaw PN (2011) Chapter 17, The biomechanics of the anterior cruciate ligament and its reconstruction. In: Klika V (ed) Theoretical biomechanics. InTech. Available from http://www.intechopen.com/books/theoretical-biomechanics/the-biomechanics-of-the-anteriorcruciate-ligament-and-its-reconstruction

Jonsson H, Riklund-Åhlmstrom K, Lind J (2004) Positive pivot shift after ACL reconstruction later predicts osteoarthrosis. 63 patients followed 5–9 years after surgery. Acta Orthop Scand 75(5):594–599

Kamath GV, Redfern JC, Greis PE et al (2011) Revision anterior cruciate ligament reconstruction. Am J Sports Med 39:199–217

Karlsson J, Irrgang JJ, van Eck CF et al (2011) Anatomic single- and double-bundle anterior cruciate ligament reconstruction, part 2. Clinical application of surgical technique. Am J Sports Med 39:2016–2026

Kaseta MK, DeFrate LE, Charnock BL et al (2008) Reconstruction technique affect femoral tunnel placement in ACL reconstruction. Clin Orthop 466:1467

Kato Y, Ingham SJ, Kramer S et al (2010) Effect of tunnel position for anatomic single-bundle ACL reconstruction on knee biomechanics in a porcine model. Knee Surg Sports Traumatol Arthrosc 18(1):2–10

Kato Y, Maeyama A, Lertwanich P et al (2013) Biomechanical comparison of different graft positions for single-bundle anterior cruciate ligament reconstruction. Knee Surg Sports Traumatol Arthrosc 21:816–823

Kim MK, Lee BC, Park JH (2011) Anatomic single bundle anterior cruciate ligament reconstruction by the two anteromedial portal method: the comparison of transportal and transtibial technique. Knee Surg Relat Res 23(4):213–219

Kim JG, Chang MH, Lim HC et al (2013) Computed tomography analysis of the femoral tunnel position and aperture shape of transportal and outside–in ACL reconstruction. Am J Sports Med 41:2512–2520

Kocher MS, Steadman JR, Briggs KK, Sterett WI, Hawkins RJ (2004) Relationships between objective assessment of ligament stability and subjective assessment of symptoms and function after anterior cruciate ligament reconstruction. Am J Sports Med 32:629–634

Koga H, Nakamae A, Shima Y et al (2010) Mechanism of anterior cruciate ligament injuries: knee kinematics in 10 injury situations from female team handball and basketball. Am J Sports Med 38(11):2218–2225

Kondo E, Merican AM, Yasuda K (2011) Biomechanical comparison of anatomic double-bundle, anatomic single-bundle, and nonanatomic single-bundle anterior cruciate ligament reconstruction. Am J Sports Med 39:279–287

Kongcharoensombat W, Ochi M, Abouheif M, Adachi N et al (2011) The transverse ligament as a landmark for tibial sagittal insertions of the anterior cruciate ligament: a cadaveric study. Arthroscopy 27(10):1395–1399

Kopf S, Musahl V, Tashman S et al (2009) A systematic review of the femoral origin and tibial insertion morphology of the ACL. Knee Surg Sports Traumatol Arthrosc 17:213–219

Kopf S, Forsythe B, Wong AK et al (2010) Nonanatomic tunnel position in traditional transtibial single-bundle anterior cruciate ligament reconstruction evaluated by three-dimensional computed tomography. J Bone Joint Surg 92-A:1427–1431

Kopf S, Pombo MW, Szczodry M, Irrgang JJ, Fu FH (2011) Size variability of the human anterior cruciate ligament insertion sites. Am J Sports Med 39(1):108–113

Kopf S, Forsythe B, Wong AK et al (2012) Transtibial ACL reconstruction technique fails to position drill holes anatomically in vivo 3D CT study. Knee Surg Sports Traumatol Arthrosc 20:2200–2207

Krosshaug T, Nakamae A, Boden BP et al (2007) Mechanisms of anterior cruciate ligament injury in basketball: video analysis of 39 cases. Am J Sports Med 35(3):359–367

Larson AI, Bullock DP, Pevny T (2012) Comparison of 4 femoral tunnel drilling techniques in anterior cruciate ligament reconstruction. Arthroscopy 28(7):972–979

Lee MC, Seong SC, Lee S et al (2007) Vertical femoral tunnel placement results in rotational knee laxity after anterior cruciate ligament reconstruction. Arthroscopy 23:771–778

Lind M, Menhert F, Pedersen AB (2012) Incidence and outcome after revision anterior cruciate ligament reconstruction: results from the Danish registry of knee ligament reconstructions. Am J Sports Med 40:1551–1557

Loh JC, Fukuda Y, Tsuda E et al (2003) Knee stability and graft function following anterior cruciate ligament reconstruction: comparison between 11 o'clock and 10 o'clock femoral tunnel placement. Arthroscopy 19(3):297–304

Lubowitz JH (2009) Anteromedial portal technique for the anterior cruciate ligament femoral socket: pitfalls and solutions. Arthroscopy 25(1):95–101

Magnussen RA, Lawrence TR, West RL et al (2012) Graft size and patient age are predictors of early revision after anterior cruciate ligament reconstruction with hamstring autograft. Arthroscopy 28:526–531

Marchant B, Noyes F, Barber-Westin S et al (2010) Prevalence of nonanatomical graft placement in a series of failed anterior cruciate ligament reconstruction. Am J Sports Med 38:1987–1996

McCulloch PC, Lattermann C, Boland AL et al (2007) An illustrated history of anterior cruciate ligament surgery. J Knee Surg 20(2):95–104

Miyasaka KC, Daniel DM, Stone ML, Hirschman P (1991) The incidence of knee ligament injuries in the general population. Am J Knee Surg 4:43–48

Moisala AS, Jarvela T, Harilainen A et al (2007) The effect of graft placement on the clinical outcome of the anterior cruciate ligament reconstruction: a prospective study. Knee Surg Sports Traumatol Arthrosc 15:879–887

Musahl V, Plakseychuk A, VanScyoc A et al (2005) Varying femoral tunnels between the anatomical footprint and isometric positions: effect on kinematics of the anterior cruciate ligament-reconstructed knee. Am J Sports Med 33:712–718

Nakamura M, Deie M, Shibuya H et al (2009) Potential risks of femoral tunnel drilling through the far anteromedial portal: a cadaveric study. Arthroscopy 25(5):481–487

Noyes FR (2009) The function of the human anterior cruciate ligament and analysis of single- and double-bundle graft reconstructions. Sports Health 1(1):66–75

Olsen OE, Myklebust G, Engebretsen L et al (2004) Injury mechanisms for anterior cruciate ligament injuries in team handball: a systematic video analysis. Am J Sports Med 32(4):1002–1012

Otani M, Nozaki M, Kobayashi M et al (2011) Comparative risk of common peroneal nerve injury in far anteromedial portal drilling and transtibial drilling in anatomical double-bundle ACL reconstruction. Knee Surg Sports Traumatol Arthrosc 20(5):838–843

Park SY, Oh H, Park S et al (2012) Factors predicting hamstring tendon graft diameters and resulting failure rates after anterior cruciate ligament reconstruction. Knee Surg Sports Traumatol Arthrosc 21:1111–1118

Petersen W, Zantop T (2007) Anatomy of the anterior cruciate ligament with regard to its two bundles. Clin Orthop 454:35–47

Piasecki DP, Bach BR, Espinoza Orias AA et al (2011) Anterior cruciate ligament reconstruction: can anatomic femoral placement be achieved with a transtibial technique? Am J Sports Med 39(6):1306–1315

Purnell ML, Larson AI, Clancy W (2008) Anterior cruciate ligament insertions on the tibia and femur and their relationships to critical bony landmarks using high-resolution volume-rendering computed tomography. Am J Sports Med 36:2083–2090

Ristanis S, Stergiou N, Siarava E et al (2009) Effect of femoral tunnel placement for reconstruction of the anterior cruciate ligament on tibial rotation. J Bone Joint Surg Br 91(9):2151–2158

Robert H, Bouguennec N, Vogeli D, Berton E, Bowen M (2013) Coverage of the anterior cruciate ligament femoral footprint using 3 different approaches in single-bundle reconstruction. A cadaveric study analyzed by 3-dimensional computed tomography. Am J Sports Med 41:2375–2403

Sadoghi P, Kröpfl A, Jansson V et al (2011) Impact of tibial and femoral tunnel position on clinical results after anterior cruciate ligament reconstruction. Arthroscopy 27:355–364

Sapega AA, Moyer RA, Schneck C, Komalahiranya N (1990) Testing for isometry during reconstruction of the anterior cruciate ligament. J Bone Joint Surg 72-A:259–267

Sasaki N, Ishibashi Y, Tsuda E et al (2012) The femoral insertion of the anterior cruciate ligament: discrepancy between macroscopic and histological observations. Arthroscopy 28:1135–1146

Schindler OS (2012) Surgery for anterior cruciate ligament deficiency: a historical perspective. Knee Surg Sports Traumatol Arthrosc 20:5–47

Scopp JM, Jasper LE, Belkoff SM (2004) The effect of oblique femoral tunnel placement on rotational constraint of the knee reconstructed using patellar tendon autografts. Arthroscopy 20:294–299

Shin Y-S, Ro K-H, Lee J-H, Lee D-H (2013) Location of the femoral tunnel in single-bundle anterior cruciate ligament reconstruction: comparison of the transtibial, anteromedial portal, and outside–in techniques. Am J Sports Med 41:2533–2539

Shino K, Suzuki T, Iwahashi T et al (2010) The resident's ridge as an arthroscopic landmark for anatomical femoral tunnel drilling in ACL reconstruction. Knee Surg Sports Traumatol Arthrosc 18:1164–1168

Siddles JA, Larson RV, Garbini JL, Downey DJ, Matsen FA (1988) Ligament length relationships in the moving knee. J Orthop Res 6:593–610

Siebold R (2011) The concept of complete footprint restoration with guidelines for single- and double-bundle ACL reconstruction. Knee Surg Sports Traumatol Arthrosc 19:699–706

Silva A, Sampaio R, Pinto E (2012) ACL reconstruction: comparison between transtibial and anteromedial portal techniques. Knee Surg Sports Traumatol Arthrosc 20:896–903

Silvers HJ, Mandelbaum BR (2007) Prevention of anterior cruciate ligament injury in the female athlete. Br J Sports Med 41(Supplement 1):i52–i59

Sommer C, Friederich NF, Müller W (2000) Improperly placed anterior cruciate ligament graft: correlation between radiological parameters and clinical results. Knee Surg Sports Traumatol Arthrosc 8:207–213

Staubli HU, Rauschning W (1994) Tibial attachment area of the anterior cruciate ligament in the extended knee position. Anatomy and cryosections in vitro complemented by magnetic resonance arthrography in vivo. Knee Surg Sports Traumatol Arthrosc 2:138–146

Steiner ME, Battaglia TC, Heming JF et al (2009) Independent drilling outperforms conventional transtibial drilling in anterior cruciate ligament reconstruction. Am J Sports Med 37(10):1912–1919

Stergiou N, Ristanis S, Moraiti C, Georgoulis AD (2007) Tibial rotation in anterior cruciate ligament (ACL)-deficient and ACL-reconstructed knees: a theoretical proposition for the development of osteoarthritis. Sports Med 37:601–613

Strauss EJ, Barker JU, McGill K, Cole BJ, Bach BR, Verma NN (2011) Can anatomic femoral tunnel placement be achieved using a transtibial technique for hamstring anterior cruciate ligament reconstruction? Am J Sports Med 39:1263–1269

Tompkins M, Milewski MD, Brockmeier SF, Gaskin CM, Hart JM, Miller MD (2012) Anatomic femoral tunnel drilling in anterior cruciate ligament reconstruction. Use of an accessory medial portal versus traditional transtibial drilling. Am J Sports Med 40(6):1313–1321

Tompkins M, Milewski MD, Carson EW et al (2013) Femoral tunnel length in primary anterior cruciate ligament reconstruction using an accessory medial portal. Arthroscopy 29:238–24

Trojani C, Sbihi A, Dijan P et al (2011) Causes for failure of ACL reconstruction and influence of meniscectomies after revision. Knee Surg Sports Traumatol Arthrosc 19:196–201

Tsukada H, Ishibashi Y, Tsuda E et al (2008) Anatomical analysis of the anterior cruciate ligament femoral and tibial footprints. J Orthop Sci 13:122–129

van Eck CF, Morse KR, Lesniak BP et al (2010) Does the lateral intercondylar ridge disappear in ACL deficient patients? Knee Surg Sports Traumatol Arthrosc 18(9):1184–1188

van Eck CF, Lesmiak BP, Schreiber VM et al (2011) Anatomic single- and double-bundle anterior cruciate ligament reconstruction flowchart. Arthroscopy 26:258–268

Wang H, Fleischli JE, Zheng N (2013) Transtibial versus anteromedial portal technique in single-bundle anterior cruciate ligament reconstruction. Outcomes of knee kinematics during walking. Am J Sports Med 41(8):1847–1856

Wetzler MJ, Getelman MH, Friedman MJ et al (1998) Revision anterior cruciate ligament surgery: etiology of failures. Oper Tech Sports Med 6:64–70

Whitehead TS (2013) Failure of anterior cruciate ligament reconstruction. Clin Sports Med 32:177–20

Wright RW, Huston LJ, Spindler KP et al (2010) Descriptive epidemiology of the multicenter ACL revision study (MARS) cohort. Am J Sports Med 38:1979–1986

Yagi M, Wong EK, Kanamori A et al (2002) Biomechanical analysis of an anatomic anterior cruciate ligament reconstruction. Am J Sports Med 30:660–666

Yamamoto Y, Hsu WH, Woo SL et al (2004) Knee stability and graft function after anterior cruciate ligament reconstruction: a comparison of a lateral and an anatomical femoral tunnel placement. Am J Sports Med 32:1825–1832

Yaru NC, Daniel DM, Penner D (1992) The effect of tibial attachment site on graft impingement in an anterior cruciate ligament reconstruction. Am J Sports Med 20(2):217–220

Yasada K, van Eck CF, Hoshino Y et al (2011) Anatomic single- and double-bundle anterior cruciate ligament reconstruction, part 1, basic science. Am J Sports Med 39:1789–1799

Zampeli F, Ntoulia A, Giotis D et al (2012) Correlation between anterior cruciate ligament graft obliquity and tibial rotation during dynamic pivoting activities in patients with anatomic anterior cruciate ligament reconstruction: an in vivo examination. Arthroscopy 28(2):234–246

Zantop T, Peterson W (2008) Rupture pattern and injury mechanism. In: Fu FH, Cohen SB (eds) Current concepts in ACL reconstruction, 1st edn. Slack, Thorofare, pp 99–110

Zantop T, Herbort M, Raschke MJ et al (2007) The role of the anteromedial and posterolateral bundles of the anterior cruciate ligament in anterior tibial translation and internal rotation. Am J Sports Med 35(2):223–227

Ziegler CG, Pietrini SD, Westerhaus BD et al (2011) Arthroscopically pertinent landmarks for tunnel positioning in single-bundle and double-bundle anterior cruciate ligament reconstructions. Am J Sports Med 39:743–752

Meniscal Allografts: Indications and Results

95

René Verdonk, Karl F. Almqvist, and Peter Verdonk

Contents

R. Verdonk (✉)
Faculty of Medicine, Ghent State University, Ghent, Belgium
e-mail: rene.verdonk@ugent.be

K.F. Almqvist
Department of Orthopaedic Surgery, Ghent University Hospital, Ghent, Belgium
e-mail: karlfredrikalmqvist@gmail.com

P. Verdonk
Antwerp Orthopaedic Center, Monica Hospitals Antwerpen, Antwerpen, Belgium

Department of Orthopaedic Surgery and Traumatology, Ghent University Hospital, Ghent, Belgium
e-mail: pverdonk@yahoo.com

M.N. Doral, J. Karlsson (eds.), *Sports Injuries*,
DOI 10.1007/978-3-642-36569-0_74

Abstract

Meniscal allograft transplantation has emerged as a useful treatment for carefully selected patients. Almost all studies, from short to long term (>10 years of follow-up), report patient satisfaction and improvement in pain and function. Physical examination findings are improved objectively in the majority of patients. Radiologically, joint space narrowing is only significantly progressive at long-term follow-up. On magnetic resonance imaging (MRI), shrinkage is seen after some years, but more in lyophilized allografts. Histologically, incomplete repopulation of the graft is noticed. Second-look arthroscopy usually shows good healing of the capsule. In a recent long-term study, progression of cartilage degeneration according to MRI and radiological criteria was halted in a number of patients, indicating a chondroprotective effect.

However, there still is a lack of consensus on how the success of a meniscal transplantation should be evaluated, which makes it difficult to compare study outcomes. According to our experiences, radiographic measurement of joint space narrowing and changes in meniscal allograft MR signal are the best assessment tools, but the use of a good clinical evaluation system, such as the International Knee Documentation Committee (IKDC) and the Hospital for Special Surgery (HSS) scoring system, remains essential.

Indications

According to current recommendations, meniscal allograft transplantation is indicated in three specific clinical settings:

1. Young patients with a history of **meniscectomy** who have pain localized to the meniscus-deficient compartment, a stable knee joint, no malalignment, and articular cartilage with only minor evidence of osteochondral degenerative changes (no more than grade 3 according to the International Cartilage Repair Society (ICRS) classification system (Table 1)) are considered ideal candidates for this procedure. Some studies (Cameron and Saha 1997; Noyes and Barber-Westin 1995; Verdonk et al. 2005; Ryu et al. 2002; Stone et al. 2006; Bhosale et al. 2007) have shown that meniscal allografts can survive in an osteoarthritic joint (Outerbridge grades 3–4), with significant improvement in pain and function. Because of the more rapid deterioration in the lateral compartment (Walker and Erkman 1975), a relatively common indication for meniscal transplantation would be a symptomatic, meniscus-deficient, lateral compartment.
2. Anterior cruciate ligament (ACL)-deficient patients who have had previous medial meniscectomy with concomitant ACL reconstruction and who might benefit from the increased stability afforded by a functional medial meniscus. It is the authors' conviction that an ACL graft is significantly protected by the meniscus allograft as much as the meniscus is protected by an ACL graft.

Table 1 International Cartilage Repair Society Cartilage Lesion Evaluation System

Grade 0	Normal
Grade 1	Superficial lesions, softening, fissures, or cracks
Grade 2	Lesions, erosion, or ulceration of less than 50 %
Grade 3	Partial-thickness defect of more than 50 %, but less than 100 %
Grade 4	Ulceration and bone exposure

3. In an effort to avert early **joint degeneration**, some also consider young, athletic patients who have had total meniscectomy as candidates for meniscal transplantation prior to the onset of symptom (Johnson and Bealle 1999). However, the results obtained so far still preclude a return to high-impact sports.

Contraindications

Advanced chondral degeneration is considered a contraindication to meniscal allograft transplantation, although some studies suggest that cartilage degeneration is not a significant risk factor for failure (Cole et al. 2003). In general, greater than grade 3 articular cartilage lesions, according to the ICRS classification system, should be of limited surface area and localized. Localized chondral defects may be treated concomitantly, as meniscus transplantation and cartilage repair or restoration may benefit each other in terms of healing and outcome (Rodeo 2001). Chondrocyte transplantation or osteochondral grafting procedures should be performed after completion of the meniscal transplantation in order to prevent accidental damage to the patch or graft during meniscal allograft insertion (Cole and Cohen 2000). Radiographic evidence of significant osteophyte formation or femoral condyle flattening is associated with inferior postoperative results because these structural modifications alter the morphology of the femoral condyle (Rijk 2004). Generally, patients over age 50 have excessive cartilage lesions and are suboptimal candidates. Axial malalignment tends to exert abnormal pressure on the allograft leading to loosening, degeneration, and failure of the graft (Rijk 2004). A corrective osteotomy should be considered in patients with more than two degrees of deviation toward the involved compartment, as compared with the mechanical axis of the contralateral limb. Varus or valgus deformity may be managed with either staged or concomitant high tibial or distal femoral osteotomy (Cole and Cohen 2000). However, as in any situation in which procedures are combined, it is unclear which aspect of the procedure is implicated in resolution of symptoms, such as relief of pain (Rijk 2004). Other contraindications to meniscal transplantation are obesity, skeletal immaturity, instability of the knee joint (which may be addressed in conjunction with transplantation), synovial disease, inflammatory arthritis and previous joint infection, and obvious squaring of the femoral condyle.

Technique for Meniscal Transplantation

Preoperative Considerations

In contrast to the use of deep-frozen allografts, a strict time schedule from harvest to transplantation is mandatory for **viable allografts**. The transplantation of viable meniscal allografts implies the availability of *viable* donor tissues, cultured in vitro immediately following harvest. Sizing of the graft is critical for correct implantation. For deep-frozen allografts, the mediolateral and anteroposterior lengths of the tibial plateau of the receptor are measured on a calibrated X-ray and transferred to the tissue bank. Since viable meniscal allografting is more limited in size options due to the fact that there is only one donor and a limited number of acceptors, the most appropriate acceptor is chosen based on corresponding donor-acceptor height and weight criteria. Once a patient is deemed to be a candidate for this type of procedure, 30–50 ml of autologous serum is prepared and frozen at −21 °C. The waiting time for a viable meniscal allograft averages 2 months – ranging from 14 days to 6 months – at our institution. Once an appropriately sized meniscal allograft is harvested, the patient is notified and an operation is planned within the next 14 days.

Surgical Technique

Introduction

The purpose of this technical chapter is to present medial and lateral meniscal allograft transplantation (1) as an open procedure or (2) as an arthroscopically assisted procedure. Both techniques use primarily soft tissue fixation of the allograft to the native meniscal rim. Additional transosseous fixation of the anterior and posterior horn is used in the arthroscopic technique, while a tag on the anterior horn is used in the open procedure for soft tissue-bone fixation.

Anesthesia and Surgical Preparation

These items are identical for the open and arthroscopic procedure. The choice of anesthesia is made in consultation between the surgeon, the anesthesiologist, and the patient and depends on patient's age, comorbidity, and history with regard to previous anesthesia. General anesthesia is preferred at our institution.

The patient is then positioned supine on the operating table. A lateral leg holder is positioned at the height of the tourniquet with the leg positioned in 90° of flexion. A foot holder is used to hold the leg in 90 and 110° of flexion as needed. Previous skin incisions are marked. The limb is exsanguinated and the tourniquet is inflated. The limb is then prepared with chlorhexidine gluconate-alcohol solution (Hibitane, Regent Medical Overseas Limited, Manchester, UK) and draped at the mid-thigh level.

Allograft Preparation for the Open Procedure

As previously described elsewhere, the allograft is positioned and fixed on a specially designed corkboard with three 25 gauge needles (Verdonk et al. 2006). With a scalpel, the residual synovial tissue is dissected from the allograft meniscus at the meniscosynovial junction level and discarded. The upper side of the allograft is marked with a methylene blue skin marker. Horizontal 2/0 polydioxanone surgical sutures (PDS II mounted on a double small needle, Ethicon, Somerville, NJ, USA) or 2/0 nonabsorbable polypropylene sutures (Prolene mounted on a double small needle, Ethicon, Somerville, NJ, USA) are placed every 3–5 mm through the posterior horn, the body, and the anterior horn of the allograft and fixed onto a specially designed suture holder (holder A). The senior surgeon (RV) prefers the use of 2/0 Prolene sutures for the posterior horn since this suture material comes with slightly smaller needles and therefore has easier surgical handling in the more narrow posterior joint space. The sutures are fixed onto the suture holder in sequence from posteriorly to anteriorly. Generally, 6–8 sutures are needed to cover the complete allograft.

Open Meniscal Allograft Transplantation

A medial or lateral parapatellar incision of approximately 8 cm is made with the knee in 90° of flexion to gain access to the involved compartment of the knee joint. The joint capsule is then opened, and the anterior horn of the meniscus remnant is transsected.

For the lateral procedure, the iliotibial band is released subperiosteally from its distal attachment. To further open up the lateral compartment, the insertion of the lateral collateral ligament (LCL) and popliteus tendon (PT) is detached with a curved osteotomy on the femoral side (Fig. 1). The center of the osteotomy bone block is first predrilled with a 2.7 mm drill. This facilitates subsequent refixation with a screw and washer. The osteotomy is done in a clockwise direction from the 8 o'clock position to the 4 o'clock position and is approximately 1.5 cm deep and conically shaped. The bone block is gently folded out using a bone clamp, and then the osteotomy is completed inferiorly from the 4 o'clock to the 8 o'clock position using the osteotome. The lateral joint space can now be opened up easily 1–2 cm by placing the knee in the figure-of-four position in 70–90° of flexion with the index foot positioned across the contralateral limb.

For the medial procedure, the medial collateral ligament is detached on the femoral side with an osteotomy (Goble et al. 1999). A flake osteotomy (0.5–1 cm in thickness) is done with a straight osteotome at the level of the medial femoral epicondyle. The soft tissues posterior to the medial collateral ligament are left in continuity. By gently placing the knee in a valgus position, the medial compartment can now be opened up in a controlled fashion.

The meniscus remnant is trimmed preferably to a stable meniscal rim with a scalpel anteriorly and with arthroscopic instruments posteriorly.

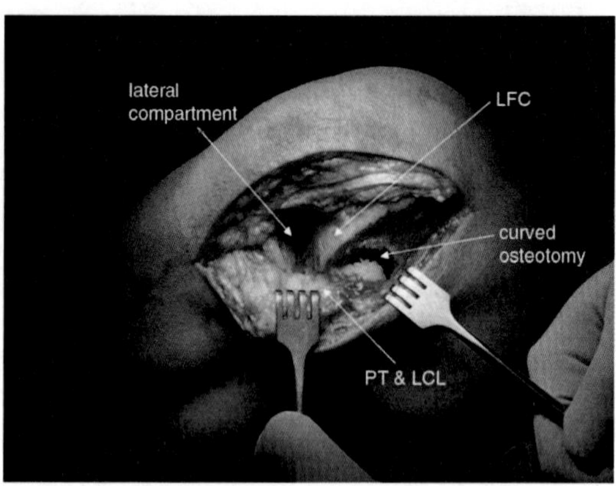

Fig. 1 Open meniscal allograft transplantation. To further open the lateral compartment, the LCL and PT are detached with a curved osteotomy on the femoral side

Most often, the insertion of the posterior horn is still intact and in continuity with the tibial plateau. The insertion of the posterior horn is also trimmed to fit the allograft. The meniscal rim deserves surgical attention, as it serves as a strong envelope encapsulating the medial or lateral compartment of the knee.

The meniscal remnant level is then marked with a small mosquito clamp anteriorly as a landmark for the correct level of subsequent fixation of the allograft. Next, the previously prepared viable meniscal allograft is introduced into the knee compartment. The sutures are taken from the holder in the correct sequence from posteriorly to anteriorly and driven through the meniscal rim one by one in an all-inside fashion from inferiorly to superiorly and transferred to a second suture holder (holder B), again in a sequence from posteriorly to anteriorly. The lateral allograft is also sutured to the popliteus tendon. The follow-up arthroscopies revealed that the popliteal hiatus will recreate itself naturally. The insertion of the anterior horn of the meniscus is not yet sutured at this stage of the operation. Once the sequence of suture transfer from holder A through the meniscal rim (and the popliteus tendon) to holder B is completed, the allograft is introduced into the compartment by gently pulling on each suture in a sequence from posteriorly to anteriorly. Generally, this procedure has to be performed progressively to establish a secure fit of the allograft to the

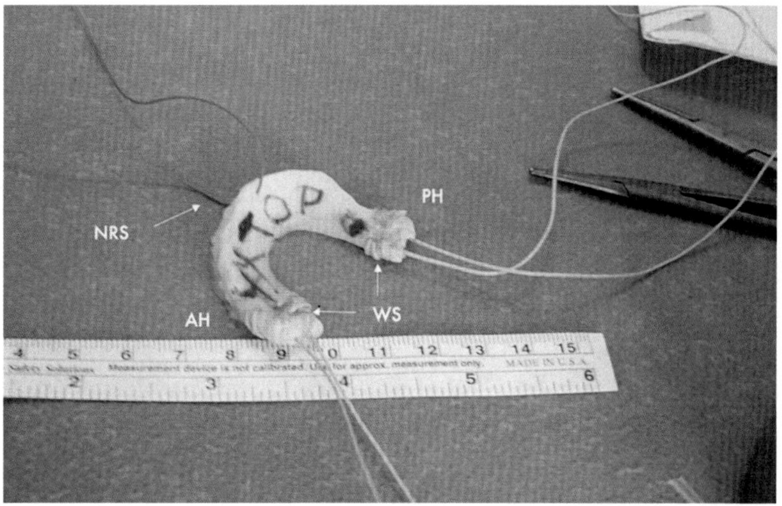

Fig. 2 Prepared lateral meniscal allograft for arthroscopic meniscal transplantation. Whipstitches(*WS*) on the inner and outer rim of anterior (*AH*) and posterior horn (*PH*). A vertical non-resorbable suture (*NRS*) is placed on the posterolateral corner, just anteriorly of the PT hiatus

meniscal rim. The suture knots are then securely tied and cut. A fine-tipped suture driver and a knot pusher are frequently required to securely tighten the posterior sutures. The knee is now positioned again in a normal 90° flexed position. The bone block of the collateral ligament and popliteus tendon is repositioned and fixed using a 35 or 40 mm 2.9 AO cancellous screw with a spiked washer. The anterior horn of the allograft is then fixed to the tibia using an anchor (GII, DePuy Mitek, Raynham, Massachusetts, USA). The Hoffa fat pad and knee capsule are closed using interrupted Vicryl 1/0 (Ethicon, Somerville, NJ, USA) cross-stitches after hemostasis.

Allograft Preparation for the Arthroscopic Procedure

The allograft is positioned and fixed on a specially designed corkboard with three 25 gauge needles. With a scalpel, the residual synovial tissue is dissected from the allograft meniscus at the meniscosynovial junction level and discarded. The upper side of the allograft is marked with a methylene blue skin marker.

Non-resorbable high-strength (Fiber wire, Arthrex, Naples, USA) sutures are placed in the anterior and posterior horn of the allograft. Generally, three whipstitches are placed on the inner and outer rim of the horn of the allograft. An additional vertical non-resorbable suture (Ethibond 2/0, Somerville, NJ, USA) is placed at the posteromedial or posterolateral corner of the medial or lateral allograft, respectively. For the lateral allograft, the posterolateral suture is positioned just anteriorly to the popliteus tendon hiatus as this will serve as a landmark during arthroscopy (Fig. 2).

Arthroscopically Assisted Lateral Meniscal Allograft Transplantation

The classic anteromedial and anterolateral portals are made. An additional anteromedial portal is positioned very medially to gain easy instrumental access for the debridement and resection of the anterior portion of the native lateral meniscus. Using shaver and punch, the remnant meniscus is debrided to the level of the meniscal rim.

A modified ACL aiming device, with a low-profile tip, is inserted through the medial portal and positioned at the anatomical posterior horn of the lateral meniscus just posterior to the ACL (Fig. 3). A guide pin is drilled first and subsequently overdrilled by a 4.5 mm cannulated drill. A double-looped metal wire is introduced through the tunnel from outside-in and picked up intra-articularly with an arthroscopical grasper and pulled out through the lateral portal. Subsequently, a suture passer (Acupass, Smith and Nephew, Memphis, Tennessee, USA) is introduced twice from outside-in just anterior to the lateral collateral ligament and the popliteus tendon into the joint: one just below and the second

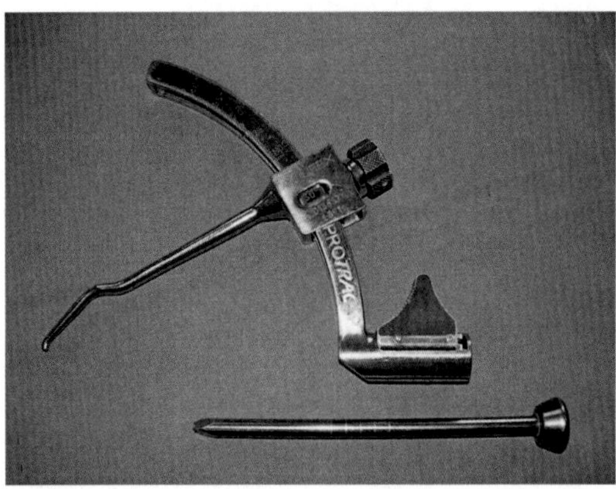

Fig. 3 Modified ACL aiming device, with low-profile tip. This device is positioned at the anatomical posterior horn of the lateral meniscus, just posterior to the ACL

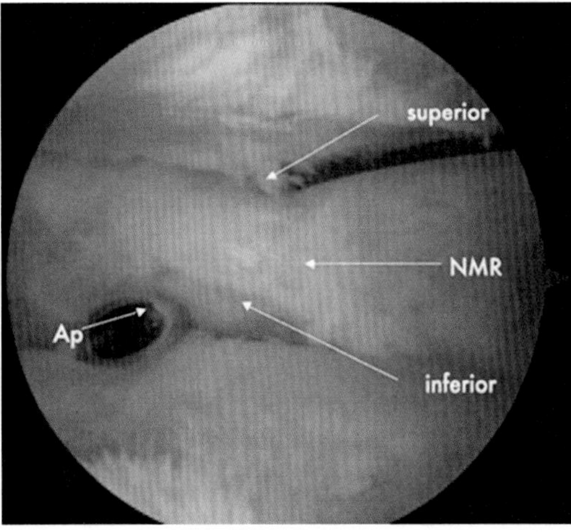

Fig. 4 A suture passer (Acupass® Ap) is introduced twice from outside-in, just anterior to the LCL and the PT, superior and inferior of the native meniscal rim (NMR)

above the native meniscal rim (Fig. 4). The looped wires are picked up and pulled out again through the lateral portal. Next, the posterior horn pull suture and the posterolateral pull suture are pulled through using the double-looped metal wire and the double-looped suture pass wire. The prepared lateral allograft is subsequently introduced into the lateral compartment throughout an enlarged lateral portal by pulling progressively on the posterolateral pull suture and the posterior horn pull suture. Care should be taken that the graft does not flip upon introduction and that pull wires do not intertwine. Risk for intertwining wires is greatly reduced by using a double-looped metal wire for the posterior horn.

The posterior horn is now positioned correctly. Its position can be slightly modified more toward the posterolateral corner or more toward the posterior horn by pulling more on the posterolateral or posterior horn traction wire. One or two all-inside meniscal fixation devices (Fastfix, Smith and Nephew, Memphis, Tennessee, USA) are used to fix the allograft to the meniscal rim. Fixation should be started in the posterolateral corner. Subsequently inside out horizontal Ethibond 2/0 sutures are used for fixing the body of the allograft. The anterior horn is fixed using outside-in PDS or Ethibond 2/0 sutures.

Prior to making the sutures knots, the anterior horn is introduced into the knee joint, and the anatomical insertion site is identified and prepared in the same manner as for the posterior tunnel. If necessary, its position can be slightly adapted to the graft position. Similar to the procedure of the posterior horn, the anterior tunnel is prepared and the traction suture is pulled through.

First, the meniscal inside out sutures are knotted. Subsequently, the anterior and posterior horn traction sutures are knotted to each other over a bone bridge on the anteromedial side of the tibia. This procedure reduces the possibly stretched capsule and native meniscal rim tied to the meniscal allograft, by pulling on the anterior and posterior horn by a transosseus suture fixation.

Arthroscopically Assisted Medial Meniscal Allograft Transplantation

A similar procedure as for the lateral allograft transplantation is performed for the medial allograft transplantation. However, some steps are different and will be highlighted in this section.

Additional to the classic anteromedial and anterolateral portal, a posteromedial portal should be used to identify the original posterior horn attachments of the native meniscus (Fig. 5). Using the same drill guide, the transosseus tunnels can be prepared. These tunnels should be prepared starting on the anterolateral side of the tibia. This direction is more in line with the forces on the traction sutures.

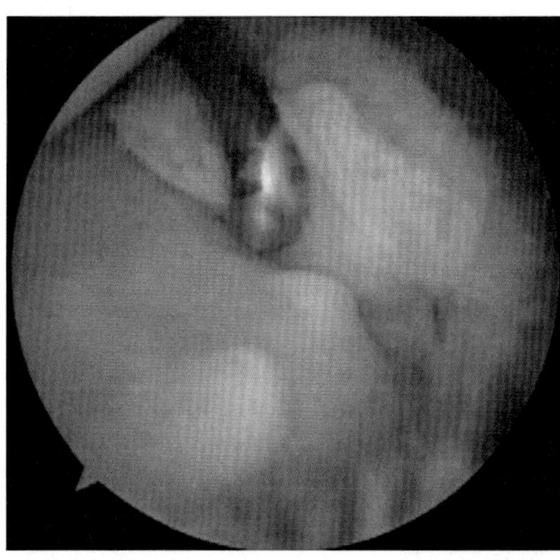

Fig. 5 Arthroscopic view of the posteromedial portal used in arthroscopically assisted medial meniscal allograft transplantation. The custom ACL guide in introduced through the intercondylar notch on the anatomical posterior horn insertion of the native medial meniscus

A posteromedial traction suture is used, as in accordance to the lateral allograft. On the medial side, however, a clear anatomical landmark such as the popliteal hiatus on the lateral side is lacking.

The anterior horn of the native medial meniscus may in some cases be very anterior on the tibial plateau resulting in a very short transosseus anterior tunnel.

Special note on soft tissue versus bone block fixation (Messner and Verdonk 1999, Paletta et al. 1997, Huang et al. 2003, Chen et al. 1996, Alhalki et al. 1999):

Biomechanical cadaver studies have shown the superiority of a bony fixation over a soft tissue fixation technique, although a recent cadaver study showed comparable results. Bony fixation, however, has also been shown to be associated with increased risk for cartilage lesions if implanted incorrectly and an increased immunological potential due to the presence of allogeneic bone. It is the authors' experience that perfect allograft size matching is essential if bony fixation is to be used. A malpositioned bone block or plugs can inflict damages to the overlying cartilage. Too small a graft will result in a need to overtension the inside out sutures and possible failure of the soft tissue fixation. Therefore, limited oversizing of the graft is commonly advocated using bone plugs or blocks. Separate bone plugs have the potential advantage that the implantation can be somewhat more variable compared to a single bone block. In addition, on the lateral side, a straight bone block sometimes induces the need to sacrifice some posterolateral fibers of the ACL.

Today, clinical and/or radiological differences have not been shown between soft tissue and bone block fixation.

Rehabilitation

Rehabilitation is initially focused on providing mobility to the joint without endangering ingrowth and healing of the graft. Therefore, 3 weeks of non-weight bearing is prescribed followed by 3 weeks of partial weight bearing (50 % of body weight). Progression to full weight bearing is allowed from week 6 on to week 10 postoperatively. The use of a knee brace is not strictly necessary and depends on the morphology and profile of the patient. For the same reasons, range of motion is limited during the first 2 weeks from 0 to 30, to increase by 30° each 2 weeks.

Isometric muscle tonification and co-contraction exercises are prescribed from day 1 postsurgery onward. Straight leg raise, however, is prohibited during the first 3 weeks. Proprioception training is started after week 3.

Swimming is allowed after week 6, biking after week 12, and running is progressively promoted starting at week 20.

Conclusion

In conclusion, ample evidence has been presented to support meniscus allograft transplantation in meniscectomized painful knees, with observance of the proper indications. Significant relief of pain and improvement in function have been achieved in a high percentage of patients. These improvements appear to be long lasting in 70 % of patients. Based on plain radiology and MRI, a subset of patients does not show further cartilage degeneration, indicating a potential chondroprotective effect. The lack of a conservatively treated control group is considered a fundamental flaw in the reported studies, making it difficult to establish the true chondroprotective effect of this type of treatment. Based on the presented results, meniscus allograft transplantation should no longer be considered as an experimental surgery for the meniscectomized painful knee.

Cross-References

▶ Arthroscopic Repair of the Meniscus Tears
▶ Human Meniscus: From Biology to Tissue Engineering Strategies
▶ Meniscal Substitutes: Polyurethane Meniscus Implant: Technique and Results
▶ Meniscectomy
▶ Meniscus Reconstruction Using a New Collagen Meniscus Implant

References

Alhalki MM, Howell SM, Hull ML (1999) How three methods for fixing a medial meniscal autograft affect tibial contact mechanics. Am J Sports Med 9 (27):320–328

Bhosale AM, Myint P, Roberts S, Menage J, Harrison P, Ashton B, Smith T, McCall I, Richardson JB (2007) Combined autologous chondrocyte implantation and allogenic meniscus transplantation: a biological knee replacement. Knee 14(5):361–368

Cameron JC, Saha S (1997) Meniscal allograft transplantation for unicompartmental arthritis of the knee. Clin Orthop 337:164–171

Chen MI, Branch TP, Hutton WC (1996) Is it important to secure the horns during lateral meniscal transplantation? A cadaveric study. Arthroscopy 12:174–181

Cole BJ, Cohen B (2000) Chondral injuries of the knee. A contemporary view of cartilage restoration. Orthop Spec Ed 6:71–76

Cole BJ, Carter TR, Rodeo SA (2003) Allograft meniscal transplantation: background, techniques, and results. Instr Course Lect 52:383–396

Goble EM, Verdonk R, Kohn D (1999) Arthroscopic and open surgical techniques for meniscus replacement–meniscal allograft transplantation and tendon autograft transplantation. Scand J Med Sci Sports 9(3):168–176

Huang A, Hull ML, Howell SM (2003) The level of compressive load affects conclusions from statistical analyses to determine whether a lateral meniscal autograft restores tibial contact pressure to normal: a study in human cadaveric knees. J Orthop Res 21:459–464

Johnson DL, Bealle D (1999) Meniscal allograft transplantation. Clin Sports Med 18:93–108

Messner K, Verdonk R (1999) It is necessary to anchor the meniscal transplants with bone plugs? A mini-battle. Scand J Med Sci Sports 9(3):186–187

Noyes FR, Barber-Westin SD (1995) Irradiated meniscus allografts in the human knee: a two to five year follow-up. Orthop Trans 19:417

Paletta GA Jr, Manning T, Snell E, Parker R, Bergfeld J (1997) The effect of allograft meniscal replacement on intraarticular contact area and pressures in the human knee. A biomechanical study. Am J Sports Med 25:692–698

Rijk PC (2004) Meniscal allograft transplantation – part I: background, results, graft selection and preservation, and surgical considerations. Arthroscopy 20:728–743

Rodeo SA (2001) Meniscal allografts – where do we stand? Am J Sports Med 29:246–261

Ryu RK, Dunbar VWH, Morse GG (2002) Meniscal allograft replacement: a 1-year to 6-year experience. Arthroscopy 18:989–994

Stone KR, Walgenbach AW, Turek TJ, Freyer A, Hill MD (2006) Meniscus allograft survival in patients with moderate to severe unicompartmental arthritis: a 2- to 7-year followup. Arthroscopy 22(5):469–478

Verdonk PC, Demurie A, Almqvist KF, Veys EM, Verbruggen G, Verdonk R (2006) Transplantation of viable meniscal allograft. Surgical technique. J Bone Joint Surg Am 88:109–118

Verdonk PCM, Demurie A, Almqvist KF, Veys EM, Verbruggen VR (2005) Transplantation of viable meniscal allograft: survivorship analysis and clinical outcome of one hundred cases. J Bone Joint Surg Am 87:715–724

Walker PS, Erkman MJ (1975) The role of the menisci in force transmission across the knee. Clin Orthop 109:184–192

Meniscal Substitutes: Polyurethane Meniscus Implant: Technique and Results

96

René Verdonk, Peter Verdonk, and Eva Lisa Heinrichs

Contents

R. Verdonk (✉)
Faculty of Medicine, Ghent State University, Ghent, Belgium
e-mail: rene.verdonk@ugent.be

P. Verdonk
Antwerp Orthopaedic Center, Monica Hospitals Antwerpen, Antwerpen, Belgium

Department of Orthopaedic Surgery and Traumatology, Ghent University Hospital, Ghent, Belgium
e-mail: pverdonk@yahoo.com; peter.verdonk@ugent.be

E.L. Heinrichs
Tissue Therapies Europe, Tissue Therapies Europe Ltd – Global Med Affairs, Daresbury Cheshire, UK
e-mail: heinrichsel@aol.com

M.N. Doral, J. Karlsson (eds.), *Sports Injuries*,
DOI 10.1007/978-3-642-36569-0_75

Abstract

Pain and other short- and long-term sequelae of irreparable meniscal tears remain a challenge for the orthopedic community, and there is a genuine need for an approach which will offer patients and surgeons new acceptable treatment options (Gilbert and Ashwood, Trauma 9:189–194, 2007).

Orteq Ltd. (London, UK) has developed a polyurethane scaffold, Actifit® (Welsing et al., Am J Sports Med 36:1978-1989, 2008), for blood vessel ingrowth and meniscal tissue regeneration (Tienen et al., Am J Sports Med 34:64-71, 2006) intended for the treatment of irreparable, painful meniscus tears and meniscal tissue defects. It is available in the medial and lateral configurations (Fig. 1). Criteria for use include an intact meniscal rim and sufficient tissue in the anterior and posterior horns to permit fixation of the scaffold. Other requirements include a well-aligned and stable knee joint, an ICRS classification grade ≤ 3, a body mass index <35 kg/m^2, and the non-presence of systemic disease or infection sequelae (Arnosky andWarren, Am J Sports Med 10:90–95, 1982).

Introduction

Pain and other short- and long-term sequelae of irreparable meniscal tears remain a challenge for the orthopedic community, and there is a genuine

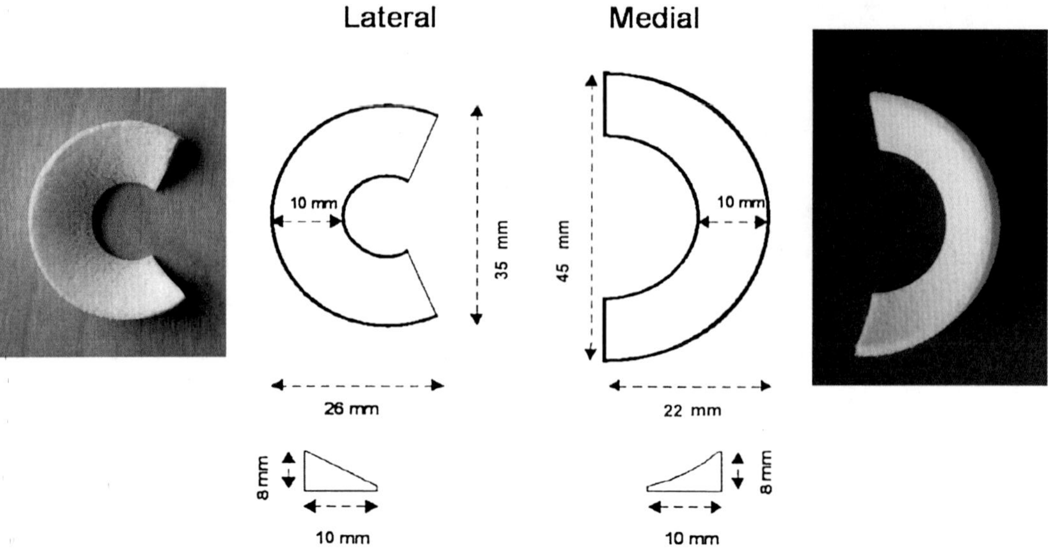

Fig. 1 The Actifit® meniscal scaffold comes in medial and lateral configurations

need for an approach which will offer patients and surgeons new acceptable treatment options (Gilbert and Ashwood 2007).

Orteq Ltd (London, UK) has developed a polyurethane scaffold, Actifit® (Welsing et al. 2008), for blood vessel ingrowth and meniscal tissue regeneration (Tienen et al. 2006) intended for the treatment of irreparable, painful meniscus tears and meniscal tissue defects. It is available in the medial and lateral configurations (Fig. 1). Criteria for use include an intact meniscal rim and sufficient tissue in the anterior and posterior horns to permit fixation of the scaffold. Other requirements include a well-aligned and stable knee joint, an ICRS classification grade ≤ 3, a body mass index <35 kg/m^2, and the absence of systemic disease or infection sequelae (Arnoczky and Warren 1982; Verdonk et al. 2008).

Implantation Procedure, Postoperative Care, and Rehabilitation

Implantation Procedure

Implantation of the Actifit® meniscal scaffold is performed arthroscopically using standard surgical arthroscopic knee procedures and equipment. Detailed instructions and related warnings and precautions are set out in the Instructions for Use accompanying the device.

Using spinal or general anesthesia, at the discretion of the orthopedic surgeon, the implantation of the Actifit® meniscal scaffold is usually performed under tourniquet conditions. Thigh fixation may be used for appropriate valgus stress positioning.

Prior to implantation of either the medial or the lateral scaffold, cartilage status and meniscal wall remnant status and integrity should be assessed. In the case of the lateral meniscus, meniscal wall integrity across the hiatus popliteus is essential for secure fixation and optimal tissue regeneration. All pathological cartilage and ligamentous findings should be carefully recorded.

In the case of a tight medial compartment, the medial collateral ligament (MCL) can be distended using the outside-in puncture method. Under valgus stress, and directed by the inside arthroscopic light, the surgeon is able to place a needle in the posteromedial side of the knee joint into the joint. The MCL is sensed and allows for progressive pie-crusting of the ligament until the appropriate opening is obtained.

The inside-out pie-crusting release technique as described by Steadman can also be used. Under

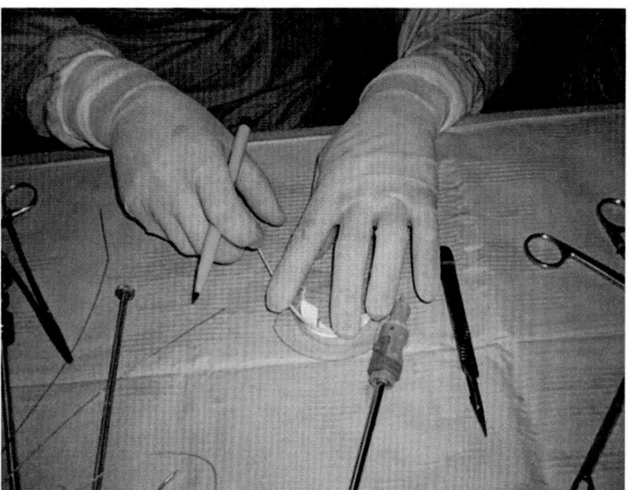

Fig. 2 The Actifit meniscal scaffold is tailored using a scalpel for a snug fit to the meniscus defect

arthroscopic control, the posteromedial corner of the knee joint is visualized. Using the Steadman pick or a spinal needle, the MCL can be reached and progressively disrupted in order to open the knee joint appropriately until visualization is obtained.

In the lateral compartment progressive pie-crusting release techniques as described above and used in the medial compartment are not possible because of anatomical considerations; however, lateral compartment narrowing is rare.

To facilitate healing, the meniscal rim can be punctured for vascular access channels and gentle rasping of the synovial lining is recommended. After debridement and preparation, the defect should reach into the red-red or red-white zone, approximately 1–2 mm from the synovial border. The defect should thereafter be measured along its inner margin using the meniscal ruler and meniscal ruler guide which accompany the Actifit® device.

The Actifit® meniscal scaffold should be measured and cut using a scalpel (Fig. 2). Sterility should be continually maintained. Care should be taken not to undersize the device. For the purpose of achieving a snug fit into the defect, the length of the scaffold should be oversized by approximately 10 %, i.e., 3 mm for small defects (<3 cm) and approximately 5 mm for large defects (≥3 cm). It is recommended that the anterior side be cut at an angle of 30–45° for easier suturing (Fig. 3).

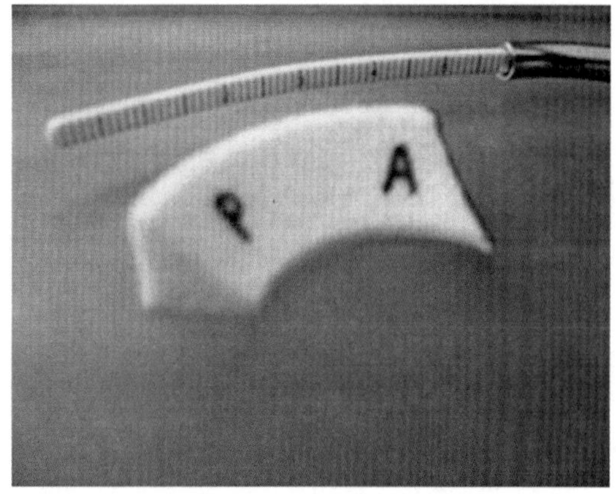

Fig. 3 The anterior side should cut at an angle of 30–45° for easier suturing

For the implantation two to three small incisions for anteromedial and anterolateral portals are needed. An arthroscopic central transpatellar tendon portal is optional. For easy insertion of the scaffold, it is recommended that the relevant portal is sized sufficiently to approximately the size of the little finger. In addition, a posteromedial or posterolateral incision may be required if an inside-out meniscal suture fixation technique is used.

Although the Actifit® material is easy to manipulate and is strong and flexible, it should be handled with care. The tailored Actifit® scaffold can be introduced into the knee joint through the anteromedial or anterolateral portal using a non-cannulated tissue tension grasper such as the Acufex Grasper Tissue Tensioner™ (Smith & Nephew) (Fig. 4). Marking the cranial and caudal scaffold surface helps to avoid problems in positioning. The Actifit® scaffold should be clamped at the posterior part of the scaffold and placed into the knee joint through the anteromedial or anterolateral portal. To ensure a good initial position of the scaffold and facilitate fixation, a vertical holding suture may be placed in the native meniscus tissue to bring the scaffold through the eye of this holding suture.

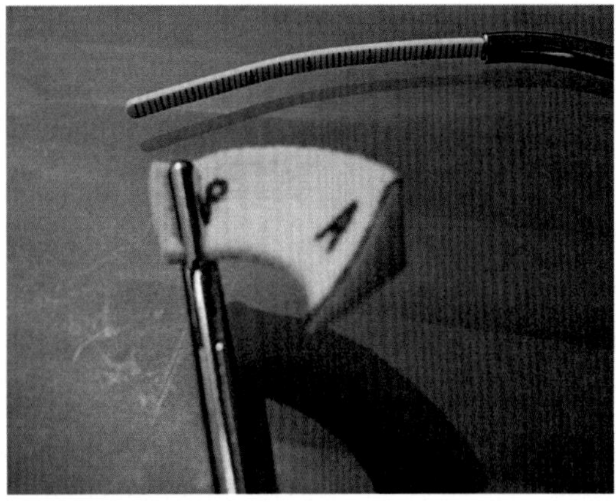

Fig. 4 The scaffold device should be manipulated using a blunt nose grasper. It is useful to mark the cranial and caudal meniscal scaffold surface

Fixation of Actifit® is accomplished by suturing the scaffold to the native meniscus tissue. Standard commercially available size 2.0 non-resorbable sutures, such as polyester or polypropylene and braided or monofilament sutures, are recommended. Which suturing techniques are used depends on the location of the defect and the surgeon's experience and preference (Hardeman et al. 2013). All-inside suturing is commonly used for the posterior horn and posterior part of the rim. All-inside, inside-out, and outside-in techniques may be used for the middle and anterior part of the rim. Horizontal sutures with an outside-in technique are commonly used for the anterior horn.

Fixation should start with a horizontal all-inside suture from the posterior edge of the scaffold to the native meniscus. Suturing should be secure; however, sutures must not be overtightened because they may alter and indent the surface of the scaffold. The distances between the sutures should be kept to approximately 0.5 cm (Fig. 5a). Each suture should be placed at one-third to one-half of the scaffold's height, as determined from the lower surface of the scaffold (Fig. 5b). Suturing through the popliteus tendon is not detrimental to later function (De Coninck et al. 2013a).

Once sutured in place if required, the scaffold may be further trimmed and fine-tuned intra-articularly using a basket punch. Stability of the fixation is tested using a probe and carefully moving the knee through a range of motion (0–90°).

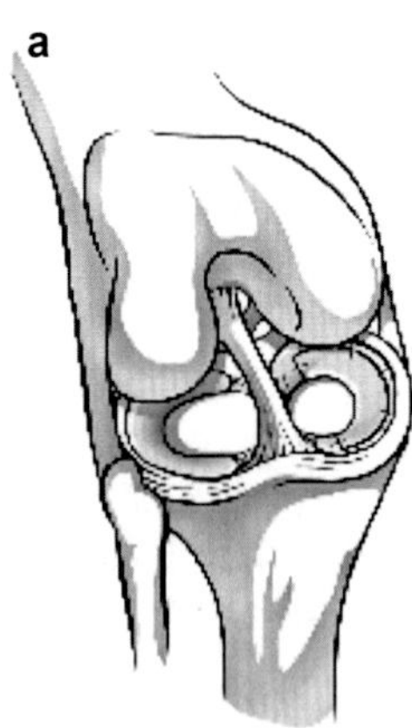

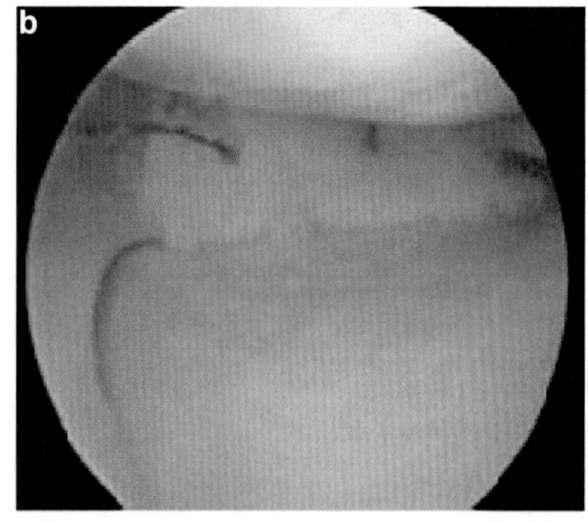

Fig. 5 (**a**) The distances between the sutures should approximately 0.5 cm. (**b**) Each suture should be placed at one-third to one-half of the scaffold height determined from the lower surface of the scaffold in order to allow proper fixation

Postoperative Care

Following implantation of the Actifit® scaffold, pain and thromboprophylactic medications are administered at the surgeon's discretion and would be those typically administered following classic meniscal suturing.

Dependent upon the meniscal scaffold stability as determined at the end of the surgical procedure, a rigid removable brace may be used over a compression bandage in the first week postimplantation.

Postoperative Rehabilitation

Following implantation of the Actifit® scaffold, the recommended postoperative rehabilitation protocol should be strictly followed to ensure optimum conditions for healing and to protect the newly formed fragile tissue from potentially harmful stresses while tissue remodeling and maturation processes are ongoing during the first 3 months postsurgery. It is important that the rehabilitation protocol is reviewed and approved to be suitable for the patient in question by the responsible orthopedic surgeon and carried out under the supervision of a professional physiotherapist.

Non-weight-bearing is recommended until 4 weeks postsurgery. Partial weight-bearing is permitted from 4 weeks onward with a gradual increase in loading up to 100 % load at 9 weeks postimplantation, at a rate of 10 kg per week for patients weighing ≤60 kg and 15 kg per week for patients weighing ≤90 kg, and without the use of the unloader brace from week 14 onward.

Under the rehabilitation protocol, motion is initiated immediately after implantation, with bending up to 30° with full extension permitted in weeks 1 and 2. Flexion is increased to 60° in week 3, and to 90° in weeks 4 and 5. From week 6 onward, flexion is further increased until a full range of motion is achieved; however, forceful movements should be avoided. Light exercise, including isometric quadriceps exercises, mobilization of the patella, heel slides, quad sets, anti-equinus foot exercises, and Achilles tendon stretching, is advised from week 1. After 9 weeks, additional exercises, including increased closed hamstring exercises, lunges between 0 and 90°, proprioception exercises, dynamic quadriceps exercises, and use of a home trainer, are indicated. Increased open and closed exercises, jogging on level ground, plyometrics, and sports-related exercises without pivoting are recommended from week 14 onward. Hydrotherapy and swimming (crawl stroke and headstroke) can commence 24 weeks postimplantation. Gradual resumption of other sports is generally commenced as of 6 months at the discretion of the responsible orthopedic surgeon; however, contact sports should be resumed only after 9 months.

Clinical Results

Safety, performance, and efficacy results to support use of the Actifit® scaffold in the treatment of painful irreparable meniscal defects were obtained from a prospective, nonrandomized, single-arm, clinical investigation conducted at nine orthopedic centers of excellence located throughout Europe. Patients recruited ($N = 52$) had an irreparable medial or lateral meniscus tear or partial meniscus loss, intact rim, both horns, and a stable well-aligned knee.

Thirty-four patients were treated with a medial meniscal scaffold and 18 patients were treated with a lateral meniscal scaffold. Demographics and baseline characteristics were representative of the population for which Actifit® is intended. The mean patient age was 30.8 ± 9.4 years and 75 % were male. The mean longitudinal defect length was 47.1 ± 10.0 mm.

The study follow-up period was 24 months and the study has been reported in the American Journal of Sports Medicine (Verdonk et al. 2012; De Coninck et al. 2013b).

Safety Results

Nine index knee-related Serious Adverse Events (SAEs) were reported in the study (five in the medial and four in the lateral indication). Three of these in the medial indication and three in the lateral indication resulted in removal. Four of the nine SAEs were reported as unrelated to the scaffold and to the procedure; four were reported as procedure related; none were reported as having a definite, probable, or possible relationship to the Actifit® scaffold.

One SAE was reported as having an unknown relationship to the Actifit® scaffold and to the procedure. This was the removal of an almost completely nonintegrated scaffold, which took place at the protocol-stipulated relook arthroscopy. The patient was asymptomatic, and importantly no signs of inflammatory reaction to the scaffold and no evidence of cartilage damage were observed during gross examination. A biopsy specimen taken from the meniscus rim post removal of the nonintegrated scaffold material showed cell-populated scaffold material integrated with tissue. No inflammatory reaction to the scaffold was observed in the biopsy. It was concluded that the integration failure was most likely due to the lack of biological response.

Cartilage scores in the index compartment were assessed at 3, 12, and 24 months postimplantation using anatomical MRI scans. Stable or improved cartilage status at 24 months was demonstrated in 92.5 % (37/40) of patients compared with baseline status.

Efficacy Results

Pain and functionality were assessed using validated clinical outcome scores. The Visual Analog Scale (VAS) was used for knee pain at 3, 6, 12, and 24 months postimplantation. The International Knee Documentation Committee (IKDC), the Lysholm score, as well as the Knee and Osteoarthritis Outcome Score (KOOS) were used to assess functionality.

For functionality on IKDC and Lysholm scores and for pain (VAS), statistically and clinically significant improvements from baseline to 24 months were reported at 3, 6, 12, and 24 months postimplantation ($p < 0.05$).

Statistically and clinically significant improvements ($p < 0.05$) were also reported for the five KOOS subcomponents: for pain, for activities of daily living and quality of life at 3, 6, 12, and 24 months, and for sports/recreation and symptoms at 6, 12, and 24 months postimplantation.

Evidence of New Tissue Formation

Tissue ingrowth into the Actifit® scaffold was assessed during the protocol-stipulated relook arthroscopy at 12 months ($n = 44$) by gross examination and histological examination of biopsies from the inner free edge of the implanted scaffold. The presence of vital tissue with no necrosis or cell death and hence consistent with biocompatibility of the scaffold was observed in all 44 biopsies at 12 months. Moreover, the histology data suggested an ongoing process of regeneration, remodeling, and maturation toward tissue resembling the human meniscus.

Tissue ingrowth was also assessed at 3 months postimplantation by evidence of vascularization in the scaffold using diagnostic contrast-enhanced MRI (DCE-MRI) ($n = 43$). All scans were assessed for neovascularization in the peripheral half of the scaffold meniscus.

At 3 months postimplantation, early evidence of tissue ingrowth was observed on DCE-MRI in the peripheral half of the scaffold, in 35 of 43(81.4 %) patients.

Conclusions

No safety concerns, other than those generally acknowledged with this type of surgery, were identified. Importantly, no safety issues related to the device, including cartilage damage or inflammatory reaction to the Actifit® scaffold or its degradation products, were observed. Efficacy data showed significant (statistical and clinical) improvement from preoperative status for the subjective clinical outcome scores as of 3 months to 24 months postimplantation. The 24-month clinical results provide strong evidence of the safety and efficacy of the Actifit® scaffold treatment option for a patient group for whom currently only restricted treatment options are available. In addition, compared to partial meniscectomy, treatment of irreparable meniscus defects with the

Actifit® scaffold has the benefit of promoting new tissue regeneration (Verdonk et al. 2008; Maher et al. 2009). The 5-year evaluation of the patients with Actifit meniscal implantation shows strong clinical evidence of good function and long-term pain relief in the indexed compartment. These findings are supported by well-positioned implant at MRI imaging at 5 years, however, still not comparable to the normal contrast of the physiological meniscus appearance.

References

Arnoczky SP, Warren RF (1982) Microvasculature of the human meniscus. Am J Sports Med 10:90–95

De Coninck T, Huysse W, Verdonk P et al (2013a) Open versus arthroscopic meniscus allograft transplantation: magnetic resonance imaging study of meniscal radial displacement. Arthroscopy 29(3):514–521. doi:10.1016/j.arthro.2012.10.029

De Coninck T, Huysse W, Verdonk P et al (2013b) Two-year follow-up study on clinical and radiological outcomes of polyurethane meniscal scaffolds. Am J Sports Med 41(1):64–72

Gilbert R, Ashwood N (2007) Meniscal repair and replacement: a review of efficacy. Trauma 9:189–194

Hardeman F, Corten K, Verdonk P et al (2013) What is the best way to fix a polyurethane meniscal scaffold? A biomechanical evaluation of different fixation modes. Knee Surg Sports Traumatol Arthrosc. [Epub ahead of print]

Maher SA, Doty SB, Rosenblatt L et al (2009) Evaluation of a meniscal repair scaffold in an ovine model. Poster presented at the 55th Annual Meeting of the Orthopaedic Research Society, Las Vegas, 22–25 February 2009

Tienen TG, Heijkants RG, de Groot JH et al (2006) Replacement of the knee meniscus by a porous polymer implant: a study in dogs. Am J Sports Med 34:64–71

Verdonk PCM, Van Laer MEE, Verdonk R (2008) Meniscus replacement: from allograft to tissue engineering. Sports Orthop Traumatol 24:78–82

Verdonk P, Beaufils P, Verdonk R, Actifit Study Group et al (2012) Successful treatment of painful irreparable partial meniscal defects with a polyurethane scaffold: two-year safety and clinical outcomes. Am J Sports Med 40(4):844–853

Welsing RT, van Tienen TG, Ramrattan N et al (2008) Effect on tissue differentiation and articular cartilage degradation of a polymer meniscus implant: a 2-year follow-up study in dogs. Am J Sports Med 36:1978–1989

Meniscectomy

97

Mahmut Nedim Doral, Gazi Huri, Kadir Büyükdoğan, Özgür Ahmet Atay, Alp Bayramoglu, and Egemen Turhan

Contents

Abstract

The menisci have several functions in the knee joint. They distribute load over the tibia and absorb the shock within the joint. They contribute to stability and proprioception and aid the lubrication and nutrition of the articular cartilage. Therefore, complete or partial loss of a meniscus can have damaging effects on a knee, leading to serious long-term problems. This chapter summarizes the body of evidence in the literature in terms of meniscus anatomy, function, tears, and surgical technique and reviews the consequences of meniscectomy.

M.N. Doral (✉)
Department of Orthopaedics and Traumatology and Department of Sports Medicine, Hacettepe University, Istanbul, Turkey
e-mail: ndoral@hacettepe.edu.tr

G. Huri
Department of Orthopaedics and Traumatology, Hacettepe University, Ankara, Turkey

Division of Shoulder Surgery, Department of Orthopaedic Surgery, Johns Hopkins University, Baltimore, MD, USA
e-mail: gazihuri@hacettepe.edu.tr

K. Büyükdoğan • E. Turhan
Faculty of Medicine, Department of Orthopaedics and Traumatology, Hacettepe University School of Medicine, Ankara, Sihhiye, Turkey
e-mail: kadirbuyukdogan@gmail.com; dregementurhan@yahoo.com

Ö.A. Atay
Faculty of Medicine, Department of Orthopaedics and Traumatology, Hacettepe University, Ankara, Sihhiye, Turkey
e-mail: oaatay@hacettepe.edu.tr

A. Bayramoglu
Faculty of Medicine, Department of Anatomy, Acibadem University School of Medicine
e-mail: info@acibadem.edu.tr

M.N. Doral, J. Karlsson (eds.), *Sports Injuries*,
DOI 10.1007/978-3-642-36569-0_71

Introduction

The meniscus is one of the essential structures for knee joint stabilization. It acts as a secondary anteroposterior stabilizer of the knee joint, aids in proprioception, and contributes to the lubrication and nutrition of the articular cartilage (Zimny et al. 1988; Hollis et al. 2000).

Among all musculoskeletal tendinous and ligamentous injuries, meniscal injuries are the most common type of injuries with an incidence of 23.8/100,000 per year and may cause knee pain and functional impairment (Clayton and Court-Brown 2008). They may result either from acute knee trauma or by a joint degeneration process. Improving the function, pain relief, and prevention of knee joint degeneration are the main goals of treatment. Currently, there are several treatment options for meniscal injuries such as conservative treatment, meniscectomy, repair, and transplantation (McCarty et al. 2002). Understanding of the substantial function and biology of the meniscus, literature encourages repairs rather than meniscectomies (Fairbank et al. 1984; Xu and Zhao 2013). However, not all meniscal tears can be repaired and meniscectomy is unavoidable in many cases. The incidence of meniscectomy in the population is reported to be 61 in 100,000 per year (Baker et al. 1985).

In this chapter, the anatomical properties and biomechanics of the meniscus and review of the literature about principles and indications of meniscectomy were discussed.

Clinical Anatomy, Histology, and Function

The meniscus separates the tibia and femur to decrease the contact area between the bones and serves as a shock absorber reducing the peak contact force experienced (Seedhom et al. 1974). It has a chondroprotective function by reducing friction between the two bones to allow smooth movement in the knee and distribute load during movement (Voloshin and Wosk 1983). Furthermore, the meniscus provides secondary stabilization to the knee joint and contributes to proprioception by type 3 mechanoreceptors and enhances articular cartilage nutrition (Zimny et al. 1988; Renstrom and Johnson 1990). Reduction of proprioception and knee muscular ability in partial meniscectomized knees compared to the nonoperated leg was reported in the literature (Malliou et al. 2012).

The meniscus is relatively avascular excluding the peripheral rim. This limited blood supply originates predominantly from the lateral and medial inferior and middle geniculate arteries. Branches from these vessels form a perimeniscal capillary plexus within the synovial and capsular tissues and enter the meniscus particularly from anterior and posterior horns (Day et al. 1985). Regarding the degree of vascularization, the meniscus can be classified into three zones; the red-red, red-white, and white-white zones (Arnoczky and Warren 1982). In addition to the dense vascular plexus, the meniscal tissue is also richly innervated. Most of the larger nerves course in a circumferential manner and are closely associated with vessels. Smaller nerves and single axons run radially, in convoluted patterns, toward the outer one-third of the meniscus. The inner two-thirds has no nerve fibers (Day et al. 1985).

The medial meniscus is a C-shaped, fibrocartilage semicircular band that is located between the medial condyle of the femur and the tibia. Because of its strong attachments to tibia via meniscotibial bands (coronary ligaments), it is less mobile and more prone to tear than the lateral meniscus (Greis et al. 2002). In addition to the anterior cruciate ligament (ACL), it contributes to sagittal and coronal plane stability of knee joint. Therefore, it is more vulnerable to tear in ACL-deficient knees. Compared to the medial meniscus, the lateral meniscus is more circular in shape and covers a larger portion of the articular surface than the medial. It is attached to medial femoral condyle via the ligaments of Humphrey (the anterior meniscofemoral ligament) and Wrisberg (posterior meniscofemoral ligament). Unlike the medial meniscus, there is no attachment to its adjacent collateral ligament and has loose attachments via fascicles to the popliteus tendon. Therefore, it is more mobile compared to the medial meniscus.

Histologically, meniscal cartilage consists of a fibrocartilaginous tissue, which synthesizes fibrocartilage matrix, rather than hyaline cartilage matrix. Predominantly, it is composed of type 1 collagen fibers (98 %) and extracellular matrix (water, glycoproteins, and elastin). The parallel orientation of the collagen fibers to the peripheral border provides stiffness and strength. It resists compression, tension, and shear forces by these fibers. The meniscus can occasionally be injured or torn by twisting the knee or applying direct force, as seen in contact sports (Greis et al. 2002).

Evaluation and Diagnosis

The evaluation for meniscal tears is based on a thorough history, physical examination, and radiologic assessment. Pain along the joint line, swelling, locking, and catching are the most common symptoms. Furthermore, loss of extension of the knee might be an indicator of a displaced bucket handle meniscal tear. Subsequently, careful physical examination of the extremity should be done to figure out the meniscal pathologies. The presence of a joint effusion, quadriceps muscle atrophy/weakness, and joint line tenderness should be checked during examination. Specific tests such as McMurray and Apley tests are also useful in the diagnosis of meniscal tears. Evans et al. reported a high specificity (98 %) of the McMurray test in the diagnosis of the meniscal tears (Evans et al. 1993). On the other hand, Medlar et al. reported lower specificity and sensitivities for this test ranging from 30 % to 50 % (Medlar et al. 1980). Moreover, joint line tenderness was reported as the best predictor of a meniscal tear with a 74 % sensitivity (Weinstabl et al. 1997). In spite of poor sensitivity and specificity of these specific tests, the physical examination still remains a very useful tool in the diagnosis of meniscal tears.

There is correlation between ACL injuries and meniscal tears. Lateral meniscus tears occur more frequently in patients with acute ACL injury, whereas medial meniscus tears are more prevalent in chronic ACL-deficient knees (Duncan et al. 1995).

Among the imaging modalities, magnetic resonance evaluation is a powerful tool in the detection of the meniscal pathologies. Regarding the improved technology in visualization systems, the accuracy, sensitivity, and specificity are considered to be 95 %, 88 %, and 57 %, respectively (Raunest et al. 1991; Muellner et al. 1997; Aydingoz et al. 2003).

Classification of Meniscal Tears

Considering the pattern of meniscal tear that is observed during arthroscopy, it could be classified as vertical longitudinal, oblique, circumferential, complex, radial, and horizontal cleavage tears (Greis et al. 2002). Among all, the radial tears (Fig. 1) are the most common types, whereas the vertical longitudinal tears (bucket handle tears) are mostly associated with an acute ACL tear (Shelbourne and Dersam 2004). Because of strong attachments to the tibia, the medial meniscus is more prone to injury than the lateral side. Incomplete posterior horn tears are generally asymptomatic and may be diagnosed incidentally. The posterior and middle thirds of the medial meniscus are the most common side for tears.

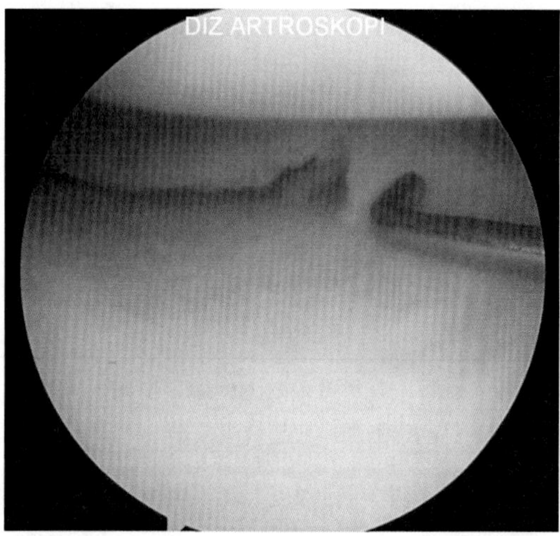

Fig. 1 Radial tear of the medial meniscus

Both flap/oblique and radial tears are typically located at that region of the meniscus.

Degenerative complex tears that generally start from the posterior horn are common in older patients. They are often associated with degenerative changes of the knee.

The type, size, and location of meniscal tears are important determinants to predict the healing capacity. The stable vertical longitudinal tears less than 10 mm, stable partial tears (less than 50 % of the meniscus thickness), and superficial tears are reported to heal spontaneously (Henning et al. 1988). However, most meniscal tears do not heal spontaneously. Regarding the vascular supply, the location of a tear can be the red-red, red-white, or white-white zone. Arnoczky and Warren demonstrated that almost only one-third of the meniscal body is vascular (Arnoczky and Warren 1982). The red-red zone tears have an excellent healing prognosis, whereas the white-white zone that is completely avascular has a poorer prognosis (Brindle et al. 2001).

Indications

There are several approaches described for the of meniscal tears such as conservative treatment, meniscectomy (total/partial), meniscus repair, and meniscal transplantation. However, the role of conservative treatment is limited. In order to decide on the best treatment option, the surgeon must consider the patient's age, activity level, and localization and type of the meniscal tear (DeHaven 1990). The indications for meniscectomy are (Greis et al. 2002):

- Symptoms refractory to conservative treatment
- Mechanical symptoms (locking, catching, and giving way)
- Avascular zone tears
- Irreducible or degenerative bucket handle tears
- Meniscal tears coexisting lower limb malalignment
- Degenerative changes of the articular cartilage
- Patient-related factors (age and level of activity, obesity, and quadriceps atrophy, etc.)

Meniscectomy

The intention of achieving long-term patient benefits leads many surgeons to develop meniscal repair techniques. In some instances, however, meniscectomy is still required and is the appropriate treatment. There are two types of meniscectomy described as partial and total. The aim is to remove the torn fragment that restricts the joint movement and avoid the friction and wear of articular cartilage due to torn edges.

Total Meniscectomy

Initially, total meniscectomy was defined as a standard treatment option of meniscus tears regarding its excellent short-term results (Perey 1962). However, following studies about potential risks of total meniscectomy, this procedure has fallen out of favor (Fairbank 1948; Jorgensen et al. 1987; Wroble et al. 1992). It was shown that there is a significant increase in contact pressure of adjacent articular surfaces after total meniscectomy (Krause et al. 1976; Baratz et al. 1986). The increased load leads to overload of the articular cartilage, which results in proteoglycan loss and disaggregation and promotes degeneration (Lanzer and Komenda 1990). There are also several publications about unsatisfactory long-term results after total meniscectomy (Tapper and Hoover 1969; Yocum et al. 1979). Tapper et al. reported the outcomes for 10–30 years after total meniscectomy and found less favorable results with a rate of only 38 % patients asymptomatic (Tapper and Hoover 1969). In addition, Yocum et al. reported that only half of 26 patients had satisfactory results at 7 years after meniscectomy (Yocum et al. 1979). Considering the disappointing results after total meniscectomy, alternative treatment options such as partial meniscectomy and repair have been recommended to preserve the meniscus as much as possible and avoid these complications. Recently partial meniscectomy has been a reasonable option when repair is not possible.

Partial Meniscectomy

Partial meniscectomy has become a preferable option over total meniscectomy since it was firstly introduced by Ikeuchi (1979). It provides a stable rim that prevents over pressuring as well as cartilage damage and affords for a more rapid return to activities of daily living. There are several publications that imply better clinical outcomes of partial meniscectomy compared to total (Northmore-Ball et al. 1983; Benedetto and Rangger 1993; McNicholas et al. 2000). In a retrospective study, the authors compared the results of three different types of meniscectomy in 219 knees, with a mean follow-up of 4.3 years, and they found better results after partial meniscectomy compared to total meniscectomy (Northmore-Ball et al. 1983). Similarly, Burks et al. studied outcomes of partial meniscectomy with a nearly 15-year follow-up. They reported a high rate of good or excellent clinical outcome with minimal degenerative changes compared with the untreated knee (Burks et al. 1997). Furthermore, Jaureguito et al. reported that 90 % of patients obtained good or excellent results and 85 % of the patients could resume their pre-injury-level activities at 2 years after partial meniscectomy (Jaureguito et al. 1995). Partial meniscectomy is also recommended as a treatment option for the treatment of meniscus variants. Atay et al. reported good and excellent results of partial lateral meniscectomy in the management of discoid meniscus tears after a mean of 5-year follow-up (Atay et al. 1997; Atay et al. 2003). However, there are still debates about long-term results and its effectivity in degenerative tears. The authors reported that knees which underwent partial meniscectomy are more prone to degeneration compared with the contralateral side at long-term follow-up (Fauno and Nielsen 1992; Rangger et al. 1995). Additionally, the amount of meniscus removed and grade of degeneration at the time of the meniscectomy have a noticeable influence on long-term functional results. Especially meniscectomy that includes over 50 % of meniscus reported to have worse radiographic changes (Higuchi et al. 2000). A multicentric study demonstrated that there is no additional benefit from arthroscopic partial meniscectomy on pain and function in the group of patients with a degenerative meniscus tear (Hare et al. 2013). Likewise, Yim et al. did not find significant difference between arthroscopic meniscectomy and nonoperative management for degenerative tears with a mean of 2-year follow-up (Yim et al. 2013).

Partial meniscectomy appears to be less favorable for treatment of lateral meniscus tears. A comparative study of medial versus lateral arthroscopic partial meniscectomy with a 10-year minimum follow-up revealed significantly worse radiologic results after lateral meniscectomy (Chatain et al. 2003). In an in vivo study, the investigators showed that the peak contact stress in articular cartilage increased 200 % more after a lateral meniscectomy than a medial meniscectomy (Pena et al. 2006).

Surgical Technique

Standard anterolateral and anteromedial portals are created in order to position the instruments and perform the diagnostic arthroscopy. For an accurate diagnostic arthroscopy, the scope is inserted in the lateral portal (viewing portal), whereas the probe is placed through the medial (working portal). However, in further steps, based on the pathology, the locations of the portals may change. For instance, in order to visualize the posterior horn lesion of medial and lateral menisci, lateral and medial portals are preferred as viewing portals, respectively. Moreover, the medial portal provides a great visualization of the lesion at the anterior horn of medial meniscus, whereas the lateral portal is good to identify the mid-third of the body of lateral meniscus (Jeong et al. 2012).

The goals of the partial meniscectomy are (Newman et al. 1993):

- To remove all damaged, abnormal, or unstable meniscal tissue

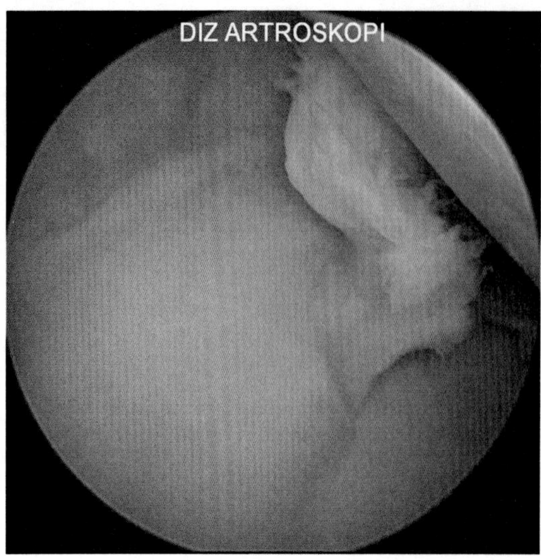

Fig. 2 Oblique/displaced tear of the medial meniscus

- To preserve as much normal meniscus as possible in order to preserve the load transmission properties of the remaining rim

Principles and surgical approaches for treatment of meniscal tears differ individually according to the type of tear. In the treatment of **oblique tears** (Newman et al. 1993; Doral et al. 2010) (Fig. 2), morsalization of the fragment is the first step of the surgery. Then, the longitudinal component is resected by arthroscopic scissors and removed using a grasper. Subsequently, the anterior and posterior edges of the meniscus are trimmed to prevent stress risers in the remaining meniscal rim (Fig. 3). Resection of **vertical longitudinal tears** (Newman et al. 1993; Doral et al. 2010) starts with reduction of the displaced fragment. Partial synovectomy may be required in order to expose

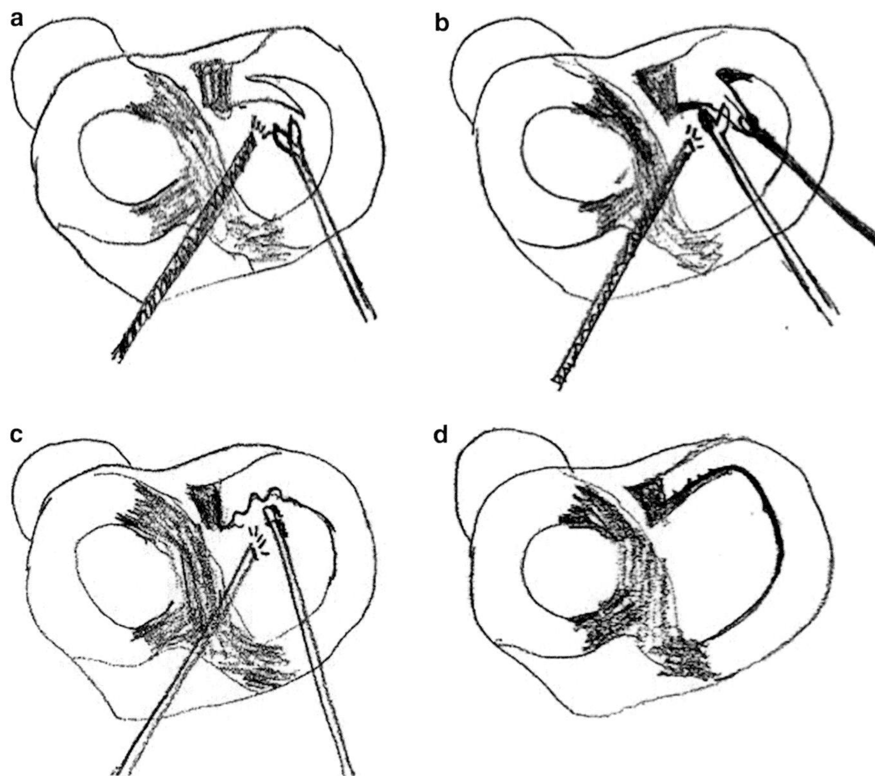

Fig. 3 Illustration of surgical technique for oblique tear of the meniscus

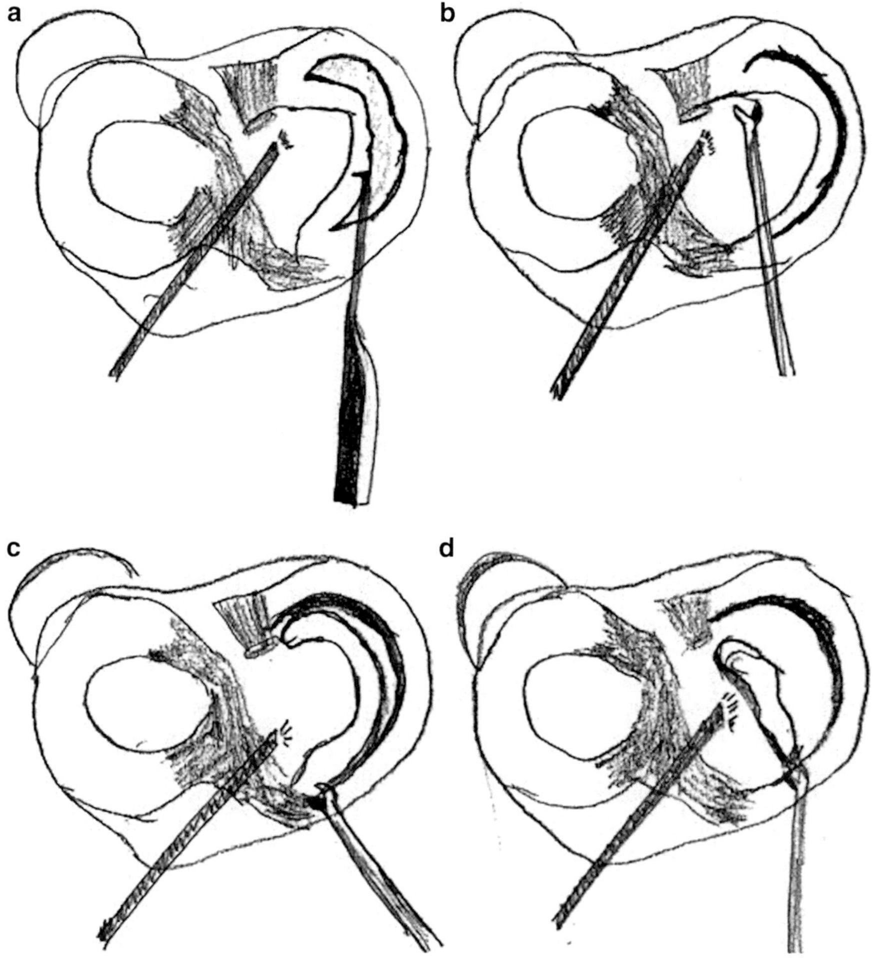

Fig. 4 Illustration of surgical technique for longitudinal tear of the meniscus

the anterior horn. Then, the posterior attachment is excised first followed by excision of the anterior attachment. After removal of the central fragment, the anterior and posterior attachment sites are trimmed to recreate a smooth, tapered inner margin. Finally, the central fragment should be checked for an existence of a hidden tear behind the fragment (Fig. 4). The approach to **radial tears** (Newman et al. 1993) is quite challenging. Prior to resection, identify the meniscal tear size with a probe. Then, resect the tear using basket forceps with different angels. Ensure that enough meniscal tissue has been excised to recreate a smooth, tapering C-shaped central edge (Fig. 5). In the case of **horizontal cleavage tears**, careful evaluation with a probe is necessary to indicate the amount of the resection as well as to address the unstable leaf or leaves. Following the resection of the unstable leaf (s), probing should be done once again to assess mobility of the remaining meniscal rim. Then the peripheral rim is trimmed to achieve a smooth edge (Fig. 6).

A **complex tear of the meniscus** is usually a combination of an oblique flap with peripheral horizontal extension. A partial excision of the tear since providing a stable rim is adequate in the majority of cases. However, care should be taken to still preserve as much peripheral tissue (including the meniscocapsular junction) as possible (Fig. 7).

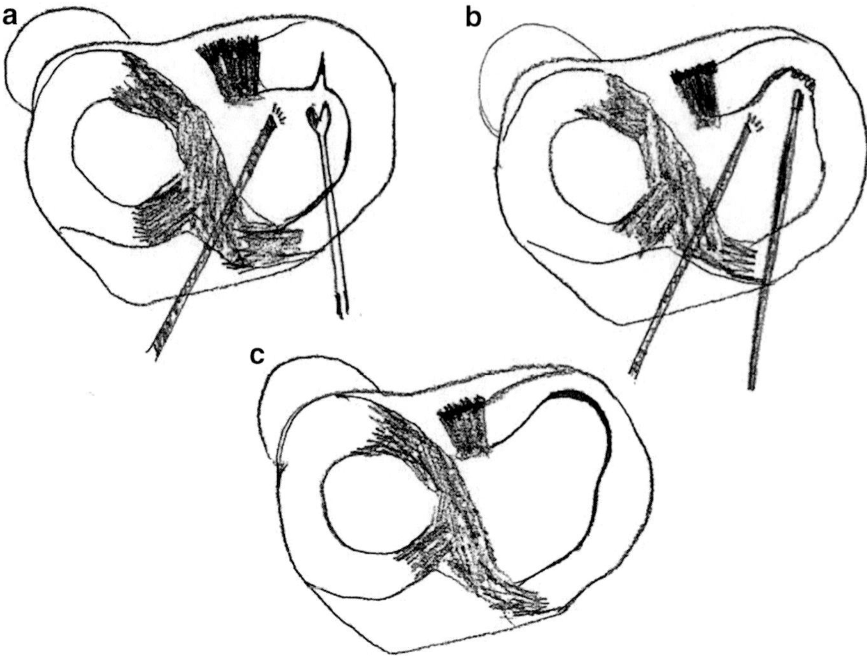

Fig. 5 Illustration of surgical technique for radial meniscus tear

In general, arthroscopic meniscectomy is a very effective surgery. However, like any surgical procedure, it can be comprised by complications. Overresection, iatrogenic articular cartilage damage, neurovascular injury, persistent drainage from portals, infection, persistent pain, and arthrofibrosis are the main complications after procedure. They can exist due to the failures in recognizing concomitant injuries, malposition of the portals, or misidentification of the components of a meniscus tear (Kinsella and Carey 2013).

Rehabilitation

Rehabilitation following a partial medial or lateral meniscectomy can usually progress as tolerated, with no contraindications or limitations due to the fact that there is no anatomic structure that must be protected. The goals are early control of pain and edema, immediate weight bearing, obtaining and maintaining a full range of motion, and regaining proper quadriceps strength. Physical therapy associated with home exercises shown to be effective in improving the knee function and range of motion (Dias et al. 2013).

Conclusion and Future

There is still no agreement about the ideal treatment option for meniscal tears. However, the only consensus is that meniscal tear treatment should be performed with a focus on meniscal function preservation. Therefore, recently meniscus repairs are preferentially being performed over meniscectomies (Abrams et al. 2013). On the other hand, partial meniscectomy is still gold standard for irreparable tears. It provides good clinical improvement and lessens the risk of degenerative changes when it is performed using an appropriate surgical technique for preservation of the remaining meniscus on particularly selected patients.

Recently, tissue engineering and replacement strategies provide a novel approach for the

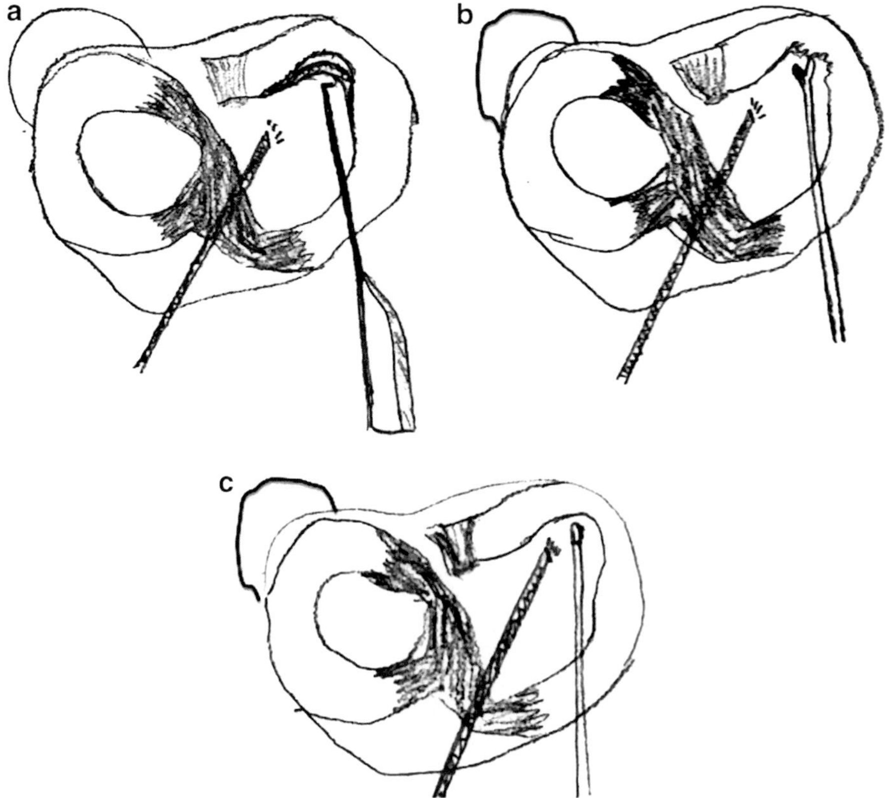

Fig. 6 Illustration of surgical technique for horizontal cleavage tear

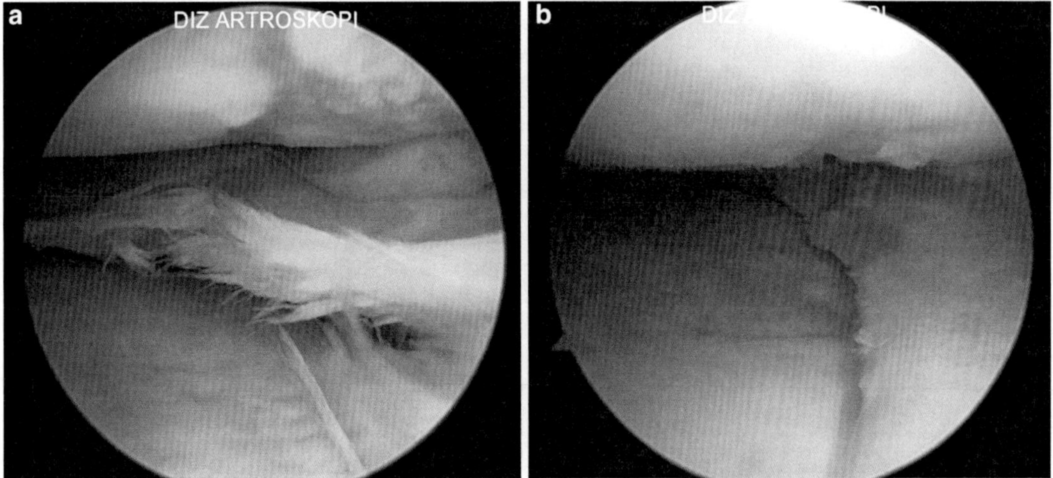

Fig. 7 (**a**) Complex tear of the medial meniscus, (**b**) the view of the medial meniscus after partial meniscectomy

treatment of severe meniscus injury. Many different concepts and approaches have been tried and tested, such as the application of natural and synthetic scaffolds, mesenchymal stem cells, growth factors, fibrin glue, and more (Welsing et al. 2008). Although they are not commonly used practically, we believe that tissue engineering and gene therapy will be the one of the most important and promising issues on the treatment of meniscal lesions.

References

Abrams GD, Frank RM, Gupta AK et al (2013) Trends in meniscus repair and meniscectomy in the United States, 2005–2011. Am J Sports Med 41:2333–2339

Arnoczky SP, Warren RF (1982) Microvasculature of the human meniscus. Am J Sports Med 10:90–95

Atay OA, Doral MN, Aksoy MC et al (1997) Arthroscopic partial resection of the discoid meniscus in children. Turk J Pediatr 39:505–510

Atay OA, Doral MN, Leblebicioglu G et al (2003) Management of discoid lateral meniscus tears: observations in 34 knees. Arthroscopy 19:346–352

Aydingoz U, Firat AK, Atay OA et al (2003) MR imaging of meniscal bucket-handle tears: a review of signs and their relation to arthroscopic classification. Eur Radiol 13:618–625

Baker BE, Peckham AC, Pupparo C et al (1985) Review of meniscal injury and associated sports. Am J Sports Med 13:1–4

Baratz ME, Fu FH, Mengato R (1986) Meniscal tears: the effect of meniscectomy and of repair on intraarticular contact areas and stress in the human knee. A preliminary report. Am J Sports Med 14:270–275

Benedetto KP, Rangger C (1993) Arthroscopic partial meniscectomy: 5-year follow-up. Knee Surg Sports Traumatol Arthrosc 1:235–238

Brindle TJ, Nyland J, Johnson DL (2001) The meniscus: review of basic principles with application to surgery and rehabilitation. J Athl Train 36:160–169

Burks RT, Metcalf MH, Metcalf RW (1997) Fifteen-year follow-up of arthroscopic partial meniscectomy. Arthroscopy 13:673–679

Chatain FP, Adeleine P, Chambat P, Neyret P (2003) A comparative study of medial versus lateral arthroscopic partial meniscectomy on stable knees: 10-year minimum follow-up. Arthroscopy 19:842–849

Clayton RA, Court-Brown CM (2008) The epidemiology of musculoskeletal tendinous and ligamentous injuries. Injury 39:1338–1344

Day B, Mackenzie WG, Shim SS et al (1985) The vascular and nerve supply of the human meniscus. Arthroscopy 1:58–62

DeHaven KE (1990) Decision-making factors in the treatment of meniscus lesions. Clin Orthop Relat Res 49–54

Dias JM, Mazuquin BF, Mostagi FQ et al (2013) The effectiveness of postoperative physical therapy treatment in patients who have undergone arthroscopic partial meniscectomy: systematic review with meta-analysis. J Orthop Sports Phys Ther 43:560–576

Doral MN, Donmez G, Bilge O et al (2010) Meniscectomy. Tech Knee Surg 9:150–158

Duncan JB, Hunter R, Purnell M et al (1995) Meniscal injuries associated with acute anterior cruciate ligament tears in alpine skiers. Am J Sports Med 23:170–172

Evans PJ, Bell GD, Frank C (1993) Prospective evaluation of the McMurray test. Am J Sports Med 21:604–608

Fairbank TJ (1948) Knee joint changes after meniscectomy. J Bone Joint Surg (Br) 30B:664–670

Fairbank JC, Pynsent PB, van Poortvliet JA et al (1984) Mechanical factors in the incidence of knee pain in adolescents and young adults. J Bone Joint Surg (Br) 66:685–693

Fauno P, Nielsen AB (1992) Arthroscopic partial meniscectomy: a long-term follow-up. Arthroscopy 8:345–349

Greis PE, Bardana DD, Holmstrom MC et al (2002) Meniscal injury: I. Basic science and evaluation. J Am Acad Orthop Surg 10:168–176

Hare KB, Lohmander LS, Christensen R et al (2013) Arthroscopic partial meniscectomy in middle-aged patients with mild or no knee osteoarthritis: a protocol for a double-blind, randomized sham-controlled multicentre trial. BMC Musculoskelet Disord 14:71

Henning CR, Clark JR, Lynch MA et al (1988) Arthroscopic meniscus repair with a posterior incision. Instr Course Lect 37:209–221

Higuchi H, Kimura M, Shirakura K et al (2000) Factors affecting long-term results after arthroscopic partial meniscectomy. Clin Orthop Relat Res 161–168

Hollis JM, Pearsall AW, Niciforos PG (2000) Change in meniscal strain with anterior cruciate ligament injury and after reconstruction. Am J Sports Med 28:700–704

Ikeuchi H (1979) Meniscus surgery using the Watanabe arthroscope. Orthop Clin N Am 10:629–642

Jaureguito JW, Elliot JS, Lietner T et al (1995) The effects of arthroscopic partial lateral meniscectomy in an otherwise normal knee: a retrospective review of functional, clinical, and radiographic results. Arthroscopy 11:29–36

Jeong HJ, Lee SH, Ko CS (2012) Meniscectomy. Knee Surg Relat Res 24:129–136

Jorgensen U, Sonne-Holm S, Lauridsen F et al (1987) Long-term follow-up of meniscectomy in athletes. A prospective longitudinal study. J Bone Joint Surg (Br) 69:80–83

Kinsella SD, Carey JL (2013) Complications in brief: arthroscopic partial meniscectomy. Clin Orthop Relat Res 471:1427–1432

Krause WR, Pope MH, Johnson RJ et al (1976) Mechanical changes in the knee after meniscectomy. J Bone Joint Surg Am 58:599–604

Lanzer WL, Komenda G (1990) Changes in articular cartilage after meniscectomy. Clin Orthop Relat Res 41–48

Malliou P, Gioftsidou A, Pafis G et al (2012) Proprioception and functional deficits of partial meniscectomized knees. Eur J Phys Rehabil Med 48:231–236

McCarty EC, Marx RG, DeHaven KE (2002) Meniscus repair: considerations in treatment and update of clinical results. Clin Orthop Relat Res 122–134

McNicholas MJ, Rowley DI, McGurty D et al (2000) Total meniscectomy in adolescence. A thirty-year follow-up. J Bone Joint Surg (Br) 82:217–221

Medlar RC, Mandiberg JJ, Lyne ED (1980) Meniscectomies in children. Report of long-term results (mean, 8.3 years) of 26 children. Am J Sports Med 8:87–92

Muellner T, Weinstabl R, Schabus R et al (1997) The diagnosis of meniscal tears in athletes. A comparison of clinical and magnetic resonance imaging investigations. Am J Sports Med 25:7–12

Newman AP, Daniels AU, Burks RT (1993) Principles and decision making in meniscal surgery. Arthroscopy 9:33–51

Northmore-Ball MD, Dandy DJ, Jackson RW (1983) Arthroscopic, open partial, and total meniscectomy. A comparative study. J Bone Joint Surg (Br) 65:400–404

Pena E, Calvo B, Martinez MA et al (2006) Why lateral meniscectomy is more dangerous than medial meniscectomy. A finite element study. J Orthop Res 24:1001–1010

Perey O (1962) Follow-up results of meniscectomy with regard to the working capacity. Acta Orthop Scand 32:457–460

Rangger C, Klestil T, Gloetzer W et al (1995) Osteoarthritis after arthroscopic partial meniscectomy. Am J Sports Med 23:240–244

Raunest J, Oberle K, Loehnert J et al (1991) The clinical value of magnetic resonance imaging in the evaluation of meniscal disorders. J Bone Joint Surg Am 73:11–16

Renstrom P, Johnson RJ (1990) Anatomy and biomechanics of the menisci. Clin Sports Med 9:523–538

Seedhom BB, Dowson D, Wright V (1974) Proceedings: functions of the menisci. A preliminary study. Ann Rheum Dis 33:111

Shelbourne KD, Dersam MD (2004) Comparison of partial meniscectomy versus meniscus repair for bucket-handle lateral meniscus tears in anterior cruciate ligament reconstructed knees. Arthroscopy 20:581–585

Tapper EM, Hoover NW (1969) Late results after meniscectomy. J Bone Joint Surg Am 51:517–526 passim

Voloshin AS, Wosk J (1983) Shock absorption of meniscectomized and painful knees: a comparative in vivo study. J Biomed Eng 5:157–161

Weinstabl R, Muellner T, Vecsei V et al (1997) Economic considerations for the diagnosis and therapy of meniscal lesions: can magnetic resonance imaging help reduce the expense? World J Surg 21:363–368

Welsing RT, van Tienen TG, Ramrattan N et al (2008) Effect on tissue differentiation and articular cartilage degradation of a polymer meniscus implant: a 2-year follow-up study in dogs. Am J Sports Med 36:1978–1989

Wroble RR, Henderson RC, Campion ER et al (1992) Meniscectomy in children and adolescents. A long-term follow-up study. Clin Orthop Relat Res 180–189

Xu C, Zhao J (2013) A meta-analysis comparing meniscal repair with meniscectomy in the treatment of meniscal tears: the more meniscus, the better outcome? Knee Surg Sports Traumatol Arthrosc

Yim JH, Seon JK, Song EK, Choi JI et al (2013) A comparative study of meniscectomy and nonoperative treatment for degenerative horizontal tears of the medial meniscus. Am J Sports Med 41:1565–1570

Yocum LA, Kerlan RK, Jobe FW et al (1979) Isolated lateral meniscectomy. A study of twenty-six patients with isolated tears. J Bone Joint Surg Am 61:338–342

Zimny ML, Albright DJ, Dabezies E (1988) Mechanoreceptors in the human medial meniscus. Acta Anat (Basel) 133:35–40

Meniscus Reconstruction Using a New Collagen Meniscus Implant

98

Maurilio Marcacci, Alberto Grassi, Giulio Maria Marcheggiani Muccioli, Marco Nitri, and Stefano Zaffagnini

Contents

M. Marcacci (✉) • A. Grassi • G.M.M. Muccioli
II Clinica Ortopedica e Traumatologica, Istituto Ortopedico Rizzoli, Bologna, Italy
e-mail: m.marcacci@biomec.ior.it; alberto.grassi@ior.it; marcheggianimuccioli@me.com

M. Nitri
Biomechanics Laboratory, Sports Traumatology Department, Istituto Ortopedico Rizzoli, Bologna, Italy
e-mail: marco.nitri@gmail.com

S. Zaffagnini
Clinica Ortopedica e Traumatologica II, Laboratorio di Biomeccanica e Innovazione Tecnologica, Università di Bologna, Bologna, Italy
e-mail: s.zaffagnini@biomec.ior.it; stefano.zaffagnini@unibo.it

M.N. Doral, J. Karlsson (eds.), *Sports Injuries*,
DOI 10.1007/978-3-642-36569-0_76

Abstract
Meniscal tears are the most common knee injuries, and for years meniscectomy has been considered the gold-standard treatment. As it is now well-known that even partial deficiency of the meniscus could be destructive for the knee joint in the long-term, meniscal substitution has gained popularity. The collagen meniscus implant (CMI) is a resorbable collagen template that supports ingrowth of new tissue and finally regeneration of lost meniscus tissue. The surgical technique is arthroscopic and the post-operative care following CMI resembles that of meniscal suture, with restricted weight-bearing and cautious joint mobilization. Often, complex cases involve a combined procedure such as anterior cruciate ligament (ACL) reconstruction, corrective osteotomy or cartilage treatment, as demonstrated by the high rate of concurrent procedures reported in the literature. The results for both lateral and medial meniscal substitution are generally good in most patients, with evidence of scaffold resorption and in-growth of meniscus-like tissue. The chondroprotective effect of the CMI has not been completely demonstrated, despite encouraging evidence suggesting a reduction of the degenerative changes in the articular cartilage.

Introduction

Meniscal tears are the most common knee injuries, with a reported annual incidence of 61 per 100,000 people (Baker et al. 1985). For years, meniscectomy has been considered the gold-standard treatment for meniscal lesions, due to a lack of knowledge regarding the role of the meniscus and the long-term effects of its deficiency. In fact, it is now well-known that even partial deficiency of the meniscus can be destructive for the knee joint in the long-term. It has been reported that meniscectomy increases the risk of developing knee osteoarthritis after 10 years in approximately 20 % of patients for the medial meniscus and 40 % for the lateral meniscus (Chatain et al. 2003). This is due to the important and irreplaceable functions of the meniscus: increasing congruity of the joint, reducing contact stresses, shock absorption, stabilization, proprioception, and cartilage lubrification and nutrition (McBride and Reid 1988; McDevitt and Webber 1990). For these reasons, the management of meniscal tears has changed dramatically over the years, from aggressive management towards more conservative strategies. Therefore, meniscal substitution using allografts and, more recently, scaffolds has been proposed in cases involving irreparable lesions.

Rationale and Development

The collagen meniscus implant (CMI) is a resorbable collagen template that supports ingrowth of new tissue and, finally, regeneration of lost meniscus tissue (Stone et al. 1992; Fig. 1). It is a porous collagen–glycosaminoglycan (GAG) matrix of defined geometry, density,

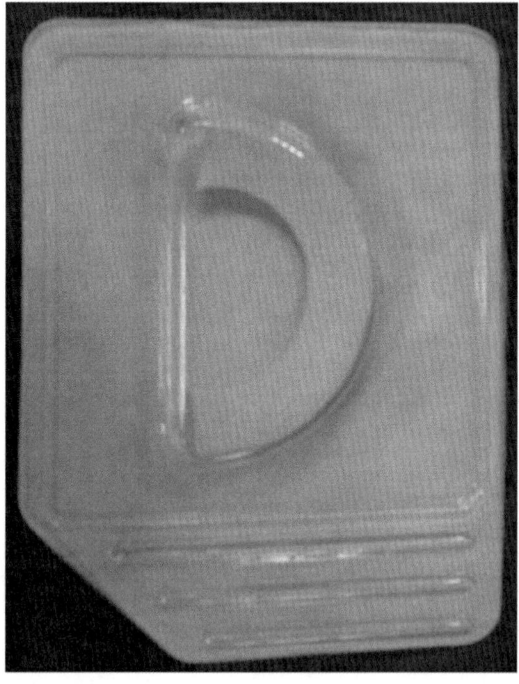

Fig. 1 Packed collagen meniscus implant

thermal stability, and mechanical strength (Li et al. 2002), composed of approximately 97 % purified type I collagen. The remaining portion of the CMI consists of GAGs, including chondroitin sulfate and hyaluronic acid. The type I collagen is isolated and purified from bovine Achilles tendon, then the collagen–GAG complex is chemically cross-linked to improve in vivo stability, handling, and implantation.

The suture pull-out strength of the fully hydrated CMI at 3 mm from the edge is greater than 20 N, permitting the implant to be properly positioned in the joint and fixed with sutures to the host meniscus remnant (Li et al. 2002).

In vitro studies have supported cellular ingrowth. The CMI has been tested on animal models, initially showing no evidence of cartilage wear or damage, and then signs of tissue regeneration (Stone et al. 1990, 1992). Later, animal studies confirmed these findings, showing healing of the implant-regenerated tissue to the host meniscus rim, and increasing amounts of tissue invasion and resorption of the CMI over time. This suggested a complete CMI resorption and replacement at 6 months in a canine model. Furthermore, magnetic resonance imaging (MRI) provided excellent correlation with the gross and histological observations, supporting the findings of continued tissue ingrowth and maturation over time.

These findings confirmed the safety of the device and showed the growth of meniscal-like tissue substituting the collagen CMI structure, allowing the possibility to implant CMI in humans.

Patient Selection and Pre-Operative Evaluation

Surgery for the meniscus-deficient knee should be considered only after a period of non-surgical treatment. When such treatment fails to provide relief of symptoms or to prevent joint space narrowing, CMI may be considered.

Accurate selection of patients and both clinical and radiological evaluation are mandatory in order to obtain a good result and prevent early failure.

Indication

CMI can be suggested in a patient who meets all of the following criteria:

- Prior loss of meniscus tissue
- Irreparable meniscus tears requiring partial meniscectomy
- Either traumatic or chronic post-traumatic meniscus tear
- Meniscus damage requiring more than 25 % removal
- Intact anterior and posterior attachments of the meniscus
- Intact rim over the entire circumference (except for the area of popliteal hiatus for lateral meniscus) of the involved meniscus
- Anterior cruciate ligament (ACL) deficiencies corrected within 12 weeks of CMI surgery
- Patients willing to follow a post-operative rehabilitation program
- Patients should be capable of understanding and following the doctor's instructions.

Treatment of an acute meniscal lesion with CMI is still a debated topic, as a multicentric study by Rodkey et al. (2008) reported no difference between CMI and partial meniscectomy for acute meniscal lesions at mid-term follow-up.

Contraindications

The main contraindications for CMI surgery are as follows:

- Concomitant posterior cruciate ligament insufficiency of the involved knee
- Grade IV degenerative cartilage disease in the affected joint
- Uncorrected malalignment of the involved knee
- Allergy to collagen of animal origin
- Allergy to chondroitin sulfate of animal origin
- Systemic or local infection
- History of anaphylactoid reaction

- Systemic administration of any type of corticosteriod, antineoplastic, immunostimulating or immunosuppressive agent within 30 days of surgery
- Evidence of osteonecrosis in the involved knee
- Medical history that is positive for, but not restricted to, the following diseases:
  - Rheumatoid arthritis
  - Severe degenerative osteoarthrosis.

Generally, the most common contraindication to CMI is advanced chondral degeneration, characterized by cartilage wear and radiographic evidence of osteophytes and femoral condyle flattening. Localized chondral defects may be addressed concomitantly with chondrocyte transplantation, osteochondral grafting, or synthetic scaffolds.

Malalignment is also reported to cause abnormal pressure on the affected compartment; therefore, a corrective osteotomy should be considered in the case of malalignment.

The lack of symptoms remains a controversial issue, as prophylactic CMI is not routinely recommended. In fact, the rehabilitation program after CMI is substantially different from that following partial meniscectomy. Furthermore, there is little evidence in favor of long-term prevention of arthrosis (Zaffagnini et al. 2011a).

Clinical Evaluation

An accurate history regarding knee trauma, injuries, and surgical procedures should be obtained. Knee pain, swelling, and mechanical symptoms exacerbated by physical activity are often present.

A physical examination should be performed and height, weight, and body mass index measured. With the patient standing, lower limb alignment is also evaluated. Range of motion (ROM) and ligament laxity are then assessed both for the affected and contralateral knee. Pain and tenderness should be reported for the affected compartment and ipsilateral quadriceps strength and circumference should be documented.

Radiological Evaluation

Accurate radiological planning is mandatory to correctly prepare for the surgery. Weight-bearing anteroposterior radiographs of both knees in full extension and a non-weight-bearing 45° flexion lateral radiograph are required. Rosenberg's view (45° flexion weight-bearing posteroanterior radiograph) can be helpful to detect subtle joint space narrowing, while mechanical axis radiography is necessary in case of low limb malalignment. MRI should be performed whenever possible, to evaluate the meniscal defect, ligament lesions, subchondral bone pathology, and cartilage status.

Surgical Technique

CMI is a surgical procedure that is mainly performed arthroscopically; therefore, good surgical skills are required in order to achieve correct placement and fixation of the device and positive outcomes. Although medial and lateral CMI are different in shape and size, and lateral and medial compartments present different anatomical features, the surgical technique is similar.

Patient Position

The patient is positioned supine, with the knee flexed to 90°. A leg holder is placed 5 cm proximal to the superior pole of the patella in order to allow valgus stress to open the medial compartment, while opening of lateral compartment is achieved by flexing the leg over the contralateral knee in the "figure-of-four" position.

Arthroscopic Setting

A medial suprapatellar portal is usually performed for water inflow, while routine anteromedial (AM) and anterolateral (AL) portals are made for the scope and instruments. The AL portal is placed distally to the patella in the soft spot, about 1–2 cm lateral to the patellar tendon; the AM portal is placed at the same level, about

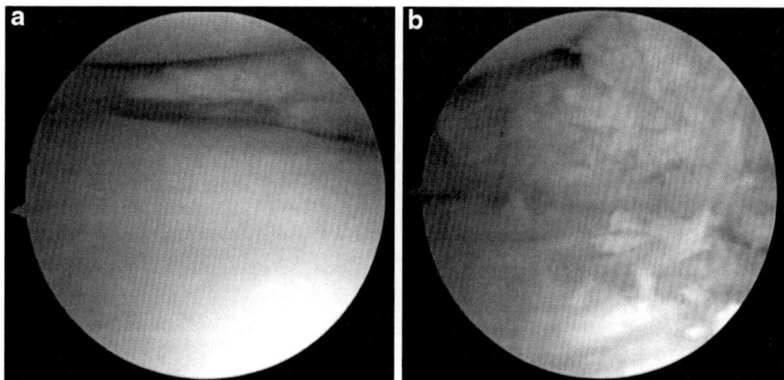

Fig. 2 The meniscal lesion is identified arthroscopically (**a**) and any degenerate or unstable meniscal tissue is removed in order to obtain a full-thickness defect with a stable meniscal rim over the entire length (**b**)

1–2 cm medial to the patellar tendon. When performing a lateral CMI, this portal is usually performed slightly above the joint line. Accessory portals may be required for a better view or access.

Once portals are established, a thorough arthroscopic examination is mandatory (Fig. 2a). Furthermore, ACL and cartilage status are controlled in order to correctly plan additional procedures.

Preparation of the Implant Bed

Any degenerate or unstable meniscal tissue is removed in order to obtain a full-thickness defect with a stable meniscal rim over the entire length using basket forceps and a motorized shaver (Fig. 2b). The meniscal rim should maintain a uniform width and extend to the red–red zone. When the defect reaches the white–red zone, bleeding is obtained by making puncture holes in the rim with a microfracture awl. The anterior and posterior attachments should be trimmed square (radially) to better match the CMI and improve fixation stability.

If the medial compartment is too tight for proper visualization, medial release with outside-in needle punctures and varus stress can be performed without the risk of any residual laxity. In contrast, tightness of the lateral compartment and not being able to place the CMI into the defect represent an intraoperative contraindication to a CMI, as secondary complications, poor healing, and lateral laxity are issues when lateral collateral ligament release is performed.

Preparation of the Collagen Meniscus Implant (CMI)

Once the implant bed is prepared, the defect is measured using a specially designed measuring device through the ipsilateral portal, starting from the posterior aspect of the lesion (Fig. 3a). The obtained measurement should be oversized by approximately 10 % when sizing the CMI in order to obtain a good press-fit and better stability. In case of disruption of the meniscus tissue at the popliteal hiatus, the measure should be oversized by 15–20 %, since the CMI may recess into the hiatus during fixation.

Once the correct size has been established, the dry CMI is removed from the sterile package and trimmed using a fresh scalpel (Fig. 3b). Care should be taken to match the shape of the CMI perfectly with the angles of the meniscal defect.

CMI Fixation

Once the device is adequately prepared, it is mounted on a curved atraumatic vascular clamp and directly inserted into the joint through the corresponding portal, which should be enlarged enough to accommodate the tip of the fifth finger (Fig. 4a). The device is then released in the proper position and the clamp retrieved without damaging cartilage surfaces (Fig. 4b). A blunt probe can also be useful to manipulate the implant into the correct position.

When the device is in the correct position, suturing to the capsule is performed. The

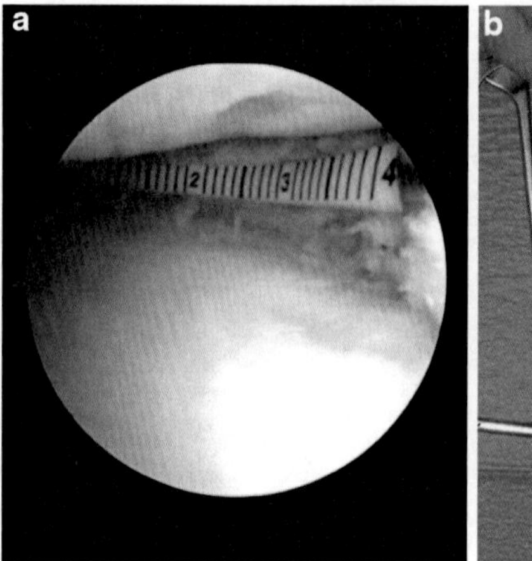

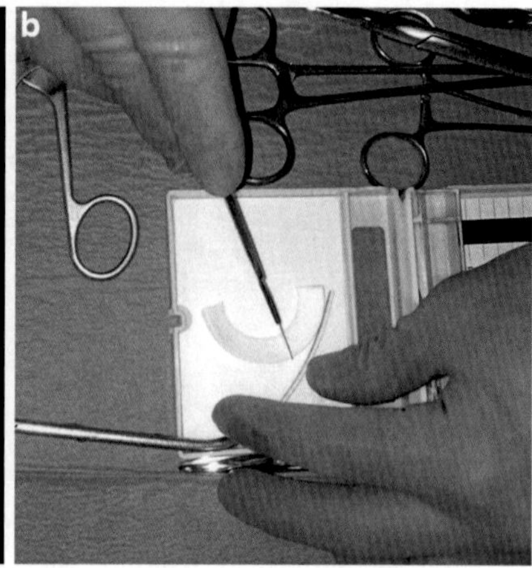

Fig. 3 A specially designed measuring device is inserted in the knee joint in order to exactly measure the length of the meniscal defect (**a**). With a scalpel the CMI is then trimmed according to the correct size previously measured (**b**)

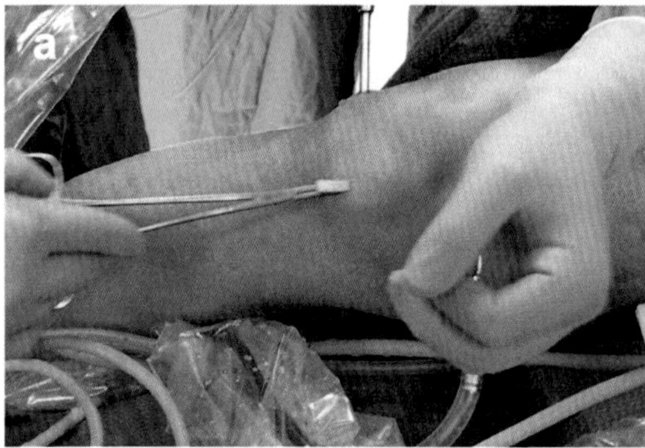

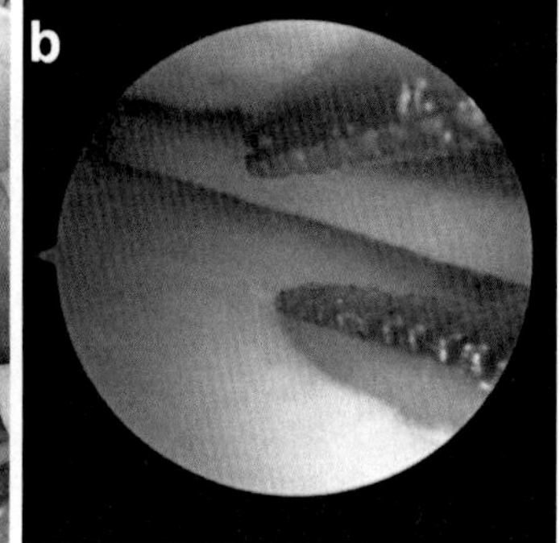

Fig. 4 The CMI is mounted on a curved clamp and directly inserted into the joint through the corresponding portal (**a**) and then released in the proper position (**b**)

new-generation meniscal repair takes the advantages of both the all-inside technique and the biomechanical proprieties of sutures. Sutures are placed vertically using a standard technique every 10–15 mm along the periphery of the device (Fig. 5), while the anterior and posterior borders are fixed using two horizontal sutures. This all-inside method is particularly indicated for the posterior third of the meniscus. When required, an inside-out suture placed every 5 mm could be used alone or in combination with the all-inside technique. This method, although more versatile, requires the execution of posterolateral or posteromedial approaches to retrieve the sutures. When performing lateral CMI, care should be taken while suturing the area of the popliteal hiatus, to avoid placing sutures directly through the popliteal tendon, because the physiological micromotion of this tendon might damage the still immature scaffold. If a 1–2 mm gap has been developed between anterior and posterior horns and the sutured CMI, a microfracture owl is used to scarify the synovium to stimulate a proliferative response at the gap interface. If the gap is more than 2 mm, the implant should be replaced.

Once the CMI is sutured, its stability is checked with a probe, the tourniquet is released, and a drain (if used) is positioned with no suction.

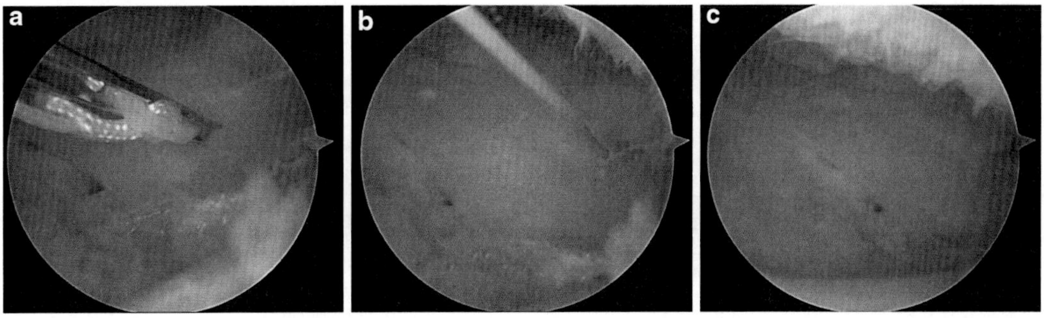

Fig. 5 The tip of the suturing device is inserted through the CMI (**a**) and the first "anchor" is released. Then the capsule is pinched just above the first passage of the stitch. After the release of the second "anchor" of the device, the stitch is pulled and locked (**b**). Finally the remaining suture is cut, obtaining a vertical stitch (**c**)

Concurrent Procedures

Anterior Cruciate Ligament Reconstruction

ACL reconstruction is the most frequent procedure associated with CMI. Concomitant ACL reconstruction has been reported to create a more favorable environment for healing of the meniscus (Koski et al. 2000), and therefore combined ACL reconstruction and CMI are recommended. In such cases, CMI insertion and fixation should be performed before definitive fixation of the graft, in order to allow better medial or lateral joint opening during stress maneuvers. For the same reason, if the procedures are staged, CMI should be performed first. However, ACL reconstruction can be delayed no more than 12 weeks after CMI, as knee instability could compromise the healing of the scaffold.

Osteotomy

As lower limb malalignment is a contraindication to a CMI procedure, any axial deformity should be corrected before or concurrently with CMI. Closing wedge lateral high tibial osteotomy (HTO) (Marcacci et al. 2007) to correct varus deformity, which has been demonstrated to reduce tibial slope, reducing stress on native or reconstructed ACL (Ducat et al. 2012; Zaffagnini et al. 2013; Feucht et al. 2013), and closing wedge medial distal femoral osteotomy (DFO) to correct valgus deformity are recommended. When concurrent CMI and HTO or DFO are performed, the arthroscopic step and device implant should be performed first.

Cartilage Treatment

Advanced cartilage damage represents a contraindication to CMI, and therefore no clear recommendations regarding cartilage treatment and CMI are available. Generally, cartilage treatment, such as microfractures, osteochondral transplantation, or autologous chondrocyte implant (ACI), should be performed before CMI, in order to try to preserve the CMI device.

Rehabilitation

The main issue related to rehabilitation after a CMI is caution during the physiotherapy program, which is fundamental in order to allow CMI healing and promote good outcomes. The program covers a period of 6 months and offers a balanced combination of strengthening and motion exercises, providing protection to the newly formed tissue throughout the delicate process of regeneration. Although guidelines suggest return to full unrestricted sporting activity, the rehabilitation program should be tailored to the patient's specific needs, expectations, and concurrent procedures.

Day 1–Day 30:

Brace: full extension, remove only for motion exercises
Motion: passive motion exercises using a continuous passive motion (CPM) machine (0–60°)
Weight-bearing: no weight-bearing (week 1), 30 % partial weight-bearing (week 2), 50 % partial weight-bearing (weeks 3–4)
Exercises: leg raises 30 × 2 (daily)

Week 5–Week 6:

Brace: full extension, remove only for motion exercises
Motion: passive motion exercises on CPM machine (0–90°)
Weight-bearing: 90 % partial weight-bearing
Exercises: leg raises 30 × 2 (daily)

Week 7–Week 8:

Brace: 0–90°, remove only for motion exercises
Motion: active motion exercises (increase ROM as tolerated)
Weight-bearing: full weight-bearing, abandon crutches
Exercises: leg raises 30 × 2 (daily), cycling without resistance (to a maximum 45 min)

Week 9–Week 16:

Brace: none
Motion: unrestricted full ROM
Weight-bearing: unrestricted full weight-bearing
Exercises: shallow knee bends from 0° to 90° 20 × 2 (daily), cycling with increased resistance (to a maximum 45 min), water exercises

Month 5–Month 6:

Brace: none
Motion: unrestricted full ROM
Weight-bearing: unrestricted full weight-bearing.
Exercises: lateral agility exercises 20–50 × 2 (daily)

Return to Sport:

Generally, return to sport is achieved after 6 months, although patient-specific issues or concurrent surgery such as cartilage treatment can lead to a prolonged rehabilitation period. In order to optimize the outcome, strict adherence to the program is mandatory, even when the patient feels able to return to his/her activities sooner than expected.

Risks and Complications

The risks related to a CMI are mainly produced by a less than perfect surgical technique. Nerve injuries have been reported after medial CMI, as a possible consequence of suture placement; also, laxity of the knee has been described, which could be produced by excessive medial or lateral release being performed to allow the opening of the affected compartment (Rodkey et al. 2008). Furthermore, when dealing with lateral meniscal substitution, improper scaffold fixation could entrap the popliteus tendon. Other complications such as pain, swelling, wound infection, and deep vein thrombosis have been reported in the literature, with incidences ranging from 0 % to 32 %.

These complications can produce failure of the implant, requiring reoperation. The failure rate ranges between 0 % and 12.5 %, and in the largest series of 160 medial CMIs (Rodkey et al. 2008) it was almost 10 %. The main causes of reoperation are persistent pain, swelling, infection, or mechanical failure of the scaffold.

Results

Clinical Results

A recent systematic review reported that satisfactory outcomes are achieved in approximately 70 % of patients treated with CMI (Harston et al. 2011), while 30 % did not receive any benefit; this is in contrast with studies that reported good/excellent results in more than 90 % of patients (Zaffagnini et al. 2012). The cornerstone study of CMI surgery is the randomized controlled trial performed by Rodkey et al. (2008), which compared medial CMI to medial meniscectomy at 5 years' follow-up. This study, involving about 300 patients, showed that good results and a low reoperation rate were obtained in patients with chronic meniscal deficiency treated with CMI. Regarding acute meniscal lesion, no significant difference was found compared with the control group, thus limiting the indication of CMI to patients with previous meniscectomy. As the lateral CMI was developed more than 10 years after the medial CMI, there are few reports in the current literature on the results of the lateral procedures (Zaffagnini et al. 2011b, 2012; Hirschmann et al. 2013). Outcomes similar to those of the medial CMI have been reported (Zaffagnini et al. 2007), even if no randomized controlled trials or long-term follow-up studies are yet available.

The potential chondroprotective effect of the scaffold in the long-term has been studied by Zaffagnini et al. (2011) in a controlled clinical trial. They compared medial CMI with medial meniscectomy at 10-year follow-up, showing lower signs of knee osteoarthritis and better clinical results, particularly pain and knee function, using the CMI.

Second Look and Histologic Findings

Besides clinical results, several studies have focused their attention on the intra-articular behavior of the implanted CMI (Fig. 6). Stone et al. (1997) reported the presence of regenerated tissue similar to the fibrous composition of meniscal cartilage after 6 months. These findings were confirmed by Rodkey et al. (1999) at 24 months' follow-up, when reduction of osteoarthritic degeneration was also noted. As suggested by these previous studies, Bulgheroni et al. (2010) showed a progressive resorption of the scaffold, with implant remnants visible at 3 years' follow-up and complete absence of the implant at 5 years. Analogously, Rodkey et al. (2008) reported that only 10–25 % of the original implant was still present at the 1-year follow-up. These findings, similar to those reported by animal studies, suggest a progressive resorption of the scaffold, which is colonized and substituted by a fibrocartilaginous tissue similar to the meniscus.

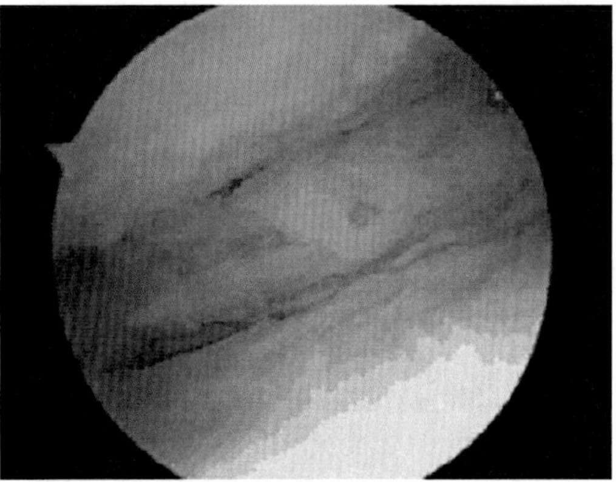

Fig. 6 Medial CMI 6 months after the implant

Magnetic Resonance Imaging Findings

The behavior of the CMI has also been widely studied with MRI (Figs. 7 and 8). Genovese et al. (2007) developed an MRI score in order to assess the signal intensity and size of the scaffold. Various reports have shown that the scaffold tends to reduce its size over time, with a consistent reduction after 1 year that slowly progresses until 10 years. Regarding the signal intensity, the MRI findings showed a reduction of the implant signal that slowly tended to become isointense to the signal of native meniscus. However, this process, which suggests implant maturation, appears to be almost complete in only a small percentage of implants. In fact, most devices assume a signal that is slightly hyperintense compared to the native meniscus, and which is more similar to the newly implanted scaffold (Bulgheroni et al. 2010; Monllau et al. 2011; Zaffagnini et al. 2011, 2012).

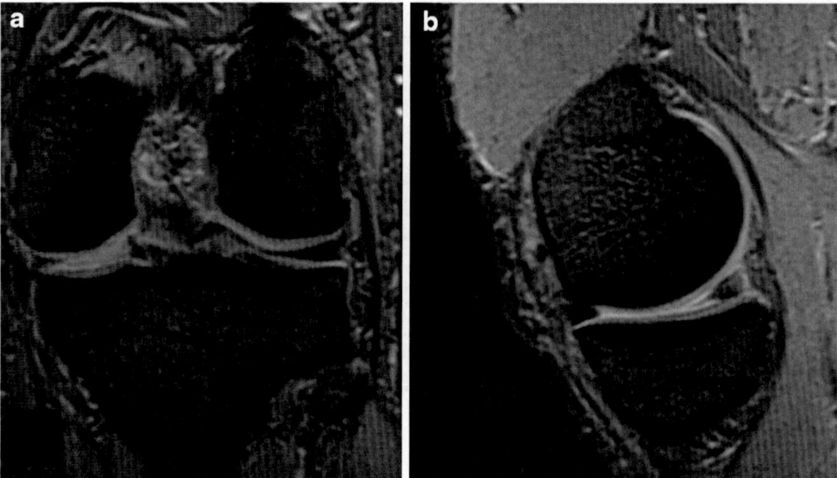

Fig. 7 MRI appearance of a medial CMI 10 years after the implant on coronal (**a**) and sagittal (**b**) view. The scaffold is still clearly visible but with a reduced size and slightly higher signal compared with the native meniscus

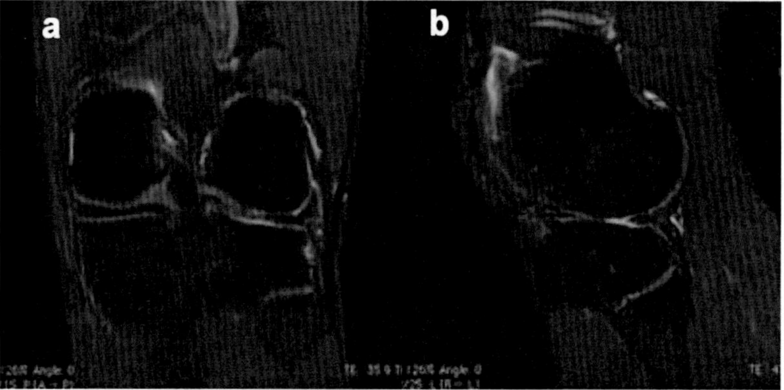

Fig. 8 MRI appearance of a lateral CMI 3 years after the implant on coronal (**a**) and sagittal (**b**) view. In this case the scaffold presents a good signal intensity, although the size appears slightly reduced compared to a normal meniscus

Results of Associated Procedures

CMI is often combined with other surgical procedures; in fact, the rate of concomitant surgery ranges from 11 % to 79 %. The main procedures performed are to address knee stability, malalignment, or cartilage pathology. As a result, it is not easy to evaluate the real effect of the CMI when additional procedures are performed, as the results could be biased by their combination.

Hirschmann et al. (2013) reported a case series of 67 patients, 53 of whom were treated with medial or lateral CMI combined with ACL reconstruction. Those patients showed more bone marrow edema and fewer good clinical results, measured by the Lysholm score, than with isolated CMI at 1 year of follow-up.

Linke et al. (2006) performed a controlled study involving 60 patients with varus morphotype and medial meniscus loss. The control group underwent high tibial valgus osteotomy (HTVO) while the treatment group underwent HTVO combined with medial CMI. At 2 years' follow-up, no significant differences were found between the groups in terms of knee function and pain. However, the improvement from baseline in the patients treated with CMI and HTVO was similar to that in other studies.

Due to the highly specialized and demanding procedures, reports of CMI and cartilage treatment are very few. Microfracture surgery is the most performed procedure, involving approximately 11–20 % of patients (Stone et al. 1997; Zaffagnini et al. 2011). Combined CMI and microfracture surgery does not appear to dramatically change the general outcomes, despite patients with cartilage injury requiring more careful management. Ronga et al. (2006) presented a report of a patient treated with combined medial CMI and ACL reconstruction, followed by medial femoral condyle MACI (matrix-applied characterized autologous cultured chondrocytes) 7 months later, due to a 5 cm^2 chondral lesion. The authors reported good clinical results, with reduction of pain and scaffold invasion by blood vessels and cells, and production of new collagen fibrils without any signs of inflammatory reaction after 2 years.

Conclusions

CMI represents an attractive surgical option for irreparable meniscal lesions. Although a wide range of conditions can potentially be treated with CMI, good results are dependent on correct indications. Good/excellent results have been reported in 70–90 % of cases. The most interesting finding regarding the CMI is evidence of resorption of the scaffold and its substitution with a meniscus-like tissue, which represents a basis for theories relating to the potential effect of chondroprotection. However, the protective properties of the CMI are yet to be proven, as only a few controlled trials have been conducted. While the clinical benefits of CMI in the mid-term have been demonstrated, further studies are needed to confirm the long-term outcomes and its protective effects on articular cartilage.

Cross-References

- ▶ Arthroscopic Repair of the Meniscus Tears
- ▶ Arthroscopic Treatment of Knee Osteoarthritis in Athletes
- ▶ Biomaterials in Musculoskeletal Conditions: Classification, Design, and Regulatory Aspects
- ▶ Human Meniscus: From Biology to Tissue Engineering Strategies
- ▶ Innovation in Sports Medicine
- ▶ Meniscal Substitutes: Polyurethane Meniscus Implant: Technique and Results
- ▶ Meniscectomy
- ▶ Role of Biologicals in Meniscus Surgery
- ▶ Rugby and Associated Sports Injuries
- ▶ Soccer and Associated Sports Injuries

References

Baker BE, Peckham AC, Pupparo F et al (1985) Review of meniscal injury and associated sports. Am J Sports Med 13(1):1–4

Bulgheroni P, Murena L, Ratti C et al (2010) Follow-up of collagen meniscus implant patients: clinical, radiological, and magnetic resonance imaging results at 5 years. Knee 17(3):224–229

Chatain F, Adeleine P, Chambat P et al (2003) A comparative study of medial versus lateral arthroscopic partial meniscectomy on stable knees: 10-year minimum follow-up. Arthroscopy 19(8):842–849

Ducat A, Sariali E, Lebel B et al (2012) Posterior tibial slope changes after opening- and closing-wedge high tibial osteotomy: a comparative prospective multicenter study. Orthop Traumatol Surg Res 98(1):68–74

Feucht MJ, Mauro CS, Brucker PU et al (2013) The role of the tibial slope in sustaining and treating anterior cruciate ligament injuries. Knee Surg Sports Traumatol Arthrosc 21(1):134–145

Genovese E, Angeretti MG, Ronga M et al (2007) Follow-up of collagen meniscus implants by MRI. Radiol Med 112(7):1036–1048

Harston A, Nyland J, Brand E et al (2011) Collagen meniscus implantation: a systematic review including rehabilitation and return to sports activity. Knee Surg Sports Traumatol Arthrosc 20(1):135–146

Hirschmann MT, Keller L, Hirschmann A et al (2013) One-year clinical and MR imaging outcome after partial meniscal replacement in stabilized knees using a collagen meniscus implant. Knee Surg Sports Traumatol Arthrosc 21(3):740–747

Koski JA, Ibarra C, Rodeo SA et al (2000) Meniscal injury and repair: clinical status. Orthop Clin North Am 31 (3):419–436

Li S-T, Rodkey WG, Yuen D et al (2002) Type I collagen-based template for meniscus regeneration. In: Lewandrowski K-U, Wise DL, Trantolo DJ, Gresser JD, Yaszemski MJ, Altobelli DE (eds) Tissue engineering and biodegradable equivalents. Scientific and clinical applications. Marcel Dekker, New York, pp 237–266

Linke RD, Ulmer M, Imhoff AB (2006) Replacement of the meniscus with a collagen implant (CMI)]. Oper Orthop Traumatol 18(5–6):453–62

Marcacci M, Zaffagnini S, Giordano G et al (2007) High tibial osteotomy: the Italian experience. Op Tech Orthop 17(1):1–86

McBride ID, Reid JG (1988) Biomechanical considerations of the menisci of the knee. Can J Sport Sci 13 (4):175–187

McDevitt CA, Webber RJ (1990) The ultrastructure and biochemistry of meniscal cartilage. Clin Orthop Relat Res 1990(252):8–18

Monllau JC, Gelber PE, Abat F et al (2011) Outcome after partial medial meniscus substitution with the collagen meniscal implant at a minimum of 10 years' follow-up. Arthroscopy 27(7):933–943

Rodkey WG, Steadman JR, Li ST (1999) A clinical study of collagen meniscus implants to restore the injured meniscus. Clin Orthop Relat Res (367 Suppl): S281–S292

Rodkey WG, DeHaven KE, Montgomery WH 3rd et al (2008) Comparison of the collagen meniscus implant with partial meniscectomy. A prospective randomized trial. J Bone Joint Surg Am 90(7):1413–1426

Ronga M, Grassi FA, Manelli A et al (2006) Tissue engineering techniques for the treatment of a complex knee injury. Arthroscopy 22(5):576.e1–576.e3

Stone KR, Rodkey WG, Webber RJ et al (1990) Future directions. Collagen-based prostheses for meniscal regeneration. Clin Orthop Relat Res 1990 (252):129–135

Stone KR, Rodkey WG, Webber R et al (1992) Meniscal regeneration with copolymeric collagen scaffolds. In vitro and in vivo studies evaluated clinically, histologically, and biochemically. Am J Sports Med 20(2):104–111

Stone KR, Steadman JR, Rodkey WG et al (1997) Regeneration of meniscal cartilage with use of a collagen scaffold. Analysis of preliminary data. J Bone Joint Surg Am 79(12):1770–1777

Zaffagnini S, Giordano G, Vascellari A et al (2007) Arthroscopic collagen meniscus implant results at 6 to 8 years follow up. Knee Surg Sports Traumatol Arthrosc 15 (2):175–183

Zaffagnini S, Marcheggiani Muccioli GM, Lopomo N et al (2011a) Prospective long-term outcomes of the medial collagen meniscus implant versus partial medial meniscectomy: a minimum 10-year follow-up study. Am J Sports Med 39(5):977–985

Zaffagnini S, Marcheggiani Muccioli GM, Grassi A et al (2011b) Arthroscopic lateral collagen meniscus implant in a professional soccer player. Knee Surg Sports Traumatol Arthrosc 19(10):1740–1743

Zaffagnini S, Marcheggiani Muccioli GM, Bulgheroni P et al (2012) Arthroscopic collagen meniscus implantation for partial lateral meniscal defects: a 2-year minimum follow-up study. Am J Sports Med 40 (10):2281–2288

Zaffagnini S, Bonanzinga T, Grassi A et al (2013) Combined ACL reconstruction and closing-wedge HTO for varus angulated ACL-deficient knees. Knee Surg Sports Traumatol Arthrosc 21(4):934–941

Meniscus Variations

99

Caglar Yilgor, Özgür Ahmet Atay, and Mahmut Nedim Doral

Contents

Electronic supplementary material: The online version of this chapter doi:10.1007/978-3-642-36569-0_267 contains supplementary material, which is available to authorized users.

C. Yilgor (✉) • Ö.A. Atay
Faculty of Medicine, Department of Orthopaedics and Traumatology, Hacettepe University, Ankara, Sihhiye, Turkey
e-mail: caglaryilgor@gmail.com; oaatay@hacettepe.edu.tr

M.N. Doral
Department of Orthopaedics and Traumatology and Department of Sports Medicine, Hacettepe University, Istanbul, Turkey
e-mail: mndoral@gmail.com; ndoral@hacettepe.edu.tr

M.N. Doral, J. Karlsson (eds.), *Sports Injuries*,
DOI 10.1007/978-3-642-36569-0_267

Abstract

The lateral meniscus is more variable than the medial meniscus morphologically regarding the size, thickness, shape, and mobility. The most common lateral meniscal variant is discoid in shape, which implies greater coverage of the tibia and usually increased thickness. Many stable lateral meniscal variants are asymptomatic and are found incidentally. The most common symptoms, which usually occur during childhood and adolescence, are a clunking sound with flexion of the knee, pain, a decreased range of motion, joint line tenderness, sensation of a foreign object within the knee, quadriceps atrophy, and effusion. Since it was first described, several classifications were proposed using clinical, radiologic, and arthroscopic findings. Although most of these classifications are descriptive, newer systems focus on influencing treatment. The treatment options for the various lateral meniscal variants include observation, partial meniscectomy with or without reattachment, total meniscectomy, and for a normally shaped unstable lesion reattachment to the adjacent capsule. It must be kept in mind that there may be no good treatment option; rather, the only choice may be the lesser of two evils. During arthroscopy a tear may not be visualized in some symptomatic discoid menisci. Therefore, a preoperative MRI is mandatory for all discoid menisci, because the absence and presence of shift and the direction of the shift must be carefully assessed before surgery since it alters the therapeutic approach. In the presence of a shift, the meniscus must be reduced before starting the excision. After resection, the tear in the opposite horn should be repaired with sutures. This chapter reviews the anatomy, embryology, etiology, and classification of discoid menisci as well as their clinical presentations, accompanying conditions, tears, and treatment.

History

The menisci consist of semilunar fibrocartilage, partly filling the space between the femoral and tibial bones. The most common meniscal anomaly is a discoid shape of the lateral meniscus. Other anomalies are hypoplasia, abnormal insertions, and a double-layered lateral meniscus.

Discoid lateral and medial menisci were first described in cadaver specimens (Young 1889; Watson-Jones 1930). Kroiss attributed the term "snapping knee syndrome" to it (Kroiss 1910). A more precise diagnosis and classification was made much later (Watanabe et al. 1979).

Embryology

The normal menisci differentiate within the limb bud from mesenchymal tissue early during fetal development. They are clearly defined at the 8th week of gestation and gain mature anatomical shape at the 14th week (Andrish 1996), without ever possessing a discoid shape (Kaplan 1957).

Anatomy

The lateral meniscus is somewhat more circular than the C-shaped medial meniscus. This is because the posterior and anterior horns of the lateral meniscus attach to the nonarticular area of the tibial plateau. A normal lateral meniscus forms five-sixths of a circle. It has an average width of about 12 mm and a height of 4–5 mm, although the normal anatomy varies considerably with regard to dimension and shape.

In adults, the C-shaped medial meniscus covers 50 % of the medial tibial plateau and is connected firmly to the joint capsule by coronary, meniscotibial, and deep medial collateral ligaments, whereas the lateral meniscus covers 70 % of the lateral tibial plateau and has firm anterior and posterior attachments, while its lateral joint capsule attachment is loose because there is no attachment at the popliteal hiatus and fibular collateral ligament. Therefore, the normal lateral meniscus has more mobility than the medial meniscus, allowing an increased excursion of the lateral meniscus on the lateral tibial plateau. Variably present posterior and anterior meniscofemoral ligaments (Wrisberg and Humphrey ligaments) pass from the medial aspect of the notch to the posterior horn of the lateral meniscus. The Wrisberg ligament passes posteriorly to the posterior cruciate, and the Humphrey ligament passes anteriorly. Usually, only one of these structures is present, and they vary quite markedly in size. The posterior third of the lateral meniscus receives a strong insertion from the popliteus muscle into its posterior horn, which allows the meniscus to be pulled posteriorly as the knee flexes (Johnson and Beynnon 2001). Together with the popliteus tendon, the lateral meniscus stabilizes the knee against excessive posterolateral rotational forces.

The most common lateral meniscal variant is discoid in shape, which implies greater coverage of the tibia and usually increased thickness. Formerly, it was believed that this variant may involve only part of the meniscus (in which case it was so-called an anterior or posterior megahorn (Jordan 1996)), or it may involve the entire meniscus. Recent studies suggest that these megahorns can be caused by partial tears of the relevant meniscal part and are not congenital variants. Variants can be normal in shape but hypermobile due to abnormal insertions or abnormal in shape, such as circular (ring-shaped) meniscus (Kim et al. 1995a; Monllau et al. 1998; Choi 1999; Arnold and Van Kampen 2000; Atay et al. 2002). Other anomalies of the lateral meniscus include a partially duplicated lateral meniscus and double-layered lateral meniscus (Suzuki et al. 1991; D'Lima et al. 1995; Kim et al. 1998).

Epidemiology

The actual incidence of lateral meniscus variations is difficult to estimate due to the high rate of asymptomatic patients. The reported prevalences of discoid lateral meniscus vary, depending on the method of investigation, the selection criteria, and the patient population. The Wrisberg type is considered to be less common.

Earlier studies suggested the prevalence of a discoid lateral meniscus in symptomatic patients who underwent open meniscectomy ranged from 2 % to 5 % (Smillie 1948; Watanabe et al. 1979). More recent arthroscopic studies have recorded prevalences varying from 0.4 % to 16.6 % (Fujikawa et al. 1981; Dickhaut and DeLee 1982; Ikeuchi 1982; Albertsson and Gillquist 1988; Neuschwander et al. 1992). These studies may be a more accurate representation of the true prevalence, because asymptomatic discoid menisci are also included. Cadaveric studies suggest a prevalence ranging from 0 % to 7 % (Noble 1977; Casscells 1978; Woods and Whelan 1990). Discoid menisci have been reported more frequently in Asian countries than in other regions of the world (Ikeuchi 1982; Kim et al. 1995b). Bilateral occurrence has been reported in 20 % of patients with discoid lateral menisci (Bellier et al. 1989).

Etiology

The underlying causes of lateral meniscal abnormalities are multifactorial. Several theories try to explain the etiology of the variant lateral meniscus. Smillie (1948) hypothesized that the discoid meniscus results from the lack of resorption of a central cartilaginous disk during normal development. Others (Kaplan 1957; Clark and Ogden 1983; Andrish 1996) later disputed this theory, because they could not identify a discoid meniscus at any stage of the embryonic development. The menisci are clearly defined at the 8th week of gestation and gain mature anatomical shape at the 14th week. Kaplan (1957) suggested that a normally shaped meniscus with abnormal attachments would have abnormal medial-to-lateral motion which will cause repetitive trauma that results in a change in the meniscal shape. During extension, due to the tension in the meniscofemoral ligaments, the meniscus subluxates posteromedially into the notch, and due to the pull of the popliteus and capsule, it reduces back into the joint on flexion (Kaplan 1957). The abnormal lack of a posterior tibial attachment could be a failure of formation due to phylogenetic incompletion (Le Minor 1990). A circular meniscus (Kim et al. 1995a) could be further evidence of this implication. The problem with this theory is that stable discoid menisci with normal attachments have been identified.

Some authors (Clark and Ogden 1983; Woods and Whelan 1990) favor a congenital origin. Woods and Whelan explain the unstable discoid meniscus as being a congenitally stable discoid-shaped meniscus that became unstable by posterior capsular separation due to increased shear forces. The causes of the other unstable types are even less clear. Originally, Watanabe et al. (1979) described the Wrisberg type as a normally shaped meniscus with abnormal attachments. Since then, other unstable variants have been included in this category; these probably represent several subtypes and as many different origins (Dickhaut and DeLee 1982; Ikeuchi 1982; Neuschwander et al. 1992).

Kaplan (1957) described a normally shaped meniscus with abnormal attachments due to repeated trauma. Later, a stable discoid meniscus that becomes unstable due to shear forces was described (Hayashi et al. 1988; Woods and Whelan 1990). A third possibility is a discoid meniscus without posterior tibial attachments. A fourth type as a normally shaped meniscus with lack of posterior tibial attachments was also described (Neuschwander et al. 1992). These all suggest a wide range of abnormalities leading to an unstable meniscus presenting with similar symptoms and often resulting in the "snapping knee" syndrome. It remains unclear whether all unstable types have the presence of the meniscofemoral ligament in common, which would allow subluxation and reduction to occur, accompanied by snapping (Jordan 1996). The author believes the primary pathology derives from the lack of a posterior tibial attachment in the presence of a meniscofemoral ligament attachment. The meniscofemoral ligament acts like a checkrein, allowing subluxation and reduction rather than dislocation.

Classification

The lateral meniscus is more variable than the medial meniscus morphologically regarding the size, thickness, shape, and mobility. Abnormal lateral menisci are classified as stabile or unstable according to its attachments. Less common abnormalities are hypoplasia, partial deficiency (Tetik et al. 2003), and double-layered lateral meniscus.

The traditional classification of the discoid menisci was made by Watanabe et al. (1979): (1) complete discoid meniscus, (2) incomplete discoid meniscus, and (3) Wrisberg-type meniscal variant. The authors depicted the Wrisberg type as a nearly normal-shaped meniscus but hypermobile due to the lack of posterior tibial attachments (Watanabe et al. 1979). Since then, other unstable menisci with both normal and discoid shape have been included as Wrisberg type (Kaplan 1957; Dickhaut and DeLee 1982; Woods and Whelan 1990). A lateral meniscal variant with the absence of the posterior coronary ligament that is nearly normal in morphology but lacks a posterior tibial attachment, which results in hypermobility, was described (Neuschwander et al. 1992), which nowadays can be classified within the Wrisberg type.

This traditional classification was expanded in 1998 (Monllau et al. 1998). They have added a fourth type to describe a ring-shaped meniscus characterized by a ring-shaped morphology with a normal posterior tibial attachment (Fig. 1).

Jordan (1996) proposed a new classification based on both arthroscopic and clinical findings, which describes more completely the various

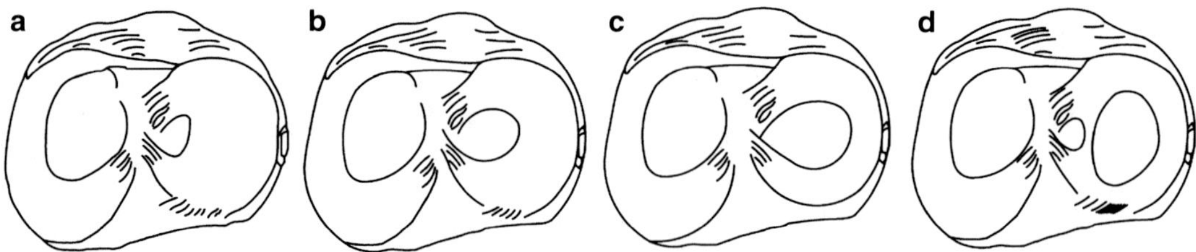

Fig. 1 Schematic drawing of modified Watanabe classification for lateral meniscal variants. (**a**) Complete discoid meniscus. (**b**) Incomplete discoid meniscus. (**c**) Wrisberg type. (**d**) Ring-shaped meniscus

Table 1 Classification of lateral meniscus variants proposed by Jordan (1996)

Classification	Correlation	Tear	Symptoms
Stable	Complete/ incomplete	Yes/ no	Yes/no
Unstable with discoid shape	Wrisberg type	Yes/ no	Yes/no
Unstable with normal shape	Wrisberg variant	Yes/ no	Yes/no

lateral meniscal types and how they influence treatment (Table 1).

A more recent article (Ahn et al. 2009) suggests a classification based on magnetic resonance imaging (MRI) findings. In their study of 82 knees, they classified the findings in four categories: (1) No shift: The peripheral portion of the discoid meniscus is not separated from the capsule, and the meniscus is not displaced. (2) Anterocentral shift: The periphery of the posterior horn is detached from the capsule, and the meniscus is displaced anteriorly or anterocentrally; as such, the anterior horn appears to be thick in sagittal sections. (3) Posterocentral shift: The periphery of the anterior horn is detached from the capsule, and the meniscus is displaced posteriorly or posterocentrally; as such, the posterior horn appears to be thick in sagittal sections. (4) Central shift: The periphery of the posterolateral portion is torn and loosens, and the entire meniscus is displaced centrally toward the notch (Ahn et al. 2009). Although a meniscus can be reduced at the time the MRI is performed and therefore a meniscus that has a peripheral tear might appear as "no shift." Nonetheless, in their study, they have found that a significantly larger number of repairs and subtotal meniscectomies were performed for the shift groups than for the no-shift group (Ahn et al. 2009). So, it can be predicted that knees with a shift on the MRI are more likely to be treated with repair or meniscectomy than knees with no shift.

Tears

Discoid menisci are more prone to mechanical trauma because of their thickness, relatively poor vascularization, and weak attachments to the posterior capsule (Hayashi et al. 1988). A recent study has shown that discoid menisci have decreased amount of collagen fibers and that the fiber is arranged heterogeneously, which may contribute to vulnerability of the discoid meniscus (Atay et al. 2007). However, patients with a tear of the discoid meniscus may not have a history of traumatic events. Tears are more common after the age of 15 (Dickason et al. 1982; Rao et al. 2001). Discoid menisci are associated with an increased incidence of tears ranging from 38 % to 88 % (Smith et al. 1999; Bin et al. 2002; Atay et al. 2003). The most common tear pattern is that of degenerative horizontal cleavage, which comprises 58–98 % of all cases of symptomatic discoid meniscal tears (Bellier et al. 1989; Aichroth et al. 1991; Pellacci et al. 1992).

Lateral meniscal variants have been classified into six tear patterns by modifying O'Connor's (Shahriaree 1992) classification (Kim et al. 2006). This classification includes six simple and comprehensive categories (Fig. 2): (1) a simple horizontal tear; (2) a combined horizontal tear, in which the major tear component is horizontal and another tear component is accompanied (Bin et al. 2002); (3) a longitudinal tear including peripheral tear; (4) a radial tear including an oblique and a flap tear; (5) a complex tear including a degenerative tear, which is a combination of two major components except a horizontal tear or a combination of three or more major tear components including a horizontal tear; and (6) a central tear which is a broad spectrum of the wear in the central portion of the discoid meniscus as a result of repeated maceration (Kim et al. 2006). Figures 3 and 4 demonstrates MRI and arthroscopic views of discoid lateral menisci from the authors' clinic with a radial and horizontal tear.

Clinical Presentation

Many stable lateral meniscal variants are asymptomatic and are found incidentally. Moreover, patients might have unilateral symptoms but have bilateral discoid menisci.

The most common symptoms, which usually occur during childhood and adolescence, are a

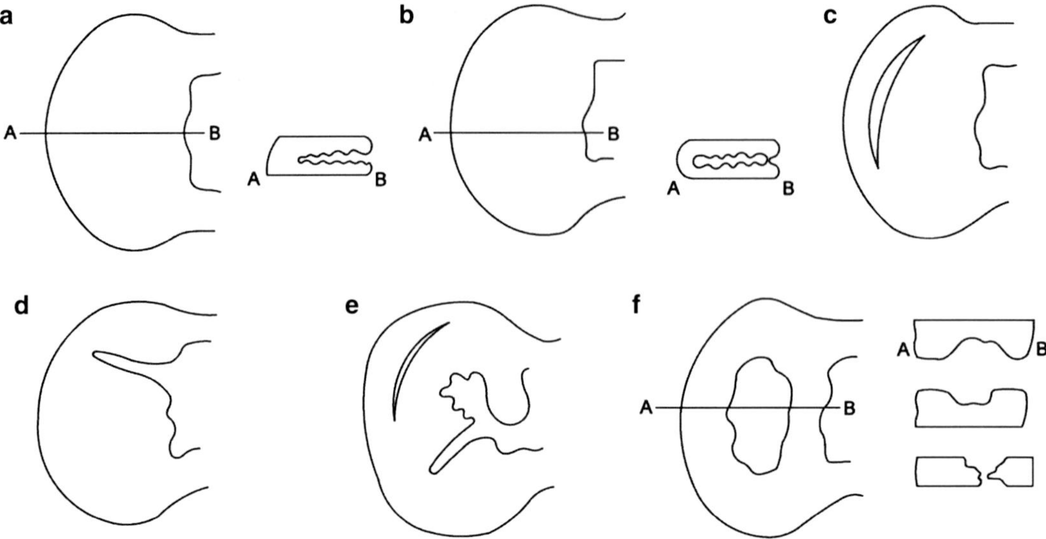

Fig. 2 Schematic drawings of the modified O'Connor's classification for lateral discoid meniscal tears: (**a**) Simple horizontal. (**b**) Combined horizontal. (**c**) Longitudinal (**d**) Radial (**e**) Complex (**f**) Central

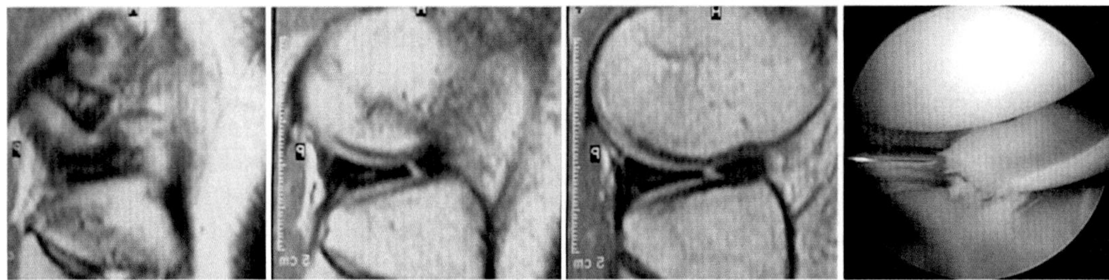

Fig. 3 MRI and arthroscopic views of a radial tear of a discoid lateral meniscus

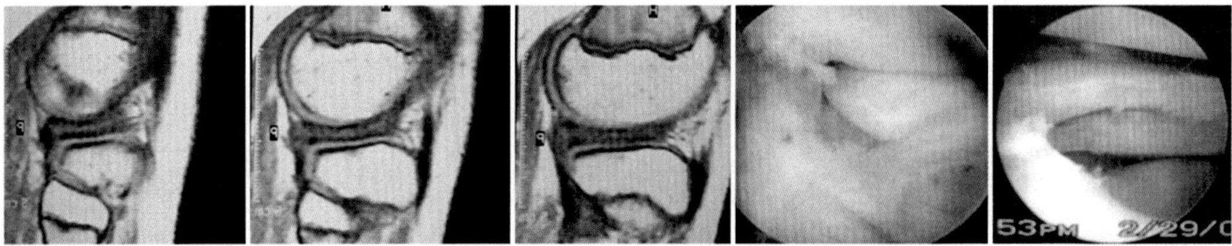

Fig. 4 MRI and arthroscopic views of a horizontal tear of a discoid lateral meniscus

clunking sound with flexion of the knee, pain, a decreased range of motion (usually lack of full extension), joint line tenderness, sensation of a foreign object within the knee, quadriceps atrophy, and effusion (Dickhaut and DeLee 1982; Ikeuchi 1982; Hayashi et al. 1988; Vandermeer and Cunningham 1989; Aichroth et al. 1991; Neuschwander et al. 1992; Washington et al. 1995; Rao et al. 2001).

The sound and feeling of this clunking and popping is attributed by the term "snapping knee syndrome" to describe a discoid meniscus

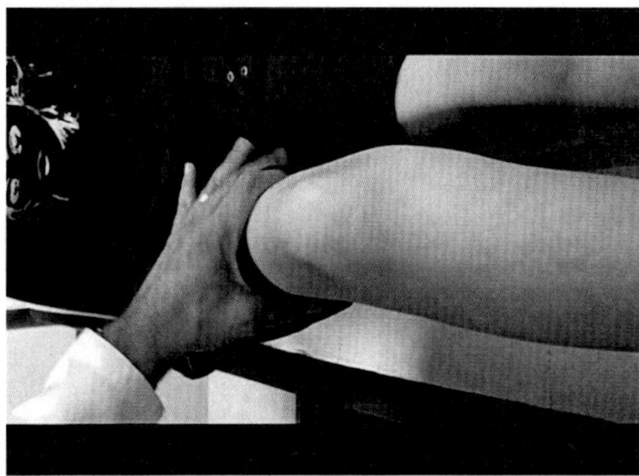

Video 1 Demonstration of snapping of the knee in flexion and extension.

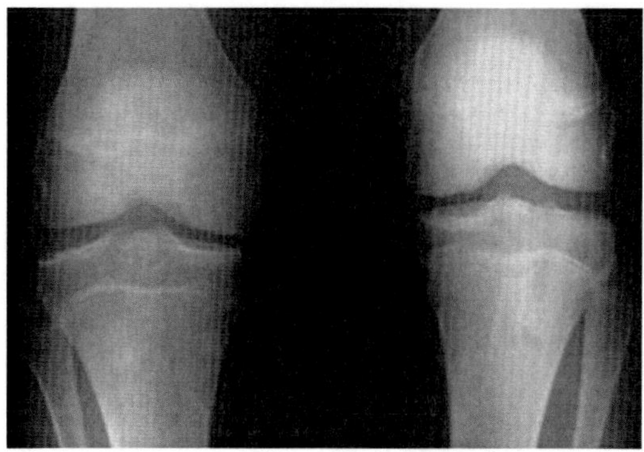

Fig. 5 Anteroposterior x-ray of a knee with bilateral discoid menisci

(Kroiss 1910) (See Video 1). Yet, pain is the predominant symptom in the majority of the cases. Pain generally begins with a minor trauma and is not always associated with a tear (Asik et al. 2003).

According to Ahn et al. (2001), the type of the discoid meniscus is associated with the clinical symptoms. In his study, he concluded that a lack of extension is more common when the anterior horn thickness is greater than 7.7 mm and extension is full when the thickness is less than 4 mm.

Accompanying Conditions

Lateral meniscal variation can be associated with other musculoskeletal anomalies. High fibular head, fibular muscular defects, hypoplasia of the lateral femoral condyle with lateral joint space widening, hypoplasia of the lateral tibial eminence, abnormally shaped lateral malleolus of the ankle, and enlarged inferior lateral geniculate artery are examples of such anomalies.

One of the most clinically demanding conditions is the association between a lateral discoid meniscus and an osteochondral lesion of the lateral femoral condyle (Irani et al. 1984). Osteochondritis dissecans of the lateral femoral condyle is relatively rare and oftentimes combined with lateral discoid meniscus and usually a torn discoid meniscus (Mizuta et al. 2001) and associated with a poorer prognosis when present. The discoid meniscus itself might produce an abnormal contact force onto the lateral femoral condyle even if the meniscus is not torn. This abnormal contact force may lead to an osteochondritis dissecans lesion in the lateral femoral condyle (Mitsuoka et al. 1999). The presence of lateral discoid meniscus was reported to occur in a majority of the osteochondritis dissecans lesions that occurred in the lateral femoral condyle (Yoshida et al. 1998). A lateral discoid meniscus tear, young age and high activity, and valgus alignment can be predisposing factors for osteochondritis dissecans of the lateral femoral condyle (Terashima et al. 2005). Partial meniscectomy is shown to permit the healing of an osteochondral lesion (Yoshida et al. 1998).

Radiology: X-ray

Standard anterior-posterior, lateral, tunnel, and skyline views contribute significantly to the establishment of diagnosis (Picard and Constantin 1964) (Figs. 5 and 6). Lateral joint space narrowing, lateral joint lipping, squaring of the lateral femoral condyle, cupping of the lateral tibial plateau, flattening of the lateral femoral condyle, tibial eminence hypoplasia, calcification of the meniscus, fibular head elevation, obliquity of the joint space, and degenerative changes may be demonstrated (Kerr 1986; Woods and Whelan 1990). These radiographic findings are present only in some cases. Associated pathologies such as osteochondritis dissecans and lateral malleolus abnormalities may also be visualized.

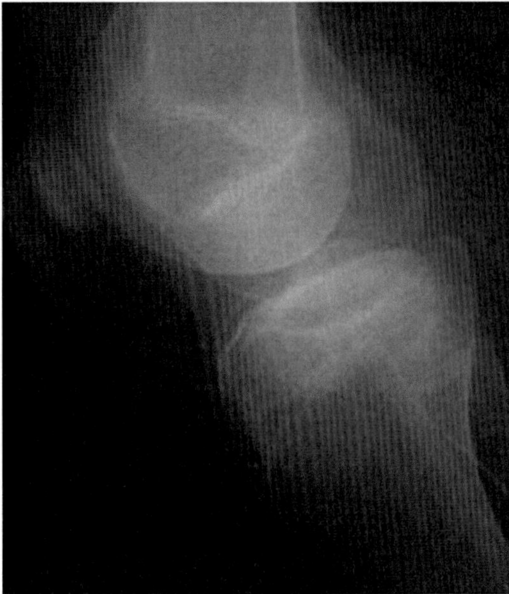

Fig. 6 Lateral x-ray of a knee with discoid menisci

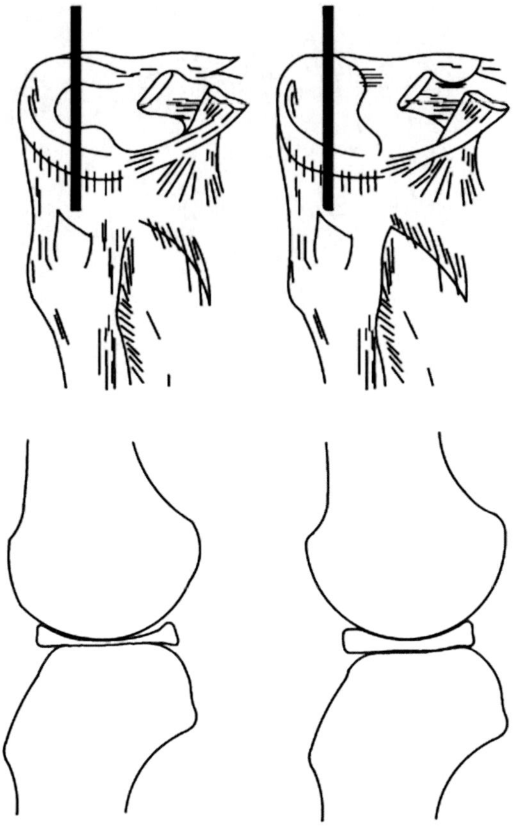

Fig. 7 Diagrammatic explanation of the bow tie appearance on sagittal MRI sections

Radiology: Ultrasonography

Ultrasonographic imaging of the menisci may demonstrate a wide and irregularly shaped lateral discoid meniscus. Sonography has been used to evaluate meniscal tears due to its availability, multi-planar capability, and economic benefit. The use of high-resolution micro-convex probes, which better fit the anatomical concavity of the popliteal fossa, achieves a better sensitivity and specificity in detecting meniscal tears (Najafi et al. 2006). The disadvantage of the use of ultrasonography is that it is an examiner-dependent tool. The sonographic criteria for diagnosis of discoid meniscus in children is reported as the absence of a normal triangular shape, the presence of an abnormally elongated and thick meniscal tissue, and the demonstration of a heterogeneous central pattern (Achour et al. 2006).

Radiology: MRI

On magnetic resonance imaging (MRI), the presence of a discoid meniscus is suggested in 5 mm sagittal sections when three or more contiguous sections demonstrate continuity of the meniscus between the anterior and posterior horns. Normally, this black "bow tie" appearance (Figs. 7 and 8) would be seen only on two contiguous sagittal sections (Silverman et al. 1989; Burk et al. 1990). Although this is a useful sign, the finding will be absent in the unstable type if the meniscus has a normal shape. The presence of a discoid shape can be further confirmed if a coronal view demonstrates increased width of the mid-anteroposterior diameter. One may also note an increase in thickness of the anterior horn, the posterior horn, or the entire meniscus. >2 mm height difference or >15 mm transverse diameter in coronal view can suggest a discoid meniscus.

MRI can also be useful for detecting intrasubstance tear and/or degeneration of lateral discoid meniscus (Hamada et al. 1994). Although

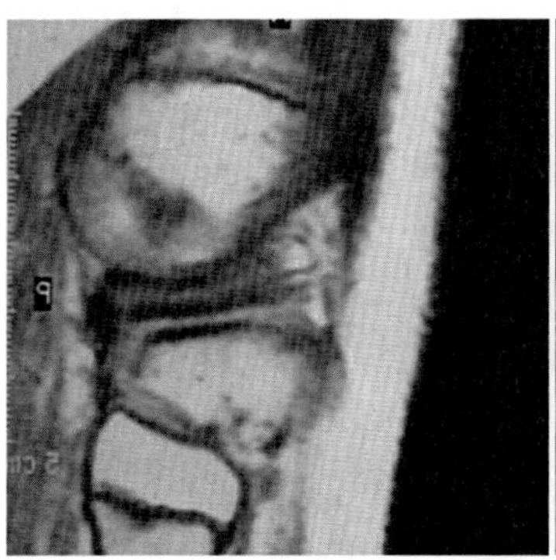
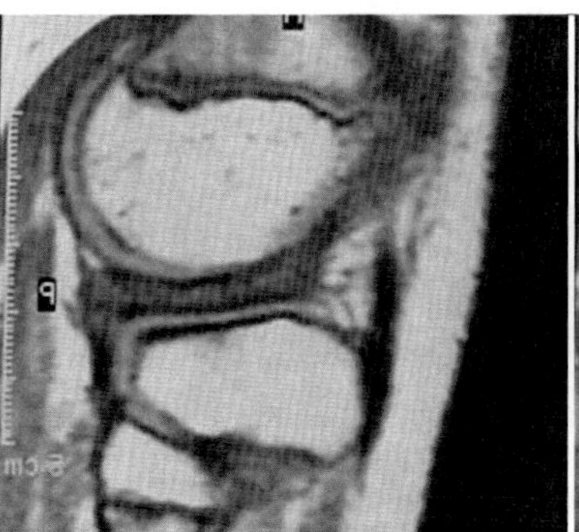
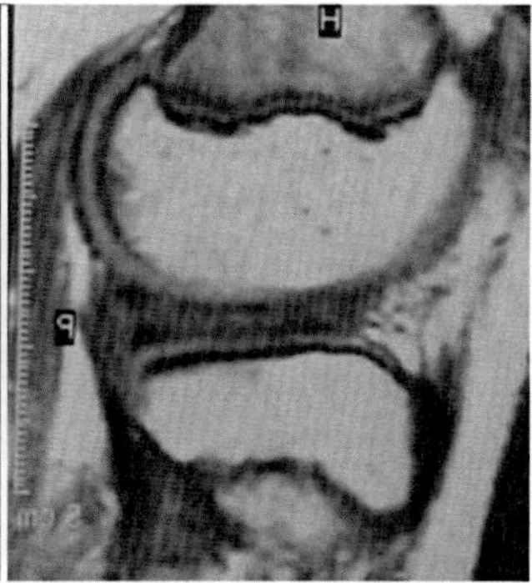

Fig. 8 Consecutive sagittal MRI sections showing bow tie appearance

valuable in the diagnosis of the discoid meniscus and tears, MRI can be insufficient in determining the type of the tear (Ryu et al. 1998).

Some authors indicate that the routine use of MRI is difficult and that arthroscopy should be used both for diagnostic and therapeutic purposes (Rao et al. 2001). A very recent study concluded that MRI is successful in determining the presence or absence of tears in discoid menisci; however, its ability to determine the tear types is questionable (Yilgor et al. 2013).

Treatment

The menisci serve in distributing loads and absorbing shock and have a role in joint stability, synovial fluid distribution, and cartilage nutrition. Partial meniscectomy of normal-shaped menisci was shown to increase the contact stresses in proportion to the amount of removed meniscus (Baratz et al. 1986). Following total meniscectomy, the contact area was decreased by up to 75 %, while contact stresses increased by 235 % (Baratz et al. 1986). A better understanding of the importance of the menisci to normal articular function has led to preservation of stable meniscal tissue as an important part of treatment planning.

Historically, the preferred treatment of a stable symptomatic lesion was open excision (Smillie 1948; Nathan and Cole 1969). However, total meniscectomy of a lateral non-discoid meniscus often leads to osteoarthritis (Fairbank 1948; Zaman and Leonard 1981; Manzione et al. 1983), and this is also true for discoid menisci in adults. In children, the risk of lateral degenerative arthritis after meniscectomy is greater than in adults; therefore, total meniscectomy for treatment of a discoid meniscus in children should be avoided whenever possible.

In order to properly choose the treatment method for the lateral meniscal variant, one must consider the age and activity level of the patient, the anatomy of the lesion, the duration and extent of the symptoms, and the amount of joint destruction. One must realize that the patient with a lateral meniscal variant usually has an abnormal knee at the outset. There may be no good treatment option; rather, the only choice may be the lesser of two evils.

The treatment options for the various lateral meniscal variants include observation, partial meniscectomy with or without reattachment, total meniscectomy, and for a normally shaped unstable lesion reattachment to the adjacent capsule. Many stable discoid menisci are found incidentally; therefore, it is reasonable to observe asymptomatic patients and inform them regarding an increased risk of having to undergo surgical treatment in the future. However, it should also be pointed out that the joint probably has adapted and could continue to function reasonably well. A snapping knee with no other symptoms and no radiographic signs of accompanying articular lesions can be followed-up and then treated should it become symptomatic. A patient may become symptomatic due to instability or a new

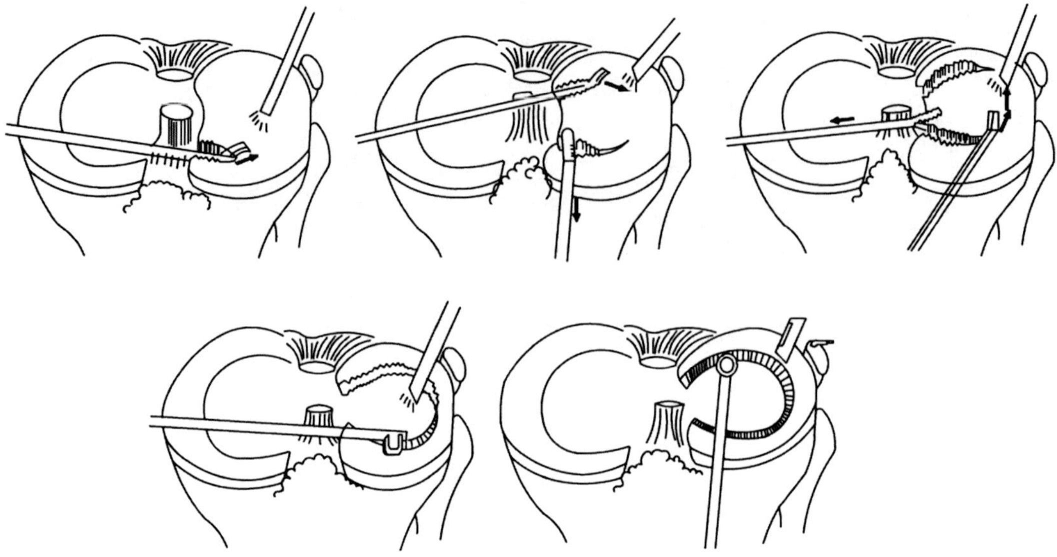

Fig. 9 Schematic explanation of one-piece excision technique

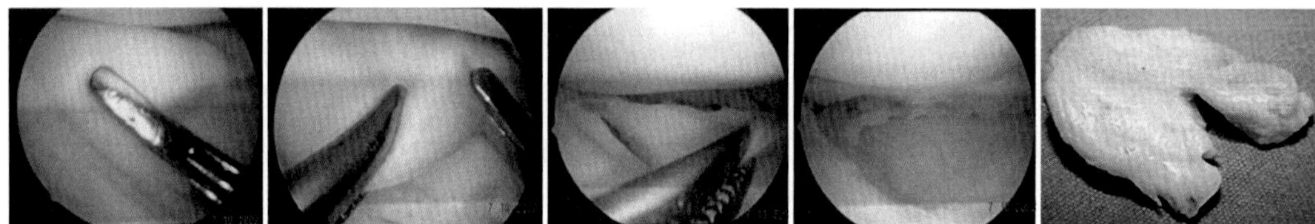

Fig. 10 One-piece excision of discoid lateral meniscus

tear of the meniscus or as the result of accompanying findings, such as osteochondral lesions to the lateral femoral condyle.

The current treatment of choice for a symptomatic stable, complete, or incomplete discoid lateral meniscus is arthroscopic partial meniscectomy (saucerization) (Ikeuchi 1982; Hayashi et al. 1988; Pellacci et al. 1992). Motorized and radiofrequency tools may be used for meniscal reshaping. In the past, some authors recommended total or subtotal meniscectomy as better than partial meniscectomy due to higher reoperation rates (Sugawara et al. 1991), because the increased thickness at the rim was thought to result in high shear forces concentrated at the resected margin due to the incongruity between meniscus and articular surface, which predisposed the abnormal meniscus rim to re-tear. Today, it is believed that a stable rim should be preserved, even though it may be composed of abnormal tissue (Fujikawa et al. 1981; Dickhaut and DeLee 1982; Bellier et al. 1989; Woods and Whelan 1990). The commonly used method for partial meniscectomy is one-piece excision that was described (Kim et al. 1996) (Fig. 9). Most authors agree that the width of the remaining peripheral rim should be between 5 and 8 mm to prevent impingement and instability of the remaining part that may lead to a future secondary meniscal tear and to decrease the rehabilitation time (Hayashi et al. 1988; Vandermeer and Cunningham 1989; Kim et al. 1995b; Smith et al. 1999). Saucerization and reattachment is also recommended for Wrisberg types (Rosenberg et al. 1987; Neuschwander et al. 1992).

During arthroscopy, a tear may not be visualized in some symptomatic discoid menisci. Therefore, a preoperative MRI is mandatory for all

Table 2 The knee rating system

Grade	Description
Excellent	No mechanical symptoms (click, locking), no pain, full range of movement
Good	No mechanical symptoms, occasional mild pain on exercise, full range of movement
Fair	Mechanical symptoms, mild to moderate pain on exercise, full range of movement
Poor	Mechanical symptoms, moderate to severe pain on exercise or pain at rest, limitation of movement

discoid menisci, because the absence and presence of shift and the direction of the shift must be carefully assessed before surgery since it alters the therapeutic approach. In the presence of a shift, the meniscus must be reduced before starting the excision (Yilgor et al. 2013). After resection, the tear in the opposite horn was repaired with sutures.

Figure 10 shows a one-piece excision performed at the authors' clinic step by step.

Treatment Outcome

The Ikeuchi rating system (Ikeuchi 1982) and Lysholm knee scale (Tegner and Lysholm 1985) are frequently used to evaluate the treatment outcome. Ikeuchi's system depends on mechanical symptoms, pain, and range of movement (Table 2). Lysholm's scale is a numerical scale where one gets points on limping, use of support, stair climbing, squatting, instability, swelling and pain of the knee, and atrophy of the thigh.

In 1991, it was reported that arthroscopic partial meniscectomy should be recommended only when the posterior attachment of the discoid meniscus is stable and that total meniscectomy is indicated for the Wrisberg ligament type of discoid meniscus with posterior instability (Aichroth et al. 1991). In the following years, results of longer follow-up studies showed that total meniscectomy results in osteoarthritic changes such as joint space narrowing and osteophytes in the lateral compartment (Washington et al. 1995; Raber et al. 1998; Aglietti et al. 1999). In 2003, excellent and good results were reported for partial meniscectomy in 85 % of their patients that had Watanabe complete- and incomplete-type discoid menisci (Atay et al. 2003). In the same year, others concluded that partial resection of discoid menisci is preferable in children, but in complete dislocation of the entire menisci, total removal may be necessary (Davidson et al. 2003). A more recent study concluded that although there were no differences in short-term follow-up for clinical results between the partial and subtotal/total meniscectomies, partial meniscectomy yielded better radiologic results for torn discoid lateral menisci in children (Lee et al. 2009). The long-term prognosis after arthroscopic meniscectomy for the torn discoid lateral meniscus was related to the volume of the meniscus removed (Good et al. 2007). Short-term results confirm that meniscal allograft transplantation after total meniscectomy could be reasonable in symptomatic patients (Kim and Bin 2006). However, long-term observations are required to evaluate these results.

Conclusion

It is suggested that there is a need for early diagnosis and greater caution in the treatment of discoid lateral menisci (Lee et al. 2009). Current classification of discoid menisci should include details about tear, symptoms, and shift besides their anatomical properties. Heightened awareness of the clinician to the possibility of discoid meniscus, its variable presentations and complications, and management considerations may improve therapeutic outcome (Yaniv and Blumberg 2007).

Cross-References

- ▶ Anatomy and Biomechanics of the Knee
- ▶ Arthroscopic Repair of the Meniscus Tears
- ▶ Asymptomatic Meniscal Tears
- ▶ Degenerative Meniscal Tears: Meniscal Cysts
- ▶ Human Meniscus: From Biology to Tissue Engineering Strategies

▶ Lateral Knee Pain
▶ Meniscal Injuries and Discoid Lateral Meniscus in Adolescent Athletes
▶ Meniscectomy
▶ Role of Biologicals in Meniscus Surgery

References

Achour NA, Tlili K, Souei MM et al (2006) Le menisque discoide chez l'enfant: aspects echographiques. J Radiol 87:35–40

Aglietti P, Bertini FA, Buzzi R et al (1999) Arthroscopic meniscectomy for discoid lateral meniscus in children and adolescents: 10-year follow-up. Am J Knee Surg 12(2):83–87

Ahn JH, Shim JS, Hwang CH et al (2001) Discoid lateral meniscus in children: clinical manifestations and morphology. J Pediatr Orthop 21(6):812–816

Ahn JH, Lee YS, Ha HC et al (2009) A novel magnetic resonance imaging classification of discoid lateral meniscus based on peripheral attachment. Am J Sports Med 37(8):1564–1569. doi:10.1177/0363546509332502

Aichroth PM, Patel DV, Marx CL (1991) Congenital discoid lateral meniscus in children. A follow-up study and evolution of management. J Bone Joint Surg 73(6):932–936

Albertsson M, Gillquist J (1988) Discoid lateral menisci: a report of 29 cases. Arthroscopy 4(3):211–214

Andrish JT (1996) Meniscal injuries in children and adolescents: diagnosis and management. J Am Acad Orthop Surg 4(5):231–237

Arnold MP, Van Kampen A (2000) Symptomatic ring-shaped lateral meniscus. Arthroscopy 16(8):852–854. doi:10.1053/jars.2000.8244

Asik M, Sen C, Taser OF et al (2003) Discoid lateral meniscus: diagnosis and results of arthroscopic treatment. Knee Surg Sports Traumatol Arthrosc 11 (2):99–104. doi:10.1007/s00167-002-0341-8

Atay OA, Aydingoz U, Doral MN et al (2002) Symptomatic ring-shaped lateral meniscus: magnetic resonance imaging and arthroscopy. Knee Surg Sports Traumatol Arthrosc 10(5):280–283. doi:10.1007/s00167-002-0292-0

Atay OA, Doral MN, Leblebicioglu G et al (2003) Management of discoid lateral meniscus tears: observations in 34 knees. Arthroscopy 19(4):346–352. doi:10.1053/jars.2003.50038

Atay OA, Pekmezci M, Doral MN et al (2007) Discoid meniscus: an ultrastructural study with transmission electron microscopy. Am J Sports Med 35 (3):475–478. doi:10.1177/0363546506294678

Baratz ME, Fu FH, Mengato R (1986) Meniscal tears: the effect of meniscectomy and of repair on intraarticular contact areas and stress in the human knee. A preliminary report. Am J Sports Med 14(4):270–275

Bellier G, Dupont JY, Larrain M et al (1989) Lateral discoid menisci in children. Arthroscopy 5(1):52–56

Bin SI, Kim JC, Kim JM et al (2002) Correlation between type of discoid lateral menisci and tear pattern. Knee Surg Sports Traumatol Arthrosc 10(4):218–222. doi:10.1007/s00167-001-0273-8

Burk DL Jr, Mitchell DG, Rifkin MD et al (1990) Recent advances in magnetic resonance imaging of the knee. Radiol Clin North Am 28(2):379–393

Casscells SW (1978) Gross pathological changes in the knee joint of the aged individual: a study of 300 cases. Clin Orthop Relat Res 132:225–232

Choi NH (1999) A ring-shaped lateral meniscus. Am J Knee Surg 12(2):109–110

Clark CR, Ogden JA (1983) Development of the menisci of the human knee joint. Morphological changes and their potential role in childhood meniscal injury. J Bone Joint Surg Am 65(4):538–547

D'Lima DD, Copp SN, Colwell CW Jr (1995) Isolated lateral ring meniscus. Case report. Am J Knee Surg 8 (3):117–118

Davidson D, Letts M, Glasgow R (2003) Discoid meniscus in children: treatment and outcome. Can J Surg J canadien de chirurgie 46(5):350–358

Dickason JM, Del Pizzo W, Blazina ME et al (1982) A series of ten discoid medial menisci. Clin Orthop Relat Res 168:75–79

Dickhaut SC, DeLee JC (1982) The discoid lateral-meniscus syndrome. J Bone Joint Surg Am 64 (7):1068–1073

Fairbank TJ (1948) Knee joint changes after meniscectomy. J Bone Joint Surg 30B(4):664–670

Fujikawa K, Iseki F, Mikura Y (1981) Partial resection of the discoid meniscus in the child's knee. J Bone Joint Surg 63-B(3):391–395

Good CR, Green DW, Griffith MH et al (2007) Arthroscopic treatment of symptomatic discoid meniscus in children: classification, technique, and results. Arthroscopy 23(2):157–163. doi:10.1016/j.arthro.2006.09.002

Hamada M, Shino K, Kawano K et al (1994) Usefulness of magnetic resonance imaging for detecting intrasubstance tear and/or degeneration of lateral discoid meniscus. Arthroscopy 10(6):645–653

Hayashi LK, Yamaga H, Ida K et al (1988) Arthroscopic meniscectomy for discoid lateral meniscus in children. J Bone Joint Surg Am 70(10):1495–1500

Ikeuchi H (1982) Arthroscopic treatment of the discoid lateral meniscus. Technique and long-term results. Clin Orthop Relat Res 167:19–28

Irani RN, Karasick D, Karasick S (1984) A possible explanation of the pathogenesis of osteochondritis dissecans. J Pediatr Orthop 4(3):358–360

Johnson R, Beynnon BD (2001) Chapman's orthopaedic surgery, 3rd edn. Lippincott Williams & Wilkins, Philadelphia

Jordan MR (1996) Lateral meniscal variants: evaluation and treatment. J Am Acad Orthop Surg 4(4):191–200

Kaplan EB (1957) Discoid lateral meniscus of the knee joint; nature, mechanism, and operative treatment. J Bone Joint Surg Am 39-A(1):77–87

Kerr R (1986) Radiologic case study. Discoid lateral meniscus. Orthopedics 9(8):1145–1147, 1142

Kim JM, Bin SI (2006) Meniscal allograft transplantation after total meniscectomy of torn discoid lateral meniscus. Arthroscopy 22(12):1344–1350 e1341. doi:10.1016/j.arthro.2006.07.048

Kim SJ, Jeon CH, Koh CH (1995a) A ring-shaped lateral meniscus. Arthroscopy 11(6):738–739

Kim SJ, Kim DW, Min BH (1995b) Discoid lateral meniscus associated with anomalous insertion of the medial meniscus. Clin Orthop Relat Res 315:234–237

Kim SJ, Yoo JH, Kim HK (1996) Arthroscopic one-piece excision technique for the treatment of symptomatic lateral discoid meniscus. Arthroscopy 12(6):752–755

Kim SJ, Lee YT, Choi CH et al (1998) A partially duplicated discoid lateral meniscus. Arthroscopy 14 (5):518–521

Kim YG, Ihn JC, Park SK et al (2006) An arthroscopic analysis of lateral meniscal variants and a comparison with MRI findings. Knee Surg Sports Traumatol Arthrosc 14(1):20–26. doi:10.1007/s00167-005-0629-6

Kroiss F (1910) Die Verletzungen der Kniegelenk Zwischenknorpel und ihrer Verbindungen. Beitr Klin Chir 66:598–801

Le Minor JM (1990) Comparative morphology of the lateral meniscus of the knee in primates. J Anat 170:161–171

Lee DH, Kim TH, Kim JM et al (2009) Results of subtotal/total or partial meniscectomy for discoid lateral meniscus in children. Arthroscopy 25(5):496–503. doi:10.1016/j.arthro.2008.10.025

Manzione M, Pizzutillo PD, Peoples AB et al (1983) Meniscectomy in children: a long-term follow-up study. Am J Sports Med 11(3):111–115

Mitsuoka T, Shino K, Hamada M et al (1999) Osteochondritis dissecans of the lateral femoral condyle of the knee joint. Arthroscopy 15(1):20–26. doi:10.1053/ar.1999.v15.015002

Mizuta H, Nakamura E, Otsuka Y et al (2001) Osteochondritis dissecans of the lateral femoral condyle following total resection of the discoid lateral meniscus. Arthroscopy 17(6):608–612. doi:10.1053/jars.2001.19979

Monllau JC, Leon A, Cugat R et al (1998) Ring-shaped lateral meniscus. Arthroscopy 14(5):502–504

Najafi J, Bagheri S, Lahiji FA (2006) The value of sonography with micro convex probes in diagnosing meniscal tears compared with arthroscopy. J Ultrasound Med Off J Am Inst Ultrasound Med 25(5):593–597

Nathan PA, Cole SC (1969) Discoid meniscus. A clinical and pathologic study. Clin Orthop Relat Res 64:107–113

Neuschwander DC, Drez D Jr, Finney TP (1992) Lateral meniscal variant with absence of the posterior coronary ligament. J Bone Joint Surg Am 74(8):1186–1190

Noble J (1977) Lesions of the menisci. Autopsy incidence in adults less than fifty-five years old. J Bone Joint Surg Am 59(4):480–483

Pellacci F, Montanari G, Prosperi P et al (1992) Lateral discoid meniscus: treatment and results. Arthroscopy 8 (4):526–530

Picard JJ, Constantin L (1964) Radiological aspects of the discoid meniscus. J Radiol Electrol Med Nucl 45:839–841

Raber DA, Friederich NF, Hefti F (1998) Discoid lateral meniscus in children. Long-term follow-up after total meniscectomy. J Bone Joint Surg Am 80 (11):1579–1586

Rao PS, Rao SK, Paul R (2001) Clinical, radiologic, and arthroscopic assessment of discoid lateral meniscus. Arthroscopy 17(3):275–277. doi:10.1053/jars.2001.19973

Rosenberg TD, Paulos LE, Parker RD et al (1987) Discoid lateral meniscus: case report of arthroscopic attachment of a symptomatic Wrisberg-ligament type. Arthroscopy 3(4):277–282

Ryu KN, Kim IS, Kim EJ et al (1998) MR imaging of tears of discoid lateral menisci. AJR Am J Roentgenol 171 (4):963–967. doi:10.2214/ajr.171.4.9762976

Shahriaree H (1992) O'Conner's textbook of arthroscopic surgery. Lippincott, Philadelphia

Silverman JM, Mink JH, Deutsch AL (1989) Discoid menisci of the knee: MR imaging appearance. Radiology 173(2):351–354

Smillie IS (1948) The congenital discoid meniscus. J Bone Joint Surg 30B(4):671–682

Smith CF, Van Dyk GE, Jurgutis J et al (1999) Cautious surgery for discoid menisci. Am J Knee Surg 12(1):25–28

Sugawara O, Miyatsu M, Yamashita I et al (1991) Problems with repeated arthroscopic surgery in the discoid meniscus. Arthroscopy 7(1):68–71

Suzuki S, Mita F, Ogishima H (1991) Double-layered lateral meniscus: a newly found anomaly. Arthroscopy 7(3):267–271

Tegner Y, Lysholm J (1985) Rating systems in the evaluation of knee ligament injuries. Clin Orthop Relat Res 198:43–49

Terashima T, Ohkoshi Y, Yamamoto K et al (2005) The pathogenesis of osteochondritis dissecans in the lateral femoral condyle associated with lateral discoid meniscus injury. Paper presented at the Biennial Congress of International Society of Arthroscopy, Knee Surgery and Orthopaedic Sports Medicine (ISAKOS), Hollywood, 3–7 Apr 2005

Tetik O, Doral MN, Atay OA et al (2003) Partial deficiency of the lateral meniscus. Arthroscopy 19(5):E42. doi:10.1053/jars.2003.50162

Vandermeer RD, Cunningham FK (1989) Arthroscopic treatment of the discoid lateral meniscus: results of long-term follow-up. Arthroscopy 5(2):101–109

Washington ER 3rd, Root L, Liener UC (1995) Discoid lateral meniscus in children. Long-term follow-up after excision. J Bone Joint Surg Am 77(9):1357–1361

Watanabe M, Takeda S, Ikeuchi H (1979) Atlas of arthroscopy, 3rd edn. Igaku-Shoin, Tokyo

Watson-Jones R (1930) Specimen of internal semilunar cartilage as a complete disc. Proc R Soc Med 23:588

Woods GW, Whelan JM (1990) Discoid meniscus. Clin Sports Med 9(3):695–706

Yaniv M, Blumberg N (2007) The discoid meniscus. J Child Orthop 1(2):89–96. doi:10.1007/s11832-007-0029-1

Yilgor C, Atay OA, Ergen B et al (2013) Comparison of magnetic resonance imaging findings with arthroscopic findings in discoid meniscus. Knee Surg Sports Traumatol Arthrosc. doi:10.1007/s00167-013-2371-9

Yoshida S, Ikata T, Takai H et al (1998) Osteochondritis dissecans of the femoral condyle in the growth stage. Clin Orthop Relat Res 346:162–170

Young R (1889) The external semilunar cartilage as a complete disc. In: Cleland J, Mackay J, Young R (eds) Memoirs and memoranda in anatomy. Williams and Norgate, London, p 179

Zaman M, Leonard MA (1981) Meniscectomy in children: results in 59 knees. Injury 12(5):425–428

Medial Patellofemoral Ligament Reconstruction: Current Concepts

100

Masataka Deie and Mitsuo Ochi

Contents

M. Deie (✉) • M. Ochi
Department of Orthopaedic Surgery, Hiroshima University, Hiroshima, Japan
e-mail: snm3@hiroshima-u.ac.jp; mochi@hiroshima-u.ac.jp; ochim@hiroshima-u.ac.jp

M.N. Doral, J. Karlsson (eds.), *Sports Injuries*,
DOI 10.1007/978-3-642-36569-0_126

Abstract

Anatomical and biomechanical studies indicate that the medial patellofemoral ligament (MPFL) is the primary restraint to lateral patellar dislocation and displacement. The MPFL lies along the second layer of the medial side components and extends from the superior two-thirds of the patellar medial edge to the femoral insertion, providing 50–60 % of the biomechanical stabilizing force for the medial patella.

In recent years, MPFL reconstruction has become an accepted surgical treatment for patellofemoral instability. The goal of such a surgical intervention should be to restore normal anatomical function and stability, and complications of MPFL reconstruction remain the major cause of technical problems with the surgery.

Quantitative stress radiography of the patella performed in the outpatient clinic may provide important information about the indications for lateral release. Furthermore, the lateral release procedure increases lateral, but not medial, instability in patients with recurrent patellar dislocation who do not exhibit medial instability prior to surgery.

The Anatomy and Biomechanics of MPFL

Anatomical and biomechanical studies revealed that the medial patellofemoral ligament (MPFL) is the primary restraint to lateral patellar dislocation and displacement (Warren and Marshall 1979; Andrish 2004; Panagiotopoulos et al 2006). The MPFL is a thin fascial band of approximately 53 mm in length (range 45–64 mm) (Tuxoe et al 2002). The anatomy of the medial side of the knee joint shows three layers: the first corresponds to the superficial retinaculum, the second to the MPFL and medial collateral ligament, and the third to the medial patellotibial ligament and the medial patellomeniscal ligament (Warren and Marshall 1979). Within this anatomical context, the MPFL extends from the superior two-thirds of the patellar medial edge to the femoral insertion, with the patellar end of the MPFL passing deep into the distal part of the vastus medialis obliquus, which overlays the MPFL at the patellar attachment and attaches to the proximal part of the patellar at the medial border. Recent anatomical studies located the femoral insertion site of the MPFL between the adductor tubercle and the medial femoral epicondyle (Nomura et al. 2000; Smirk and Morris 2003; Steensen et al. 2004; Fig. 1).

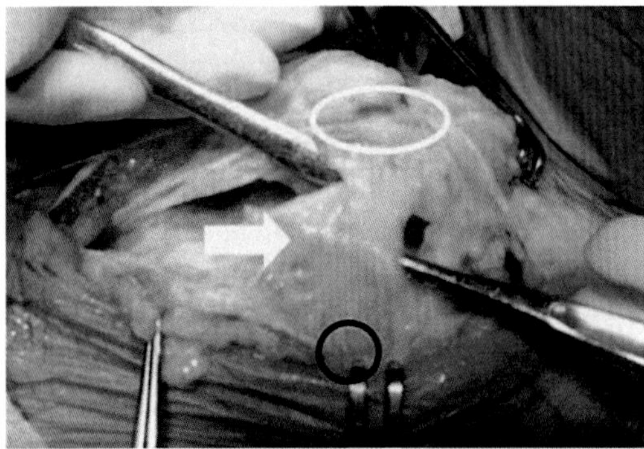

Fig. 1 Image of MPFL (*arrow*). *White circle* shows the natural MPFL attachment at the patellar site and the *black circle* shows the femoral attachment of the MPFL

Biomechanical studies show that the MPFL provides 50–60 % of the medial patella-stabilizing force (Conlan et al. 1993; Desio et al. 1998; Nomura et al. 2000). Conlan et al. (1993) further showed that the MPFL could resist 53 % of the biomechanical force needed to cause a 12.7-mm patellar lateral displacement. In a similar study, Desio et al. (1998) displaced the patella laterally at 20 % knee flexion, using a ball joint to allow patellar tilt. By sequential cutting of structures, they found that the MPFL had resisted 60 % of this force. The studies described above tested their knees near to full extension, because the patella is known from clinical experience to dislocate most commonly in a relatively extended posture. In addition, Amis et al. (2003) described that the contribution of the MPFL to resisting patellar lateral displacement was determined as the difference between the force measured at 10 mm lateral displacement before and after the MPFL was transected.

MPFL Reconstruction

MPFL reconstruction has become an accepted surgical technique for restoring patellofemoral instability over the last decade. Non-anatomical reconstruction of the MPFL can lead to non-physiological patellofemoral pressure and abnormal patellar tracking, whereas a surgical intervention should aim for anatomical reconstruction.

Femoral insertion is the critical part of an MPFL reconstruction since it allows isometric adjustments of the graft, resulting in a good clinical outcome.

The radiographic landmarks for the femoral MPFL center recommended by Schottle et al. (2007) are 1.3 mm anterior to the posterior cortex extension and 2.5 mm distal to the posterior origin of the medial femoral condyle, just proximal to the posterior point of the Blumensaat line on the lateral view (Fig. 2). On the other hand, Smirk and Morris (2003) reported that the best patellar attachment site should include the normal MPFL attachment, in the superior third of the patella, and an attachment in the middle of the patella.

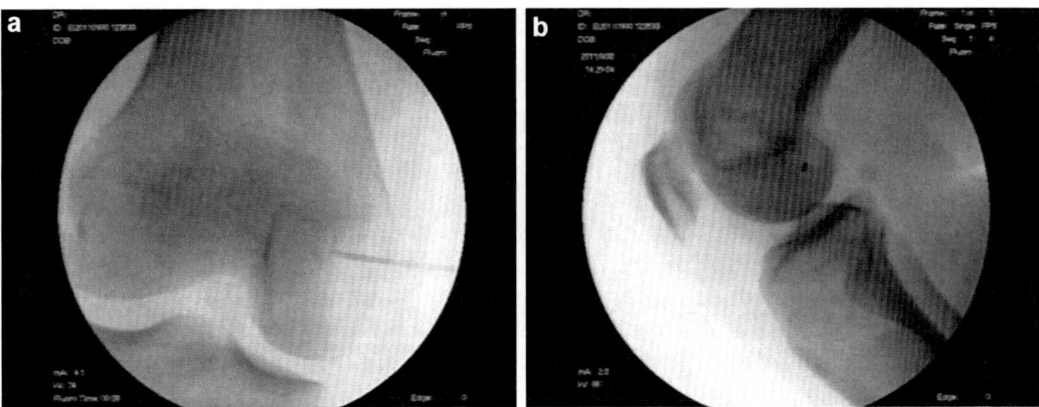

Fig. 2 Fixation point of grafted MPFL at the femoral site: (**a**) Coronal view. (**b**) Lateral view

The Surgical Procedures of MPFL Reconstruction

Many surgical procedures for MPFL reconstruction with excellent clinical results have been reported in the last two decades. In 1990, Suganuma et al. (1990) described an MPFL reconstruction method in a Japanese journal using an autograft tendon or an artificial ligament. Then, 2 years later, Ellera (1992) reported using an artificial polyester ligament that was fixed in a transverse drill hole of the patella and then fixed to the medial femoral condyle with a metal screw. Following these reports, many surgeons reported on MPFL reconstructions, with techniques including a free semitendinosus, gracilis, quadriceps, adductor tendon, a vastus medialis retinaculum autograft, and artificial ligament (Munuta et al. 1999; Cossey and Paterson 2005; Schottle et al. 2005). Fixation techniques have also varied, with femoral side fixations conducted such that the bone tunnel was made and fixed using an interference screw, the endobutton technique, direct suture, or a bone plug and staple (Muneta et al. 1999; Cossey and Paterson 2005; Schottle et al. 2005; Deie et al. 2011; Fig. 3). For children, to avoid damaging the femoral distal epiphysis, surgeons have mostly reported the tendon transfer technique whereby the graft was passed through the posterior one-third of the MCL femoral insertion, which acts as a pulley (Deie et al. 2003; Fig. 4).

The patellar site fixation was also variable, with three main techniques reported: (1) through a drill hole in the patella, (2) avoid drilling in the patella by using an anchor fixation or interference screw, and (3) suture fixation on the patellar surface with attachment to the medial site of the patella.

All techniques aimed to supply graft tissue from the medial aspect of the patella to the insertion site of the natural MPFL at the adductor tubercle of the medial femoral condyle, to reconstruct the ligament anatomically.

Complications of MPFL Reconstruction

Various complications have been reported with MPFL reconstruction including patellar fracture, recurrent lateral instability, patellofemoral arthrosis, loss of range of motion, and medial instability (Traunat and Erasmus 2009; Parikh and Wall 2011). Parikh et al. (2013) reported complications in 16.2 % of their 179 knees, with almost half resulting from technical problems. In addition, non-anatomical placement of the femoral tunnel could cause recurrent lateral instability and arthrosis of the patellofemoral joint. Female gender and bilateral cases were also reported as risk factors associated with postoperative complications. A small bone tunnel has been recommended to avoid patellar fracture after MPFL, and based on over 100 MPFL reconstructions, we recommend suture fixation on the patella.

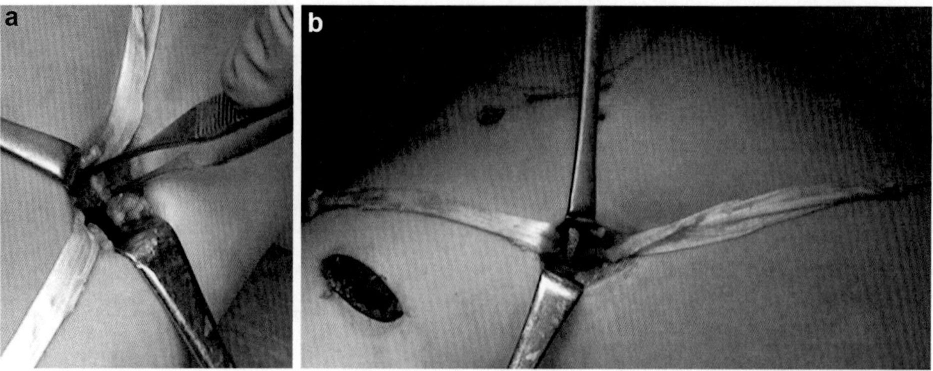

Fig. 3 Our surgical procedure – graft fixation at the femoral site. (**a**) The grafted tendon (semitendinosus tendon) was inserted at the bone tunnel and the plug was fixed. (**b**) Then, the staple was fixed over the bone plug and the grafted tendon

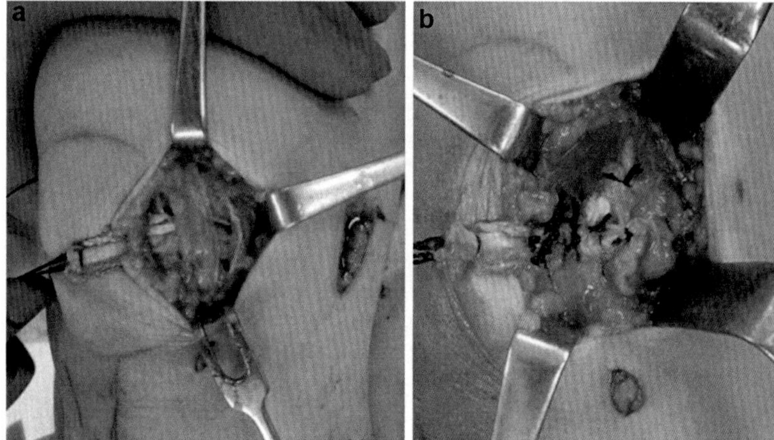

Fig. 4 Our surgical procedure – graft fixation at the patellar site. (**a**) The grafted tendon (semitendinosus tendon) was induced at the patellar surface. (**b**) The grafted tendon was then sutured at the periosteum of the patellar surface

Indication for Lateral Release with MPFL Reconstruction and Quantitative Stress Radiography of the Patella

Lateral release has been performed alone or in combination with medial tightening procedures to treat both acute and chronic lateral instability of the patellofemoral joint (Chen and Ramanathan 1984; Aglietti et al. 1989; Fithian et al 2004). Lateral release as an open or arthroscopic procedure is also performed to treat disorders of the extensor mechanism of the knee (Fulkerson and Shea 1990). Patellofemoral joint stability depends on several factors including the balance of quadriceps muscle forces, the articular geometry of the patella and femur, the retinacular structures of the MPFL, and the direction of the patellar tendon (Amis and Farahmand 1996). While MPFL reconstruction has become an accepted surgical technique to restore patellofemoral instability, there are many causes of patellar instability, making the selection of the best surgical treatment difficult. Lateral release is a surgical procedure that is sometimes performed to treat patellofemoral pain, maltracking, and instability. It is considered a relatively benign

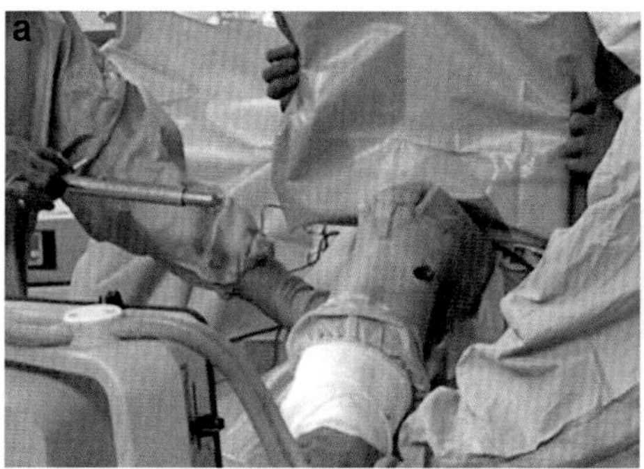

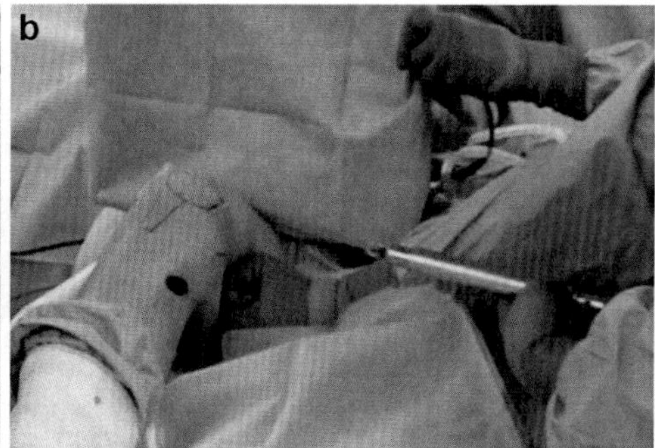

Fig. 5 Intraoperative quantitative stress radiography of the patella. Before lateral release at surgery, a soft wire (28 gauge) was inserted into the center of the patella from the lateral side to the inside, and then, 20 N stress was similarly applied from the medial to lateral direction (**a**) and from the lateral to medial direction to obtain axial images (**b**)

procedure, requiring minimal surgical intervention without the need for immobilization, and is associated with only minor complications (Henry et al. 1986; Schonholtz et al. 1987).

In the past, the importance of lateral release in the prevention of recurrent patellar dislocation has been emphasized (Chen and Ramanathan 1984). However, when lateral release is used alone as a procedure to treat patellar instability, the failure rate is unacceptably high (Aglietti et al. 1989; Kolowich et al. 1990; Shellock et al. 1990; Fithian et al. 2004). Furthermore, some reports have described medial dislocation after lateral release (Hughston et al. 1996; Clifton et al. 2010).

It is now rare for lateral release to be performed alone and usually involves an additional technique to correct the balance of the patella. However, even after MPFL reconstruction, performing lateral release can result in serious complications, including medial subluxation of the patella (Hughston et al. 1996; Clifton et al. 2010). Therefore, determining the indications for lateral release during MPFL reconstruction is very important. We have consistently performed quantitative stress radiography of the patella to make such a decision since 1988 (Ochi et al. 1992, 1993). The efficacy of this approach, which can be performed in the outpatient clinic, is valuable as an indicator for lateral release and to evaluate instability of the patella before and after lateral release.

Preoperative and Intraoperative Evaluation of Patellar Laxity

Quantitative Stress Radiography of the Patella

The recurrent dislocation patellar knees have undergone the stress radiography to detect patellar laxity. All patients were evaluated radiographically in the outpatient clinic and then again at the time of surgery before and after the lateral release procedure (detailed procedure and data, Niimoto et al., KSSTA under revision). In the outpatient clinic, patellar stress radiography views were obtained at 45° knee flexion with 20 N stress from the medial to lateral direction and from the lateral to medial direction using a pushing apparatus (Ochi et al. 1992; Clifton et al. 2010). The intraoperative stress views obtained before and after lateral release are as follows: a soft wire was inserted into the center of the patella from the lateral side to the inside (Fig. 5a) and 20 N of stress was similarly applied from the medial to lateral direction and from the lateral to medial direction to obtain axial images (Fig. 5b). Then, we evaluated the laxity of the patella.

Preoperative and intraoperative stress views were well correlated both the medial and lateral laxity. Medial laxity shows no significant differences before and after lateral release. However, the lateral laxity after lateral release significantly increased to compare the lateral laxity before lateral release.

These data gain the results from patients with recurrent patellar dislocation. In these patients, the patellar stress radiography obtained in the outpatient clinic was as useful as conventional radiography performed in anesthetized patients prior to surgery as an indicator for lateral release. In addition, the lateral instability increased significantly after the lateral release procedure, whereas there was little change in medial instability, in patients with recurrent patellar dislocation in whom lateral release was indicated on the basis of patellar stress radiography.

Ochi et al. (1993) have obtained quantitative stress radiography images of the patella when selecting the treatment strategy for patellar instability and deciding whether to perform the lateral release procedure since 1988. They described two main types of lateral dislocation: one in which the lateral retinaculum is tighter than normal and another in which the medial retinaculum is looser than normal (Ochi et al. 1993). They also highlighted that patients showing medial laxity on stress radiography before surgery would experience medial patellar dislocation with lateral release.

Although lateral release is widely used to perform worldwide, the procedure has resulted in serious complications, including medial subluxation of the patella. Even now, lateral release performed in isolation to treat patellofemoral disorders remains contentious. It is important to appreciate what can be achieved with the release of the lateral retinaculum (Clifton et al. 2010). Thus, we strongly recommend quantitative patellar stress radiography to indicate lateral release and to avoid the possible complication of patellar instability treatments.

Conclusions

1. MPFL reconstruction is now a promising surgical treatment for patellar instability.
2. The complications of MPFL reconstruction are mainly due to technical problems.
3. Quantitative stress radiography of the patella in the outpatient clinic could be very useful in determining indications for lateral release.
4. The lateral release procedure increases lateral, but not medial, laxity in patients with recurrent patellar dislocation who do not exhibit medial laxity prior to surgery.

References

Aglietti P, Pisaneschi A, Buzzi R et al (1989) Arthroscopic lateral release for patellar pain or instability. Arthroscopy 5:176–183

Amis AA, Farahmand F (1996) Biomechanics masterclass: extensor mechanism of the knee. Curr Orthop 10:102–109

Amis AA, Firer P, Mountney J, Senavongse W et al (2003) Anatomy and biomechanics of the medial patellofemoral ligament. Knee 10:215–220

Andrish J (2004) The biomechanics of patellofemoral stability. J Knee Surg 17:35–39

Chen SC, Ramanathan EBS (1984) The treatment of patellar instability by lateral release. J Bone Joint Surg Br 66:344–348

Clifton R, Ng CY, Nutton RW (2010) What is the role of lateral retinacular release? J Bone Joint Surg Br 92B:1–6

Conlan T, Garth WP Jr, Lemons JE (1993) Evaluation of the medial soft-tissue restrains of the extensor mechanism of the knee. J Bone Joint Surg Am 75:682–693

Cossey AJ, Paterson R (2005) A new technique for reconstructing the medial patellofemoral ligament. Knee 12:93–98

Deie M, Ochi M, Sumen Y et al (2003) Reconstruction of the medial patellofemoral ligament for the treatment of habitual or recurrent dislocation of the patella in children. J Bone Joints Surg Br 85:887–890

Deie M, Ochi M, Adachi N et al (2011) Medial patellofemoral ligament reconstruction fixed with a cylindrical bone plug and a grafted semitendinosus tendon at the original femoral site for recurrent patellar dislocation. Am J Sports Med 39:140–145

Desio SM, Burks RT, Bachus KN (1998) Soft tissue restrains to lateral patellar translation in the human knee. Am J Sports Med 26:59–65

Ellera Gomes JL (1992) Medial patellofemoral ligament reconstruction for recurrent dislocation of the patella: a preliminary report. Arthroscopy 8:335–340

Fithian DC, Paxton EW, Post WR et al (2004) Lateral retinacular release: a survey of the International Patellofemoral Study Group. Arthroscopy 20:463–468

Fulkerson JP, Shea KP (1990) Disorders of patellofemoral alignment. J Bone Joint Surg Am 72A:1424–1429

Henry JH, Goletz TH, Williamson B (1986) Lateral retinacular release in patellofemoral subluxation. Indications, results, and comparison to open patellofemoral reconstruction. Am J Sports Med 14:121–129

Hughston JC, Flandry F, Brinker MR et al (1996) Surgical correction of medial subluxation of the patella. Am J Sports Med 24:486–491

Kolowich PA, Paulos LE, Rosenberg TD et al (1990) Lateral release of the patella: indications and contraindications. Am J Sports Med 18:359–365

Muneta T, Sekiya I, Tsuchiya M et al (1999) A technique for reconstruction of the medial patellofemoral ligament. Clin Orthop 359:151–155

Nomura E, Horiuchi Y, Kihara M (2000) Medial patellofemoral ligament restraint in lateral patellar translation and reconstruction. Knee 7:121–127

Ochi M, Sota T, Matsuda T et al (1992) The significance of roentgenograph of patella under 2 kg stress in the skyline view (in Japanese). Bessatsu Seikeigeka 38–43

Ochi M, Deie M, Ikuta Y (1993) A new surgical procedure for recurrent patellar dislocation and subluxation. 2nd AOSSM/JOSSM trans-pacific meeting 38

Panagiotopoulos E, Strzelczyk P, Herrmann M et al (2006) Cadaveric study on static medial patellar stabilizers: the dynamizing role of the vastus medialis obliquus on medial patellofemoral ligament. Knee Surg Sports Traumatol Arthrosc 14:7–12

Parikh SN, Wall EJ (2011) Patellar fracture after medial patellofemoral ligament surgery. A report of five cases. J Bone and Joint Surg Am 93:e97(1–8)

Parikh SN, Nathan ST, Wall EJ et al (2013) Complications of medial patellofemoral ligament reconstruction in young patients. Am J Sports Med 41:1030–1038

Schonholtz GJ, Zahn MG, Magee CM (1987) Lateral retinacular release of the patella. Arthroscopy 3:269–272

Schöttle PB, Fucentese SF, Romero J (2005) Clinical and radiological outcome of medial patellofemoral ligament reconstruction with a semitendinosus autograft for patella instability. Knee Surg Sports Traumatol Arthrosc 13:516–521

Schöttle PB, Schmeling A, Rosenstiel N et al (2007) Radiographic landmarks for femoral tunnel placement in medial patellofemoral ligament reconstruction. Am J Sports Med 35:801–804

Shellock FG, Mink JH, Deutsch A et al (1990) Evaluation of patients with persistent symptoms after lateral retinacular release by kinetic magnetic resonance imaging of the patellofemoral joint. Arthroscopy 6:226–234

Smirk C, Morris H (2003) The anatomy and reconstruction of the medial patellofemoral ligament. Knee 10:221–227

Steensen RN, Dopirak RM, McDonald WG 3rd (2004) The anatomy and isometry of the medial patellofemoral ligament: implications for reconstruction. Am J Sports Med 32:1509–1513

Suganuma J, Mitani T, Suzuki N et al (1990) Reconstruction of the medial patellofemoral ligament (in Japanese). J Tokyo Knee Soc 10:137–148

Traunat M, Erasmus PJ (2009) Management of overtight medial patellofemoral ligament reconstruction. Knee Surg Sports Traumatol Arthrosc 17:480–483

Tuxoe J, Teir M, Winge S et al (2002) The medial patellofemoral ligament: a dissection study. Knee Surg Sports Traumatol Arthrosc 10:138–140

Warren LF, Marshall JL (1979) The supporting structures and layers on the medial side of the knee: an anatomical analysis. J Bone Joint Surg Am 61:56–62

Partial Anterior Cruciate Ligament Ruptures: Knee Laxity Measurements and Pivot Shift

101

Bruno Ohashi, James Ward, Paulo Araujo, Mauricio Kfuri, Hélder Pereira, João Espregueira-Mendes, and Volker Musahl

Contents

B. Ohashi (✉)
Center for Orthopaedics and Traumatology of Brasilia, Brasilia, DF, USA
e-mail: brunohashi@yahoo.com

J. Ward
Department of Orthopaedic Surgery, University of Pittsburgh Medical Center, Pittsburgh, PA, USA
e-mail: wardjp@upmc.edu

P. Araujo • M. Kfuri
Department of Biomechanics, Medicine and Rehabilitation of Locomotor System – Ribeirao Preto Medical School – São Paulo University, Brazil, São Paulo, Brazil
e-mail: pauloaraujo@hotmail.com; mauricio@kfuri.med.br

H. Pereira
3B's Research Group – Biomaterials, Biodegradables and Biomimetics, Headquarters of the European Institute of Excellence on Tissue Engineering and Regenerative Medicine, University of Minho, Taipas, Guimarães, Portugal

ICVS/3B's – PT Government Associated Laboratory, Guimarães, Portugal

Clínica Espregueira–Mendes F.C. Porto Stadium – FIFA Medical Centre of Excellence, Porto, Portugal

Orthopedic Department, Centro Hospitalar Póvoa de Varzim, Vila do Conde, Portugal
e-mail: heldermdpereira@gmail.com

J. Espregueira-Mendes
3B's Research Group – Biomaterials, Biodegradables and Biomimetics, Headquarters of the European Institute of Excellence on Tissue Engineering and Regenerative Medicine, University of Minho, Taipas, Guimarães, Portugal

Clínica Espregueira–Mendes F.C. Porto Stadium – FIFA Medical Centre of Excellence, Porto, Portugal

Orthopedic Department, Centro Hospitalar Póvoa de Varzim, Vila do Conde, Portugal

ICVS/3B's – PT Government Associated Laboratory, Braga/Guimarães, Portugal

Orthopaedic Department, Hospital S. Sebastião, Feira, Portugal
e-mail: jem@espregueira.com; joaoespregueira@netcabo.pt

M.N. Doral, J. Karlsson (eds.), *Sports Injuries*,
DOI 10.1007/978-3-642-36569-0_85

Abstract
Partial anterior cruciate ligament (ACL) tears can involve isolated injury to the anteromedial (AM) bundle, the posterolateral (PL) bundle, or ACL remnant healing to the posterior cruciate ligament (PCL). The viability and function of the partial ACL tear is assessed through history, physical examination, including laximetry utilizing new technologies, imaging, and arthroscopy. New treatment algorithms aim at individualizing treatment for partial ACL injuries to ultimately improve clinical outcomes for patients.

Introduction

Treatment algorithms for injuries of the anterior cruciate ligament (ACL) are rapidly evolving as the best available evidence from higher-level studies develops. With the increased recognition of partial tears of the ACL, new techniques for reconstruction or augmentation are being reported. Further research is defining the role of platelet-rich plasma (PRP), fibrin clot, and other growth factor augmentation techniques (Rodeo et al. 1999; Yeh et al. 2007; Kuang et al. 2010). The treating physician must be aware of the new advances in technique to provide a more complete analysis of the injury, with the aim being restoration of each patient's unique anatomy to achieve the goal of individualized ACL reconstruction.

Ruptures of either the anteromedial (AM) or posterolateral (PL) bundle in isolation have been reported to comprise between 5 % and 28 % of all injuries to the ACL. These partial tears pose new diagnostic challenges to the orthopedic surgeon. Suboptimal outcomes following ACL reconstruction can be related to an inaccurate diagnosis and poor preoperative planning. Improved diagnostic ability is necessary to select the optimal course of treatment for each patient. ACL augmentation procedures, which aim to reconstruct the AM bundle or PL bundle, are increasingly being performed and are showing good results (Ochi et al. 2006; Sonnery-Cottet et al. 2010).

Preservation of the ACL remnants may aid the biological process following an ACL reconstruction or augmentation surgery. The remnants may serve as a mechanical restraint in anterior knee stability (Crain et al. 2005). Histological studies revealed improved healing potential due to the vascular support provided by the epiligamentous tissue (Howell et al. 1995). Also, the remnants may provide a proprioceptive function due to the presence of neural mechanoreceptors (Ochi et al. 1999; Georgoulis et al. 2001; Adachi et al. 2002).

Clinical examination remains one of the most important steps when evaluating the injured knee. Ligamentous laxity is difficult to quantify and is currently graded subjectively by the examiner (Noyes et al. 1991; Kuroda et al. 2012). Hole et al. found that clinical evaluation is unreliable in the differentiation of a 75 % sectioned ligament from a completely sectioned ligament (Hole et al. 1996). To minimize this problem, objective instrumented laxity methods have been developed. The KT-1000 (MEDmetric Corp., San Diego, CA, USA) and the Rolimeter (Aircast, Vista, CA) are commonly used to quantify the Lachman test but with the limitation of measuring only anterior tibial translation. Instrumented anteroposterior laxity does not correlate with postoperative outcomes or development of osteoarthritis (Kocher et al. 2002).

The pivot shift is the most specific test for the diagnosis of an ACL rupture. It is also the most reliable test for the diagnosis of partial lesions (DeFranco and Bach 2009). It is manifested clinically by the complaint of "giving way" and as a physical sign that can be detected (Galway and MacIntosh 1980). The presence of a pivot shift has been correlated with poor subjective and objective knee scores, with rates of return to the same level of play and with the development of degenerative changes (Jonsson et al. 2004; Leitze et al. 2005). Thus, the goal of ACL reconstruction is elimination of the pivot shift.

V. Musahl
Department of Orthopaedic Surgery, University of Pittsburgh Medical Center, Pittsburgh, PA, USA

Division of Sports Medicine, Orthopaedic Surgery, University of Pittsburgh, Pittsburgh, PA, USA
e-mail: musahlv@upmc.edu

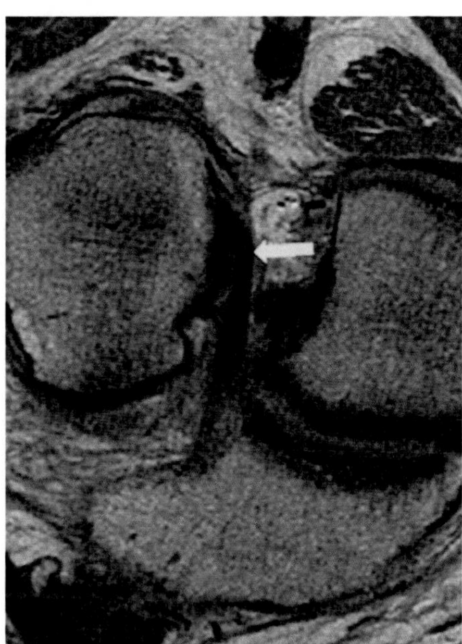

Fig. 1 Oblique coronal PD/TSE MR image showing a right knee with a partial ACL tear. The AM bundle is intact (*arrow*)

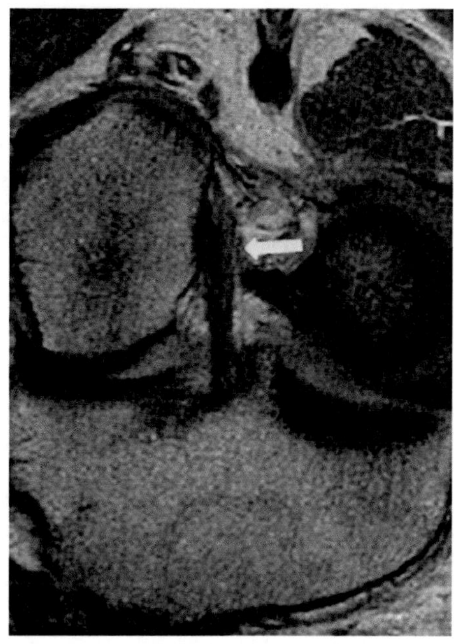

Fig. 2 Oblique coronal PD/TSE MR image showing a right knee with a partial ACL tear. The PL bundle is intact (*arrow*)

Partial Tears

Definition and Classification

A partial ACL rupture is defined as either an isolated lesion of the AM bundle or the PL bundle. The diagnosis is made by a combination of history, physical examination, advanced imaging, and arthroscopy. An isolated rupture of the AM bundle with a competent PL bundle is characterized as "PL intact" (Fig. 1). The converse is called "AM intact" (Fig. 2). The remnant of the ACL may adhere to the PCL which is called "PCL healing" (Bach and Warren 1989).

In terms of surgical versus nonsurgical treatment, it is necessary to distinguish whether the partial rupture is "functional" or "nonfunctional." Preserved bundles, which can develop tension on probing during arthroscopy, are classified as functional. If the preserved bundle shows abnormal laxity, it is classified as a "nonfunctional" partial rupture Dejour et al. (2013) (Fig. 3).

How Can the Clinical Examination Help with the Diagnosis?

Several devices are currently used to aid the clinician in the diagnosis of either a complete or a partial ACL tear. Siebold and Fu demonstrated that PL bundle ruptures showed 1–3 mm of increased laxity on KT-1000 measurements. For AM tears, the translation was greater, with a difference between 2 and 4 mm (Siebold and Fu 2008). Dejour et al. used Telos stress tests and bilateral stress radiographs and found complete tears to have a median of 9 mm of translation, 6 mm in all nonfunctional partial tears, and 4 mm in functional partial tears (Dejour et al. 2013). They were unable to differentiate between the anatomic patterns of the partial tear, i.e., AM versus PL tear. Panisset et al. studied the differences between complete and partial tears using the Rolimeter and the Telos device. The Rolimeter showed a mean side-to-side difference (SSD) of 5.3 mm for complete tears and 2.6 mm for partial tears, and the Telos device showed 7.4 mm and 4.0 mm, respectively. A threshold value of 5 mm

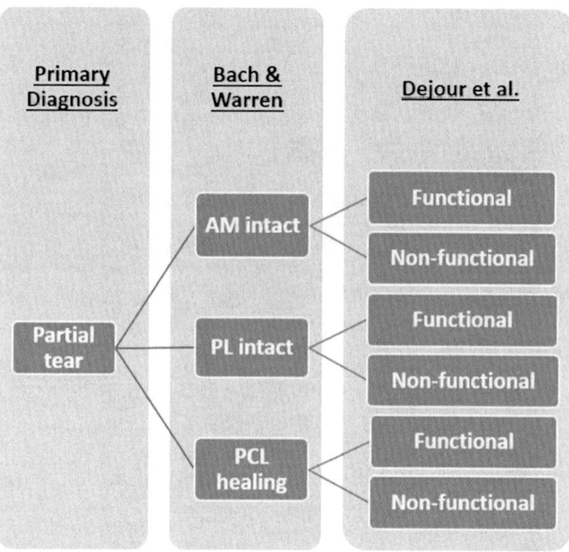

Fig. 3 Flowchart showing the classifications of partial tears according to Bach and Warren (1989) and Dejour et al. (2013)

of SSD demonstrated by the Telos device was strongly associated with the differential diagnosis of complete and partial tears of the ACL (sensitivity 80.9 %, specificity 81.8 %) (Panisset et al. 2012).

The Pivot-Shift Test

Historical Review

In 1972, Galway and MacIntosh characterized the pivot shift as anterior subluxation of the lateral tibial plateau on the femoral condyle as the knee approaches extension with spontaneous reduction in flexion (Galway and MacIntosh 1980). Losee, in 1982, stated that for the pivot shift to occur, the ACL, lateral, and posterolateral portions of the capsule have to be deficient (Losee 1982).

Many descriptions of the maneuver have been proposed. The classic description by Galway and MacIntosh is internal rotation of the foot, valgus moment on the knee by the upper hand, and during the flexion of the knee the displaced tibial plateau reduces (Galway and MacIntosh 1979). Bach et al. described a modified maneuver with the foot in external rotation, as an option to increase the sensitivity of the test. In addition, the position of the hip may influence the amount of translation during the maneuver. Placing the hip in abduction with tibial external rotation yielded the highest pivot-shift grade when compared to the hip in adduction and the tibia in external or internal rotation (Bach et al. 1988).

In 1987, Jakob and Stäubli created a method of grading the pivot shift. In their method, the maneuver is carried out with the patient's foot in three different rotations: internal, neutral, and external rotation. The system consists of three different grades: (I) the pivot shift occurs only in internal rotation with a small, gentle sliding reduction; (II) a "clunk" is felt when rotating the tibia in the neutral but mainly in internal rotation; and (III) a pronounced "clunk" occurs in neutral and external rotation, being less obvious in internal rotation. According to this method, increased grades represent involvement of different compartments of the knee, from mild anterolateral laxity in grade I through marked shift and translation in both compartments in grade III (Jakob et al. 1987).

As seen, there is a lack of agreement for the execution of the pivot-shift test. The maneuver can be executed with different speeds and forces and its grade is based on the clinician's subjective feel of the phenomenon while performing the test. Clinical grading of the pivot-shift test has low interobserver reliability (Noyes et al. 1991). In an effort to increase consistency between examiners, Musahl et al. attempted to obtain agreement on a standardized pivot-shift technique between

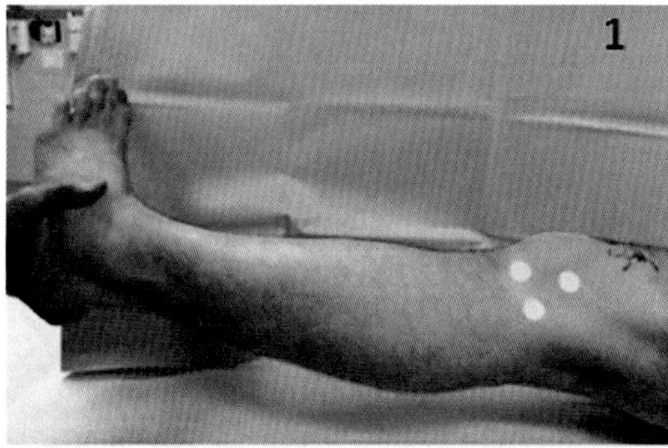

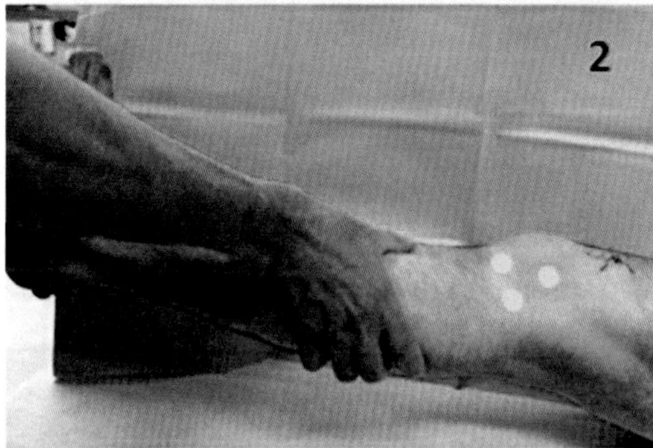

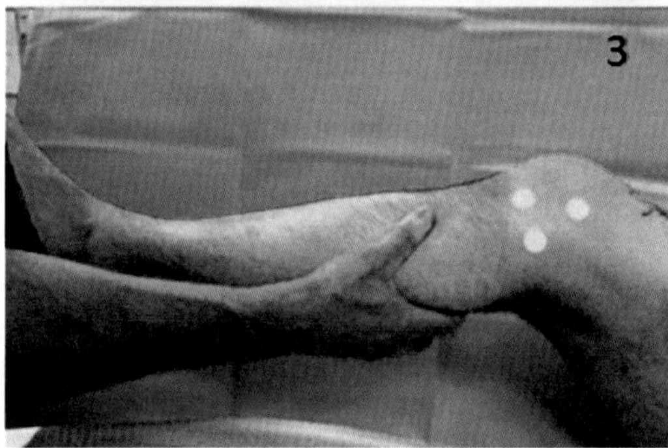

Fig. 4 Standardized technique for the pivot-shift test in three steps (Hoshino et al 2012a). The test is shown for a left knee. (1) Internal rotation applied by examiners' left hand (*top*). (2) Valgus stress applied by examiners' right hand (*middle*). (3) Knee flexion (applied by left hand) with release of the rotational stress and reduction of the tibial plateau (*bottom*)

experts and assess acceptance. The standardized maneuver consists of three steps (example for the left knee examination): (1) left hand holds the heel while internally rotating the leg; (2) with thumb up, the right hand applies a valgus moment just distal to the joint line; and (3) while flexing the knee with the left hand, rotational stress is released and the reduction is felt with the right hand (Fig. 4). Variation of acceleration between 12 expert examiners was significantly reduced when performing the standardized technique, yielding improved consistency for the test. Also, 87 % of the surgeons tested easily acquired the standardized test after instruction (Hoshino et al. 2012a).

Rotatory Knee Laxity and Pivot Shift

A major limitation of the pivot-shift test is that it is a non-weight-bearing examination and cannot mimic the true effect of rotatory knee laxity in dynamic weight-bearing conditions. The importance of rotatory knee laxity is increased with the focus on anatomic ACL reconstruction.

For the envelope of laxity of the knee, the ACL performs a primary function in preventing rotatory instability with the collateral ligaments, menisci, and joint capsule performing secondary functions (Bull et al. 2002; Bedi et al. 2010; Suero et al. 2012). The specific contributions of each structure are a point of current debate.

Bony morphology influences knee stability and the pivot-shift test. Musahl et al. described the influence of the femoral condyle and tibial plateau, concluding that smaller lateral tibial plateaus can be related to higher grade pivot-shift test results (Musahl et al. 2010a). Brandon et al. found that a higher pivot-shift grade is associated with an increased degree of posterior-inferior tibial slope (Brandon et al. 2006). Hoshino et al. using 3D-CT data and a dynamic stereo radiographic system, concluded that distal femoral geometry can influence dynamic rotatory laxity (Hoshino et al 2012d).

The function of the AM bundle concerning rotational instability has been rediscovered and increased in importance, despite the fact that the PL bundle was believed to be the primary bundle responsible for controlling rotational stability. Yasuda et al. stated that both bundles are important in both anterior and rotational laxity and the relative contributions of each bundle are dependent on the knee flexion angle (Yasuda et al. 2011). Similar findings have been echoed by other authors (Kato et al. 2013).

How Can the Pivot-Shift Test Help with the Diagnosis of a Partial Tear?

The pivot-shift test is the most important and useful test to define the extent of injury to the ACL. DeFranco and Bach determined that if damage to the ACL fibers is severe enough to produce a positive pivot-shift test, then the remaining ACL is nonfunctional (DeFranco and Bach 2009). Dejour et al. highlighted the importance of combining results of clinical tests to correctly diagnose partial tears and allowing for adequate preoperative planning. Higher grades (II or III) of pivot-shift laxity were consistent with complete tears, whereas lower grades (0 or I) were related to partial tears (Dejour et al. 2013). Van Eck et al. determined that primarily anterior laxity, but a lower-grade pivot shift, likely has an isolated AM bundle tear. Conversely, a large pivot shift with only a lower-grade Lachman test is more indicative of an isolated PL bundle rupture (Van Eck et al. 2010).

The recent interest in rotatory laxity and the pivot-shift test has made apparent the need for a reliable and noninvasive method to quantify the maneuver. Several devices designed to measure laximetry of the pivot-shift test have been developed. The goal of rotatory knee laxity testing is the development of a noninvasive, user-friendly device that provides accurate and reliable measurements.

Pivot-Shift Laximetry

There are several devices reported to measure dynamic rotatory knee laxity (Zaffagnini et al. 2006; Musahl et al. 2010b; Colombet et al. 2012; Kuroda et al. 2012; Lopomo et al. 2012; Hoshino et al. 2013). However, the pivot-shift phenomenon is a combination of motions in more than one degree of freedom. The main issue is to obtain relevant data from such a complex movement. Different techniques to analyze aspects of the pivot-shift maneuver such as tibial acceleration (Ahldén et al. 2012), lateral compartment translation (Bedi et al. 2010), velocity of translation (Labbe et al. 2011), and the "angle of p" (Lane et al. 2008) have been attempted.

Computer-Assisted Surgery and Kinematics

Computer-assisted ACL reconstruction has been used to evaluate tunnel positioning (Nakagawa et al. 2008; Voos et al. 2010). Its use in evaluating knee kinematics and laxity is also valuable. It can provide valuable data on anteroposterior translation and internal and external rotation (Plaweski et al. 2011). This invasive method requires two rigid bodies attached to pins inserted in the distal femur and proximal tibia to provide an intraoperative 3D anatomic model of the patient's knee surface geometry. The accuracy of the navigation system is reported to be ± 1 mm for linear measurements and $\pm 1^\circ$ for angular measurements and is precise in measuring laxity (Colombet et al. 2007; Lane et al. 2008). Limitations include invasiveness, use restricted to the operating room, and lack of comparison with the uninjured side.

Electromagnetic Tracking Devices

Electromagnetic measurement systems (EMS) are noninvasive and can be used in vivo, allowing six degrees of freedom of knee kinematics. The system works with transmitters attached to the skin that are digitized by a specially made stylus pen. A computer is used to collect and record data.

Hoshino et al., using the EMS, found that acceleration of tibial translation during the pivot-shift test correlated with clinical grading (Hoshino et al. 2007). Araki et al. compared partial and complete tears of the ACL using the EMS and found decreased knee laxity in patients with partial tears during the Lachman test and the pivot-shift test. Mean acceleration of tibial reduction was significantly reduced in partial tears when compared with complete tears (Araki et al. 2013).

Further studies documenting validity and accuracy of these devices must be performed prior to widely accepted usage. These devices are also bulky which results in difficulty in performing the examination in the office.

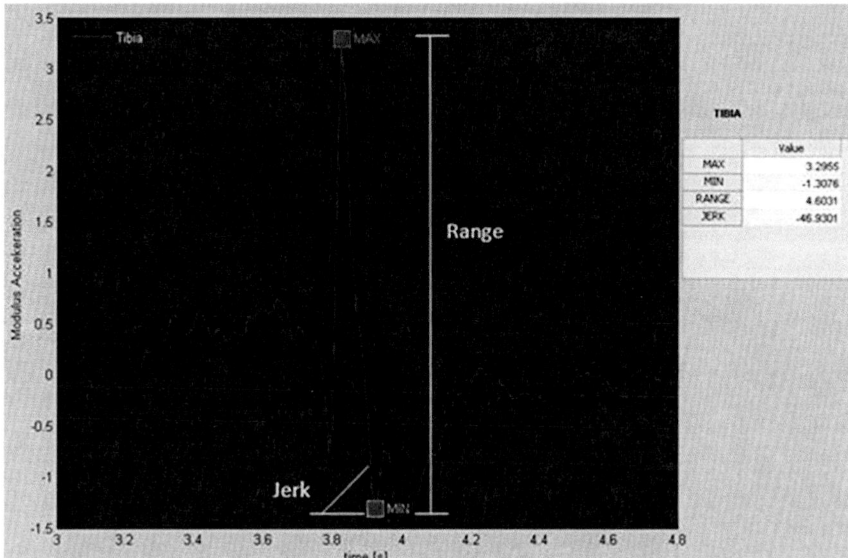

Fig. 5 Analysis of tibial acceleration by an inertial sensor. The *graph* shows tibial acceleration in m/s^2 versus time in seconds. The spike in the curve (at 3.8 s) is produced by the reduction phase of the tibia during the pivot-shift test. The results for the test are shown on the right. Range of acceleration is measured as the difference between the maximum and minimum values of acceleration (in this case 4.6 m/s^2). Jerk is a suggestion of the smoothness of the identified phenomenon (Lopomo et al. 2012)

Triaxial Accelerometer

The triaxial accelerometer for the pivot-shift test is a noninvasive tool consisting of an inertial sensor connected to a computer. The sensor is affixed to the proximal tibia and wirelessly transmits information in real time.

Studies regarding the clinical validation of the accelerometer's use on quantifying the pivot-shift test have been performed. Lopomo et al. found a probability of 70–80 % for diagnosing an ACL-deficient knee using only acceleration parameters (Lopomo et al. 2012) (Fig. 5). Ahldén et al. found that tibial acceleration during the reduction phase of the pivot shift had a good correlation with the clinical grade of the test (Ahldén et al. 2012). Araujo et al. found that the accelerometer had a moderate to good correlation with the electromagnetic system for the acceleration parameter, using the standardized pivot-shift test previously described (Araujo et al. 2012).

Mayema et al., in a sectioning study, demonstrated increased acceleration and rotational instability was observed with increased damage to the ACL (Maeyama et al. 2011). Hoshino et al. highlighted that acceleration during the reduction phase of the pivot shift is a good indicator of rotational instability, which reflects the dynamic behavior of the pivot-shift phenomenon (Hoshino et al. 2012c).

Image-Based Techniques

Dynamic Stereo Radiography (DSX)

Radiostereometric analysis (RSA) is a highly precise biplanar radiographic film technique used to obtain 3D information on knee kinematics. It is an invasive method that uses implanted tantalum spheres measuring 1.6 mm diameter in the femur and tibia. This technique is capable of tracking the markers with an accuracy of approximately 0.1 mm (Tashman and Anderst 2003). Using RSA, Tashman et al. demonstrated that rotational instability was not restored by transtibial ACL reconstruction (Tashman 2004).

DSX is a noninvasive method of measuring knee motion. It is a radiographic model-based tracking technique that measures the three-dimensional in vivo motion of the tibiofemoral

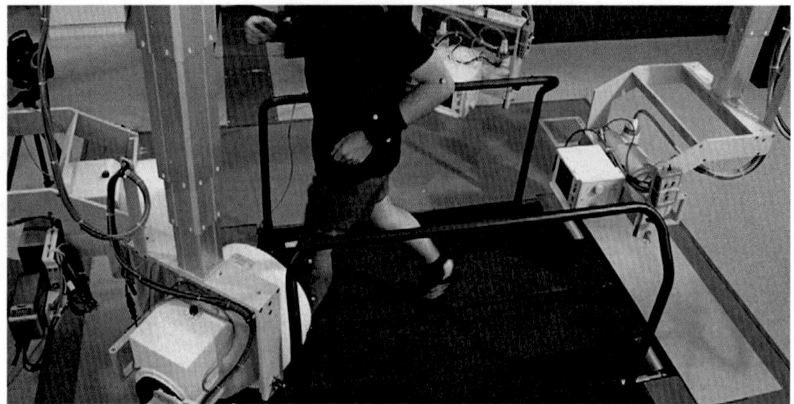

Fig. 6 A treadmill run test is shown with simultaneous biplane fluoroscopy of the knee (dynamic stereo radiography, DSX) (From Ahlden et al. (2012); **needs permission** from Springer Science and Business Media)

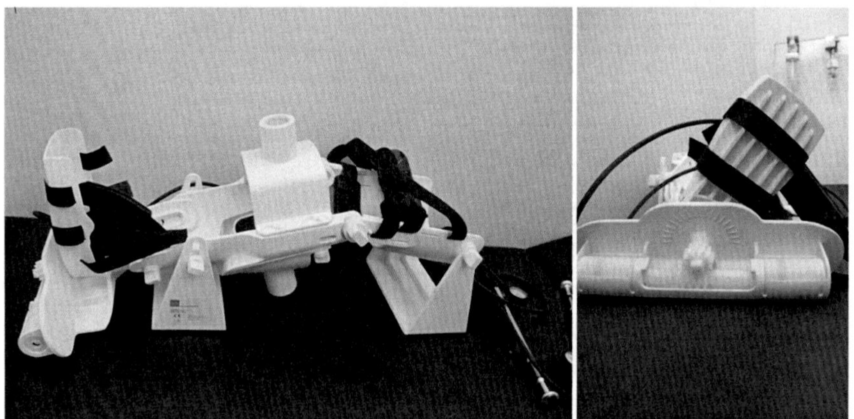

Fig. 7 Photography of PKTD® currently in clinical application

joint (Fig. 6). Precision of this method was validated when analyzing joint motion during running and was less than 1.0° for rotation and less than 1.0 mm for translation (Anderst et al. 2009). It is considered the gold standard of kinematics evaluation but requires complex tools, is labor intensive, and is expensive.

Dynamic MRI Evaluation (PKTD)

The Porto-knee testing device (PKTD) (Fig. 7) has proved to be a reliable tool in the quantification of anteroposterior translation (comparing to KT-1000) and rotatory knee laxity (compared to lateral pivot shift under anesthesia). A strong positive correlation has been found between lateral pivot-shift test under anesthesia and the difference between lateral and medial tibial translation of ACL-deficient knees (threshold level for 2+/3+ is 3.5 mm) (Espregueira-Mendes et al. 2012).

PKTD is built in polyurethane, enabling it to be used during MRI (or CT scans). The tibia is put under stress caused by the inflation of cuffs which have a standardized pressure of 46.7 kPa (load per unit area), applied in the posterior proximal calf region. It can be adjusted to different degrees of knee flexion and different degrees of external/internal rotation inflicted by the footplate. Measurements are taken considering only fix bony landmarks (Fig. 8) to overcome inherent bias of considering soft tissue (less precise) for quantification.

Partial ACL ruptures (Ochi et al. 2006; Sonnery-Cottet et al. 2010) have been recognized as difficult to identify by preoperative MRI (Van Dyck P et al. 2012). Furthermore, it is even

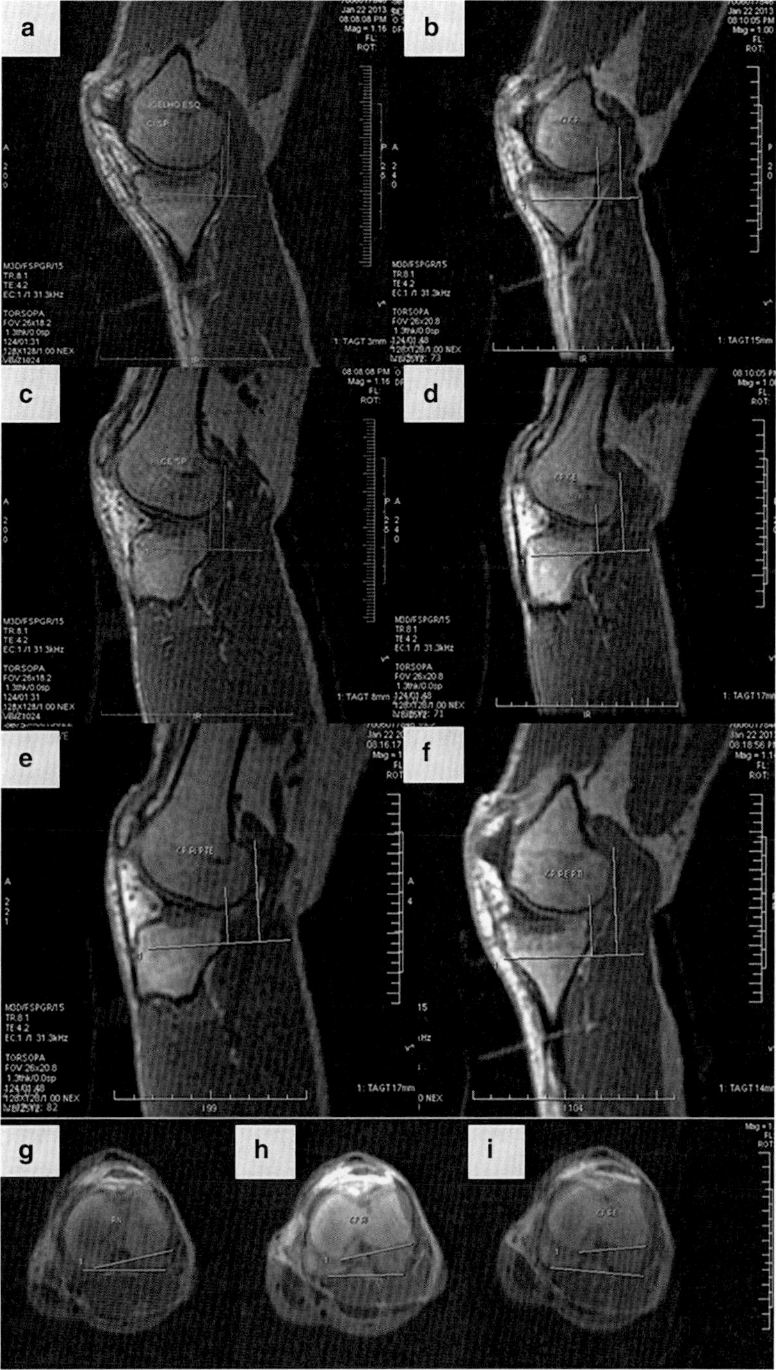

Fig. 8 Standard protocol evaluation of a case initially classified as having partial ACL rupture corresponding to AM bundle. Sagittal view with foot in neutral position without load application correspondent to medial (**a**) and lateral compartments (**c**). Result after load applications correspondent to medial (**b**) and lateral compartments (**d**). In this case the differential would be respectively of 12 mm and 9 mm. Image correspondent to load after maximum internal foot rotation in lateral compartment (**e**) and after maximum external foot rotation in medial compartment (**f**). Evaluation of angular and linear tibial dislocation from axial views: without load (**g**) and with load after internal (**h**) and external foot rotation (**i**). Evaluation confirmed global ACL insufficiency

more difficult to establish the functional behavior of the ligament's remnant. ACL injuries, initially classified by radiologists as "partial ACL ruptures," often present an instability pattern of total rupture (Fig. 8). The possibility of combining functional and anatomic evaluation helps preoperative evaluation. Patients and surgeons might be informed of other surgical options (e.g., augmentation procedure) to be considered in advance.

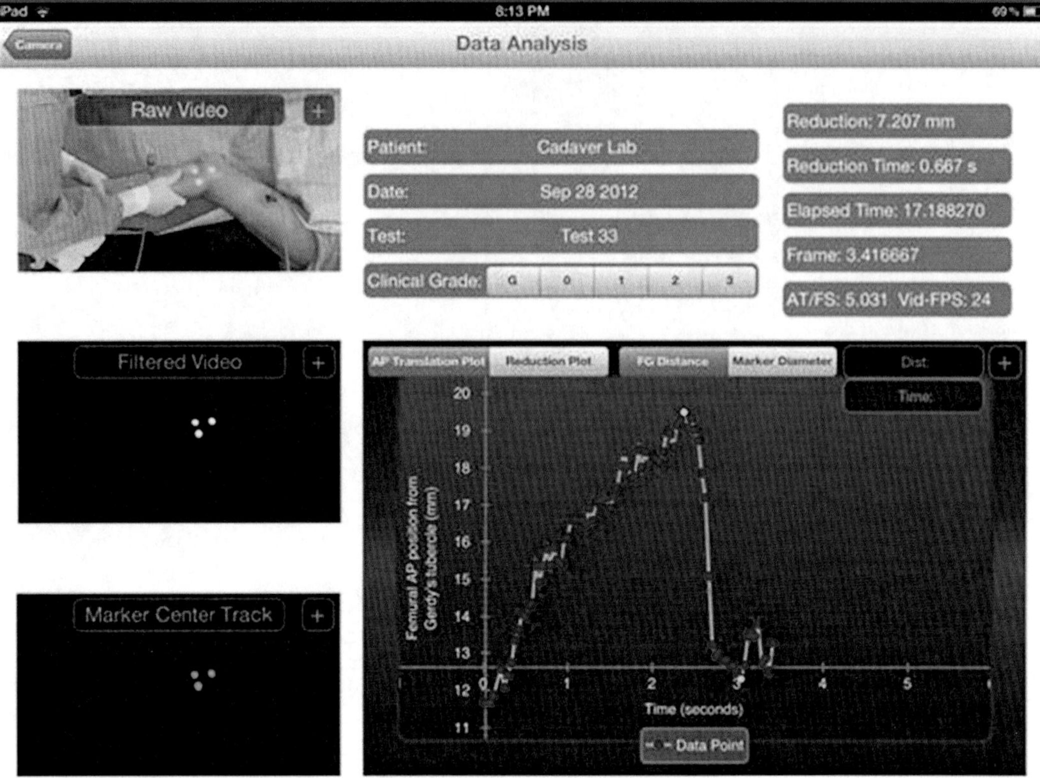

Fig. 9 The iPad app (PIVOT app) for quantitative analysis of the pivot-shift test. Three stickers are placed on Gerdy's tubercle, fibula head, and lateral epicondyle. The PIVOT app simultaneously records a video of the standardized pivot-shift test (*upper left*), filters the video (*middle left*) to track the center of three markers (*lower left*), and calculates translation (in mm) over time (in seconds; *lower right*). The data analysis is shown on the top of the screen. This example is of a cadaver lab demonstration with transection of the ACL, lateral meniscus, and lateral capsule. The reduction of the tibia during the pivot-shift test occurred at 2.5 s, the reduction time was 0.7 s, and the translation was 7.2 mm (Hoshino et al. KSSTA 2013)

More than the evaluation of the "amount of tibial translation" in a single position of the knee joint, one might test the translation in several positions considering the different kinematic roles of AM and PL bundles. By means of inducing tension on ACL during imaging acquisition, it is possible to rule out the so-called chewing gum effect, testing the mechanical behavior of ruptures initially classified as partial (Sonnery-Cottet and Chambat 2007; Lorenz et al. 2009) (Fig. 8). A flaccid ACL remnant or PCL healing might look like viable in an acceptable position on static imaging but reveal to be functionally unable to resist stress.

Despite being in the early time of its clinical application, PKTD has proved to be a valuable tool. The ability of identifying partial ruptures and the status of the remaining bundle due to its unique feature of combining anatomical and dynamic "clinical" evaluation amplified by the high resolution of MRI places the PKTD in a noticeable spot in the preoperative planning.

Image Analysis Method (iPad)

Translation of the lateral compartment during the reduction phase of the pivot-shift test can be successfully detected noninvasively using simple image analysis (Hoshino et al. 2012a, b, c). Technological improvements have allowed the development of an iPad (Apple Inc., Cupertino, CA, USA) application, allowing for near real-time image analysis. For image detection by the app, three round yellow stickers are attached to the skin over the lateral epicondyle, Gerdy's tubercle, and fibular head. The data provided generates a graphic showing the relationship between translation and time (Fig. 9).

Hoshino et al. studied 34 patients with unilateral ACL-deficient knees who underwent reconstruction. Using the iPad app, the pivot shift was measured under anesthesia in both knees, using the standardized pivot-shift maneuver described earlier. The image analysis is able to detect an increase in the lateral translation in the ACL-deficient knees compared to the contralateral knees and correlates with grading of the pivot-shift test (Hoshino et al. 2013).

The iPad app is under process of validation. A prospective international multicenter validation of outcome technology study is currently under way (PIVOT study; ISAKOS/OREF research grant). This system might be able to detect partial, complete, and combined ACL injuries. Ultimately, quantitative pivot-shift analysis will help improve the preoperative evaluation and clinical outcomes for patients.

Clinical Outcomes

Postoperative results following ACL augmentation surgery are promising. In 2000, Adachi et al. compared an augmentation procedure with "traditional" ACL reconstruction with a minimum follow-up of 2 years in 40 patients. They have shown that postoperative anterior translation was significantly less in the augmentation group. Also, the final inaccuracy of joint position sense was significantly less in the augmentation group (Adachi et al. 2000). Similar results were demonstrated by Ochi et al. in a series with 45 patients with a minimum of 2 years of follow-up. They found a significant reduction in anterior translation, measured by the KT-2000, from 3.3 $\pm$ 2.4 mm in side-to-side difference to a mean of 0.5 $\pm$ 2.7 mm. Joint position sense inaccuracy was 1.6° $\pm$ 1.8°, which improved significantly to 0.3° $\pm$ 2.0° after surgery (Ochi et al. 2009). In both studies, they highlighted the importance of preserving the remnants as a mechanism to improve proprioception.

Buda et al. analyzed 28 patients who underwent ACL augmentation surgery. Twenty-five patients were rated as excellent, three as fair. Also, a good correlation was shown between clinical results, graft integration, and graft signal on MRI examination. Yoon et al. compared 82 cases of ACL reconstruction, 40 cases of AM augmentation, and 42 cases of PL augmentation. There was no difference between the groups in postoperative measurements including range of motion, Lachman test, pivot-shift test, and KT-1000 arthrometry (Yoon et al. 2009). Sonnery-Cottet et al. performed 36 AM bundle reconstructions, achieving a significant difference in side-to-side difference between preoperative (4.8 mm, min. 3, max. 6) and postoperative (0.8 mm, min. 0, max. 2) instrumented laxity (Sonnery-Cottet et al. 2010).

Summary

Partial ACL tears, involving either the AM or the PL bundle, present a challenging diagnosis for the surgeon. Laximetry, mainly through the evaluation of rotatory knee laxity via the pivot-shift test, is the most specific clinical examination for diagnosis of partial ACL tears. New noninvasive technologies, made for daily use in the office, are being developed and may open new perspectives in knee ligament evaluation. These technologies include electromagnetic tracking devices, inertial sensors, and image analysis with the iPad. New treatment algorithms are being developed with specific and individualized treatment for partial, complete, and combined ACL injuries. Surgical reconstruction of partial ACL tears can involve preservation of the ACL stump, single-bundle reconstruction of isolated AM or PL bundle tears (under preservation of the intact bundle), or single-bundle augmentation during revision ACL reconstruction. Ultimately, improved diagnosis and treatment of partial ACL tears will lead to a more individualized surgery and improved clinical outcomes for patients.

Cross-References

- ► Anterior Cruciate Ligament Injuries and Surgery: Current Evidence and Modern Development
- ► Innovation in Sports Medicine
- ► Personalized Treatment Algorithms for Anterior Cruciate Ligament Injuries
- ► Platelet-Rich Plasma: From Laboratory to the Clinic
- ► Primary Anterior Cruciate Ligament Repair in Athletes with Mesenchymal Stem Cells and Platelet-Rich Plasma
- ► Return to Play Decision-Making Following Anterior Cruciate Ligament Reconstruction: Multi-factor Considerations
- ► Return to the Field for Football (Soccer) After Anterior Cruciate Ligament Reconstruction: Guidelines
- ► Revision Anterior Cruciate Ligament Reconstruction
- ► Role of Growth Factors in Anterior Cruciate Ligament Surgery
- ► Single Versus Double Anterior Cruciate Ligament Reconstruction in Athletes
- ► Structured Rehabilitation Model with Clinical Outcomes After Anterior Cruciate Ligament Reconstruction

References

Adachi N, Ochi M, Uchio Y et al (2000) Anterior cruciate ligament augmentation under arthroscopy. Arch Orthop Trauma Surg 120(3–4):128–133

Adachi N, Ochi M, Uchio Y et al (2002) Mechanoreceptors in the anterior cruciate ligament contribute to the joint position sense. Acta Orthop Scand 73(3):330–334

Ahlden M, Araujo P, Hoshino Y et al (2012) Clinical grading of the pivot shift test correlates best with tibial acceleration. Knee Surg Sports Traumatol Arthrosc 20 (4):708–12

Ahldén M, Hoshino Y, Samuelsson K et al (2012) Dynamic knee laxity measurement devices. Knee Surg Sports Traumatol Arthrosc 20(4):621–632

Anderst W, Zauel R, Bishop J et al (2009) Validation of three-dimensional model-based tibio-femoral tracking during running. Med Eng Phys 31(1):10–16

Araki D, Kuroda R, Matsushita T et al (2013) Biomechanical analysis of the knee with partial anterior cruciate ligament disruption: quantitative evaluation using an electromagnetic measurement system. Arthroscopy.29 (6):1053–1062 [Epub ahead of print]

Araujo P, Ahlden M, Hoshino Y et al (2012) Comparison of three non-invasive quantitative measurement systems for the pivot shift test. Knee Surg Sports Traumatol Arthrosc 20:692–697

Bach BR, Warren RF (1989) "Empty wall" and "vertical strut" signs of ACL insufficiency. Arthroscopy 5 (2):137–140

Bach BR, Warren RF, Wickiewicz TL (1988) The pivot shift phenomenon: results and description of a modified clinical test for anterior cruciate ligament insufficiency. Am J Sports Med 16(6):571–576

Bedi A, Musahl V, Lane C et al (2010) Lateral compartment translation predicts the grade of pivot shift: a cadaveric and clinical analysis. Knee Surg Sports Traumatol Arthrosc 18(9):1269–1276

Brandon ML, Haynes PT, Bonamo JR et al (2006) The association between posterior-inferior tibial slope and anterior cruciate ligament insufficiency. Arthroscopy 22(8):894–899

Bull AMJ, Earnshaw PH, Smith A et al (2002) Intraoperative measurement of knee kinematics in reconstruction of the anterior cruciate ligament. J Bone Joint Surg (Br) 84(7):1075–1081

Colombet P, Robinson J, Christel P et al (2007) Using navigation to measure rotation kinematics during ACL reconstruction. Clin Orthop Relat Res 454:59–65

Colombet P, Jenny JY, Menetrey J et al (2012) Current concept in rotational laxity control and evaluation in ACL reconstruction. Orthop Traumatol Surg Res 98 (8 Suppl):S201–S210

Crain EH, Fithian DC, Paxton EW et al (2005) Variation in anterior cruciate ligament scar pattern: does the scar pattern affect anterior laxity in anterior cruciate ligament-deficient knees? Arthroscopy 21(1):19–24

DeFranco MJ, Bach BR (2009) A comprehensive review of partial anterior cruciate ligament tears. J Bone Joint Surg Am 91(1):198–208

Dejour D, Ntagiopoulos PG, Saggin PR et al (2013) The diagnostic value of clinical tests, magnetic resonance imaging, and instrumented laxity in the differentiation of complete versus partial anterior cruciate ligament tears. Arthroscopy 29(3):491–499

Espregueira-Mendes J, Pereira H, Sevivas N, Passos C, Vasconcelos JC, Monteiro A et al (2012) Assessment of rotatory laxity in anterior cruciate ligament-deficient knees using magnetic resonance imaging with Porto-knee testing device. Knee Surg Sports Traumatol Arthrosc 20:671–678

Galway HR, MacIntosh DL (1980) The lateral pivot shift: A symptom and sign of anterior cruciate ligament insufficiency. Clin Orthop Relat Res (147):45–50

Georgoulis AD, Pappa L, Moebius U et al (2001) The presence of proprioceptive mechanoreceptors in the remnants of the ruptured ACL as a possible source of re-innervation of the ACL autograft. Knee Surg Sports Traumatol Arthrosc 9(6):364–368

Hole RL, Lintner DM, Kamaric E, Bruce J (1996) Increased tibial translation after partial sectioning of the anterior cruciate ligament. Am J Sports Med 24 (4):556–560

Hoshino Y, Kuroda R, Nagamune K et al (2007) In vivo measurement of the pivot-shift test in the anterior cruciate ligament-deficient knee using an electromagnetic device. Am J Sports Med 35(7):1098–1104

Hoshino Y, Araujo P, Ahlden M et al (2012a) Standardized pivot shift test improves measurement accuracy. Knee Surg Sports Traumatol Arthrosc 20(4):732–736

Hoshino Y, Araujo P, Irrgang JJ et al (2012b) An image analysis method to quantify the lateral pivot shift test. Knee Surg Sports Traumatol Arthrosc 20(4):703–707

Hoshino Y, Kuroda R, Nagamune K et al (2012c) Optimal measurement of clinical rotational test for evaluating anterior cruciate ligament insufficiency. Knee Surg Sports Traumatol Arthrosc 20(7):1323–1330

Hoshino Y, Wang JH, Lorenz S et al. (2012d) The effect of distal femur bony morphology on in vivo knee translational and rotational kinematics. Knee Surg Sports Traumatol Arthrosc 20(7):1331–8

Hoshino Y, Araujo P, Ahldén M et al (2013) Quantitative evaluation of the pivot shift by image analysis using the iPad. Knee Surg Sports Traumatol Arthrosc. doi:10.1007/s00167-013-2396-0. [Epub ahead of print]

Howell SM, Knox KE, Farley TE et al (1995) Revascularization of a human anterior cruciate ligament graft during the first two years of implantation. Am J Sports Med 23(1):42–49

Jakob RP, Stäubli HU, Deland JT (1987) Grading the pivot shift. Objective tests with implications for treatment. J Bone Joint Surg (Br) 69(2):294–299

Jonsson H, Riklund-Ahlström K, Lind J (2004) Positive pivot shift after ACL reconstruction predicts later osteoarthrosis: 63 patients followed 5–9 years after surgery. Acta Orthop Scand 75(5):594–599

Kato Y, Maeyama A, Lertwanich P et al (2013) Biomechanical comparison of different graft positions for single-bundle anterior cruciate ligament reconstruction. Knee Surg Sports Traumatol Arthrosc 21 (4):816–823

Kocher MS, Steadman JR, Briggs K et al (2002) Determinants of patient satisfaction with outcome after anterior cruciate ligament reconstruction. J Bone Joint Surg Am 84-A(9):1560–1572

Kuang GM, Yau WP, Lu WW et al (2010) Osteointegration of soft tissue grafts within the bone tunnels in anterior cruciate ligament reconstruction can be enhanced. Knee Surg Sports Traumatol Arthrosc 18 (8):1038–1051

Kuroda R, Hoshino Y, Araki D et al (2012) Quantitative measurement of the pivot shift, reliability, and clinical applications. Knee Surg Sports Traumatol Arthrosc 20 (4):686–691

Labbe DR, De Guise JA, Godbout V et al (2011) Accounting for velocity of the pivot shift test manoeuvre decreases kinematic variability. Knee 18(2):88–93

Lane CG, Warren RF, Stanford FC et al (2008) In vivo analysis of the pivot shift phenomenon during computer navigated ACL reconstruction. Knee Surg Sports Traumatol Arthrosc 16(5):487–492

Leitze Z, Losee RE, Jokl P et al (2005) Implications of the pivot shift in the ACL-deficient knee. Clin Orthop Relat Res 436:229–236

Lopomo N, Zaffagnini S, Signorelli C et al (2012) An original clinical methodology for non-invasive assessment of pivot-shift test. Comput Methods Biomech Biomed Engin 15(12):1323–8

Lorenz S, Illingworth KD, Fu FH (2009) Diagnosis of isolated posterolateral bundle tears of the anterior cruciate ligament. Arthroscopy 25:1203–1204, author reply 4–5

Losee RE (1982) Concepts of the pivot shift. Clin Orthop Relat Res 172:45–51

Maeyama A, Hoshino Y, Debandi A et al (2011) Evaluation of rotational instability in the anterior cruciate ligament deficient knee using triaxial accelerometer: a biomechanical model in porcine knees. Knee Surg Sports Traumatol Arthrosc 19(8):1233–1238

Musahl V, Ayeni OR, Citak M et al (2010a) The influence of bony morphology on the magnitude of the pivot shift. Knee Surg Sports Traumatol Arthrosc 18 (9):1232–1238

Musahl V, Voos JE, O'Loughlin PF et al (2010b) Comparing stability of different single- and double-bundle anterior cruciate ligament reconstruction techniques: a cadaveric study using navigation. Arthroscopy 26 (9 Suppl):S41–S48

Nakagawa T, Takeda H, Nakajima K et al (2008) Intraoperative 3-dimensional imaging-based navigation-assisted anatomic double-bundle anterior cruciate ligament reconstruction. Arthroscopy 24 (10):1161–1167

Noyes FR, Grood ES, Cummings JF et al (1991) An analysis of the pivot shift phenomenon. The knee motions and subluxations induced by different examiners. Am J Sports Med 19(2):148–155

Ochi M, Iwasa J, Uchio Y et al (1999) The regeneration of sensory neurones in the reconstruction of the anterior cruciate ligament. J Bone Joint Surg (Am) 81 (5):902–906

Ochi M, Adachi N, Deie M et al (2006) Anterior cruciate ligament augmentation procedure with a 1-incision technique: anteromedial bundle or posterolateral bundle reconstruction. Arthroscopy 22(4):463.e1–463.e5

Ochi M, Adachi N, Uchio Y et al (2009) A minimum 2-year follow-up after selective anteromedial or posterolateral bundle anterior cruciate ligament reconstruction. Arthroscopy 25(2):117–122

Panisset J-C, Ntagiopoulos P-G, Saggin PR et al (2012) A comparison of Telos™ stress radiography versus Rolimeter™ in the diagnosis of different patterns of anterior cruciate ligament tears. Orthop Traumatol Surg Res 98(7):751–758

Plaweski S, Grimaldi M, Courvoisier A et al (2011) Intraoperative comparisons of knee kinematics of double-bundle versus single-bundle anterior cruciate ligament reconstruction. Knee Surg Sports Traumatol Arthrosc 19(8):1277–1286

Rodeo S, Suzuki K, Deng XH et al (1999) Use of recombinant human bone morphogenetic protein-2 to enhance tendon healing in a bone tunnel. Am J Sports Med 27(4):476–488

Siebold R, Fu FH (2008) Assessment and augmentation of symptomatic anteromedial or posterolateral bundle tears of the anterior cruciate ligament. Arthroscopy 24 (11):1289–1298

Sonnery-Cottet B, Chambat P (2007) Arthroscopic identification of the anterior cruciate ligament posterolateral bundle: the figure-of-four position. Arthroscopy 23 (1128):e1–e3

Sonnery-Cottet B, Lavoie F, Ogassawara R et al (2010) Selective anteromedial bundle reconstruction in partial ACL tears: a series of 36 patients with mean 24 months follow-up. Knee Surg Sports Traumatol Arthrosc 18 (1):47–51

Suero EM, Njoku IU, Voigt MR et al (2012) The role of the iliotibial band during the pivot shift test. Knee Surg Sports Traumatol Arthrosc. doi:10.1007/s00167-012-2257-2. [Epub ahead of print]

Tashman S (2004) Abnormal rotational knee motion during running after anterior cruciate ligament reconstruction. Am J Sports Med 32(4):975–983

Tashman S, Anderst W (2003) In-vivo measurement of dynamic joint motion using high speed biplane radiography and CT: application to canine ACL deficiency. J Biomech Eng 125(2):238

Van Dyck P, De Smet E, Veryser J, Lambrecht V, Gielen JL, Vanhoenacker FM et al (2012) Partial tear of the anterior cruciate ligament of the knee: injury patterns on MR imaging. Knee Surg Sports Traumatol Arthrosc. 20(2): 256–261 [Epub ahead of print],

Van Eck CF, Lesniak BP, Schreiber VM, Fu FH (2010) Anatomic single- and double-bundle anterior cruciate ligament reconstruction flowchart. Arthroscopy 26 (2):258–268

Voos JE, Musahl V, Maak TG et al (2010) Comparison of tunnel positions in single-bundle anterior cruciate ligament reconstructions using computer navigation. Knee Surg Sports Traumatol Arthrosc 18 (9):1282–1289

Yasuda K, Van Eck CF, Hoshino Y et al (2011) Anatomic single- and double-bundle anterior cruciate ligament reconstruction, part 1: basic science. Am J Sports Med 39(8):1789–1799

Yeh W, Lin S, Yuan L et al (2007) Effects of hyperbaric oxygen treatment on tendon graft and tendon-bone integration in bone tunnel: biochemical and histological analysis in rabbits. J Orthop Res 25:636–645

Yoon KH, Bae DK, Cho SM et al (2009) Standard anterior cruciate ligament reconstruction versus isolated single-bundle augmentation with hamstring autograft. Arthroscopy 25(11):1265–1274

Zaffagnini S, Bignozzi S, Martelli S et al (2006) New intraoperative protocol for kinematic evaluation of ACL reconstruction: preliminary results. Knee Surg Sports Traumatol Arthrosc 14(9):811–816

Zantop T, Herbort M, Raschke MJ, Fu FH, Petersen W (2007) The role of the anteromedial and posterolateral bundles of the anterior cruciate ligament in anterior tibial translation and internal rotation. Am J Sports Med 35:223–227

Patellar Dislocations: Overview

102

Sinan Karaoğlu, Ugur Haklar, and Fatih Karaaslan

Contents

Abstract

Patellofemoral problems are common in both athletic and nonathletic individuals and this chapter describes the normal patellofemoral joint and factors that predispose patients to patellar instability. The treatment options for patellar dislocations are described. In general, most of acute dislocations should be treated nonoperatively unless the instability is associated with an osteochondral injury. But occasionally, surgical management of medial patellofemoral ligament (MPFL) injuries without loose bodies may also be taken into consideration. Future treatment modalities in patellofemoral instabilities will most probably be dominated by surgical interventions more than conservative therapy. Chronic dislocations should be treated based on an understanding of the patient's individual reason for recurrent instability.

Introduction

Patellofemoral problems are common in both athletic and nonathletic individuals. In the nonathletic population, women present more commonly with patellar disorders. One of the most common patellofemoral disorders is patellar instability due to subluxation and dislocation. Patellar instability, which includes both subluxation and complete patellofemoral dislocation, is the second most common cause of traumatic

S. Karaoğlu (✉)
Department of Orthopaedics and Traumatology, Memorial Kayseri Hospital, Kayseri, Turkey
e-mail: sinankaraoglu@hotmail.com

U. Haklar
Orthopaedics and Traumatology Department, Bahcesehir University Medical Faculty, Liv Hospital, Istanbul, Turkey
e-mail: dr.haklar@superonline.com

F. Karaaslan
Department of Orthopedics, Bozok University Medical Faculty, Yozgat, Turkey
e-mail: fkaraaslan@gmail.com

M.N. Doral, J. Karlsson (eds.), *Sports Injuries*,
DOI 10.1007/978-3-642-36569-0_124

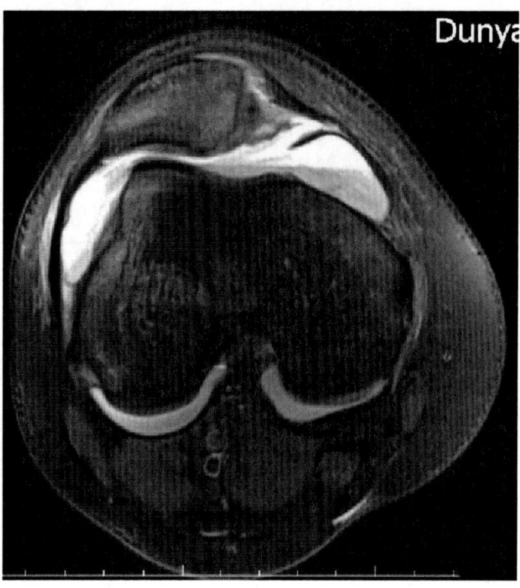

Fig. 1 Fluid–fluid levels in knee joints representing lipohemarthrosis after patellar dislocation

hemarthrosis of the knee (Fig. 1), and it accounts for approximately 3 % of all knee injuries (Ahmad et al. 2000).

Patellofemoral instability is most commonly reported in young, active individuals involved in sports activities. Patients with a first-time acute patellar dislocation have been reported to be injured mostly during sports activity (Atkin et al. 2000). For most patients, a careful history and physical examination is sufficient to make the diagnosis of patellar instability. A thorough history must contain the type of sports activities, present and past injuries, exact location of the pain, knee giving way, knee locking, or catching history. An accurate diagnosis also needs specific knowledge of patellofemoral (PF) anatomy, biomechanics, and functional behavior of the PF joint (Karaoğlu et al. 2012).

Factors Affecting Stability

In normal knees, there is a balance between active and passive structures around the patella both medially and laterally. The patella is centered into the femoral trochlea during the entire range of motion.

This fine dynamic balance is disrupted in patients presenting with objective patellar instability. For patellar instability, four major predisposing factors have been described: generalized ligament laxity, trochlear dysplasia, patella alta, patellar tilt, and increased tibial tuberosity–femoral groove distance (TT–TG). Secondary factors in patellar instability are a wide pelvis, knee recurvatum, increased femoral anteversion, valgus alignment, and external tibial torsion, but their absence does not prevent the development of patellar instability (Dejour et al. 1994; Feller et al. 2007; Panni et al. 2011; Haklar and Ulku 2012).

Stability of the patellofemoral joint involves dynamic and static stabilizers, which control movement of the patella within the trochlea, referred to as "patellar tracking." Patellar tracking can be altered by imbalances in these stabilizing forces affecting the distribution of forces along the patellofemoral articular surface, the patellar and quadriceps tendons, and the adjacent soft tissues (Reilly and Martens 1972; Karaoğlu et al. 2012). Both passive and dynamic stabilizing factors influence the position of the patella in the trochlea; the major dynamic stabilizer is the vastus medialis obliquus (VMO) muscle, and the primary ligamentous stabilizer is the MPFL. The patella functions as the fulcrum of a lever, maximizing flexion and extension with a given quadriceps force and also acts as a pulley, by changing the direction of the quadriceps force.

The ventral part of the patella is covered by articular cartilage, and a smooth median crest runs vertically in it, defining a medial and a lateral facet. The lateral facet is larger than the medial facet, and both lateral and medial facets are concave (Panni et al. 2011). The patella sits in the femoral trochlea, which is composed of the two walls joining in the median trochlear groove. The two walls are convex in the sagittal and frontal plane, but the lateral wall is normally larger, higher, and more prominent than the medial that contributes to lateral stability (Panni et al. 2011). The patella is stabilized by the lateral and medial retinacula. The lateral retinaculum is produced by the confluence of different structures divided into two layers: the superficial oblique retinaculum and the deep transverse retinaculum. The superficial retinaculum is thin and runs from the iliotibial band to the lateral aspect of the patella. The deep layer is formed by three components: the lateral patellofemoral ligament, the lateral patellotibial ligament, and the midportion of the deep transverse retinaculum (Kaplan 1962; Mariani and Caruso 1979; Fulkerson and Gossling 1980). The medial retinaculum is formed by capsular condensations and ends on the proximal two-thirds of the deep surface of the patella. It includes the medial patellofemoral ligament and the medial patellotibial ligament (Panni et al. 2011).

It is well known that the MPFL is recognized as the primary soft-tissue restraint to lateral translation. The MPFL originates on the anterior aspect of the medial epicondyle and inserts on the proximal two-thirds of the patellar medial margin (Zaffagnini et al. 2013). Cadaveric studies have documented that the MPFL provided 60 % of restraint to lateral subluxation in extension and early flexion, and the lateral retinaculum and medial patellomeniscal ligament contributed 10 % and 13 %, respectively (Desio et al. 1998). After acute dislocation of the patella, the medial retinaculum and MPFL are frequently torn in as high as 94–98 % of patients (Vainionpaa et al. 1990; Sallay et al. 1996). The mean tensile strength and stiffness of the native MPFL are 208 N and 12.5 N/mm, respectively (Conlan et al. 1993; Amis et al. 2003). Another important biomechanical concept is that of the quadriceps angle, which is a measurement used to determine patellofemoral alignment (Maquet 1976). The Q-angle is the angle formed by the intersection of a line drawn from the anterior superior iliac spine (ASIS) to the center of the patella and a line drawn from the center of the patella to the tibial tuberosity. The larger the Q-angle, the greater the resultant lateral force tending to displace the patella laterally. It has been demonstrated that an increase in the Q-angle may lead to increased lateral contact pressures or lateral patellar dislocation (Mizuno et al. 2001).

History and Physical Examination

The nature of injury and specific physical findings, including a detailed examination of the retinacular structure around the patella, will most accurately pinpoint the specific source of anterior knee pain or instability. Obtaining a thorough history of the patient's symptoms is important when establishing a diagnosis of patellar injury or dislocation. A common symptom of patellar injury and dislocation is acute pain after a direct contact or sudden change of direction with the knee close to extension. With sudden changes in direction, the femur medially rotates over the ground-stabilized tibia.

Under these conditions, athletes commonly feel the knee giving way, which is the result of quadriceps inhibition from pain, a physiologic protective mechanism. Rapid swelling, intense knee pain, and difficulty with any knee flexion angle usually exist. Other injuries with similar presentations and mechanism of injury are meniscal and ligamentous injuries, particularly injuries of the anterior cruciate ligament or medial collateral ligament.

The physical examination begins with inspection. A knee effusion is common with an acute patellar dislocation. Other observations common in patellofemoral dysfunction include abnormal femoral anteversion, patella alta, tibial torsion, genu recurvatum, genu valgum, genu varum, pes planus, and ligamentous laxity. These factors often contribute to patellar injury and dislocation.

Following inspection, the physician must palpate the knee and surrounding structures. Evaluate the patella by applying pressure to the superior and inferior pole and medial and lateral aspects of the patella. Feel for changes in the quality of movement. Applying pressure to the superior pole allows the physician to palpate for tenderness along the inferior, medial, and lateral aspects of the patella.

The examination must include an assessment of medial and lateral structures. Relative weakness of the VMO and tightness of the lateral soft-tissue structures may result in lateral patellar tilt; this tightness may manifest as decreased medial patellar glide. In patients with an acute dislocation, significant tenderness medially near the medial retinaculum suggests a torn structure, often the MPFL. Individuals with patellofemoral pathology often experience pain with medial palpation. Tenderness noted superolaterally suggests a chondral injury after dislocation. In the event of traumatic dislocation, soft-tissue lesions of the knee are commonly associated with intra-articular fractures and chondral injuries. These concomitant injuries contribute to the patient's acute pain. Additionally, assess for tightness of the hamstrings (popliteal angle), quadriceps (**Ely's tests**), and iliotibial band (**Ober's test**). Muscular tightness affects patellar motion and function.

"The patellar apprehension test," also referred to as the "Fairbanks apprehension test," can be used with the patient lying supine and relaxed (Karaoğlu et al. 2012). The physician uses one hand to push the patient's patella as lateral as possible, in order to obtain a lateral patellar glide. Starting with the knee flexed at 30°, the physician grasps the leg at the ankle/heel with the other hand and performs a slow, combined flexion in the knee and hip. This lateral glide is sustained throughout the test. The test is considered positive when it reproduces the patient's pain or when apprehension is noted. The apprehension can manifest itself in a number of ways, ranging from verbal expressions of anxiety over grabbing the knee to involuntary quadriceps muscle contractions (to prevent further knee flexion) (Malanga et al. 2003; Karaoğlu et al. 2012). Assessing lateral patellar tracking with knee motion is an important part of the examination for patellofemoral dysfunction. A positive J sign indicates lateral patellar tracking. A positive J sign is observed as the patella tracking laterally when the patient brings the knee from flexion to extension (i.e., the patella moves notably laterally at terminal knee extension). This can be visualized well if the physician places a digit on both the medial and lateral aspects of the superior patella. A healthy patella moves mostly superiorly and slightly laterally at terminal knee extension.

The Q-angle should be assessed in patients with patellar injury or dislocations. The Q-angle is the angle measured from the ASIS to the patella to the tibial tuberosity. The Q-angle is measured in full extension and normal values for males <13° and in females <18° in knee flexion. The Q-angle should be <8° and this value is called dynamic Q-angle. Typically, the Q-angle is quantified statically using a goniometer. However, it has been recently proposed that segmental motions of the lower extremity during dynamic tasks may increase Q-angle and the lateral force acting on the patella (dynamic Q-angle) (Zhu et al. 2013). Standard Q-angle measurements are 10° for males and 15° for females. Some causes of increased Q-angle are genu valgum, high femoral anteversion, medial tibial torsion, laterally positioned tuberositas tibiae (TT), tight lateral retinaculum, weakness of VMO, and patella alta.

The tubercle–sulcus angle is also important to make a decision for treatment. Palpation must enclose all landmarks of PF joint including tibial tuberosity, patellar tendon and patella borders, crepitus with active range of motion (AROM), patellar mobility, medial and lateral retinaculum, infrapatellar fat pad, quadriceps tendon, distal IT band and Gerdy's tubercle, and the medial plica.

Knee posture is also important. Valgum, varum, and recurvatum deformities and foot deformities must be checked. Examinations of flexion and extension are also important for patellofemoral crepitus and patellar tracking. Examination of the lateral retinaculum must be applied carefully (tenderness, patellar tilt, and evaluations of patellar mobility). Quadriceps strength and hamstring tightness must be checked (Karaoğlu et al. 2012).

Eccentric step test. For the eccentric step test, the patient performs the testing in bare feet and stands on top of a 15 cm platform. The patient is asked to step forward and down toward the floor. After the patient performs the test with the unaffected leg, the test is repeated with the involved side. A positive test is one where the patient reports knee pain during test performance.

Clark's Sign

The physician must apply this test when patient is lying supine with the knee in 30°of flexion, placing one hand on top of the patella and applying gentle downward pressure, asking the patient to contract the quadriceps muscle while applying a downward pressure on the patella, and this test is repeated with the knee flexed to 60°. If the patient experiences patellofemoral pain and cannot hold the contraction, a positive test can implicate chondromalacia patella. The physician must apply this test with stabilization of the patella during a quads set. A positive result occurs if the patient has PF pain and an instability to contract the quadriceps group. Many false-positive results can be found (Malanga et al. 2003; Karaoğlu et al. 2012).

Patellar Glide Tests

The patient is supine and fully relaxed with the involved knee placed on a bolster so that it is flexed to about 30°, and the physician glides the patella medially and laterally, taking care to avoid tilting the patella during the assessment according to shift quantity of patella mobility in both sides; there may be hypomobile patella (<0.5 quadrant) or hypermobile patella (>2 quadrants) (Malanga et al. 2003; Karaoğlu et al. 2012).

Patellar tilt test. Grasp the patella with the index finger and thumb and elevate the lateral border and depress the medial. If tilting is 0–15°, it is considered normal, over 15° is considered hypermobile, while below 0° is considered a hypomobile patella (Malanga et al. 2003; Karaoğlu et al. 2012).

Radiology

Radiographs should include an axial view of the patella and a precise AP/lateral radiograph. Radiographs can demonstrate varus or valgus alignment, accessory ossification centers, osteochondral fractures, and patellar relationship like alta or baja. When acute patellar dislocation is suspected, a radiographic evaluation should be performed to rule out osteochondral fragments within the joint. Anteroposterior, lateral, and Merchant views should be obtained (Kaplan 1962). The Merchant view is obtained by having the patient lie supine with the knee flexed to 45°. The radiograph is taken with the radiographic beam aimed 30° to the floor. A similar view is the sunrise view, which is obtained by having the patient lie prone with the knee flexed (Haklar and Ulku 2012). For determination of sagittal positioning of the patella, the Blackburne–Peel ratio can be used more reliably than Insall–Salvati ratio (Haklar and Ulku 2012).

Computed tomography is the easiest way to determine tilt and subluxation. Images must be taken at 15°, 30°, and 45° of flexion, and serial images must show normal patellar tracking which means the patella is centered in the trochlea without tilt at 15° of flexion. The patellar tilt angle is the angle between the line along the lateral facet of the patella and the line along posterior condyle (normal >12º). Also axial computerized tomography images at different positions of lower limb can provide three-dimensional images of the patellofemoral joint, and the highest point of tibial tuberosity from the deepest point of trochlea can be assessed easily. A distance between the tibial tuberosity and the trochlear groove (TT–TG) exceeding 20 mm is nearly always associated with patellar instability (Haklar and Ulku 2012).

Magnetic resonance imaging also can be done to obtain information on soft tissues such as MPFL. MRI is also more sensitive for bony and cartilaginous pathology. MRI findings that are consistent with an acute patellofemoral dislocation are focal impaction injuries of the lateral femoral condyle, osteochondral injuries to the medial facet of the patella, and medial retinacular ligament injuries (Fig. 2). Associated osteochondral injuries are an indication for surgical repair; if this type of injury is missed, the patient's outcome is likely to be poor (Quinn et al. 1993; Elias and White 2004; Karaoğlu et al. 2012).

Ultrasonography is another diagnostic tool for the evaluation of medial side injuries. The most significant findings were the correlation of free fluid around the medial collateral ligament (Malanga et al. 2003) with avulsion of the femoral attachment of the MPFL and the presence of avulsed fragments of bone from the medial border

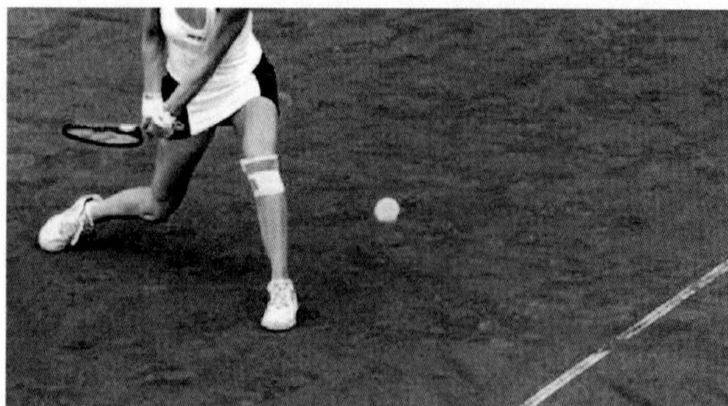

Fig. 2 Even though a tennis player is exposed to the same mechanism hundreds of times during a game, dislocation never occurs if no etiologic factors exist

of the patella. Visualization of loose bodies and localization of osteochondral lesions are made possible by the use of ultrasonography, and with the use of dynamic modification, it is even possible to assess the functional status of the MPFL precisely (Haklar and Ulku 2012).

Treatment

Treatment of Acute Dislocation

Based on a systematic review article (Stefancin and Parker 2007), nonoperative treatment has been recommended for the management of a first-time traumatic dislocation except in several specific circumstances. Exceptions include the presence of an osteochondral fracture, substantial disruption of the medial patellar stabilizers, a laterally subluxated patella with normal alignment of the contralateral knee, or a second dislocation, or in patients not improving with appropriate rehabilitation (Sillanpaa and Maenpaa 2012).

Nonoperative Treatment

Patients with acute patellar dislocation may present after spontaneous reduction of the injury, which results in a diagnostic challenge for the clinician. However, in the on-field situation or emergency department, a closed reduction may need to be performed (Fig. 3).

With the knee in extension, gentle lateral-to-medial pressure is applied to reduce the patella. Occasionally, intravenous sedation is required to help the patient relax enough for the reduction maneuver to work. Acute swelling and pain are typically managed with icing, gentle compression, and nonsteroidal anti-inflammatory drugs (NSAIDs). Nonoperative treatment has been historically suggested for patients with a primary patellar dislocation. A short immobilization period is used for patient comfort and is followed by different physiotherapy programs. The optimal conservative management has yet to be established, and there are different physiotherapy interventions in the literature (Bustos and Cosgarea 2006; Smith et al. 2010; Sillanpaa and Maenpaa 2012). Acute primary patellar dislocation is painful. The hemarthrosis can be aspirated for pain relief. There is no clear evidence that the knee should be immobilized after a primary dislocation. Studies have poorly described the

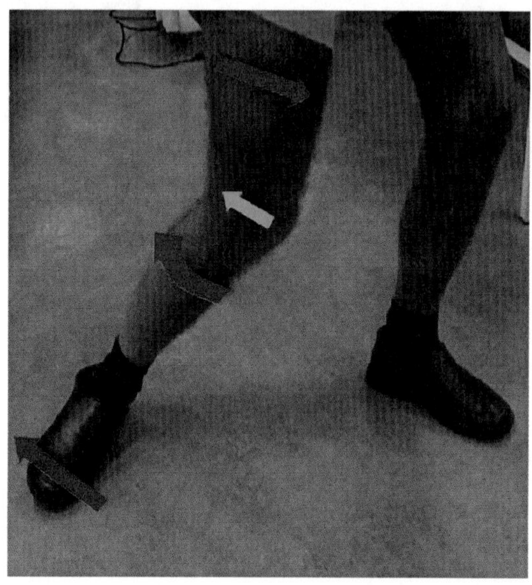

Fig. 3 Injury mechanism of indirect patella dislocation

primary and recurrent nature of the patellar dislocation, and the immobilization period has varied widely between 0 to 6 weeks (Bustos and Cosgarea 2006; Sillanpaa and Maenpaa 2012). In a prospective randomized study in which immediate mobilization was compared with flexion restriction with a patellar brace, Maenpaa et al. reported that there was no difference at 2 years (Maenpaa et al. 2010).

The aims of physiotherapy are to restore knee range of motion and to strengthen the quadriceps muscles to restore the dynamic part of the patellar soft-tissue stabilizers (Bustos and Cosgarea 2006; Greiwe et al. 2010; Sillanpaa and Maenpaa 2012). Patients should be encouraged to perform quadriceps setting exercises with the presence of tolerable pain and after a few weeks, strenuous exercises should be started aimed at normalizing quadriceps strength and control. At 4–6 weeks, by which point walking and knee range of motion have been normalized, exercises continue with more extensive extension raises, proprioceptive activities, and core stability training. Return to full activity can be suggested at 3 months. Avoiding chronic muscle weakness and imbalance is the main rehabilitation goal. A variety of different clinical outcomes have been reported in patients after physiotherapy management after a lateral patellar dislocation (Bustos and Cosgarea 2006; Smith et al. 2010).

Surgical Treatment

Surgery is an option for symptomatic patients who have failed conservative management or for initial treatment of patients with an acute dislocation with a concomitant injury, such as osteochondral fracture, meniscal tear, or a loose body (Fig. 4). Current emphasis is on anatomic reconstruction of the MPFL, although in the presence of malalignment or articular pathology of the patella, a distal bony realignment may be added (Bustos and Cosgarea 2006; Figs. 5 and 6).

MPFL Repair

The number of recent studies of surgical management for acute patellofemoral instability reflects a growing interest in the surgical treatment of young active patients who have a torn MPFL (Arendt and Dejour 2013). In acute dislocations, it may be possible to repair the MPFL. This is true only at first dislocations that are addressed with immediate surgery. Therefore, some surgeons are advocating immediate surgery after an initial patella dislocation to repair the MPFL, despite the fact that this has not been shown to decrease the chance of repeat dislocation. Some authors described the results of immediate surgical

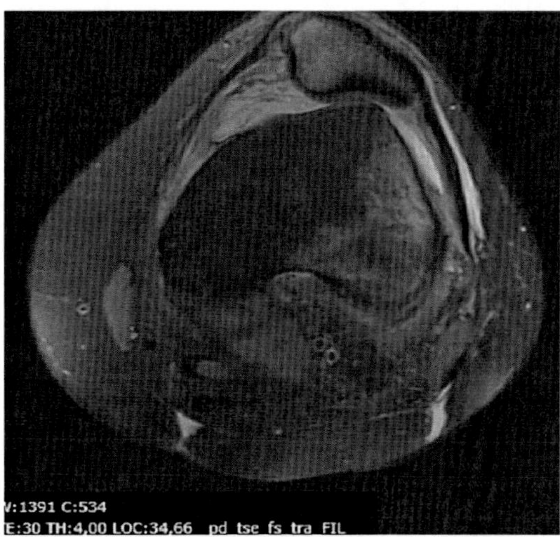

Fig. 4 Bony edema of the lateral femoral condyle and medial part of the patella after patellar dislocation

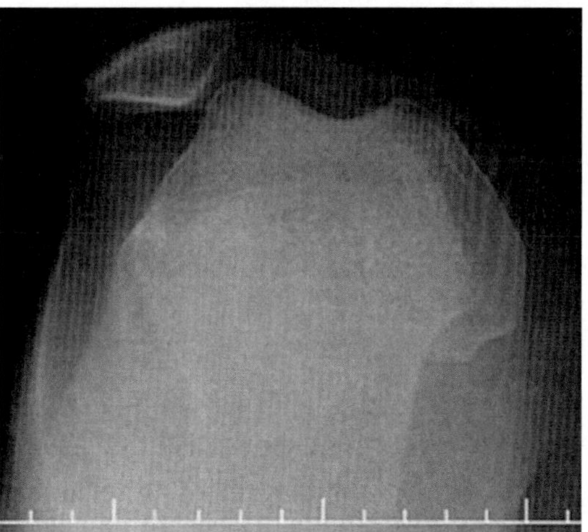

Fig. 5 Dislocated patella

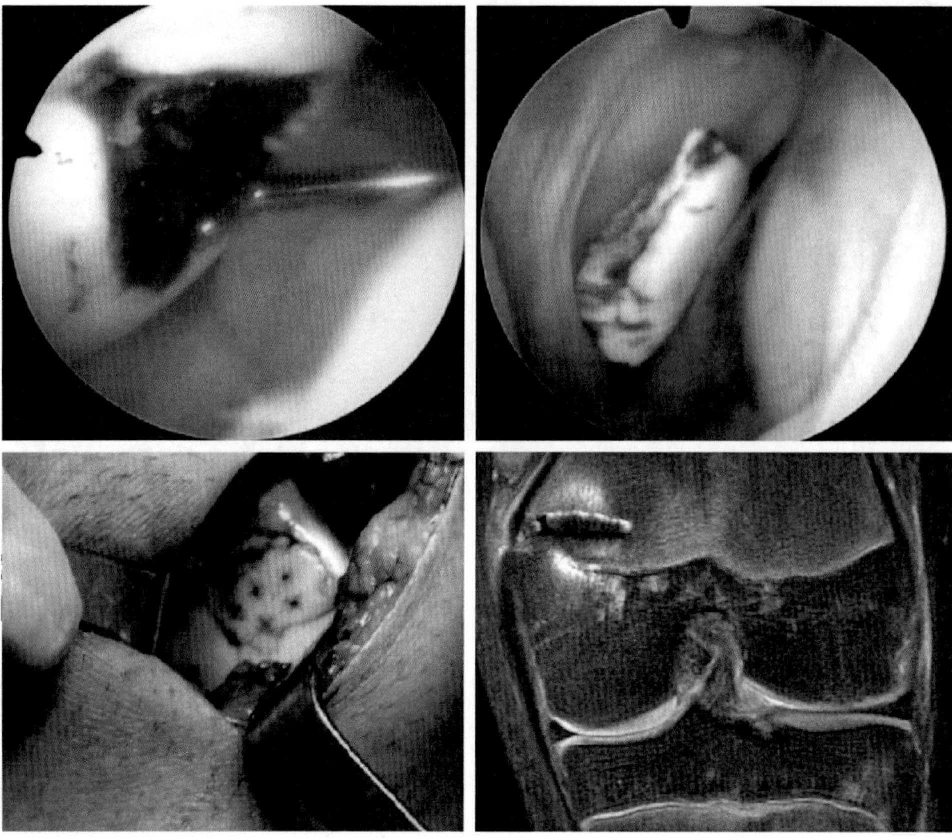

Fig. 6 An osteochondral fragment from lateral femoral condyle after acute patellar dislocation, its fixation with PLLA darts, and postoperative MRI scans

intervention for acute primary dislocations with clinical and radiographic evidence of MPFL injury in active people. They performed open repair of the MPFL. No cases of recurrent instability were noted, and 58–100 % of patients returned to preinjury activity level in those studies (Sallay et al. 1996; Ahmad et al. 2000; Owens et al. 2005). In a retrospective study, 126 patients were examined at a mean of 8.1 years after initial treatment for primary traumatic patellar dislocation; 63 patients were treated conservatively, and 63 had some form of surgery (i.e., arthroscopy only, fixation of concomitant osteochondral fractures, or repair of the MPFL) (Buchner et al. 2005). The authors reported no significant difference between the two groups with respect to recurrent instability, activity level, and functional outcomes as expressed by Lysholm scores. In a randomized controlled trial, Bitar et al. (2012) concluded that treatment with MPFL reconstruction produced better results, based on the analyses of posttreatment recurrences and the better final results of the Kujala questionnaire after a minimum follow-up period of 2 years. A recent review article also concluded that current evidence suggests that not all primary dislocations should undergo the same treatment. Authors noted MPFL reconstruction may theoretically be more reliable than repair, but the optimal time to perform additional bony corrections is not known. A normal or minor dysplastic patellofemoral joint may be suitable for nonoperative treatment, whereas a higher grade of trochlear dysplasia or other significant abnormalities may benefit from surgical treatment (Sillanpaa and Maenpaa 2012).

Treatment of Recurrent Instability

Nonoperative Treatment

Although nonsurgical management protocols vary widely, patients with recurrent instability may benefit from an initial course of physical therapy. Physical therapy should focus on quadriceps strengthening (especially of the VMO) and stretching. Occasionally, bracing during sports activity will help reduce the instability episodes. In the current literature, nonsurgical management of patellar dislocations has resulted in redislocation rates of 15–44 % with persistent symptoms of anterior knee pain, instability, and limitations of activity affecting more than 50 % of patients (Hawkins et al. 1986; Tuxoe et al. 2002; Andrish 2008).

Surgical Treatment

More than 100 different surgical procedures have been described to treat patellofemoral instability (Brown et al. 1984; Letts et al. 1999; Myers et al. 1999). In the case of recurrent instability, careful identification of the underlying pathology is critical. Once the site of pathology is identified, surgical treatment is considered.

Surgical regimens have been one of three types: proximal realignment, distal realignment, or combination of the two. In studies comparing efficacy of proximal versus distal alignment, distal shows no benefit over proximal. Lateral retinacular release as an isolated procedure for patellar instability has been shown to have inferior outcomes.

Studies comparing surgical and nonsurgical treatment of patellar instability have failed to show superior long term clinical results with surgical treatment. Some studies of surgical treatment have shown an increased risk of developing patellofemoral arthrosis despite the reduction in dislocations after surgery (Andrish 2008).

Surgical Treatment Options for Acute and Recurrent Patellar Dislocations

- Proximal realignment
  - MPFL repair
  - MPFL reconstruction
  - Medial reefing of VMO
- Distal realignment
  - Bony procedures
    - Medialization
    - Anteromedialization
  - Soft-tissue procedures
  - Roux–Goldthwait procedure
  - Elmslie–Trillat procedure
- Combined procedures

Complications

It is possible to run across iatrogenic medial subluxation due to performed medialization procedures and patellar fractures after opened tunnels for MPFL reconstruction. However, all known complications of knee surgery, including arthrofibrosis which is more frequently seen in early cases, are valid for these patients, too.

Overview

Patellar dislocation occurs as a result of the presence of pathologies in soft-tissue restraints, patellofemoral geometry, patellofemoral alignment or lower extremity alignment, and gait. Yet, there is no consensus for treating most of the pathologies. But treatment modalities continue to evolve. Generally, nonoperative treatment with patellar bracing is recommended for primary patellar dislocations without a loose body. However, if the patient already has loose bodies after dislocation, arthroscopic removal or possible fixation of the loose body is recommended with simultaneously medial repair.

Once these pathoanatomies have been identified for the individual patient, a systematic approach to surgical realignment and the determination of the components of appropriate surgical intervention are then possible.

Nowadays the presence of loose bodies is a reported indication for surgical intervention. But management of MPFL injuries without loose bodies surgically should also be taken into consideration. Future treatment modalities in patellofemoral instabilities will most probably be dominated by surgical interventions more than conservative therapy.

Cross-References

- ▶ Arthroscopic Patellar Instability Surgery
- ▶ Knee Dislocations
- ▶ Medial Patellofemoral Ligament Reconstruction: Current Concepts
- ▶ Patellofemoral Problems in Adolescent Athletes
- ▶ Prevention of Knee Injuries in Soccer Players
- ▶ Reconstruction of the Medial Patellofemoral Ligament: A Surgical Technique Perspective from an Orthopedic Surgeon

References

Ahmad CS, Stein BE et al (2000) Immediate surgical repair of the medial patellar stabilizers for acute patellar dislocation. A review of eight cases. Am J Sports Med 28(6):804–810

Amis AA, Firer P et al (2003) Anatomy and biomechanics of the medial patellofemoral ligament. Knee 10(3): 215–220

Andrish J (2008) The management of recurrent patellar dislocation. Orthop Clin North Am 39(3):313–327, vi

Arendt EA, Dejour D (2013) Patella instability: building bridges across the ocean a historic review. Knee Surg Sports Traumatol Arthrosc 21(2):279–293

Atkin DM, Fithian DC et al (2000) Characteristics of patients with primary acute lateral patellar dislocation and their recovery within the first 6 months of injury. Am J Sports Med 28(4):472–479

Bitar AC, Demange MK et al (2012) Traumatic patellar dislocation: nonoperative treatment compared with MPFL reconstruction using patellar tendon. Am J Sports Med 40(1):114–122

Brown DE, Alexander AH et al (1984) The Elmslie-Trillat procedure: evaluation in patellar dislocation and subluxation. Am J Sports Med 12(2):104–109

Buchner M, Baudendistel B et al (2005) Acute traumatic primary patellar dislocation: long-term results comparing conservative and surgical treatment. Clin J Sport Med 15(2):62–66

Bustos JC, Cosgarea AJ (2006). Patellofemoral instability. In: Cosgarea AJ (ed) Orthopaedic sports medicine board review manual, vol 2. Turner White Communications, Wayne, pp 1–11

Conlan T, Garth WP Jr et al (1993) Evaluation of the medial soft-tissue restraints of the extensor mechanism of the knee. J Bone Joint Surg Am 75(5):682–693

Dejour H, Walch G et al (1994) Factors of patellar instability: an anatomic radiographic study. Knee Surg Sports Traumatol Arthrosc 2(1):19–26

Desio SM, Burks RT et al (1998) Soft tissue restraints to lateral patellar translation in the human knee. Am J Sports Med 26(1):59–65

Elias DA, White LM (2004) Imaging of patellofemoral disorders. Clin Radiol 59(7):543–557

Feller JA, Amis AA et al (2007) Surgical biomechanics of the patellofemoral joint. Arthroscopy 23(5):542–553

Fulkerso JP, Gossling HR (1980) Anatomy of the knee joint lateral retinaculum. Clin Orthop Relat Res 153:183–188

Greiwe RM, Saifi C, Ahmad CS et al (2010) Anatomy and biomechanics of patellar instability. Oper Tech Sports Med 18(2):62–67

Haklar U, Ulku T (2012) Overview of patellar dislocations in athletes. In: Doral MN (ed) Sports injuries. Springer, Berlin/Heidelberg, pp 585–596

Hawkins RJ, Bell RH et al (1986) Acute patellar dislocations. The natural history. Am J Sports Med 14(2): 117–120

Kaplan EB (1962) Some aspects of functional anatomy of the human knee joint. Clin Orthop 23:18–29

Karaoğlu S, Aygül V, Karagöz Z (2012) Patellofemoral pain syndrome. In: Doral MN (ed) Sports injuries. Springer, Berlin/Heidelberg, pp 565–569

Letts RM, Davidson D et al (1999) Semitendinosus tenodesis for repair of recurrent dislocation of the patella in children. J Pediatr Orthop 19(6):742–747

Maenpaa H, Sillanpaa PJ, Paakkala A (2010) A prospective, randomized trial following conservative treatment in acute primary patellar dislocation with special reference to patellar braces. Knee Surg Sports Traumatol Arthrosc 18(suppl 1):119

Malanga GA, Andrus S et al (2003) Physical examination of the knee: a review of the original test description and scientific validity of common orthopedic tests. Arch Phys Med Rehabil 84(4):592–603

Maquet P (1976) Advancement of the tibial tuberosity. Clin Orthop Relat Res 115:225–230

Mariani PP, Caruso I (1979) An electromyographic investigation of subluxation of the patella. J Bone Joint Surg Br 61-B(2):169–171

Mizuno Y, Kumagai M et al (2001) Q-angle influences tibiofemoral and patellofemoral kinematics. J Orthop Res 19(5):834–840

Myers P, Williams A et al (1999) The three-in-one proximal and distal soft tissue patellar realignment procedure. Results, and its place in the management of patellofemoral instability. Am J Sports Med 27(5): 575–579

Owens BD, Nelson BJ, Taylor DC (2005) Surgical treatment of primary traumatic patellar dislocations. Tech Knee Surg 4:140–146

Panni AS, Cerciello S et al (2011) Patellar shape can be a predisposing factor in patellar instability. Knee Surg Sports Traumatol Arthrosc 19(4):663–670

Quinn SF, Brown TR et al (1993) MR imaging of patellar retinacular ligament injuries. J Magn Reson Imaging 3(6):843–847

Reilly DT, Martens M (1972) Experimental analysis of the quadriceps muscle force and patello-femoral joint reaction force for various activities. Acta Orthop Scand 43(2):126–137

Sallay PI, Poggi J et al (1996) Acute dislocation of the patella. A correlative pathoanatomic study. Am J Sports Med 24(1):52–60

Sillanpaa PJ, Maenpaa HM (2012) First-time patellar dislocation: surgery or conservative treatment? Sports Med Arthrosc 20(3):128–135

Smith TO, Davies L et al (2010) Clinical outcomes of rehabilitation for patients following lateral patellar dislocation: a systematic review. Physiotherapy 96(4): 269–281

Stefancin JJ, Parker RD (2007) First-time traumatic patellar dislocation: a systematic review. Clin Orthop Relat Res 455:93–101

Tuxoe JI, Teir M et al (2002) The medial patellofemoral ligament: a dissection study. Knee Surg Sports Traumatol Arthrosc 10(3):138–140

Vainionpaa S, Laasonen E et al (1990) Acute dislocation of the patella. A prospective review of operative treatment. J Bone Joint Surg Br 72(3):366–369

Zaffagnini S, Colle F, Lopomo N, Sharma B, Bignozzi S, Dejour D, Marcacci M (2013) The influence of medial patellofemoral ligament on patellofemoral joint kinematics and patellar stability. Knee Surg Sports Traumatol Arthrosc 21:2164–2171

Zhu Z, Zhang Y, Shao H, Ding H, Wang G (2013) An in vivo study of the dynamic Q angle of the knee joint during flexion. In: Long M (ed) World congress on medical physics and biomedical engineering 26–31 May 2012, Beijing, vol 39. Springer, Berlin/Heidelberg, pp 234–237

Patellar Tendinopathy

103

Peter U. Brucker and Andreas B. Imhoff

Contents

Abstract

Patellar tendinopathy – also known as the jumper's knee – represents a clinically relevant lesion in orthopedic sports medicine and can be commonly seen in recreational as well as in professional sports performing repetitive jumping and landing activities. Many different treatment modalities have been suggested; however, there is yet no consensus for the optimal treatment regime of patellar tendinopathy. This chapter defines the term "patellar tendinopathy", describes its pathogenetic mechanisms, summarizes diagnostics including clinical and imaging-based findings as well as conservative and operative treatment options by focusing on evidence-based levels in the treatment of patellar tendinopathy.

Abbreviations

ESWT	Extracorporeal shock wave therapy
MMP	Matrix metalloproteinase
PrP	Platelet-rich plasma
MRI	Magnetic resonance imaging
BMI	Body mass index

Introduction

There is a general agreement that the patellar tendon is particularly vulnerable to injury and to overuse and not infrequently difficult to manage successfully as defined by complete pain relief and healing. Patellar tendinopathy is usually

P.U. Brucker (✉) • A.B. Imhoff
Department of Orthopaedic Sports Medicine, Klinikum rechts der Isar, Technical University of Munich, Munich, Germany
e-mail: peter.brucker@lrz.tu-muenchen.de

M.N. Doral, J. Karlsson (eds.), *Sports Injuries*,
DOI 10.1007/978-3-642-36569-0_68

activity related with recurrent, chronic, or acute overloading of the patellar tendon. Therefore, patellar tendinopathy can be either acute, acute on chronic, or chronic.

Definition and Pathogenesis

Tendinopathies of the patella represents a commonly and relevantly clinical problem in sports medicine. Human (Rees et al. 2006) and animal studies (Warden 2007) have demonstrated a degenerative underlying pathology, but not an inflammatory process, even though abnormal neovascularization can be found in patellar tendinopathy (Weinberg et al. 1998). Therefore, patellar tendinopathy corresponds more to a tendinotic rather than a tendinitic alteration (Khan et al. 2002). However, it is also suggested that patellar tendinopathy includes a pathology continuum starting with an inflammatory, reactive stage and progresses to a degenerative stage, which still may have the potential of reversibility (Cook and Purdam 2009). Overall, a tendinosis or tendinopathy of the proximal patellar tendon is well known as the "jumper's knee", firstly described by Blazina et al. in 1973 (Blazina et al. 1973). In addition, structural alterations of the patellar tendon may also occur in the midsubstance or at the distal part. Recent basic research has shown that autocrine and paracrine effects of neurotransmitters (glutamate, substance P) as well as nerve-related cholinergic pathways are the main pathologic mechanisms in chronic patellar tendinosis (Danielson et al. 2006) ("▶ Chap. 184, Tendinopathies in Sports: From Basic Research to the Field").

Internal risk factors of patellar tendinopathy include lower flexibility of the quadriceps and the hamstrings muscles, higher body weight and body mass index (BMI), increased waist-to-hip ratio, leg-length difference, reduced ankle dorsiflexion, arch height of the foot, and overall vertical jump performance, whereas large increases in training load represent the major external risk factor (James et al. 2014; van der Worp et al. 2011). Training load for jumping and landing activities is usually dependent on the specific requirement profile of the sports discipline, level of sports performance, and the individual position of the athlete in team sports, which results in unequal expositions of typical training activities.

Diagnosis

Specific symptoms of a patellar tendinopathy include anterior knee pain with a localized pain center at the inferior patella pole usually during or following knee extensor loading activities, but decreases after a period of rest. However, the clinical symptoms may vary with respect to pain and activity level. Ferretti and colleagues (Ferretti et al. 2002) described a modified classification of Blazina et al. (1973) with special focus on the occurrence of symptoms at different activity levels (Table 1). In addition, the active extension is usually painful with or without resistance. Overall, these symptoms may occur in various athletic activities, but jumping athletes are predisposed. Local tenderness on palpation, sometimes combined with focal swelling, is the main clinical finding.

Imaging-based diagnostic tools include gray-scale ultrasonography, color or power Doppler sonography, radiography, and magnetic resonance imaging (MRI) (Fig. 1). Gray-scale ultrasonography and color or power Doppler sonography are noninvasive and cost-effective imaging

Table 1 Clinical classification of patellar tendinopathy (jumper's knee) according to the levels of symptoms (according to Ferretti et al. (2002))

Stage	Level of symptoms
0	No pain
1	Pain only after intense sports activity; no undue functional impairment
2	Pain at the beginning and after sports activity; still able to perform at a satisfactory level
3	Pain during sports activity; increasing difficulty in performing at a satisfactory level
4	Pain during sports activity; unable to participate in sport at a satisfactory level
5	Pain during daily activity; unable to participate in sport at any level

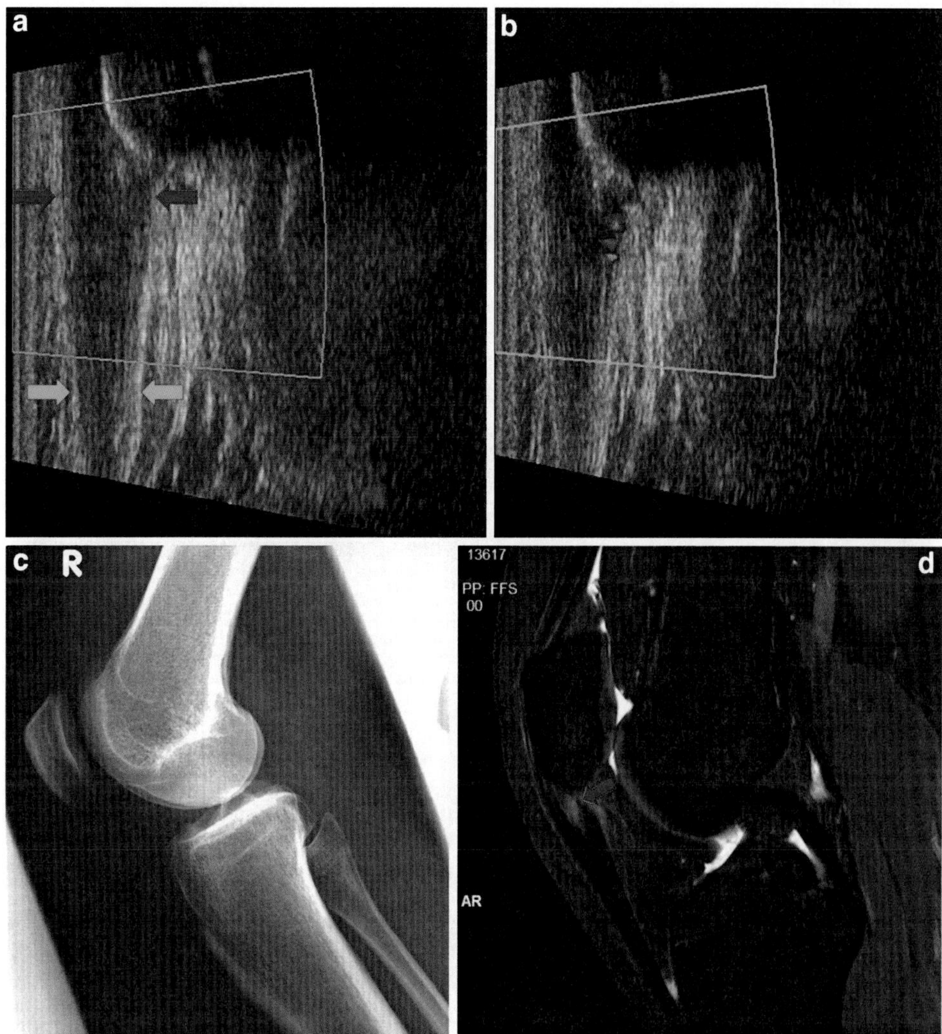

Fig. 1 Imaging techniques in patellar tendinopathy: (**a**) gray-scale ultrasonography (*red arrows* show a pathologic thickening and partial hypoechogenicity of the proximal patellar tendon, *green arrows* indicate normal patellar tendon structure and shape); (**b**) color Doppler sonography highlights pathologic neovascularization areas; (**c**) conventional radiography (*lateral view*) with regular osseous findings and absent calcifications of the patellar tendon; (**d**) magnetic resonance imaging (MRI) (*red arrow* demonstrates pathologic areas at the proximal patellar tendon as well as concomitant partial patellar tendon rupture)

techniques, which are usually performed within one diagnostic session and which immediately can confirm the clinical diagnosis. Typical pathologic findings in gray-scale ultrasonography for patellar tendinopathy are abnormal thickening of the tendon with irregular structure of the tendon fibers and hypoechogenic tendon areas closely or directly adjacent to the patellar tendon insertion site (Fig. 1a) (Terslev et al. 2001). In color or power Doppler sonography, occurrence of neovessels within the altered tendon areas is characteristic for patellar tendinopathy (Fig. 1b) (Alfredson and Ohberg 2005; Weinberg et al. 1998). Lateral views in regular radiography (Fig. 1c) provide additional information of osseous abnormalities, e.g., osteophytes, at the inferior patella pole, calcifications of the patellar tendon itself, patellofemoral osteoarthrosis, and/or additional growth disturbances of the apophyses in M. Sinding-Larsen at the inferior patella as well as in M. Osgood-Schlatter at the tibial tuberosity (Ostlere 2013; Thomas et al. 2014) ("▶ Chap. 209, Patellofemoral Problems in Adolescent Athletes"). MRI gives an excellent illustration with respect to quantitative and qualitative dimensions of the tendinopathy and potential concomitant partial ruptures of the patellar tendon within the tendinopathic area (Fig. 1d) (Ostlere 2013; Thomas et al. 2014).

Therapy

Various conservative and operative treatment strategies have been reported in the literature. Overall, conservative treatment concepts without or with injection therapies are commonly accepted as first- or second-line treatment, whereas operative therapies were usually performed following initial conservative treatment regimes in chronic, recurrent, or refractory cases.

Conservative Treatment

Conservative treatment injection therapies include rest, ice, anti-inflammatory medication, electrotherapy, physical therapy, physiotherapy, eccentric training, low-intensity pulsed ultrasound, and extracorporeal shock wave therapy (ESWT) (Frohm et al. 2007; Jonsson and Alfredson 2005; Larsson et al. 2012; Purdam et al. 2004; van Leeuwen et al. 2009; Visnes and Bahr 2007; Warden et al. 2008; Young et al. 2005; Zwerver et al. 2010) ("▶ Chap. 107, Physiotherapy in Patellofemoral Pain Syndrome"). Eccentric training has nowadays become the first-line conservative treatment and therefore the treatment of choice for patellar tendinopathy due to mostly consistent good results and overall successful clinical outcome (Frohm et al. 2007; Jonsson and Alfredson 2005; Larsson et al. 2012; Purdam et al. 2004; Visnes and Bahr 2007; Young et al. 2005). Interestingly, modulation of the eccentric training technique itself also influences the clinical result, since a decline eccentric squat technique on an oblique base has shown superior outcome compared to a standard eccentric technique on a flat ground (Purdam et al. 2004). However, the optimal eccentric training program in consideration of frequency, load, and dosage has yet to be determined. In addition to eccentric training, temporally limited, but adequate rest of causative loading activities and patterns may represent another key factor for successful treatment of patellar tendinopathy, even though there is no high-quality evidence for supporting a strategy of withdrawal from concomitant sportive activities during eccentric training programs (Saithna et al. 2012).

Focused ESWT may represent a second-line conservative treatment in chronic patellar tendinopathy after eccentric training has failed (Rodriguez-Merchan 2013). It seems to be both effective and safe with positive effects on pain level and function; however, a common agreement on a specific treatment protocol for the focused ESWT also cannot be made so far (van Leeuwen et al. 2009).

Conservative Treatment with Minimal-Invasive Injection Therapies

Different injection treatment options are available and increasingly used for patellar tendinopathy: platelet-rich plasma (PRP) (Fig. 2) ("▶ Chap. 261, Platelet-Rich Plasma: From Laboratory to the Clinic"), polidocanol, corticosteroids, and aprotinin (van Ark et al. 2011). These substances vary in their effects and target areas within the patellar tendon and the tendinopathic zone (Table 2) as well as in their efficacy (van Ark et al. 2011). Contrary to other injection substances, a relapse of symptoms in the long-term follow-up can be often seen in corticosteroids (van Ark et al. 2011).

Furthermore, novel cell-based treatment strategies with autologous skin-derived tendon-like cells (Clarke et al. 2011) or bone marrow mononuclear cells (Pascual-Garrido et al. 2012) were applied for refractory patellar tendinopathy. All aforementioned substances as well as selected cell suspensions can be injected under ultrasonographic guidance for correct placement within the (peri)tendinous target area. Generally, injection

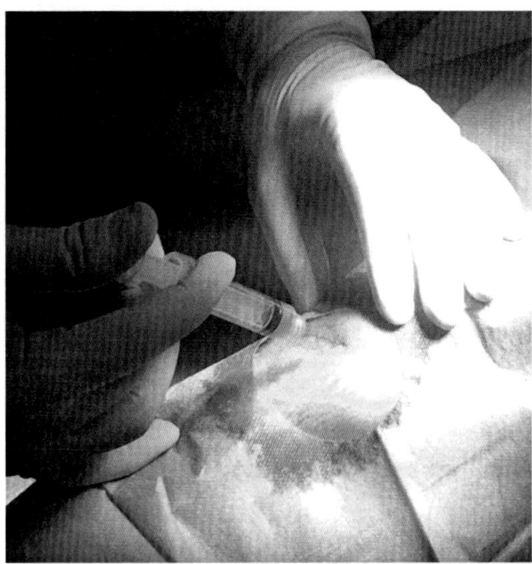

Fig. 2 Transtendinous injection of platelet-rich plasma (autologous conditioned plasma (ACP®), Arthrex, Munich, GER) at the superior patella insertion site posteriorly under sterile conditions. During the injection, the patella is fixed with the other hand. Optionally, ultrasonography may be used for defining the correct injection zone

Table 2 Injection substances and their effects and target areas (Baksh et al. 2013; Cáceres et al. 2008; Katler and Weissmann 1977; van Ark et al. 2011)

Substance	Effects and target areas
Platelet-rich plasma	Local enhancement of autologous growth factors, additional influence and modulation of cell adhesion, cell migration, and cell differentiation by autocrine and/or paracrine cellular pathways
Polidocanol	Chemical destruction of neovessels and their accompanying nerves channeling pain signals
Corticosteroids	Inhibition of inflammatory processes by upregulating the expression of anti-inflammatory proteins and downregulating the expression of proinflammatory proteins through interaction with the glucocorticoid receptors
Aprotinin	Inhibition of collagenase and matrix metalloproteinases (MMPs) by inhibition of the plasmin-activation pathway

therapies can be combined with other conservative treatment options (e.g., rest, ice, physical therapy, physiotherapy, eccentric training); however, the combination of a multimodal conservative approach is actually not standardized and therefore not evaluated with respect to enhanced synergistic effects and optimized clinical outcome.

Operative Treatment

Operative therapies of patellar tendinopathy encompass arthroscopic and open surgical techniques. Arthroscopic techniques imply denervation or resection of the inferior patella pole, debridement of the patellar tendon, patellar release, and scraping (Coleman et al. 2000; Cucurulo et al. 2009; Cuéllar and Mina 2007; Maier et al. 2013; Ogon et al. 2006), whereas in open techniques drilling of the inferior patella pole or resection of the inferior patella pole with or without additional resection of the central third of the patellar tendon have been described (Blazina et al. 1973; Coleman et al. 2000; Cucurulo et al. 2009; Cuéllar and Mina 2007; Fritschy and Wallensten 1993). Approaches in open techniques include central transtendinous or paramedian incisions medially or laterally to the patellar tendon. In transtendinous techniques, the patellar tendon is incised along with the fiber arrangement (Cucurulo et al. 2009).

Preoperatively, it may be helpful to mark the most symptomatic region of the patellar tendon. For arthroscopic techniques, usually a standard high anterolateral and a high anteromedial portal were used, with both portals placed approximately 1 cm more laterally and medially, respectively, compared to a regular position of the arthroscopic portals (Maier et al. 2013). A needle can be applied for subsequent optimal portal placement (Fig. 3a). During diagnostic arthroscopy, synovial overgrowth of the retropatellar cartilage by neovessels might be visible as a pathognomonic sign for chronic patellar tendinopathy (Maier et al. 2013).

In the preferred arthroscopic technique, so-called "patellar release" technique, exposure

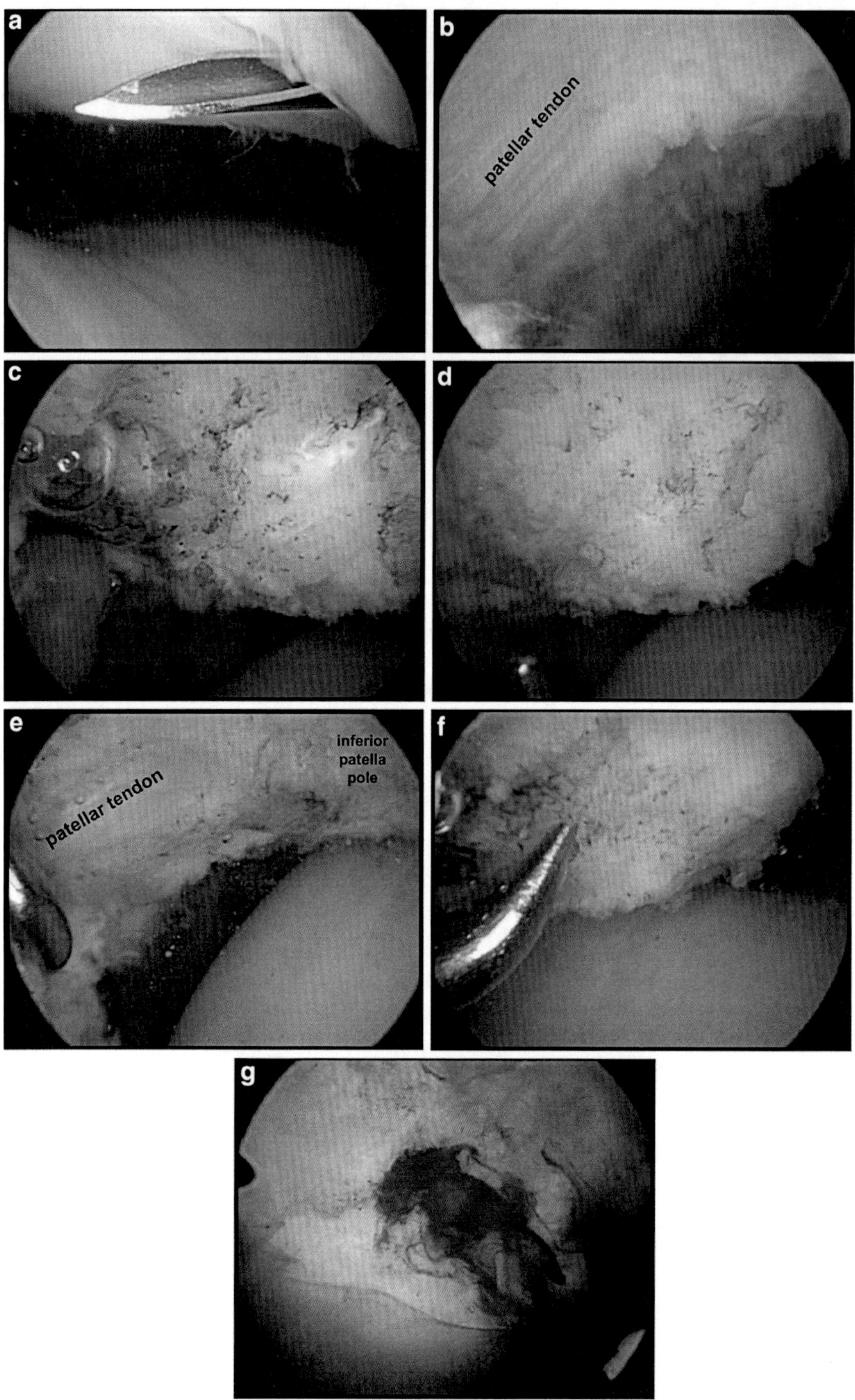

Fig. 3 Arthroscopic "patellar release" technique and additive arthroscopic microfracture of the inferior patella pole: (**a**) correct positioning of the secondary portal using a needle; (**b**) visualization of the posterior aspect of the proximal patellar tendon; (**c**) arthroscopic debridement and denervation of the peritendinous soft tissue; (**d**) finalized debridement and denervation of the inferior patella pole; (**e**) scraping of the posterior aspect of the proximal patellar tendon; (**f**) microfracture of the inferior patella pole; (**g**) bleeding due to microfracture following temporarily opened tourniquet

and visualization of the inferior patella pole as well as the posterior part of the proximal patellar tendon is realized by arthroscopic removal of the hypertrophic synovial membrane and parts of the infrapatellar (Hoffa) fat pad (Fig. 3b) utilizing an electrosurgical device (e.g., Opes®, Arthrex, Munich, GER) (Fig. 3c). Two needles are positioned transdermally for arthroscopic determination of the mediolateral extension of the symptomatic proximal patellar tendon area. Then, a denervation procedure of the non-articulating part of the inferior patella pole between the retropatellar cartilage border and the patellar tendon insertion site is performed (Fig. 3d) (Maier et al. 2013). Additionally, the so-called scraping techniques target the region with pathologically high blood flow (Alfredson 2011) by mechanically destroying and disrupting the peritendinous system of neovessels and accompanying nerval fibers (Fig. 3e). Microfracture of the already denervated inferior patella pole may be performed as an additive procedure (Fig. 3f). Temporary opening of the tourniquet demonstrates sufficient depths of the microfracture channels (Fig. 3g). In cases of additional inferior osteophytes or spurs at the patella, osseous resection may be necessary.

A comparison of arthroscopic and open techniques for patellar tendinopathy in a multicenter study revealed a success rate of more than 80 % independently of the surgical technique in an athletic study population with initial, but unsuccessful conservative treatment (Cucurulo et al. 2009). In another retrospective comparative study, arthroscopic patellar tenotomy was as successful as a traditional open technique. However, even demonstrating symptomatic benefit in all patients, only approximately half of the patients who underwent either open or arthroscopic patellar tenotomy were later competing at their former sporting level (Coleman et al. 2000).

Evidence

Both conservative and operative treatment modalities provide overall good results; however, there is still a relevant number of nonresponders to either treatment strategy. Even though prospective randomized trials have been already published (Larsson et al. 2012), the literature still lacks a sufficient number of high-quality studies comparing the different therapy strategies and their potential combination for enhancing as well as for optimizing the clinical outcome.

From an evidence-based view, the following consequences can be already drawn due to high-level prospective, randomized controlled trials comparing different treatment modalities:

Eccentric Training Versus Surgery

A 12-week eccentric training program did not result in inferior clinical results in patellar tendinopathy compared to open patellar tenotomy with wedge-shaped full-thickness excision of the proximal patellar tendon (Bahr et al. 2006). Therefore, eccentric training should be performed for at least 12 weeks before open tenotomy is considered as a therapeutic option for patellar tendinopathy.

Sclerosing Polidocanol Versus Surgery

A treatment with sclerosing polidocanol injections demonstrated inferior clinical results compared to arthroscopic shaving of the region with high blood flow for mechanical disruption of the neovessels and nerves. For correct intervention performance, both treatment modalities were guided by color Doppler ultrasonography (Willberg et al. 2011).

Conclusion

Overall, patellar tendinopathy or jumper's knee seems more a degenerative than an inflammatory alteration of the patellar tendon. The diagnosis of patellar tendinopathy includes typical anamnesis, clinical examination, and multimodal imaging-based analysis. Multiple treatment concepts have been described for patellar tendinopathy. Many of these treatment methods (eccentric training,

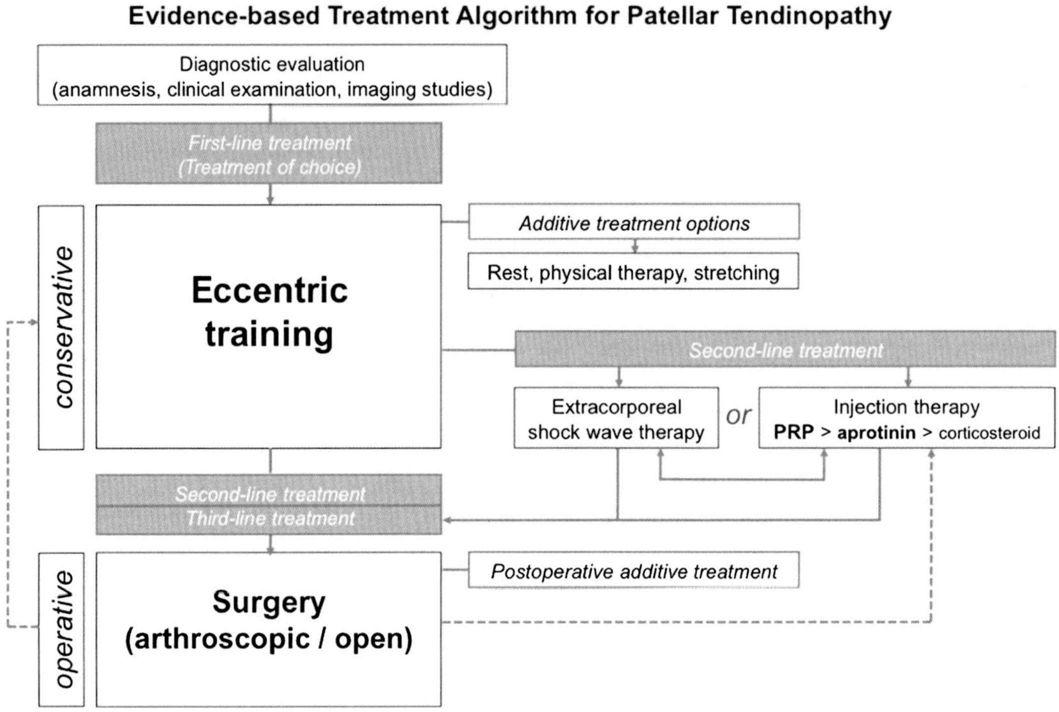

Evidence-based Treatment Algorithm for Patellar Tendinopathy

Diagnostic evaluation (anamnesis, clinical examination, imaging studies)
First-line treatment (Treatment of choice)
conservative
Eccentric training
Additive treatment options
Rest, physical therapy, stretching
Second-line treatment
Extracorporeal shock wave therapy
or
Injection therapy
PRP > aprotinin > corticosteroid
Second-line treatment
Third-line treatment
operative
Surgery (arthroscopic / open)
Postoperative additive treatment

Fig. 4 Proposed evidence-based treatment algorithm for patellar tendinopathy demonstrating first-, second-, and third-line treatment options and potential combination of additive therapeutic modalities. Second-line conservative treatment (injection therapy vs. extracorporeal shock wave therapy) may be performed in an alternating way or subsequently. Dotted arrows represent additive or combined therapeutic strategies in prolonged courses following surgery or after surgical failure. (*Abbreviation*: *PRP* platelet-rich plasma)

sclerosing polidocanol, surgical debridement, scraping, tendon release) address the pathologic “neoneurovascularization” process by applying shear forces and mechanical irritation to the pathologic vascularization site, hereby destroying and disrupting the neovessels as well as the accompanying nerves, which are responsible for pain signaling.

To date, strong evidence can be only stated for the use of eccentric training in patellar tendinopathy. However, the optimal frequency, load, and dosage of eccentric exercises have yet to be investigated. Only limited evidence exists for surgery (either open or arthroscopic), sclerosing injections, and ESWT. Novel treatment options, e.g., PRP injections, may offer further starting points of enhanced healing capacities, but are scientifically not sufficiently validated so far. In the future, the lack of high-level, well-designed studies with adequate numbers of patients as well as long-term follow-ups must be counteracted to finally draw stronger conclusions. Based on the current evidence levels, a structured treatment algorithm was developed and proposed for a stepwise treatment of patellar tendinopathy (Fig. 4). However, knowledge of internal as well as the external risk factors and prevention strategies represents another essential field to even prohibit patellar tendinopathy in the athletes at risk (“► Chap. 254, Injury Prevention in Different Sports”).

Cross-References

- ► Injury Prevention in Different Sports
- ► Patellofemoral Problems in Adolescent Athletes
- ► Physiotherapy in Patellofemoral Pain Syndrome

- ▶ Platelet-Rich Plasma: From Laboratory to the Clinic
- ▶ Tendinopathies in Sports: From Basic Research to the Field

References

Alfredson H (2011) Ultrasound and Doppler-guided mini-surgery to treat midportion Achilles tendinosis: results of a large material and a randomised study comparing two scraping techniques. Br J Sports Med 45:407–410

Alfredson H, Ohberg L (2005) Neovascularisation in chronic painful patellar tendinosis–promising results after sclerosing neovessels outside the tendon challenge the need for surgery. Knee Surg Sports Traumatol Arthrosc 13:74–80

Bahr R, Fossan B, Loken S, Engebretsen L (2006) Surgical treatment compared with eccentric training for patellar tendinopathy (Jumper's Knee). A randomized, controlled trial. J Bone Joint Surg Am 88:1689–1698

Baksh N, Hannon CP, Murawski CD, Smyth NA, Kennedy JG (2013) Platelet-rich plasma in tendon models: a systematic review of basic science literature. Arthroscopy 29:596–607

Blazina ME, Kerlan RK, Jobe FW, Carter VS, Carlson GJ (1973) Jumper's knee. Orthop Clin North Am 4:665–678

Cáceres M, Hidalgo R, Sanz A, Martínez J, Riera P, Smith PC (2008) Effect of platelet-rich plasma on cell adhesion, cell migration, and myofibroblastic differentiation in human gingival fibroblasts. J Periodontol 79:714–720

Clarke AW, Alyas F, Morris T, Robertson CJ, Bell J, Connell DA (2011) Skin-derived tenocyte-like cells for the treatment of patellar tendinopathy. Am J Sports Med 39:614–623

Coleman BD, Khan KM, Kiss ZS, Bartlett J, Young DA, Wark JD (2000) Open and arthroscopic patellar tenotomy for chronic patellar tendinopathy. A retrospective outcome study. Victorian Institute of Sport Tendon Study Group. Am J Sports Med 28:183–190

Cook JL, Purdam CR (2009) Is tendon pathology a continuum? A pathology model to explain the clinical presentation of load-induced tendinopathy. Br J Sports Med 43:409–416

Cucurulo T, Louis ML, Thaunat M, Franceschi JP (2009) Surgical treatment of patellar tendinopathy in athletes. A retrospective multicentric study. Orthop Traumatol Surg Res 95:S78–S84

Cuéllar EC, Mina NZ (2007) Jumper's knee. Surgery and arthroscopic treatment with scraping and povidone collagen in high-performance athletes. Acta Ortop Mex 21:234–238

Danielson P, Alfredson H, Forsgren S (2006) Immunohistochemical and histochemical findings favoring the occurrence of autocrine/paracrine as well as nerve-related cholinergic effects in chronic painful patellar tendon tendinosis. Microsc Res Tech 69:808–819

Ferretti A, Conteduca F, Camerucci E, Morelli F (2002) Patellar tendinosis: a follow-up study of surgical treatment. J Bone Joint Surg Am 84-A:2179–2185

Fritschy D, Wallensten R (1993) Surgical treatment of patellar tendinitis. Knee Surg Sports Traumatol Arthrosc 1:131–133

Frohm A, Saartok T, Halvorsen K, Renstrom P (2007) Eccentric treatment for patellar tendinopathy: a prospective randomised short-term pilot study of two rehabilitation protocols. Br J Sports Med 41:e7

James LP, Kelly VG, Beckman EM (2014) Injury risk management plan for volleyball athletes. Sports Med 44(9):1185–95

Jonsson P, Alfredson H (2005) Superior results with eccentric compared to concentric quadriceps training in patients with jumper's knee: a prospective randomised study. Br J Sports Med 39:847–850

Katler E, Weissmann G (1977) Steroids, aspirin, and inflammation. Inflammation 2:295–307

Khan KM, Cook JL, Kannus P, Maffulli N, Bonar SF (2002) Time to abandon the "tendinitis" myth. BMJ 324:626–627

Larsson ME, Kall I, Nilsson-Helander K (2012) Treatment of patellar tendinopathy – a systematic review of randomized controlled trials. Knee Surg Sports Traumatol Arthrosc 20:1632–1646

Maier D, Bornebusch L, Salzmann GM, Südkamp NP, Ogon P (2013) Mid- and long-term efficacy of the arthroscopic patellar release for treatment of patellar tendinopathy unresponsive to nonoperative management. Arthroscopy 29:1338–1345

Ogon P, Maier D, Jaeger A, Suedkamp NP (2006) Arthroscopic patellar release for the treatment of chronic patellar tendinopathy. Arthroscopy 22(462):e461–e465

Ostlere S (2013) The extensor mechanism of the knee. Radiol Clin North Am 51:393–411

Pascual-Garrido C, Rolon A, Makino A (2012) Treatment of chronic patellar tendinopathy with autologous bone marrow stem cells: a 5-year-followup. Stem Cells Int 2012:953510

Purdam CR, Jonsson P, Alfredson H, Lorentzon R, Cook JL, Khan KM (2004) A pilot study of the eccentric decline squat in the management of painful chronic patellar tendinopathy. Br J Sports Med 38:395–397

Rees JD, Wilson AM, Wolman RL (2006) Current concepts in the management of tendon disorders. Rheumatology (Oxford) 45:508–521

Rodriguez-Merchan EC (2013) The treatment of patellar tendinopathy. J Orthop Traumatol 14:77–81

Saithna A, Gogna R, Baraza N, Modi C, Spencer S (2012) Eccentric exercise protocols for patella tendinopathy: should we really be withdrawing athletes from sport? A systematic review. Open Orthop J 6:553–557

Terslev L, Qvistgaard E, Torp-Pedersen S, Laetgaard J, Danneskiold-Samsoe B, Bliddal H (2001) Ultrasound and power doppler findings in jumper's knee – preliminary observations. Eur J Ultrasound 13:183–189

Thomas S, Rupiper D, Stacy GS (2014) Imaging of the patellofemoral joint. Clin Sports Med 33:413–436

van Ark M, Zwerver J, van den Akker-Scheek I (2011) Injection treatments for patellar tendinopathy. Br J Sports Med 45:1068–1076

van der Worp H, van Ark M, Roerink S, Pepping GJ, van den Akker-Scheek I, Zwerver J (2011) Risk factors for patellar tendinopathy: a systematic review of the literature. Br J Sports Med 45:446–452

van Leeuwen MT, Zwerver J, van den Akker-Scheek I (2009) Extracorporeal shockwave therapy for patellar tendinopathy: a review of the literature. Br J Sports Med 43:163–168

Visnes H, Bahr R (2007) The evolution of eccentric training as treatment for patellar tendinopathy (jumper's knee): a critical review of exercise programmes. Br J Sports Med 41:217–223

Warden SJ (2007) Animal models for the study of tendinopathy. Br J Sports Med 41:232–240

Warden SJ, Metcalf BR, Kiss ZS, Cook JL, Purdam CR, Bennell KL, Crossley KM (2008) Low-intensity pulsed ultrasound for chronic patellar tendinopathy: a randomized, double-blind, placebo-controlled trial. Rheumatology (Oxford) 47:467–471

Weinberg EP, Adams MJ, Hollenberg GM (1998) Color Doppler sonography of patellar tendinosis. AJR Am J Roentgenol 171:743–744

Willberg L, Sunding K, Forssblad M, Fahlstrom M, Alfredson H (2011) Sclerosing polidocanol injections or arthroscopic shaving to treat patellar tendinopathy/jumper's knee? A randomised controlled study. Br J Sports Med 45:411–415

Young MA, Cook JL, Purdam CR, Kiss ZS, Alfredson H (2005) Eccentric decline squat protocol offers superior results at 12 months compared with traditional eccentric protocol for patellar tendinopathy in volleyball players. Br J Sports Med 39:102–105

Zwerver J, Dekker F, Pepping GJ (2010) Patient guided Piezo-electric extracorporeal shockwave therapy as treatment for chronic severe patellar tendinopathy: a pilot study. J Back Musculoskelet Rehabil 23:111–115

104 Posterior Cruciate Ligament Reconstruction: New Concepts

Waqas M. Hussain, Brett W. McCoy, Michael J. Griesser, and Lutul Farrow

Contents

W.M. Hussain (✉)
ORA Orthopedics, Moline, IL, USA
e-mail: waqasmhussain@gmail.com

B.W. McCoy
Southwest Orthopaedics Inc., Parma, OH, USA
e-mail: brettmccoy216@gmail.com

M.J. Griesser
Performance Orthopaedics and Sports Medicine, Clinton Memorial Hospital, Wilmington, OH, USA
e-mail: michaeljgriesser@gmail.com

L. Farrow
Cleveland Clinic Sports Health Center, Garfield Heights, OH, USA
e-mail: lutulfarrowmd@yahoo.com

M.N. Doral, J. Karlsson (eds.), *Sports Injuries*,
DOI 10.1007/978-3-642-36569-0_108

Abstract

Although injuries to the posterior cruciate ligament (PCL) are uncommon and have been infrequently studied, the anatomy of the structure including its origin, attachment, and surrounding structures has been well characterized. Based on the severity of the mechanism of injury, other adjacent structures may be affected and a careful physical examination is important. Additionally, imaging including x-rays, MRI, and CT can provide important information. Many PCL injuries can be treated without surgery, but recent studies have demonstrated that patients are at a greater predisposition for developing degenerative changes. Surgery is performed for instability and combined ligamentous injuries and may include single-bundle and double-bundle reconstructions and transtibial and tibial-inlay techniques, either through open or arthroscopic methods. In the chapter, the authors have outlined their preferred method of the open, tibial-inlay technique with accompanying pearl and pitfalls for this technique.

Introduction

Injuries to the posterior cruciate ligament (PCL) are not uncommon. However, they occur less frequently and have been studied less often than injuries to other ligaments of the knee. The true incidence of PCL injury is much higher than previously believed, and increased clinical suspicion coupled with better physical examination and imaging techniques has led to improved diagnosis.

It is estimated that the incidence of PCL injury in the general population comprises 3 % of all acute knee injuries (Miyasaka et al. 1991). The incidence of PCL injury in the trauma population is reported to be as high at 37 % (Fanelli 1993; Fanelli and Edson 1995). Posterior cruciate ligament injuries typically occur in the second and third decades of life. Miyasaka et al. have previously reported that these injuries are most common in individuals aged 15–29 (Miyasaka et al. 1991). Isolated PCL injuries occur much less frequently than other ligamentous injuries of the knee and also have been studied less, which has resulted in fewer high level evidence studies in the medical literature.

The appropriate definitive treatment of isolated PCL tears is a topic of frequent debate. Traditionally, they have been treated nonoperatively. Bergfeld et al. have demonstrated that the majority of athletes with isolated tears of the PCL were able to return to athletic activity following rehabilitation exercises (Parolie and Bergfeld 1986). Studies pertaining to the natural history of PCL-deficient knees have prompted some to recommend increased surgical management of these injuries.

Evaluation

The history should focus on the patient's injury mechanism, activity level, occupation, and symptoms. The examiner should attempt to determine the severity of injury and any concomitant pathology. Acutely, PCL injuries may present with mild swelling, pain, and an antalgic gait. The classic audile "pop" or sudden, massive effusion described with ACL injuries occurs less frequently with isolated PCL injuries. However, it is uncommon for patients with multiple injured ligaments to be asymptomatic. Acutely, these patients present with marked pain, swelling, and stiffness. As this initial pain and swelling subside, pain and instability become the predominant complaints.

Physical examination begins with careful evaluation of lower extremity alignment and gait. The patient's affected knee should be evaluated for the presence of any increased recurvatum and varus or valgus malalignment. Any abnormal varus thrust with ambulation should be noted, as this may be indicative of concomitant injury to the posterolateral corner. The posterior drawer examination is the gold standard for diagnosis of PCL injury (Clancy et al. 1983; Grood et al. 1988; Harner and Hoher 1988; Covey and Sapega 1993; Bergfeld et al. 2001a). The patient is positioned supine with the knee in 90° of flexion. The examiner then places a posteriorly directed force on the proximal tibia while monitoring the step-off between the anteromedial tibial plateau and the medial femoral condyle. The amount of displacement and quality of the endpoint are assessed. Normally, there is a 1 cm anterior step-off between the anteromedial tibial plateau and the medial femoral condyle. The severity of PCL injury can be graded depending on the amount of posterior translation. In grade I injuries, there is abnormal posterior translation of the tibial plateau with maintenance of the anterior step-off (translation <5 mm). Grade II injuries occur when the plateau displaces 5–10 mm posteriorly and becomes flush with the medial femoral condyle. When the examiner is able to translate the plateau posterior to the medial femoral condyle (>10 mm), the injuries are classified at grade III.

Multiple special tests have been described for the diagnosis of PCL injuries. Posterior tibial sag is assessed at 90° of knee and hip flexion with the patient supine on the examination table. This test is positive when the normal prominence of the tibial tubercle is not seen as gravity subluxes the tibia posteriorly (Fig. 1). When posterior tibial sag is seen in full extension, this may be indicative of a combined PLC injury (Fig. 2). The quadriceps active test is positive when contraction of the quadriceps restores the normal contour of the tibial tubercle. This test is performed with the patient supine and the knee in 60° of flexion. The examiner holds pressure on the foot and asks the patient to contract the quadriceps muscle. The test is

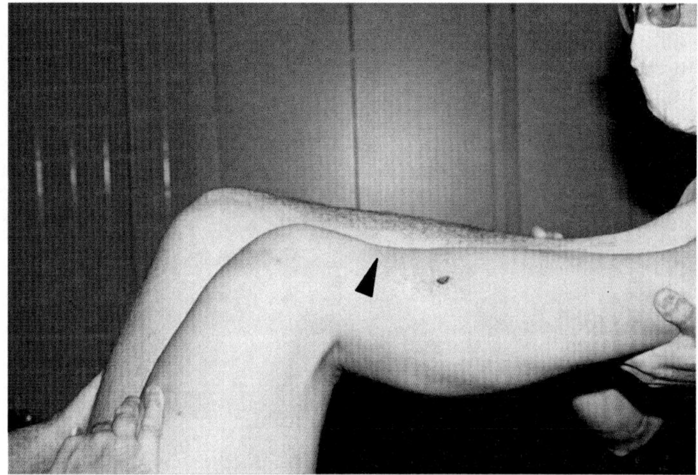

Fig. 1 Posterior tibial sag. Loss of tibial tubercle prominence (*arrow*)

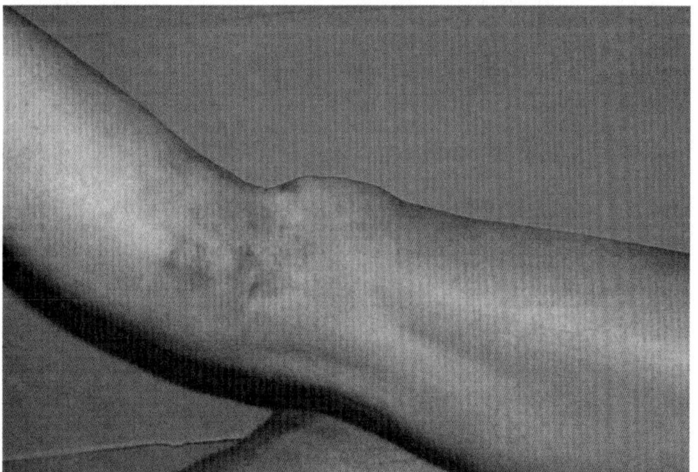

Fig. 2 Extension recurvatum

positive when the quadriceps mechanism pulls the posteriorly subluxed tibia to a reduced position, restoring the normal prominence of the tibial tubercle. Alternatively, the test can be performed by instructing the patient to try and slide his/her foot distally on the examining table. This maneuver effectively causes contraction of the quadriceps and may be easier for the patient to understand.

Careful assessment for PLC injury is important and may significantly alter treatment. The dial test can be performed in the prone or supine position (Fig. 3). An external rotation force is applied to the leg with the knee in 30° and 90° of flexion and compared to the contralateral limb. Increased rotation of the tibia only at 30° of flexion suggests a PLC injury. When rotation is increased >10° only at 90°, an isolated PCL injury is suspected. When rotation is increased at both angles, combined PCL and PLC injuries may be present. Severe medial knee injuries may also have a positive dial test at both 30° and 90°. Griffith et al. noted that the primary external rotation stabilizer is the distal division of the superficial medial collateral ligament at 30° of knee flexion (Griffith et al. 2009).

The varus stress test also can be an important indicator of injury. A varus stress is applied to the knee at 0° and 30° of flexion. Varus laxity at 30° of flexion is an indication of PLC injury, and laxity at both full extension and 30° of flexion indicates injury to both the PLC and PCL. Another

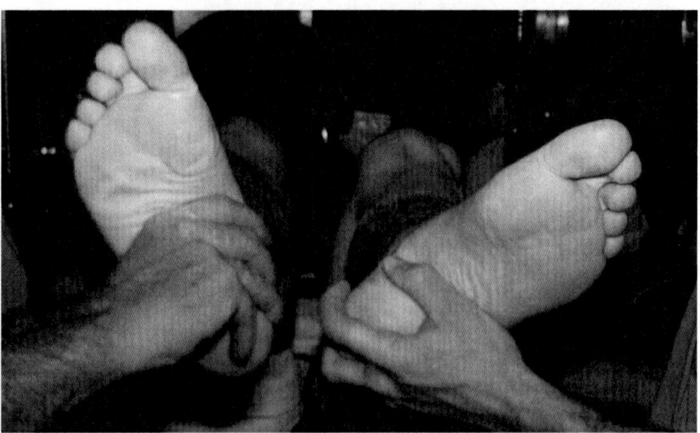

Fig. 3 Increased external tibial rotation at 90° of knee flexion

important test is the posterolateral drawer test. This test is performed with the knee flexed to 80°, and the foot is externally rotated while a posterior load is applied. A positive result occurs when the lateral tibial plateau rotates posteriorly and externally relative to the medial tibial plateau.

Diagnostic Imaging

Radiographic evaluation should include plain radiographs of the contralateral knee to allow for comparison of both extremities and detection of subtle radiographic changes. The authors prefer performing a weight-bearing posteroanterior (PA) view in 45° of flexion. Rosenberg et al. noted that cartilage wear most commonly involves the contact zones from 30° to 60° of knee flexion, and this view more accurately demonstrates subtle joint space narrowing that is commonly underestimated by standard AP radiographs performed in full extension (Rosenberg et al. 1988). Additionally, a 45° non-weight-bearing lateral view and bilateral axial views of the patellae, as described by Merchant, are obtained (Merchant et al. 1974). Standing hip-knee-ankle films on a long cassette may also be obtained to evaluate coronal plane limb alignment.

PCL stress x-rays may also be a useful adjunct in evaluating PCL injuries. This course of imaging can help a clinician differentiate between a partial PCL tear, a complete PCL tear, and a complete PCL tear with concomitant ligamentous injury. Margheritini et al. demonstrated that x-rays performed in 90° of flexion allowed for easier quantification of displacement and resultant laxity (Margheritini et al. 2003). Sekiya et al. noted that a grade III posterior drawer combined with more than 10 mm of displacement on stress radiography correlated with a PLC injury in addition to an underlying PCL tear (Sekiya et al. 2008).

Magnetic resonance imaging (MRI) can provide important diagnostic information. MRI can delineate the exact location and severity of the PCL injury. Determination of injury location may have important implications with respect to treatment. For example, femoral "peel-off" injuries or tibial-sided avulsions may occasionally be amenable to primary repair (Fig. 4). MRI also allows for the evaluation of the articular surfaces. Specifically, special cartilage sequences allow evaluation of associated chondral injury. The severity of chondral injury is important, as advanced cartilage injury may be a contraindication to reconstruction of the PCL. Injuries to the menisci and concomitant ligamentous injury can also be accurately delineated with MRI and may have implications with respect to treatment and prognosis. In the setting of an osseous tibial avulsion, a computed tomography (CT) scan may be utilized to assess both the size and displacement of the bony piece. This bony detail may be visualized better on CT as opposed to MR imaging. The size and amount of displacement may help guide fixation options and make a determination between operative and nonoperative

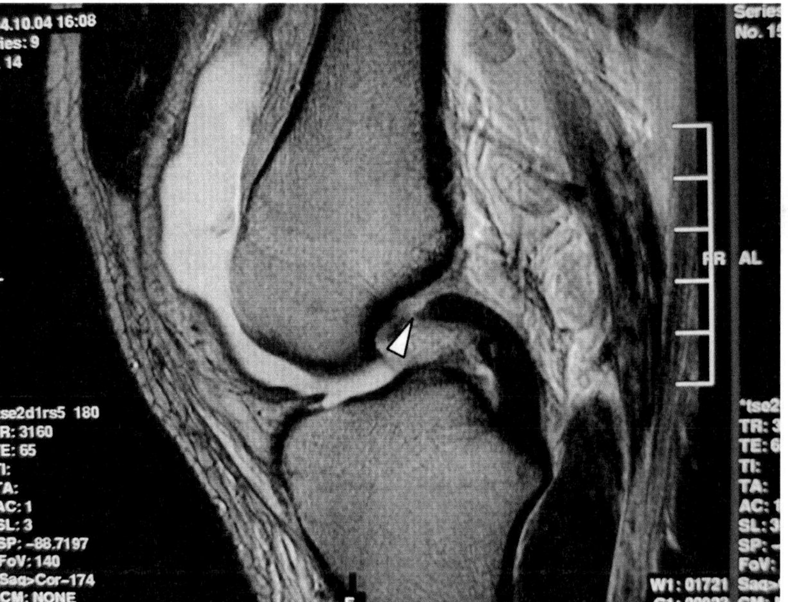

Fig. 4 MRI with proximal avulsion of PCL (*arrow*)

treatment, respectively. Finally, a bone scan may be helpful for the evaluation of patients with chronic PCL injuries. In patients with relatively normal plain radiographs but painful knees following long-standing PCL injury, a bone scan can be obtained to appreciate subtle degenerative changes. In the absence of uptake, further conservative management is recommended.

Operative Indications

Several factors influence the decision to operatively treat PCL injuries. The primary indications for PCL reconstruction are persistent pain and symptomatic instability. One of the clearest indications for PCL reconstruction is combined ligamentous injury. Injury to the PCL in combination with injuries to the ACL, medial collateral ligament (MCL), and/or the PLC complex are potentially devastating injuries that typically present with marked knee instability. These combined ligamentous injuries require surgical intervention to restore proper knee function and kinematics.

Controversy exists concerning the management of isolated tears of the PCL. Most surgeons address acute bony avulsion injuries of the PCL attachment sites with surgical fixation, and grade III injuries of the PCL involving more than 8 mm of posterior tibial displacement are typically considered for surgical reconstruction. Symptomatic, isolated grade II tears of the PCL with less than 8 mm of posterior tibial displacement accompanied by further decrease in posterior tibial translation with internal rotation of the tibia in the young, active patient present a treatment dilemma. Currently, most surgeons would not recommend operative management of PCL injuries in this acute subgroup of patients. Those patients with continued pain and/or instability following an adequate course of conservative management may be counseled for operative intervention.

When studying outcomes in pediatric and adolescent patients undergoing operative management for PCL injuries, Kocher et al. noted that in 14 patients treated with surgical repair or ligament reconstruction, all knees achieved full or near-full range of motion with no evidence of growth arrest or angular deformity. However, patients who sustained knee dislocations demonstrated worse outcomes when compared to those who had not dislocated. The authors thus concluded that PCL reconstruction is a safe option in children and adolescents with multiligamentous knee injuries or in isolated injuries who have failed nonoperative management (Kocher et al. 2012).

Surgical Techniques

Multiple surgical techniques are available for reconstruction of the PCL. Despite these options, clinical results following PCL reconstruction are not as predictable as outcomes following reconstruction of the ACL. Controversy exists regarding the optimal positioning for the tibial and femoral tunnels and the number of bundles utilized for reconstruction. Multiple biomechanical studies have been published to evaluate these variables. Unfortunately, no prospective, randomized studies exist to compare various reconstruction techniques in vivo. Regardless of technique, the primary goal of PCL reconstruction is to restore normal knee anatomy and kinematics.

Graft Selection

Multiple graft options exist for PCL reconstruction. Graft options vary with respect to anatomic donor site as well as choice of allograft versus autograft tissues. Allograft tissues avoid donor side morbidity improving postoperative rehabilitation. Allografts may also avoid insult to the quadriceps mechanism, a dynamic inhibitor of posterior tibial translation (Hoher et al. 2003). In the knee with a multiple ligamentous injury, allograft tissues theoretically avoid further insult to an already compromised knee joint. Also, allograft tissue potentially shortens total operative time by eliminating the time required for harvest and allowing preparation prior to patient arrival in the operative theater.

A common concern with allograft tissue is the potential for bacterial contamination and disease transmission. Although potentially devastating, both of these complications are rare. The development of improved donor screening and testing procedures has all but eliminated the risk of disease transmission. The risk of bacterial contamination has also been lessened by contemporary techniques of aseptic graft harvest, antibiotic preparation, and sterilization techniques. Furthermore, the most commonly used techniques for graft sterilization do not appear to significantly alter the biomechanical properties of the allograft tissue. Allograft tissue cost may be prohibitive and should be carefully considered.

Autograft tissues are more cost effective and avoid the potential complication of disease transmission. Autograft tissues also incorporate more quickly than allograft tissues. The principle drawback to autograft tissue is the associated donor site morbidity. Anterior knee pain, quadriceps weakness, and patella fracture have all been documented following harvest of bone patellar bone autograft. Likewise, with concomitant ligamentous injury, autograft may provide an additional insult to an already compromised extremity.

Some authors advocate the use of mixed grafts consisting of a semitendinosus and gracilis autograft combined with tibialis anterior allograft. Yang et al. studied the outcomes of PCL reconstructions comparing mixed grafts to Achilles tendon allografts in terms of knee function, posterior instability, and graft appearance with a second look arthroscopic assessment. Satisfactory results were obtained for both the mixed and allograft groups, but more complications were encountered with the use of the Achilles tendon allograft with a higher rate of partial tear and less synovialization of the graft at the femoral aperture (Yang et al. 2012). Controversy continues to surround the choice of graft tissue with the necessity of additional well-constructed clinical and laboratory studies.

Single-Bundle Versus Double-Bundle Reconstruction

Single-bundle reconstruction techniques attempt to reconstruct the stronger anterolateral bundle of the PCL. Multiple authors have reported residual posterior laxity following this technique (Race and Amis 1998; Clancy and Bison 1999; Petrie and Harner 1999; Harner et al. 2000). In an attempt to eliminate this laxity, some authors promote anatomic reconstruction of both bundles. Harner et al. demonstrated in biomechanical specimens that the double-bundle technique more effectively restored normal knee kinematics throughout the entire range of motion compared to singe-bundle reconstruction, and posterior tibial translation also decreased (Harner et al. 2000). Several other biomechanical studies have also confirmed these findings (Race and Amis 1998; Clancy and Bison 1999; Petrie and Harner 1999; Wijdicks et al. 2013). The double-bundle technique may provide a theoretical advantage of providing a larger graft tissue than single-bundle reconstructions, which may potentially explain the biomechanical advantages of this technique. To eliminate this factor, Bergfeld et al. utilized same-sized grafts for double-bundle and single-bundle reconstructions (Bergfeld et al. 2001b). This biomechanical model demonstrated that there were no differences in translation between the single- and double-bundle reconstructions (Bergfeld et al. 2001b). Fanelli et al. compared single- and double-bundle arthroscopic transtibial tunnel PCL reconstruction using allograft and noted that both techniques provided successful results when evaluated by stress radiography, arthrometer measurements, and rating scales (Fanelli et al. 2012). In a recently published randomized controlled trial, Yoon et al. evaluated double-bundle and single-bundle reconstruction of the PCL using Achilles allograft. Although they noted a statistically significant difference with greater stability with double-bundle reconstruction, it was unclear whether this difference was clinically significant especially in the context of similar subjective outcome scores (Yoon et al. 2011). Also, Spiridonov et al. evaluated 39 patients undergoing endoscopic PCL reconstruction with double-bundle allograft and demonstrated significant improvements in subjective and objective outcome scores and stability (Spiridonov et al. 2011). Likewise, creating additional femoral and tibial tunnels for double-bundle reconstruction makes an already complex procedure markedly more complicated. Furthermore, clinical studies comparing double-bundle and single-bundle PCL reconstruction are still lacking. Therefore, the authors do not recommend routine double-bundle reconstruction for the PCL-deficient knee.

Transtibial Versus Tibial-Inlay Reconstruction

Another major operative variable relates to the tibial footprint. The PCL tibial attachment can be recreated utilizing either the transtibial or tibial-inlay technique. The transtibial approach reconstructs the PCL tibial attachment arthroscopically through a tibial tunnel. The tibial attachment site can be visualized with a 70° scope, and a posteromedial arthroscopic portal is established to aid with debridement and preparation of the tibial footprint. Under image intensification, a guide pin is placed into the distal and lateral aspect of the PCL footprint with the aid of a PCL guide, and a reamer is passed over the guide wire to create the tibial tunnel. Special care must be taken to protect the posterior neurovascular structures.

The tibial-inlay approach addresses the PCL tibial attachment through an open technique (Berg 1995). The authors prefer the tibial-inlay technique and the approach is described in detail below. Bergfeld et al. have demonstrated that the tibial-inlay technique has significantly decreased posterior laxity from 30° to 90° when compared to the tibial tunnel technique (Bergfeld et al. 2001b). Furthermore, the tibial tunnel technique displayed increased BTB graft thinning at the anterior aperture of the tibial tunnel under cyclic load (Bergfeld et al. 2001b). In the tibial tunnel technique, the BTB graft makes a short, acute pass around the proximal posterior tibia referred to as the "killer turn." The authors hypothesized that the increased thinning and fraying seen at this area may be responsible for clinical failure when utilizing this technique. No tibial-inlay specimens in this study demonstrated increased fraying or thinning under cycle load. While biomechanical evidence illustrates the advantages of the tibial-inlay technique over the tibial tunnel technique, there are no prospective, randomized studies comparing both reconstructions. It should be noted however that posterior tibial translation was decreased to within 2 mm of the contralateral limb and patellofemoral scores improved in the small series by Berg (1995).

Also, in a systematic review by Panchal and Sekiya comparing the open tibial-inlay versus arthroscopic transtibial PCL reconstruction, the authors noted no biomechanical difference or increased stability with open inlay reconstructions, and they observed graft degradation associated with the killer turn following arthroscopic transtibial reconstruction questioning the advantage of this technique. They concluded that the arthroscopic tibial-inlay technique may provide the benefits of both open and arthroscopic techniques with comparable stability according to biomechanical studies (Panchal and Sekiya 2011).

Arthroscopic Tibial-Inlay Technique

Specific limitations and concerns surrounding the open tibial-inlay technique and arthroscopic transtibial PCL reconstruction have been well documented leading to the development of the arthroscopic tibial-inlay technique. In the arthroscopic technique, a recipient tibial socket is created by utilizing a retrograde drilling device for tunnel placement. An appropriately sized bone plug from an Achilles allograft is then seated within the tibial tunnel in a press fit fashion allowing for increased stability and is augmented with sutures passed anteriorly through the tibia tied over a post or button. This bone-to-bone healing and the avoidance of attenuation of the graft at the killer turn have been proposed as potential benefits allowing for improved stability and earlier rehabilitation (Salata and Sekiya 2011).

Studies comparing the arthroscopic tibial inlay to open and transtibial techniques are sparse but have demonstrated promising results. In a clinical study published by Kim et al. comparing the arthroscopic double-bundle inlay, single-bundle inlay, and transtibial techniques, the authors noted a significant decrease in posterior tibial translation when using the arthroscopic double-bundle inlay compared to the transtibial technique (Kim et al. 2010). However, no studies to date have directly compared the arthroscopic transtibial and arthroscopic tibial-inlay techniques.

One potential benefit of this technique focuses on the potential of earlier bone-to-bone healing in the tibial tunnel allowing earlier rehabilitation. Previously, early and aggressive rehabilitation following reconstruction with the transtibial technique has been viewed negatively due to the potential for the development of increased instability (Fanelli 2008). This laxity is thought to be due in part to the acute angles at which the graft emerges and inserts on the tibia and femur leading to thinning and resultant tissue compromise. Thus, avoiding a threshold of knee cycles above which the graft may thin has been encouraged until the graft has sufficiently healed in place. With the use of the arthroscopic tibial-inlay technique, Salata and Sekiya advocate an earlier rehabilitation protocol based on an 8-week healing time for the tibial plug by minimizing stress at the tibial site (Salata and Sekiya 2011).

Another potential advantage of the arthroscopic tibial-inlay technique is its application in PCL reconstruction with skeletally immature patients. Bovid et al. reported a case of an 11-year-old child in which the femoral tunnel was placed entirely within the epiphysis and the tibial tunnel was minimally crossed with a small drill hole and suture material. At 17 months following surgery, there was no radiographic evidence of growth arrest or angular deformity (Bovid et al. 2010).

Arthroscopic tibial-inlay PCL reconstruction has also briefly been studied in the context of revision PCL reconstruction. Lee et al. studied revision PCL reconstruction with a modified arthroscopic tibial-inlay double-bundle technique. They noted the most common probable causes of failure of primary PCL reconstructions included undiagnosed posterolateral rotatory instability and improper graft tunnel placement. They also concluded that arthroscopic revision PCL reconstruction with use of a modified tibial-inlay double-bundle technique improved knee stability and outcomes compared to preoperative measures (Lee et al. 2012).

Author's Preferred Method

A combined femoral sciatic nerve block may be performed in the preoperative holding area. This peripheral nerve block lessens the need for

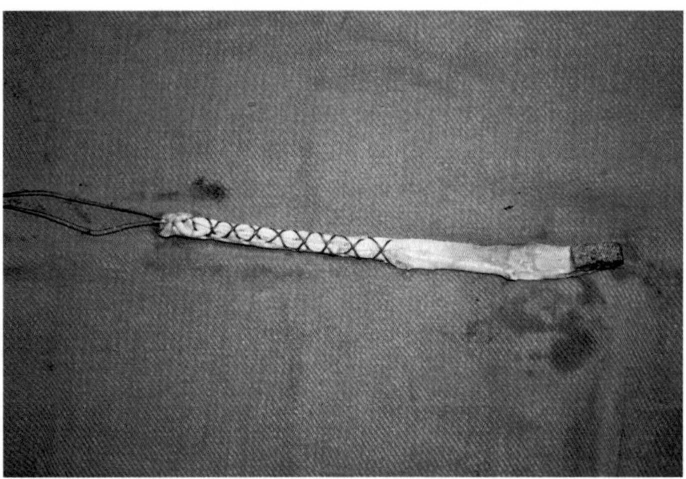

Fig. 5 Prepared Achilles tendon allograft

intraoperative narcotics and sedation which may result in less nausea and a faster recovery postoperatively. Formal intubation is preferable, as a laryngeal mask or facemask may not provide reliable control of the airway when the patient is turned to the prone position. For the start of the case, the patient is placed in the supine position on a standard operating table. A non-sterile tourniquet is placed as proximal on the operative thigh as possible. The unaffected limb is then placed into a well-padded well-leg holder with the peroneal nerve free from pressure, while the operative extremity is placed into an arthroscopic leg holder. The end of the operative table is then maximally flexed, leaving the operative limb freely suspended.

Standard anterolateral and anteromedial arthroscopic portals are established. A small incision is made just above the superolateral pole of the patella, and a rigid outflow cannula is placed into the suprapatellar pouch. Diagnostic arthroscopy proceeds in a methodical, orderly fashion. The patellofemoral articulation is examined for chondral damage because this articulation may experience advanced degenerative changes with PCL deficiency. Next, the arthroscope is brought into the lateral gutter. Here the popliteus tendon is identified, and the arthroscope is pushed gently along its course to identify any injury to this structure. At this time, the arthroscope is passed into the lateral compartment as a varus force is applied to the knee. Injury to the posterolateral ligamentous complex may manifest as excessive joint space opening when in this position (LaPrade 1997). Residual PCL fibers are debrided with a large-bore shaver. In some cases one of the meniscofemoral ligaments may be intact. Great effort should be made to retain the meniscofemoral ligaments because they contribute significant resistance to posterior tibial translation.

An Achilles allograft is preferred for reconstruction of the PCL. The calcaneal bone block is fashioned to be approximately 25 mm in length, 10–12 mm wide, and 5 mm thick. The bone block is then prepared to accept a 6.5 mm cancellous screw used for lag-type tibial fixation. The tendinous portion of the graft should be approximately 10–11 mm wide and 70 mm in length. The distal 3–4 cm is then tubularized with a #5 Ethibond in a whipstitch fashion. The tubularized tendon should fit snugly through a 10–11 mm sizing tube (Fig. 5).

Traditionally, the femoral tunnel during single-bundle PCL reconstruction should be placed at the 11 o'clock position in the right knee (1 o'clock in the left knee), reconstructing the larger anterolateral (AL) bundle of the PCL. Various anatomic landmarks exist that assist with tunnel placement. Ideally, the guide pin should be placed in the center of the residual anterolateral bundle fibers. Alternatively, two osseous landmarks also exist for reference (Farrow et al. 2007; Lopes et al. 2008; Anderson et al. 2012). The medial

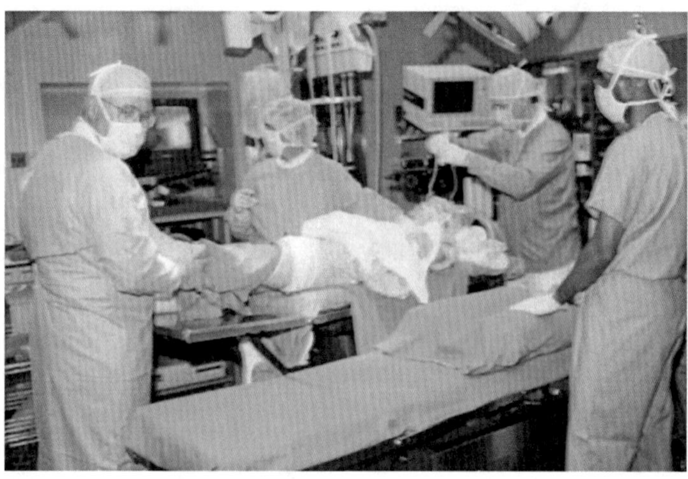

Fig. 6 Operative personnel in place and prepared for patient turn onto second operative table

intercondylar ridge described by Farrow et al. represents the posterior border of the native PCL (Farrow et al. 2007). As such the femoral tunnel should lie just anterior to this landmark. The second osseous landmark, the medial bifurcate ridge, defines the junction between the PCL anterolateral (ALB) and posteromedial (PMB) bundles (Lopes et al. 2008). The PCL ALB lies superior to this landmark. The vastus medialis oblique is identified and elevated, and the femoral tunnel is drilled from outside-in over a guide pin.

After preparation of the femoral tunnel, the knee is prepared for repositioning. A DePuy graft passer (DePuy Mitek, Raynham, MA) is placed antegrade through the femoral tunnel, into the intercondylar notch, and passed into the posterior compartment adjacent to the medial border of the PCL tibial insertion. The external portion of the graft passer is laid against the skin and secured with Coban, a sterile self-adhering wrap (3 M Inc., St. Paul, MN). A sterile, impervious stockinet is then placed over the extremity and overwrapped to the mid-thigh with an additional sterile Coban. At this time, all drapes are removed and the patient is placed into the prone position. This typically requires assistance from at least four people – the anesthesiologist to maintain the head and neck, two assistants on either side to facilitate the turn, and one person to manage the lower extremities (Fig. 6). In a smaller individual, the turn can be accomplished on the same operating room table. However, in most individuals, it is necessary to turn the patient onto a second operating table.

After the patient has been re-prepped and draped, then a posterior approach is begun. The popliteal crease is identified and marked at this time. The limb is exsanguinated, and the tourniquet is inflated. Starting at the popliteal crease, a 4 cm vertical incision is made distally along the medial border of the medial head of the gastrocnemius muscle. The interval between the gastrocnemius and semimembranosus is developed bluntly with finger dissection. The gastrocnemius is then retracted laterally to expose the posterior joint capsule (Fig. 7). Lateral retraction of the gastrocnemius protects the popliteal artery, which lies lateral to the muscle. The PCL facet is then palpated just proximal to the superior border of the popliteus muscle belly. A window is made in the overlying posterior capsule with electrocautery. A curved osteotome is then used to make a 20 mm by 10 mm by 5 mm cortical window at the footprint of the PCL tibial attachment (Fig. 8). The graft passer is retrieved through the posterior capsular window and then used to pull the tendinous graft into the joint and through the femoral tunnel. The Achilles bone block is now keyed into the cortical window with a 30 mm partially threaded 6.5 mm cancellous screw with a washer. The tourniquet is then deflated, the wound is carefully

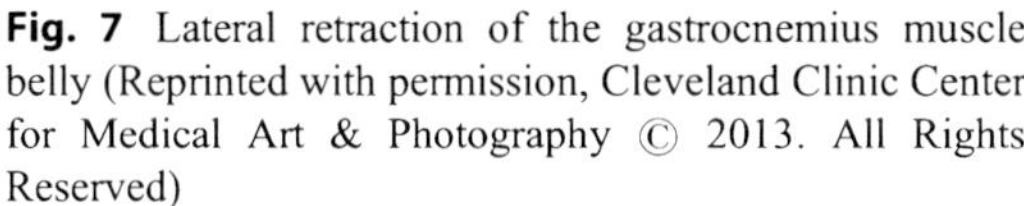

Fig. 7 Lateral retraction of the gastrocnemius muscle belly (Reprinted with permission, Cleveland Clinic Center for Medical Art & Photography © 2013. All Rights Reserved)

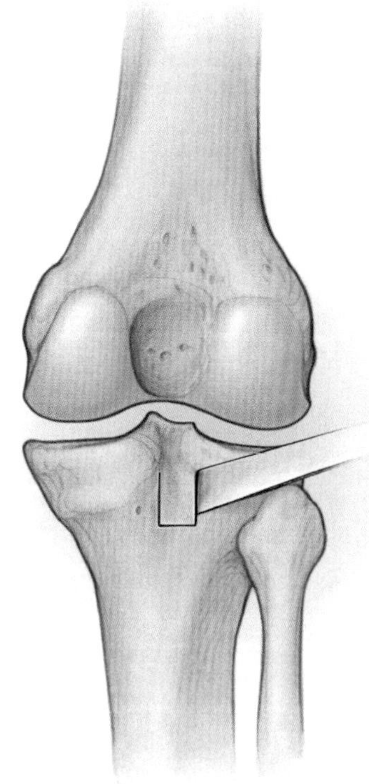

Fig. 8 Creating posterior cortical window (Reprinted with permission, Cleveland Clinic Center for Medical Art & Photography © 2013. All Rights Reserved)

examined for bleeding, and electrocautery is used to obtain meticulous hemostasis. At this time, the posterior capsulotomy is closed with one Vicryl suture. The investing fascia and then the skin are closed with interrupted nonabsorbable sutures. The extremity is then prepared for the turn and return to the prone position as described above.

Once the patient is turned to the supine position, the limb is again placed into an arthroscopic leg holder and prepped and draped. Proper graft placement is confirmed arthroscopically. A soft tissue interference screw is placed into the femoral tunnel from outside-in, while an anterior drawer is applied to the tibia and the graft is tensioned at 70° of knee flexion (Fig. 9). At this time the knee is taken through a range of motion to ensure that full range of motion is present after graft fixation. The arthroscopic portals and medial incision are closed in the usual fashion, and the wounds are dressed sterilely.

Postoperative Rehabilitation

Postoperatively the patient is placed into a full-leg, hinged knee brace locked in extension for 4 weeks. Partial weight bearing is allowed initially and advanced to full weight bearing as tolerated. Isometric quadriceps exercises are begun immediately. From 4 to 8 weeks postoperatively, the patient is advanced to active-assisted range of motion. Isotonic quadriceps exercises are added at this time, and bicycling is encouraged. Closed kinetic chain exercises are begun at 8 weeks post surgery. From week 12 to week 20, sideboard exercises are progressed to agility exercises. Likewise, fast walking is progressed to jogging at 16–20 weeks. A knee brace with block to extension at 15° is continued for exercise. At weeks 20–28, running and full speed agility exercises are incorporated, and following this advance, the brace is discontinued for activity. At 28 weeks

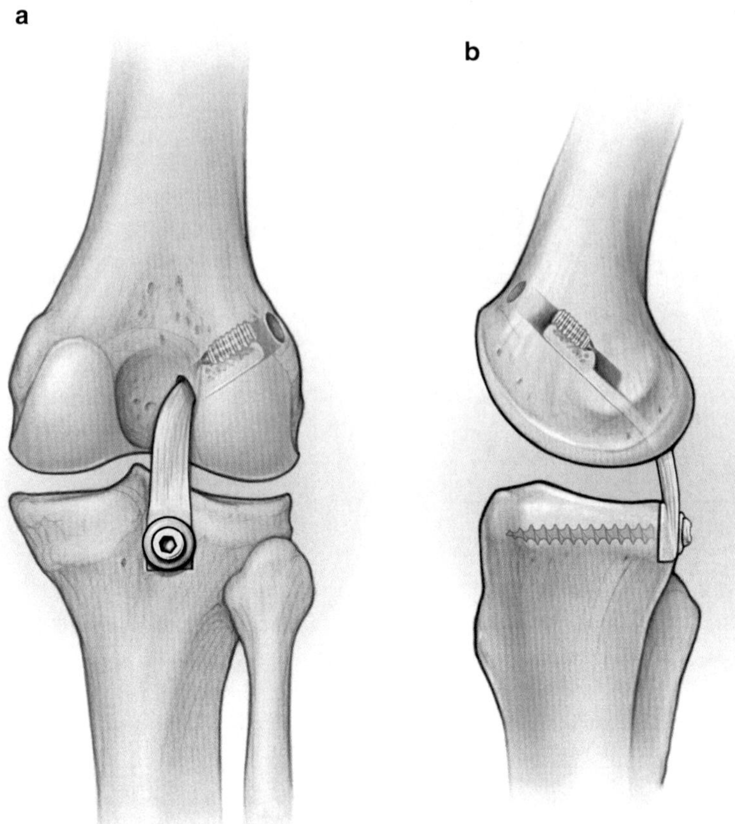

Fig. 9 Posterior (**a**) and lateral (**b**) views of secured allograft tendon (Reprinted with permission, Cleveland Clinic Center for Medical Art & Photography © 2013. All Rights Reserved)

post surgery, the patient is allowed to return to full activity without restriction.

A recent article by Pierce et al. reviewed PCL rehabilitation protocols and revealed that rehabilitation should focus on progressive weight bearing, strengthening the quadriceps muscles, and preventing posterior sag. One particular strategy to enhance rehabilitation includes the incorporation of prone passive range of motion to prevent placing undue stress on the reconstructed graft or healing ligament (Pierce et al. 2013).

Pearls

1. Reduction of posterior tibial sag may help with passage of the graft passer into the posterior compartment next to the remnant of the PCL tibial attachment. Avoid placement of the passer beneath the meniscus. Make a concerted effort to maintain the meniscofemoral ligaments of Humphrey and Wrisberg, and thread the passer between the intervals created by these two structures if possible.
2. Lateral retraction of the medial head of the gastrocnemius is facilitated with slight flexion of the knee and internal rotation of the tibia.
3. Gynecological retractors (i.e., vaginal retractors) are long and narrow and aid with visualization during the posterior approach.
4. Once retracted, the medial head of the gastrocnemius can be temporarily held in position with a Steinman pin placed into the lateral aspect of the proximal tibia. This provides for a wide field of view for tibial preparation and graft fixation.
5. The slide board during rehabilitation is a great tool for transitioning to jogging and running.
6. Posterior tibial inlay can be difficult without turning the patient. The authors feel that the additional 15–20 min of operative time is well

worth the effort considering the ease of posterior visualization.

Pitfalls

1. Malposition of the distal femoral incision may prohibit accurate placement of the femoral guide pin. It is important to place the incision one-third the distance from the medial femoral epicondyle and the medial border of the patella. This will allow the vastus medialis to be elevated rather than splitting the muscle fibers, which may lead to quadriceps inhibition in the early postoperative period.
2. Injuries to the posterolateral ligament complex are commonly associated with PCL injuries. Reconstruction of the PCL could fail if posterolateral rotatory instability is not addressed. In this case, a varus high tibial osteotomy should be considered.
3. There is a potential for osteonecrosis or subchondral collapse if the femoral tunnel is placed too close to the articular surface. The distal border of the femoral tunnel should be 3–4 mm away from the articular cartilage border and aimed away from the joint.
4. The femoral tunnel starting point at the medial aspect of the femoral metaphysis should not start too far proximal to the medial articular border. More proximal starting position will lead to a more acute angle for graft passage.
5. One must be aware of aberrant branches of the posterior tibial artery overlying the posterior tibial footprint of the PCL.

Cross-References

▶ Allografts in Posterior Cruciate Ligament Reconstructions
▶ Anatomy and Biomechanics of the Knee
▶ Combined Anterior and Posterior Cruciate Ligament Injuries
▶ Current Concepts in the Treatment of Posterior Cruciate Ligament Injuries
▶ Reconstruction of the Posterolateral Corner of the Knee

References

Anderson CJ, Ziegler CG, Wijdicks CA, Engebretsen L, LaPrade RF (2012) Arthroscopically pertinent anatomy of the anterolateral and posteromedial bundles of the posterior cruciate ligament. J Bone Joint Surg Am 94:1936–1945

Berg EE (1995) Posterior cruciate ligament tibial inlay reconstruction. Arthroscopy 11:69–76

Bergfeld JA, McAllister DR, Parker RD, Valdevit AD, Kambic H (2001a) The effects of tibial rotation on posterior translation in knees in which the posterior cruciate ligament has been cut. J Bone Joint Surg Am 83-A:1339–1343

Bergfeld JA, McAllister DR, Parker RD, Valdevit AD, Kambic HE (2001b) A biomechanical comparison of posterior cruciate ligament reconstruction techniques. Am J Sports Med 29:129–136

Bovid KM, Salata MJ, Vander Have KL, Sekiya JK (2010) Arthroscopic posterior cruciate ligament reconstruction in a skeletally immature patient: a new technique with case report. Arthroscopy 26:563–570

Clancy WG Jr, Bison LJ (1999) Double bundle technique for reconstruction of the posterior cruciate ligament. Oper Tech Sports Med 7:110–117

Clancy WG Jr, Shelbourne KD, Zoellner GB, Keene JS, Reider B, Rosenberg TD (1983) Treatment of knee joint instability secondary to rupture of the posterior cruciate ligament. Report of a new procedure. J Bone Joint Surg Am 65:310–322

Covey CD, Sapega AA (1993) Injuries of the posterior cruciate ligament. J Bone Joint Surg Am 75:1376–1386

Fanelli GC (1993) Posterior cruciate ligament injuries in trauma patients. Arthroscopy 9:291–294

Fanelli GC (2008) Posterior cruciate ligament rehabilitation: how slow should we go? Arthroscopy 24:234–235

Fanelli GC, Edson CJ (1995) Posterior cruciate ligament injuries in trauma patients: part II. Arthroscopy 11:526–529

Fanelli GC, Beck JD, Edson CJ (2012) Single compared to double-bundle PCL reconstruction using allograft tissue. J Knee Surg 25:59–64

Farrow LD, Chen MR, Cooperman DR, Victoroff BN, Goodfellow DB (2007) Morphology of the femoral intercondylar notch. J Bone Joint Surg Am 89:2150–2155

Griffith CJ, LaPrade RF, Johansen S, Armitage B, Wijdicks C, Engebretsen L (2009) Medial knee injury: part 1, static function of the individual components of the main medial knee structures. Am J Sports Med 37:1762–1770

Grood ES, Stowers SF, Noyes FR (1988) Limits of movement in the human knee. Effect of sectioning the posterior cruciate ligament and posterolateral structures. J Bone Joint Surg Am 70:88–97

Harner CD, Hoher J (1988) Current concepts: evaluation and treatment of posterior cruciate ligament injuries. Am J Sports Med 26:471–482

Harner CD, Vogrin TM, Hoher J, Ma CB, Woo SL (2000) Biomechanical analysis of a posterior cruciate ligament reconstruction. Deficiency of the posterolateral structures as a cause of graft failure. Am J Sports Med 28:32–39

Hoher J, Scheffler S, Weiler A (2003) Graft choice and graft fixation in PCL reconstruction. Knee Surg Sports Traumatol Arthrosc 11:297–306

Kim SJ, Kim SH, Kim SG, Kung YP (2010) Comparison of the clinical results of three posterior cruciate ligament reconstruction techniques: surgical technique. J Bone Joint Surg Am 92(Suppl 1 Pt 2):145–157

Kocher MS, Shore B, Nasreddine AY, Heyworth BE (2012) Treatment of posterior cruciate ligament injuries in pediatric and adolescent patients. J Pediatr Orthop 32:553–560

LaPrade RF (1997) Arthroscopic evaluation of the lateral compartment of knees with grade 3 posterolateral knee complex injuries. Am J Sports Med 25:596–602

Lee SH, Jung YB, Lee HJ, Jung HJ, Kim SH (2012) Revision posterior cruciate ligament reconstruction using a modified tibial-inlay double-bundle technique. J Bone Joint Surg Am 94:516–522

Lopes OV Jr, Ferretti M, Shen W, Ekdahl M, Smolinski P, Fu FH (2008) Topography of the femoral attachment of the posterior cruciate ligament. J Bone Joint Surg Am 90:249–255

Margheritini F, Mancini L, Mauro CS, Mariani PP (2003) Stress radiography for quantifying posterior cruciate ligament deficiency. Arthroscopy 19:706–711

Merchant AC, Mercer RL, Jacobsen RH, Cool CR (1974) Roentgenographic analysis of patellofemoral congruence. J Bone Joint Surg Am 56:1391–1396

Miyasaka KC, Daniel DM, Stone ML, Hirshman P (1991) The incidence of knee ligament injuries in the general population. Am J Knee Surg 4:3–8

Panchal HB, Sekiya JK (2011) Open tibial inlay versus arthroscopic transtibial posterior cruciate ligament reconstructions. Arthroscopy 27:1289–1295

Parolie JM, Bergfeld JA (1986) Long-term results of nonoperative treatment of isolated posterior cruciate ligament injuries in the athlete. Am J Sports Med 14:35–38

Petrie RS, Harner CD (1999) Double bundle posterior cruciate ligament reconstruction technique: University of Pittsburgh approach. Oper Tech Sports Med 7:118–126

Pierce CM, O'Brien L, Griffin LW, Laprade RF (2013) Posterior cruciate ligament tears: functional and postoperative rehabilitation. Knee Surg Sports Traumatol Arthrosc 21:1071–1084

Race A, Amis AA (1998) PCL reconstruction. In vitro biomechanical comparison of 'isometric' versus single and double-bundled 'anatomic' grafts. J Bone Joint Surg Br 80:173–179

Rosenberg TD, Paulos LE, Parker RD, Coward DB, Scott SM (1988) The forty-five-degree posteroanterior flexion weight-bearing radiograph of the knee. J Bone Joint Surg Am 70:1479–1483

Salata MJ, Sekiya JK (2011) Arthroscopic posterior cruciate ligament tibial inlay reconstruction: a surgical technique that may influence rehabilitation. Sports Health 3:52–58

Sekiya JK, Whiddon DR, Zehms CT, Miller MD (2008) A clinically relevant assessment of posterior cruciate ligament and posterolateral corner injuries. Evaluation of isolated and combined deficiency. J Bone Joint Surg Am 90:1621–1627

Spiridonov SI, Slinkard NJ, LaPrade RF (2011) Isolated and combined grade-III posterior cruciate ligament tears treated with double-bundle reconstruction with use of endoscopically placed femoral tunnels and grafts: operative technique and clinical outcomes. J Bone Joint Surg Am 93:1773–1780

Wijdicks CA, Kennedy NI, Goldsmith MT, Devitt BM, Michalski MP, Aroen A et al (2013) Kinematic analysis of the posterior cruciate ligament, part 2: a comparison of anatomic single- versus double-bundle reconstruction. Am J Sports Med 41:2839–2848

Yang JH, Yoon JR, Jeong HI, Hwang DH, Woo SJ, Kwon JH et al (2012) Second-look arthroscopic assessment of arthroscopic single-bundle posterior cruciate ligament reconstruction: comparison of mixed graft versus achilles tendon allograft. Am J Sports Med 40:2052–2060

Yoon KH, Bae DK, Song SJ, Cho HJ, Lee JH (2011) A prospective randomized study comparing arthroscopic single-bundle and double-bundle posterior cruciate ligament reconstructions preserving remnant fibers. Am J Sports Med 39:474–480

105 Perioperative and Postoperative Anterior Cruciate Ligament Rehabilitation Focused on Soft Tissue Grafts

John Nyland, Jeff Wera, Kenneth G. W. Mackinlay, and David N. M. Caborn

Contents

J. Nyland (✉)
Kosair Charities College of Health and Natural Sciences, Spalding University, Louisville, USA
e-mail: jnyland@spalding.edu

J. Wera • K.G.W. Mackinlay
Division of Sports Medicine, Department of Orthopaedic Surgery, University of Louisville, Louisville, KY, USA
e-mail: jeff.c.wera@gmail.com; kgmack01@louisville.edu

D.N.M. Caborn
JPG – Shea Orthopaedic Group, Orthopedic Surgery, University of Louisville, Kentucky OneHealth, Louisville, KY, USA
e-mail: david.caborn@louisville.edu

M.N. Doral, J. Karlsson (eds.), *Sports Injuries*,
DOI 10.1007/978-3-642-36569-0_103

Abstract

When the athlete arrives at the clinic following ACL reconstruction, it may seem too late to implement a primary knee injury prevention plan. However, primary prevention of a similar injury to the contralateral knee is of the utmost importance in addition to secondary prevention of injury to the reconstructed knee. Having a sound understanding of the pathomechanics that lead to the primary knee injury and any potentially related trunk and lower extremity dysfunction history is essential when designing a post-ACL reconstruction rehabilitation plan. Equally important is understanding the athlete's expectations in regard to sport competitive level, intensity, and volume. To optimize the likelihood for the patient returning effectively to the athlete role and safely returning to competitive sport, the therapeutic exercise and movement activity delivery mode may be as important as the selected tasks at each phase of recovery. The therapeutic exercise environment should serve as the forum for patient education about postural alignment and neuromuscular control influences on knee forces and torques. The rehabilitation clinician must understand specific movement tasks common to the athlete's sport, the position played within the sport(s), the team and athlete's style of play, and the athlete's role on the team.

Introduction

Initiation of the psychobehavioral role transition from patient to returned athlete is as important as correcting knee range of motion deficits, neuromuscular strength, power, control impairments, and functional limitations. A dilemma exists in that the patient may display impatience and anxiety regarding delays in returning to the athletic field, potentially returning before they have reestablished consistently strong performance capability, neuromuscular control, and adequate fatigue resistance. Rehabilitation programs often display poor physiological system preparation without adequate consideration for maintaining and improving short- and longer-term anaerobic and aerobic energy system function in a sport- and position-specific manner. Over the course of rehabilitation following ACL injury and reconstruction, there is a tendency for the athlete's lean body mass to decrease and body fat percentage to increase. There is also a tendency for fast twitch muscle fibers to display inhibition and atrophy particularly in the quadriceps femoris and gastrocnemius muscles.

Successfully returning an injured athlete to competitive sport requires rehabilitation program planning prior to surgery. Since many factors may change between the athlete's index ACL injury, surgery, and return to competitive play, it is important to understand that both the athlete and the rehabilitation team are chasing a moving target. While it is known that a minimum of several months will pass prior to consideration of safe return to competitive play, less is known about the dynamics of the team to which they will be returning, expectations regarding their performance contributions, and the "all or none" perception of return to play readiness.

To optimize the likelihood for an effective return to the athlete role and safe return to competitive sport, the therapeutic exercise and movement activity delivery mode may be as important as the selected tasks at each phase of recovery. The rehabilitation clinician must understand specific movement tasks common to the athlete's sport(s), the position played within the sport(s) the athlete will be returning to, the team and athlete's style of play, and the athlete's role on the team. The therapeutic exercise environment should serve as the forum for patient education regarding postural alignment and neuromuscular influences on knee forces and torques. This chapter focuses on the rehabilitation of athletes following ACL reconstruction when soft tissue grafts are used. Within this context, the focus of this chapter is placed on experiences when tibialis tendon allografts, hamstring tendon autografts, and quadriceps tendon autografts without bone components are used for ACL reconstruction. General rehabilitation program guidelines are listed in Table 1.

Table 1 General rehabilitation program guidelines

1.	Reestablish normal or non-impaired joint mobility (particularly at the knees, hips, and ankles)
2.	Correct or minimize the influence of any associated impairments, deficits, or functional limitations throughout the body
3.	Continue progressive resistance single-leg leg press progression initiated during terminal rehabilitation
4.	Begin sport-specific functional movement task performance in an active learning environment using social cognitive theory principles
5.	Demonstrate proficient eccentric neuromuscular performance capability during functional movements in a small-to-large amplitude, slow-to-fast velocity progression
6.	Focus on neuromuscular control and postural alignment training during sudden single lower extremity landings and running directional changes
7.	Integrate exteroceptive denial activities during select functional movement tasks to enhance somatosensory position sense acuity
8.	Focus on movement form, smoothness, and general quality throughout each session, never substituting intensity or speed at the expense of appropriate technique and postural alignment
9.	Athlete must pass a scripted field test including specific form, dynamic knee stability, lower extremity power, agility-reaction time, and consistent, endurant speed/skill components prior to being released to full conditioning activities and structured team practice progressions that necessitate consistently appropriate postural alignment

Soft Tissue Graft Selection: Rehabilitation Differences Should Exist

From a purely rehabilitation perspective, programmatic differences should exist when soft tissue allografts or autografts are used for ACL reconstruction. For example, based on harvest-site concerns that increase the potential for arthrofibrosis following graft harvest, early motion, early weight bearing, and early neuromuscular electrical stimulation use may be more important during the acute care period when autograft tendons are used for ACL reconstruction (Wright et al. 2008). Based on concerns related to delayed and less complete graft remodeling/ligamentization and greater potential for graft slippage within the tunnel and/or graft elongation, closed kinetic chain exercises may be preferred to open kinetic chain exercises when soft tissue allografts are used. Since allograft use is not associated with early postsurgical pain and effusion from soft tissue graft harvest-site irritation, these patients may be better able to perform an independent home program during the early postoperative phase with proper guidance. This would ultimately save limited insurance-reimbursed outpatient physical therapy visits for the later phases of rehabilitation when key functional progression decisions must be made generally between 12 and 26 weeks postsurgery. The need for functional knee bracing following ACL reconstruction is debatable and should be related to the status of the secondary stabilizers such as medial collateral ligament biomechanical integrity. The soft tissue allograft group may benefit more from functional knee brace use over the initial year or more post-ACL reconstruction (Giotis et al. 2011) because of greater concerns related to graft slippage, elongation, less complete and more variable remodeling/ligamentization, and greater concerns related to delayed laxity and sudden failure (Claes et al. 2011). Grafts that possess a bony component may more closely restore time zero construct stiffness and reduce early graft-tunnel slippage concerns. Patients who have undergone ACL reconstruction with any soft tissue graft, but particularly allografts, should undergo a slightly delayed rehabilitation progression particularly regarding lower extremity impact loading through the knee. These patients may also benefit from greater use of secondary, extra-tunnel tibial graft fixation. Experience suggests that early patience regarding soft tissue graft use pays great dividends regarding later function. Animal studies using an ovine model have described hamstring autograft (Scheffler et al. 2008), hypercellularity and intense revascularization between 4 and 12 weeks post-ACL reconstruction, and ligamentization from 6 months through >2 years with gradually increasing collagen synthesis and changes in crimp pattern (Scheffler et al. 2008; Claes et al. 2011). In a review of rabbit model studies, Gulotta and Rodeo (2007) reported that at 1 week post-ACL reconstruction, fibrovascular tissue is observed between the graft and the bone tunnel. However, by 12–26 weeks postsurgery, histological evidence of a more "normal" tendon, unmineralized fibrocartilage, mineralized fibrocartilage, and bone continuum can be observed. Using a canine model to evaluate hamstring graft-bone tunnel fixation, Rodeo et al. (1993) reported the biomechanical failure mode to be tendon pullout from mechanical grips rather than tunnel slippage or graft elongation by as early as 12 weeks postsurgery. However, the systematic review of Claes et al. (2011) suggests a slower, more variable, and less predictable human soft tissue graft integration, remodeling, and ligamentization timetable. When soft tissue allografts are used, the rehabilitation clinician should be vigilant in monitoring for early effusion and have greater concerns regarding delays in the timing and extent of complete graft-bone socket or tunnel integration and ligamentization. In summary, soft tissue allografts display a greater chance of delayed laxity, positive pivot shift testing, and sudden failure. In addition to harvest-site considerations, when quadriceps tendon autografts are used for ACL reconstruction, the rehabilitation clinician must be vigilant regarding the progressive restoration of complete non-impaired active and passive knee flexion in combination with hip extension, the likelihood of prolonged quadriceps femoris muscle inhibition, and the potential for compromised hip flexor strength and hip-knee kinesthesia. When hamstring autografts are used, concerns exist regarding terminal active knee flexion range of motion, strength, and medial side dynamic knee stability (particularly if the gracilis tendon is also harvested for graft use).

Tunnel-Socket Drilling Method, Anatomic vs. Nonanatomic Placement, and Fixation

ACL reconstruction trends are moving toward greater use of anatomically placed soft tissue grafts using extra-tunnel fixation. Based on registry information of more than 9,000 ACL reconstruction patients, anteromedial portal use to achieve more anatomical femoral tunnel graft placement has recently been associated with a greater need for revision ACL reconstruction compared to more conventional transtibial tunnel drilling (Rahr-Wagner et al. 2013). However, information regarding surgeon experience level, bone tunnel or socket depth, fixation method, rehabilitation progression, and release to full activity timing are lacking, making direct cause-effect relationships impossible to establish. Greater details are needed before definitive conclusions can be made from these data.

Intra-tunnel fixation increases graft construct stiffness and decreases bungee and windshield wiper effects. Extra-tunnel fixation increases construct ultimate failure load and enhances intra-tunnel healing. An innovative extra-cortical and bone socket aperture graft fixation approach can provide double-bundle ACL function in single tibial and femoral sockets with an all-inside technique using a soft tissue graft with interpositional PEEK wedges (Arthrex, Naples, FL, USA) (Fig. 1) to simulate double-bundle graft function (Fig. 2) (Nyland et al. 2014). Extra-cortical fixation optimizes failure load resistance without compromising graft-socket healing, while aperture fixation decreases the likelihood of socket widening and decreases bungee and windshield wiper graft movements.

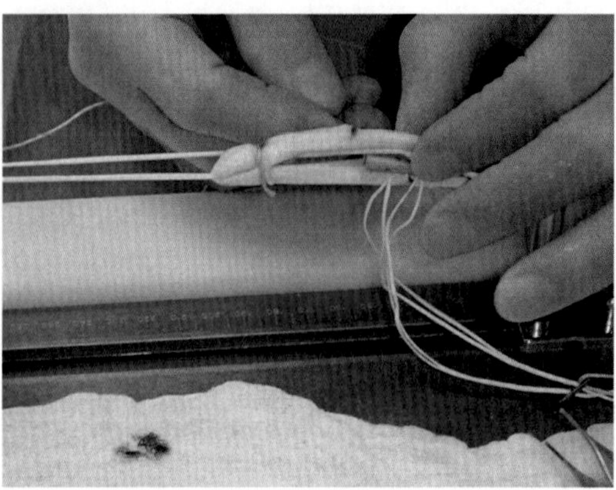

Fig. 1 Soft tissue graft suturing with PEEK wedges to simulate double-bundle function

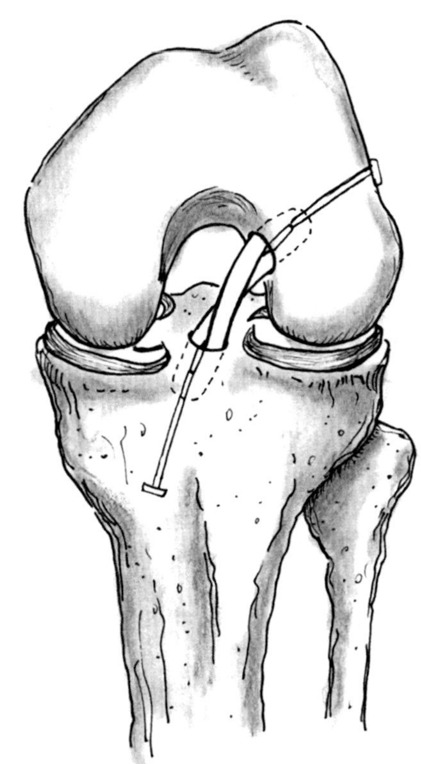

Fig. 2 Schematic depicting soft tissue graft placement with aperture fixation provided by PEEK wedges and extra-cortical fixation provided via titanium buttons

Concerns related to soft tissue graft-bone tunnel fixation have also prompted some knee surgeons to incorporate platelet concentrates to improve the structural integrity of the graft-tunnel interface. However, scant evidence supports this practice (Vavken et al. 2011; Mirzatolooei et al. 2013).

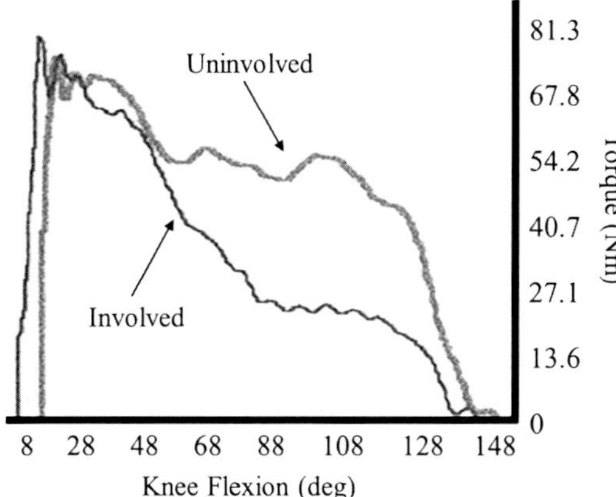

Fig. 3 Involved knee flexor strength impairment at >90° knee flexion compared to the noninvolved, contralateral knee during prone isokinetic testing at >2 years post-ACL reconstruction using semitendinosus-gracilis autograft (Elmlinger et al. 2006)

Mirzatolooei et al. (2013) failed to observe significant group tunnel widening differences when platelet-rich plasma was applied to hamstring autografts used for double-bundle ACL reconstruction. In addition to harvest-site considerations when hamstring autografts are used, concerns exist regarding active knee flexion end range of motion and strength between 90 and ≥135° particularly when the knee is evaluated in positions of function with the hip extended (Fig. 3) (Elmlinger et al. 2006). In a systematic review of level I–II studies, Han et al. (2012) reported that patients displayed similar activity levels, knee function restoration, and return to sport timing at ≥2 year follow-up regardless if primary ACL reconstruction used intra-tunnel or extra-tunnel hamstring autograft fixation. The intra-tunnel fixation group however initiated full weight bearing and jogging/running earlier (Han et al. 2012).

Therapeutic Exercise Selection and Delivery Mode: Basic Concepts

In addition to therapeutic exercise selection, the mode of delivery is of particular importance. Use of social cognitive theory principles gradually empowers the athlete with great decision-making responsibility (Bandura 2001). Rehabilitation clinicians need to advance the intervention beyond merely assigning therapeutic exercises based solely on physiological and biomechanical factors. Instead they should create a more active learning environment for the patient-athlete. An optimized therapeutic exercise "learning environment" needs to drive positive cognitive appraisal, affect, and psychobehavioral changes (Winett et al. 2009). It would be beneficial for the rehabilitation clinician to reflect about what lesson the patient-athlete learned on any given day during therapeutic exercise performance. Rehabilitation clinicians need to steer the therapeutic exercise program design focus towards functionally relevant movements that serve more than one purpose, such as strength-balance and power-coordination activities, that also possess a postural alignment educational requirement. The design philosophy for therapeutic exercise programs should resemble a rigorous educational curriculum. Therapeutic exercises progress from less complicated, low-velocity and small-amplitude, primarily low-intensity uniplanar movements to more complex, high-velocity and larger-amplitude, multi-planar movements where the patient-athlete functions on the edge of being in control of the movement ("on the edge of chaos") (Nyland 2012a). Of particular importance is the focus on progressive resistance eccentric exercises to improve gluteus maximus, hamstring, quadriceps femoris, and gastrocnemius-soleus muscle strength, hypertrophy, and function as contributors to the lower extremity neuromuscular stretch-shortening cycle and instantaneous movement decelerators (Gerber et al. 2007). Specific criteria must be established that provide an objective basis for safe advancement through latter rehabilitation phases to more intensive conditioning, sport-specific training, return to sport practice, and eventual release to competition. In addition to reestablishing non-impaired lower extremity joint range of motion, muscle strength, power and endurance, balance and postural control (Howells et al. 2011), and perceived functional levels, of growing concern is the patient-athlete's state of psychobehavioral readiness for returning to their sport. While certain elite athletes may have genetic or psychobehavioral predispositions that make returning to their pre-injury level more achievable, others may have considerable difficulty given the changes in self-efficacy, kinesiophobia, and motivation that normally occurs between adolescence and early to mid-adulthood. In either scenario, successfully completing any return to sport criteria is not the end itself. As long as the athlete who has undergone ACL injury, reconstruction, and rehabilitation desires to pursue competitive athletics, they must commit to maintaining neuromuscular control and postural alignment training. The rehabilitation progression must also be transitional helping the patient safely advance from the clinic environment to the athletic field, transformational in also helping them move from the patient role to the athlete role, and timely in regard to progressively greater exercise intensity, frequency, and total volume applications. The progression should also be cognizant of the Specific Adaptations to Imposed Demands (SAID) principle, titrated with periodization, to reflect multiple short-term treatment goals that change with the rehabilitation program phase. Lastly, the therapeutic exercise progression should be translational helping the patient ascend from being a patient to matching or exceeding their expectations returning to their former level of athletic participation. Rest periods should increase as session intensity increases. However, prior to returning to sport, movement challenges performed while the athlete experiences slight peripheral and central neuromuscular fatigue should be included as a training stimulus to better prepare them for sport- and position-specific demands.

Acute Care: Reestablish Independent Activity of Daily Living Function (0–4 Weeks)

While progressive resistance exercises, neuromuscular control, and sensorimotor training are involved in all rehabilitation phases, during the acute care phase, there needs to be a sensorimotor training bias. Control of knee pain and effusion are essential during this phase. With all soft tissue grafts, concerns exist regarding early elongation, tunnel or socket slippage, or both. With growing trends toward extra-articular soft tissue graft fixation, enabling greater circumferential graft-tunnel integration, it is imperative that the rehabilitation team provide progressive, functionally relevant weight-bearing exercises that minimize the loads that may induce graft elongation or tunnel slippage. Minimizing quadriceps femoris muscle inhibition is essential and of particular concern when a quadriceps tendon is harvested for autograft use.

Regardless of soft tissue graft selection, the progressive restoration of full active and passive knee flexion-extension range of motion in positions of function is essential. Particular attention should be placed on restoring the extensibility of muscles or muscle groups with pelvic attachments as they influence lumbopelvic region, hip, and knee position and function (Nyland et al. 2010a). Terminal knee flexion restoration should be evaluated with the patient in prone with the hip slightly extended. Terminal knee extension restoration should also be evaluated while the patient is supine with the hip slightly flexed. These positions enable more valid representations of true active knee flexion and extension function than postures which completely remove musculotendinous tension.

To facilitate effective cognitive appraisal and emotional responses to knee injury, ACL reconstruction, and rehabilitation, the clinician needs to serve as a guide and advocate in addition to being a caregiver. They must help the patient transition back to athlete status through positive psychobehaviors, decreased depression, increased self-efficacy and resilience, reduced kinesiophobia, and realistic reinjury fear beliefs. The therapeutic exercise environment is the ideal location to implement social cognitive theory principles of progressive task mastery, vicarious learning, social persuasion, modeling, and reciprocal determinism to develop self-efficacy and positive psychobehavioral changes (Bandura 2001). The rehabilitation environment should attempt to create the ideal situation for tissue healing, regeneration, motor learning, and education. During the acute phase (0–4 weeks), more

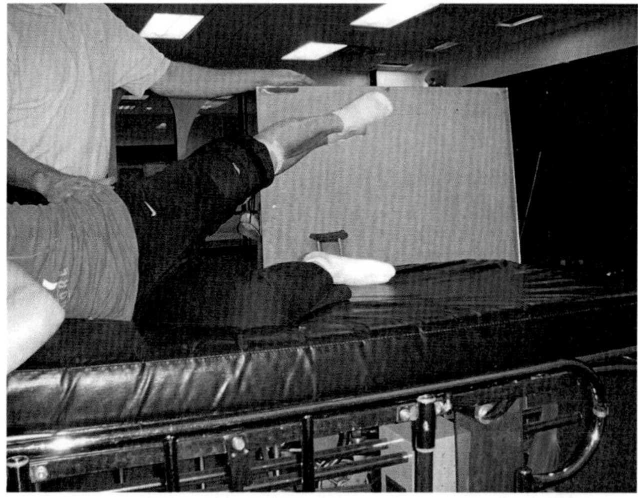

Fig. 4 Side-lying hip abduction-active knee extension with tactile feedback

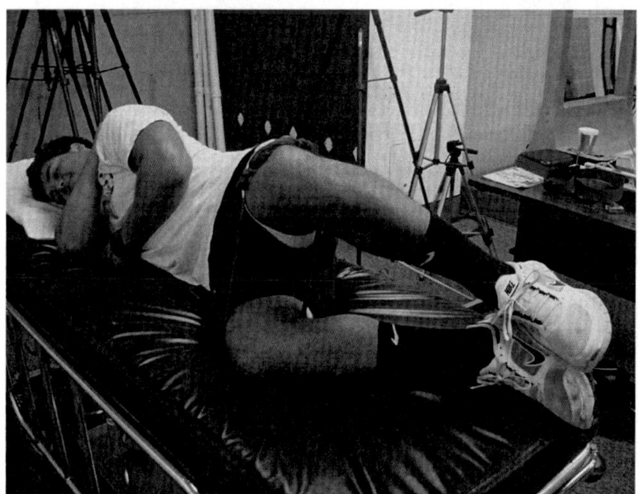

Fig. 5 Side-lying hip abduction-external rotation with resistance band

exercises are performed with limited or no weight bearing including multidirectional progressive resistance straight leg raises (Fig. 4), side-lying hip abduction-external rotation (Fig. 5), and posterior pelvic tilt-hip abduction-external rotation-supine bridges (Fig. 6). There is no better resistance training exercise to isolate quadriceps femoris activation throughout full active knee range of motion than the seated knee extension. To optimize proficiency with this exercise, however, progressively higher-amplitude quadriceps femoris activation and hamstring muscle group inhibition are needed to enable successful terminal knee extension against greater resistance. This factor, in combination with the long resistance lever arm between the support pad placed over the distal leg and the center of rotation at the lateral femoral epicondyle, increases the possibility of anterior tibial translatory forces during terminal knee extension. This may increase the risk for soft tissue graft elongation or bone tunnel slippage. Since the majority of evidence regarding soft tissue graft remodeling and integration is based on animal models, not human studies (Claes et al. 2011), athletes are encouraged to perform active seated knee extensions during the acute care phase in combination with hip adduction during both extension and flexion movements without distal resistance. For this reason and because of early concerns regarding quadriceps or hamstring autograft harvest-site irritation, the majority of therapeutic exercises during the early acute care phase include non-weight-bearing progressive resistance exercises that focus primarily on hip and ankle movements while maintaining isometric knee positioning, or range-specific progressive weight-bearing exercises that focus on eccentric neuromuscular activation such as the Eccentron (BTE, Hanover, MD, USA (Fig. 7). Although beneficial for patients who have undergone ACL reconstruction with any type of soft tissue graft, progressive resistance exercises that focus on eccentric neuromuscular activation such as the Eccentron might be especially beneficial for patients who receive a soft tissue allograft because it combines a method of increasing quadriceps femoris, hamstring, and gluteus maximus hypertrophy, strength, and functional performance capability in a closed kinetic chain mode (Gerber et al. 2007).

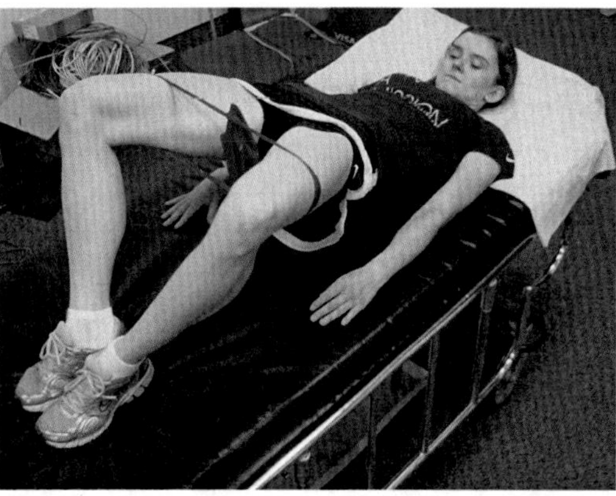

Fig. 6 Supine bridges with posterior pelvic tilt while abducting and externally rotating bilateral hips against resistance band

Intermediate Rehabilitation Transitioning From "Patient" To "Athlete" Role (5–26 Weeks)

This phase blends progressive resistance exercises with neuromuscular control training activities. As concerns related to acute knee pain, effusion, and graft harvest-site irritation decrease over the initial month postsurgery, more emphasis is placed on achieving integrated and balanced hip-knee-ankle function, albeit with greater emphasis on weight-bearing movements with appropriate hip-knee-ankle postural alignment to effect balanced lower extremity neuromuscular control. Movement examples include progressive resistance multidirectional lunges (Fig. 8), single-leg lateral step-ups (Fig. 9), single-leg squats (Fig. 10), matrix movements (Fig. 11), and progressive resistance single-leg leg pressing. In addition to progressive resistance and lower extremity joint movement amplitude, movement velocity is also

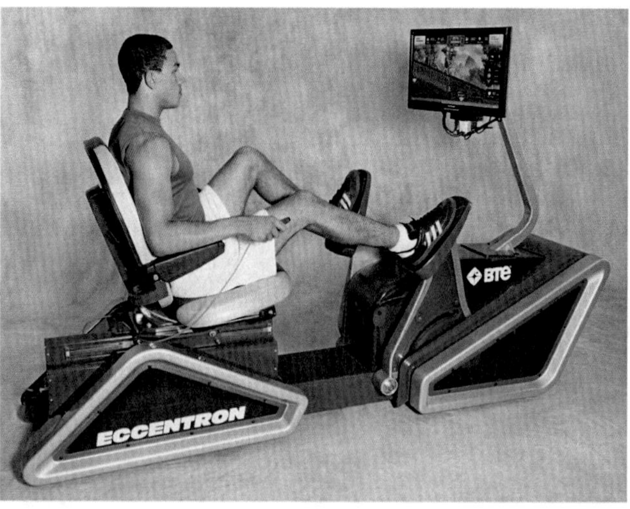

Fig. 7 Lower extremity eccentric muscle activation training on the Eccentron device

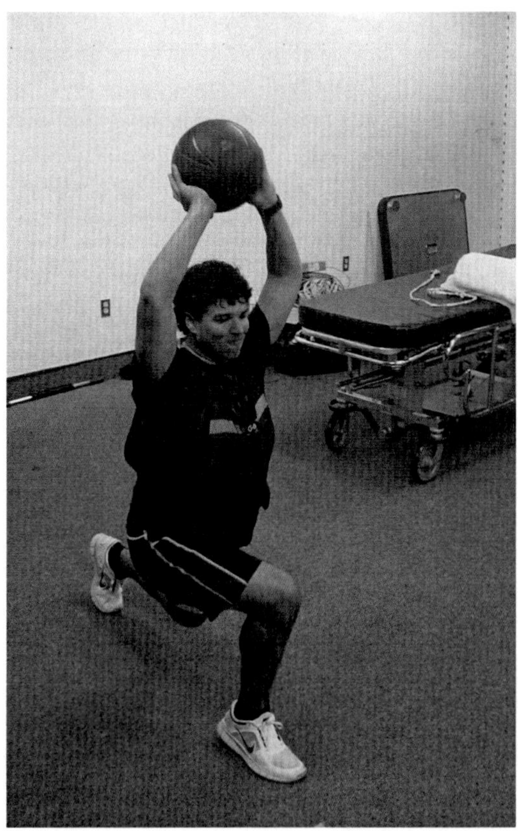

Fig. 8 Forward bounce-back lunge with weighted vest and 12 lb (5.4 kg) medicine ball

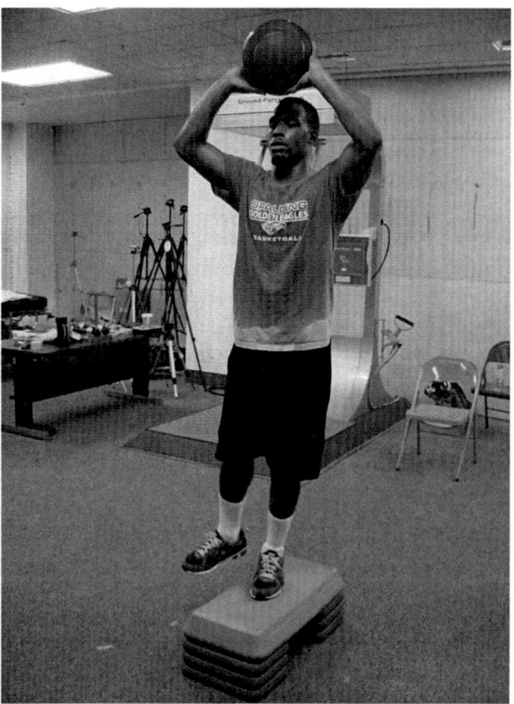

Fig. 9 Single-leg lateral step-ups on 10 inch (25.4 cm) step using a 12 lb (5.4 kg) medicine ball

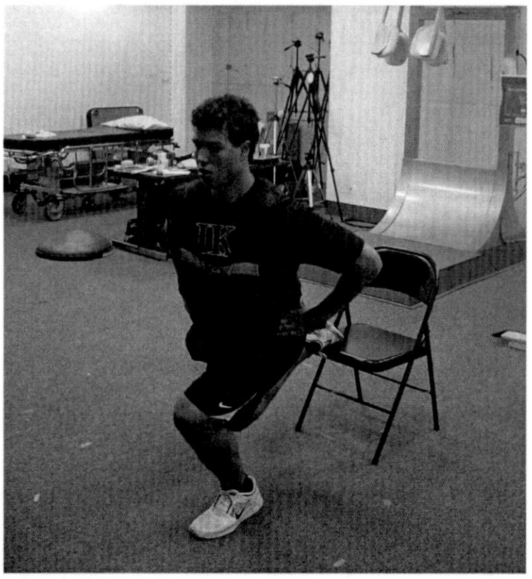

Fig. 10 Single-leg squats with weighted vest

progressively increased (plyometrics). Whether performing slow-velocity, low-impact stepping or higher-velocity, high-impact plyometric training, the patient must focus on high-quality movement form. Smooth, symmetrical upper and lower extremity movements with the head erect and the trunk slightly flexed are required, while also avoiding excessive frontal and sagittal plane trunk lean (Herrington et al. 2013). At the lower extremity, symmetrical, moderate hip flexion-internal rotation; symmetrical, knee-leg alignment with moderate knee flexion; and symmetrical foot alignment with moderate ankle dorsiflexion should all occur during soft jump landings (Paterno et al. 2007). The athlete is often required to hold a medicine ball or another object overhead to better challenge hip and lumbopelvic region muscle control of appropriate trunk alignment when progressing from basic limp-free walking gait with active neuromuscular knee extension control to multidirectional running-cutting and hopping or jumping movements. With increased progressive resistance and movement speed, however, it is essential to revisit functional lower extremity musculotendinous extensibility from positions of function, both on a treatment plinth (Fig. 12) and during weight-bearing movements such as backstep-"butt" kick (Fig. 13), extremely slow-speed carioca (Fig. 14), slow-speed lateral stepping (Fig. 15), supine bridge-heel walking (Fig. 16), crab crawl (Fig. 17), and form run simulation with long-axis transverse plane rotation of the trunk and hips with exaggerated arm movements (Fig. 18). Slow-speed movements are valuable for several reasons: (1) If the athlete has pain, they can easily stop before they go too far, too fast, decreasing pain and injury risk. (2) They allow for a prolonged period of single-leg support and balance challenge at the surgical side lower extremity than quicker movements, allowing sufficient time for neuromuscular responses to develop at the impaired joint. (3) They provide greater time for the rehabilitation clinician to distinguish correct from incorrect postural alignment and movement patterns and provide appropriate instructional feedback. (4) They provide the rehabilitation clinician greater time to identify segmental movement performance deficiencies, such as surgical lower extremity knee extensor weakness, and maladaptive compensations such as excessive hip extensor muscle group compensation. (5) They remove the opportunity for the patient to conceal true functional impairments by using momentum generated through adjacent non-impaired lower extremity joints such as the ankle and hip or increased use of the contralateral lower extremity to enable successful movement

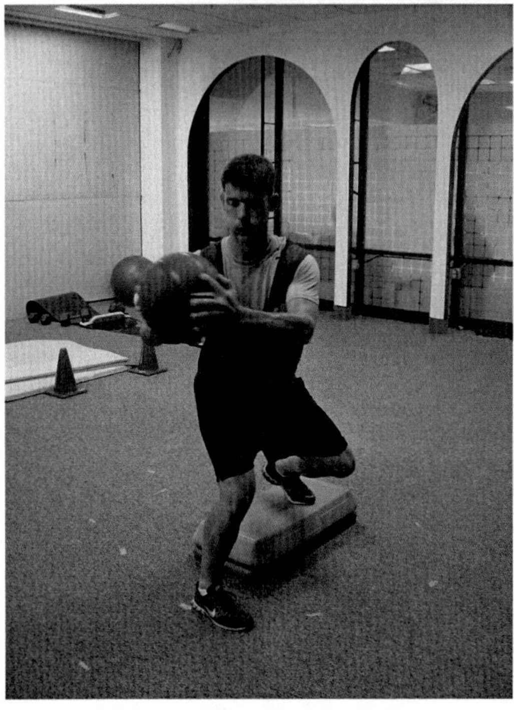

Fig. 11 Matrix exercise on a 6 in (15.2 cm) step using a weighted vest and a 12 lb (5.4 kg) medicine ball

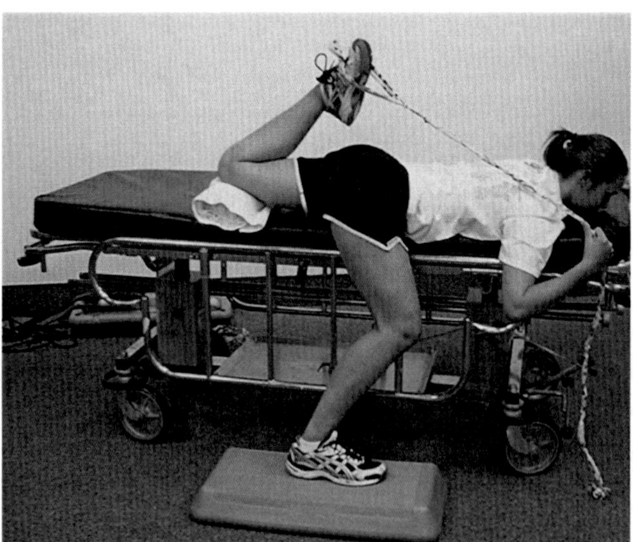

Fig. 12 Prone left lower extremity quadriceps femoris stretch with hip extended and right lower extremity hamstring stretch

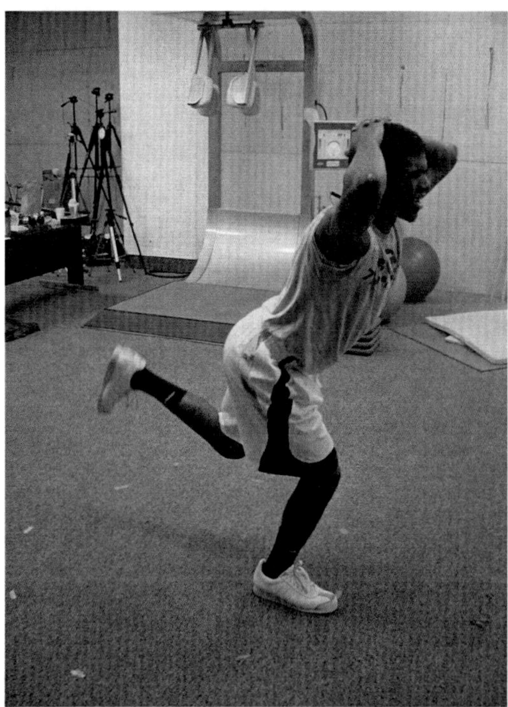

Fig. 13 Slow-speed, backstep-"butt" kick

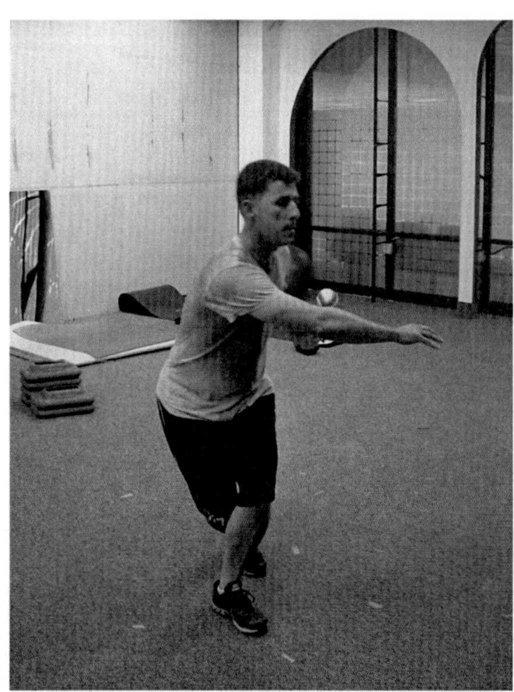

Fig. 14 Slow-speed carioca

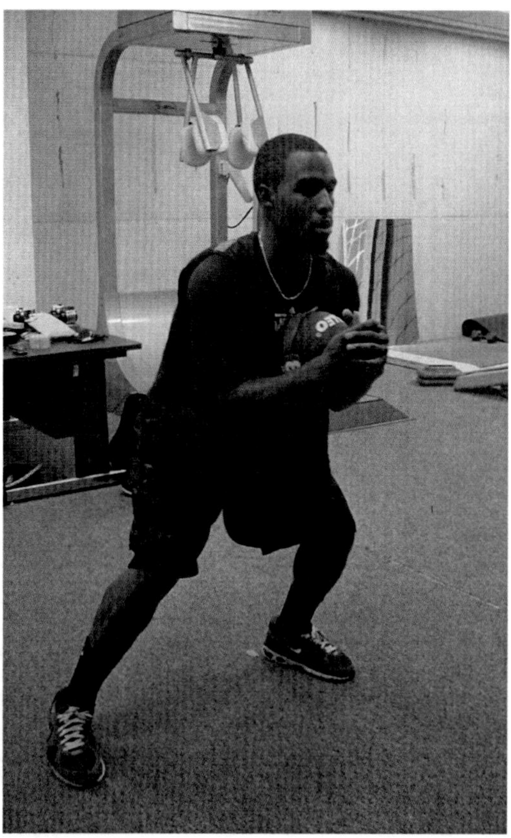

Fig. 15 Slow-speed lateral stepping with weighted vest and 8 lb (3.63 kg) medicine ball

performance. Slower movements also help the rehabilitation clinician ensure that neuromuscular functions as well as postural control and balance improvements are occurring within functional postures representative of non-impaired musculotendinous extensibility.

During this phase, weight-bearing functional therapeutic exercises are beneficial. This includes multidirectional lunges with resistance provided by a weighted body vest and medicine ball (18–26 weeks postsurgery). Functional therapeutic exercises begin with slow-speed movements allowing the patient to perform sequence learning to develop improved postural awareness and sensorimotor adaptations (2–12 weeks postsurgery), setting the stage for transfer of learning to more sport-specific tasks. The patient progresses to more exploratory movements with chaotic instances created by sudden movement path

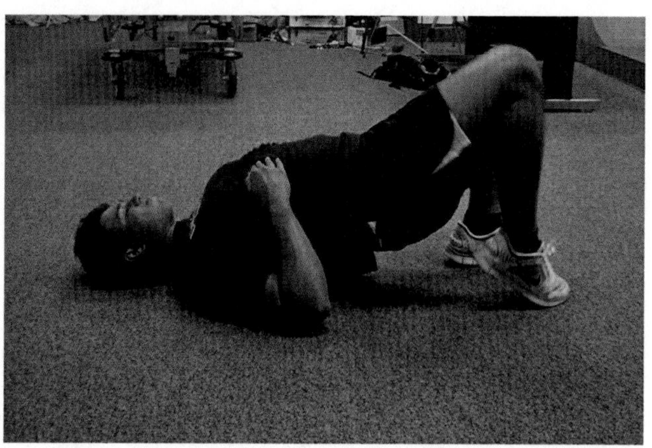

Fig. 16 Supine bridge-heel walking

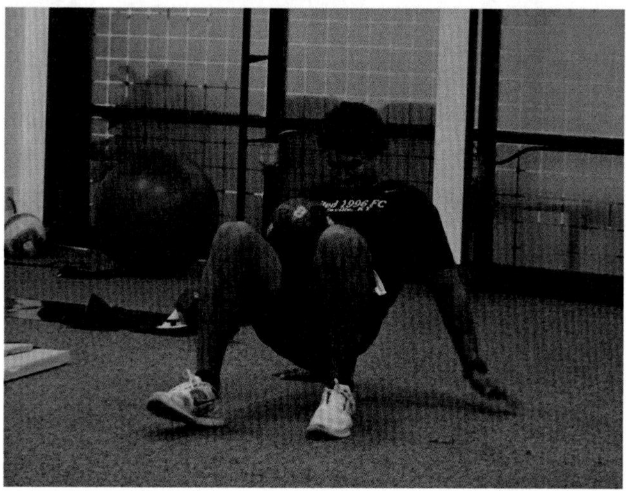

Fig. 17 Crab crawling with 8 lb (3.63 kg) medicine ball

perturbations (12–20 weeks postsurgery) to more performance-based skilled movements, translating the clinical experience to more sport-specific tasks (20–26 weeks postsurgery) (Nyland 2012a). Following participation in an exercise progression that has been described previously (Nyland et al. 2010a) and progressive resistance strength training to rule out lower extremity or core strength impairments, the athlete eventually progresses to sport-specific training and objective field testing.

Functional therapeutic exercises simulate the weight-bearing and non-weight-bearing components of daily activities in a manner that replicates three-dimensional function within joint ranges of motion and velocities that facilitate the desired physiological and biomechanical responses (Nyland et al. 2005). Before consideration of a return to intense conditioning or sport-specific training, the rehabilitation clinician and athlete must be confident that during single-leg landings the athlete can consistently withstand intense three-dimensional lower extremity loading involving contralateral pelvic drop, femoral internal rotation, knee valgus, tibial internal rotation, and foot pronation (Hewett and Myers 2011). The rehabilitation program has progressive milestones, including non-impaired knee extension (within 0–2 weeks postsurgery), quadriceps femoris neuromuscular control during walking (within 0–2 weeks postsurgery), full active and passive knee flexion (within 8 weeks postsurgery), reestablishing normal core and lower extremity strength and power (within

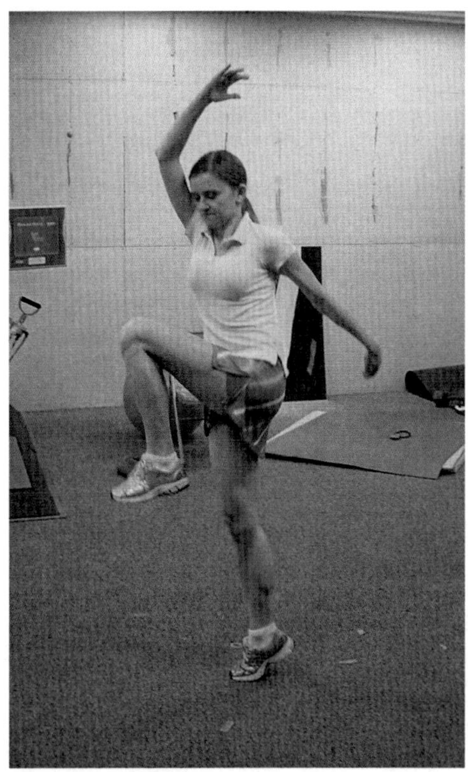

Fig. 18 Form run simulation holding peak ankle plantar flexion position for 2–3 seconds

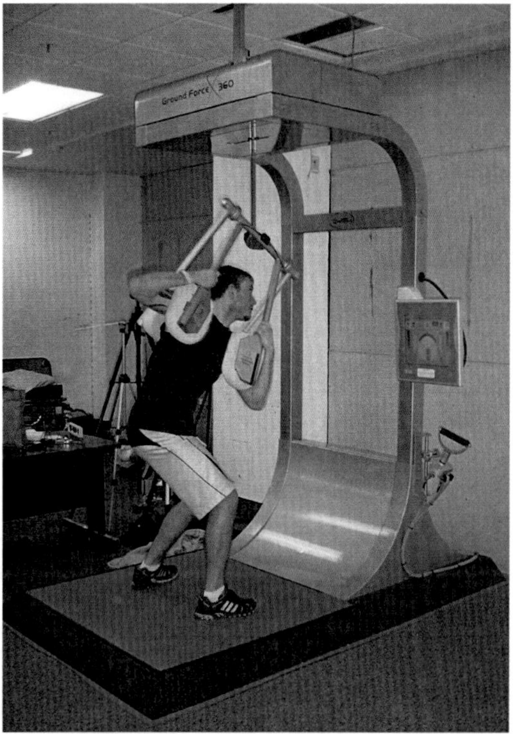

Fig. 19 Whole body, long-axis rotational training on the Ground Force 360 Device

12–14 weeks postsurgery), and consistent evidence of dynamic knee stability during clinical single-leg hop testing (within 14–18 weeks postsurgery) (Nyland 2012a). When these milestones are met, sport-specific training may begin.

Sport-Specific Training with Neuromuscular Training Bias (27–36 Weeks)

The sport-specific training phase has a strong neuromuscular control training bias. Innovative devices like the Ground Force 360 (Fig. 19) (Nyland et al. 2010b) provide a useful environment to apply variable movement, multi-planar progressive resistance and velocity concentric-eccentric neuromuscular training that translates earlier clinical exercise experiences to higher-intensity, more sport-specific applications (Nyland 2012a). Once the athlete has approximately 80 % bilaterally equivalent single-leg leg pressing capability following the progression shown in Table 2, more aggressive single-leg hopping and jumping tasks are implemented such as chop step – single-leg hop – stabilization (Fig. 20), double- and single-leg crossover hop over a variable height tape (Fig. 21), "V" single- and double-leg hop progression (Fig. 22), and single-leg flexed knee stabilization with ball toss on unstable-firm (Fig. 23) and unstable-soft (Fig. 24) surfaces.

The surgical side lower extremity single-leg double hop deficiency is approximately 20 % greater than the surgical side lower extremity single-leg leg press deficiency when compared to the nonsurgical lower extremity. Restoration of 80 % bilateral single-leg leg press equivalency suggests that only 60 % bilateral single-leg double hop equivalency exists. Therefore, rehabilitation clinicians should proceed with caution as they progress the athlete to more intense plyometric

Table 2 Single-leg leg press weekly resistance progression

Set	Repetition goal	Nonsurgical lower extremity (kg)	Surgical lower extremity (example beginning with 50 % of nonsurgical lower extremity resistance at week 1) (kg)	Increase resistance by a minimum of 10 % each week (example at end of week 8) (kg). Desire to achieve 110 % capability if the injured knee involves the preferred or dominant stance lower extremity
1	12	18.2	9.1	18.2
2	12	27.2	13.6	27.2
3	10	36.3	18.2	36.3
4	10	45.4	22.7	45.4
5	8	54.4	27.2	54.4
6	8	63.5	31.8	63.5

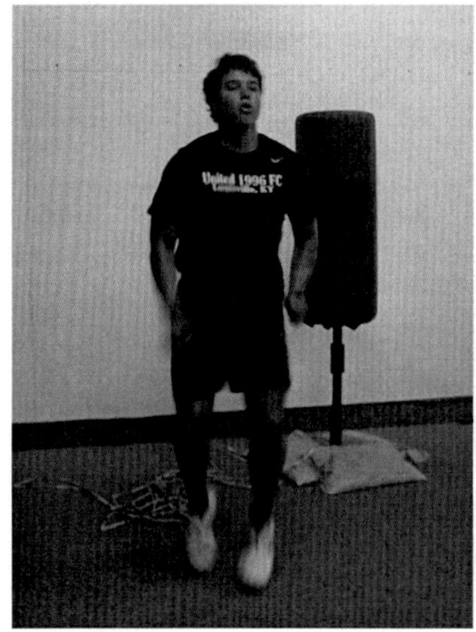

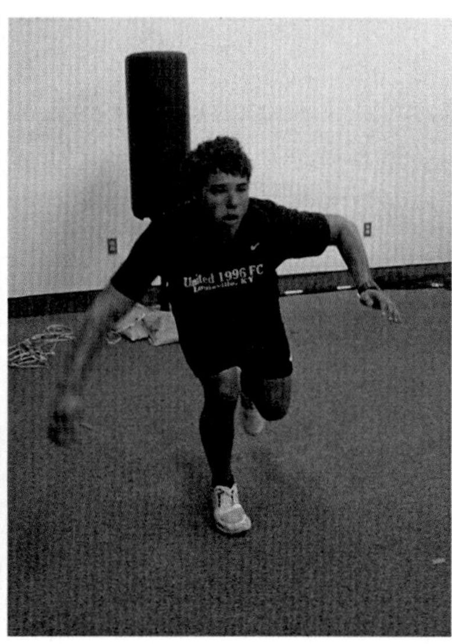

Fig. 20 Chop step, single-leg hop stabilization holding stability position for 2–3 seconds before repeating to the opposite side

movements. Using a three-dimensional dynamic knee model, Shin et al. (2009) reported that peak ACL strain increased nonlinearly with increasing peak valgus knee moments. They concluded that although greater magnitude knee valgus moments increased peak ACL strain during single-leg landing, increased knee valgus moments alone were not sufficient to induce an isolated ACL tear. An ACL tear only occurred with coupled tibial external rotation associated with medial collateral ligament (MCL) impairment. Increasing strain on a healthy MCL prevented proportional increases in ACL strain at higher-magnitude knee valgus moments. Postural alignment and neuromuscular control training that reduces the external knee valgus moment can reduce both ACL and MCL strain. Ma et al. (2000) reported that the ACL graft is subjected to significantly greater in situ forces with concomitant MCL deficiency with valgus loading. They concluded that the ACL reconstructed knee with combined ACL and MCL injury should be protected from high valgus moments during early healing to avoid excessive graft loading. Joseph et al. (2008) reported that as little as a 5° medial rearfoot post decreased drop jump landing initial contact knee valgus and decreased peak knee valgus among healthy female college athletes.

Returning to Sport Practice Shared Decision-Making (37–52 Weeks or More)

Following release from outpatient physical therapy, the following eight-session program is implemented (1 session/week for 8 weeks with supplemental, once weekly single-leg leg pressing). The following progression is generally followed. Prior to beginning the program, the athlete completes the Knee Outcome Survey – Sports Activity Scale (KOS-SAS). Session #1 focuses on movement education and reviewing the athlete's goals to determine their appropriateness and the likelihood of balancing satisfaction with realistic expectations. Session #2 introduces a weighted vest beginning at approximately 10 % bodyweight during movement tasks consisting primarily of slow-speed, multidirectional stepping tasks. Session #3 introduces progressive intensity two-legged hops and jumps and the athlete is instructed to perform a 3.2 km jog-run once/week. Session #4 introduces progressive intensity single-leg hops and jumps. The nonsurgical lower extremity single-leg leg press for eight-repetition maximum is reevaluated at week #4 to reset surgical side percentage goals. Session #5 introduces progressive intensity agility maneuvers and the athlete is instructed to begin progressive effort (50–100 %) 18.3–36.6–54.9 m straight sprints for three repetitions each once/week. Sessions #6–#8 increase training volume to improve general conditioning with a focus on areas of perceived deficiency and agility maneuvers like the cutting "circuit board" (Fig. 25a, b) and intense cutting-pivoting maneuvers while sprinting. When the athlete meets the following goals, approximately 95–110 % bilateral single-leg leg press equivalency, 90–100 % KOS-SAS score, and bilateral equivalence with active and passive knee flexion-extension range of motion, they are ready to participate in a structured objective field

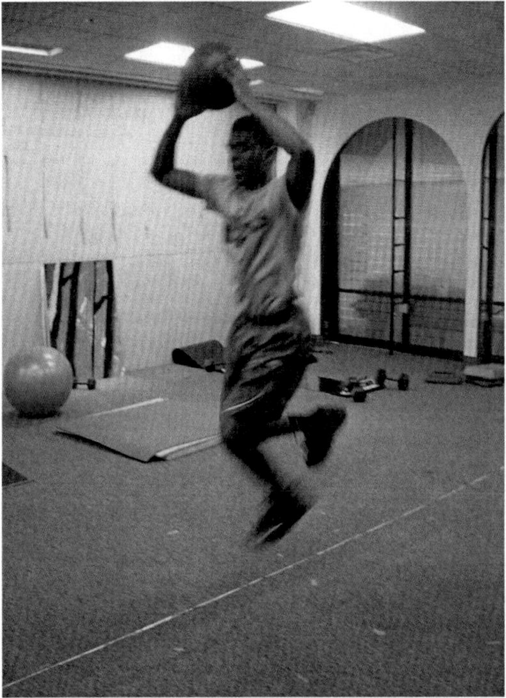

Fig. 21 Double-leg crossover hop over caution tape using a 12 lb (5.4 kg) medicine ball

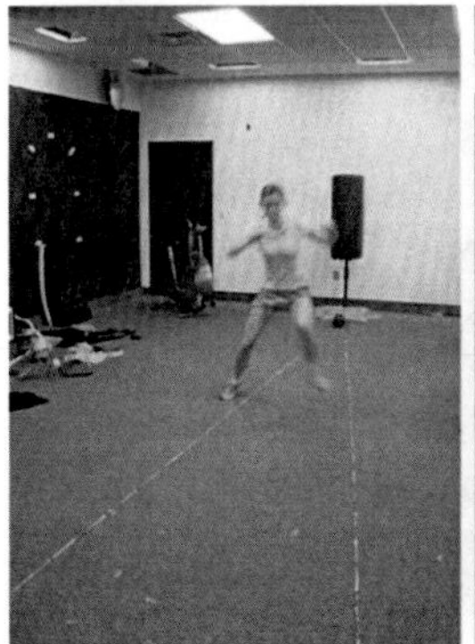
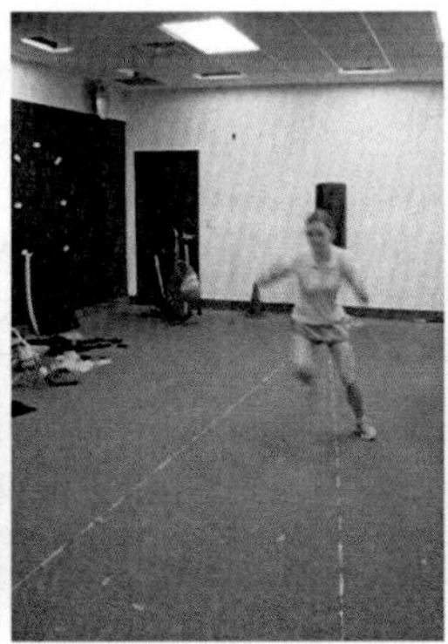
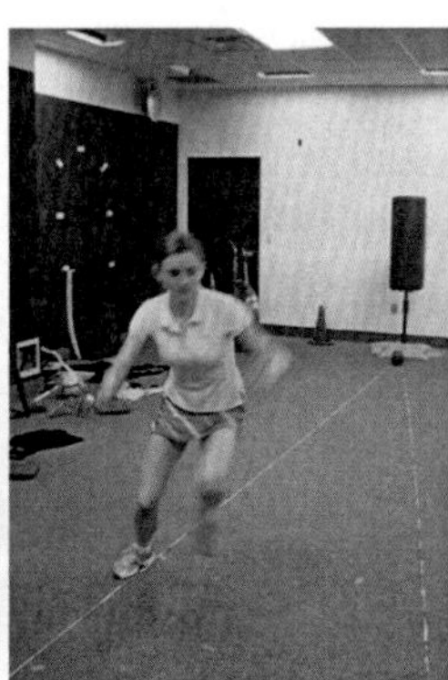
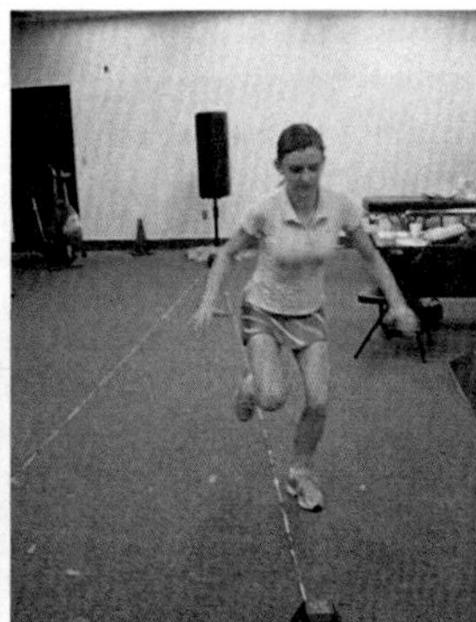

Fig. 22 "V" pattern hop progression

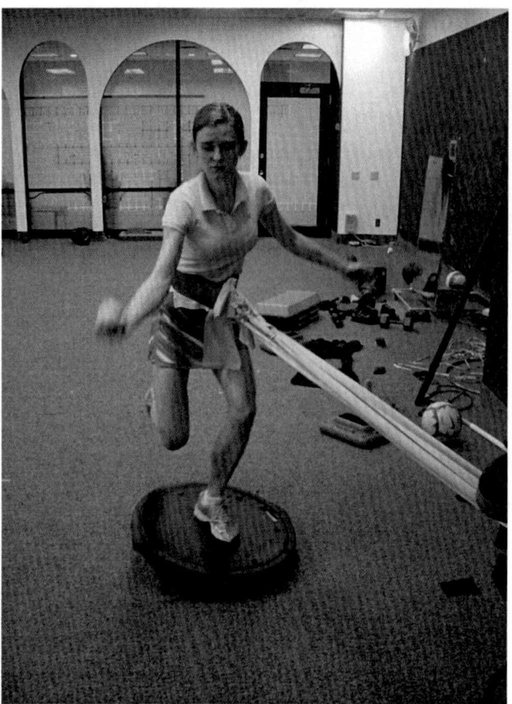

Fig. 23 Single-leg postural control training on unstable, firm surface

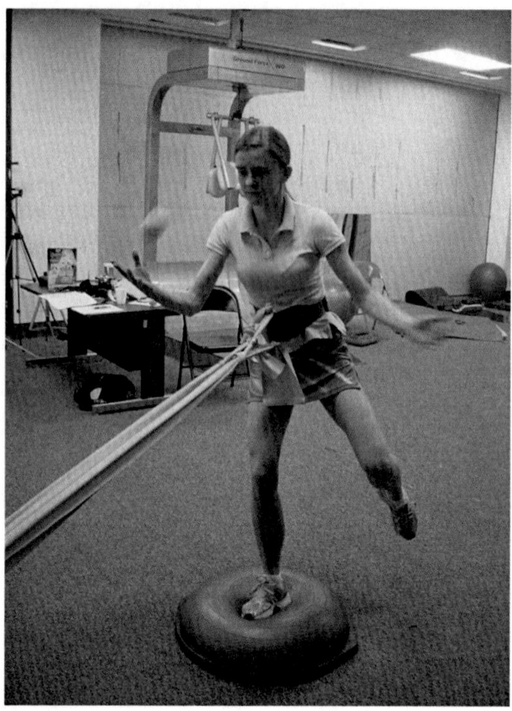

Fig. 24 Single-leg postural control training on unstable soft surface

test that will lead to return to sport practice consideration. Field testing should match important return to competitive sport criteria. The program includes five categories: form, dynamic knee stability, lower extremity power, agility-reaction time, and consistent and endurant skills during the performance of high speed sport specific movements speed skills. Within these categories five or six tasks are selected that display sport-specific and position-specific relevance as well as consideration for the style or tempo of team play. Following two jogging-running laps around the athletic field periphery and volitional static and ballistic stretching, the test is initiated alternating tasks between more difficult dynamic knee stability, lower extremity power, and agility-reaction time maneuvers with the active rest provided by slower, lower intensity form-focused movements. After passing the test, a formal report is sent to the treating surgeon, the athlete (and/or their parents), the team athletic trainer, and if approved by the athlete, to their coach. To pass the field test, the athlete must pass each movement test. Since restoration of pre-injury levels of anaerobic and aerobic conditioning are generally not achieved by this point in their recovery, the form movement category serves as a dynamic warm-up, active rest, and confirmation of non-impaired lower extremity musculotendinous extensibility juxtaposed between more intense single-leg stabilization, power, agility, reaction time, and sport skill tasks. Upon passing the field test, the athlete is permitted to return to unrestricted full sport conditioning, structured and supervised sport practices, but not competition. If the athlete is able to successfully complete two full weeks of practice without complaint, without any signs of knee dysfunction such as limping, pain, or effusion, and when the team athletic trainer, sport physiotherapist, team physician, coach, parents, and the athlete mutually agree that the athlete is ready, they are permitted to return to competition. This type of shared decision-making is essential to increase the likelihood of a successfully integrated

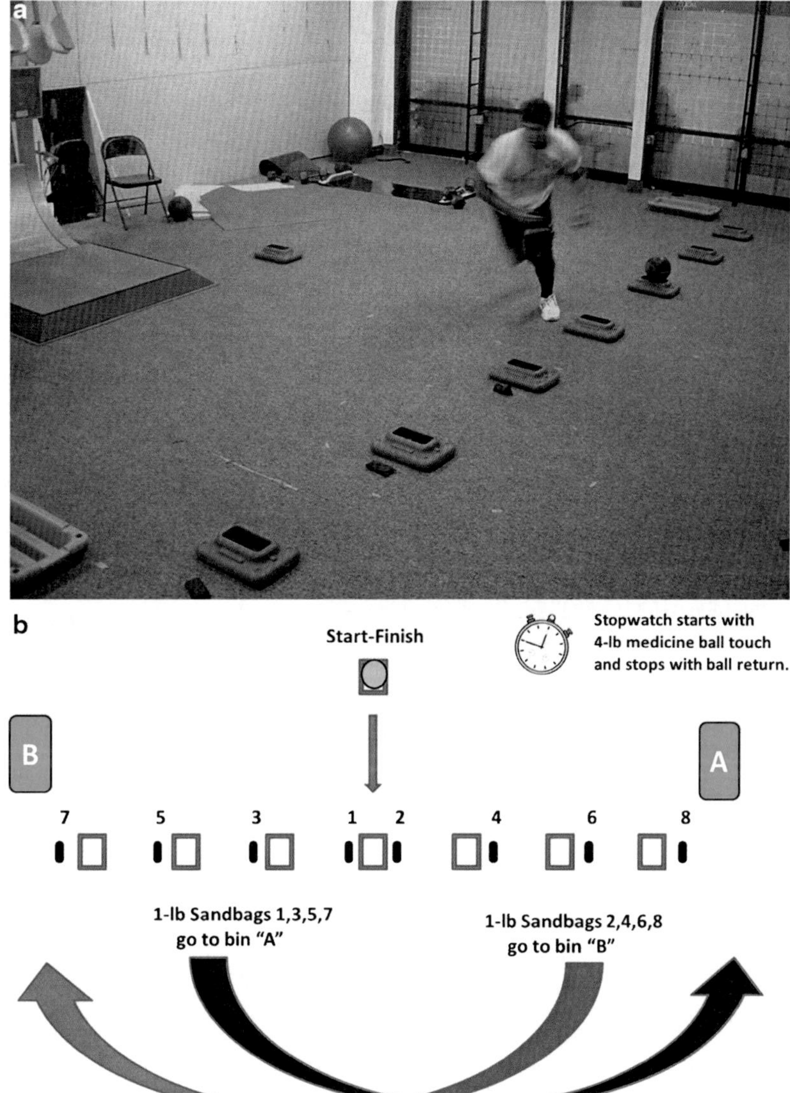

Fig. 25 "Circuit board cutting drill" After picking up a 4 lb (1.8 kg) medicine ball from its starting position and sprinting straight ahead to place it within a plastic socket, the subject transfers its associated sandbag (1) into the scoring bin (**a**). After this the subject moves as quickly as possible to carry another sandbag (2) into its scoring bin (**b**). Following this, the medicine ball must be moved progressively side-to-side to each socket before each sandbag is transferred to its respective bin. When all sandbags have been transferred the subject returns the medicine ball to the starting position. Quicker time to task completion indicates improving agility, rapid acceleration-deceleration, and cutting function

return to competitive sport and reduced risk of surgical side reinjury or injury to the contralateral knee. With these guidelines applied, a pilot study of 50 athletes was performed (Nyland et al. 2013). Subjects (20.2 ± 7.7 years of age) had sustained their knee injury from soccer ($n = 15$), American football ($n = 11$), basketball ($n = 9$), and other sport including gymnastics, lacrosse, baseball, field hockey, wrestling, volleyball, downhill skiing, and badminton. At time of testing 96 % (48/50) reported improved overall knee function during sport, 56 % (28/50) had a two-level perceived overall sport activity knee function improvement (from abnormal to normal), 84 % (42/50) displayed ≥90 % hop-go-stop (double hop) bilateral equivalence, 84 % (42/50) displayed ≥90 % single-leg hop timing bilateral equivalence, and 80 % (40/50) displayed ≥90 % single-leg timed crossover hop timing. By 3 ± 1.3 years (minimum of 2 years) return to sport, only 1 of 50 (2 %) patients had sustained another knee injury (patella dislocation following primary medial patellofemoral ligament repair at 15 years of age).

Summary

The process of returning the patient to the athlete role begins with preoperative planning. Each rehabilitation phase has distinct short- and long-term performance and educational goals. Sport-specific training provides the ideal scenario for the recovering athlete to truly evaluate their functional readiness. Shared decision-making by all key "stakeholders" in the athlete's life increases the soundness of the return to play decision-making process and increases its likelihood for success.

Cross-References

- ▶ Factors Affecting Return to Sport After Anterior Cruciate Ligament Reconstruction
- ▶ Medial Collateral Ligament and Anterior Cruciate Ligament Synergy: Functional Interdependence
- ▶ Structured Rehabilitation Model with Clinical Outcomes After Anterior Cruciate Ligament Reconstruction

References

Bandura A (2001) Health promotion from the context of social cognitive theory. In: Norman P, Abraham C, Conner M (eds) Understanding and changing health behavior: from health beliefs to self-regulation. Academic, Netherlands, pp 299–337

Claes S, Verdonk P, Forsyth R et al (2011) The "ligamentization" process in anterior cruciate ligament reconstruction: what happens to the human graft a systematic review of the literature. Am J Sports Med 39(11):2476–2483

Elmlinger BS, Nyland JA, Tillett ED (2006) Knee flexor function 2 years after anterior cruciate ligament reconstruction with semitendinosus-gracilis autografts. Arthroscopy 22(6):650–655

Gerber JP, Marcus RL, Dibble LE et al (2007) Effects of early progressive eccentric exercise on muscle structure after anterior cruciate ligament reconstruction. J Bone Joint Surg Am 89(3):559–570

Giotis D, Tsiaras V, Ristanis S et al (2011) Knee braces can decrease tibial rotation during pivoting that occurs in high demanding activities. Knee Surg Sports Traumatol Arthrosc 19(8):1347–1354

Gulotta LV, Rodeo SA (2007) Biology of autograft and allograft healing in anterior cruciate ligament reconstruction. Clin Sports Med 26(4):509–524

Han DL, Nyland J, Kendzior M et al (2012) Intratunnel versus extratunnel fixation of hamstring autograft for anterior cruciate ligament reconstruction. Arthroscopy 28(10):1555–1566

Herrington L, Myer G, Horsley I (2013) Task based rehabilitation protocol for elite athletes following anterior cruciate ligament reconstruction: a clinical commentary. Phys Ther Sport 14:188–198

Hewett TE, Myer GD (2011) The mechanistic connection between the trunk, hip, knee, and anterior cruciate ligament injury. Exerc Sport Sci Rev 39:161–166

Howells BE, Ardern CL, Webster KE (2011) Is postural control restored following anterior cruciate ligament reconstruction? A systematic review. Knee Surg Sports Traumatol Arthrosc 19:1168–1177

Joseph M, Tiberio D, Baird JL et al (2008) Knee valgus during drop jumps in National Collegiate Athletic Association Division I female athletes: the effect of a medial post. Am J Sports Med 36(2):285–289

Ma CB, Papageorgiou CD, Debski RE et al (2000) Interaction between the ACL graft and MCL in a combined ACL + MCL knee injury using a goat model. Acta Orthop Scand 71(4):387–393

Mirzatolooei F, Alamdari MT, Khalkhali HR (2013) The impact of platelet-rich plasma on prevention of tunnel widening in anterior cruciate ligament reconstruction using quadrupled autologous hamstring tendon. J Bone Joint Surg 95B:65–69

Nyland J (2012a) Therapeutic strategies for developing neuromuscular control in the kinetic chain. Orthopaedic section independent study course 22.1.4 education and interventions for musculoskeletal injuries: a biomechanics approach. Orthopaedic Section, APTA, Inc

Nyland J, Brand E, Fisher B (2010a) Update on rehabilitation following ACL reconstruction. Open Access J Sports Med http://www.dovepress.com/update-on-rehabilitation-following-acl-reconstruction-peer-reviewed-article-OAJSM

Nyland J, Burden R, Krupp R et al (2010b) Whole body, long-axis rotational training improves lower extremity neuromuscular control during single leg drop landing and stabilization. Clin Biomech 26:363–370

Nyland J, Fisher B, Brand E et al (2010c) Osseous deficits after anterior cruciate ligament injury and reconstruction: a systematic review with suggestions to improve osseous homeostasis. Arthroscopy 26:1248–1257

Nyland J, Klein S, Caborn DN (2010d) Lower extremity compensatory neuromuscular and biomechanical adaptations 2 to 11 years after anterior cruciate ligament reconstruction. Arthroscopy 26:1212–1225

Nyland J, Krupp R, Caborn DNM (2013) Knee re-injury prevention program following rehabilitation improves sports performance and patient outcomes. Abstract #866, 60th ACSM annual meeting and 4th world congress on exercise is medicine. Indianapolis, 28 May–1 June 2013

Nyland J, Lachman N, Kocabey Y et al (2005) Anatomy, function and rehabilitation of the popliteus musculotendinous complex. J Orthop Sports Phys Ther 35(3):165–179

Nyland J, Lee YH, McGinnis M et al (2014) ACL double bundle linked cortical-aperture tibial fixation: A technical note. Arch Orthop Trauma Surg 134(6):835–842

Paterno MV, Ford KR, Myer GD et al (2007) Limb asymmetries in landing and jumping 2 years following anterior cruciate ligament reconstruction. Clin J Sport Med 17:258–262

Rahr-Wagner L, Thillemann TM, Pedersen AB et al (2013) Increased risk of revision after anteromedial compared with transtibial drilling of the femoral tunnel during primary anterior cruciate ligament reconstruction: results from the Danish knee ligament reconstruction register. Arthroscopy 29(1):98–105

Rodeo SA, Arnoczky SP, Torzilli PA et al (1993) Tendon-healing in a bone tunnel. A biomechanical and histological study in the dog. J Bone Joint Surg Am 75 (12):1795–1803

Scheffler SU, Schmidt T, Gangey I et al (2008) Fresh-frozen free-tendon allografts versus autografts in anterior cruciate ligament reconstruction: delayed remodeling and inferior mechanical function during long-term healing in sheep. Arthroscopy 24 (4):448–458

Shin CS, Chaudhari AM, Andriacchi TP (2009) The effect of isolated valgus moments on ACL strain during single-leg landing: a simulation study. J Biomech 42 (3):280–285

Vavken P, Sadoghi P, Murray MM (2011) The effect of platelet concentrates on graft maturation and graft-bone interface healing in anterior cruciate ligament reconstruction in human patients: a systematic review of controlled trials. Arthroscopy 27 (11):1573–1583

Winett RA, Williams DM, Davy BM (2009) Initiating and maintaining resistance training in older adults: a social cognitive theory-based approach. Br J Sports Med 43:114–119

Wright RW, Preston E, Fleming BC et al (2008) A systematic review of anterior cruciate ligament reconstruction rehabilitation: Part I: continuous passive motion, early weight bearing, postoperative bracing, and home-based rehabilitation. J Knee Surg 21(3):217–224

Personalized Treatment Algorithms for Anterior Cruciate Ligament Injuries

106

Burak Demirağ and Cenk Ermutlu

Contents

Abstract

A standardized treatment algorithm for ACL rupture may not be suitable for everybody because individuals may present with different characteristics. Social and physiological differences and different injury patterns necessitate an individualized treatment plan. This chapter focuses on factors such as gender, age, work and activity level, osteoarthritis, chronicity, associated lesions, anatomy, and tear morphology to develop an individualized approach to ACL rupture. A thorough understanding of these factors is necessary to develop an individualized algorithm, both for diagnosis and treatment of ACL rupture.

Introduction

Anterior cruciate ligament (ACL) rupture is the most frequent ligamentous injury of the knee (Griffin et al. 2000). ACL tears are more prevalent among people involved in sports or heavy labor. It is a serious injury and the instability caused by a torn ACL makes other structures of the knee prone to additional damage and predisposes to future osteoarthritis.

Reconstruction of the ACL is a common orthopedic procedure with standardized algorithms. However, several factors such as age, gender, work, level of sports activities, lifestyle, concomitant knee injuries, tear morphology, degree of instability, time lapse between injury and surgery,

B. Demirağ (✉)
Department of Orthopaedics and Traumatology, Uludağ University Faculty of Medicine, Bursa, Turkey
e-mail: burakdemirag@hotmail.com

C. Ermutlu
Department of Orthopaedics and Traumatology, İstanbul Training and Research Hospital, İstanbul, Turkey
e-mail: cermutlu@hotmail.com

M.N. Doral, J. Karlsson (eds.), *Sports Injuries*,
DOI 10.1007/978-3-642-36569-0_84

knee anatomy, and presence of osteoarthritis (OA) need to be considered when planning the treatment. In contrast to conventional treatment algorithms where a "one size fits all" philosophy may apply, individualized ACL treatment takes these factors into consideration and allows for the customization of the treatment algorithm.

This chapter focuses on how surgical indications, graft-fixation methods, and surgical techniques may differ among individuals, based upon the authors' clinical experience and evidence in the literature. Identifying the individual characteristics of a patient will help to prevent the possible pitfalls and complications and will serve to achieve stable knees with potentially improved clinical outcomes.

Age

Age, whether physiological or chronological, is an important determining factor when individualizing the treatment of a patient with an ACL tear. When considering ACL reconstruction, the term "older" is used to define patients over 40 years old, whereas males younger than 16 and females younger than 14 are usually considered "skeletally immature." Treatment algorithms of these age groups need to be individualized, beginning with the question of proceeding to ACL reconstruction or following nonsurgical therapy.

For years, the general approach for patients older than 40 has been to consider those with sedentary lifestyle for nonsurgical therapy. However, the activity level of this age group has risen recently, and an increased number of older individuals participate in recreational sports. This has led to a greater frequency of injuries in this age group and increasing patients' expectations from treatment. Rather than determining the treatment method for patients by classifying them as either sedentary or active, their activity levels, occupations, and posttreatment expectations should be taken into consideration.

Nonsurgical treatment and bracing may be an option for "older" patients with lower activity levels who participate in low-impact sports and whose lifestyles and occupations do not require significant knee stability. However, reliance on a brace to return to pre-injury level of activity with continuing knee instability may lead to significant rates of instability recurrence (Seng et al. 2008).

The treatment of ACL injuries in older athletes remains controversial. Although accompanying osteochondral and meniscal pathologies are usually thought to be age related, patients in this age group may have a delay in surgical intervention and may be susceptible to longer periods of knee instability, which may be the reason for these concomitant lesions (Legnani et al. 2011). Surgical intervention in older patients should address the joint environment, malalignment, contracture, cartilage loss, inflammation, and pain to ensure optimal clinical results. The patient's activity level, overall health status, expectations, and possible complications should be considered.

An alternative to ACL reconstruction in the older age group is the "healing response" technique (Steadman et al. 2012). It has been reported to be applicable to an unstable knee joint with a proximal tear of the ACL. This technique is basically an application of the microfracture procedure on the proximal footprint of the ACL in order to generate a healing response. It is technically undemanding, is performed arthroscopically, and does not impede future ACL reconstruction. Postoperative care involves brace use and a customized rehabilitation protocol.

Several studies in the literature report successful outcomes for ACL reconstruction in patients over 40 years old and even in those over 55 (Arbuthnot and Brink 2010; Gee et al. 2013). Reconstruction of the ACL with autograft has been reported to provide stabile knees with high knee scores, with complication rates similar to those of younger patients. The clinical outcome for these patients is directly related to concomitant osteochondral and meniscal lesions, rather than the type of autograft used (Brown et al. 2013). Although no graft is demonstrated to be superior, diminished blood supply and inadequate inflammatory response in the elderly raise concerns about the biological integration of the allografts.

The rate of complications such as infection, re-rupture of the graft, laxity, and arthrofibrosis is similar to other age groups (Gee et al. 2013).

Exercises for range of motion (ROM), quadriceps strengthening, and patellar mobility are particularly important to avoid arthrofibrosis, the most devastating complication.

Incidence of sports injury cases has been increasing among pediatric and adolescent patients. Surgical intervention on these skeletally immature patients carries the risk of growth plate disruption and may lead to premature closure, angular deformities, and limb-length discrepancy. Delaying surgery to avoid these complications prolongs the unstable period and makes the knee potentially susceptible to additional meniscal and chondral injuries.

The first step in the treatment of this group of patients is to document the physical maturation of the patient using the chronological age, Tanner charts, and wrist age determination. The history is particularly important in the diagnosis of ACL rupture in this age group. The child may abstain from telling the details of the injury or deny the injury itself. Physical examination is the most reliable method to diagnose an ACL tear in the child. The presence of a joint effusion or hemarthrosis must alert the orthopedist for ligamentous injury to the knee joint.

The diagnostic value of MRI has been reported to be limited because the ACL in a child has different signal characteristics, and standard sequences may fail to show an ACL tear (McConkey et al. 2011), and interpretation of the different sequences by an experienced musculoskeletal radiologist may be necessary.

The treatment algorithm following the diagnosis is critical. Surgical techniques may be grouped as physis sparing extra-articular or intra-articular techniques, partial physis sparing techniques, and transphyseal techniques. There are common critical points in all of these techniques: The tunnels must be as narrow as possible, must traverse the physis as perpendicular as possible, and must be placed close to the center of the growth plate in the transverse and coronal planes. Excessive tensioning of the graft must be avoided. Fixation devices placed inside the tunnel must not cross the growth plate. Patellar tendon or quadriceps grafts with bony plugs should not be used unless only the soft tissue tendon grafts cross the physes inside the tunnels.

Children with ACL tears respond to nonsurgical treatment well (Fabricant et al. 2013). This includes absolute avoidance of pivoting and cutting activities, functional bracing during sports activities, and extensive rehabilitation.

Many articles in the literature report good results and no angulation or limb discrepancy with transphyseal intervention in patients in the early Tanner stage of development if certain pitfalls are avoided (Hui et al. 2012; Kim et al. 2012). The success of these methods in providing knee stability in adulthood and in prevention of OA needs to be assessed.

Gender

The incidence of ACL injury is several times higher in females than in males (Sutton and Bullock 2013). Possible reasons for this difference include both extrinsic factors, such as muscle strength and landing biomechanics, and intrinsic factors such as joint laxity and notch dimensions.

The female knee has been reported to have distinct intrinsic anatomical characteristics. The notch dimensions are probably the most widely evaluated anatomical differences between men and women. The notch width is narrower in women, and notch stenosis is more prevalent (LaPrade and Burnett 1994). Women have an increased quadriceps angle and posterior tibial slope that could predispose to ACL injury. Females also have a smaller ACL cross-sectional area and a lower ratio of ACL width to femoral intercondylar notch width. These anatomical differences may require special surgical considerations, such as performing routine notchplasty and performing an anatomic single-bundle ACL reconstruction versus a double-bundle surgery when reconstructing female knees.

There is some evidence to support the hypothesis that the mechanical properties of the ACL are subject to change throughout the menstrual cycle, becoming more lax during the preovulatory phase. Similarly, ACL injury rate is reported to increase during the ovulatory phase (Belanger et al. 2013).

Female and male athletes appear to land differently. The type of landing patterns may be significant when screening for injury risk factors. Females who land with the knees in inadequate flexion and in greater-than-normal valgus and external rotation are at increased risk of ACL injury (Butler et al. 2013). When limited to a contact injury mechanism, females are more likely to injure the ACL in their supporting leg, whereas males tend to injure their kicking leg. This research suggests that limb dominance serve as an etiological factor for ACL injuries sustained while playing soccer (Brophy et al. 2010).

Following ACL reconstruction female athletes are more likely than male athletes to rupture the contralateral ACL. However, the re-rupture risk of the reconstructed knee is similar between males and females (Shelbourne et al. 2009). No single factor has been strongly correlated to increased ACL tears in women. Further studies on gender differences are necessary to develop specific rehabilitation protocols or to modify surgical techniques.

Although self-reported outcomes in the first 2 years following reconstruction with soft tissue allografts are worse for females than males, longer-term studies demonstrate no difference between males and females (Paterno et al. 2012).

Female patients have greater knee laxity following an ACL reconstruction with a hamstring autograft compared with males who underwent a similar procedure. These results are derived from lower-level evidence, because no randomized central trials have answered this question (Sutton and Bullock 2013).

It has been shown by Wu et al. that the ACL femoral footprint size and gender are not correlated. It is therefore concluded that gender must not be regarded as a critical factor when deciding whether to perform a double-bundle ACL reconstruction or not (Wu et al. 2011).

Work and Activity

The majority of patients following an ACL injury will have static and dynamic instability and will be symptomatic. Dynamic stability has been defined as the ability of a joint to remain stable when subjected to rapidly shifting loads during motion. Only a small number of patients will achieve dynamic stability without surgical intervention. Following a proper ACL reconstruction, static stability of the knee is restored. Evidence of dynamic stability restoration and return to pre-injury levels of activity is missing.

In the beginning of the 1980s, Noyes reported that some patients with ACL tears would compensate well and described the "rule of thirds" (Noyes et al. 1983). This rule simply states that one third of the patients will compensate well and return to sports activities with sudden cutting and pivoting, one third will avoid symptoms of instability through modification or substitution of activities, and one third will deteriorate and require reconstructive surgery.

Eastlack et al. have developed a similar classification, grouping patients as "potential copers" and "non-copers" (Eastlack et al. 1999). Potential copers are individuals who have the ability to restore dynamic stability through rehabilitation and are candidates for conservative treatment (Fitzgerald et al. 2000). Several authors have attempted to define certain characteristics to identify potential copers and non-copers. Such identification would aid in deciding on indications for nonsurgical treatment and will improve the outcome of nonsurgical treatment.

Patients' "potential coper" or "non-coper" status seems to be affected by not only the results of nonsurgical treatment but also has bearing on postoperative clinical results. The important issue is to determine the adequacy and limitations of the scanning tests. "Non-coper" patients may regain static stability after surgery to the extent that their postoperative results in certain tests are indicative of "coper" status. It has not been possible to prove that this is a condition of actual dynamic stability and patients are restored to pre-injury activity level and that they will not experience further problems in activities with sudden cutting and pivoting. These conditions have been the subject of many studies in the 2000s, but need to be reexamined with the current advanced surgical techniques in mind.

Reconstruction of ACL restores knee mechanic stability and facilitates biointegration and reinnervation of the graft, which is important in providing dynamic stability via providing afferent proprioceptive signals that can trigger protective signals. Failure of this proprioceptive recovery theoretically interrupts the dynamic responses, causing a delay in muscle response to anterior translation forces. Static stability of the reconstructed knee may be inadequate to resist repetitive forces, making the knee susceptible to laxity, re-rupture, or loss of function.

In the Tegner and Lysholm activity scales, the patients' activity level is graded according to sports participation and work. Occupational activity is grouped as work sedentary, work light labor, work moderately, and work heavy labor, whereas sports activities are grouped as competitive or recreational sports. Indications for ACL reconstruction should be evaluated on the basis of patient's activity level, degree of instability, and desire to continue vigorous physical activity. Recreational and competitive activities are further subdivided according to specific sports involved. These different sports and occupations require different activity levels. The problems posed by an unstable knee and the minimum activity level required following surgery vary among those different occupations and sports. Some authors base their graft type and fixation techniques according to the patient's activity level and sports participation.

Patellar tendon grafts should be preferred for athletes involved in sports where hamstring injury is common (football, sprinting). Soft tissue tendon grafts are reported to be suitable for sports which include kneeling. Hamstring tendons must be preferred for athletes subjected to patellar tendon pathologies (basketball, volleyball, tennis). Hamstring tendons are associated with slightly increased anterior–posterior laxity, and patellar tendons are associated with increased kneeling pain as a result of donor site morbidity (Steiner et al. 2008).

Harvesting the hamstring graft causes graft site morbidity similar to muscle sprain and may pose problems for sports like sprint and weight lifting. Mark Miller prefers patellar tendon graft for American football players, ballet dancers, gymnasts, sprinters, hurdlers, and high-profile athletes and hamstring graft for athletes involved in jumping sports (Miller and Hart 2010). Some authors state that patellar tendon graft should be used if return to pre-injury activity level is crucial (Macaulay et al. 2012).

Osteoarthritis

ACL tears are reported to accelerate joint degeneration and lead to osteoarthritis in a high proportion of patients. ACL tears, whether treated surgically or not, are clearly associated with an increased osteoarthritis incidence in former soccer players, and ACL reconstruction has not been shown to conclusively reduce OA risk (Ahldén et al. 2012). Altered knee biomechanics, meniscal, chondral, and other soft tissue injuries and patient factors all contribute to an accelerated development of OA after ACL injury. Osteoarthritis after ACL reconstruction is related to increased intra-articular pressure after surgery, bone marrow edema and partially resolved biomechanical defects, and presence of concomitant meniscal, chondral, and other internal joint lesions. Following ACL reconstruction, failure to regain full ROM, especially in extension, predisposes the patient to osteoarthritis and poor clinical outcome (Shelbourne et al. 2007).

Long-term retrospective studies point to the success of ACL reconstruction with patellar tendon autograft in providing knee stability and return to sports. However, early development of osteoarthritis in knees with concomitant ACL reconstruction and meniscectomy remains unsolved. Improved rotational stability claimed by supporters of the double-bundle technique may be a potential reason to prefer this method in knees with meniscectomy to prevent osteoarthritis in the long term.

Radiological evaluation of an arthritic knee with ACL rupture needs to be done on a compartmental basis. Radiological morphological changes such as femoral notch narrowing and prominent eminences are specific to chronic ACL rupture and are not related to osteoarthritis.

If patellofemoral osteoarthritis is present, many surgeons avoid using a patellar tendon autograft, usually preferring allograft. Isolated medial compartment osteoarthritis caused by malalignment necessitates addition of high tibial valgus osteotomy to ACL reconstruction. Cases with long-term ACL deficiency and unsatisfactory conservative treatment present with multiple compartment osteoarthritis, diminished ROM, and evidence of moderate osteoarthritis during arthroscopy. Surgeons should abstain from reconstructing these knees as degenerative process accelerates in such cases following surgical intervention.

Early or Late Reconstruction

The timing of ACL reconstruction has long been debated. The standard approach is the one stated by Shelbourne, which is to delay surgery until clinical signs of inflammation subside. There must be minimal or no swelling, no hyperemia, and full range of motion. This period is usually 3 weeks. Shelbourne et al. reported increased risk of arthrofibrosis and loss of range of motion, particularly extension, in knees operated in the first week following injury. Loss of range of motion is a serious predisposing factor to osteoarthritis (Shelbourne et al. 2012).

In contrast, Bottoni et al. reported very good results with early ACL reconstruction in their randomized prospective trial and stated that those standard criteria for timing of surgery, no swelling, full range of motion, and diminished pain do not necessarily apply to all cases (Bottoni et al. 2008). The rationale in this approach was that surgery in a recovered knee following acute phase of the injury delivered a second blow. Early ACL reconstruction rendered the surgical trauma into the acute phase of the injury. Furthermore, additional meniscal and chondral injuries caused by recurring episodes of instability are prevented. Also, meniscal repair has a higher chance of success if performed in the early period. Delaying the surgery causes simple lesion that could be treated with simple partial meniscectomy to turn into complicated degenerative lesions.

Numerous studies evaluate the results of chronic ACL tear reconstruction, accompanying injuries, and their effect on the outcome (Tandogan et al. 2004; Demirağ et al. 2011). Long-term ACL deficiency causes morphological changes in the notch and the eminences. Drilling through these eminences carries the risk of blowout fracture of the tibial cortex around the tunnel opening and irregular tunnel widening. To prevent this, smaller diameter tunnels may be drilled first and dilators can be used. The altered anatomy of these areas makes it harder to identify ACL footprints on tibia and femur. In such cases, distance from the posterior and inferior sides of the intercondylar notch is more reliable.

Delaying the surgery decreases the success of meniscal repair and causes simple lesions that could be treated with simple partial meniscectomy to turn into complicated degenerative lesions. Focal chondral lesions also tend to turn into diffuse pathologies that cannot be treated arthroscopically. The presence of these chondral and meniscal lesions causes repeating episodes of knee swelling.

Associated Lesions

Low-grade (1–2) cartilage lesions associated with ACL tears usually do not need any treatment. Full-thickness, focal lesions necessitate treatment with autologous transplantation, which is a more aggressive treatment method when compared to microfracture and debridement. When using this method, any interaction with the tunnels must be carefully assessed around the notch and the superolateral cartilage, where the graft is harvested.

Meniscus tears accompanying low-grade cartilage lesions can usually be treated with simple debridement. The patients should be informed about higher incidence of osteoarthritis following concomitant meniscectomy and ACL reconstruction.

Meniscal tears repaired during ACL reconstruction surgery are reported to heal well. Both procedures complement each other. A well-repaired functional meniscus is essential to restore joint stability. Meniscal repair together with ACL reconstruction can be accomplished in a single tourniquet time. Inflating the tourniquet only at times when a clear view of the joint is necessary will prevent exceeding the tourniquet time. Another option if the repair is complicated is to repair the meniscus first and to perform the ACL reconstruction approximately 1 month later. The time until the second surgery should not be delayed to prevent occurrence of additional injuries and prolonged rehabilitation period.

ACL reconstruction in knees with additional ligament injuries requires a different approach. If there is additional MCL injury because both ligaments are disrupted, the knee can become unstable in several planes of function. ACL reconstruction should be delayed till inflammation subsides and ROM is restored, in order to prevent arthrofibrosis. Third degree instabilities require simultaneous repair or reconstruction of the MCL. Bracing following ACL reconstruction can treat I° and II° degree lesion. Massive uncontrolled valgus stress during the surgery should be avoided since it will cause additional tension on the already damaged MCL. A patellar tendon graft is preferable as harvesting the hamstring tendons, secondary medial stabilizers of the knee joint, will diminish the already compromised medial support.

Another important lesion is the posterolateral corner (PLC) injury. The varus stress and dial tests are valuable when diagnosing these lesions. PLC injury accompanying ACL rupture should definitely be reconstructed. Otherwise, the outcome of ACL injury is poor and in the long term ligament laxity develops (LaPrade et al. 1999). Presence of additional ligament injuries frequently prompts use of allograft materials.

Anatomy

The patellar tendon should have a width of at least 3 cm, otherwise either the graft harvested will be less than 10 mm in width or the remaining patellar tendon will have insufficient medial and lateral tissue with weaker bony attachments. MRI can evaluate the patellar tendon width preoperatively. If preoperative MRI reveals a width of less than 3 cm, hamstring tendon grafts should be used. Sometimes this situation is evident only after surgical exploration. In such cases, the skin incision needs to be extended and soft tissue grafts must be harvested.

In cases with patellofemoral osteoarthritis, patellar tendon grafts should be avoided. Similarly, the sequelae of Osgood–Schlatter's disease may cause deformity of the tibial tuberosity.

The risk of tunnel–graft mismatch increases if patellar tendon graft is longer than 100 mm. Solutions such as staple fixation of the tibial end of the graft may be required.

If one chooses a transtibial ACL reconstruction, the distal orifice of the tibial tunnel must lie inside the triangle formed by MCL, tibial joint line, and patellar tendon (Steiner et al. 2008). Drilling the tunnel as close to MCL as possible will allow for an ideal horizontal graft angle. Attention must be paid to avoid disrupting the MCL, especially in smaller knees. The tip of the internal tibial tunnel guide must be placed medial to the anterior horn of the lateral meniscus. Displacing the tunnel posteriorly or toward PLC may be accepted; anterior translation should be avoided. Such adjustments are relatively hard in smaller knees.

If the medial plateau is depressed and wineglass shaped, drilling a close to the horizontal tunnel may result in a tunnel roof that is too thin and may injure the anterior horn of the medial meniscus or cause the tibial plateau to blow out.

Knees with narrow notches and short AP distance may be suitable for single-bundle ACL anatomic reconstruction. If the notch is relatively wide and tibial plateau is circular in the transverse plane rather than elliptical, the double-bundle technique may be more suitable. The authors believe that single-bundle reconstruction with horizontal graft placement is able to provide better rotational stability if the plateau is elliptic in the transverse plane.

In knees with a decreased lateral femoral condyle height, a horizontal femoral tunnel leaves a short bone segment lateral to the tunnel. Cortical-cancellous fixation materials may protrude through the lateral wall of the femur, irritating the iliotibial band and lateral patellar retinaculum during knee motion. Patients with such anatomical characteristics should be considered for other graft-fixation methods such as loop fixation or interference screws.

Tear Morphology

Injury to the ACL may result in total disruption of tendon integrity or in partial tear with some ligamentous tissue remaining intact. Pattern of injury, along with other factors as age, gender, and work, depicts the mode of treatment. Partial tear of ACL is a common injury with its incidence ranging from 10 % to 28 %. The simplest form of a partial tear results from low-energy knee sprain. Despite elongation and stretching, ligament integrity is preserved, a reactive synovial tissue forms covering the ligament, and small bleeding foci appear along the damaged fibers. Partial lesions used to be defined according to the percentage of the ligament remaining intact. Because such a precise percentage is subjective and always hard to diagnose with arthroscopy, it may be simplified by referring to those with more than 50 % damage as high-grade and those with less than 50 % as low-grade partial tears (Hong et al. 2003). Double-bundle supports tend to describe the lesion by referring to the specific bundle that is ruptured as if anteromedial (AMB) or posterolateral (PLB) bundle. Defining the injury as present in either the AMB or PLB is important to develop an appropriate treatment plan.

The history of a patient with a partial tear of the ACL is similar to complete ACL tears. The patient usually describes a feeling of a pop inside the knee during a twisting motion, followed by acute swelling and pain. The force of trauma may be less compared to complete ACL tears, and some patients are able to continue the sports activity immediately after the injury. The clinical picture of motion restriction, effusion, pain, and spasm of hamstring muscles, defined as "angry knee" by some authors, is much less dramatic and usually is shorter. Patient history may help to identify the torn bundle, because the AMB is injured usually with the knee flexed, whereas PLB is torn with the knee in extension and internal rotation (Girgis et al. 1975, Furman et al. 1976).

The Lachman, anterior drawer, and pivot shift tests are valuable to diagnose a partial tear. Instrumented laxity tests such as KT-1000 are useful to objectively quantify the amount of laxity; however, increased muscle tension in a painful and swollen knee may result in inaccurate results. Instrumented laxity tests on partial ACL tears may reveal 3–5 mm of difference in anterior translation between the intact and the injured knee. It is widely accepted that laxity tests of a partial tear are mildly positive compared to a complete tear, with a relatively hard end point. The Lachman and anterior drawer tests may fail to detect laxity if more than 25 % of the ligament is intact (Hole et al. 1996). A lack of anterior translation and an increased internal rotation in isolated PLB tears cause negative anterior drawer and Lachman tests, whereas the pivot shift is positive. On the contrary, rupture of the AMB causes marked anterior translation, especially during the Lachman test (Christel et al. 2012). However it is not valuable in differentiating between AMB or PLB tears.

Although imaging tests are useful, the diagnosis of a partial tear is almost always confirmed arthroscopically. A careful and thorough assessment is necessary to evaluate the functionality of the remaining ligament and to identify if the tear is diffuse or limited to a single bundle. If the remaining ligament is adequate to provide stability, no intervention is necessary and other intraarticular pathologies are addressed. In cases with knee instability, partial or standard ACL reconstruction is performed.

It is not possible to clinically diagnose simple partial tears as long as the knee is functionally stable. Increased intrasubstance signal intensity in MRI and arthroscopic demonstration of hemorrhage on the tendon fibers may indicate a partial tear. It is important to differentiate a partial tear from mucoid degeneration on MRI. Although acute partial tears are easier to recognize, chronic cases may also present with isolated AMB or PLB injuries. Careful debridement of torn fibers aids in identifying the nature of injury. The mass of remnant ligament, direction of the fibers, tension of the ligament observed at various knee flexion angles, and physical examination under general anesthesia are important factors when planning the treatment method. Sometimes the injury is not isolated in a single bundle, and a diffuse pattern of damage is present on both bundles. This results in the formation of a pathological tissue mass where injured fibers, remnant ligament, and elongated fibers merge as a single unit. In such cases where ligament injury is not limited to a single-bundle, morphological properties of the remaining intact tissue are as important as the disrupted portion in indicating treatment (Ochi et al. 2006). Crain et al. have defined three types of scar morphology following complete ACL tear (Crain et al. 2005). The torn ligament may adhere onto the PLC, roof of the intercondylar notch, or anterior distal to the proximal footprint. This last pattern is important because it provides a small degree of anterior stability.

Macroscopic and microscopic anatomy of a partially torn ACL is disrupted whether the injury is diffuse or isolated to a single bundle. The synovial cover disappears and epiligamentous circulation is diminished. This causes circulatory compromise of a portion of the intact fibers and results in partial necrosis. Repetitive traumas or episodes of instability may increase the extent of injury. Certain intra-articular cytokines and biological agents diffuse through ACL and disrupt the structural properties of the ligament. Following these, a partial tear may progress to a complete tear (Dye 1996).

Partial ACL tears may present with three different scenarios: following an acute injury, in chronic cases with symptoms of instability, or as incidental findings where arthroscopy is performed to address a different intra-articular pathology. Prolonged pain and instability in the chronic phase is indicative for surgical intervention. Possible surgical interventions include surgical reconstruction of a single anteromedial or posterolateral bundle with tendon graft if the remaining bundle is intact and functional, augmentation with preservation of the remnant part, and standard single- or double-bundle ACL reconstruction following resection of the remaining intact fibers. The last approach is technically the same as standard reconstruction, and it is suitable when the remaining ligamentous tissue is shown to be clinically nonfunctional.

Conclusion

Anatomical and biological properties of ACL differ between individuals. Similarly, patient expectations and activity levels vary greatly. All these factors should be considered before ACL reconstruction. The main aim of ACL reconstruction is to restore tendon anatomy and biology and patients' activity levels as close to pre-injury state as possible. This requires a detailed preoperative planning based on individual characteristics of the patient. Factors which make a difference in diagnosis, treatment, and postoperative rehabilitation need to be clearly defined in order to improve the outcome. A thorough understanding of these factors is necessary to develop an individualized algorithm, both for diagnosis and treatment of ACL rupture.

References

Ahldén M, Samuelsson K, Sernert N, Forssblad M, Karlsson J, Kartus J (2012) The Swedish National Anterior Cruciate Ligament Register: a report on baseline variables and outcomes of surgery for almost 18,000 patients. Am J Sports Med 40(10):2230–2235

Arbuthnot JE, Brink RB (2010) The role of anterior cruciate ligament reconstruction in the older patients, 55 years or above. Knee Surg Sports Traumatol Arthrosc 18(1):73–78

Belanger L, Burt D, Callaghan J, Clifton S, Gleberzon BJ (2013) Anterior cruciate ligament laxity related to the menstrual cycle: an updated systematic review of the literature. J Can Chiropr Assoc 57(1):76–86

Bottoni CR, Liddell TR, Trainor TJ, Freccero DM, Lindell KK (2008) Postoperative range of motion following anterior cruciate ligament reconstruction using autograft hamstrings: a prospective, randomized clinical trial of early versus delayed reconstructions. Am J Sports Med 36(4):656–662

Brophy R, Silvers HJ, Gonzales T, Mandelbaum BR (2010) Gender influences: the role of leg dominance in ACL injury among soccer players. Br J Sports Med 44(10):694–697

Brown CA, McAdams TR, Harris AH, Maffulli N, Safran MR (2013) ACL reconstruction in patients aged 40 years and older: a systematic review and introduction of a new methodology score for ACL studies. Am J Sports Med 41(9):2181–2190

Butler RJ, Willson JD, Fowler D, Queen RM (2013) Gender differences in landing mechanics vary depending on the type of landing. Clin J Sport Med 23(1):52–57

Christel PS, Akgun U, Yasar T, Karahan M, Demirel B (2012) The contribution of each anterior cruciate ligament bundle to the Lachman test: a cadaver investigation. J Bone Joint Surg Br 94(1):68–74

Crain EH, Fithian DC, Paxton EW, Luetzow WF (2005) Variation in anterior cruciate ligament scar pattern: does the scar pattern affect anterior laxity in anterior cruciate ligament-deficient knees? Arthroscopy 21(1):19–24

Demirağ B, Aydemir F, Daniş M, Ermutlu C (2011) Incidence of meniscal and osteochondral lesions in patients undergoing delayed anterior cruciate ligament reconstruction. Acta Orthop Traumatol Turc 45(5):348–352

Dye SF (1996) The future of anterior cruciate ligament restoration. Clin Orthop Relat Res 325:130–139

Eastlack ME, Axe MJ, Snyder-Mackler L (1999) Laxity, instability, and functional outcome after ACL injury: copers versus noncopers. Med Sci Sports Exerc 31:210–215

Fabricant PD, Jones KJ, Delos D, Cordasco FA, Marx RG, Pearle AD, Warren RF, Green DW (2013) Reconstruction of the anterior cruciate ligament in the skeletally immature athlete: a review of current concepts: AAOS exhibit selection. J Bone Joint Surg Am 95(5):e28

Fitzgerald GK, Axe MJ, Snyder-Mackler L (2000) A decision-making scheme for returning patients to high level activity with nonoperative treatment after anterior cruciate ligament rupture. Knee Surg Sports Traumatol Arthrosc 8:76–82

Furman W, Marshall JL, Girgis FG (1976) The anterior cruciate ligament. A functional analysis based on postmortem studies. J Bone Joint Surg Am 58:179–185

Gee AO, Kinsella S, Huffman GR, Sennett BJ, Tjoumakaris FP (2013) Anterior cruciate ligament reconstruction in patients aged >40 years: a case-control study. Phys Sportsmed 41(1):30–34

Girgis FG, Marshall JL, Monajem A (1975) The cruciate ligaments of the knee joint. Anatomical, functional and experimental analysis. Clin Orthop Relat Res 106:216–231

Griffin LY, Agel J, Albohm MJ et al (2000) Noncontact anterior cruciate ligament injuries: risk factors and prevention strategies. J Am Acad Orthop Surg 8(3):141–150

Hole RL, Lintner DM, Kamaric E, Moseley JB (1996) Increased tibial translation after partial sectioning of the anterior cruciate ligament. The posterolateral bundle. Am J Sports Med 24(4):556–560

Hong SH, Choi JY, Lee GK, Choi JA, Chung HW, Kang HS (2003) Grading of anterior cruciate ligament injury. Diagnostic efficacy of oblique coronal magnetic resonance imaging of the knee. J Comput Assist Tomogr 27:814–819

Hui C, Roe J, Ferguson D, Waller A, Salmon L, Pinczewski L (2012) Outcome of anatomic transphyseal anterior cruciate ligament reconstruction in Tanner stage 1 and 2 patients with open physes. Am J Sports Med 40(5):1093–1098

Kim SJ, Shim DW, Park KW (2012) Functional outcome of transphyseal reconstruction of the anterior cruciate ligament in skeletally immature patients. Knee Surg Relat Res 24(3):173–179

LaPrade RF, Burnett QM 2nd (1994) Femoral intercondylar notch stenosis and correlation to anterior cruciate ligament injuries. A prospective study. Am J Sports Med 22(2):198–202

LaPrade RF, Resig S, Wentorf F, Lewis JL (1999) The effects of grade III posterolateral knee complex injuries on anterior cruciate ligament graft force. A biomechanical analysis. Am J Sports Med 27(4):469–475

Legnani C, Terzaghi C, Borgo E, Ventura A (2011) Management of anterior cruciate ligament rupture in patients aged 40 years and older. J Orthop Traumatol 12(4):177–184

Macaulay AA, Perfetti DC, Levine WN (2012) Anterior cruciate ligament graft choices. Sports Health 4(1):63–68

McConkey MO, Bonasia DE, Amendola A (2011) Pediatric anterior cruciate ligament reconstruction. Curr Rev Musculoskelet Med 4(2):37–44

Miller MD, Hart J (2010) Overview of evaluation & technical pearls. In: Lieberman JR, Berry DJ, Azar FM (eds) Advanced reconstruction: knee. American Academy of Orthopaedic Surgeons, Rosemont

Noyes FR, Matthews DS, Mooar PA, Grood ES (1983) The symptomatic anterior cruciate-deficient knee. Part II: the results of rehabilitation, activity modification, and counseling on functional disability. J Bone Joint Surg Am 65:163–174

Ochi M, Adachi N, Deie M, Kanaya A (2006) Anterior cruciate ligament augmentation procedure with a 1-incision technique: anteromedial bundle or posterolateral bundle reconstruction. Arthroscopy 22(4):463e1–463e5

Paterno MV, Weed AM, Hewett TE (2012) A between sex comparison of anterior-posterior knee laxity after anterior cruciate ligament reconstruction with patellar tendon or hamstrings autograft: a systematic review. Sports Med 42(2):135–152

Seng K, Appleby D, Lubowitz JH (2008) Operative versus nonoperative treatment of anterior cruciate ligament rupture in patients aged 40 years or older: an expected-value decision analysis. Arthroscopy 24(8):914–920

Shelbourne KD, Biggs A, Gray T (2007) Deconditioned knee: the effectiveness of a rehabilitation program that restores normal knee motion to improve symptoms and function. N Am J Sports Phys Ther 2(2):81–89

Shelbourne KD, Gray T, Haro M (2009) Incidence of subsequent injury to either knee within 5 years after anterior cruciate ligament reconstruction with patellar tendon autograft. Am J Sports Med 37(2):246–251

Shelbourne KD, Freeman H, Gray T (2012) Osteoarthritis after anterior cruciate ligament reconstruction: the importance of regaining and maintaining full range of motion. Sports Health 4(1):79–85

Steadman JR, Matheny LM, Briggs KK, Rodkey WG, Carreira DS (2012) Outcomes following healing response in older, active patients: a primary anterior cruciate ligament repair technique. J Knee Surg 25(3):255–260

Steiner ME, Murray MM, Rodeo SA (2008) Strategies to improve anterior cruciate ligament healing and graft placement. Am J Sports Med 36(1):176–189

Sutton KM, Bullock JM (2013) Anterior cruciate ligament rupture: differences between males and females. J Am Acad Orthop Surg 21(1):41–50

Tandogan RN, Taşer O, Kayaalp A, Taşkiran E, Pinar H, Alparslan B, Alturfan A (2004) Analysis of meniscal and chondral lesions accompanying anterior cruciate ligament tears: relationship with age, time from injury, and level of sport. Knee Surg Sports Traumatol Arthrosc 12(4):262–270

Wu E, Chen M, Cooperman D, Victoroff B, Goodfellow D, Farrow LD (2011) No correlation of height or gender with anterior cruciate ligament footprint size. J Knee Surg 24(1):39–43

Physiotherapy in Patellofemoral Pain Syndrome

107

Defne Kaya, John Nyland, Michael J. Callaghan, and Mahmut Nedim Doral

Contents

D. Kaya (✉)
Department of Physical Therapy and Rehabilitation, Faculty of Health Science, Biruni University, İstanbul, Turkey
e-mail: defne@hacettepe.edu.tr

J. Nyland
Kosair Charities College of Health and Natural Sciences, Spalding University, Louisville, USA
e-mail: jnyland@spalding.edu; john.nyland@louisville.edu

M.J. Callaghan
Centre for Rehabilitation Science, University of Manchester, Manchester, UK
e-mail: michael.callaghan@manchester.ac.uk

M.N. Doral
Department of Orthopaedics and Traumatology and Department of Sports Medicine, Hacettepe University, Istanbul, Turkey
e-mail: mndoral@gmail.com; ndoral@hacettepe.edu.tr

M.N. Doral, J. Karlsson (eds.), *Sports Injuries*,
DOI 10.1007/978-3-642-36569-0_122

Abstract
Patellofemoral pain syndrome (PFPS) is one of the most common lower extremity conditions seen in orthopedic practice. The source of PFPS is believed to be multifactorial. Although PFPS is recognized as one of the most common lower extremity disorders encountered in the general population, its etiology and treatment remains controversial. This chapter discusses the efficacy of differing physiotherapy interventions with consideration for proximal, local, and distal factors, taping or bracing, and quadriceps muscle strengthening for PFPS treatment.

Introduction

Patellofemoral pain syndrome (PFPS) is a common problem experienced by adolescent and active adult populations, and it is often activity related and aggravated by functional activities such as stairs climbing, running, and squatting (Post and Fulkerson 1994). Common causative factors are lower extremity weakness, especially in the quadriceps muscles, malalignment of the lower extremity, foot deformity such as hallux valgus and increased subtalar pronation, and tightness of the lateral retinaculum, iliotibial band, hamstring muscles, and tensor fascia lata muscle (Thomeë et al. 1995; Kaya et al. 2009; Yosmaoglu et al. 2013). Correct patellar alignment may depend in part upon the balance of strength and neuromuscular activation timing between the vastus medialis obliquus (VMO) and vastus lateralis (VL) muscles. A VMO and VL imbalance is one proposed mechanism for abnormal patellar tracking (Cowan et al. 2001). Generalized quadriceps muscle weakness may result in patellar malposition (Dvir et al. 1990, 1991) and altered VMO timing, suggesting that muscle length changes at activation onset will negatively influence force-producing capability (Nordin and Frankel 1989).

Prior to approximately 2005, nonsurgical interventions for PFPS focused on patient education (Clark et al. 2000); soft tissue mobilization (*passive stabilizers of the knee*); strengthening exercises (*active stabilizers of the knee*) (McConnell 1996) such as quadriceps strengthening (Arroll et al. 1997); VMO and VL neuromuscular training exercises (Cerny 1995); patellar alignment correction techniques such as taping and bracing (McConnell 1996); electrical stimulation to facilitate quadriceps femoris muscle activation, especially for the VMO and VL (Kaya et al. 2013); and modalities such as cold application to reduce both pain and edema (Shelton and Thigpen 1991).

Following the 2nd International Patellofemoral Pain Research Retreat, physiotherapy interventions for PFPS have been reclassified. The aim of this retreat was to bring together scientists and clinicians from around the world who are conducting research aimed at understanding the factors that contribute to the development and, consequently, the treatment of PFPS (Powers et al. 2012).

In light of this retreat, it was recommended that clinicians should focus on:

Considering and if necessary correcting proximal, local, and distal factors
Appropriate use of taping or bracing
Treatment of quadriceps muscle weakness

(a) **Local Factors and Treatment Options**

***Relation Between Patellar Maltracking, VMO Movement, and Quadriceps Muscle Torque*:** Patellar maltracking increases patellofemoral reaction forces 0.5 times body weight during walking (Matthews et al. 1977) and up to more than seven times body weight during squatting (Mason et al. 2008). Patellar maltracking (lateral and/or superior shifted, tilted, rotated) may cause knee pain and decrease muscle strength (Derasari et al. 2010). Patellar taping has been shown to reduce knee pain (Warden et al. 2008) and improve patellofemoral kinematics (Derasari et al. 2010). Patellar taping can correct malalignments such as lateral shift, lateral tilt, and varus rotation compared to the untaped state (Derasari et al. 2010). Additionally, the imbalance caused by atrophy and dysplasia of the oblique portion of the vastus medialis obliquus muscle (VMO) plays an important role in patellar malalignment (Cerny 1995). Vastus medialis obliquus muscle training exercises and/or a general quadriceps-strengthening program can reduce knee pain, improve function, and improve the quality of life of patients with PFPS (Syme et al. 2009). Interventions such as taping, electrical stimulation, bracing, VMO training, lower leg training, and correcting patellar maltracking should be considered in physiotherapy programming.

***Relation Between the Proprioception Deficit and Patellofemoral Pain Syndrome*:** Abnormal knee proprioception has been identified among subjects with PFPS compared to healthy control subjects (Callaghan 2011). Squats with internally and externally rotated hip positions (Balci et al. 2009), using of a hip-stabilizing orthosis, functional exercises to increase hip muscle strength (Lee et al. 2012), and patellar taping or bracing (Callaghan et al. 2012) should be rehabilitation program considerations to improve knee proprioception and dynamic postural stability.

***Metabolic Activity*:** Increased subchondral bone metabolic activity has been demonstrated in individuals with idiopathic PFPS (Naslund et al. 2005). They reported that scintigrams of 44 % of the painful knees and 52 % of the patients showed diffuse uptake (Naslund et al. 2005). Further work is needed to substantiate these deficits and better discern the efficacy of differing treatment options.

(b) **Distal Factors and Treatment Options**

An association between excessive subtalar pronation, patellar maltracking, and PFPS has been described (Tiberio 1987). Tiberio (1987) stated that to achieve knee extension in midstance, the tibia must externally rotate relative to the femur to ensure adequate motion for the screw-home mechanism of the knee. To compensate for this lack of tibial external rotation, the femur would have to internally rotate on the tibia such that the tibia is in a position of relative external rotation. Compensatory internal rotation of the femur would therefore permit the necessary screw-home mechanics needed to enable knee extension during midstance (Tiberio 1987).

The delayed peak rearfoot eversion and a greater amount of rearfoot eversion at heel strike during walking and running and less rearfoot eversion range during running were shown in patients with PFPS (Barton et al. 2009). However, the possible association between the kinematic variations, patellofemoral joint loading, pain, and subsequent pathology is still unclear. Additionally, peak rearfoot eversion and peak tibia internal rotation are positively correlated in patients with PFPS (Barton et al. 2012).

The traditional paradigm that foot orthoses work via mechanical alterations has been expanded to include alternative paradigms of shock attenuation, neuromuscular effects, proprioceptive input, or placebo (Powers et al. 2012). Custom-made foot orthoses (Munuera and Mazoteras-Pardo 2011), medially wedged foot orthoses (minimal effect) (Boldt et al. 2013), unmodified prefabricated foot orthoses (Barton et al. 2011), off-the-shelf foot orthoses, and flat inserts (Collins et al. 2009) should be given physiotherapy program consideration to improve lower extremity function and decrease knee pain among patients with PFPS.

Although several studies have provided data displaying prolonged or excessive subtalar pronation in patients with PFPS, the presence of hallux valgus in this group of patients has only recently been described (Kaya et al. 2009). Kaya et al. (2009) reported that 84 out of 99 patients had an abnormal hallux valgus angle on the affected side and 78 out of 99 patients had an abnormal hallux valgus angle on the unaffected side. This study revealed a significant difference between the hallux valgus angles of patients with unilateral PFPS and their asymptomatic limb (Kaya et al. 2009). Further comprehensive biomechanical studies are warranted to analyze the relationship between hallux valgus angle and PFPS and pain pathways.

(c) **Proximal Factors and Treatment Options**

Patellofemoral pain syndrome is associated with decreased hip strength, specifically at the abductors and external rotators (Powers 2010; Souza et al. 2010). An association between increased dynamic quadriceps angle, increased patellofemoral joint stress, and excessive hip adduction during weight-bearing activities is well-known (Powers 2010). Additionally, a direct relationship between excessive femur internal rotation during weight-bearing activities and patellar maltracking has been described in patients with PFPS (Souza et al. 2010).

An association between decreased hip strength and PFPS has also been reported (Meira and Brumitt 2011). Because the hip muscles help control frontal plane femur position, thereby assisting with the control of knee valgus, increasing their strength may help patients with PFPS. Specifically, hip abductor strengthening can positively influence knee valgus alterations.

Strengthening programs include simple more isolated isometric exercises (prone heel squeezes), to exercises that integrate the knee and hip such as manual perturbations in side lying, standing hip abduction against a resistance band, side-to-side walking with a resistance band around the ankles ("monster walking"), eccentric exercises, pelvic drop exercises, lateral step-ups, depth squats, single-leg squats on a physioball, modified single-leg squats, side bridges, and lunges while twisting (Meira and Brumitt 2011).

***Interesting Approach*: Lumbo-pelvic Manipulation:** Correction of sacroiliac joint dysfunction may facilitate knee extensor muscle activation among patients with PFPS patients (Suter et al. 1999). Sacroiliac joint or lumbo-pelvic region manipulation may help decrease quadriceps inhibition in the involved knees of patients with PFPS (Suter et al. 1999; Iverson et al. 2008).

Treatment of Quadriceps Muscle Weakness for the Treatment of the PFPS

Because the contact area between the patella and the femur changes throughout knee flexion and extension, the quadriceps-strengthening exercise prescription for patients with PFPS must be well designed. *Open kinetic chain exercises* are performed typically where the foot is free to move. These exercises are essentially non-weight bearing, with the movement occurring at the knee. If there is any resistance applied, it is applied to the distal lower extremity (Miller and Croce 2007). During open kinetic chain activities such as seated knee extensions, patellofemoral joint reaction forces increase as the knee moves from 90° flexion to full knee extension (Lieb and Perry 1971). The most dramatic increase in patellofemoral joint reaction forces occurs from 30° knee flexion to full extension (McConnell and Fulkerson 1996). *Closed kinetic chain exercises* are performed where the foot is fixed on the ground. The foot remains in constant contact with the surface, usually the ground or the base of an exercise device such as a leg press. These exercises are typically weight-bearing exercises, where the patient uses his or her own body weight and/or external resistance. Since closed kinetic chain exercises involve multi-joint movements, they are often labelled as being more sport-specific exercise (Miller and Croce 2007). During closed kinetic chain activities such as squats, patellofemoral joint reaction forces increase with increasing knee flexion, especially between 30° knee flexion and full knee flexion (McConnell and Fulkerson 1996).

Safe Ranges for Exercises: Doucette and Child reported improved patellofemoral joint congruence angles during closed kinetic chain exercises between 0° and 20° knee flexion and open kinetic chain exercises from 30° flexion to full knee flexion (Doucette and Child 1996). These findings are consistent with the report of Steinkamp et al. which suggested that the optimal range for open kinetic chain exercise peripatellar muscle strengthening such as a seated knee extension was from 90° to 60°, while the best range during closed kinetic chain exercise such as a seated leg press was from 0° to 30° flexion (Steinkamp et al. 1993). These range of motion limits created the lowest patellofemoral joint reaction forces.

Open Kinetic Chain Exercise

Isometric Quadriceps Exercise

Pain-free quadriceps exercises are important when treating patients with PFPS (Malone et al. 2002). Isometric quadriceps exercises have been advocated for patients with PFPS and eccentric muscle activations (Möller et al. 1986). Comparatively isolated vastus medialis muscle training in conjunction with functional lower extremity training has also been recommended (Doucette and Goble 1992).

Isometric quadriceps exercises such as straight leg raises can facilitate quadriceps activation without stressing the patellofemoral joint while minimizing patellofemoral joint reaction forces, because the patella has no contact with the femoral condyles in the full extension position (McMullen et al. 1990).

It is widely known that patients with PFPS can benefit from isometric quadriceps exercises and straight leg raise exercises, particularly during the acute care period (Eburne and Bannister 1996; Roush et al. 2000; Thomeé 1997). Roush et al. investigated the effects of modified straight leg raise exercises ("Muncie method") in the treatment of patients with PFPS (Roush et al. 2000). They evaluated pain, functional level, and isokinetic strength of the quadriceps muscle at the beginning and end of treatment (Roush et al. 2000). They found that patients who performed quadriceps-strengthening home exercise program with modified straight leg raise exercises had significantly less pain and improved function (Roush et al. 2000). These results showed that patients with PFPS can benefit from isometric quadriceps-strengthening and straight leg raise exercises. A physiotherapy program that includes isometric and straight leg raise exercises, particularly during the acute care phase, can positively enhance function in patients with PFPS.

Isokinetic Exercise

Isokinetic exercises differ from isometrics in that they allow subjects to move the tibia over the femur through a selected range of motion and velocity. Closed-chain exercises are safest in the 0–45° range. In contrast to closed-chain exercises, open-chain exercises (leg curls and seated knee extensions) are most safely performed from 25° to 90° for patients with PFPS (Steinkamp et al. 1993; Stiene et al. 1996; Grelsamer and Klein 1998). These researchers agree with the potential for excessive patellofemoral contact forces when performing resisted open-chain knee extension exercises near terminal knee extension.

Using a pretest, posttest study design, Hazneci et al. (2005) compared 24 men with PFPS and 24 healthy men for isokinetic knee muscle strength. An isokinetic exercise protocol was performed at angular velocities of 60° and 180°/s. These sessions were repeated three times/week for 6 weeks. After isokinetic exercise protocol intervention, peak torque and total quadriceps and hamstring work improved significantly in the PFPS group. They suggested that improved knee muscle strength and work capacity also had positive effects on passive knee joint position sense. Their finding showed that isokinetic exercise prescription in rehabilitation protocols for patients with PFPS not only improves knee stabilization but also proprioceptive acuity (Hazneci et al. 2005).

McMullen et al. (1990) designed a 2-phase isokinetic program for patients with chondromalacia patella. Phase 1 included low-speed 30°, 60°, 90°, and 120°/s angular velocities performed in a short range of motion arc (30° to 0°). When patients could perform Phase 1 exercises without pain, they progressed to Phase 2 which included high-speed 180°, 240°, and 300°/s angular velocities through a larger range of motion arc (90° to 0°). They reported that some patients did not tolerate an aggressive isokinetic program (McMullen et al. 1990).

Werner and Eriksson (1993) evaluated the effect of eccentric quadriceps training in patients with unilateral PFPS and compared them to the effects of eccentric and concentric quadriceps training in patients with bilateral PFPS. Fifteen patients and nine age- and sex-matched healthy controls participated in this study. Nine patients with unilateral PFPS performed eccentric exercises, while six with bilateral PFPS trained one knee eccentrically and one knee concentrically. Quadriceps muscle training was performed on a Kin-Com dynamometer at 90° and 120°/s angular velocity twice a week for 8 weeks. Before and after the treatment period, thigh muscle torques were measured at 60°, 90°, 120° and 180°/s for quadriceps and at 60° and 180°/s for hamstrings. For functional evaluation, a functional knee score was calculated before training, after 8 weeks of training and at a mean of 3.4 years after completion of the training. After 8 weeks of training and at follow-up times of 1 and 3.4 years, the patients were also questioned regarding whether or not they felt improvement from the training program. Knee pain magnitude was measured using the Borg Pain Scale. This study reported that, compared with control subjects, patients with PFPS had a significantly lower knee extensor torque in their painful leg at all test velocities. The greatest difference was found during eccentric quadriceps activations. After training, the eccentrically trained group of patients with PFPS displayed improvements in both eccentric and concentric knee extensor torque. Of the six patients in the bilateral training group, there were five who increased concentric knee extensor torque and three who increased eccentric torque. Patients in both groups reported no pain or mild pain during the training sessions (Werner and Eriksson 1993).

Results from these studies verified that patients with PFPS can benefit from isokinetic exercises if they perform all exercises in a pain-free range of knee motion.

Closed Kinetic Chain Exercise

In closed kinetic chain exercises, more selective vastus medialis obliquus activation can be obtained at 60° of knee flexion (Tang et al. 2001). Maximal vastus medialis obliquus/vastus lateralis ratio was also observed at this knee flexion angle, and muscle contraction intensity was also greatest at this angle (Tang et al. 2001).

Witvrouw et al. compared the efficacy of open kinetic chain versus closed-chain exercises in patients with PFPS (Witvrouw et al. 2000). Sixty patients were separated randomly into two groups: an open kinetic chain exercise group or a closed kinetic chain exercise group. Patients performed their exercise program over a 5-week duration. Isokinetic muscle strength, Kujala patellofemoral score, and flexibility and functional tests were evaluated pretreatment, posttreatment, and 3 months following treatment. Although patients improved functionally, the authors did not find any difference between the open kinetic chain and closed kinetic chain exercise group (Witvrouw et al. 2000). Their study showed that both open and closed kinetic chain exercise programs lead to an improved subjective and clinical outcome in patients with PFPS. Superior performance during functional tests such as the triple jump for distance among the closed kinetic chain group suggests that this type of program may be slightly better than a primarily open kinetic chain program in the treatment of patients with PFPS (Witvrouw et al. 2000).

In a later study, Witvrouw et al. (2004) followed up on these patients at approximately 5 years posttreatment finding that both groups maintained the good subjective and functional outcomes they had achieved immediately after conservative treatment. Significant group differences were not observed at the 5-year follow-up for the majority of the examined parameters. However, on 3 of the 18 visual analogue scale measures (pain during descending stairs, pain during jumping, and pain during sports), the open kinetic chain group showed fewer complaints than the closed kinetic chain group. The authors concluded that both open kinetic chain and closed kinetic chain exercise programs lead to equally successful long-term functional outcomes among PFPS patients (Witvrouw et al. 2004).

Stiene et al. evaluated the results of closed kinetic chain exercises versus isokinetic exercises performed over an 8-week period among patients with patellofemoral joint dysfunction (Stiene et al. 1996). At approximately 1-year post-program participation, both groups had significant improvements in peak isokinetic knee extensor torque at all angular velocities, but only the closed kinetic chain group showed significant improvement in closed kinetic chain testing and perceived functional status. They concluded that closed kinetic chain training may be more effective than joint isolation exercise in restoring function such as step-up performance in patients with patellofemoral dysfunction (Stiene et al. 1996).

Thomeé (1997) found no difference between isometric exercises and open- and closed-chain exercises for treatment of PFPS. Patients in the isometric group performed quadriceps isometric contractions. Patients in the other group performed open and closed kinetic chain exercises that focused on eccentric quadriceps activation. After 12 weeks, the researchers found that pain level decreased and functional level and muscle strength increased in both groups (Thomeé 1997); results of the aforementioned studies suggest that closed kinetic chain exercises may be more tolerable than open kinetic chain exercises for patients with PFPS.

Weight-Bearing Versus Non-Weight-Bearing Exercises

Both weight-bearing and non-weight-bearing exercises are considered appropriate for strengthening the quadriceps and can be considered as key elements in the treatment of PFPS (for examples of functional neuromuscular and functional proprioceptive exercises, see Tables 1 and 2).

Table 1 Functional neuromuscular exercises for patients with patellofemoral pain syndrome

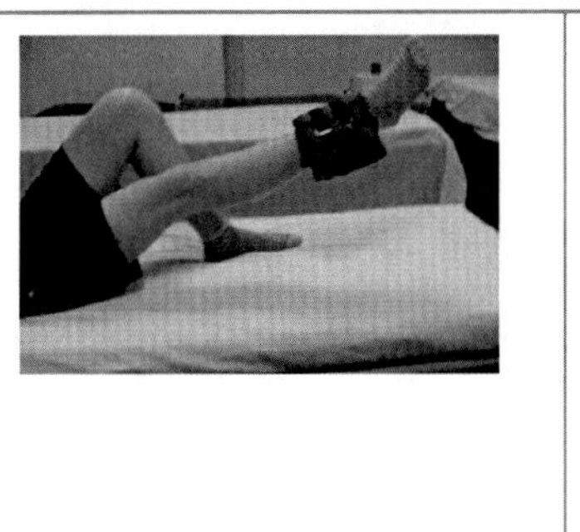	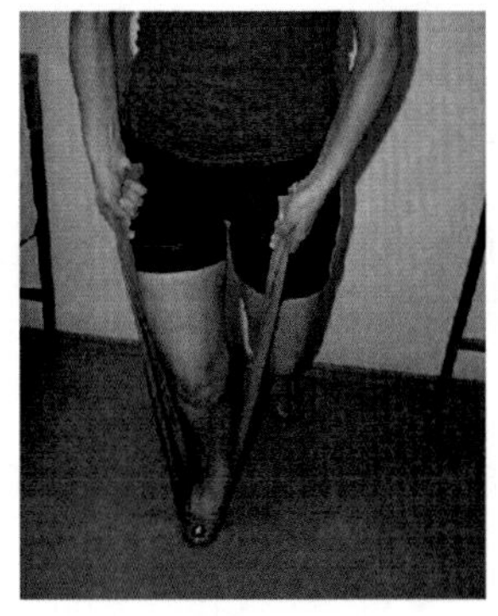	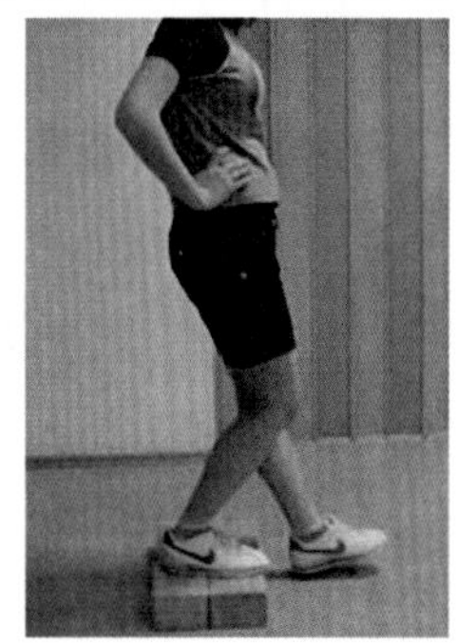
Fig. 1 Straight leg raises	Fig. 2 Terminal extension during squat	Fig. 3 Eccentric exercises
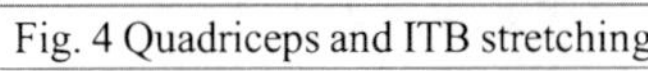	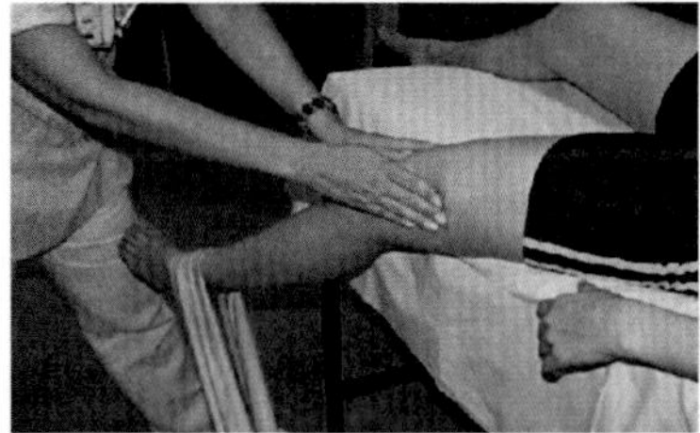	
Fig. 4 Quadriceps and ITB stretching	Fig. 5 Pin stretching	
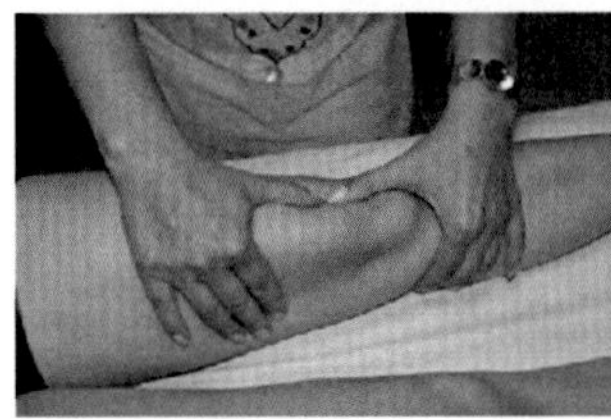	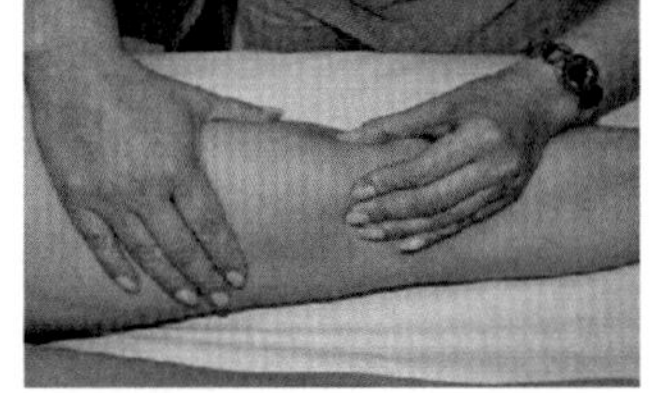	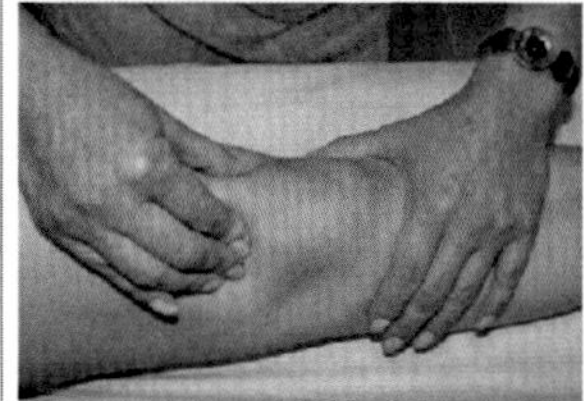
Fig. 6 Patellar mobilization (medial and superior and inferior)		

Herrington and Al-Sherhi (2007) designed a randomized controlled trial to compare the efficacy of single-joint non-weight-bearing quadriceps exercise versus multiple-joint weight-bearing quadriceps exercise for individuals with PFPS. Forty-five patients with PFPS between 18 and 35 years of age were randomized into one of three groups. Patients in group 1 performed knee extension exercises, patients in group 2 performed seated leg press exercises, and patients in group 3 (control group) received no treatment. Subjective symptoms, knee extensor muscle strength, and functional performance were evaluated at the time of the initial examination and at the end of 6-week treatment period. Patients in both exercise groups demonstrated a statistically significant decrease in pain and an increase in muscle strength and functional performance, as compared to the control group. Significant group differences were not observed. Their study demonstrates that both weight-bearing and non-weight-bearing quadriceps exercises can

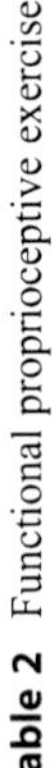

Table 2 Functional proprioceptive exercises

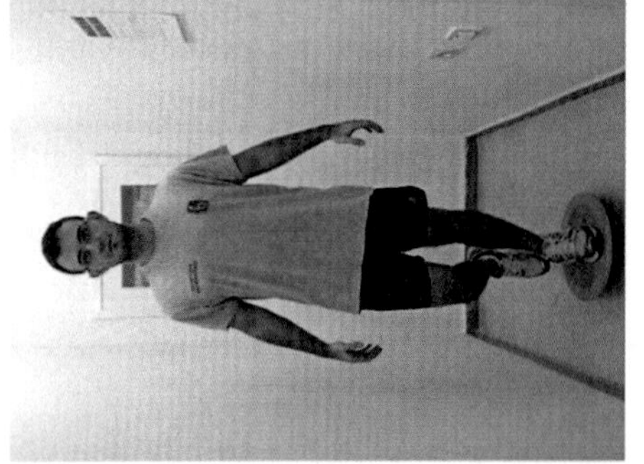	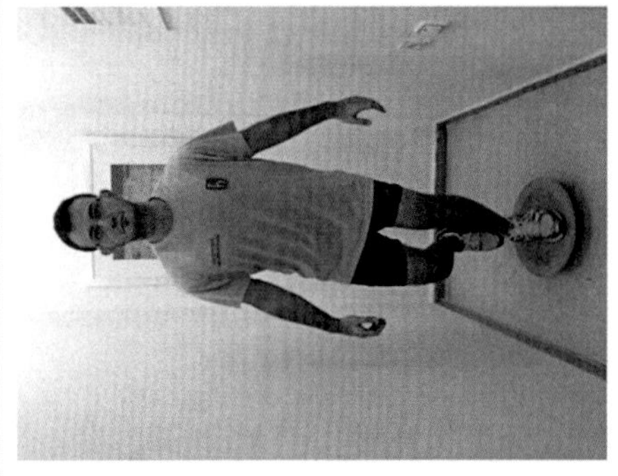	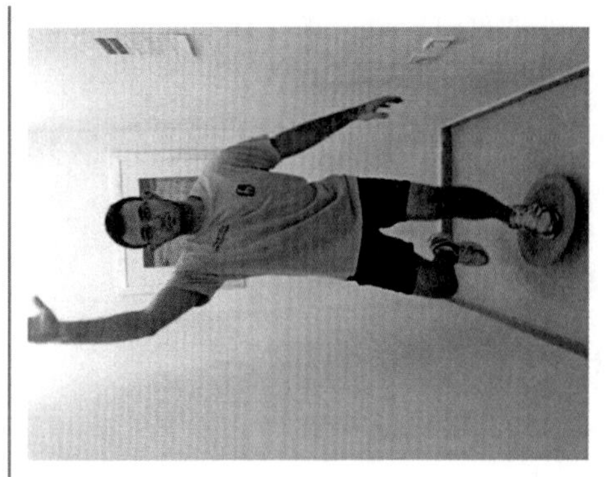
A:One-legged knee flexion		A
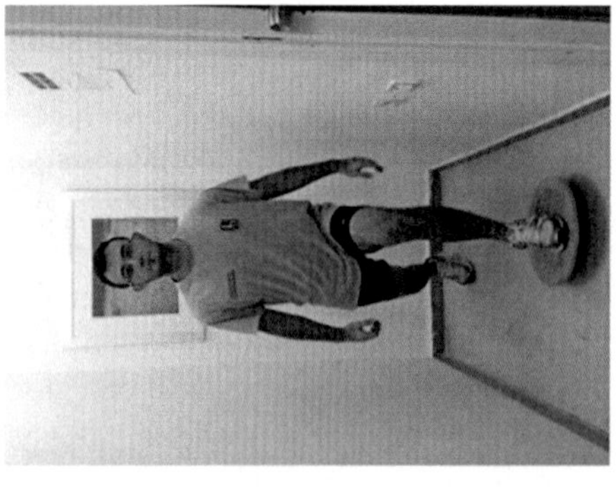	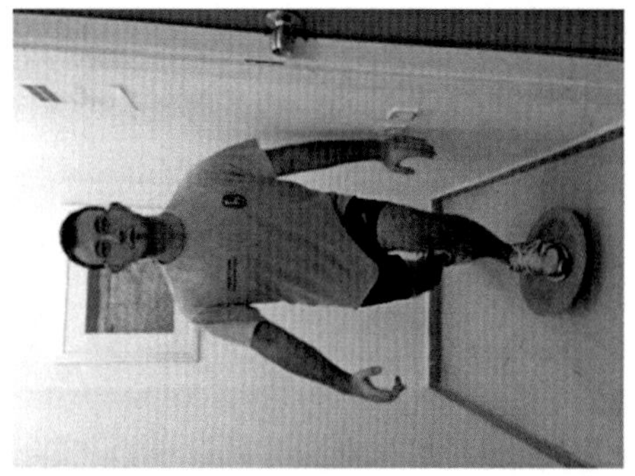	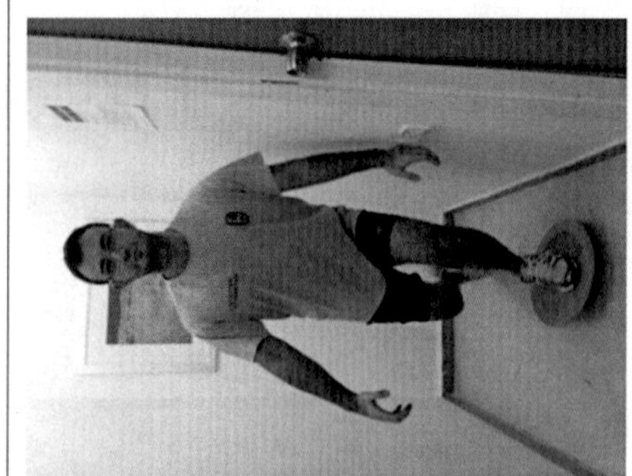
B:One-legged stance		B

(continued)

Table 2 (continued)

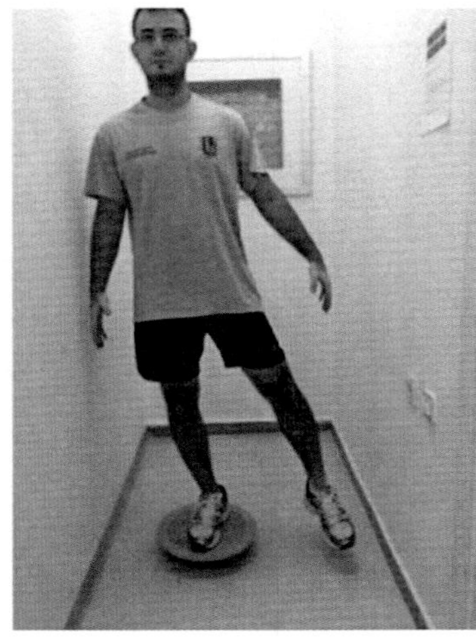	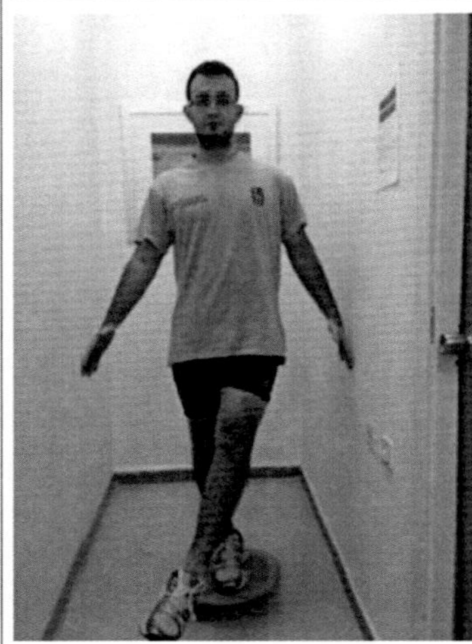	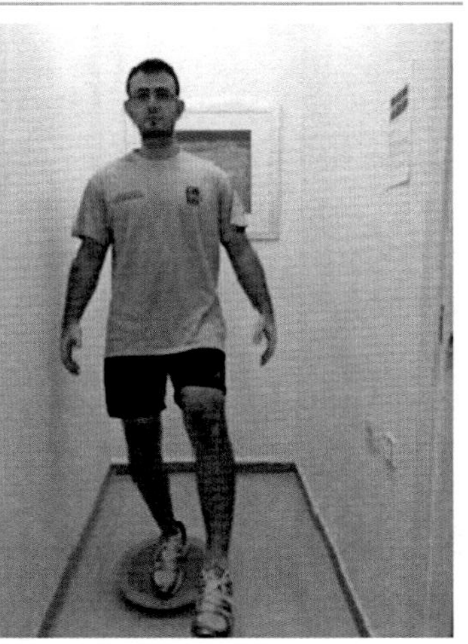 C
C:Crossed leg sway		

significantly improve subjective and clinical outcomes in patients with PFPS (Herrington and Al-Sherhi 2007).

Using a pretest-posttest study design, Boling et al. (2006) evaluated the effects of a weight-bearing rehabilitation program on quadriceps electromyographic activity, pain, and function in subjects diagnosed with PFPS. Fourteen patients diagnosed with PFPS and 14 healthy control subjects volunteered to participate in their study. Patients participated in a 6-week rehabilitation program. The rehabilitation program consisted of weight-bearing exercises that focused on strengthening the quadriceps. Electromyographic onsets of the VMO and vastus lateralis were collected during a stair-stepping task. A visual analogue scale (VAS) and Functional Index Questionnaire (FIQ) were administered at pretest and posttest and during each week of the intervention. They found that vastus lateralis and VMO onset timing differences (vastus lateralis electromyographic onset minus VMO electromyographic onset) and VAS and FIQ scores significantly improved in patients diagnosed with PFPS. Vastus lateralis and VMO onset timing in the patients were significantly different from those in the control group at baseline and were not significantly different from the control group after the intervention. They concluded that patients with PFPS responded favorably and quickly to a therapeutic exercise program that incorporated quadriceps strengthening (Boling et al. 2006).

Steinkamp et al. (1993) reported that patellofemoral joint reaction forces are minimized when closed kinetic chain exercises such as the seated leg press are performed from 0° to 40° knee flexion. Because of this, patients with PFPS may be better able to tolerate movements between 0°–40° knee flexion than open kinetic chain exercises such as the seated knee extension where patellofemoral joint reaction forces and stresses are greater within the same range.

Conclusions

Patellofemoral pain syndrome is a multifactorial problem that requires careful consideration of local, proximal, and distal factors during rehabilitation treatment planning. Carefully designed, longitudinal, prospective studies are needed to better discern etiology, pain source, and the efficacy of different physiotherapy interventions.

Acknowledgments Authors would like to thank Prof. Inci Yuksel, PT, PhD, and Yigitcan Karanfil, MD, for taking photographs.

Cross-References

- ▶ Patellar Dislocations: Overview
- ▶ Patellofemoral Problems in Adolescent Athletes
- ▶ Return to Play after Acute Patellar Dislocation
- ▶ Structured Rehabilitation Model for Patients with Patellofemoral Pain Syndrome

References

Arroll B, Ellis-Pegler E, Edwards A, Sutcliffe G (1997) Patellofemoral pain syndrome. A critical review of the clinical trials on nonoperative therapy. Am J Sports Med 25:207–212

Balci P, Tunay VB, Baltaci G, Atay AO (2009) The effects of two different closed kinetic chain exercises on muscle strength and proprioception in patients with patellofemoral pain syndrome. Acta Orthop Traumatol Turc 43(5):419–425

Barton CJ, Levinger P, Menz HB, Webster KE (2009) Kinematic gait characteristics associated with patellofemoral pain syndrome: a systematic review. Gait Posture 30:405–416

Barton CJ, Menz HB, Crossley KM (2011) Effects of prefabricated foot orthoses on pain and function in individuals with patellofemoral pain syndrome: a cohort study. Phys Ther Sport 12(2):70–75

Barton C, Levinger P, Crossley K, Webster K, Menz H (2012) The relationship between rearfoot, tibial, and femoral kinematics in individuals with patellofemoral pain syndrome. J Orthop Sports Phys Ther 42:A32

Boldt AR, Willson JD, Barrios JA, Kernozek TW (2013) Effects of medially wedged foot orthoses on knee and hip joint running mechanics in females with and without patellofemoral pain syndrome. J Appl Biomech 29(1):68–77

Boling MC, Bolgla LA, Mattacola CG, Uhl TL, Hosey RG (2006) Outcomes of a weight-bearing rehabilitation program for patients diagnosed with patellofemoral pain syndrome. Arch Phys Med Rehabil 87:1428–1435

Callaghan MJ (2011) What does proprioception testing tell us about patellofemoral pain? Man Ther 16(1):46–47

Callaghan MJ, McKie S, Richardson P, Oldham JA (2012) Effects of patellar taping on brain activity during knee joint proprioception tests using functional magnetic resonance imaging. Phys Ther 92(6):821–830

Cerny K (1995) Vastus medialis oblique/vastus lateralis muscle activity ratios for selected exercises in persons with and without patellofemoral pain syndrome. Phys Ther 75:672–683

Clark DI, Downing N, Mitchell J, Coulson L, Syzpryt EP, Doherty M (2000) Physiotherapy for anterior knee pain: a randomised controlled trial. Ann Rheum Dis 59:700–704

Collins N, Crossley K, Beller E, Darnell R, McPoil T, Vicenzino B (2009) Foot orthoses and physiotherapy in the treatment of patellofemoral pain syndrome: randomised clinical trial. Br J Sports Med 43(3):169–171

Cowan SM, Bennell KL, Hodges PW, Crossley KM, McConnell J (2001) Delayed onset of electromyographic activity of vastus lateralis compared to vastus medialis obliquus in subjects with patellofemoral pain syndrome. Arch Phys Med Rehabil 82:183–189

Derasari A, Brindle TJ, Alter KE, Sheehan FT (2010) McConnell taping shifts the patella inferiorly in patients with patellofemoral pain: a dynamic magnetic resonance imaging study. Phys Ther 90:411–419

Doucette SA, Child DP (1996) The effect of open and closed chain exercise and knee joint position on patellar tracking in lateral compression syndrome. J Orthop Sports Phys Ther 23:104–110

Doucette SA, Goble EM (1992) The effect of exercise on patellar tracking in lateral patellar compression syndrome. Am J Sports Med 20:434–440

Dvir Z, Halperin N, Shklar A, Robinson D, Weissman I, Ben-Shosan I (1990) Concentric and eccentric torque variations of the quadriceps femoris in patello-femoral pain syndrome. Clin Biomech 5:68–72

Dvir Z, Halperin N, Shklar A, Robinson D (1991) Quadriceps function and patellofemoral pain syndrome. Part I: pain provocation during concentric and eccentric isokinetic activity. Isokinet Exerc Sci 11:26–30

Eburne J, Bannister G (1996) The McConnell regimen versus isometric quadriceps exercises in the management of anterior knee pain. A randomised prospective controlled trial. Knee 3:151–153

Grelsamer RP, Klein JR (1998) The biomechanics of the patellofemoral joint. J Orthop Sports Phys Ther 28:286–298

Hazneci B, Yildiz Y, Sekir U, Aydin T, Kalyon TA (2005) Efficacy of isokinetic exercise on joint position sense and muscle strength in patellofemoral pain syndrome. Am J Phys Med Rehabil 84:521–527

Herrington L, Al-Sherhi A (2007) A controlled trial of weight-bearing versus non-weight-bearing exercises for patellofemoral pain. J Orthop Phys Ther 37:155–160

Iverson CA, Sutlive TG, Crowell MS, Morrell RL, Perkins MW, Garber MB et al (2008) Lumbopelvic manipulation for the treatment of patients with patellofemoral pain syndrome: development of a clinical prediction rule. J Orthop Sports Phys Ther 38:297–309

Kaya D, Atay OA, Callaghan MJ, Cil A, Caglar O, Citaker S, Yuksel I, Doral MN (2009) Hallux valgus in patients with patellofemoral pain syndrome. Knee Surg Sports Traumatol Arthrosc 17:1364–1367

Kaya D, Yüksel I, Callaghan MJ, Güney H, Atay OA, Çıtaker S, Huri G, Bilge O, Doral MN (2013) High voltage pulsed galvanic stimulation adjunct to rehabilitation program for patellofemoral pain syndrome: a prospective randomized controlled trial. Turk J Physiother Rehabil 24(1):1–8

Lee SP, Souza RB, Powers CM (2012) The influence of hip abductor muscle performance on dynamic postural stability in females with patellofemoral pain. Gait Posture 36(3):425–429

Lieb FJ, Perry J (1971) Quadriceps function: an electromyographic study under isometric conditions. J Bone Joint Surg Am 53:749–758

Malone TR, Davies GJ, Walsh WM (2002) Muscular control of the patella. Clin Sports Med 21:349–362

Mason JJ, Leszko F, Johnson T, Komistek RD (2008) Patellofemoral joint forces. J Biomech 41:2337–2348

Matthews LS, Sonstegard DA, Henke JA (1977) Load bearing characteristics of the patello-femoral joint. Acta Orthop Scand 48:511–516

McConnell J (1996) Management of patellofemoral problems. Man Ther 1:60–66

McConnell J, Fulkerson J (1996) The knee: patellofemoral and soft tissue injuries. In: Zachazewski JE, Magee DJ, Quillen WS (eds) Athletic injuries and rehabilitation, 1st edn. W.B. Saunders, Philadelphia, pp 693–728

McMullen W, Roncarati A, Koval P (1990) Static and isokinetic treatments of the chondromalacia patella: a comparative investigation. J Orthop Sports Phys Ther 12:256–266

Meira EP, Brumitt J (2011) Influence of the hip on patients with patellofemoral pain syndrome: a systematic review. Sports Health 3(5):455–465

Miller JP, Croce RV (2007) Analysis of isokinetic and closed chain movements for hamstring reciprocal coactivation. J Sport Rehabil 16:319–325

Möller BN, Krebs B, Tideman-Dal C, Aaris K (1986) Isometric contractions in the patellofemoral pain syndrome: an electromyographic study. Arch Orthop Trauma Surg 105:24–27

Munuera PV, Mazoteras-Pardo R (2011) Benefits of custom-made foot orthoses in treating patellofemoral pain. Prosthetics Orthot Int 35(4):342–349

Naslund JE, Odenbring S, Naslund UB, Lundeberg T (2005) Diffusely increased bone scintigraphic uptake in patellofemoral pain syndrome. Br J Sports Med 39:162–165

Nordin M, Frankel V (1989) Basic biomechanics of the musculoskeletal system. Lippincott Williams & Wilkins, London

Post MD, Fulkerson MD (1994) Knee pain diagrams: correlation with physical examination findings in patients with anterior knee pain. Arthroscopy 10:618–623

Powers CM (2010) The influence of abnormal hip mechanics on knee injury: a biomechanical perspective. J Orthop Sports Phys Ther 40:42–51

Powers CM, Bolgla LA, Callaghan MJ, Collins N, Sheehan FT (2012) Patellofemoral pain: proximal, distal, and local factors, 2nd international research retreat. J Orthop Sports Phys Ther 42(6):A1–A54

Roush MB, Sevier TL, Wilson JK, Jenkinson DM, Helfst RH, Gehlsen GM, Al B (2000) Anterior knee pain: a clinical comparison of rehabilitation methods. Clin J Sports Med 10:22–28

Shelton GL, Thigpen LK (1991) Rehabilitation of patellofemoral dysfunction: a review of the literature. J Orthop Sports Phys Ther 14:243–249

Souza RB, Draper CE, Fredericson M, Powers CM (2010) Femur rotation and patellofemoral joint kinematics: a weight-bearing magnetic resonance imaging analysis. J Orthop Sports Phys Ther 40:277–285

Steinkamp LA, Dillingham MF, Markel MD, Hill JA, Kaufman KR (1993) Biomechanical considerations in patellofemoral joint rehabilitation. Am J Sports Med 21:438–444

Stiene HA, Brosky T, Reinking MF, Nyland J, Mason MB (1996) A comparison of closed kinetic chain and isokinetic joint isolation exercise in patients with patellofemoral dysfunction. J Orthop Sports Phys Ther 24:136–141

Suter E, McMorland G, Herzog W, Bray R (1999) Decrease in quadriceps inhibition after sacroiliac joint manipulation in patients with anterior knee pain. J Manip Physiol Ther 22:149–153

Syme G, Rowe P, Martin D, Daly G (2009) Disability in patients with chronic patellofemoral pain syndrome: a randomised controlled trial of VMO selective training versus general quadriceps strengthening. Man Ther 14(3):252–263

Tang SF, Chen CK, Hsu R, Chou SW, Hong WH, Lew HL (2001) Vastus medialis obliquus and vastus lateralis activity in open and closed kinetic chain exercises in patients with patellofemoral pain syndrome: an electromyographic study. Arch Phys Med Rehabil 82:1441–1445

Thomeé R (1997) A comprehensive treatment approach for patellofemoral pain syndrome in young women. Phys Ther 77:1690–1703

Thomeë R, Renstrom P, Karlsson J, Grimby G (1995) Patellofemoral pain syndrome in young women, II: muscle function in patients and healthy controls. Scand J Med Sci Sports 5:245–251

Tiberio D (1987) The effect of excessive subtalar joint pronation on patellofemoral joint mechanics: a theoretical model. J Orthop Sports Phys Ther 9:160–169

Warden SJ, Hinman RS, Watson MA Jr, Avin KG, Bialocerkowski AE, Crossley KM (2008) Patellar taping and bracing for the treatment of chronic knee pain: a systematic review and meta-analysis. Arthritis Rheum 59:73–83

Werner S, Eriksson E (1993) Isokinetic quadriceps training in patients with patellofemoral pain. Knee Surg Sports Traumatol Arthrosc 1:162–168

Witvrouw E, Lysens R, Bellemans J, Peers K, Vanderstraeten G (2000) Open versus closed kinetic chain exercises for patellofemoral pain. A prospective, randomized study. Am J Sports Med 28:687–694

Witvrouw E, Danneels L, Van Tiggelen D, Willems TM, Cambier D (2004) Open versus closed kinetic chain exercises in patellofemoral pain: a 5-year prospective randomized study. Am J Sports Med 32:1122–1130

Yosmaoglu HB, Kaya D, Guney H, Nyland J, Baltaci G, Yuksel I, Doral MN (2013) Is there a relationship between tracking ability, joint position sense, and functional level in patellofemoral pain syndrome? Knee Surg Sports Traumatol Arthrosc 21:2564–2571

Prevention of Knee Injuries in Soccer Players

108

Eduard Alentorn-Geli, Jurdan Mendiguchía, and Gregory D. Myer

Contents

E. Alentorn-Geli (✉)
Department of Orthopaedic Surgery and Traumatology, Parc de Salut Mar, Hospital del Mar & Hospital de l'Esperança, Universitat Autonoma de Barcelona (UAB), Barcelona, Spain
e-mail: ealentorngeli@gmail.com

J. Mendiguchía
Department of Physical Therapy, Zentrum Rehab and Performance Center, Barañain, Navarre, Spain
e-mail: jurdan24@hotmail.com

G.D. Myer
Division of Sports Medicine, Cincinnati Children's Hospital Medical Center, Cincinnati, OH, USA
e-mail: greg.myer@cchmc.org

M.N. Doral, J. Karlsson (eds.), *Sports Injuries*,
DOI 10.1007/978-3-642-36569-0_81

Abstract

Soccer is a very popular sport in the world, but the incidence of anterior cruciate ligament (ACL) and other **knee** injuries is high. **Knee** injuries account for high short-, mid-, and long-term health impairment to **soccer** players and have high economic costs as well. The purpose of this chapter is to provide a review of the existing literature regarding studies investigating the effects of **prevention** programs on the incidence of **knee** and ACL injuries in **soccer** players. This review demonstrates that (1) there is no definitive evidence to suggest that **prevention** programs are effective at reducing **knee** injuries in general or specific ACL injuries in male **soccer** players; (2) there is evidence to suggest that **prevention** programs are not effective at reducing **knee** injuries in female **soccer** players; and (3) however, there is evidence to suggest that **prevention** programs are effective at reducing specific **knee** injury such as injury to the ACL in female **soccer** players. More studies are needed to investigate the effects of **prevention** programs on elite male and female **soccer** players.

Introduction

Soccer is the most popular sport in the world. While it can be considered a relatively safe activity, the rate of injuries is high (Junge and Dvorak 2004). **Knee** injuries are among the most common problems in **soccer** (Morgan and Oberlander 2001; Agel et al. 2007; Dick et al. 2007). It has been estimated that **soccer** players may suffer a **knee** injury at a rate of 2.61 injuries per 1,000 h of exposure in female players (Dick et al. 2007) and 2.07 injuries per 1,000 h of exposure in male players (Hawkins et al. 2001; Agel et al. 2007). **Knee** injuries in athletes account for high health and economic costs (Gottlob et al. 1999; Gottlob and Baker 2000; Lohmander et al. 2004, 2007). Therefore, **prevention** of these injuries, including anterior cruciate ligament (ACL) injuries, is a topic of high relevance in sports.

The purpose of this chapter is to provide a review of the existing literature regarding studies investigating the effects of **prevention** programs on the incidence of **knee** and ACL injuries in **soccer** players.

Review of Evidence

A systematic electronic literature search was conducted using the PubMed (MEDLINE) database from 1975 to September 2012, the EMBASE database from 1980 to September 2012, and The Cochrane Library from 1980 to September 2012. An updated literature search was conducted through PubMed (MEDLINE) in April 2013. From 3,322 references initially identified, 57 corresponded to **prevention** programs aimed to reduce injury rates or modify risk factors for **knee** or ACL injuries in athletes of any sport. From these, five were included in this review. After the updated literature search and the review of reference lists of articles, a total of 16 articles met the final inclusion criteria. Studies were included if they applied **prevention** programs aimed to reduce **knee** injuries in **soccer** players, including studies involving males and females.

Male Players

Seven studies applied **prevention** programs aimed to reduce **knee** injuries in male **soccer** players (Ekstrand et al. 1983; Caraffa et al. 1996; Junge et al. 2002; Malliou et al. 2004; Engebretsen et al. 2008; Grooms et al. 2013; Van Beijsterveldt et al. 2012). These studies involved a total sample of 2,028 **soccer** players, and three were randomized controlled trials (Ekstrand et al. 1983; Engebretsen et al. 2008; Van Beijsterveldt et al. 2012), three were prospective nonrandomized controlled trials (Caraffa et al. 1996; Junge et al. 2002; Malliou et al. 2004), and one was prospective cohort study (Grooms et al. 2013). Nine hundred ninety-eight players underwent an injury **prevention** program, whereas 1,030 served as matched controls. Only two of these studies were applied in professional or high-level players (Malliou et al. 2004; Engebretsen et al. 2008). The characteristics of the **prevention** programs were preseason (Caraffa et al. 1996; Engebretsen et al. 2008), in-season (Junge et al. 2002; Malliou et al. 2004; Grooms et al. 2013; Van Beijsterveldt et al. 2012), and undetermined (Ekstrand et al. 1983); three programs were applied as a warm-up (Junge et al. 2002; Grooms et al. 2013; Van Beijsterveldt et al. 2012), and some of them were applied two to three times per week (Malliou et al. 2004; Engebretsen et al. 2008; Van Beijsterveldt et al. 2012) for 20 min each session (Caraffa et al. 1996; Malliou et al. 2004; Grooms et al. 2013; Van Beijsterveldt et al. 2012) approximately; most of them applied balance/proprioception training (Caraffa et al. 1996; Junge et al. 2002; Malliou et al. 2004; Grooms et al. 2013; Van Beijsterveldt et al. 2012); three of them applied the F-MARC 11+ program (Junge et al. 2002; Grooms et al. 2013; Van Beijsterveldt et al. 2012). In terms of **knee** injuries in general, the principal results were as follows: three **prevention** programs were effective at preventing **knee** injuries in male **soccer** players (Ekstrand et al. 1983; Malliou et al. 2004; Van Beijsterveldt et al. 2012), and three others were not (Junge et al. 2002; Engebretsen et al. 2008; Grooms et al. 2013). Regarding specific ACL injuries, the principal results were as follows: one **prevention** program was effective at preventing ACL injuries in male **soccer** players (Caraffa et al. 1996), and another one was not (Grooms et al. 2013). Table 1 summarizes the

Table 1 Summary of studies with prevention programs aimed to reduce knee injuries in male soccer players

Reference	Intervention	Design	Participants	Sport – level of competition	Prevention program	Results	Conclusions
Ekstrand et al. 1983	Compare the incidence of injuries between experimental (prevention program) (group A) and control groups (group B)	Prospective randomized controlled trial	N: 180 (12 teams, 6 in each group) Age: Gr A 24.3 years (SD 3.7), Gr B 24.7 years (SD 4.1) Height: NR Weight: NR BMI: NR	Male soccer – Swedish senior division	Duration: NR Frequency: NR Session duration: NR Type of exercise: program based on 7 parts – correction of training, optimum equipment, prophylactic ankle taping, controlled rehabilitation, exclusion of knee instability, information, and expert supervision	Total number of injuries: 23 in experimental group vs. 93 in control group ($p < 0.001$) Knee sprains: 1 in experimental group vs. 17 in control group ($p < 0.05$)	Prevention programs significantly reduce knee injuries in soccer players
Caraffa et al. 1996	Compare the incidence of ACL injury between experimental (proprioception training) and control groups	Prospective controlled study (3 seasons)	N: 600 (40 teams, 20 in each group) Age: NR Height: NR Weight: NR BMI: NR	Male soccer – semiprofessional and amateur (Italy)	Duration: at least 30 days (preseason) Frequency: daily Session duration: 20 min Type of exercise: balance/ proprioception training	Experimental group: 10 ACL injuries; 0.15 injuries per team/ season Control group: 70 ACL injuries; 1.15 injuries per team/ season ($p < 0.001$)	Proprioception training can significantly reduce the incidence of ACL injuries in soccer players
Junge et al. 2002	Compare the incidence of injuries between experimental (prevention program) and control groups	Prospective controlled trial	N: 263. After dropouts, 101 in experimental group, 93 in control group Age: 16.7 years in experimental group, 16.3 years in control group ($p < 0.005$) Height: NR Weight: NR BMI: NR	Male soccer – amateur from Switzerland	Duration: 1 year in-season Frequency: NR Frequency: NR Type of exercise: general intervention (to improve warm-up, cooldown, taping of unstable ankle, adequate rehabilitation) + F-MARC Bricks (exercises to improve ankle and knee stability, flexibility, and strength training (for the trunk, hip, and legs), coordination, reaction time, and endurance)	Intervention: 0.76 injuries x player/year. Control: 1.18 injuries x player/year ($p < 0.01$). Greatest reduction in mild, overuse, and in-training injuries and in low-skill than in high-skill teams Knee injuries in experimental vs. control groups: 0.11 injuries/player/ year vs. 0.19 (N.S.)	Prevention programs can significantly reduce injuries in male soccer players, especially in low-skill players, but not specific knee injuries

(continued)

Table 1 (continued)

Reference	Intervention	Design	Participants	Sport – level of competition	Prevention program	Results	Conclusions
Malliou et al. 2004	Compare the incidence of injuries between experimental (balance/ proprioception training) and control groups	Prospective controlled trial	N: 100, 50 for each group Age: 16.7 years (SD 0.5) in experimental group, 16.9 years (SD 0.7) in control group Height: 1.7 m (SD 4.1) in experimental group, 1.7 m (7.3) in control group Weight: 65.9 kg (SD 7.9) in experimental group, 63.5 kg (SD 5.3) in control group BMI: NR	Male soccer – young championship of the 1st Greek division	Duration: 1 season Frequency: 2 times a week Session duration: 20 min/day Type of exercise: balance/ proprioception training through Biodex Stability System, mini trampoline, and balance boards	Training improved balance parameters within experimental group (no changes in control) 60 lower limb injuries in experimental group, 88 in control group (no p value) Knee ligament strains in experimental vs. control groups: 14 (28 %) vs. 28 (56 %) (no p value)	Balance training can prevent lower limb injuries, including knee injuries, in young male soccer players

Engebretsen et al. 2008	Compare the incidence of injuries between experimental (prevention program) and control groups composed of high-risk subjects	Prospective randomized controlled trial	N: 388, 193 in experimental group, 195 in control group Age: NR Height: NR Weight: NR BMI: NR	Male soccer – professional and semiprofessional players (1st, 2nd, and 3rd Norwegian divisions)	Duration: 10 weeks (preseason) Frequency: 3 times/week Session duration: NR Duration: 10 weeks (preseason)	Total injury incidence: 5.3 (95 % CI 4.6–6) in high-risk experimental group, 4.9 (4.3–5.6) in high-risk control group (N.S.) Knee injuries: incidence 0.5 (95 % CI 0.1–0.9) in experimental group, 0.5 (0.2–0.9) in control group (N.S.)	No influence of prevention program on knee injuries in male soccer players (although compliance was poor)
Grooms D et al. 2012	Assess the incidence of lower extremity injuries in subjects undergoing standard 1-season (2009) warm-up program and specific 1-season (2010) warm-up program aimed to reduce injuries	Prospective cohort study	N: 41 Age: 20.1 years (SD 2) Height: 1.77 m (SD 6.1) Weight: 73.6 kg (SD10.1) BMI: 23.4	Male soccer – National Collegiate Athletic Association Division III	Duration: 1 year Frequency: 5–6 per week Session duration: 20 min Type of exercise: F-MARC 11+ program (2010) – structured warm-up program with core stability, balance, dynamic stabilization (plyometrics), and eccentric hamstring strength	No ACL injuries in either season No ACL injuries in either season	No effect of F-MARC 11+ warm-up program on the prevention of knee and ACL injuries in male soccer players (low number of injuries observed)

(continued)

Table 1 (continued)

Reference	Intervention	Design	Participants	Sport – level of competition	Prevention program	Results	Conclusions
Van Beijsterveldt et al. 2012	Compare the incidence of injuries between experimental (prevention program) and control groups	Prospective randomized controlled trial	N: 456, 223 in experimental group, 233 in control group Age: 24.4 years (SD 4.1) in experimental group, 25.1 years (SD 4.3) in control group (N.S.) Height: 1.85 m (SD 0.1) in experimental group, 1.82 m (0.1) in control group ($p < 0.05$) Weight: 79.1 kg (SD 7.4) in experimental group, 77.4 kg (SD 7.4) in control group ($p < 0.05$) BMI: 23.2 (SD 1.8) in experimental group, 23.3 (SD 1.8) in control group (N.S.)	Male soccer – Dutch high-level amateur players	Duration: 1 season – Frequency: 2–3 per week Session duration: 20 min Type of exercise: F-MARC 11+ program – structured warm-up program with core stability, balance, dynamic stabilization (plyometrics), and eccentric hamstring strength Frequency: 2–3 per week	Injury incidence: 9.6 per 1,000 soccer hours (95 % CI 8.4–11) in experimental group, 9.7 (8.5–11.1) in control group (N.S.) No significant differences in injury severity, recurrence of injury, or days of sport absenteeism Knee injuries: 11.7 % in experimental group, 19.8 % in control group ($p < 0.05$)	Prevention program (F-MARC 11+) significantly reduced the incidence of knee injuries in male amateur soccer players

seven studies investigating the effects of **prevention** programs on **knee** injuries in male **soccer** players.

The characteristics of the **prevention** program in the four studies that found a significant effect at reducing **knee** injuries in male players are as follows (Ekstrand et al. 1983; Caraffa et al. 1996; Malliou et al. 2004; Van Beijsterveldt et al. 2012): (1) duration of the program, 1 month (one study), one season (two studies), and undetermined (one study); (2) weekly frequency, daily (one study), two to three times per week (two studies), and undetermined (one study); and (3) duration of each session, 20 min (three studies) and undetermined (one study).The main characteristics of the **prevention** program are balance/proprioception (three studies), eccentric strength training (one study), core stability (one study), and plyometric strength training (one study).

Female Players

Nine studies applied **prevention** programs aimed to reduce **knee** injuries in female **soccer** players (Heidt et al. 2000; Söderman et al. 2000; Mandelbaum et al. 2005; Gilchrist et al. 2008; Soligard et al. 2008; Steffen et al. 2008; Emery and Meeuwisse 2010; Kiani et al. 2010; Walden et al. 2012). One study included both males and females, and the results were not specified according to gender (Emery and Meeuwisse 2010). These studies involved a total sample of 15,628 **soccer** players, and seven were randomized controlled trials (Heidt et al. 2000; Söderman et al. 2000; Gilchrist et al. 2008; Soligard et al. 2008; Steffen et al. 2008; Emery and Meeuwisse 2010; Walden et al. 2012), and two prospective nonrandomized controlled trials (Mandelbaum et al. 2005; Kiani et al. 2010). Seven thousand five hundred fifty-one players underwent an injury **prevention** program, whereas 8,077 served as matched controls. All studies involved high school, collegiate, or amateur **soccer** players. The characteristics of the **prevention** programs were preseason (Heidt et al. 2000) and in-season (Söderman et al. 2000; Mandelbaum et al. 2005; Gilchrist et al. 2008; Soligard et al. 2008; Steffen et al. 2008; Emery and Meeuwisse 2010; Kiani et al. 2010; Walden et al. 2012); six programs were applied as a warm-up (Mandelbaum et al. 2005; Gilchrist et al. 2008; Soligard et al. 2008; Steffen et al. 2008; Kiani et al. 2010; Walden et al. 2012), and many of them were applied two to three times per week (Heidt et al. 2000; Söderman et al. 2000; Mandelbaum et al. 2005; Gilchrist et al. 2008; Kiani et al. 2010; Walden et al. 2012) for 20 min each session (Söderman et al. 2000; Mandelbaum et al. 2005; Gilchrist et al. 2008; Soligard et al. 2008; Steffen et al. 2008; Kiani et al. 2010; Walden et al. 2012) approximately; most of them applied balance/proprioception training (Söderman et al. 2000; Soligard et al. 2008; Steffen et al. 2008; Emery and Meeuwisse 2010; Kiani et al. 2010; Walden et al. 2012). In terms of **knee** injuries in general, the principal results were as follows: two **prevention** programs were effective at preventing **knee** injuries in male **soccer** players (Soligard et al. 2008; Kiani et al. 2010), and six others were not (Heidt et al. 2000; Söderman et al. 2000; Gilchrist et al. 2008; Steffen et al. 2008; Emery and Meeuwisse 2010; Walden et al. 2012). Three studies found that **prevention** programs were effective at reducing ACL injuries in female **soccer** players (Mandelbaum et al. 2005; Gilchrist et al. 2008). Table 2 summarizes the nine studies investigating the effects of **prevention** programs on **knee** injuries in female **soccer** players.

The characteristics of the **prevention** program in the five studies that reported a significant effect at reducing **knee** injuries in female players are as follows (Mandelbaum et al. 2005; Gilchrist et al. 2008; Soligard et al. 2008; Kiani et al. 2010; Walden et al. 2012): (1) duration of the program, 3 months (one study), one season (three studies), and years (one study); (2) weekly frequency, two to three times per week (four studies) and undetermined (one study); and (3) duration of each session, 20 min (five studies). The main characteristics of the **prevention** program are balance/proprioception (three studies), eccentric strength training (four studies), core stability (four studies), stretching (three studies), and plyometric strength training (four studies).

Table 2 Summary of studies with prevention programs aimed to reduce knee injuries in female soccer players

Reference	Intervention	Design	Participants	Sport – level of competition	Prevention program	Results	Conclusions
Heidt et al. 2000	Compare the incidence of injuries between experimental (preseason conditioning) and control groups	Prospective randomized controlled trial	N: 300 (42 in experimental group; rest served as controls) Age: 14–18 years Height: NR Weight: NR BMI: NR	Female soccer – competitive high school (USA)	Duration: 7 weeks (preseason) Frequency: 3 times a week Session duration: NR Duration: 7 weeks (preseason)	Total number of injuries: 14 % in experimental group vs. 33.7 % in control group ($p <$ 0.009) Knee injuries: 43 % of all injuries in experimental group vs. 32 % in control group (no p value); 7 % of all subjects in experimental group vs. 11 % in control group (no p value) Experimental vs. control groups: ACL 2.4 % vs. 3.1 %, Medial Collateral Ligament sprain or tear 2.4 % vs. 2.3 %, chondromalacia patellae 0 % vs. 2.3 %, meniscal tear 0 % vs. 1.2 %, contusion 0 % vs. 1.2 %, bursitis 2.4 % vs. 0 %, patellar subluxation or dislocation 0 % vs. 0.8 % (no p values)	Preseason conditioning prevention program reduces lower extremity injuries, but not specific knee injuries, in female soccer players
Soderman et al. 2000	Compare the incidence of injuries between experimental (balance/ proprioception training) and control groups	Prospective randomized controlled trial	N: 221 (121 in intervention and 100 in control groups); after dropouts 62 and 78, respectively Age: 20.4 years (SD 4.6) in experimental	Female soccer – 2nd and 3rd Swedish division	Duration: 7 months Frequency: 3 times a week Session duration: 10–15 min/day Type of exercise: balance/proprioception training through a balance board with	No differences between groups for lower extremity injuries Higher incidence of major injuries in experimental group Knee injuries in experimental vs. control groups: total 13 % vs.	Balance training was not effective at the prevention of lower extremity injuries, including knee injuries, in female soccer players

			group, 20.5 years in control group (5.4) Height: 165 cm (5.7) in experimental group, 167 cm (4.7) in control group Weight: 60 kg (5.9) in experimental group, 61 kg (6.6) in control group BMI: NR		exercises of increasing difficulty Duration: 7 months	7.7 %, ACL 4.8 % vs. 1.3 %, ACL + Medial Collateral Ligament 1.6 % vs. 0 %, MCL 1.6 % vs. 1.3 %, Lateral Collateral Ligament 3.2 % vs. 0 %, contusion 1.6 % vs. 5.1 % (no p value)	
Mandelbaum et al. 2005	Compare the incidence of ACL injuries between experimental (neuromuscular/ proprioception training) and control groups	Prospective controlled trial	N: 2,946, 1,041 in experimental group, 1,905 in control group Age: range 14–18 years in experimental group Height: NR Weight: NR BMI: NR	Female soccer – nonprofessional soccer (Coast Soccer League of Southern California, USA)	Duration: 2 years Frequency: 2–3 times/ week Session duration: 20 min Type of exercise: PEP program before regular training – 3 basic warm-up activities, 5 stretching techniques of the trunk and lower extremity, 3 strengthening exercises, 5 plyometric activities, and 3 soccer-specific agility drills	Significant decrease in ACL injuries in experimental compared to control groups: 88 % in 1st season and 74 % in 2nd season ACL injuries per 1,000 players: 3.18 in experimental group, 17.6 in control group ($p <$ 0.001)	Neuromuscular and proprioception programs decrease the incidence of ACL injuries in female soccer players
Gilchrist et al. 2008	Compare the incidence of ACL injuries between experimental (neuromuscular/ proprioception training) and control groups	Prospective randomized controlled trial	N: 1,435, 583 in experimental group, 852 in control group Age: mean 19.8 years in experimental group, 19.8 years in control group	Female soccer – National Collegiate Athletic Association Division I (USA)	Duration: 12 weeks Frequency: 3 times/ week Session duration: 20 min Type of exercise: PEP program before regular training – 3 basic warm-up activities, 5 stretching techniques of the trunk	Total knee injuries: 1.1 per 1,000 athletic exposures in experimental group, 1.09 in control group (N.S.) Total noncontact ACL injuries: 0.05 per 1,000 athletic exposures in experimental group, 0.19	Prevention programs may help reduce the risk of noncontact ACL injuries, but not knee injuries in general, in female soccer players

(continued)

Table 2 (continued)

Reference	Intervention	Design	Participants	Sport – level of competition	Prevention program	Results	Conclusions
			(N.S.) Height: 1.6 m in experimental group, 1.6 m in control group (N.S.) Weight: 61.9 kg in experimental group, 62 kg in control group (N.S.) BMI: 22.3 in experimental group, 22.3 in control group (N.S.)		and lower extremity, 3 strengthening exercises, 5 plyometric activities, and 3 soccer-specific agility drills	in control group = 3.3 times lower ($p = 0.066$) No differences in the incidence of knee injuries or noncontact ACL injuries between groups in early or late season Significantly lower number of noncontact ACL injuries in experimental compared to control group if previous ACL injury ($p = 0.04$)	
Soligard et al. 2008	Compare the incidence of injuries between experimental (comprehensive warm-up program) and control groups	Prospective randomized controlled trial	N: 1,892, 1,055 in experimental group, 837 in control group Age: mean 15.4 years (SD 0.7) in both groups (N.S.) Height: NR Weight: NR BMI: NR	Female soccer – Norwegian 15–16-year-old divisions	Duration: 8 months Frequency: NR Session duration: 20 min Type of exercise: comprehensive warm-up program to improve strength, awareness, and neuromuscular control during static and dynamic movements	All injuries: 13 % in experimental group vs. 19.8 % in control group ($p = 0.04$) Lower extremity injuries: 11.5 % in experimental group vs. 17.1 % in control group ($p = 0.07$) Knee injuries: incidence 0.7 injuries per 1,000 played hours in experimental group, 1.3 in control group ($p = 0.005$) Severe and overuse injuries significantly lower in the experimental group	Structured warm-up program can reduce knee injuries in female soccer players

Steffen et al. 2008	Compare the incidence of injuries between experimental (prevention program) and control groups	Prospective randomized controlled trial	N: 2,020, 1,073 in experimental group, 947 in control group Age: mean 15.4 years (SD 0.8) in both groups (N.S.) Height: NR BMI: NR	Female soccer – Norwegian under-17 league	Duration: 8 months Frequency: NR Session duration: 20 min Type of exercise: F-MARC 11+ – structured warm-up program with core stability, balance, dynamic stabilization (plyometrics), and eccentric hamstring strength	No differences between both groups for overall injury incidence and acute injuries during matches and practices Knee injuries: incidence 0.5 (95 % CI 0.3–0.6) injuries per 1,000 h of exposure in experimental group vs. 0.6 (0.4–0.7) in control group (N.S.)	No influence of prevention program to decrease the risk of knee injuries in female soccer players (compliance was poor)
Emery and Meeuwisse 2010	Compare the incidence of injuries between experimental (neuromuscular prevention program) and control groups	Prospective randomized controlled trial	N: 744, 380 in experimental group, 364 in control group Age: U13–U15 47 % in experimental group, 49 % in control group; U16–U18 53 % in experimental group, 51 % in control group (N.S.) Height: 1.6 m in both groups (N.S.) Weight: 55 kg in experimental group, 54 kg in control group (N.S.) BMI: 19.9 in experimental group, 20.4 in control group (N.S.)	Male and female indoor soccer – Calgary Minor Soccer Association clubs (under 13 to under 18, tiers 1 or 2)	Duration: 20 weeks Frequency: NR Session duration: 30 min (15 min was home based) Type of exercise: soccer-specific neuromuscular training program – dynamic stretching, eccentric strength, agility, jumping, and balance	Injury rate (injuries per 1,000 player-hours): all injuries 3.35 in experimental group vs. 2.08 in control group ($p = 0.04$); acute injuries 3.05 vs. 1.75 ($p = 0.018$); lower extremity injuries 2.54 vs. 1.75 (N.S.); knee sprain 0.34 vs. 0.12 (N.S.). All analyses adjusted by previous injury and age	Neuromuscular prevention program decreases the total number of injuries, but not specific knee sprains, in young soccer players

(*continued*)

Table 2 (continued)

Reference	Intervention	Design	Participants	Sport – level of competition	Prevention program	Results	Conclusions
Kiani et al. 2010	Compare the incidence of injuries between experimental (prevention program) and control groups	Prospective controlled trial	N: 1,506, 777 in experimental group, 729 in control group Age: 14.7 years in experimental group, 15 years in control group (N.S.) Height: NR Weight: NR BMI: NR	Female soccer – Swedish regional soccer, between 13 and 19 years	Duration: 1 year Frequency: 2 per week (preseason) and 1 per week (regular season) Session duration: 20–25 min Type of exercise: HarmoKnee prevention program (improve awareness, provide adequate warm-up, and improve motion patterns) – warm-up, muscle activation, balance, strength, and core stability	Knee injuries: 3 (incidence 0.04 per 1,000 player-hours) in experimental group, 13 (incidence 0.2 per 1,000 player-hours) in control group (no p value). Contact injuries: 2 of 3 in experimental group, 3 of 13 in control group (no p value) Prevention program reduced incidence of knee injuries in 77 % (crude rate ratio 0.23 (95 % CI 0.04–0.83)) Noncontact knee injury incidence 90 % lower in experimental group (crude rate ratio 0.1 (0–0.7)) ACL injuries: 0 in experimental group, 5 in control group (no p value)	Knee injuries can be reduced with prevention programs in young female soccer players

Walden et al. 2012	Compare the incidence of injuries between experimental (neuromuscular prevention program) and control groups	Prospective randomized controlled trial	N: 4,564, 2,479 in experimental group, 2,085 in control group Age: 14 years (SD 1.2) in experimental group, 14.1 years (SD 1.2) in control group (N.S.) Height: 1.63 m (SD 0.06) in experimental group, 1.63 m (0.06) in control group (N.S.) Weight: 53 kg (SD 8.6) in experimental group, 53 kg (SD 8.4) in control group (N.S.) BMI: NR	Female soccer – Swedish Football Association (under 14 to under 18 years)	Duration: 1 season Frequency: 2 per week Duration: 1 season Type of exercise: neuromuscular warm-up program – core stability, balance, proper knee alignment	ACL injuries: 64 % reduction in rate of ACL tear with the prevention program; 0.28 % in experimental group, 0.67 % in control group (rate ratio 0.36, 95%CI 0.15–0.85) ($p = 0.02$) Severe knee injuries: 1.05 % in experimental group, 1.49 % in control group (rate ratio 0.7, 95 % CI 0.42–1.18) ($p = 0.18$)	Neuromuscular warm-up prevention program significantly reduced ACL injuries, but not overall severe knee injuries, in female soccer players

Discussion

The principal findings of this review are as follows: (1) there is no definitive evidence to suggest that **prevention** programs are effective at reducing **knee** injuries in general or specific ACL injuries in male **soccer** players; (2) there is evidence to suggest that **prevention** programs are not effective at reducing **knee** injuries in female **soccer** players; and (3) there is evidence to suggest that **prevention** programs are effective at reducing ACL injuries in female **soccer** players. These conclusions are based on studies with a high level of evidence (10 of 16 studies were prospective randomized controlled trials – level I evidence).

The number of studies and evidence regarding risk factors and **prevention** programs for **knee** and ACL injuries differs considerably between males and females (Griffin et al. 2006; Hewett et al. 2006a, b; Renstrom et al. 2008; Alentorn-Geli et al. 2009a, b, 2014a, b; Posthumus et al. 2011; Dai et al. 2012a, b). Thus, it is needed to differentiate between those programs applied in a male or female sample, and, consequently, both sexes should not be included in the same study unless results are specified by gender. Although the level of evidence in the included studies is high, there are some limitations and considerations that should be discussed. Studies by Engebretsen and coworkers (2008) and Steffen and coworkers (2008) found no efficacy of **prevention** programs to reduce **knee** injuries in male and female **soccer** players, respectively. Unfortunately, the compliance with the preventive program was poor, with 29 % and 24 %, respectively (Engebretsen et al. 2008; Steffen et al. 2008). It is crucial that the compliance of **prevention** programs is as high as possible to know the real effects on injury rates. Recent reports indicate an inverse dose-response relationship between compliance with neuromuscular training programs and incidence of ACL injury (Sugimoto et al. 2012a). Thus, the authors concluded that attending and completing neuromuscular sessions appears to be an important factor for preventing ACL injuries (Sugimoto et al. 2012a). Ideally, compliance should not be less than 70 % (Aaltonen et al. 2007). Another very important consideration when analyzing the existing data is the number of **knee** or ACL injuries suffered by **soccer** players in either the experimental or the control group. Some studies demonstrate small sample of **knee** or ACL injuries in male (Engebretsen et al. 2008; Grooms et al. 2013) and female **soccer** players (Heidt et al. 2000; Söderman et al. 2000; Emery and Meeuwisse 2010; Walden et al. 2012), which increases the risk of type II error in cases where no significant differences were found between both the experimental and control groups (Heidt et al. 2000; Söderman et al. 2000; Engebretsen et al. 2008; Emery and Meeuwisse 2010; Grooms et al. 2013; Walden et al. 2012). Interestingly, when only considering articles with a large sample, seven of the nine studies (for both male and female **soccer** players) were able to find a significant efficacy of **prevention** programs to reduce **knee** or ACL injuries (Caraffa et al. 1996; Mandelbaum et al. 2005; Gilchrist et al. 2008; Soligard et al. 2008; Kiani et al. 2010; Van Beijsterveldt et al. 2012; Walden et al. 2012). If only considering studies without significant efficacy of **prevention** programs to reduce **knee** or ACL injuries, five of seven were among those studies with a smaller sample (Heidt et al. 2000; Söderman et al. 2000; Junge et al. 2002; Engebretsen et al. 2008; Grooms et al. 2013). It has to be kept in mind that the sample size will have a strong influence on the total number of injuries suffered by the included players. Therefore, although the sample size may not be apparently small in some studies (Ekstrand et al. 1983; Söderman et al. 2000; Junge et al. 2002; Engebretsen et al. 2008), a limited sample size can lead to a low number of total injuries taking into account the general incidence of expected **knee** or ACL injuries in **soccer** players. Therefore, it is essential to perform a power analysis before commencement of an intervention study in this field (Söderman et al. 2000). Sugimoto and coworkers suggested that a strategy to reduce the numbers needed to treat and improve the efficiency of ACL injury **prevention** programs would be to develop a screening system to identify and target at-risk athletes with neuromuscular training (Sugimoto et al. 2012b). A limiting factor to conduct **prevention** studies is that they often involve many **soccer** teams and different professionals, which increases difficulty with control of compliance, dropout rates, and data collection. Although it is difficult to include a large and homogeneous sample of **soccer** players in this kind of studies, it has to be stated that the results may clearly depend on the sample size. Thus, a big effort is encouraged whenever investigating the effects of **prevention** programs on **knee** injuries in athletes so that authors include as many subjects as possible. Last, but not least, some studies did not report some anthropometric characteristics of the subjects (Ekstrand et al. 1983; Caraffa et al. 1996; Heidt et al. 2000; Junge et al. 2002; Mandelbaum et al. 2005; Engebretsen et al. 2008; Soligard et al. 2008; Steffen et al. 2008; Kiani et al. 2010) or some of the characteristics of the **prevention** programs such as the length of the program, weekly frequency, or duration of the session (Ekstrand et al. 1983; Heidt et al. 2000; Junge et al. 2002; Engebretsen et al. 2008; Steffen et al. 2008; Emery and Meeuwisse 2010). It is assumed that all the reviewed studies involved a homogeneous sample and applied **prevention** programs with similar characteristics, but these parameters should be always reported in this kind of studies.

Studies concluding that **prevention** programs were effective at reducing **knee** injuries in male and female **soccer** players share some characteristics: applied throughout the whole season, at a frequency of two to three times per week for 20 min each session, and including balance/proprioception exercises, eccentric and plyometric strength exercises, core stability exercises, and stretching exercises. However, no clear conclusions can be drawn on the higher efficacy of these characteristics, as studies with similar parameters were not able to demonstrate a significant effectiveness of **prevention** programs at reducing **knee** injuries in **soccer** players. The use of video-based awareness programs to reduce the rate of injuries in **soccer** players has not demonstrated adequate preventive effects (Arnason et al. 2005).

There is a special consideration for the **prevention** of ACL injuries in the female athlete. A recent meta-analysis was conducted to assess the influence of age of neuromuscular implementation on the effectiveness for reduction of ACL injury incidence in the female athlete (Myer et al. 2013). The authors found an age-related association between neuromuscular **prevention** programs and reduction of ACL incidence (Myer et al. 2013). They stated that the potential window of opportunity for optimized ACL injury risk reduction through neuromuscular **prevention** programs may be during early adolescence, before the onset of neuromuscular deficits and peak **knee** injury incidence in female athletes (Myer et al. 2013).

It is important to note that the lack of significant differences in injury rates between experimental and control groups may be also explained by the fact that many regular training programs in **soccer** (those programs applied to control subjects) may have some of the characteristics of the **prevention** programs. This is a potential problem difficult to control, as it is not possible to modify the normal training protocol in teams when conducting an investigation. In addition, it is sometimes difficult to include **prevention** programs in the regular schedule of practice in **soccer** teams. Nonetheless, programs have been especially designed to facilitate its inclusion in regular training of teams, as they last for 20 min (easy to fit in regular trainings) and also have been designed as warm-up exercises so that they can be easily included before the match as well.

Conclusions

- There is no definitive evidence to suggest that **prevention** programs are effective at reducing **knee** injuries in general or specific ACL injuries in male **soccer** players.
- There is evidence to suggest that **prevention** programs are not effective at reducing **knee** injuries in general in female **soccer** players.
- There is evidence to suggest that **prevention** programs are effective at reducing ACL injuries in female **soccer** players.

- More studies are needed to investigate the effects of **prevention** programs on professional male and female **soccer** players.

Cross-References

- ▶ Anterior Cruciate Ligament Injuries and Surgery: Current Evidence and Modern Development
- ▶ Anterior Cruciate Ligament Injuries: Prevention Strategies
- ▶ Anterior Cruciate Ligament Injuries with Concomittant Meniscal Pathologies
- ▶ Prevention in Soccer Injuries
- ▶ Prevention of Childhood Sports Injuries
- ▶ Prevention of Hamstring Muscle Injuries in Sports
- ▶ Soccer and Associated Sports Injuries
- ▶ Sports Participation and Risk of Knee Osteoarthritis: A Critical Review of the Literature

References

Aaltonen S, Karjalainen H, Heinonen A, Parkkari J, Kujala UM (2007) Prevention of sports injuries: systematic review of randomized controlled trials. Arch Intern Med 167:1585–1592

Agel J, Evans TA, Dick R, Putukian M, Marshall SW (2007) Descriptive epidemiology of collegiate men's soccer injuries: National Collegiate Athletic Association Injury Surveillance System, 1988–1989 through 2002–2003. J Athl Train 42:270–277

Alentorn-Geli E, Myer GD, Silvers HJ, Samitier G, Romero D, Lazaro-Haro C, Cugat R (2009a) Prevention of non-contact anterior cruciate ligament injuries in soccer players. Part 1: mechanisms of injury and underlying risk factors. Knee Surg Sports Traumatol Arthrosc 17:705–729

Alentorn-Geli E, Myer GD, Silvers HJ, Samitier G, Romero D, Lazaro-Haro C, Cugat R (2009b) Prevention of non-contact anterior cruciate ligament injuries in soccer players. Part 2: a review of prevention programs aimed to modify risk factors and to reduce injury rates. Knee Surg Sports Traumatol Arthrosc 17:859–879

Alentorn-Geli E, Mendiguchia J, Samuelsson K, Musahl V, Karlsson J, Cugat R, Myer GD (2014a) Prevention of anterior cruciate ligament injuries in sports. Part I: systematic review of risk factors in male athletes. Knee Surg Sports Traumatol Arthrosc. 2014;22:3–15

Alentorn-Geli E, Mendiguchia J, Samuelsson K, Musahl V, Karlsson J, Cugat R, Myer GD (2014b) Prevention of non-contact anterior cruciate ligament injuries in sports. Part II: systematic review of prevention programs in male athletes. Knee Surg Sports Traumatol Arthrosc. 2014;22:16–25

Arnason A, Engebretsen L, Bahr R (2005) No effect of a video-based awareness program on the rate of soccer injuries. Am J Sports Med 33:77–84

Caraffa A, Cerulli G, Projetti M, Aisa G, Rizzo A (1996) Prevention of anterior cruciate ligament injuries in soccer. A prospective controlled study of proprioceptive training. Knee Surg Sports Traumatol Arthrosc 4:19–21

Dai B, Herman D, Liu C, Garrett WE Jr, Yu B (2012a) Prevention of ACL injury, part I: injury characteristics, risk factors, and loading mechanism. Res Sports Med 20:180–197

Dai B, Herman D, Liu H, Garrett WE Jr, Yu B (2012b) Prevention of ACL injury, part II: effects of ACL injury prevention programs on neuromuscular risk factors and injury rate. Res Sports Med 20:198–222

Dick R, Ferrara MS, Agel J, Courson R, Marshall SW, Hanley MJ, Reifsteck F (2007) Descriptive epidemiology of collegiate women's soccer injuries: National Collegiate Athletic Association Injury Surveillance System, 1988–1989 through 2003–2004. J Athl Train 42:221–233

Ekstrand J, Gillquist J, Liljedahl SO (1983) Prevention of soccer injuries. Supervision by doctor and physiotherapist. Am J Sports Med 11:116–120

Emery CA, Meeuwisse WH (2010) The effectiveness of a neuromuscular prevention strategy to reduce injuries in youth soccer: a cluster-randomised controlled trial. Br J Sports Med 44:555–562

Engebretsen AH, Myklebust G, Holme I, Engebretsen L, Bahr R (2008) Prevention of injuries among male soccer players. A prospective, randomized intervention study targeting players with previous injuries or reduced function. Am J Sports Med 36:1052–1060

Gilchrist J, Mandelbaum BR, Melancon H, Ryan GW, Silvers HJ, Griffin LY, Watanabe DS, Dick RW, Dvorak J (2008) A randomized controlled trial to prevent noncontact anterior cruciate ligament injury in female collegiate soccer players. Am J Sports Med 36:1476–1483

Gottlob CA, Baker CL (2000) Anterior cruciate ligament reconstruction: socioeconomic issues and cost effectiveness. Am J Orthop (BelleMead NJ) 29:472–476

Gottlob CA, Baker CL, Pellissier JM, Colvin L (1999) Cost effectiveness of anterior cruciate ligament reconstruction in young adults. Clin Orthop Relat Res 367:272–282

Griffin LY, Albohm MJ, Arendt EA, Bahr R, Beynnon BD, DeMaio M, Dick RW, Engebretsen L, Garrett WE Jr, Hannafin JA, Hewett TE, Huston LJ, Ireland ML, Johnson RJ, Lephart S, Mandelbaum BR, Mann BJ, Marks PH, Marshall SW, Myklebust G, Noyes FR, Powers C, Shields C Jr, Shultz SJ, Silvers H, Slauterbeck J, Taylor DC, Teitz CC, Wojtys EM, Yu B (2006) Understanding and preventing noncontact anterior cruciate ligament injuries: a review of the Hunt Valley II meeting, January 2005. Am J Sports Med 34:1512–1532

Grooms D, Palmer T, Oñate J, Myer GD, Grindstaff T (2013) Soccer-specific warm-up and lower extremity injury rates in collegiate male soccer players. J Athl Train 48:782–789

Hawkins RD, Hulse MA, Wilkinson C, Hodson A, Gibson M (2001) The association football medical research programme: an audit of injuries in professional football. Br J Sports Med 35:43–47

Heidt RS Jr, Sweeterman LM, Carlonas RL, Traub JA, Tekulve FX (2000) Avoidance of soccer injuries with preseason conditioning. Am J Sports Med 28:659–662

Hewett TE, Ford KR, Myer GD (2006a) Anterior cruciate ligament injuries in female athletes: part 2, a meta-analysis of neuromuscular interventions aimed at injury prevention. Am J Sports Med 34:490–498

Hewett TE, Myer GD, Ford KR (2006b) Anterior cruciate ligament injuries in female athletes: part 1, mechanisms and risk factors. Am J Sports Med 34:299–311

Junge A, Dvorak J (2004) Soccer injuries: a review on incidence and prevention. Sports Med 34:929–938

Junge A, Rosch D, Peterson L, Graf-Baumann T, Dvorak J (2002) Prevention of soccer injuries: a prospective intervention study in youth amateur players. Am J Sports Med 30:652–659

Kiani A, Hellquist E, Ahlqvist K, Gedeborg R, Michaëlsson K, Byberg L (2010) Prevention of soccer-related knee injuries in teenaged girls. Arch Intern Med 170:43–49

Lohmander LS, Ostenberg A, Englund M, Roos H (2004) High prevalence of knee osteoarthritis, pain, and functional limitations in female soccer players twelve years after anterior cruciate ligament injury. Arthritis Rheum 50:3145–3152

Lohmander LS, Englund PM, Dahl LL, Roos EM (2007) The long-term consequence of anterior cruciate ligament and meniscus injuries: osteoarthritis. Am J Sports Med 35:1756–1769

Malliou P, Gioftsidou A, Pafis G, Beneka A, Godolias G (2004) Proprioceptive training (balance exercises) reduces lower extremity injuries in young soccer players. J Back Musculoskelet Rehabil 17:101–104

Mandelbaum BR, Silvers HJ, Watanabe DS, Knarr JF, Thomas SD, Griffin LY, Kirkendall DT, Garrett W Jr (2005) Effectiveness of a neuromuscular and proprioceptive training program in preventing anterior cruciate ligament injuries in female athletes: 2-year follow-up. Am J Sports Med 33:1003–1010

Morgan BE, Oberlander MA (2001) An examination of injuries in major league soccer. The inaugural season. Am J Sports Med 29:426–430

Myer GD, Sugimoto D, Thomas S, Hewett TE (2013) The influence of age on the effectiveness of neuromuscular training to reduce anterior cruciate ligament injury in female athletes: a meta-analysis. Am J Sports Med 41:203–215

Posthumus M, Collins M, September AV, Schwellnus MP (2011) The intrinsic risk factors for ACL ruptures: an evidence-based review. Phys Sportsmed 39:62–73

Renstrom P, Ljungqvist A, Arendt E, Beynnon B, Fukubayashi T, Garrett W, Georgoulis T, Hewett TE, Johnson R, Krosshaug T, Mandelbaum B, Micheli L, Myklebust G, Roos E, Roos H, Schamasch P, Shultz S, Werner S, Wojtys E, Engebretsen L (2008) Non-contact ACL injuries in female athletes: an International Olympic Committee current concepts statement. Br J Sports Med 42:394–412

Söderman K, Werner S, Pietila T, Engstrom B, Alfredson H (2000) Balance board training: prevention of traumatic injuries of the lower extremities in female soccer players? A prospective randomized intervention study. Knee Surg Sports Traumatol Arthrosc 8:356–363

Soligard T, Myklebust G, Steffen K, Holme I, Silvers H, Bizzini M, Junge A, Dvorak J, Bahr R, Andersen TE (2008) Comprehensive warm-up programme to prevent injuries in young female footballers: cluster randomised controlled trial. BMJ 337:a2469

Steffen K, Myklebust G, Olsen OE, Holme I, Bahr R (2008) Preventing injuries in female youth football – a cluster-randomized controlled trial. Scand J Med Sci Sports 18:605–614

Sugimoto D, Myer GD, Bush HM, Klugman MF, Medina McKeon JM, Hewett TE (2012a) Compliance with neuromuscular training and anterior cruciate ligament injury risk reduction in female athletes: a meta-analysis. J Athl Train 47:714–723

Sugimoto D, Myer GD, McKeon JM, Hewcsmett TE (2012b) Evaluation of the effectiveness of neuromuscular training to reduce anterior cruciate ligament injury in female athletes: a critical review of relative risk reduction and numbers-needed-to-treat analyses. Br J Sports Med 46:979–988

Van Beijsterveldt AMC, Van de Port IGL, Krist MR, Schmikli SL, Stubbe JH, Frederiks JE, Backx FJG (2012) Effectiveness of an injury prevention programme for adult male amateur soccer players: a cluster-randomised controlled trial. Br J Sports Med 46:1114–1118

Walden M, Atroshi I, Magnusson H, Wagner P, Hagglund M (2012) Prevention of acute knee injuries in adolescent female football players: cluster randomised controlled trial. BMJ 344:e3042

Anterior Cruciate Ligament Injuries: Prevention Strategies

109

Grethe Myklebust and Kathrin Steffen

Contents

Abstract

ACL injuries are a major challenge in many sports and the need for effective and efficacious prevention tools is essential. Most ACL injuries are noncontact in nature and being a female participating in a pivoting sport is a major risk factor. The main injury mechanisms are a cutting movement and a one-leg landing after a jump. Several prevention programs have successfully reduced the number of ACL injuries in different sports. The prevention programs consist of neuromuscular training, including lower extremity strength and balance exercises, in combination with core and trunk control. The chapter will present several prevention programs and discuss the future challenges in relation to ACL prevention.

Introduction

Severe knee injuries, such as ACL injuries, constitute a serious problem. Unfortunately, they are frequent in many sports. The knowledge regarding ACL injuries has improved substantially in the last 10–15 years. Knowledge about who is injured, how the athlete gets injured, and in many sports how to prevent ACL injuries is available. This chapter will briefly present ACL injury epidemiology, injury mechanism, and risk factors. The main focus will be to present the knowledge on how athletes can be prevented from having an

G. Myklebust (✉) • K. Steffen
Department of Sports Medicine, Oslo Sport Trauma Research Center, Norwegian School of Sport Sciences, Norwegian University of Sport and Physical Education, Oslo, Norway

IOC Medical & Scientific Department, Lausanne, Switzerland
e-mail: grethe.myklebust@nih.no; kathrin.steffen@nih.no

M.N. Doral, J. Karlsson (eds.), *Sports Injuries*,
DOI 10.1007/978-3-642-36569-0_82

ACL injury and touch upon the future challenges in ACL prevention.

Epidemiology: Who Is Injured?

In soccer, as in other team sports characterized by sudden changes of direction and pivoting accelerations and decelerations, ACL injuries are a particular concern, especially among female athletes. Studies have shown that female soccer and basketball players have a two to three times higher ACL injury risk compared to their male counterparts (Prodromos et al. 2007). In handball and wrestling females have a four times higher risk than male athletes (Myklebust et al. 1997; Prodromos et al. 2007), while no gender differences in knee injury risk were identified among World Cup alpine skiers (Bere et al. 2014).

Most ACL injuries occur in patients in the late teens and early 20s, and the differences between the sexes is apparent already in the beginning of the puberty (Walden et al. 2011; Sutton and Bullock 2013). Most athletes want to have an ACL reconstruction so they can continue playing their sport with a stable knee. Another argument for performing a reconstruction is that it may reduce the risk of further damage to knee, like meniscal tears and development of early osteoarthritis (OA). However, so far there is no evidence that ACL reconstructed patients develop less OA than patients treated nonoperatively.

The treatment algorithms after an ACL injury differ between different countries. In the USA it has been estimated that approximately 90–95 % of ACL injuries get reconstructed, while in the Scandinavian countries about 50 % are nonoperatively treated (Magnussen et al. 2010). However, it is a general agreement that if athletes desire to return to high-level pivoting sports, a reconstruction of the ACL is recommended.

Risk Factors

There is solid evidence that being a female athlete in a pivoting sport is a major risk factor for an ACL tear. The reasons for the obvious gender gap in the risk of ACL injury are not completely clear. Various researchers have suggested differences in anatomy and hormonal and neuromuscular function as potential reasons for the higher injury risk in women than in men. To date, however, there is little evidence linking all these potential intrinsic risk factors to noncontact ACL injuries, and a great deal of controversy exists on the relative importance of the different factors (Renstrom et al. 2008; Dai et al. 2012). In addition, recent studies have suggested that a history of knee ligament injury is a predominant risk factor for a subsequent injury, either a re-rupture of the ACL graft, an ACL rupture to the contralateral knee, or another severe knee injury (Hagglund et al. 2006; Steffen et al. 2008).

The main external risk factor that has been found is the effect of friction between shoes and the playing surface. Investigations from Australian rules football and handball suggest that a high shoe–surface friction is associated with an increased risk of ACL injury; for example, with high friction, the foot can abruptly stop in a cutting or turning maneuver. This will cause the knee to twist suddenly at foot strike and collapse (Olsen et al. 2003; Meyers and Barnhill 2004).

In addition, participating in a game appears to be a strong risk factor for knee injury. Studies from handball have shown that the relative risk of sustaining an ACL injury is up to 30 times higher in competition than in training (Myklebust et al. 1997, 2003). However, the exact reasons for the large difference are not determined. It will be necessary to assess playing situation and player/opponent behavior to improve our understanding.

Injury Mechanisms

ACL injuries are most commonly noncontact situations in nature (approximately 70 % of the injuries) and often occur in a cutting maneuver or in one-leg landing after a jump (Hewett et al. 2006). Even if there is no direct player contact to the knee, many cases involve some sort of perturbation by an opponent (e.g., being pushed slightly off balance prior to the occurrence of the injury). The mechanisms for noncontact

ACL injuries are widely debated. What seems clear from several studies from various team sports and even alpine skiing is that knee valgus (where the knee collapses inward into a "knock-knee" position) is an important factor in many cases. This implies that avoiding valgus knee motion is important for preventing injuries.

Prevention of ACL Injuries

Multiple studies have that acute knee injuries in general and more specific ACL injuries can be prevented (Myklebust et al. 2003; Olsen et al. 2005; Gilchrist et al. 2008; Walden et al. 2012). The successful prevention programs attempt to alter the quality of the movement in the lower leg to increase core and lower limb stability and raise awareness of the knee position in relation to the foot. One essential part of the programs is to emphasize the "hip–knee–toe in line position" in all types of exercises, both in balance and strength exercises. The primary goal of this strategy is to maintain posture and lower limb balance in an attempt to correct knee positioning as far as possible.

How? What Type of Exercises?

Most of the prevention programs are designed as structured warm-up programs to ensure that all players are exposed to the preventive effects on a regular basis. Studies from various sports show that proper warm-up on a regular basis can reduce the risk of ACL and lower extremity injuries by 30–50 % (Myklebust et al 2003; Olsen et al. 2005; Pasanen et al. 2008; Soligard et al 2008).

The "11+" program of the International Federation of Association Football (FIFA) is a good example of a multifaceted preventive program that includes core stability, balance, strength, and running exercises (Fig. 1) (Soligard et al. 2008). The exercises emphasize neuromuscular control and hip control and knee alignment that avoid excessive knee valgus during both static and dynamic movements. The program is divided into three parts: part I begins with running exercises; part II involves six exercises with three levels of increasing difficulty to improve strength, balance, muscle control, and core stability; part III concludes the program with further running exercises. The staged levels of difficulty increase the program's effectiveness and allow coaches and players to individually adapt the program to their needs. The program is a 20 min program and replaces the usual warm-up before training. The 11+ program was primarily developed to reduce lower limb injuries in youth and amateur football. However, similar multifaceted warm-up programs exist for other sports such as floorball and handball, and the same concept can be applied to other sport settings as well (Olsen et al. 2005; Pasanen et al. 2009).

In the Randomized Controlled Trial study by Olsen et al. among youth female and male handball players, they showed that a structured warm-up program including running exercises with and without ball, technique training focusing on planting and cutting movements and two-foot landings after jump shots, balance training, and strength and power exercises resulted in a 50 % reduction of acute lower extremity injuries. In addition, an 80 % reduction in severe knee ligament injuries was found among players in the intervention group compared to the control group (Olsen et al. 2005).

In the study by Myklebust et al. (2003), a five-phase neuromuscular training program was tried out among female top three level handball players (Fig. 2). The program consisted of three different balance exercises focusing on neuromuscular control and planting and landing skills. Though this program seems to focus on balance, there are also strength elements included, such as two- and one-leg squats. During an initial training period of 5–7 weeks, the exercise should be done a minimum of three times per week, with training for 15 min per session. Maintenance training once or twice a week continues throughout the competitive season.

Most of the exercises were partner exercises and the players were encouraged to be focused and conscious of the quality of their movements to improve awareness and knee control during standing, cutting, jumping, and landing. An important

The 11+
PART 1 RUNNING EXERCISES · 8 MINUTES
1 RUNNING STRAIGHT AHEAD
2 RUNNING HIP OUT
3 RUNNING HIP IN
4 RUNNING CIRCLING
5 RUNNING RUNNING & JUMPING
6 RUNNING QUICK RUN
PART 2 STRENGTH · PLYOMETRICS · BALANCE · 10 MINUTES
LEVEL 1
LEVEL 2
LEVEL 3
7 THE PLANK BOTH LEGS - 3 sets
7 THE PLANK ALTERNATE LEGS - 3 sets
7 THE PLANK ONE LEG LIFT - 3 sets
8 SIDE PLANK STATIC - 3 sets on each side
8 SIDE PLANK DYNAMIC - 3 sets on each side
8 SIDE PLANK WITH LEG LIFT - 3 sets on each side
9 HAMSTRINGS NORDIC HAMSTRINGS - 1 set
9 HAMSTRINGS NORDIC HAMSTRINGS - 1 set
9 HAMSTRINGS NORDIC HAMSTRINGS - 1 set
10 SINGLE-LEG BALANCE HOLD THE BALL - 2 sets
10 SINGLE-LEG BALANCE THROWING BALL WITH PARTNER - 2 sets
10 SINGLE-LEG BALANCE TEST YOUR PARTNER - 2 sets
11 SQUATS WITH TOE RAISE - 2 sets
11 SQUAT WALKING LUNGES - 2 sets
11 SQUATS ONE-LEG SQUATS - 2 sets on each leg
12 JUMPING VERTICAL JUMPS - 2 sets
12 JUMPING LATERAL JUMPS - 2 sets
12 JUMPING BOX JUMPS - 2 sets
PART 3 RUNNING EXERCISES · 2 MINUTES
13 RUNNING OVER THE PITCH
14 RUNNING BOUNDING RUN
15 RUNNING RUNNING & CUTTING
KNEE POSITION CORRECT
KNEE POSITION INCORRECT
Oslo Sports Trauma RESEARCH CENTER
F-MARC FOOTBALL FOR HEALTH
FIFA

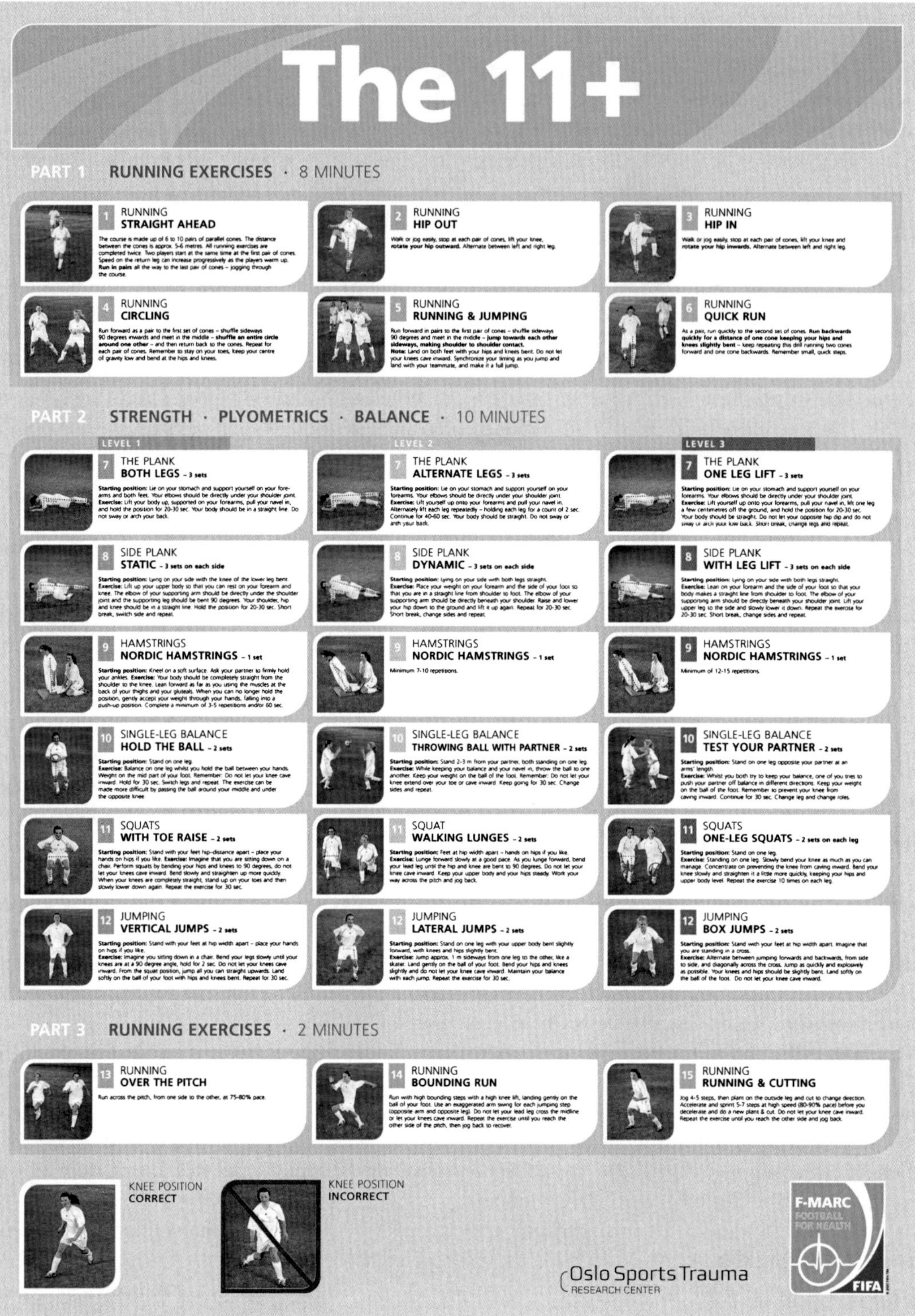

Fig. 1 The 11+ exercise program developed by the International Federation of Association Football (FIFA). http://f-marc.com/11plus/11plus/

Prevention of ACL injuries in team sport athletes
Right
Wrong
Level 1
Floor exercises
Running and planting, partner running backwards and giving feedback on the quality of the movement, change position after 20 s.
Mat exercises
Two players standing on one leg on the mat throwing to each other.
Wobble board exercises
Two players standing two legged on the board throwing to each other.
Level 2
Floor exercises
Jumping exercise–right leg–right leg over to left leg–left leg and finishing with a two-foot landing with flexion in both hips and knees.
R L R R L L L R L
Mat exercises
Jump shot from a box (30–40 cm high) with a two-foot landing with flexion in hip and knees.
Wobble board exercises
Squats on two legs, then on one leg.
Level 3
Floor exercises
Running and planting (as in week 1), now doing a full plant and cut movement with the ball, focusing on knee position.
Mat exercises
"Step" down from box with one-leg landing with flexion in hip and knee.
Wobble board exercises
Two players throwing to each other, one foot on the board.
Level 4
Floor exercises
Two and two players together two-leg jump forward and backwards, 180° turn and the same movement backwards; partner tries to push the player out of control but still focusing on landing technique.
Mat exercises
Two players both standing on balance mats trying to push partner out of balance, first on two-legs, then on one leg.
Wobble board exercises
One foot on the board, bounding the ball with their eyes shut.
Level 5
Floor exercises
Expanding the movement from week 3 to a full plant and cut, then a jump shot with two-legged landing.
Mat exercises
The players jump on a mat catching the ball, then take a 180° turn on the mat.
Wobble board exercises
Two players, both standing on balance boards trying to push partner out of balance, first on two legs, then on one leg.
Squats: Imagine that you are sitting down on a chair. Perform squats by bending your hips and knees to 90 degrees, do not let your knees cave inward. Bend slowly and straighten up more quickly.
Nordic Hamstrings: Your body should be completely straight from the shoulder to the knee. Lean forward as far as you can by using the hamstring muscles to resist the forward falling motion.
Squat-walking lunges: As you lunge forward, bend your lead leg until the hip and knee are bent to 90 degrees. Do not let your knee cave inward. Keep your upper body and hips steady.
Lateral jumps: Jump approx. 1m sideways from one leg to the other, like a skater. Land gently on the ball of your foot. Bend your hips and knees slightly and do no let your knee cave inward.
Sprunglauf: Spring as high and far as possible off the supporting leg. Bring the knee of the trailing leg up as high as possible and the opposite arm in front of the body.
Oslo Sports Trauma
RESEARCH CENTER
©www.skadefri.no
Skadefri!

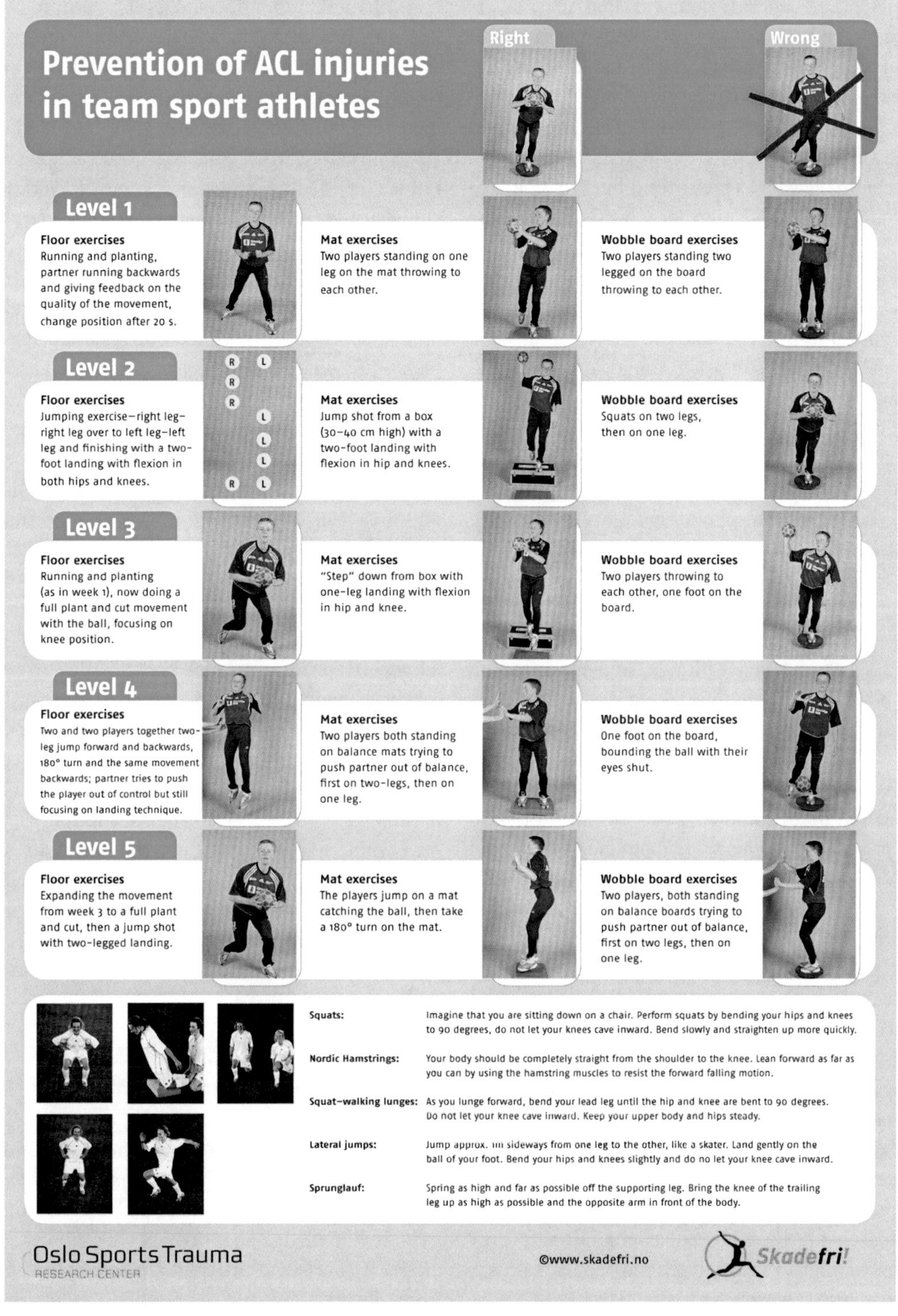

Fig. 2 Prevention of ACL injuries in team sport (Myklebust et al. 2003)

aspect of the intervention was that the players should give feedback to each other on their movement quality. Emphasis was given to core stability and hip and knee position in relation to the foot (the "knee over toe" position). The intervention gave a significant reduction of ACL injuries from the control season to the second intervention season among the elite players who completed the program, and they also found a significant reduction in the risk of noncontact ACL injuries (Myklebust et al. 2003). A video presentation of the prevention programs of Olsen et al. and Myklebust et al. studies is found at www.ostrc.no and at www.skadefri.no.

The neuromuscular warm-up program "Knäkontroll" ("knee control") significantly reduces the rate of ACL injuries among adolescent female football players (Walden et al. 2012). "Knäkontroll" contains exercises focusing on knee control and core stability similar to other programs in, for example, handball. The six exercises are one-leg knee squat, pelvic lift, two-leg knee squat, the bench, lunge, and exercises on jump/landing technique. Each exercise is subdivided into four steps of progressive difficulty (Fig. 3). The exercises are to be preceded by 5 minutes of low intensity running and take about 15 min to complete after familiarization. In the project, the teams were instructed to conduct the exercises during the warm-up at two training sessions a week throughout the whole season. All players started on the first level of difficulty and proceeded to the next level when exercises were performed with good control as assessed by the coach.

Evidence from research on recreational alpine skiers shows that an educational program to increase awareness of high-risk situations and of how to appropriately modify behavior can prevent ACL injuries. Although currently there are no prevention programs for skiers, it might be reasonable to assume that conditioning programs similar to those described for team sports might also work for alpine skiers (Bere et al. 2014).

As described, multifaceted warm-up programs all include balance and jumping exercises. These programs focus on strength, balance, coordination, jumping, and agility training. As known from injury statistics in many sports, it is vital to avoid high-risk positions for the knee joint. Hence, athletes should be instructed to land on both feet, because two-leg landings reduce the forces affecting each knee and thereby reduce the loading on the knee joints. In addition, studies of the injury mechanisms of knee injuries have shown that a landing with flexed knees and hips helps avoid knee valgus by better absorbing the landing forces. It is also stated that athletes in cutting sports should avoid a wide sidestep cutting technique, since it will increase knee valgus and the knee abduction moments, which gives a potentially harmful joint loading (Kristianslund et al. 2014).

ACL injury prevention works. However, there is still a lack of knowledge to optimize injury prevention programs to make them time efficient, which exercises are the "right ones," or the "perfect ones," if such exercises exist at all. Another important challenge is to convince coaches and athletes to use the present knowledge. "Are the exercises really worth doing? It takes 20 min; is it necessary to do this program every training session?" This is only some of the skepticism that is heard from the field. A future goal is to find the minimal effective dose to reduce the number of ACL injuries effectively; hopefully two to four exercises 5–10 min two to three times a week will be sufficient. Hopefully ongoing ACL risk factor studies will give an answer on the type of exercises and the dose needed to reduce ACL injury risk.

Who Should Be Targeted?

Most prevention programs today are made as one-size-fits all package, to be performed by all athletes. Hopefully, future studies will give more specific knowledge about which type of exercises different sports and different athletes should perform. Further evidence is needed to determine whether a preseason functional testing, e.g., by a drop jump or single-leg squat test, can be used to identify athletes with higher risk, e.g., poor knee control.

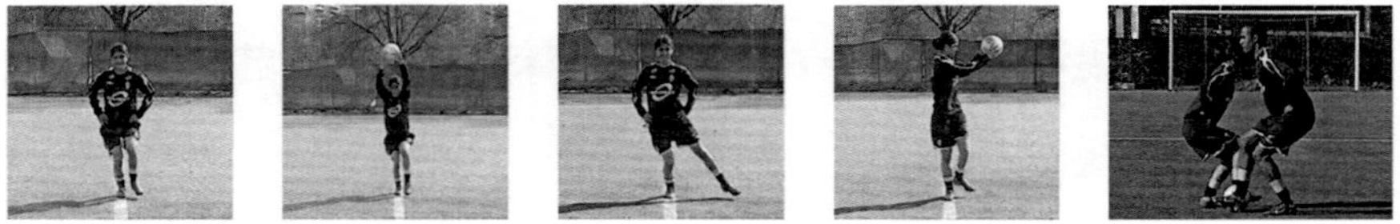

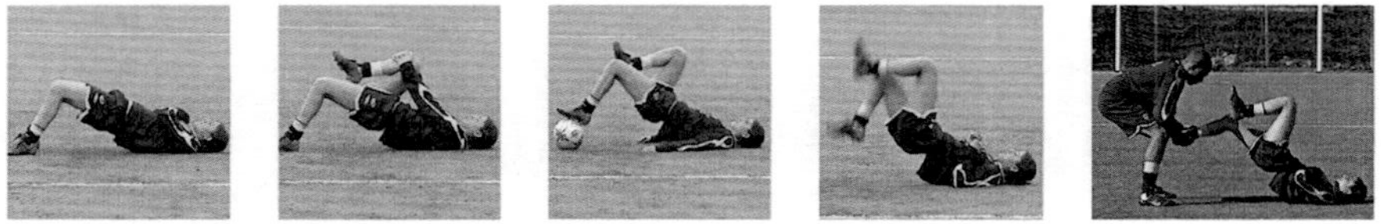

Exercise	Instructions	Repetitions/duration
1. One-legged knee squat	Slow movement with a smooth turn, horizontal pelvis and non-supporting foot in front of the body with slightly flexed hip and knee.	
Level A	Hands on the hips.	3 x 8-15 reps
Level B	Hold a ball over the head with straight arms.	3 x 8-15 reps
Level C	Hands on the hips. Mark with the non-supporting foot just above the ground at the 12-02-04-06 o'clock positions.	3 x 5 reps
Level D	Bend down while holding a ball and let the ball touch the ground outside the supporting foot. Make a diagonal movement upwards and raise the ball over the head with straight arms on the contralateral side.	3 x 8-15 reps
Pair-exercise	Teammate stands slightly oblique in front of you and a ball is pressed between the lateral sides of the feet of the non-supporting legs.	3 x 5-10 reps
2. Pelvic lift	Supine position. Lift the pelvis from the ground while keeping the back straight.	
Level A	Both feet on the ground and hands across the chest.	3 x 8-15 reps
Level B	One foot on the ground and the contralateral leg flexed in the hip and knee 90 degrees with both hands on the knee.	3 x 8-15 reps
Level C	One foot on a football and the contralateral leg flexed in the hip and knee 90 degrees with the arms on the ground alongside the body.	3 x 8-15 reps
Level D	One foot on the ground and the other in the air. Keep the upper arms on the ground with the elbows flexed 90 degrees. Push away the supporting foot and land on the other foot.	3 x 8-15 reps
Pair-exercise	Teammate stands with flexed knees and supports the heel of one of your feet in her hands. Hands across the chest and lift the pelvis.	3 x 8-15 reps
3. Two-legged knee squat	Slow movement with a smooth turn, back in a straight position and feet shoulder-wide apart with the soles in contact with the ground.	
Level A	Hold a ball in front of the body with straight arms.	3 x 8-15 reps
Level B	Hands on the hips.	3 x 8-15 reps
Level C	Hold a ball over the head with straight arms.	3 x 8-15 reps
Level D	Same as Level C but continue the movement and rise up on the toes after returning to the starting position and stay briefly in that position.	3 x 8-15 reps
Pair-exercise	Teammate stands next to you approximately 1 meter away, face opposite directions. Hold a ball between you with one hand and the other hand on the hip. Apply slight pressure on the ball while performing the knee squat.	3 x 8-15 reps

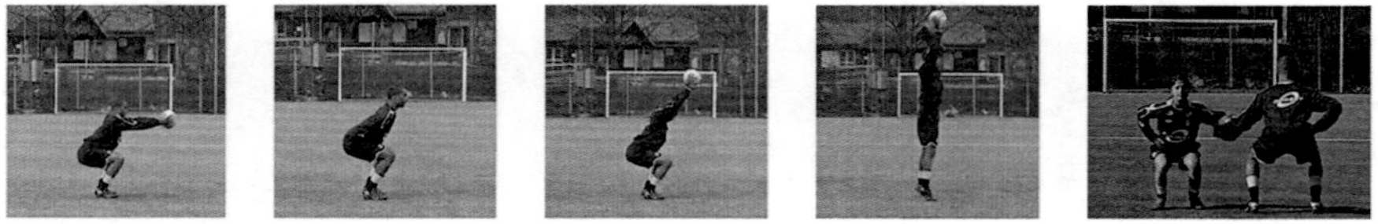

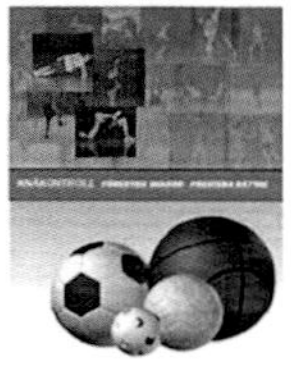

Waldén M, Atroshi I, Magnusson H, Wagner P, Hägglund M. Prevention of acute knee injuries in adolescent female football players: cluster randomised controlled trial. BMJ 2012;344:e3042 doi: 10.1136/bmj.e3042.
Waldén M, Atroshi I, Magnusson H, Wagner P, Hägglund M. Republished research: Prevention of acute knee injuries in adolescent female football players: cluster randomised controlled trial. Br J Sports Med. 2012 Oct;46(13):904.

Fig. 3 (continued)

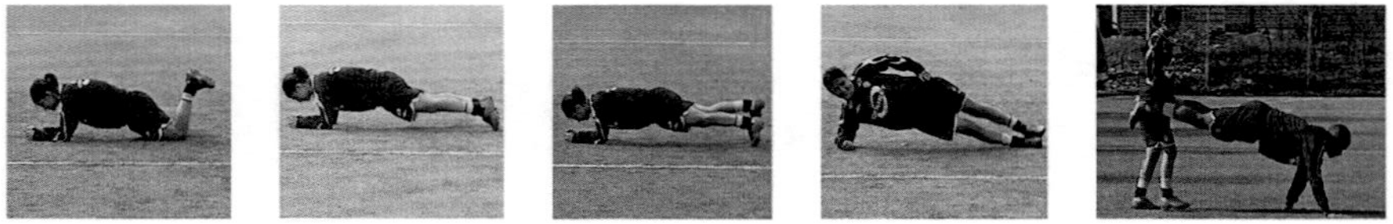

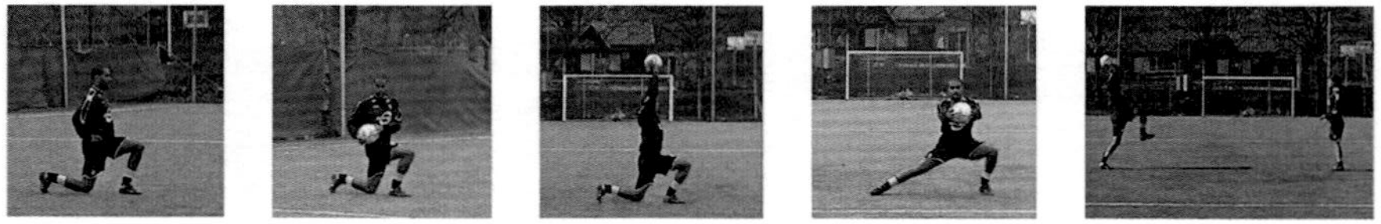

Exercise	Instructions	Repetitions/duration
4. The bench	Lift the body and keep it in a straight line.	
Level A	Prone position. Support on the knees and on the lower arms with the elbows kept under the shoulders.	15-30 sec
Level B	Same as Level A but with support on the tip of the feet.	15-30 sec
Level C	Same as Level B, but move the foot to the side and back to the starting position. Alternate sides.	15-30 sec
Level D	Lie sideways with support on the foot and the lower arm with the elbow kept under the shoulder and the other hand on the hip. Lift the hip off the ground and stay briefly in that position with good control before slowly returning to the starting position.	5-10 reps
Pair-exercise	Teammate stands behind you and holds your feet or lower legs. Lift the body and walk forward by using the hands on the ground.	15-30 sec
5. The lunge	Take a deep step with a marked knee lift and a soft landing. The rear knee should not touch the ground.	
Level A	Hands on the hips. Move forward with each step.	3 x 8-15 reps
Level B	Hold a ball in front of the body with straight arms. Rotate the upper body while stepping forward and position the ball laterally of the front leg. Move forward with each step and alternate sides.	3 x 8-15 reps
Level C	Hold a ball over the head with straight arms. Perform a forward lunge and push back with the front leg and return to the starting position.	3 x 8-15 reps
Level D	Hold a ball in front of the body with straight arms. Perform a sideway lunge and return to the starting position.	3 x 8-15 reps
Pair-exercise	Teammate stands in front of you 5-10 meters away. Perform a forward lunge while making a throw-in with a ball.	3 x 8-15 reps
6. Jump/landing	Make a jump with a soft landing. Stay briefly in the landing position.	
Level A	Stand on one leg with the knee slightly bent and hands on the hips. Make a short forward jump and land on the same foot. Jump backwards to the starting position.	3 x 8-15 reps
Level B	Stand on two legs shoulder-wide apart with the hands on the back. Make a sideways jump and land on one foot. Alternate sides.	3 x 8-15 reps
Level C	Take a few quick steps on the same spot and make a short jump straight forward landing on one foot.	3 x 5 reps
Level D	Same as level C, but change direction and jump to one side (90 degrees turn). Alternate sides.	3 x 5 reps
Pair-exercise	Teammate stands in front of you approximately 5 meters away. Make a two-legged jump while heading a football and land on two legs.	3 x 8-15 reps

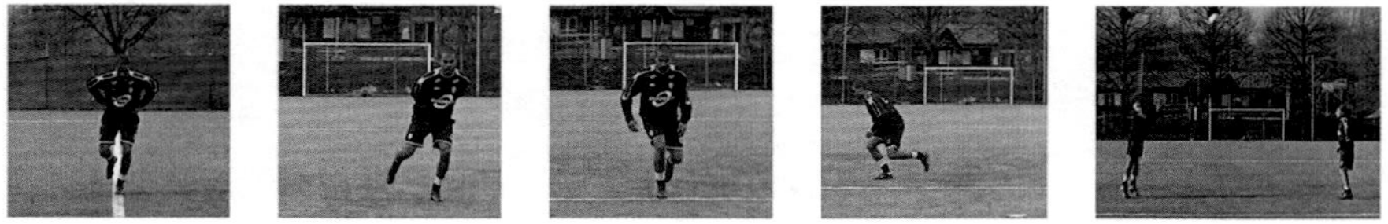

SvFF

Folksam

SISU Idrottsutbildarna

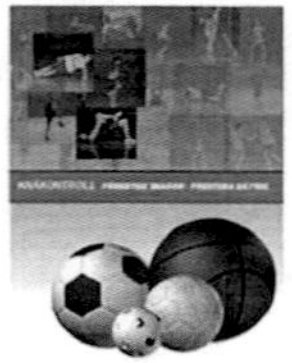

FOTBOLL

Waldén M, Atroshi I, Magnusson H, Wagner P, Hägglund M. Prevention of acute knee injuries in adolescent female football players: cluster randomised controlled trial. BMJ 2012;344:e3042 doi: 10.1136/bmj.e3042.
Waldén M, Atroshi I, Magnusson H, Wagner P, Hägglund M. Republished research: Prevention of acute knee injuries in adolescent female football players: cluster randomised controlled trial. Br J Sports Med. 2012 Oct;46(13):904.

Fig. 3 Knäkontroll study ("Knee control") (Waldén et al. 2012)

Effective prevention of sport injuries also requires successful implementation of efficacious interventions. This, in turn, requires knowledge about the implementation context, including how people, their attitudes, and their safety (or risk) behavior interact with these interventions. In other words, true injury prevention can only be achieved if some form of behavioral change occurs in all those involved with an athlete's safety and health (e.g., the athlete, coach, parents, and referee). Therefore, one of the major goals should be to establish sound habits for injury prevention early in life.

When to Start?

When giving recommendations in relation to the right age for implementing prevention exercises, most authors suggest starting as soon as children start participating in organized sports. From a motor learning development aspect, this age (6–12) might be important in relation to develop "good habits" and less vulnerable movement patters, in addition to establish correct playing technique and fair play. However, the youngest age groups are actually at low risk for injury; soccer is a safe sport for children. This is the conclusion in a study where the authors examined the risk of injuries in children 6–16 years old playing organized soccer. They presented injury data as relative injury risk (injury per 1,000 playing hours) and absolute injury risk (total number of injuries to a player or team during a season) and compared the numbers with injury data from elite soccer players. Interestingly, the comparison showed that elite players had an absolute injury risk which was 11 and 30 times higher than girls' ages 13–16 years and 6–12 years, respectively. Therefore, spending time on specific injury prevention programs among the youngest, who perhaps train once or twice a week, is probably neither realistic nor necessary. The results of Froholdt et al. (2009) support the notion that most efforts are required into prevention from 12 to 14 years. This is supported by the results from a meta-analysis by Myer and coworkers which revealed an age-related association between NMT implementation and reduction of ACL incidence. The data indicate that the potential window of opportunity for optimized ACL injury risk reduction may be before the onset of neuromuscular deficits and peak knee injury incidence in female athletes. Specifically, it may be optimal to initiate integrative NMT programs during early adolescence, before the period of altered mechanics that increase injury risk (Myer et al. 2013).

Prevention Works, also in the Long Run?

The studies presented in this chapter have shown that success in ACL injury prevention in the short run is possible. The interventions work when they are conducted, especially if the compliance with the program is sufficient. The intervention's efficacy (that the intervention is capable of producing the desired effect) is promising; however, their efficiency (whether the desired effect occurs under real-life conditions) is barely investigated. However, that an intervention is efficient in a controlled trial does not mean that it will be widely adopted and have an impact on public health. Finch (2006) emphasizes that only research that can and will be adopted by the participants, the coaches, and the sporting bodies will succeed in the long run.

In a study among Swiss amateur soccer players, a countrywide campaign to prevent soccer injuries was proven effective after implementing "The 11." More than 5,000 coaches were trained, and 4 years later the number of injuries among teams performing "The 11" was 10.7 % (matches) and 25.4 % (training) lower than teams not using the program (Junge et al. 2011). Another study in female handball wanted to investigate if the ACL injury prevention initiative taken in Norway during the last decade had been successful in the long run. The ACL incidence was followed 10 years after the ACL prevention study (Myklebust et al. 2003) was finished. After the intervention it was up to the teams and coaches to continue doing the prevention program; however, the post-intervention incidence surveillance from

2001 to 2005 showed that the ACL incidence gradually increased after the intervention and the teams and players did not continue to do the exercises. As a consequence several initiatives were started in the following years; in a series of regional coach seminars, at the end of the seminar, every attendee received a DVD including video clips of the preventing exercises. A new prevention study in handball showing an 80 % reduction in knee ligament injuries among the intervention group was published and received a lot of attention in the media and among the handball players and coaches (Olsen et al. 2005). These efforts were effective and a substantial reduction of the ACL numbers was seen in 2006. To continue the knowledge translation activities, the Oslo Sport Trauma Research Center launched a new website in 2008 to provide information on prevention programs in a format targeting coaches and athletes, including videos of different prevention programs (www.skadefri.no). A new ACL surveillance was performed in 2010–2011 and the low ACL incidence from 2006 was kept low (Myklebust et al. 2013). These studies show that the ACL injury rate can be kept low through nationwide preventive initiatives and focusing on the coach as the key partner.

Coach as a Key Partner

Winning and performance are the key factors for coaches and players. Therefore, motivating coaches and players to follow exercise programs is easier if they do not only prevent injuries but there also is a direct performance benefit. Coach education is the key. Knowledge of sport injuries, injury prevention, and attitudes and beliefs to the importance of injury prevention training is quite varied among coaches. This was confirmed in a study among female soccer coaches in the USA. In a survey, they found that only 20 % of the coaches had implemented the ACL prevention programs. Successful implementation was associated with performance- enhancing benefits of ACL prevention programs; education of the program should be required for licensure and ACL prevention programs should be driven by the soccer organizations (Joy et al. 2013). Well-trained coaches will be able to deliver a new exercise program in the correct way. Without doubt, injury prevention should be mandatory as part of the coach education and certification at all levels.

Conclusion

It is possible to prevent ACL injuries; however, much research is still needed. A better understanding on ACL injury risk factors and mechanisms may optimize current injury prevention programs and consequently result in fewer serious knee injuries and lower costs for the public health system. New prevention studies are not needed to confirm that the existing programs work; however, the current knowledge needs to be spread out, and coaches, athletes, and sport federations have to be convinced that ACL prevention is possible. Establish warm-up routines, stop talking about "injury prevention programs" or "special programs," and call them "exercises that improve performance and reduce injuries." This will make it an easier sell!

References

Bere T, Florenes TW, Nordsletten L et al (2014) Sex differences in the risk of injury in World Cup alpine skiers: a 6-year cohort study. Br J Sports Med. 2014 Jan;48(1):36–40

Dai B, Herman D, Liu H et al (2012) Prevention of ACL injury, part I: injury characteristics, risk factors, and loading mechanism. Res Sports Med 20:180–197

Finch C (2006) A new framework for research leading to sports injury prevention. J Sci Med Sport 9:3–9

Froholdt A, Olsen OE, Bahr R (2009) Low risk of injuries among children playing organized soccer: a prospective cohort study. Am J Sports Med 37:1155–1160

Gilchrist J, Mandelbaum BR, Melancon H et al (2008) A randomized controlled trial to prevent noncontact anterior cruciate ligament injury in female collegiate soccer players. Am J Sports Med 36:1476–1483

Hagglund M, Walden M, Ekstrand J (2006) Previous injury as a risk factor for injury in elite football: a prospective study over two consecutive seasons. Br J Sports Med 40:767–772

Hewett TE, Myer GD, Ford KR (2006) Anterior cruciate ligament injuries in female athletes: part 1, mechanisms and risk factors. Am J Sports Med 34:299–311

Joy E, Taylor JR, Novak M et al (2013) Factors influencing the implementation of ACL injury prevention strategies by girls soccer coaches. J Strength Cond Res 27:2263–2269

Junge A, Lamprecht M, Stamm H et al (2011) Countrywide campaign to prevent soccer injuries in Swiss amateur players. Am J Sports Med 39:57–63

Kristianslund E, Faul O, Bahr R et al (2014) Sidestep cutting technique and knee abduction loading: implications for ACL prevention exercises. Br J Sports Med. 2014 May;48(9):779–83

Magnussen RA, Granan LP, Dunn WR et al (2010) Cross-cultural comparison of patients undergoing ACL reconstruction in the United States and Norway. Knee Surg Sports Traumatol Arthrosc 18:98–105

Meyers MC, Barnhill BS (2004) Incidence, causes, and severity of high school football injuries on FieldTurf versus natural grass: a 5-year prospective study. Am J Sports Med 32:1626–1638

Myer GD, Sugimoto D, Thomas S et al (2013) The influence of age on the effectiveness of neuromuscular training to reduce anterior cruciate ligament injury in female athletes: a meta-analysis. Am J Sports Med 41:203–215

Myklebust G, Maehlum S, Engebretsen L et al (1997) Registration of cruciate ligament injuries in Norwegian top level team handball. A prospective study covering two seasons. Scand J Med Sci Sports 7:289–292

Myklebust G, Engebretsen L, Braekken IH et al (2003) Prevention of anterior cruciate ligament injuries in female team handball players: a prospective intervention study over three seasons. Clin J Sport Med 13:71–78

Myklebust G, Skjolberg A, Bahr R (2013) ACL injury incidence in female handball 10 years after the Norwegian ACL prevention study: important lessons learned. Br J Sports Med 47:476–479

Olsen OE, Myklebust G, Engebretsen L et al (2003) Relationship between floor type and risk of ACL injury in team handball. Scand J Med Sci Sports 13:299–304

Olsen OE, Myklebust G, Engebretsen L et al (2005) Exercises to prevent lower limb injuries in youth sports: cluster randomised controlled trial. BMJ 330:449

Pasanen K, Parkkari J, Pasanen M et al (2008) Neuromuscular training and the risk of leg injuries in female floorball players: cluster randomised controlled study. BMJ 337:295

Pasanen K, Parkkari J, Pasanen M et al (2009) Effect of a neuromuscular warm-up programme on muscle power, balance, speed and agility: a randomised controlled study. Br J Sports Med 43:1073–1078

Prodromos CC, Han Y, Rogowski J et al (2007) A meta-analysis of the incidence of anterior cruciate ligament tears as a function of gender, sport, and a knee injury-reduction regimen. Arthroscopy 23:1320–1325

Renstrom P, Ljungqvist A, Arendt E et al (2008) Non-contact ACL injuries in female athletes: an International Olympic Committee current concepts statement. Br J Sports Med 42:394–412

Soligard T, Myklebust G, Steffen K et al (2008) Comprehensive warm-up programme to prevent injuries in young female footballers: cluster randomised controlled trial. BMJ 337:a2469

Steffen K, Myklebust G, Andersen TE et al (2008) Self-reported injury history and lower limb function as risk factors for injuries in female youth soccer. Am J Sports Med 36:700–708

Sutton KM, Bullock JM (2013) Anterior cruciate ligament rupture: differences between males and females. J Am Acad Orthop Surg 21:41–50

Walden M, Hagglund M, Werner J et al (2011) The epidemiology of anterior cruciate ligament injury in football (soccer): a review of the literature from a gender-related perspective. Knee Surg Sports Traumatol Arthrosc 19:3–10

Walden M, Atroshi I, Magnusson H et al (2012) Prevention of acute knee injuries in adolescent female football players: cluster randomised controlled trial. BMJ 344:e3042

Primary Anterior Cruciate Ligament Repair in Athletes with Mesenchymal Stem Cells and Platelet-Rich Plasma

110

Alberto Gobbi, Dnyanesh G. Lad, Georgios Karnatzikos, and Sukeshrao Sankineni

Contents

A. Gobbi (✉) • D.G. Lad • G. Karnatzikos
Orthopaedic Arthroscopic Surgery International (O.A.S.I.) Bioresearch Foundation, Gobbi Onlus, Milan, Italy
e-mail: gobbi@cartilagedoctor.it; sportmd@tin.it; dnyaneshlad@gmail.com; fellow@oasiortopedia.it; giokarnes@gmail.com

S. Sankineni
Sports Medicine, OASI Bioresearch Foundation Gobbi NPO, Orthopaedic Arthroscopic Surgery International, Milan, Italy
e-mail: sukeshrao.sankineni@gmail.com

M.N. Doral, J. Karlsson (eds.), *Sports Injuries*,
DOI 10.1007/978-3-642-36569-0_262

Abstract

Anterior cruciate ligament (ACL) injuries are very common, affecting a young, active population and shrouded in controversy regarding the appropriate treatment. New and alternative treatment options need to be investigated to address acute partial ACL tears. There are numerous advantages in repairing the ACL rather than reconstructing it. With bone marrow healing stimulation, introduction of platelet-rich plasma injections, and availability of synthetic and biologic scaffolds, repair of the ACL is no longer an impossible task. Current treatment strategy for ACL rupture, although satisfactory, can be improved in the case of partial tears.

Introduction

Rupture of the anterior cruciate ligament (ACL) is one of the most common knee injuries with an incidence of 1 in 3,000 (Frank and Jackson 1997). As a result of increased participation in recreational and competitive sporting activities, the number of knee ligament injuries has been on a steady rise in the past few decades. According to an ongoing study in the United States, an estimated 200,000 ACL reconstructions (ACLR) are performed annually (National Institutes of Health (NIH) et al. 2011). The sequelae of chronic anterior tibial instability have been well described and documented, including episodic pain and instability, chondral and meniscal injury, and early-onset osteoarthritis. The treatment of acute ACL injury is an area of considerable controversy, although sports medicine has seen rapid advances in the recent years. Despite having a high success rate of 80 %, ACL reconstruction with tendon graft still has some disadvantages. Reduced proprioception, postoperative tendon weakness, inability to restore normal knee kinematics, and premature onset of osteoarthritis are some of the reported shortcomings following ACLR (Gobbi et al. 2005; Lohmander et al. 2007). Considering the fact that ACL tears most commonly affect young people, leading to significant morbidity, newer and alternative therapeutic options should be investigated to effectively address acute partial ACL lesions.

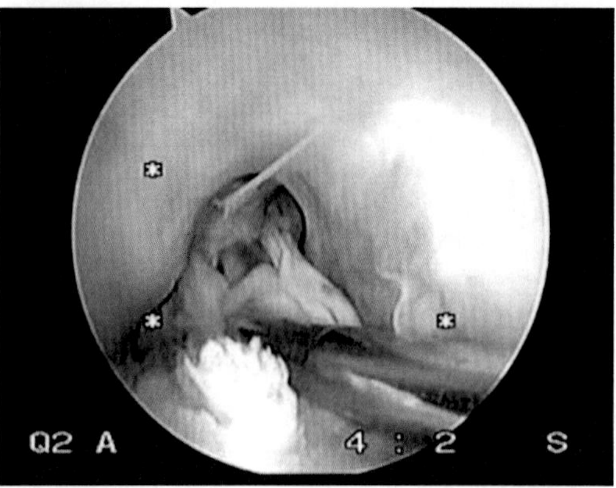

Fig. 1 Torn ACL

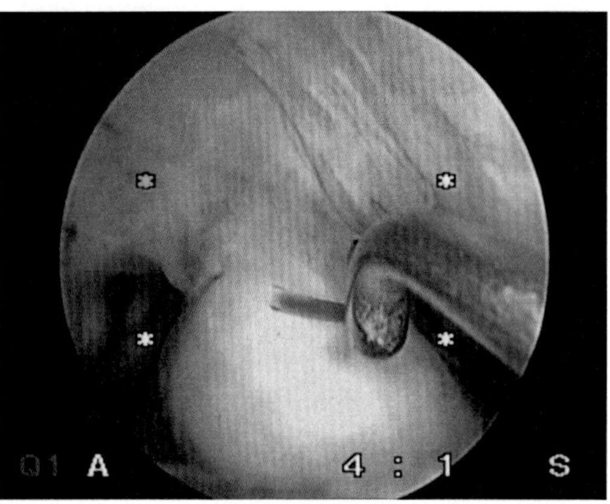

Fig. 2 The healed ACL following primary suture of the ligament augmented with the use of growth factors and bone marrow-derived multipotent, mesenchymal stem cells

ACL Repair

Suture repair of the torn ACL was first described in 1895; but it was O' Donoghue who popularized this technique in the 1950s (O'Donoghue 1950). Long-term follow-up studies showed that these techniques presented failure rates up to 90 % and were therefore abandoned (Feagin and Curl 1976). Despite reports of poor healing potential of the ACL in the past, recent investigations have demonstrated the possibility of ACL healing after primary suture of the ligament augmented with the use of growth factors and bone marrow-derived multipotent, mesenchymal stem cells (BMSCs) (Kaplan et al. 1990; Steadman et al. 2006; Murray et al. 2009) (Figs. 1 and 2). The potential advantage of repair over reconstruction technique is the preservation of the anatomy and kinematics of the ACL, proprioception of the knee, absence of donor-site morbidity, and potentially decreased muscular weakness.

Cellular therapies offer an interesting option in the treatment of the injured ACL by addressing the defect in healing at a molecular level and leading to a more biological way of healing. Steadman's "healing response therapy" (Steadman et al. 2006) was one of the earliest treatments described which extolled the role of BMSCs in aiding the healing of a ruptured ACL in human subjects. The results of this therapy were reported as encouraging and were based on the multipotent nature of the bone marrow cells. The recent finding of similarity between ACL outgrowth cells and BMSCs (Steinert et al. 2011) has presented the possibility to modulate these cells to enhance the healing of a repaired ACL. Bioactive proteins and growth factors play an important role in tissue healing because they can regulate key processes in tissue repair, including cell proliferation, chemotaxis, migration, cellular differentiation, and extracellular matrix synthesis (Gobbi et al. 2012). Platelet-rich plasma (PRP) contains many important growth factors, and recent studies have proven the beneficial effects of PRP in augmenting the healing of ACL (Murray et al. 2007; Cheng et al. 2010).

For repair of the ACL, therapies can be broadly classified into three methods: cellular, structural, and composite solutions.

Cellular Therapies

Bone Marrow Healing Stimulation

The ideal source of cells for use in an ACL engineering paradigm should provide cells that are readily available for clinical use, show robust proliferation, and possess the potential to elaborate extracellular matrix (ECM) in an organized fashion (Petrigliano et al. 2006). Early studies established the capacity of fibroblasts originating from various mesenchymal tissues to proliferate, synthesize collagen, and respond to mechanical and biochemical growth factors making them a potential source for ligament engineering. Although adult fibroblasts retain many of the phenotypic qualities necessary for collagen synthesis, they are relatively quiescent and have limited potential for further differentiation (Van Eijk et al. 2004). Bone marrow stromal cells (BMSC) are an attractive candidate for ligament engineering because they have the potential to differentiate into cells of multiple mesenchymal lineages, the synthetic and proliferative systems of these cells are robust, and they have the potential to readily adapt to their local niche. BMSC can be easily accessed in most patients without significant additional surgery or the risk of immune reaction (Vunjak-Novakovic et al. 2004). A comparative evaluation of goat BMSCs, ACL fibroblasts, and skin fibroblasts was undertaken by Van Eijk et al. (Van Eijk et al. 2004) to evaluate the optimal cell source for ACL engineering. The cells were seeded onto a degradable suture material and cultured for a maximum of 12 days. Each of the cell types attached, proliferated, and synthesized ECM rich in type I collagen. However, the scaffolds seeded with BMSCs showed the highest DNA content and collagen production.

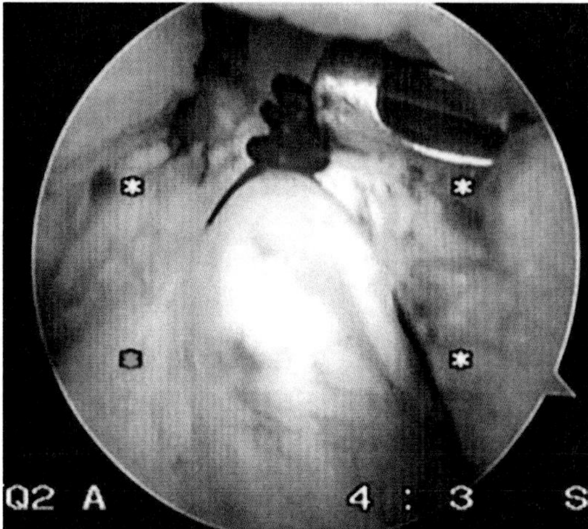

Fig. 3 Primary repair of ACL, suture seen in situ

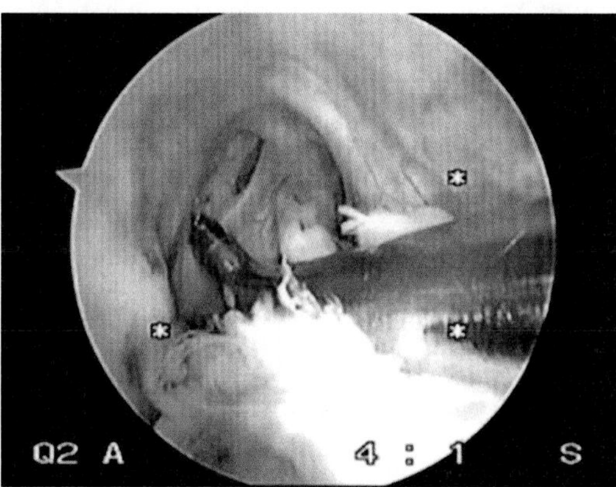

Fig. 4 Microfracture at the ACL insertion to facilitate healing stimulation

In 2009, an article published in the American Journal of Sports Medicine showed that primary ACL repair combined with bone marrow healing stimulation could restore satisfactory knee stability and function in athletes with acute ACL incomplete tears (Gobbi et al. 2009) (Figs. 3 and 4).

Platelet-Rich Plasma (PRP) and Growth Factors

PRP is defined as the volume of the plasma fraction from autologous blood with a platelet concentration above the baseline count

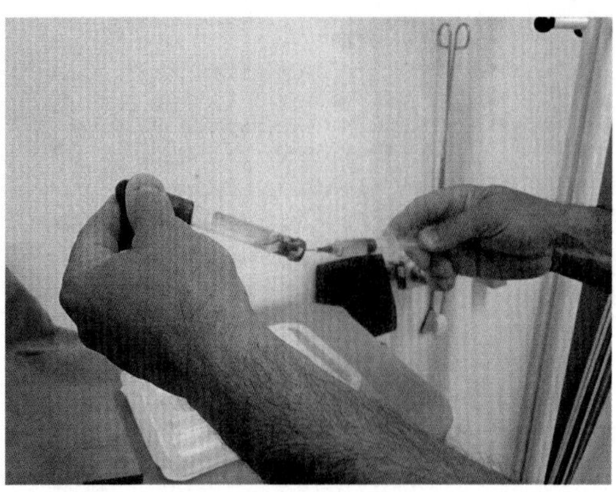

Fig. 5 PRP being aspirated into a syringe after its preparation

(200,000 platelets/μL). Platelets contain many important bioactive proteins and growth factors (GFs). These factors regulate key processes in tissue repair, including cell proliferation, chemotaxis, migration, cellular differentiation, and extracellular matrix synthesis. The rationale for the use of PRP is to stimulate the natural healing cascade and tissue regeneration by a "supraphysiologic" release of platelet-derived factors directly at the site of treatment.

Autologous PRP can be obtained from simple blood extraction with a commercially available kit. Once the blood is collected into a tube containing anticoagulant, it undergoes a centrifugation process to produce PRP (Fig. 5). For PRP gel preparations, platelets are normally activated by thrombin (autologous or animal derived), calcium chloride, or procoagulant enzyme (i.e., batroxobin), which works as a fibrinogen-cleaving enzyme inducing rapid fibrin clot formation. When PRP solutions are injected directly for topical treatment, platelets are activated by endogenous thrombin and/or intra-articular collagen. Based on the preparation methods, PRP can be referred to as leukocyte-rich PRP, leukocyte-poor PRP (LP-PRP), or platelet-poor PRP (PPP) (Dohan Ehrenfest et al. 2008). A PRP preparation rich in growth factors is the preferred preparation to aid in tendon healing and improving functional outcomes in patients. As per the absolute number of platelets obtained, method of activation, and presence or absence of white blood cells (PAW) classification system, the PRP obtained was classified as P2 Bβ (P2 = platelets > baseline levels to 750,000 platelets/*u*L, B = WBCs below or equal to baseline level, β = neutrophils equal or below baseline, if activated "x" is added) (DeLong et al. 2012). PRP is rich in growth factors such as platelet-derived growth factor (PDGF), transforming growth factor-β (TGF-β), and IGF-1 which are known to have a role in the biological healing process.

However, researchers have questioned the beneficial effects of isolated PRP use in tissue healing. Murray et al. (Murray et al. 2009) contested the role of PRP in ACL healing following their results in skeletally immature animals. They performed ACL repair in 15 pigs and ACL repair with PRP injection in another 15 pigs, but the addition of PRP to the suture repairs did not improve AP knee laxity maximum tensile load or linear stiffness of the ACL repairs after 14 weeks in vivo. However, the use of collagen-platelet composites has been reported to have beneficial effects (Vunjak-Novakovic et al. 2004). Growth factors have been proven in in vitro studies to enhance cellular proliferation and migration and increase collagen production. Among the growth factors, PDGF, fibroblast growth factor (FGF), bone morphogenic protein (BMP), and TGF-β have shown to enhance the healing of ligaments. Kobayashi et al. (Kobayashi et al. 1997) noted improved healing and vascularity following instillation of FGF in the canine ACL, while Aspenberg and Forslund (Aspenberg and Forslund 1999) reported the use of BMP 14 in the Achilles tendon and showed improved healing. These growth factors can be used along with synthetic scaffolds to enhance the process of repair of ACL. Chen (Chen 2009) reported the use of BMP 2 along with hydrogel and periosteum to stimulate tendon-bone healing in an ACL reconstruction model. Moreau et al. (Moreau et al. 2005) have attempted to establish specific media formulations and growth factor combinations that support BMSC differentiation toward a fibroblast phenotype. They reported that media supplemented with ascorbate-2-phosphate was potent in promoting BMSC proliferation, and they cited three growth factors and media combinations that enhanced fibroblast differentiation: (1) EGF and TGF, (2) bFGF and TGF, and (3) growth factor-free advanced Dulbecco's minimal essential medium (ADMEM).

Experience with Cellular Therapies

In a study conducted at Orthopaedic Arthroscopic Surgery International (OASI) Bioresearch Foundation, Milan, 50 athlete patients were prospectively followed up for 5 years. All of them underwent an arthroscopic primary ACL repair combined with BMS technique and growth factors after an acute partial ACL injury. Included in this study were patients less than 40 years old presenting with a documented acute ACL injury (<4 weeks from the time of trauma), with a history of giving away sensation, and positive Lachman and pivot shift tests. Exclusion criteria were lesions not amenable to primary repair, mid-substance ACL tears, associated chondral lesions > grade 3 on the ICRS classification system, partial or complete tears of the lateral (fibular) collateral ligament (LCL) or posterior cruciate ligament (PCL), grade 3 medial collateral ligament (MCL) injury, patients with contralateral knee ligament injury, severe lower limb malalignment, and history of previous surgery on the same knee. Anterior translation of the knee was objectively assessed with the use of Rolimeter® (Aircast ®, Boca 100 Raton, FL, USA), and the pivot shift was measured before surgery under anesthesia according to the IKDC objective knee score. Knee function and activity level were assessed using Marx, Noyes, Tegner, single assessment numeric evaluation (SANE), Lysholm, and IKDC objective scoring systems which were assessed preoperatively and followed up at 1, 2, and 5 years. ACL repair was performed by passing No. 1 polydioxanone (PDS) sutures (Ethicon, Piscataway, New Jersey) using a Clever Hook or Express suture passer (DePuy Mitek, Raynham, Massachusetts) through the torn portions of the ACL and tied using a Duncan loop. The aim of this step was re-approximation of the torn ends of the ligament, thereby reducing the gap between the residual ends and providing continuity to the ligament, allowing the BMSCs recruited from the penetration of the bone marrow to promote healing. Using a 45° microfracture awl, several holes (1.5 mm in diameter, 3–4 mm apart, and 3 mm deep) were made around the anatomic femoral insertion of the ACL. Bleeding was confirmed under direct visualization. PRP glue was then injected at the repaired site to biologically augment the healing process. In cases of a partial tear of both the AM and PL bundles, a microfracture was performed around the femoral insertion of the ACL followed by pasting the PRP glue along the tendon; no suture repair was performed in these lesions. The rehabilitation protocol was standardized for all patients.

Four patients had a re-tear during sporting activity and underwent ACL reconstruction within 2 years from primary repair surgery; their last evaluation scores at 2 years follow-up were included in the final results. Three patients out of the four were involved in high-risk sports. One patient presented with loss of ROM greater than 15° at final follow-up. One patient had episodes of giving away of the operated knee despite a lack of any significant injury, but an MRI revealed an intact but lax ligament. Anterior translation was significantly reduced (<3 mm side to side difference) at 5 years follow-up. Pre-injury and final Tegner scores were comparable, while the final SANE score was significantly lower than the pre-injury value. The final Marx, Noyes, and Lysholm scores were similar to the preoperative values. The final IKDC objective score was normal in 78 % of patients, nearly normal in 20 %, and severely abnormal in 2 %. Thirty-nine patients (78 %) fully resumed sport activity. The return to sport was reached at a mean of 5.9 (SD = 1.3) months after surgery. Eleven patients (22 %) did not return to sport at pre-injury level; in four of them, this was a personal choice. A second look arthroscopy was performed in six out of 50 patients and revealed a healed ACL which was stable on probing and had minimal fibrous tissue.

It was concluded that primary ACL repair with BMS and growth factors represents an effective procedure in the treatment of acute partial ACL tears. However, careful patient selection, accurate surgical technique, and proper functional rehabilitation are essential to achieve good results. This treatment does not burn any bridges so that conversion to a standard ACLR can be done in the event of a failure.

Structural Therapies

Supplementing a ruptured ACL with a scaffold is an interesting method to aid in the healing of the ACL. An ideal scaffold must be biocompatible with the cell source and recipient, while allowing for cell adhesion and proliferation. The scaffold must be strong enough to withstand mechanical stress, yet it must degrade over time and yield to the progress of native tissue ingrowth. Moreover, the scaffold structure will influence the transport of nutrients, metabolites, and regulatory molecules to and from the cells seeded within the scaffold (Gobbi et al. 2009) (Fig. 6). Many varieties of scaffold materials have been considered, including biologic materials such as collagen, silk, and biodegradable polymers and composite materials (Lin et al. 1999; Steadman et al. 2006). Collagen received a great deal of early interest and has been in clinical use for decades. Although the fibrous collagen scaffolds support cell attachment, spreading, and fiber coverage with ECM, the capacity of the construct to support mechanical loading decreases over time (Goulet et al. 1997). This has led investigators to study alternative scaffold materials. Molecules such as hyaluronic acid, chitosan, and alginate, which have inherent biocompatibility and cell-adhesion properties, have been modified to make them more appropriate for ligament engineering applications (Majima et al. 2005). Wiig et al. (Wiig et al. 1990) reported the use of intra-articular hyaluronic acid as a scaffold in a central defect rabbit model with a ruptured ACL and reported a greater angiogenic response, more pronounced repair, and higher type III collagen when compared to saline-treated controls. However, the biomechanical strength of the healing tendons was not assessed in their study. In recent times, use of hydrogel either as a scaffold alone or as a composite with collagen, platelet-rich plasma (PRP) (Moreau et al. 2005), and periosteum (Majima et al. 2005) has shown good outcomes in experimental studies. The results of the clinical application of this product in humans are awaited.

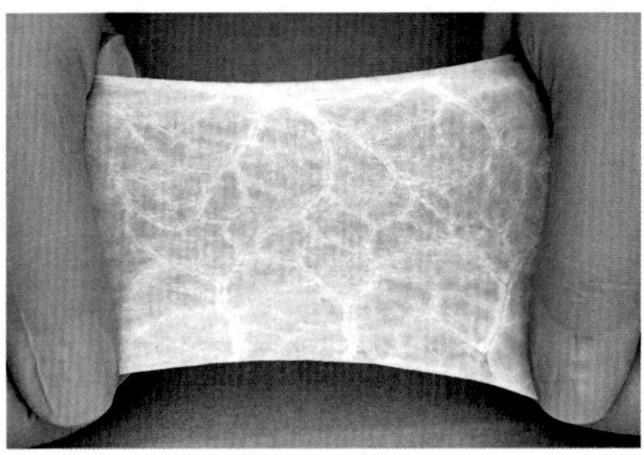

Fig. 6 Collagen-based scaffold

Cell Scaffold Composites

A combination of cell therapy embedded in a scaffold seems to be a promising treatment of ACL rupture. This is based on the premise that while PRP/BMSCs from the bone marrow will act as the source of growth factors and precursor cells, the scaffold would act both as a matrix in the cellular process and as a biomechanical support following primary repair of ACL and provide a secure environment for the cells away from the effects of plasmin. In an in vitro study by Cheng et al. (Cheng et al. 2010), the addition of PRP to collagen hydrogel enhanced ACL cell viability, metabolic activity, and collagen synthesis and has been purported to stimulate ACL healing. In an experimental study conducted by Murray et al. (Murray et al. 2009), supplementation of suture repair with collagen-platelet composite resulted in the formation of a large scar mass in the region of the ACL in a porcine ACL model. Load at yield, maximum load, and ACL tangent modulus were all significantly higher in the suture repairs augmented with collagen-platelet composite than in repairs performed with suture alone. Other laboratory studies have also supported this concept and elucidated the potential benefits of the cell-scaffold composites (Fan et al. 2008).

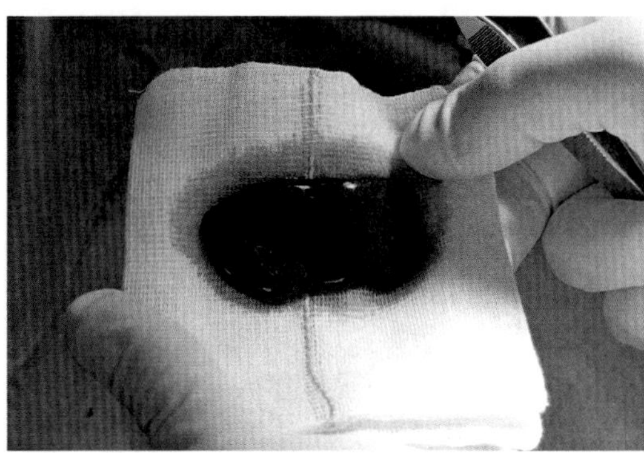

Fig. 7 Appearance of BMAC once prepared and ready for use

After conducting laboratory studies in Sweden, the OASI Bioresearch Foundation is starting a new project where a group of patients will undergo primary ACL repair augmented with a synthetic slowly degradable scaffold enriched with bone marrow aspirate concentrate (BMAC) embedded in platelet-rich plasma (Fig. 7). The BMAC is expected to act as a source of BMSCs and PRP as a source of growth factors, and the biodegradable scaffold should augment the repaired ligament and provide a matrix for the tissue ingrowth giving both cellular and biomechanical support to the injured tissue.

Conclusions

With the modern emphasis on fitness and athleticism, the prevalence of ACL injuries is on the rise, and patients' expectations have also increased. The current strategies applied to ACL reconstruction are satisfactory. However, the goal should remain to improve this procedure further and eliminate its associated complications. ACL primary repair and a healing stimulation technique can be a viable treatment in acute partially torn ACL. Careful patient selection and proper functional rehabilitation are essential to achieve good results. Current research has found that natural and synthetic scaffolds can sustain cell adhesion, growth, and matrix deposition under appropriate conditions and that growth factors and mechanical stimuli have a role in modulating cellular response. Although these advancements are promising, many obstacles persist. Only through perseverance and human trials will we succeed in this endeavor to achieve successful ACL repairs.

Cross-References

▶ Anterior Cruciate Ligament Augmentation in Partial Ruptures
▶ Anterior Cruciate Ligament Injuries and Surgery: Current Evidence and Modern Development
▶ Arthroscopic Repair of Partial Anterior Cruciate Ligament Tears: Perspective from an Orthopedics Surgeon

References

Aspenberg P, Forslund C (1999) Enhanced tendon healing with GDF 5 and 6. Acta Orthop Scand 70(1):51–54

Chen CH (2009) Strategies to enhance tendon graft-bone healing in anterior cruciate ligament reconstruction. Chang Gung Med J 32(5):483–493

Cheng M, Wang H, Yoshida R et al (2010) Platelets and plasma proteins are both required to stimulate collagen gene expression by anterior cruciate ligament cells in three-dimensional culture. Tissue Eng Part A 16(5):1479–1489

DeLong J, Ryan R, Mazzocca A (2012) Platelet-rich plasma: the PAW classification system. Arthrosc J Arthrosc Relat Surg 28(7):998–1009

Dohan Ehrenfest DM, Rasmusson L, Albrektsson T (2008) Classification of platelet concentrates: from pure platelet-rich plasma (P-PRP) to leukocyte- and platelet-rich fibrin (L-PRF). Trends Biotechnol 27(3):158–167

Fan H, Liu H, Wong EJ et al (2008) In vivo study of anterior cruciate ligament regeneration using mesenchymal stem cells and silk scaffold. Biomaterials 29(23):3324–3337

Feagin JA Jr, Curl WW (1976) Isolated tear of the anterior cruciate ligament: 5-year follow-up study. Am J Sports Med 4:95–100

Frank CB, Jackson DW (1997) The science of reconstruction of the anterior cruciate ligament. J Bone Joint Surg Am 79:1556–1576

Gobbi A, Domzalski M, Pascual J et al (2005) Hamstring anterior cruciate ligament reconstruction: is it necessary to sacrifice the gracilis? Arthroscopy 21(3):275–280

Gobbi A, Bathan L, Boldrini L (2009) Primary repair combined with bone marrow stimulation in anterior cruciate ligament lesions: results in a group of athletes. Am J Sports Med 37(3):571–578

Gobbi A, Karnatzikos G, Mahajan V et al (2012) Platelet-rich plasma treatment in symptomatic patients with knee osteoarthritis: preliminary results in a group of active patients. Sports Health 4(2):162–172

Goulet F, Germaine L, Rancourt D et al (1997) Tendons and ligaments. In: Lanza RP, Langer R, Chick W (eds) Principles of tissue engineering, 2nd edn. Landes/Academic, San Diego, pp 711–721

Kaplan N, Wickiewicz TL, Warren RF (1990) Primary surgical treatment of anterior cruciate ligament ruptures. A long-term follow-up study. Am J Sports Med 18(4):354–358

Kobayashi D, Kurosaka M, Yoshiya S et al (1997) Effect of basic fibroblast growth factor on the healing of defects in the canine anterior cruciate ligament. Knee Surg Sports Traumatol Arthrosc 5(3):89–194

Lin VS, Lee MC, O'Neal S et al (1999) Ligament tissue engineering using synthetic biodegradable fiber scaffolds. Tissue Eng 5:443–452

Lohmander LS, Englund PM, Dahl LL et al (2007) The long-term consequence of anterior cruciate ligament and meniscus injuries: osteoarthritis. Am J Sports Med 35(10):1756–1769

Majima T, Funakosi T, Iwasaki N et al (2005) Alginate and chitosan polyion complex hybrid fibers for scaffolds in ligament and tendon tissue engineering. J Orthop Sci 10:302–307

Moreau JE, Chen J, Bramono DS et al (2005) Growth factor induced fibroblast differentiation from human bone marrow stromal cells in vitro. J Orthop Res 23:164–174

Murray MM, Spindler KP, Abreu E et al (2007) Collagen-platelet rich plasma hydrogel enhances primary repair of the porcine anterior cruciate ligament. J Orthop Res 25(1):81–91

Murray MM, Palmer M, Abreu E et al (2009) Platelet-rich plasma alone is not sufficient to enhance suture repair of the ACL in skeletally immature animals: an in vivo study. J Orthop Res 27(5):639–645

National Institutes of Health (NIH), National Institute of Arthritis and Musculoskeletal and Skin Diseases (NIAMS), Vanderbilt University, United States (2011) Prognosis and Predictors of ACL Reconstruction – A Multicenter Cohort Study. Available at: http://clinicaltrials.gov/ct2/show/NCT00463099

O' Donoghue DH (1950) Surgical treatment of fresh injuries to the major ligaments of the knee. J Bone Joint Surg Am 32(A: 4):721–738

Petrigliano F, McAllister D, Wu B (2006) Tissue engineering for anterior cruciate ligament reconstruction: a review of current strategies. Arthroscopy 22(4):441–451

Steadman JR, Cameron-Donaldson ML, Briggs KK et al (2006) A minimally invasive technique ("healing response") to treat proximal ACL injuries in skeletally immature athletes. J Knee Surg 19(1):8–13

Steinert AF, Kunz M, Prager P et al (2011) Mesenchymal stem cell characteristics of human anterior cruciate ligament outgrowth cells. Tissue Eng Part A 17(9–10):1375–1388

Van Eijk F, Saris DB, Riesle J et al (2004) Tissue engineering of ligaments: a comparison of bone marrow stromal cells, anterior cruciate ligament, and skin fibroblasts as cell source. Tissue Eng 10:893–903

Vunjak-Novakovic G, Altman G, Horan R et al (2004) Tissue engineering of ligaments. Annu Rev Biomed Eng 6:131–156

Wiig ME, Amiel D, VandeBerg J et al (1990) The early effect of high molecular weight hyaluronan (hyaluronic acid) on anterior cruciate ligament healing: an experimental study in rabbits. J Orthop Res 8(3):425–434

Proximal Tibiofibular Syndesmotic Disruptions in Sport

111

Madi El-Haj and Yoram A. Weil

Contents

Abstract

The proximal tibiofibular joint (PTFJ) is a highly stabilized ligamentous arthroidal synovial joint, creating a continuum between the knee and ankle motion unit. PTFJ instability is a rare pathologic entity which is a commonly overlooked diagnosis, especially in the setting of high-energy trauma. The most common Ogden-type dislocation is anterolateral; other types are associated with a high incidence of common peroneal nerve injury. Patients may present with complaints of pain rather than instability. Although soft tissue reconstruction of the joint can be considered especially in athletic young patients, arthrodesis can be another potential treatment option, especially for chronic instability, posttraumatic arthrosis, or failed prior surgery.

Overview

Proximal tibiofibular joint (PTFJ) dislocation is an extremely uncommon injury, which may be easily missed during the initial assessment and on plain radiographs (Ellis 2003; Laing et al. 2003). The PTFJ is a stable joint, due to its strong ligamentous support (Levy et al. 2006). Although the most common PTFJ injury mechanism is usually hyperflexion of the knee with an inverted and extended foot (Ogden 1974b; Falkenberg and Nygaard 1983), resulting in the anterior dislocation of the fibular head, other mechanisms exist

M. El-Haj
Department of Orthopaedics, Hadassah Hebrew University Hospital, Jerusalem, Israel
e-mail: madi@hadassah.org.il

Y.A. Weil (✉)
Department of Orthopaedic Surgery, Orthopaedic Trauma Service, Hadassah Hebrew University Hospital, Jerusalem, Israel
e-mail: weily@hadassah.org.il; yoramweil@gmail.com

M.N. Doral, J. Karlsson (eds.), *Sports Injuries*,
DOI 10.1007/978-3-642-36569-0_133

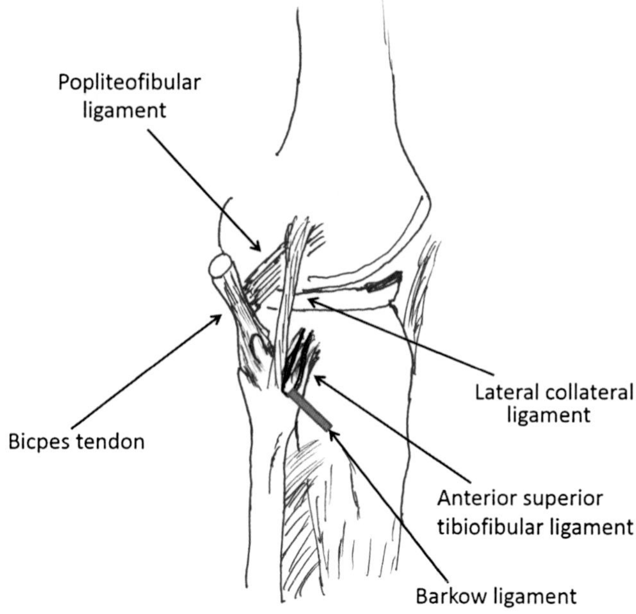

Fig. 1 Schematic drawing of the right knee illustrating the Ligamentous attachment around the PTFJ the bold line represent the ligament of Barkow

involving high injury trauma. The following chapter will discuss the anatomy, joint biomechanics, injury mechanisms, and treatment options.

Anatomy

Bony anatomy of the fibula: The fibula is attached to the tibia by the capsule of the superior tibiofibular articulation and an interosseous membrane that pass obliquely to blend with the inferior syndesmosis. The latter is comprised of the anterior and posterior tibiofibular ligament and the interosseous ligament.

The proximal fibula lies posterior to the central weight-bearing portion of the lateral tibial condyle, and the upper head (***capitulum fibulœ***) is a quadrilateral surface projecting upward, forward, and medially. The styloid process is the most proximal part of the fibular head and serves for the attachment of the popliteofibular ligament (Brinkman et al. 2005; Fig. 1). The cross-sectional diameter of the fibula is triangular in the upper, trapezoidal in the middle, and elliptical at the lower part of the bone (Brinkman et al. 2005).

Muscular and ligamentous attachments: The long head of the biceps divides distally into a direct arm that inserts into the posterolateral edge of the fibular head, and an anterior arm crossing lateral to the fibular collateral ligament, and separated by a bursa, on its way to attach to the lateral edge of the fibular head (Terry and LaPrade 1996b; Fig. 1).

The short head of the biceps divides into six insertions distally (Terry and LaPrade 1996b), of which only the direct arm is attached to the superior edge of the fibular head, posterior and lateral to the styloid process and posterior and medial to the fibular collateral ligament (Terry and LaPrade 1996b).

The fibular collateral ligament originates as a fan-shaped structure from the lateral femoral epicondyle and supracondylar ridge of the femur. It then runs distally where its medial fibers attach the lateral fibular edge and the medial fibers continue distally and blend with the superficial fascia of the peroneal compartment (Fig. 1).

Other ligamentous attachments include the fabellofibular ligament, the popliteofibular ligament, and the popliteus muscle which inserts onto the styloid process of the proximal fibula (Terry and LaPrade 1996a, b).

Proximal tibiofibular joint (PTFJ): The proximal tibiofibular joint is a small gliding synovial joint. It has several biomechanical roles including transmission of about one sixth of the compressive static force applied to the ankle (Lambert 1971). However, it is suggested that the joint functions mainly in the dissipation of the tensile forces generated by the lateral tibial bending moment (Espregueira-Mendes and da Silva 2006). This is supported by some biomechanical evidence demonstrating that the proximal and middle third of the fibula withstand the highest tensile forces other than any other skeletal bone (Evans and Band 1966).

The PTFJ is an arthroidal sliding synovial joint covered by hyaline cartilage formed of fibular facet of different shapes overhanging the corresponding facet in the posterolateral edge of the lateral tibial condyle. Different shapes of the articular facets have been described including planar, trichoid, double trichoid, condylar, trochlear, ball and socket, and saddle (Eichenblat and Nathan 1983; Bozkurt et al. 2003; Espregueira-Mendes and da Silva 2006; Fig. 2).

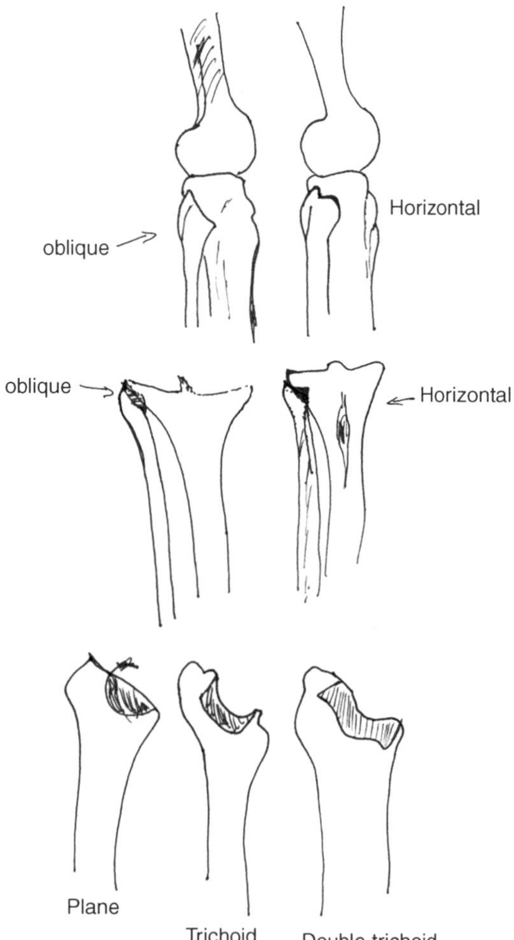

Fig. 2 Different shapes of fibular facet including oblique, horizontal. In the inferior panel planar trichoid and double trichoid shapes

The articular inclination ranges from 5 to 80° (Ogden 1974a; Falkenberg and Nygaard 1983; Ellis 2003; Laing et al. 2003); the horizontal is more common than oblique inclination and is associated with increased articular surface area and rotator mobility. The contour of the articular facets is elliptical, circular, and triangular, and there is no clear relationship between the facet shape and development of early osteoarthritis although osteoarthritic changes have been reported in the oblique–trichoid shape (Espregueira-Mendes and da Silva 2006).

The capsule of the joint is thickened anteriorly, invaginating into the joint, separated from each bone by fat pad lined with a synovial membrane; in 10 % of the cases, it is continuous with the synovial membrane of the knee joint (Lambert 1971; Espregueira-Mendes and da Silva 2006).

The ligamentous stabilization of the joint is provided mainly by the anterior and posterior tibiofibular ligaments, representing thickenings of the joint capsule (Laing et al. 2003), and the ligament of Barkow (Terry and LaPrade 1996b; Ellis 2003; Laing et al. 2003). The latter was found to be present in about 95 % of the cases, acting in the same manner as the anterior and posterior tibiofibular ligament. Additional stabilization is provided by the fibular collateral ligament and the short and long head of biceps (Figs. 1 and 3).

Neurovascular structures: The peroneal artery originates from the tibial artery in most of the cases. However, in 5 % of the cases, it originates directly from the popliteal artery. The distance from the fibular head to the peroneal artery origin ranges from 3.5 to 9.5 mm (Brinkman et al. 2005). The common peroneal nerve arises from the sciatic nerve at the level of popliteal fossa. It travels distally and laterally traverses the interval between the short head of the biceps femoris muscle posteriorly and the lateral head of the gastrocnemius muscle anteriorly. It then hooks around the fibular head laterally entering the anterolateral

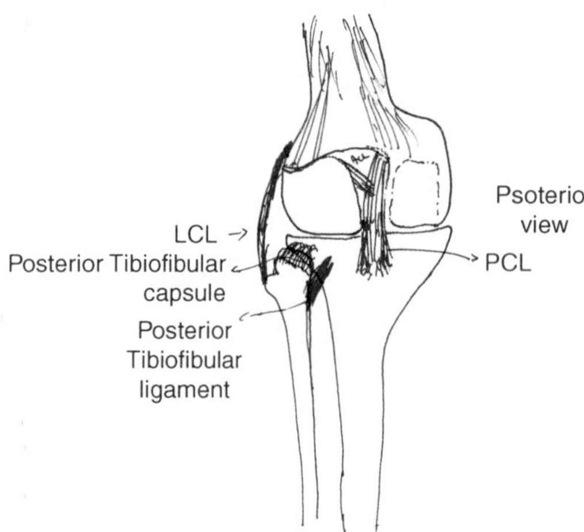

Fig. 3 Posterior view of the proximal tibiofibular joint demonstrates the posterior tibiofibular ligament and capsule

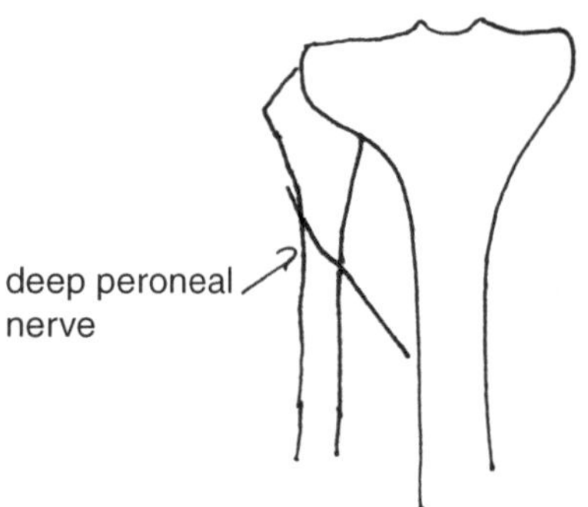

Fig. 4 Schematic anterior view of a right proximal tibiofibular joint. The common peroneal; recurrent anterior branch for the proximal tibiofibular joint, deep and the superficial peroneal nerve.

aspect of the leg deep to the peroneus longus muscle, where the nerve splits into deep and superficial peroneal branches. Clinically the coursing superficially around the fibular head makes the peroneal nerve vulnerable to traumatic injury from proximal tibiofibular joint dislocation, proximal fibular fracture, or compression by the origin of the peroneus longus or ganglion cyst (Spinner et al. 2009; Donovan et al. 2010; Fig. 4).

Joint Biomechanics

The proximal tibiofibular joint and the interosseous membrane are considered as an integral unit of the ankle joint. The major biomechanical function of the fibula is maximizing ankle stability during the different phases of ankle motion. As the ankle joint widens during dorsiflexion, the fibula external rotates, excurse superiorly and bend medially, causing the oblique fibers of the interosseous membrane to become horizontal. The vertical downward movement of the fibula becomes more important during the strike phase of running when the forces applied are three to six times than the body weight, and the above fibular dynamics enables deepening the ankle mortise and converting the compressive forces into tension forces across the interosseous membrane and tibiofibular ligaments, hence providing a shock absorber function (Weinert et al. 1973).

Specifically, the PTFJ externally rotates during dorsiflexion of the ankle (Ogden 1974b; Eichenblat and Nathan 1983; Bozkurt et al. 2003; de Seze et al. 2005) which is more accentuated in horizontal fibular joint's facet variants compared to the oblique variants (Ogden 1974a). These movements enable the dissipation of torsional stresses applied at the ankle joint (Lambert 1971).

However the PTFJ also participates in knee joint biomechanics where the fibular head translates in the anterior-posterior plane as a function of knee flexion (Ogden 1974a; Andersen 1985). As the knee flexes, the proximal fibula moves anteriorly with relative relaxation of the fibular collateral ligament and the biceps femoris while with knee extension, these structures become taut and pull the fibula posteriorly (Ogden 1974a; Andersen 1985). In internal rotation of the knee the tensile forces are transmitted by the fibular collateral ligament to the fibular head causing the posterior translation, while in external rotation the PTFJ motion is directed anteriorly (Scott et al. 2007).

PTFJ Dislocation and Subluxation

Subluxation may be idiopathic or traumatic acute or chronic; while first reported by Nelaton in 1874 (Ogden 1974b; Turco and Spinella 1985; Weinert and Raczka 1986; Harvey and Woods 1992), it is an uncommon problem in orthopedics occurring in <1 % of knee injury cases (Harvey and Woods 1992). Idiopathic subluxation usually is part of a more generalized ligamentous laxity, muscular dystrophy, or Ehlers–Danlos syndrome. It is more common in females and it is usually bilateral. Patients usually have lateral pain that increases with direct pressure over the fibular head, decreasing pain intensity as approaching skeletal maturity (Ogden 1974a; Semonian et al. 1995; Sekiya and Kuhn 2003); however, atraumatic proximal fibular subluxation in otherwise healthy individuals is extremely rare but exists (Klaunick 2010; Morrison et al. 2011).

Mechanism of Injury and Classification

The mechanism of injury results usually from twisting, hyperextension (contact and noncontact), and anterior blow to a flexed knee, or a valgus force on a flexed knee (LaPrade and Terry 1997). Harrisson and Hindenach (1959) described four types of proximal tibiofibular dislocations: anterolateral, posteromedial, superior, and subluxation. Later, in 1974, Ogden (1974b) reviewed the literature and used the same classification on 108 cases (Fig. 4a).

Anterior dislocation: This is the commonest type and usually is the result of an athletic injury (Veth et al. 1981; Harvey and Woods 1992; Fallon et al. 1994). The mechanism is usually hyperflexion injury with an inverted and extended foot creating an anterior and lateral pressure on the fibular head resulting in anterior dislocation (Ogden 1974b; Falkenberg and Nygaard 1983; Fig. 5a).

Posteromedial dislocation: It is usually as a direct blow to the knee forcing the fibular head posteriorly and medial such as in a car bumper injury (Fig. 5b).

Superior dislocation: It is usually associated with tibia shaft fracture, as a result of axial loading, e.g., falling from height (Harrison and Hindenach 1959; Gabrion et al. 2003; Fig. 5c).

Further two types were recognized (Fig. 4b) including:

Posterolateral: It is very rare and may be often overlooked in high-energy trauma (Nikolaides et al. 2007).

Inferior dislocation: The mechanism of inferior proximal tibiofibular dislocation is avulsion of the leg resulting in neurovascular lesions (Gabrion et al. 2003).

Clinical Presentation

Acute dislocation: The clinical presentation of patients with acute dislocations is more variable; typical symptoms include lateral knee swelling and pain with ankle motion, locking episodes, and inability to bear weight (Falkenberg and Nygaard 1983; Thomason and Linson 1986). However, especially for acute PTFJ dislocation, a painful lateral knee mass presents with exacerbation during dorsiflexion and eversion of the foot. An additional physical sign is the tense cord formed by the stretched biceps femoris tendon, providing a useful clue in the diagnosis (Ogden 1974b). Associated injury to the common peroneal nerve is most common with the posteromedial tibiofibular dislocation (Sekiya and Kuhn 2003). However, the functional status of the peroneal nerve should be documented with any type of tibiofibular dislocations.

Chronic dislocation: The differential diagnoses of lateral knee pain and/or instability include a lateral meniscus injury, peroneal nerve entrapment (Donovan et al. 2010; Dong et al. 2012), snapping biceps femoris (Kristensen et al. 1989), and iliotibial band syndrome (Barber and Sutker 1992). Nonspecific clinical symptoms exist that mimic lateral meniscus injury, with complaints of lateral knee popping, clicking, and catching (Turco and Spinella 1985; Thomason and Linson 1986). However, a history of worsening pain with twisting motions further suggests lateral meniscus tears (Owen 1968; Giachino 1986). In suspected chronic PTFJ injuries or patients with atraumatic subluxation, it is vital to examine the presence of increased translation of the fibular head compared with the opposite normal knee. For this purpose, two specific tests exist; the apprehension test is done with the knee flexed to 90° to relax the fibular collateral ligament and biceps femoris; an anterior–posterior translatory force is then applied

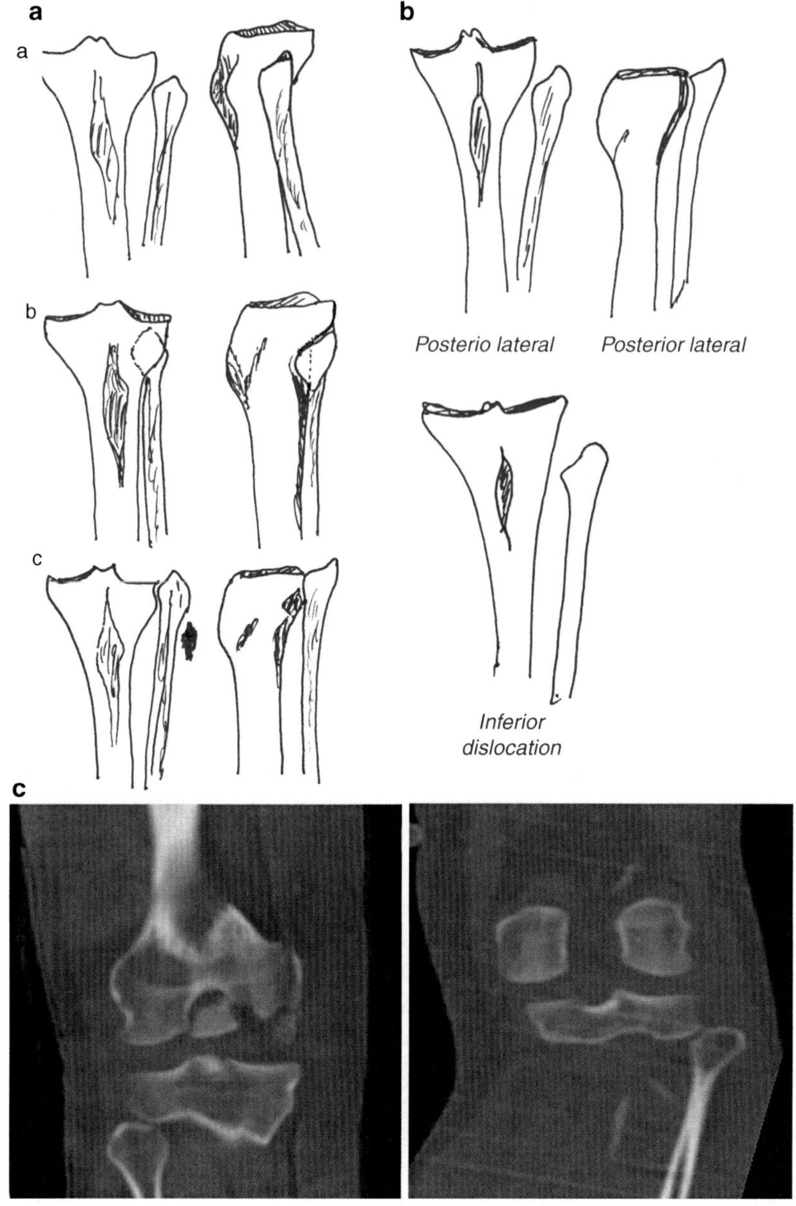

Fig. 5 (**a**) Classification scheme of the proximal tibiofibular joint dislocation according to Ogden. A. Anterolateral dislocation - the The dislocation occurs proceed from lateral to anterior. B. Posteromedial dislocation – the fibula slides posteriorly then medially. C. Superior dislocation - the upward displacement is with associated varying degree of lateralization. (**b**) Two rare dislocation: posterolateral and inferior dislocation of the proximal tibiofibular joint dislocation. (**c**) 53 years old injured during pedestrian motor vehicle accident, suffered from traumatic amputation of the left leg, initial CT demonstrated superior left PTFJ dislocation of the amputated leg as compared to the right PTFJ

to the fibular head while assessing for apprehension and motion (Sijbrandij 1978). The other test is the Radulescu test; since the PTFJ is usually stable with an extended knee, the test is performed in the prone, flexed position. While the knee flexed to 90°, one hand is stabilizing the thigh while internally rotating the leg in an attempt to subluxate or dislocate the fibula anteriorly (Baciu et al. 1974).

Radiographic Evaluation

Radiographic assessment of the PTFJ should include supine and weight-bearing anterior–posterior and lateral radiographs of both the injured and noninjured knees in order to detect changes in the position of the proximal fibula relative to the tibia.

X-ray images of proximal tibiofibular joint should consist of true anterior–posterior and lateral views of both knees (Resnick et al. 1978).

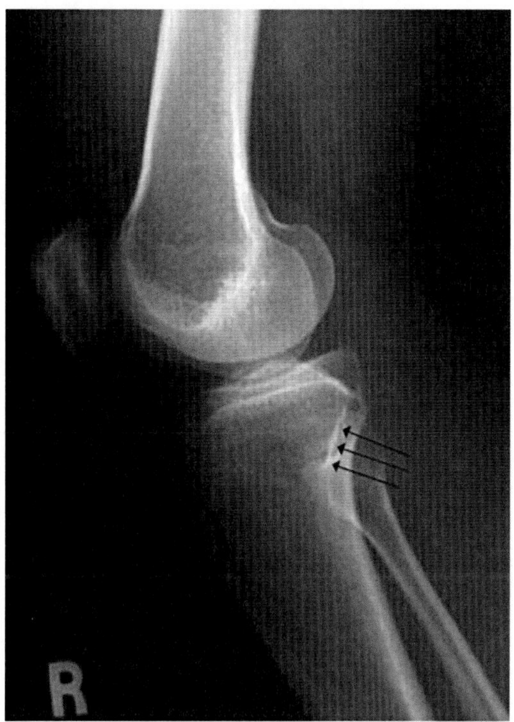

Fig. 6 Resnicks line: Lateral radiograph showing fibular head overlying posterior border of tibia. Increased radiodensity (arrowheads) which identifies most posteromedial portion of lateral tibial condyle, which projected over midportion of fibular head

Resnick et al. defined the most posteromedial portion of the lateral tibial condyle as a radio-dense line on lateral view, at which the middle third of the fibula head should be over this line. With anterolateral dislocation, almost the entire fibular head projects anterior to the Resnick's line, whereas in posteromedial dislocation there is minimal overlap between the proximal tibia and fibula (Fig. 6).

Axial computed tomography is far more accurate than radiographs in establishing the diagnosis (Keogh et al. 1993). MRI is particularly useful for its high-resolution depiction of the soft tissues and changes in the bone such as marrow edema patterns after trauma.

Treatment of Proximal Tibiofibular Instability

Treatment of PTFJ injuries depends on the mechanism of injury, chronicity, and clinical symptoms and associated injuries.

Acute traumatic dislocation: A simple closed reduction may be attempted. In an anterolateral dislocation, the knee is flexed (80–110°) and the foot dorsiflexed and externally rotated, and pressure is applied over the fibular head while the injury mechanism is reversed, until a "pop" is heard. The reduction should be followed by meticulous examination of other associated soft tissue injuries with an emphasis on the common peroneal nerve, fibular collateral ligament, and a complete posterolateral corner injury. Then, cast or brace immobilization should be applied with protected weight bearing followed by full weight bearing for six weeks. In the presence of pain in ankle dorsiflexion and eversion, ankle motion should be restricted (Aladin et al. 2002). Posteromedial and superior dislocations, along with failed closed reduction of anterolateral injuries, are repaired by open reduction and internal fixation (Wheeless 2005 Proximal tibiofibular joint injuries; Original text by Clifford R. Wheeless, III, MD. Last updated by Data Trace Staff on Friday, August 31, 2012 1:23 p.m.).

Surgical treatments include primary repair of the anterior and posterior tibiofibular ligaments, screw fixation, Kirschner-wire fixation, fixation using the TightRope syndesmosis device, and fixation using tendons of the biceps femoris (Miettinen et al. 1999) and gracilis (Sekiya and Kuhn 2003; Horst and LaPrade 2010). Hardware should be removed after 6–12 weeks, similar to a syndesmosis injury of the ankle (Andersen 1985; Turco and Spinella 1985) (Fig. 7).

Atraumatic subluxations: They are usually managed nonoperatively with a supportive strap or bandage placed 1 cm below the fibular head (Hernandez et al. 1996). Physical therapy, nonsteroidal anti-inflammatory medications, and limitation of activities that evoke pain should result in resolution of symptoms.

Chronic dislocations: Treatment options include fibular head resection, partial resection arthroplasty, arthrodesis, soft tissue reconstruction, and midshaft fibular resection.

Fibular head resection: It should be considered in patients with arthritis changes; however, partial resection arthroplasty is biomechanically more preferred although no conclusive evidence on

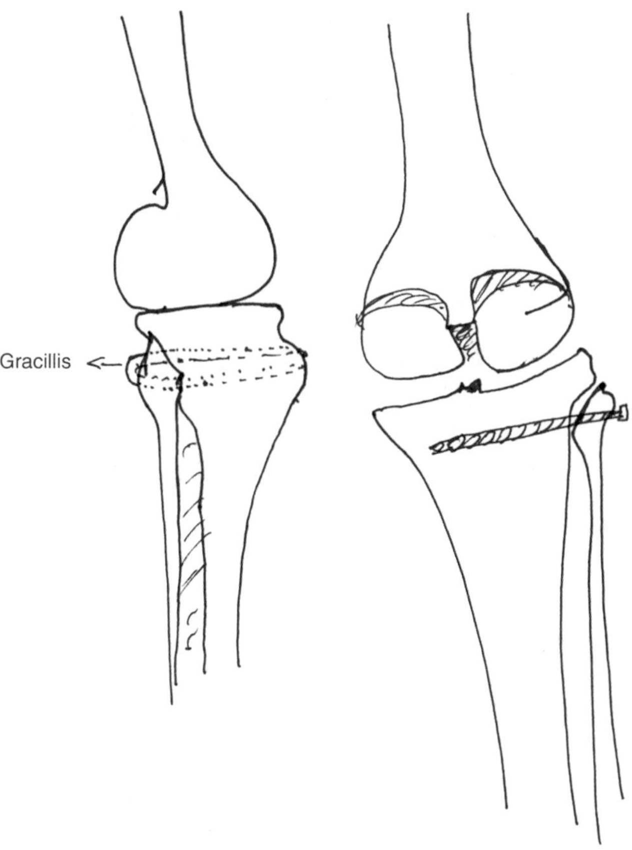

Fig. 7 Schematic view of proximal tibiofibular joint reconstruction using Gracills graft and syndemsotic screw

gait function precludes fibular head resection as good treatment option (Draganich et al. 1991; Agarwal et al. 2012). Complications include chronic knee pain, lateral knee instability, and ankle pain (Draganich et al. 1991; Halbrecht and Jackson 1991) and are contraindicated in athletes (Sekiya and Kuhn 2003).

Arthrodesis

This may be offered as good option for chronic instability in either the presence or absence frank arthritic changes. However, since the proximal fibula externally rotates during dorsiflexion of the ankle (Ogden 1974b; Eichenblat and Nathan 1983; Bozkurt et al. 2003; de Seze et al. 2005) and has motion in both the anterior–posterior direction with knee flexion, increased stress may be transferred to the ankle following PTFJ arthrodesis potentially leading to pain at the ankle (Baciu et al. 1974; Ogden 1974a, b). Uncoupling the proximal fibula and ankle by resecting a small segment of the fibula at the junction of the proximal and middle thirds may prevent the transmission of abnormal stresses to the distal fibula and ankle enabling a more functionally acceptable arthrodesis.

Soft tissue reconstructions using the biceps tendon, deep fascia, iliotibial band, and autogenous semitendinosus tendon with interference screws have also been described and are attempted in traumatic cases especially in younger patients (Horst and LaPrade 2010), However, they are technically demanding and success may be limited in cases where osteoarthritis is already present.

Summary

The proximal tibiofibular joint is a highly stabilized ligamentous arthroidal synovial joint, creating a continuum between the knee and ankle motion unit. PTFJ instability is a rare pathologic entity, which commonly goes with overlooked diagnosis, especially in the setting of high-energy trauma. The most common Ogden-type dislocation is anterolateral; other types are associated with a high incidence of common peroneal nerve injury. Although soft tissue reconstruction of the joint should be considered, especially in athletic young patients, arthrodesis may be an option, especially for chronic instability, posttraumatic arthrosis, or failed prior surgery.

References

Agarwal DK, Saseendar S et al (2012) Outcomes and complications of fibular head resection. Strategies Trauma Limb Reconstr 7(1):27–32

Aladin A, Lam KS et al (2002) The importance of early diagnosis in the management of proximal tibiofibular dislocation: a 9- and 5-year follow-up of a bilateral case. Knee 9(3):233–236

Andersen K (1985) Dislocation of the superior tibiofibular joint. Injury 16(7):494–498

Baciu CC, Tudor A et al (1974) Recurrent luxation of the superior tibio-fibular joint in the adult. Acta Orthop Scand 45(5):772–777

Barber FA, Sutker AN (1992) Iliotibial band syndrome. Sports Med 14(2):144–148

Bozkurt M, Yilmaz E et al (2003) The proximal tibiofibular joint: an anatomic study. Clin Orthop Relat Res 406:136–140

Brinkman JM, Schwering PJ et al (2005) The insertion geometry of the posterolateral corner of the knee. J Bone Joint Surg (Br) 87(10):1364–1368

de Seze MP, Rezzouk J et al (2005) Anterior innervation of the proximal tibiofibular joint. Surg Radiol Anat 27(1):30–32

Dong Q, Jacobson JA et al (2012) Entrapment neuropathies in the upper and lower limbs: anatomy and MRI features. Radiol Res Pract 2012:230679

Donovan A, Rosenberg ZS et al (2010) MR imaging of entrapment neuropathies of the lower extremity. Part 2. The knee, leg, ankle, and foot. Radiographics 30(4):1001–1019

Draganich LF, Nicholas RW et al (1991) The effects of resection of the proximal part of the fibula on stability of the knee and on gait. J Bone Joint Surg Am 73(4):575–583

Eichenblat M, Nathan H (1983) The proximal tibiofibular joint. An anatomical study with clinical and pathological considerations. Int Orthop 7(1):31–39

Ellis C (2003) A case of isolated proximal tibiofibular joint dislocation while snowboarding. Emerg Med J 20(6):563–564

Espregueira-Mendes JD, da Silva MV (2006) Anatomy of the proximal tibiofibular joint. Knee Surg Sports Traumatol Arthrosc 14(3):241–249

Evans FG, Band S (1966) Physical and histological differences between human fibular and femoral compact bone. In: Evans FG (eds) Studies on the anatomy and function of bone and joints. Springer, Berlin Heidelberg New York, pp 142–155

Falkenberg P, Nygaard H (1983) Isolated anterior dislocation of the proximal tibiofibular joint. J Bone Joint Surg (Br) 65(3):310–311

Fallon P, Virani NS et al (1994) Delayed presentation: dislocation of the proximal tibiofibular joint after knee dislocation. J Orthop Trauma 8(4):350–353

Gabrion A, Jarde O et al (2003) Inferior dislocation of the proximal tibiofibular joint: a report on four cases. Acta Orthop Belg 69(6):522–527

Giachino AA (1986) Recurrent dislocations of the proximal tibiofibular joint. Report of two cases. J Bone Joint Surg Am 68(7):1104–1106

Halbrecht JL, Jackson DW (1991) Recurrent dislocation of the proximal tibiofibular joint. Orthop Rev 20(11):957–960

Harrison R, Hindenach JC (1959) Dislocation of the upper end of the fibula. J Bone Joint Surg (Br) 41-B(1):114–120

Harvey GP, Woods GW (1992) Anterolateral dislocation of the proximal tibiofibular joint: case report and literature review. Todays OR Nurse 14(3):23–27

Hernandez JA, Rius M et al (1996) Snapping knee from anomalous biceps femoris tendon insertion: a case report. Iowa Orthop J 16:161–163

Horst PK, LaPrade RF (2010) Anatomic reconstruction of chronic symptomatic anterolateral proximal tibiofibular joint instability. Knee Surg Sports Traumatol Arthrosc 18(11):1452–1455

Keogh P, Masterson E et al (1993) The role of radiography and computed tomography in the diagnosis of acute dislocation of the proximal tibiofibular joint. Br J Radiol 66(782):108–111

Klaunick G (2010) Recurrent idiopathic anterolateral dislocation of the proximal tibiofibular joint: case report and literature review. J Pediatr Orthop B 19(5):409–414

Kristensen G, Nielsen K et al (1989) Snapping knee from biceps femoris tendon. A case report. Acta Orthop Scand 60(5):621

Laing AJ, Lenehan B et al (2003) Isolated dislocation of the proximal tibiofibular joint in a long jumper. Br J Sports Med 37(4):366–367

Lambert KL (1971) The weight-bearing function of the fibula. A strain gauge study. J Bone Joint Surg Am 53(3):507–513

LaPrade RF, Terry GC (1997) Injuries to the posterolateral aspect of the knee. Association of anatomic injury patterns with clinical instability. Am J Sports Med 25(4):433–438

Levy BA, Vogt KJ et al (2006) Maisonneuve fracture equivalent with proximal tibiofibular dislocation.

A case report and literature review. J Bone Joint Surg Am 88(5):1111–1116

Miettinen H, Kettunen J et al (1999) Dislocation of the proximal tibiofibular joint. A new method for fixation. Arch Orthop Trauma Surg 119(5–6):358–359

Morrison TD, Shaer JA et al (2011) Bilateral, atraumatic, proximal tibiofibular joint instability. Orthopedics 34(2):133

Nikolaides AP, Anagnostidis KS et al (2007) Inferior dislocation of the proximal tibiofibular joint: a new type of dislocation with poor prognosis. Arch Orthop Trauma Surg 127(10):933–936

Ogden JA (1974a) The anatomy and function of the proximal tibiofibular joint. Clin Orthop Relat Res 101:186–191

Ogden JA (1974b) Subluxation and dislocation of the proximal tibiofibular joint. J Bone Joint Surg Am 56(1):145–154

Owen R (1968) Recurrent dislocation of the superior tibiofibular joint. A diagnostic pitfall in knee joint derangement. J Bone Joint Surg (Br) 50(2):342–345

Resnick D, Newell JD et al (1978) Proximal tibiofibular joint: anatomic-pathologic-radiographic correlation. AJR Am J Roentgenol 131(1):133–138

Scott J, Lee H et al (2007) The effect of tibiofemoral loading on proximal tibiofibular joint motion. J Anat 211(5):647–653

Sekiya JK, Kuhn JE (2003) Instability of the proximal tibiofibular joint. J Am Acad Orthop Surg 11(2):120–128

Semonian RH, Denlinger PM et al (1995) Proximal tibiofibular subluxation relationship to lateral knee pain: a review of proximal tibiofibular joint pathologies. J Orthop Sports Phys Ther 21(5):248–257

Sijbrandij S (1978) Instability of the proximal tibio-fibular joint. Acta Orthop Scand 49(6):621–626

Spinner RJ, Hebert-Blouin MN et al (2009) Clock face model applied to tibial intraneural ganglia in the popliteal fossa. Skeletal Radiol 38(7):691–696

Terry GC, LaPrade RF (1996a) The biceps femoris muscle complex at the knee. Its anatomy and injury patterns associated with acute anterolateral-anteromedial rotatory instability. Am J Sports Med 24(1):2–8

Terry GC, LaPrade RF (1996b) The posterolateral aspect of the knee. Anatomy and surgical approach. Am J Sports Med 24(6):732–739

Thomason PA, Linson MA (1986) Isolated dislocation of the proximal tibiofibular joint. J Trauma 26(2):192–195

Turco VJ, Spinella AJ (1985) Anterolateral dislocation of the head of the fibula in sports. Am J Sports Med 13(4):209–215

Veth RP, Klasen HJ et al (1981) Traumatic instability of the proximal tibiofibular joint. Injury 13(2):159–164

Weinert CR Jr, Raczka R (1986) Recurrent dislocation of the superior tibiofibular joint. Surgical stabilization by ligament reconstruction. J Bone Joint Surg Am 68(1):126–128

Weinert CR Jr, McMaster JH et al (1973) Dynamic function of the human fibula. Am J Anat 138(2):145–149

Radiologic Criteria in Patellar Dislocations

112

Paulo Renato Fernandes Saggin and David Dejour

Contents

P.R. Fernandes Saggin (✉)
Instituto de Ortopedia e Traumatologia de Passo Fundo, Passo Fundo, RS, Brazil
e-mail: paulosaggin@yahoo.com.br

D. Dejour
Department of Knee Surgery & Sports Traumatology, Lyon-Ortho-Clinic; Clinique de la Sauvegarde, Lyon, France
e-mail: corolyon@wanadoo.fr; dr.dejour@lyon-ortho-clinic.com

M.N. Doral, J. Karlsson (eds.), *Sports Injuries*,
DOI 10.1007/978-3-642-36569-0_120

Abstract

Imaging of ***patellofemoral instability*** allows the recognition of the disturbances of shape and congruence leading to dislocations. The key to adequate imaging is complete evaluation of the underlying factors leading to instability. This chapter discusses the radiographic signs of these factors involved in the genesis of instability, which are trochlear dysplasia, patella alta, abnormal tibial tuberosity-trochlear groove distance, and lateral patellar tilt. Additionally, the acute signs of patellar dislocation are reviewed.

Introduction

Imaging of the patellofemoral articulation is of great interest since it allows the recognition of the disturbances of shape and stability. Accurate diagnosis and treatment are dependent on the correct interpretation of the radiologic data obtained from the individuals being investigated. To achieve this purpose, the factors determining instability must be identified, quantified, and classified. In general terms, these factors are ***trochlear dysplasia***, ***patella alta***, excessive ***tibial tuberosity-trochlear groove (TT-TG) distance***, and ***patellar tilt*** associated with insufficiency of the medial restraints (though these may be a consequence of the previous parameters). The alignment of the lower limb has to be analyzed including torsional abnormalities.

Together with individual variations, the various factors affecting patellofemoral joint stability sometimes make the definition of abnormality difficult. For this chapter's purpose, the definition of patellofemoral joint abnormality will be based on the available literature, but one should be aware that patellofemoral instability results from a complex interplay of factors, and simple deviations from the patterns defined as normal can be present in normal individuals.

Trochlear Dysplasia

Trochlear dysplasia is the single factor most associated with patellar instability (Dejour et al. 1994). Instead of being concave, the trochlea is flat or convex. The normal trochlear bony constraint to lateral patellar displacement is diminished and as a consequence dislocations can occur.

The diagnosis is classically made on X-ray using a perfect lateral view. To achieve perfect superimposition of the posterior aspects of both femoral condyles, fluoroscopy is recommended if one's radiology technicians have difficulty in obtaining this view. The diagnostic feature is the ***crossing sign***. The normal projection of the trochlear groove line does not cross the projection of the facets, but remains posterior to them and occasionally blends with the anterior cortex proximally; in dysplastic trochleae, the projection of the groove line crosses or reaches the projection of the facets, determining the "crossing sign" (Maldague and Malghem 1985; Dejour et al. 1994). On lateral radiographic views, two other typical features of trochlear dysplasia can often be identified: the supratrochlear spur (a proximal and lateral osseous protuberance) and the double-contour sign (the medial hypoplastic facet projection seen posterior and distal to the crossing sign and the groove projection) (Fig. 1).

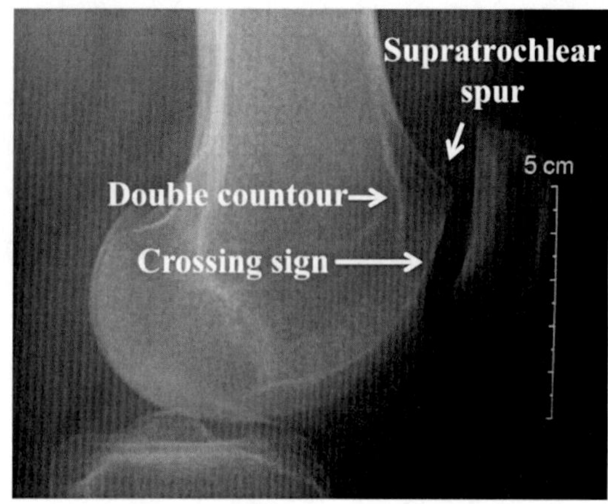

Fig. 1 Trochlear dysplasia findings. The three findings defining trochlear dysplasia on lateral projections: crossing sign, supratrochlear spur, and double contour

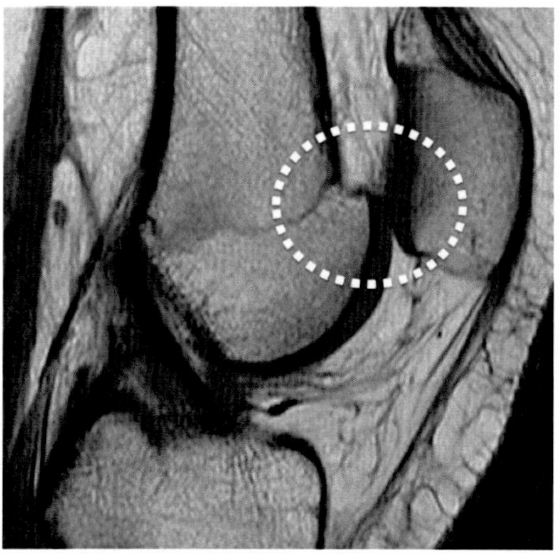

Fig. 2 MR midsagittal image. Nipple-like prominence suggestive of trochlear dysplasia

On magnetic resonance (MR) midsagittal images, the presence of a nipple-like anterior prominence at the superior border of the trochlea is highly suggestive of dysplasia, while rare in normal trochleae. A sharp steplike transition from the anterior femoral cortex to the trochlea is found, while normal knees usually present a smooth transition (Pfirrmann et al. 2000; Fig. 2).

The trochlear groove may be anterior, posterior, or flush with the anterior femoral cortex (estimated by a line drawn tangential to the most distal 10 cm of the anterior femoral cortex, called "line X"). Quantitative assessment of the trochlear prominence is obtained measuring the translation from the floor of the groove to the line "X." This distance is called "trochlear bump." In normal knees this measurement is negative or close to zero (mean −0.8 ± 2.9 mm), while in dysplastic trochleae, it is positive (mean 3.2 ± 2.4 mm) (Dejour et al. 1994; Fig. 3). A similar measurement may be obtained from midsagittal MR images. Pfirrmann et al. (2000) analyzed 16 patients with trochlear dysplasia and 23 controls and reported that a "ventral trochlear prominence" greater than 8 mm could diagnose trochlear dysplasia with 75 % sensitivity and 83 % specificity (Fig. 4).

The trochlear depth is the distance from the anterior (ventral) projection of the facets to the bottom of the groove, along a line subtended 15° from a perpendicular to the tangent of the posterior femoral cortex. In Dejour's study, in a control group, it was 7.8 ± 1.5 mm, while in patients with patellofemoral instability, it was 2.3 ± 1.8 mm (Dejour et al. 1994; Fig. 5).

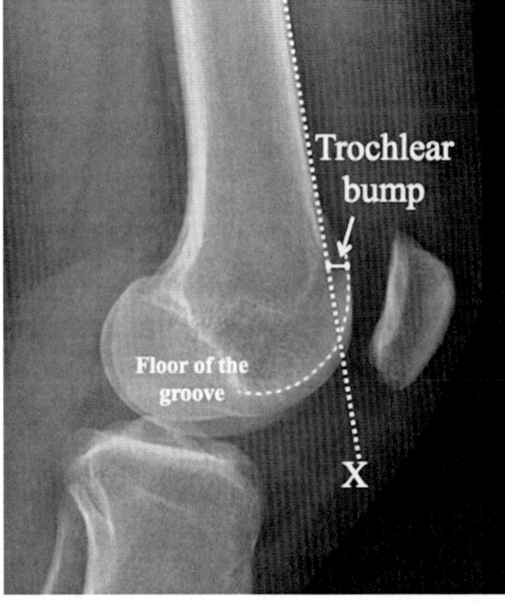

Fig. 3 Trochlear bump. The distance of the bottom of the groove from the "X" line

Axial radiographic views are another way to evaluate trochlear dysplasia. Normal trochleae are concave, but dysplastic trochleae are shallower than normal ones, flat, or even convex.

The sulcus angle (Brattstroem 1964) is calculated from the bottom of the groove (vertex) and projected to the highest point of both the medial and lateral facets. Brattstroem (1964) defined its normal value as 142° (SD ± 0,6°) investigating X-rays obtained at an angle of approximately 25° between the beam and the longitudinal axis of the femur. Merchant (Merchant et al. 1974) defined its normal values as ranging from 126° to 150° (average 138°) on axial X-rays obtained with the knee at 45° of flexion (Fig. 6).

Axial cuts from magnetic resonance imaging (MRI) or computed tomography (CT) have the ability to image the proximal part of the trochlea, where the dysplasia is more evident. This part of the trochlea is not adequately imaged on axial radiographs, explaining why sometimes dysplasia is missed on this imaging modality (Fig. 7). On axial cuts obtained with MRI, the lateral trochlear inclination (LTI) angle can be measured (Carrillon et al. 2000): Two lines are drawn, one connecting the posterior aspect of the femoral condyles (reference line) and another tangential to the lateral facet. Below a threshold value set at

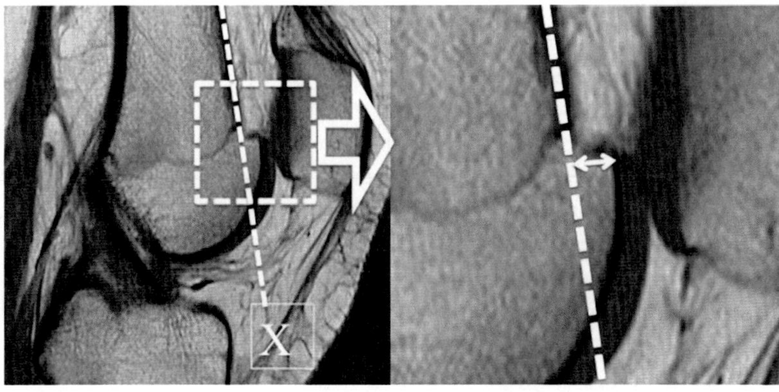

Fig. 4 Ventral trochlear prominence. A value above 8 mm is indicative of dysplasia

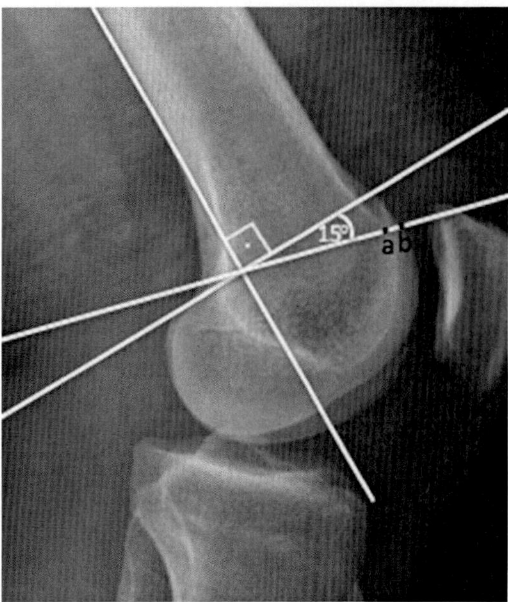

Fig. 5 Trochlear depth. Distance from "a" to "b"

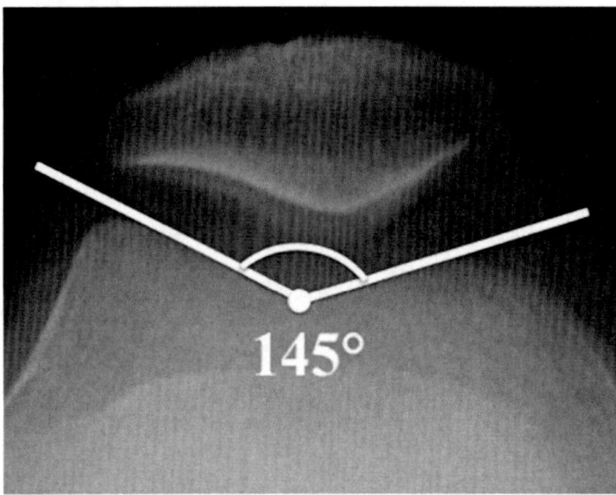

Fig. 6 Sulcus angle

11°, LTI has demonstrated to be an excellent indicator of patellofemoral instability with an accuracy of 90 %, therefore also indicating the presence of trochlear dysplasia (Fig. 8).

On MR transverse images 3 cm proximal to the joint line, trochlear depth may be measured subtracting the anteroposterior distance between the deepest point of the trochlear groove and the line paralleling the posterior outlines of the femoral condyles from the mean of the maximal anteroposterior distance of the medial and lateral condyles to the same posterior line (Fig. 9). In Pfirrmann's study, dysplastic knees showed a mean of −0.6 mm (range −6.5 to −2.7 mm) while controls showed a mean of 5.2 mm (range 2.4–10.5 mm). If a threshold was set at 3 mm, they reported that a specificity of 100 % and sensitivity of 96 % could be expected (Pfirrmann et al. 2000). In the same study, facet asymmetry (medial facet/lateral facet) inferior to 40 % provided similar specificity and sensitivity to dysplasia diagnosis (Fig. 9).

The combined analysis of standard radiographs and CT slice imaging allowed ***trochlear dysplasia* to be classified** into four types (Dejour et al. 1998; DeJour and Saggin 2010):

- Type A: The presence of a crossing sign on the true lateral view. The trochlea is shallower than normal, but still symmetric and concave.
- Type B: Crossing sign and trochlear spur. The trochlea is flat in axial images. There is prominence of all the trochleae.
- Type C: The crossing and double-contour signs are present on the lateral view. There is no trochlear prominence and, in axial views, the lateral facet is convex and the medial hypoplastic.
- Type D: Combines all the mentioned signs – crossing sign, supratrochlear spur, and double-contour sign. On the axial view, there is clear asymmetry of the height of the facets, also referred as a cliff pattern (Fig. 10).

Since the lateral radiographic view can underestimate the severity of the trochlear dysplasia, a two-grade analysis (low grade, corresponding to type A, and high grade, corresponding to types B, C, and D) based on MRI scans has reported better interobserver and intra-observer agreement (Lippacher et al. 2012).

Patella Alta

In normal knees, patellar engagement with the trochlea occurs at around 20° of knee flexion. Patella alta refers to an abnormally high riding

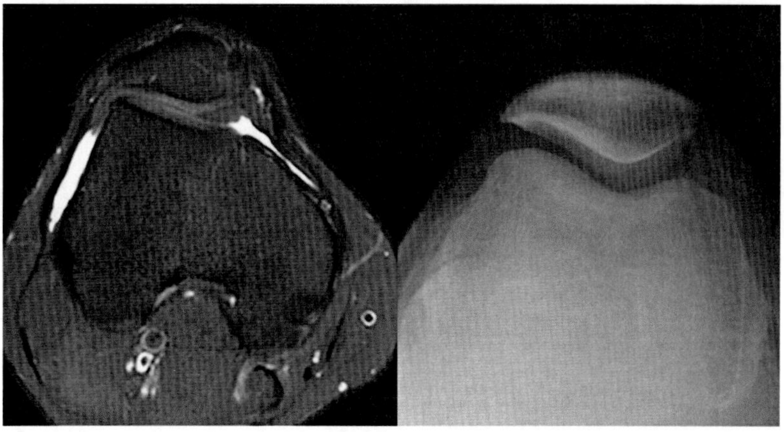

Fig. 7 Trochlear dysplasia in extension. The MR image exhibits the flat trochlea not identified on the flexed axial X-ray which images the lower part of the trochlea

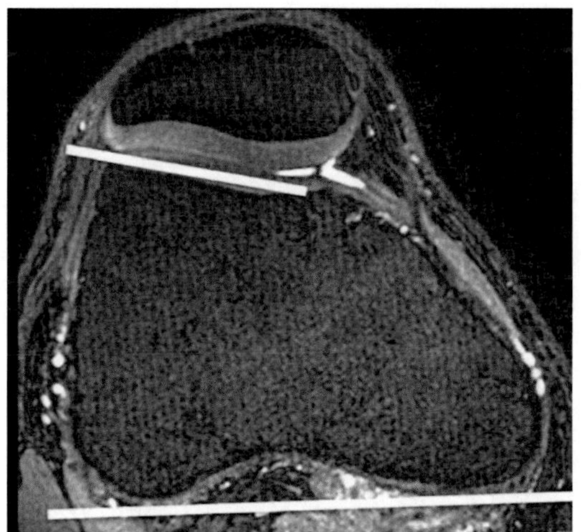

Fig. 8 Lateral trochlear inclination angle

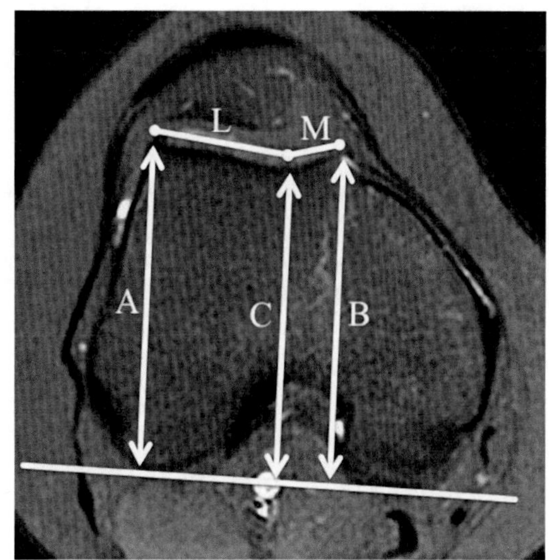

Fig. 9 Trochlear depth on MR axial images ((A + B)/2 – C). Facet asymmetry in percentage (M/L × 100)

patella that engages the osseous restraint to dislocation (the trochlear groove) later in flexion, increasing the patellar "free" arc of movement which can facilitate dislocation.

Lateral radiographic views are the key to the diagnosis of patella alta. Several methods of assessing patellar height have been proposed. The most popular ones are performed on lateral-views and use the tibia as reference. The three main ones are:

- Caton and Deschamps (Caton et al. 1982; Caton 1989): Is the ratio between the distance from the lower edge of the patellar articular surface to the anterosuperior angle of the tibia outline (AT) and the length of the articular surface of the patella (AP). A ratio (AT/AP) of 0.6 and smaller determines patella infera and a ratio greater than 1.2 indicates patella alta.
- Insall and Salvati (1971): Is the ratio between the length of the patellar tendon (LT) and the longest sagittal diameter of the patella (LP). Insall determined that this ratio (LT/LP) was normally one. A ratio smaller than 0.8

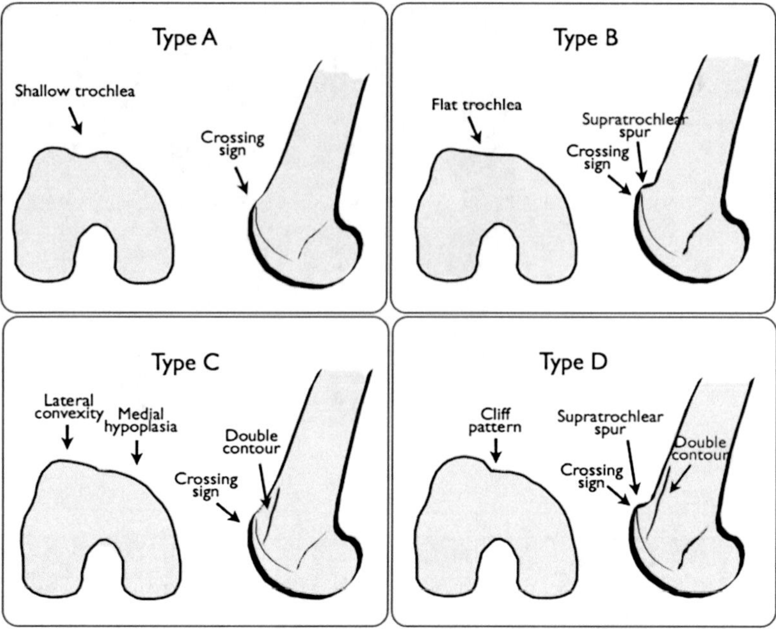

Fig. 10 Trochlear dysplasia classification

indicates patella infera (baja) and a ratio greater than 1.2 indicates patella alta.

– Blackburne-Peel (1977): Is the ratio between the length of the perpendicular line drawn from the tangent to the tibial plateau to the inferior pole of the articular surface of the patella (A) and the length of the articular surface of the patella (B). The normal ratio (A/B) was defined as 0.8. In patella infera it is smaller than 0.5, and in patella alta it is greater than 1.0 (Fig. 11).

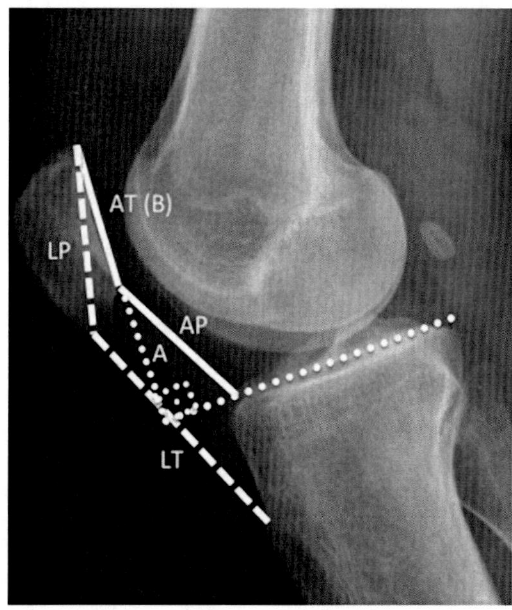

Fig. 11 Patellar height measurement (popular methods using the tibia as reference)

MR sagittal images have also proved to be a reliable tool to the diagnosis of patella alta. Miller et al. (1996) applied the Insall-Salvati method to 46 knees and compared MRI and radiographs. Good-to-excellent correlation between the values was reported, and they concluded that patellar height can be reliably assessed on sagittal MR imaging. With this method, patella alta was suggested at values greater than 1.3. Neyret et al. (2002) measured with radiographs and MRI the patellar tendon length in 42 knees with a history of patellar dislocation and 51 control knees. On MR images, the mean patellar tendon length was 44 mm in controls and 52 mm in the dislocation group. The distance between the tibial plateau and the point of tendon insertion was also measured and found to be 28 and 29 mm in the control and dislocation groups, respectively. They concluded that patella alta is caused by a long patellar tendon rather than by its

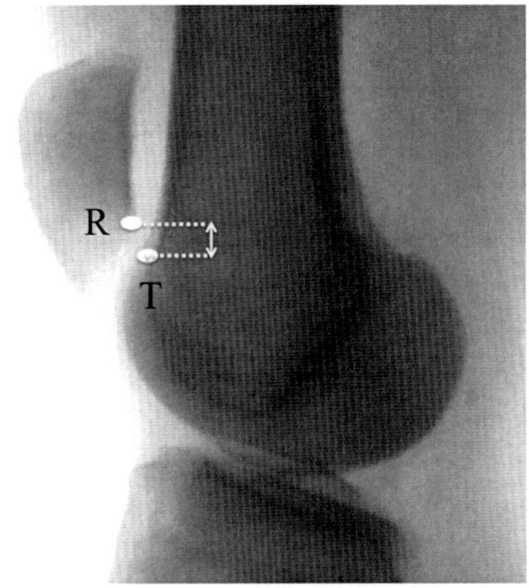

Fig. 12 Patellar height measurement according to Bernageau. Patella alta is defined if "R" is more than 6 mm above "T"

abnormal insertion into the tibia. Additionally, they did not report any significant differences between radiographic and MRI tendon length measurements.

Instead of the tibia, the trochlea can be used as the reference point for patellar height assessment. Bernageau et al. (1975) described a method on lateral X-rays with the knee in extension and the quadriceps contracted. If the inferior edge of the articular surface of the patella (R) was more than 6 mm proximal to the superior limit of the trochlea (T), patella alta was present, and if R was more than 6 mm distal to T, there was patella infera (Fig. 12).

Biedert and Albrecht (2006) described the patellotrochlear index on sagittal cuts of MRI, performed with the knees in extension, the foot 15° externally rotated, and the quadriceps consciously relaxed. To calculate the index, first the length of the articular cartilage of the patella (baseline patella, BLp) must be measured. The second measure is the length from the trochlear most superior aspect to the most inferior part of the trochlea facing the patellar articular cartilage (BLt). The ratio BLt/BLp is calculated in percentages, and values above 50 % indicate patella infera, while values inferior to 12.5 % indicate patella alta (Fig. 13).

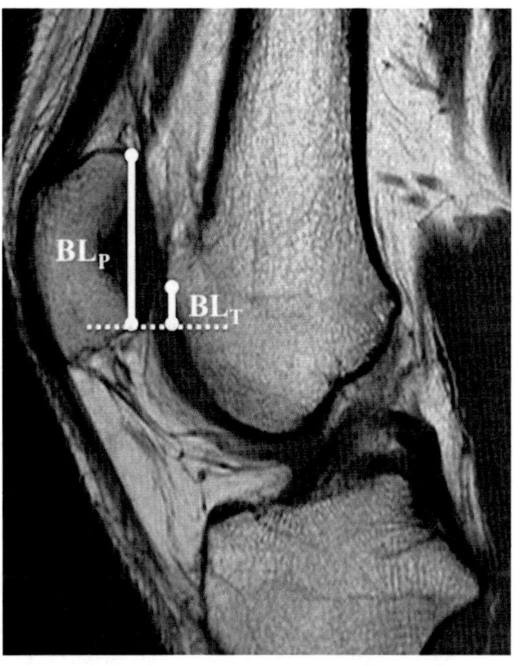

Fig. 13 Patellar height measurement according to Biedert and Albrecht. The ratio BLt/BLp is calculated in percentages. Patella alta is indicated if the ratio is inferior to 12.5 %

Abnormal Tibial Tuberosity-Trochlear Groove Distance (and Torsional Abnormalities)

The coronal valgus alignment of the extensor apparatus and the forces produced by femoral internal and tibial external torsion produce a lateral vector acting on the patella that can be estimated and measured by the tibial tuberosity-trochlear groove (TT-TG) distance. The TT-TG was described first by Goutallier et al. (1978) in 1978 on radiographic axial views at 30° of knee flexion to quantify the coronal alignment of the extensor mechanism (or what is called in clinical evaluation the "Q-angle").

Nowadays, the TT-TG is measured more reliably on CT images, since its value is increased at the end-stage extension of the knee (Dietrich et al. 2012). It is measured with two CT superimposed cuts and expressed in millimeters (Dejour et al. 1994). The first cut is through the proximal trochlea. It is the first cut with cartilage, identified by a slight condensation of the lateral facet and by the shape of the notch, which is rounded and looks like a Roman arch (called the "reference cut"). The second cut goes through the proximal part of the tibial tubercle. These two cuts are then superimposed. The deepest point of the trochlear groove and the central point of the tibial tubercle are projected on a line tangential to the posterior femoral condyles. The distance between both points is measured. The normal value in a control population is 12 mm; in the population with objective patellar dislocation, the value is greater than 20 mm in 56 % of the cases (Dejour et al. 1994). Values above 20 mm are considered abnormal (Fig. 14).

The TT-TG can be reliably determined on MRI using either cartilage or bony landmarks. Schoettle et al. (2006) evaluated the reliability of the TT-TG on MRI compared to CT scan in 12 knees with patellofemoral instability or anterior knee pain. The mean TT-TG referenced on bony landmarks was 14.4 ± 5.4 mm on CT scans and 13.9 ± 4.5 mm on MR images. The mean TT-TG referenced on cartilaginous landmarks was 15.3 ± 4.1 mm on CT scans and 13.5 ± 4.6 mm on MR images. They found excellent interperiod (bony vs. cartilaginous TT-TG) and intermethod (CT vs. MRI measurement) reliabilities, 91 % and 86 %, respectively.

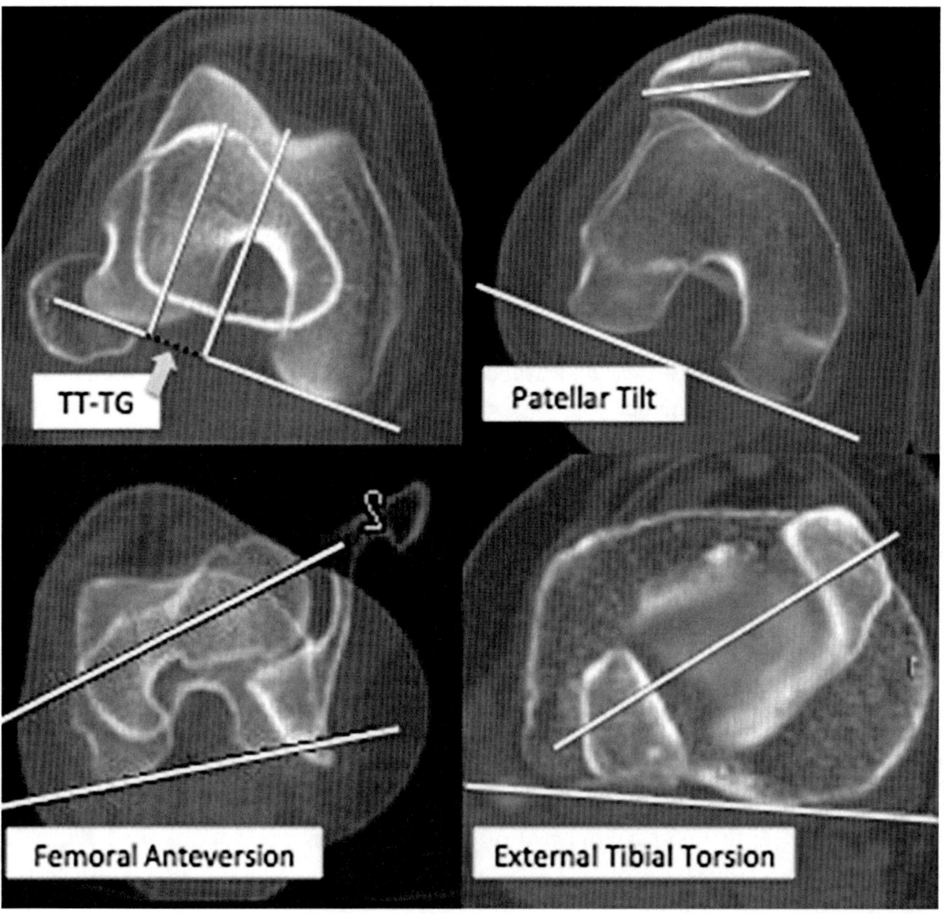

Fig. 14 The Lyon protocol for patellar instability assessment. All four parameters are obtained from superimposition of CT axial cuts

Another important contribution of CT produced by the superimposition of images is the assessment of torsional deformities, such as femoral anteversion and external tibial torsion. Femoral anteversion is defined as the angle formed between the axis of the femoral neck and a line tangential to the posterior condyles. Tibial torsion is the angle calculated between a line tangent to the posterior tibial plateau and another through the bimalleolar axis (Fig. 14).

Femoral anteversion is increased in patients with patellar instability (15.6 ± 9 vs. 10.8 ± 8.7 in normal knees), although some overlap of values may exist. External tibial torsion has shown too much variability between individuals to have any particular significance. Combined with tilt and TT-TG, these constitute the Lyon protocol for CT analysis (Dejour et al. 1994) (Fig. 14). Similar results have been reported recently on MRI. Diederichs et al. (2013) investigated patients with patellar dislocations and controls and found a 1.56-fold higher femoral anteversion on the first group (20.3° ± 10.4° vs. 13.0° ± 8.4°). External tibial torsion differences were not significant regardless of the method used.

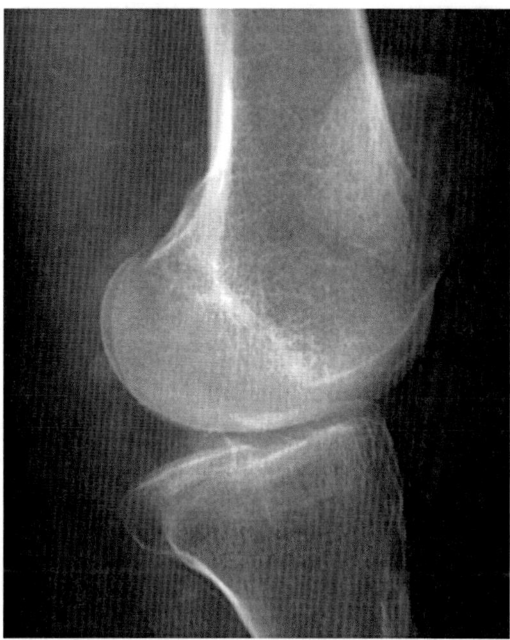

Fig. 15 Severe patellar tilt. The femur is visualized in profile while the patellar projection is almost an "anteroposterior"

Lateral Patellar Tilt (and Subluxation)

Patellar tilt and subluxation refer to the abnormal position of the patella in relation to the trochlear groove. While tilt means increased lateral inclination of the transverse diameter of the patella, subluxation refers primarily to abnormal mediolateral displacement of the patella in relation to the trochlea.

Tilt was formerly believed to be one of the leading factors in the genesis of instability, theorized to be caused by *vastus medialis obliquus* insufficiency. Actually, it seems to be the result of a complex interplay of factors, including trochlear and patellar shape and congruence, medial restraint insufficiency, and possible lateral retinacular tightness. Whether the cause or consequence of instability, tilt must be considered for diagnosis and adequate treatment of instability.

On the lateral radiographic view, the shape of the patella is dependent on its tilt. Normally, the lateral facet is anterior to the crest. Mild tilt occurs when both lines (lateral facet and crest) are superimposed, and severe tilt is when the crest is anterior to the lateral facet (Maldague and Malghem 1985; Fig. 15).

Methods of evaluating tilt and subluxation have been described for radiographic axial views:

- The *congruence angle* is measured on X-rays at 45° of knee flexion. After measuring the sulcus angle (used to access trochlear shape), two other lines are drawn from its vertex: one bisecting the sulcus angle (reference line) and another to the apex of the patella. The angle between these two lines is the congruence angle, considered positive if the line to the patellar apex is lateral to the reference line. The average congruence angle is −6° (SD ± 11°), and it measures primarily subluxation (Merchant et al. 1974; Fig. 16).
- The *lateral patellofemoral angle* is formed by one line connecting the highest points of the medial and lateral facets of the trochlea and another tangent to the lateral facet of the

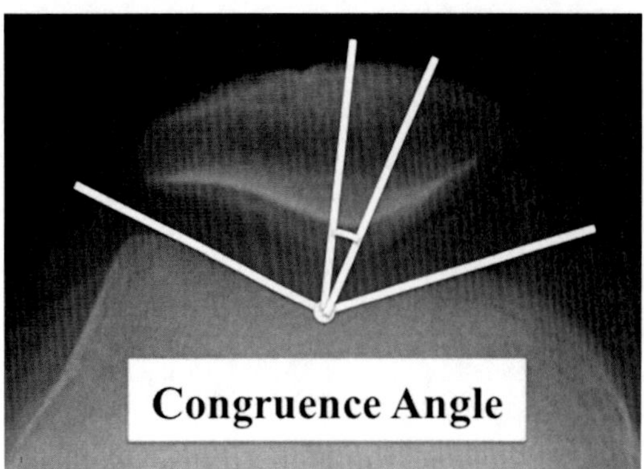

Fig. 16 Congruence angle. Two lines are drawn from the vertex of the *sulcus angle* – one bisecting the angle (reference line) and another to the apex of the patella

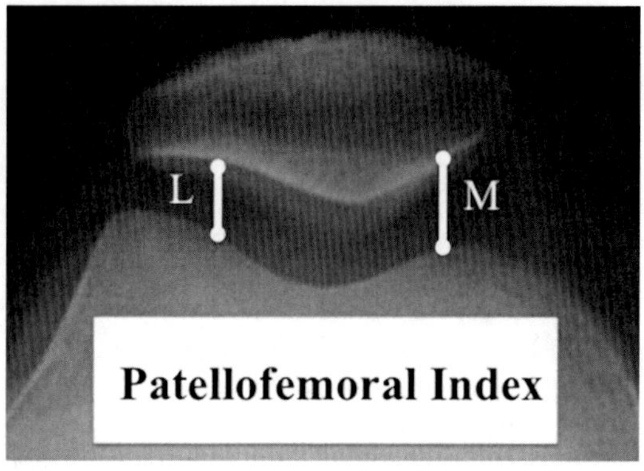

Fig. 18 Patellofemoral index. The ratio (M/L) between the thickness of the medial joint space (*M*) and the lateral joint space (*L*)

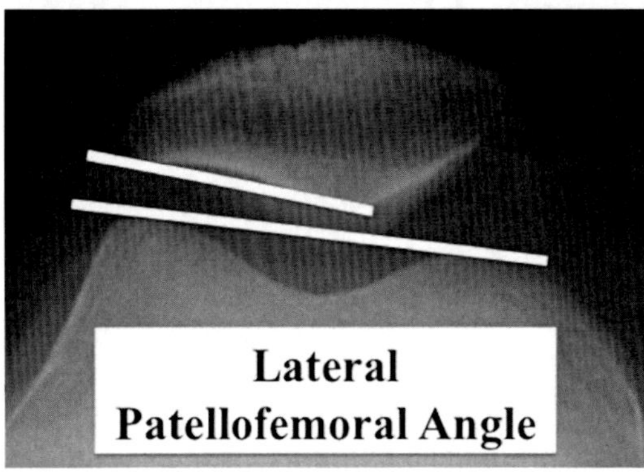

Fig. 17 Lateral patellofemoral angle. One line connecting the highest points of the medial and lateral facets of the trochlea and another tangent to the lateral facet of the patella

patella, drawn on 20° of knee flexion axial views. In normal knees this angle should open laterally (except in 3 % of the normal population in which it can be parallel). Medial opening was not demonstrated in normal individuals in a series of 100 patients. It demonstrates primarily tilt (Laurin et al. 1978, 1979; Fig. 17).

- The *patellofemoral index* is the ratio (M/L) between the thickness of the medial joint space (M) and the lateral joint space (L), measured on 20° axial views. It should measure 1.6 or less (Laurin et al. 1978, 1979; Fig. 18).

Malghem and Maldague described one radiographic view obtained at 30° of knee flexion while one examiner pulls the forefoot laterally –30° lateral rotation (LR) view (Malghem and Maldague 1989). The cassette is held over the patient's thighs, and the X-ray beam is directed cranially. The patellar position (centered or subluxated) is defined according to the congruence angle. In their series, the 30°LR view was superior to standard 45° axial views in detecting patellar subluxation. In 27 knees operated on for patellar instability, 45° routine views depicted subluxation in only seven cases, while 30°LR views demonstrated it in all cases. Additionally, when both views showed signs of instability, the degree of subluxation was greater in the 30°LR view.

CT scans allow for measurement of tilt in complete extension, which increases sensitivity because as the knee flexes, trochlear engagement of the patella reduces or corrects tilt and subluxation (Fig. 19). Another important contribution of CT scans is that they allow tilt measurements to be performed with a constant reference – the posterior femoral condyles (versus the variable trochlear shape in the instability population observed in X-rays). According to the Lyon protocol (Dejour et al. 1994), patellar tilt is the angle formed by the transverse axis of the patella and a line tangent to the posterior femoral condyles. It must be measured with and without quadriceps contraction, and this can be accomplished either with two superimposed cuts or with a single cut that images both references. Values above 20° are considered abnormal (Fig. 14).

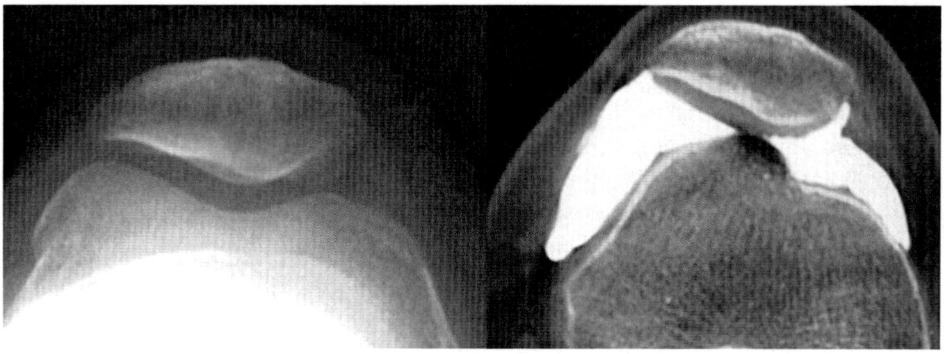

Fig. 19 Subluxation is missed during flexion (*left*) but clearly identified in imaging modalities performed in extension (*right*)

Grelsamer et al. (2008) described their results using a MRI tilt angle similar to that proposed by Dejour et al. in the Lyon protocol, using a line connecting the medial and lateral borders of the patella and the posterior femoral condyles as a reference. Thirty patients with tilt and 51 patients without tilt were evaluated. Patients with significant tilt on the physical examination could be expected to have an MRI tilt angle that was 10° or greater, whereas an angle of less than 10° was associated with the absence of significant tilt on the physical examination.

Since patellar tilt is dependent on the degree of the knee flexion (even in normal knees) and quadriceps contraction, the analysis of tilt and subluxation with variable conditions adds important information to the understanding of patellar tracking and to the determination of any abnormalities. Delgado-Martins (1979), comparing extension CT images and axial radiographs at 30, 60, and 90° of flexion in normal knees, reported that in complete extension with the quadriceps relaxed, only 13 % of the patellae were centered in the trochlea (the median crest corresponded exactly with the intercondylar groove), while this rate increased to 29 % at 30°, 63 % at 60°, and 96 % at 90° of flexion. Schutzer et al. (1986) also found in healthy subjects a mild degree of lateral shifting and tilting from 0 to 5° of flexion, while a central or medialized patella at 10° of flexion. The study of Martinez et al. (1983) did not corroborate these findings; 19 of 20 patients had the patella well centered in the trochlear groove in complete extension with the quadriceps relaxed.

In the Lyon protocol, tilt is measured with and without quadriceps contraction providing dynamic information of the stability of the patella. In H. Dejour's study, 83 % of the objective patellar dislocation group have patellar tilt superior to 20° compared to 3 % in the reference normal group. If instead of using only the relaxed quadriceps measure a mean is calculated between the measures performed with the quadriceps relaxed and in contraction and the threshold value remains the same, sensitivity and specificity are improved. Ninety percent of the objective patellar dislocation population have presented values over this, while the same remains true for only 3 % of controls (Dejour et al. 1994).

Dynamic MR imaging of the patellofemoral joint has been described to evaluate tracking during early flexion (Shellock et al. 1988, 1989). Axial images are acquired sequentially with increments of flexion. These images can be analyzed individually or as a cine-loop display, thus facilitating interpretation and recognition of abnormal tracking (Brossmann et al. 1994). In normal tracking, the ridge of the patella is situated over the center of the trochlea (the groove), and this relation is maintained through increments of knee flexion, as the patella moves distally in the vertical plane. Quantitative assessments have also been described (Kujala et al. 1989), but despite all the studies produced, no consensus on measurement protocols and abnormal values exist. At the moment, dynamic MRI remains as a promising procedure, but without a well-defined clinical application.

Acute Dislocations

Imaging of acute dislocations is useful to confirm the diagnosis and define treatment.

Radiographs are useful to identify severe instability and incongruence. Anteroposterior, lateral, and axial views are complementary and must be performed. Fragments of the patella or the lateral femoral condyle can be identified after acute dislocations and may indicate surgical treatment (Fig. 20). CT findings in acute dislocations are similar to the X-ray ones, but with increased accuracy. Smaller osseous fragments can be identified and better measured.

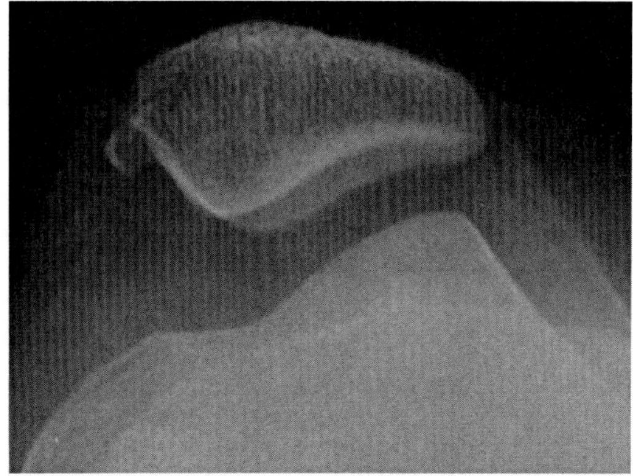

Fig. 20 Osseous avulsion from the medial border of the patella. Additionally, patellar tilt and subluxation are present and trochlear dysplasia can be identified

Patellar dislocation may not be suspected before MRI examination in up to 50–75 % of cases (Lance et al. 1993; Kirsch et al. 1993). MR imaging is particularly helpful in acute dislocations for the recognition and evaluation of associated lesions. The mechanism of the injury explains most of the abnormalities seen on MRI. These acute findings include (Kirsch et al. 1993; Virolainen et al. 1993; Elias et al. 2002; Diederichs et al. 2010):

- Joint effusion: Although unspecific, this seems to be the single finding most present in acute patellar dislocations (Virolainen et al. 1993).
- Injury/disruption of the medial patellofemoral ligament: Present in almost every case of acute dislocation, the MPFL tear may show variable patterns (at the patellar insertion, femoral insertion, midsubstance, or combined locations) (Balcarek et al. 2010). Injuries at the femoral origin that could be missed on arthroscopy are adequately identified on MRI (Balcarek et al. 2011). Injury of the medial retinaculum at its patellar attachments or midsubstance and tearing of the distal belly of the *vastus medialis obliquus* can be associated findings.
- Lateral femoral condyle/trochlear contusion and/or osteochondral lesion.
- Medial patellar facet contusion and/or osteochondral lesion, sometimes with osteochondral fragment avulsion.
- Patellar tilt and subluxation (Fig. 21).

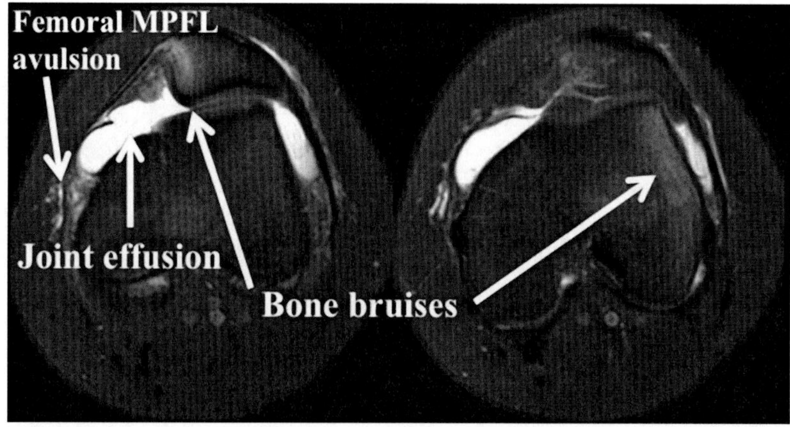

Fig. 21 Several findings indicating acute dislocation of the patella

Conclusion

Adequate imaging of patellofemoral instability allows the recognition of the disturbances of shape and congruence leading to dislocations. The heterogeneity of the methods of assessment of these abnormalities and the vast nomenclature described make a standardized approach difficult. Ultimately, most described methods intend to demonstrate similar abnormalities, which can be grouped in the four main factors of instability previously discussed.

Cross-References

- ▶ Anatomy and Biomechanics of the Knee
- ▶ Arthroscopic Patellar Instability Surgery
- ▶ Medial Patellofemoral Ligament Reconstruction: Current Concepts
- ▶ Patellar Dislocations: Overview
- ▶ Patellofemoral Problems in Adolescent Athletes

References

Balcarek P, Ammon J, Frosch S et al (2010) Magnetic resonance imaging characteristics of the medial patellofemoral ligament lesion in acute lateral patellar dislocations considering trochlear dysplasia, patella alta, and tibial tuberosity–trochlear groove distance. Arthroscopy 26:926–935. doi:10.1016/j.arthro.2009.11.004

Balcarek P, Walde TA, Frosch S et al (2011) MRI but not arthroscopy accurately diagnoses femoral MPFL injury in first-time patellar dislocations. Knee Surg Sports Traumatol Arthrosc 20:1575–1580. doi:10.1007/s00167-011-1775-7

Bernageau J, Goutallier D, Debeyre J, Ferrané J (1975) New exploration technic of the patellofemoral joint. Relaxed axial quadriceps and contracted quadriceps. Rev Chir Orthop Réparatrice Appar Mot 61(Suppl 2):286–290

Biedert RM, Albrecht S (2006) The patellotrochlear index: a new index for assessing patellar height. Knee Surg Sports Traumatol Arthrosc Off J ESSKA 14:707–712. doi:10.1007/s00167-005-0015-4

Blackburne JS, Peel TE (1977) A new method of measuring patellar height. J Bone Joint Surg (Br) 59:241–242

Brattstroem H (1964) Shape of the intercondylar groove normally and in recurrent dislocation of patella. A clinical and x-ray-anatomical investigation. Acta Orthop Scand Suppl 68(Suppl 68):1–148

Brossmann J, Muhle C, Büll CC et al (1994) Evaluation of patellar tracking in patients with suspected patellar malalignment: cine MR imaging vs arthroscopy. AJR Am J Roentgenol 162:361–367

Carrillon Y, Abidi H, Dejour D et al (2000) Patellar instability: assessment on MR images by measuring the lateral trochlear inclination-initial experience. Radiology 216:582–585

Caton J (1989) Method of measuring the height of the patella. Acta Orthop Belg 55:385–386

Caton J, Deschamps G, Chambat P et al (1982) Patella infera. Apropos of 128 cases. Rev Chir Orthop Réparatrice Appar Mot 68:317–325

DeJour D, Saggin P (2010) The sulcus deepening trochleoplasty—the Lyon's procedure. Int Orthop 34:311–316. doi:10.1007/s00264-009-0933-8

Dejour H, Walch G, Nove-Josserand L, Guier C (1994) Factors of patellar instability: an anatomic radiographic study. Knee Surg Sports Traumatol Arthrosc Off J ESSKA 2:19–26

Dejour D, Reynaud P, Lecoultre B (1998) Douleurs et Instabilité Rotulienne, Essai de Classification. Méd Hyg 56:1466–1471

Delgado-Martins H (1979) A study of the position of the patella using computerised tomography. J Bone Joint Surg (Br) 61-B:443–444

Diederichs G, Issever AS, Scheffler S (2010) MR imaging of patellar instability: injury patterns and assessment of risk factors. Radiogr Rev Publ Radiol Soc N Am Inc 30:961–981. doi:10.1148/rg.304095755

Diederichs G, Köhlitz T, Kornaropoulos E et al (2013) Magnetic resonance imaging analysis of rotational alignment in patients with patellar dislocations. Am J Sports Med 41:51–57. doi:10.1177/0363546512464691

Dietrich TJ, Betz M, Pfirrmann CWA et al (2012) End-stage extension of the knee and its influence on tibial tuberosity-trochlear groove distance (TTTG) in asymptomatic volunteers. Knee Surg Sports Traumatol Arthrosc Off J ESSKA. doi:10.1007/s00167-012-2357-z

Elias DA, White LM, Fithian DC (2002) Acute lateral patellar dislocation at MR imaging: injury patterns of medial patellar soft-tissue restraints and osteochondral injuries of the inferomedial patella. Radiology 225:736–743

Goutallier D, Bernageau J, Lecudonnec B (1978) The measurement of the tibial tuberosity. Patella groove distanced technique and results (author's transl). Rev Chir Orthop Réparatrice Appar Mot 64:423–428

Grelsamer RP, Weinstein CH, Gould J, Dubey A (2008) Patellar tilt: the physical examination correlates with MR imaging. Knee 15:3–8. doi:10.1016/j.knee.2007.08.010

Insall J, Salvati E (1971) Patella position in the normal knee joint. Radiology 101:101–104

Kirsch MD, Fitzgerald SW, Friedman H, Rogers LF (1993) Transient lateral patellar dislocation: diagnosis with MR imaging. AJR Am J Roentgenol 161:109–113

Kujala UM, Osterman K, Kormano M et al (1989) Patellar motion analyzed by magnetic resonance imaging. Acta Orthop Scand 60:13–16

Lance E, Deutsch AL, Mink JH (1993) Prior lateral patellar dislocation: MR imaging findings. Radiology 189:905–907

Laurin CA, Lévesque HP, Dussault R et al (1978) The abnormal lateral patellofemoral angle: a diagnostic roentgenographic sign of recurrent patellar subluxation. J Bone Joint Surg Am 60:55–60

Laurin CA, Dussault R, Levesque HP (1979) The tangential x-ray investigation of the patellofemoral joint: x-ray technique, diagnostic criteria and their interpretation. Clin Orthop 144:16–26

Lippacher S, Dejour D, Elsharkawi M et al (2012) Observer agreement on the Dejour trochlear dysplasia classification: a comparison of true lateral radiographs and axial magnetic resonance images. Am J Sports Med. doi:10.1177/0363546511433028

Maldague B, Malghem J (1985) Significance of the radiograph of the knee profile in the detection of patellar instability. preliminary report. Rev Chir Orthop Réparatrice Appar Mot 71(Suppl 2):5–13

Malghem J, Maldague B (1989) Patellofemoral joint: 30 degrees axial radiograph with lateral rotation of the leg. Radiology 170:566–567

Martinez S, Korobkin M, Fondren FB et al (1983) Computed tomography of the normal patellofemoral joint. Invest Radiol 18:249–253

Merchant AC, Mercer RL, Jacobsen RH, Cool CR (1974) Roentgenographic analysis of patellofemoral congruence. J Bone Joint Surg Am 56:1391–1396

Miller TT, Staron RB, Feldman F (1996) Patellar height on sagittal MR imaging of the knee. AJR Am J Roentgenol 167:339–341

Neyret P, Robinson AHN, Le Coultre B et al (2002) Patellar tendon length–the factor in patellar instability? Knee 9:3–6

Pfirrmann CW, Zanetti M, Romero J, Hodler J (2000) Femoral trochlear dysplasia: MR findings1. Radiology 216:858–864

Schoettle PB, Zanetti M, Seifert B et al (2006) The tibial tuberosity-trochlear groove distance; a comparative study between CT and MRI scanning. Knee 13:26–31. doi:10.1016/j.knee.2005.06.003

Schutzer SF, Ramsby GR, Fulkerson JP (1986) Computed tomographic classification of patellofemoral pain patients. Orthop Clin N Am 17:235–248

Shellock FG, Mink JH, Fox JM (1988) Patellofemoral joint: kinematic MR imaging to assess tracking abnormalities. Radiology 168:551–553

Shellock FG, Mink JH, Deutsch AL, Fox JM (1989) Patellar tracking abnormalities: clinical experience with kinematic MR imaging in 130 patients. Radiology 172:799–804

Virolainen H, Visuri T, Kuusela T (1993) Acute dislocation of the patella: MR findings. Radiology 189:243–246

Reconstruction of Neglected Tears of the Extensor Apparatus of the Knee

113

Nicola Maffulli, Alessio Giai Via, and Francesco Oliva

Contents

N. Maffulli (✉)
Department of Musculoskeletal Disorders, School of Medicine and Surgery, University of Salerno, Salerno, Italy

Centre for Sports and Exercise Medicine, Mile End Hospital, Queen Mary University of London, Barts and the London School of Medicine and Dentistry, London, UK
e-mail: n.maffulli@qmul.ac.uk

A. Giai Via • F. Oliva
Department of Orthopaedics and Traumatology, University of Rome "Tor Vergata", Rome, Italy
e-mail: alessiogiaivia@hotmail.it; olivafrrancesco@hotmail.com

M.N. Doral, J. Karlsson (eds.), *Sports Injuries*,
DOI 10.1007/978-3-642-36569-0_132

Abstract

The extensor apparatus of the knee consists of the quadriceps muscle and tendon, the patella, and patellar tendon. Patellar fractures are common injuries, and neglected patella fractures are exceptional, while quadriceps or patellar tendon tears may be misdiagnosed in emergency department. Patellar tendon and quadriceps tendon ruptures are serious injuries. The surgical management of chronic tears (greater than 6 weeks) may be highly demanding because of the retraction of the patella, the soft tissue retraction, and scar formation which create an irreducible gap. In these cases, primary repair is not possible. Many surgical techniques have been proposed for the treatment of neglected ruptures, but the optimal management is controversial. In this chapter two surgical techniques for reconstruction of the chronic ruptures of the quadriceps and patellar tendon are described.

Introduction

The knee extensor apparatus consists of the quadriceps muscle and tendon, the patella and patellar tendon. The quadriceps tendon (QT) is formed by the confluence of the rectus femoris, vastus intermedius, vastus lateralis, and vastus medialis tendons. It inserts in the proximal pole and on the dorsal, medial, and lateral surfaces of the patella. QT is composed of three different sheets.

The rectus femoris forms the superficial sheet, the vastus medialis and lateralis tendon form the middle sheet, and the vastus intermedius forms the deeper sheet. The synovial membrane lies just below the vastus intermedius tendon. The patellar tendon (PT) is the distal continuation of the QT, and it extends from the inferior pole of the patella to the tibial tubercle. The extensor apparatus transmits force from quadriceps to the leg, and the patella acts as a fulcrum to increase the lever moment arm of the quadriceps, increasing the efficiency of extensor apparatus of 1.5 times (Amis 2007).

Patellar fractures are six times more frequent than tendon ruptures, but while neglected patella fractures are exceptional, quadriceps or patellar tendon tears may be misdiagnosed (Saragaglia et al. 2013). In this chapter, the treatment of chronic patellar and quadriceps tendon tears will be discussed.

Chronic Patellar Tendon Rupture

Patellar tendon (PT) rupture is a serious injury. It accounts for approximately 3 % of all injuries to the tendon–ligament complex of the knee (Wiegand et al. 2013). Since most of these injuries occur in tendons with degenerative changes, such lesions are increasingly considered as evolving from asymptomatic tendinopathy (Loppini and Maffulli 2012).

In acute injuries, the tendon is typically sutured to the inferior pole of the patella or simply repaired in a tendon to tendon configuration (Enad 1999). After 2 weeks, the patella is retracted proximally, and scarring of the surrounding soft tissues makes primary repair increasingly more difficult (Maffulli et al. 2013).

The management of chronic ruptures (>6 weeks) is controversial. To deal with small gaps (2 cm or less), distal release of the quadriceps or a proximal transposition of the tibial tuberosity has been performed with good results (Casey and Tietjens 2001). Larger gaps are technically more demanding, as the debridement of the scar and degenerated tendon ends do not allow to juxtapose the tendon stumps to each other. This usually results from adhesions and quadriceps contracture or atrophy, and achieving the correct patellar height may be difficult. Some authors recommended a Z lengthening of the quadriceps tendon to adequately mobilize the patella and relocate it to its anatomical position (Mandelbaum et al. 1988). To strengthen the construct and allow earlier return to motion, tendon augmentations have been described. Autologous semitendinosus and gracilis tendon grafts, contralateral bone–patellar tendon–bone, turndown of the quadriceps tendon, lateral gastrocnemius muscle belly and part of the achilles tenedon, extensor mechanism allograft using bone–patellar tendon–bone allograft and Achilles tendon, and artificial materials have been used (Scuderi 1958; Cadambi 1992; Chiou 1997; Fukuta 2003; Milankov 2007; Lewis 2008). However, the optimal management of these lesions is still controversial.

Distal transposition of the sartorius muscle has been proposed, but the development of scar and degenerated tissue within and around the muscle fibers could impair the strength and biomechanics of the construct (Hess and Reinders 1986). The reverse gastrocnemius flap may be considered for large gaps, but its large volumes, later degeneration, and some loss in range of motion may limit its use.

Dejour et al. proposed the use of a contralateral autograft composed of a block of tibial tuberosity, middle third of the patellar tendon, patella, and quadriceps tendon (Dejour et al. 1992). The reconstruction with a Y-shaped, folded back vastus lateralis fascia flap has been proposed. The authors stated that this technique was able to restore quadriceps function, the correct hight of the patella and allowed early postoperative mobilisation (Wiegand et al. 2013). The use of semitendinosus tendon to bridge the patellar tendon gap was first described by Kelikian et al. in 1957 (Wiegand et al. 2013).

Recently, the reconstruction of the chronic ruptures of PT with ipsilateral hamstrings tendon leaving the distal insertion in situ has been proposed (Maffulli et al. 2013). This procedure offers several advantages. First, the hamstring tendons are stronger than the distal iliotibial tract, fascia lata, or quadriceps–patellar retinaculum (Tashiro et al. 2003) and ensure a strong integration to the tendon–bone interface (Chen et al. 2012). Harvesting of the tendons is relatively easy; they are strong and they are routinely used for other surgical procedures (Charalambous and Kwaees 2013). Their blood supply is at least partially maintained by preserving the distal insertion of hamstring tendons, and it could promote better tendon healing. In ACL reconstruction with semitendinosus tendon autograft with or without maintaining the tibial insertion using an animal model, Papachristou et al. showed that harvesting the semitendinosus tendon without the detachment of the tibial attachment could preserve a sufficient blood supply to keep it viable (Papachristou et al. 2007).

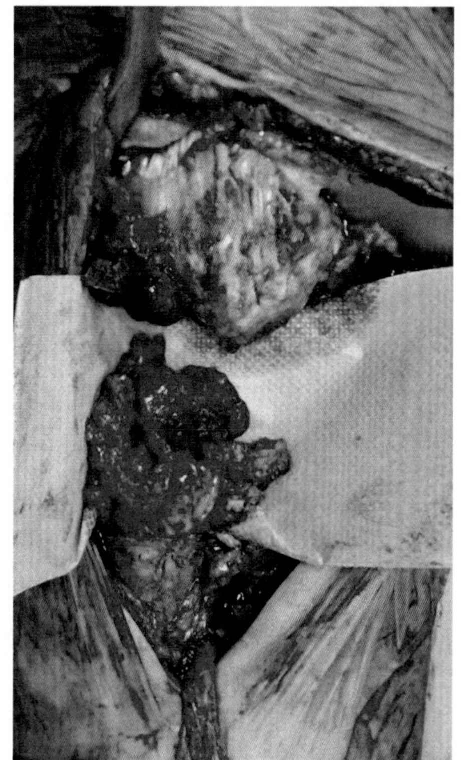

Fig. 1 Chronic patellar tendon rupture

Surgical Technique

Under general anesthesia and with the patient supine, the knee is prepped and draped in the usual sterile fashion. With the knee flexed to 90°, a midline incision is performed from the proximal pole of the patella to approximately 3 cm distal to the tibial tuberosity. The PT ends are exposed, freeing them from surrounding fibrotic and scar tissue (Fig. 1). Through the same incision, the fascia is dissected and the pes anserinus is identified. The tendons of gracilis and semitendinosus are freed of surrounding tissues and vincula. Each tendon is passed through an open tendon stripper, and it is gently advanced proximally, taking care to follow the anatomical course of the tendons. Once the proximal tendon edges of both tendons have been harvested, the proximal ends are prepared in the usual fashion using five continuous two-sided number one resorbable stitches. The distal tendon ends are left in situ, attached to the tibia, and sutured in the same way. With the knee extended, the patella is mobilized, and its distal half exposed. A tunnel in the midportion of the patella is drilled transversely with a cannulated burr over a Kirschner wire (Fig. 2), and another transverse tunnel is drilled at least 2 cm posterior to the tibial tuberosity. Both tunnels are drilled lateral to medial, and they are of equal diameter, usually 7 mm. A guidewire and a fiber wire suture are inserted into the hole to pass the tendon graft through the patellar tunnel from lateral to medial. Once the tendon ends are crossed over in a figure of eight fashion, in the same way, the graft is switched through the lower tunnel, behind the tibial tuberosity (Fig. 3). Traction is applied to the patella to try and relocate it as close as possible to its physiological position, without attempting to release the quadriceps tendon or further dissect the peripatellar tissues. The graft is secured to the patella tunnel exit holes with absorbable tendon to periosteum sutures and in the distal tunnel using a bioabsorbable 7 mm diameter interference screw. The subcutaneous fat is juxtaposed using fine absorbable sutures, the skin closed with subcuticular absorbable sutures. The leg is immobilized in full extension using a cylinder cast leaving the ankle free.

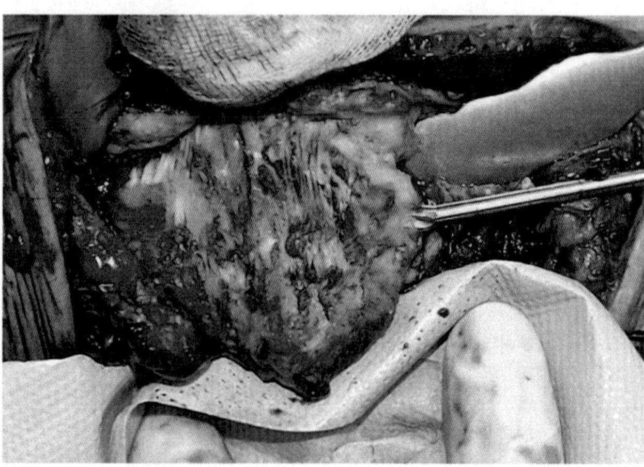

Fig. 2 Transverse tunnel in the midportion of the patella

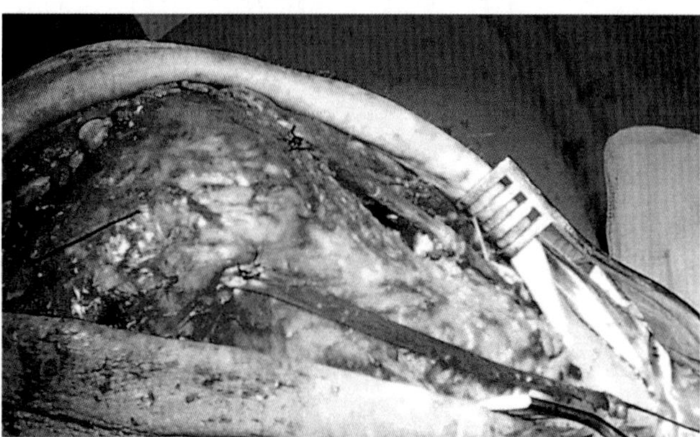

Fig. 3 Graft positioning

Postoperative Rehabilitation

Postoperative mobilization with crutches is recommended immediately, weight bearing is allowed as tolerated, and isometric exercises of the quadriceps muscles are encouraged as soon as patients can tolerate them. Active ankle flexion–extension mobilization is started immediately, and the patients are encouraged to try straight leg raise. At 2 weeks from surgery, the cylinder cast and the dressings are removed, and a removable splint is applied for another 2 weeks. Active mobilization is started at 4 weeks. Concentric exercises are started at 6 weeks, if full active and passive motions have been regained, and eccentric exercises are started after 12 weeks. Running, if desired, can be started gradually after 6 months, with the advice to progress to gentle training according to their own progress. Patients are allowed to resume sport activities at 9 months and discharged at 12 months if asymptomatic.

Complications

This technique is not without risks. Patellar fracture, tibial tuberosity fracture, infections, and hypoesthesia over the anterior aspect of the knee have been described (Tompkins 2012; Maffulli 2013). Persistent anterior knee pain has also been reported, probably related to degenerative changes to the patella.

Quadriceps Tendon Rupture

Quadriceps tendon rupture is a relative uncommon injury with an incidence of 1.37/100,000 patients per year (Clayton and Court-Brown 2008) (Fig. 4).

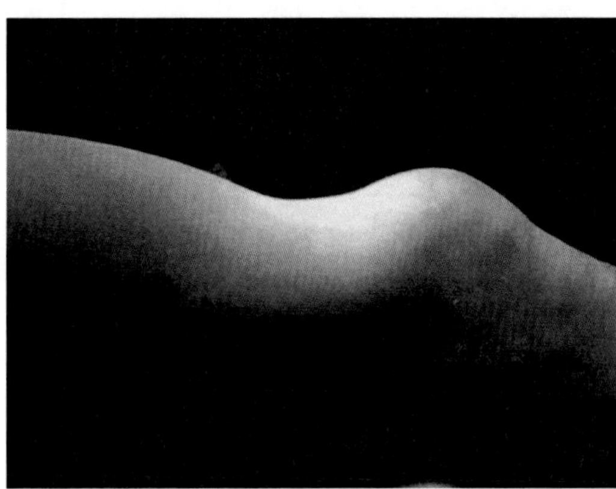

Fig. 4 Clinical examination 6 months following quadriceps tendon injury: a palpable gap proximal to the upper pole of the patella was evident

Table 1 Causes of quadriceps tendon rupture

Mechanisms of injury	Rate
Simple fall	61.5 %
Fall from stairs	23.4 %
Sport activities	6 %
Spontaneous ruptures	3.2 %
Agricultural injuries (penetrating trauma)	2.3 %
Car accident	3.2 %
Non-penetrating trauma	0.4 %

While PT rupture occurs more frequently in patients younger than 40 years, QT injuries are more common in males older than 40 years (Siwek and Rao 1981).

QT injuries may be caused by a direct trauma, or more frequently, they are associated to degenerative tendon changes. Violent eccentric contraction is the most common mechanism of injury (Scuderi 1958), but spontaneous ruptures may also occur (Table 1). Spontaneous ruptures affect people with predisposing conditions such as chronic renal failure, rheumatoid arthritis, diabetes, gout, and steroids abuse (Ciriello et al. 2012). Dobbs et al. reported a 0.1 % incidence of QT rupture after TKA (Dobbs et al. 2005). Spontaneous bilateral QT rupture is not exceptional, and and it has been reported from 6 % to 12 % of cases (Shah 2002; Ciriello 2012). A recent review reported that in more than 70 % of cases, ruptures occur at the distal portion of the QT, within 2 cm from the superior pole of the patella, while in about 12 % of cases, it involves the proximal part (Ciriello et al. 2012). Rasoul et al. found a correlation between the site of rupture and the age of patient (Rasul and Fischer 1993). In patients older than 40, ruptures occur more frequently at the tendon–bone junction, whereas in patients younger than 40 years, tears involve the mid-tendinous area.

Diagnosis is based on the triad of acute pain, sometimes accompanied by a cracking sensation, failure of active knee extension, and palpable suprapatellar gap. The inability to maintain the passively extended knee against gravity suggests an extensor mechanism injury. But despite this clinical presentation, the diagnosis of QT tears may be difficult, and a delay in diagnosis is not uncommon. This probably results from the lack of a specific test for QT rupture (Jolles et al. 2007) and because often the patient refuses to extend the knee actively because of the associated pain, causing confusing diagnosis. Missing diagnosis in the emergency department has been reported in 40–67 % of cases (Jolles 2007; Saragaglia 2013).

Anteroposterior and lateral radiographs of the knee are the initial imaging. They allow assessment of bony injury, and they can provide indirect evidence of QT rupture. Ultrasound and MRI are useful for diagnosis of QT rupture and are recommended in doubtful cases, but their use did not decrease the high rate of misdiagnosis in emergency department (Jolles et al. 2007). However, in patients with clear clinical signs, a palpable gap, and an extensor mechanism deficit, MRI is not necessary (Lee et al. 2013).

Many different surgical techniques have been described to repair a QT rupture, and as in the patellar tendon, timing was identified as the determining factor in the functional outcome. Repair should be done in the first 48–72 h post injury to achieve a successful outcome (Scuderi 1958). Patients who had delay repair had poorer functional outcomes and decreased self-reported satisfaction (Rougraff et al. 1996). Furthermore, surgical technique did not affect outcome, but delayed surgery results in poorer results (Ciriello et al. 2012). Repair of chronic ruptures is more demanding because of soft tissue retraction, muscle contraction, and scar formation which can create an irreducible gap. In these cases, a primary repair is not possible, and lengthening procedures and extensor mechanism reconstruction are needed. The Codivilla techniques are well accepted (Saragaglia et al. 2013). An inverted V full-thickness flap is made in the QT, 1.5–2 cm from the proximal edge of the tear. The edges are then sutured with several stitches of thick non-resorbable suture, the triangular tendon flap is pulled back distally as reinforcement, and the open proximal portion of the inverted V is sutured longitudinally in side-to-side fashion. Rizio and Jarmon reported good results in three cases treated with a V-Y plasty (Rizio and Jarmon 2008). They performed a V-Y lengthening without augmentation or cerclage wire for gaps smaller than 20 mm. Three locking sutures were passed through three bone tunnels into the patella and tied distally over the patella. The authors did not use additional turndown flap to avoid further compromise of the tendon. Reconstruction of chronic QT tear with ipsilateral hamstring tendons has been also described (Leopardi 2006; Nguene-Nyemb 2011; McCormick 2013).

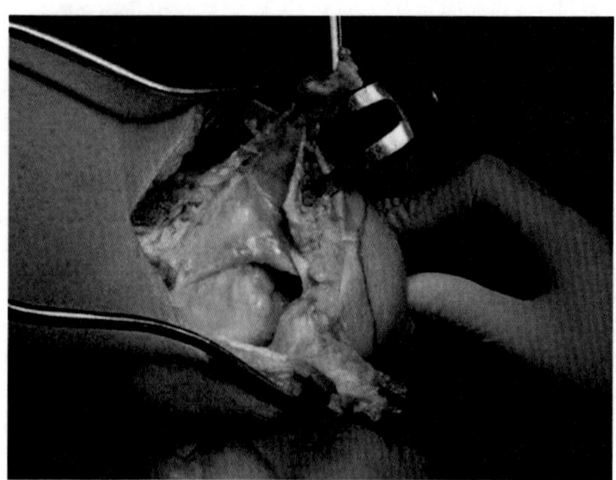

Fig. 5 Intraoperative appearance of the full-thickness defect of 10·4 cm produced after debridement

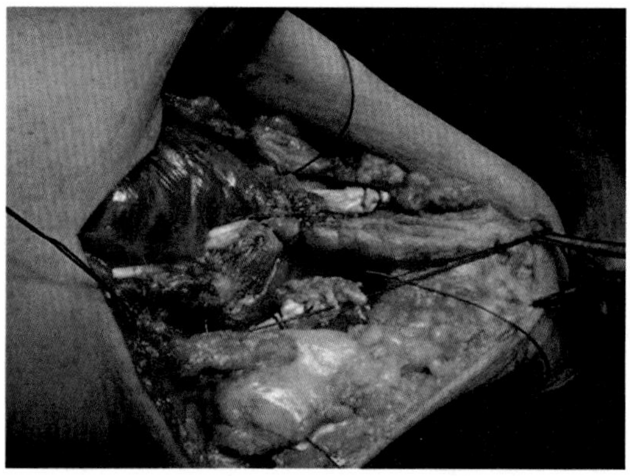

Fig. 6 Final intraoperative appearance. The free gracilis and semitendinosus graft was passed through a transverse patellar tunnel, leaving free the distal parts of the tendons, which were then passed through the quadriceps tendon several times to bridge the defect

Surgical Technique

A longitudinal 3 cm skin incision is made over the pes anserinus, and the hamstring tendons are harvested in the usual fashion. A longitudinal midline incision is made overlying the quadriceps tendon and the proximal patella to expose quadriceps tendon (Fig. 5). A 5 mm transverse tunnel is drilled through the midportion of the patella, and the graft is pulled into the patellar tunnel, leaving free the distal parts of the tendons. The free ends of the tendons are then passed through the quadriceps tendon several times to bridge the defect (Fig. 6). After the operation, patients are placed in a long-leg cast or a knee brace for 6 weeks, before starting physical therapy. Early weight bearing is usually allowed with crutch support.

Complications

The most common complications after QT repair are quadriceps atrophy and decreased muscular strength (Lee et al. 2013). They occur in 20–30 % of cases, but this does not influence patient's satisfaction (Ciriello et al. 2012). Patella baja is a frequent consequence of chronic QT rupture (Rizio and Jarmon 2008). Recently 6.9 % incidence of heterotopic ossifications, 2.5 % of pulmonary embolism, 1.2 % of superficial infection, and 1.1 % of deep infection have been reported (Ciriello et al. 2012). Reruptures (2 % of cases) and anterior knee pain may also occur (Ciriello et al. 2012).

Conclusion

Neglected rupture of the PT is a debilitating problem. Reconstruction of chronic tears of PT reconstruction using the ipsilateral hamstring gracilis and semitendinosus tendon graft leaving their distal insertion in situ is safe and effective. It allows early mobilization of the knee and patients to return to preinjury daily activities with satisfactory outcomes.

Few case report and case series are reported regarding surgical management of chronic QT ruptures. No high-quality studies are available. It is therefore difficult to choose the best evidence-based treatment. The infrequence of QT rupture is another limiting factor for well-conducted studies. Timing of surgery, more than surgical technique, seems to be the determining factor for functional outcome. For this reason, improving diagnosis and more attention in emergency department is demanding in order to decrease the high rate of misdiagnosis and improve clinical outcome.

Cross-References

► Anatomy and Biomechanics of the Knee

References

Amis AA (2007) Current concepts of anatomy and biomechanics of patellar instability. Med Arthrosc 15:48–56

Cadambi A, Engh GA (1992) Use of a semitendinosus tendon autogenous graft for rupture of the patellar ligament after total knee arthroplasty. A report of seven cases. J Bone Joint Surg Am 74:974–949

Casey MT Jr, Tietjens BR (2001) Neglected ruptures of the patellar tendon. A case series of four patients. Am J Sports Med 29:457–460

Charalambous CP, Kwaees TA (2013) Anatomical consideration in hamstring tendon harvesting for anterior cruciate ligament reconstruction. Muscles Ligaments Tendons J 2:253–257

Chen B, Li R, Zhang S (2012) Reconstruction and restoration of neglected ruptured patellar tendon using semitendinosus and gracilis tendons with preserved distal insertions: two case reports. Knee 19:508–512

Chiou HM, Chang MC, Lo WH (1997) One-stage reconstruction of skin defect and patellar tendon rupture after total knee arthroplasty. A new technique. J Arthroplasty 12:575–579

Ciriello V, Gudipati S, Tosounidis T, Soucacos PN, Giannoudis PV (2012) Clinical outcomes after repair of quadriceps tendon rupture: a systematic review. Injury 43:1931–1938

Clayton RA, Court-Brown CM (2008) The epidemiology of musculoskeletal tendinous and ligamentous injuries. Injury 39:1338–1344

Dejour H, Denjean S, Neyret P (1992) Treatment of old or recurrent ruptures of the patellar ligament by contralateral autograft. Rev Chir Orthop Reparatrice Appar Mot 78:58–62

Dobbs RE, Hanssen AD, Ewallen G, Pagnano MW (2005) Quadriceps tendon rupture after total knee arthroplasty. Prevalence, complications, and outcomes. Bone Joint Surg Am 87:37–45

Enad JG (1999) Patellar tendon ruptures. South Med J 92:563–566

Fukuta S, Kuge A, Nakamura M (2003) Use of the Leeds-Keio prosthetic ligament for repair of patellar tendon rupture after total knee arthroplasty. Knee 10:127–130

Hess P, Reinders J (1986) Transposition of the sartorius muscle for reconstruction of the extensor apparatus of the knee. J Trauma 26:90–92

Jolles BM, Garofalo R, Gillain I, Schizas C (2007) A new clinical test in diagnosing quadriceps tendon rupture. Ann R Coll Surg Engl 89:259–261

Lee D, Stinner D, Mir H (2013) Quadriceps and patellar tendon ruptures. J Knee Surg 26:301–308

Leopardi P, Vico G, Rosa D, Cigala F, Maffulli N (2006) Reconstruction of a chronic quadriceps tendon tear in a body builder. Knee Surg Sports Traumatol Arthrosc 14:1007–1011

Lewis PB, Rue JP, Bach BR Jr (2008) Chronic patellar tendon rupture: surgical reconstruction technique using 2 achilles tendon allografts. J Knee Surg 21:130–135

Loppini M, Maffulli N (2012) Conservative management of tendinopathy: an evidence-based approach. Muscle Ligament Tendons J 2:133–136

Maffulli N, Del Buono A, Loppini M, Denaro V (2013) Ipsilateral hamstring tendon graft reconstruction for chronic patellar tendon ruptures: average 5.8-year follow-up. J Bone Joint Surg Am 95:1231–1236

Mandelbaum BR, Bartolozzi A, Carney B (1988) A systematic approach to reconstruction of neglected tears of the patellar tendon. A case report. Clin Orthop Relat Res 235:268–271

McCormick F, Nwachukwu BU, Kim J, Martin SD (2013) Autologous hamstring tendon used for revision of quadriceps tendon tears. Orthopedics 36:529–532

Milankov MZ, Miljkovic N, Stankovic M (2007) Reconstruction of chronic patellar tendon rupture with contralateral BTB autograft: a case report. Knee Surg Sports Traumatol Arthrosc 15:1445–1448

Nguene-Nyemb AG, Huten D, Ropars M (2011) Chronic patellar tendon rupture reconstruction with a semitendinosus autograft. Orthop Traumatol Surg Res 97:447–450

Papachristou G, Nikolaou V, Efstathopoulos N et al (2007) ACL reconstruction with semitendinosus tendon autograft without detachment of its tibial insertion: a histologic study in a rabbit model. Knee Surg Sports Traumatol Arthrosc 15:1175–1180

Rasul AT Jr, Fischer DA (1993) Primary repair of quadriceps tendon ruptures. Results Treat Clin Orthop Rel Res 289:205–207

Rizio L, Jarmon N (2008) Chronic quadriceps rupture: treatment with lengthening and early mobilization without cerclage augmentation and a report of three cases. J Knee Surg 21:34–38

Rougraff BT, Reeck CC, Essenmacher J (1996) Complete quadriceps tendon ruptures. Orthopedics 19:509–514

Saragaglia D, Pison A, Rubens-Duval B (2013) Acute and old ruptures of the extensor apparatus of the knee in adults (excluding knee replacement). Orthop Traumatol Surg Res 99:67–76

Scuderi C (1958) Ruptures of the quadriceps tendon; study of twenty tendon ruptures. Am J Surg 95:626–634

Shah MK (2002) Simultaneous bilateral rupture of quadriceps tendons: analysis of risk factors and associations. South Med J 95:860–866

Siwek CW, Rao JP (1981) Ruptures of the extensor mechanism of the knee joint. J Bone Joint Surg Am 63:932–937

Tashiro T, Kurosawa H, Kawakami A, Hikita A, Fukui N (2003) Influence of medial hamstring tendon harvest on knee flexor strength after anterior cruciate ligament reconstruction. A detailed evaluation with comparison of single- and double-tendon harvest. Am J Sports Med 31:522–529

Tompkins M, Arendt AA (2012) Complications in patellofemoral surgery. Sports Med Arthrosc Rev 20:187–193

Wiegand N, Naumov I, Vamhidy L, Warta V, Than P (2013) Reconstruction of the patellar tendon using a Y-shaped flap folded back from the vastus lateralis fascia. Knee 20:139–143

Reconstruction of the Medial Patellofemoral Ligament: A Surgical Technique Perspective from an Orthopedic Surgeon

114

Nicola Maffulli, Alessio Giai Via, and Francesco Oliva

Contents

Abstract

Primary traumatic patellar dislocation is a common injury in young active population. The medial patellofemoral ligament (MPFL) is the primary restraint in preventing lateralization of the patella, and it is injured in most cases. Primary patellofemoral dislocation is usually managed nonoperatively, but recurrent dislocations are relatively common. A tear of the MPFL is the essential lesion of recurrent lateral patellar dislocation in patients without any predisposing factors. Many surgical procedures have been commonly used for treatment of recurrent patellar dislocation. MPFL reconstruction using an autogenous gracilis tendon through a double patellar bony tunnel is a safe and reliable technique in patients without predisposing anatomic factors. This technique does not preclude further surgical procedures when failure occurs. However, long-term studies are needed.

Introduction

Primary traumatic patellar dislocation is a common injury in young active population, and it accounts for approximately 3 % of all knee injuries (Tsai et al. 2012). It typically results from a sport injury, and its average annual incidence ranges between 5.8 and 7.0 per 100,000 person-years (Sillanpaa et al. 2008). Women are more likely to sustain a patellar dislocation than men.

N. Maffulli (✉)
Department of Musculoskeletal Disorders, School of Medicine and Surgery, University of Salerno, Salerno, Italy

Department of Orthopaedic and Traumatology, School of Medicine, University of Rome "Tor Vergata", Rome, Italy
e-mail: n.maffulli@qmul.ac.uk

A. Giai Via • F. Oliva
Department of Orthopaedic and Traumatology, University of Rome "Tor Vergata", Rome, Italy
e-mail: alessiogiaivia@hotmail.it; olivafrrancesco@hotmail.com

M.N. Doral, J. Karlsson (eds.), *Sports Injuries*,
DOI 10.1007/978-3-642-36569-0_127

Table 1 Restraint provided by medial static stabilizers to lateral patellar dislocation (Amis et al. 2003)

Ligament	Restraint provided (%)
MPFL	50–60 %
Medial patellomeniscal ligament	22 %
Medial retinaculum	11 %
Medial patellotibial ligament	5 %

Patellofemoral stability is provided by both active stabilizers, including active muscle tension, and passive stabilizers such as bony and soft tissue structures. The lateral retinaculum is an important restraint to medial dislocation, while the medial patellofemoral ligament (MPFL), the medial patellomeniscal ligament, the medial patellotibial ligament, and the medial retinaculum provide stability to lateral dislocations (Amis et al. 2003). The MPFL is the primary passive restraint to lateral patellar translation at 0–30° of knee flexion (Senavongse and Amis 2005), the angle at which lateral patellar instability most often occurs. The MPFL is a thin structure with a mean tensile strength of 208 N (Mountney et al. 2005), and cadaveric studies reported that it provides 50–60 % of the soft tissue restraint to lateral patellar translation (Conlan et al. 1993; Table 1). The MPFL is located in the second layer of the anteromedial aspect of the knee, and its femoral insertion area at the femur is between the adductor tubercle and the medial epicondyle (Nomura et al. 2005). The MPFL is formed by two bundles, an inferior-straight bundle and a superior oblique bundle (Kang et al. 2010). The angle formed between the two bundles is approximately 15°. This leads to a wide patellar insertion, with the footprint occupying approximately half of the patellar height, on average 22 mm at its proximal medial side (Kang et al. 2010). Although the two bands run in distinct directions, they are not separated and the MPFL works as a single intact structure with no functional difference between the two bands.

Tears of MPFL are common after lateral patellar dislocations. Magnetic resonance imaging studies and immediate surgical exploration in knees with acute patellar dislocation have demonstrated an MPFL injury in up to 100 % of these patients (Spritzer et al. 1997; Ahmad et al. 2000; Fig. 1). Osteochondral fractures are also common injuries after patellar dislocations, occurring in nearly 25 % of cases (Sillanpaa et al. 2008).

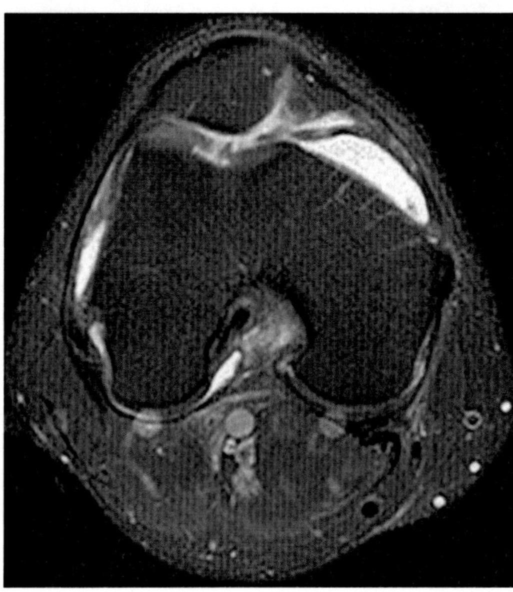

Fig. 1 An axial T2-weighted fast-spin-echo magnetic resonance imaging scan illustrates the index lesion in a patient sustaining a primary traumatic lateral dislocation of the patella

Primary patellofemoral dislocation is usually managed nonoperatively, with acute surgical repair indicated in specific cases such as chondral lesions or fractures (Palmu et al. 2008; Tsai et al. 2012). However, recurrent dislocations are relatively common, and long-term recurrence rates can be up to 45 % (Maenpaa and Lehto 1997). In up to 80 % of patients, recurrent instability is attributed to predisposing factors. Four major predisposing factors have been described: trochlear dysplasia, patella alta, patellar tilt, and increased tibial tuberosity–femoral groove distance (TT–TG) (Dejour et al. 1994). Secondary factors in patellar instability are knee recurvatum, femoral anteversion, valgus alignment, and external tibial torsion, but their absence does not prevent the development of patellar instability (Dejour et al. 1994). After careful clinical and imaging evaluations, all these conditions need to be considered to restore the biomechanics of the patellofemoral joint. Many surgical treatments attempt to correct anatomic predisposing factors, others involve a simple repair of pathologic tissue, and some techniques attempt to do both. Lateral retinacular release, proximal or disatal realignment, trochleoplasty, purely soft tissue reconstructions, and combinations of these procedures have been purposed with different results (Abraham et al. 1989; Panni et al. 2005). All these nonanatomic surgical procedures have been used also in recurrent patellar dislocation without any predisposing factor altering the patellar tracking (Aglietti et al. 1994; Nakagawa et al. 2002). Several studies reported inconsistent outcomes, recurrent dislocations, patellofemoral pain, and arthritis in up to 40 % of these patients (Muneta et al. 1999; Nakagawa et al. 2002). Since the MPFL has been demonstrated as the primary constraint in preventing lateralization of the patella, this provides biomechanical support for its reconstruction in recurrent patellar dislocation without other predisposing factors. In a cadaveric study, MPFL reconstruction showed a significant reduction in lateral displacement and ligament load compared with medial transfer of the tibial tuberosity (Ostemeier et al. 2006).

Several surgical techniques have been described. Semitendinosus, gracilis, quadriceps tendon, and synthetic grafts have been used to reconstruct the MPFL, all showing good early to midterm results (Deie et al. 2003; Schottle et al. 2005). Clear superiority of only one of these surgical techniques has not been reported to date. The authors' preferred method for an anatomic MPFL reconstruction using autologous ipsilateral gracilis tendon graft is described below (Fig. 2).

Surgical Technique

The patient is placed supine, with an above-knee tourniquet, following the administration of prophylactic antibiotics. A diagnostic arthroscopy is performed to address any intra-articular damage to the knee. The gracilis tendon is harvested and prepared in the usual fashion (Maffulli and Leadbetter 2005). If the gracilis tendon is insufficient in thickness or length (less than 15 cm), the semitendinosus tendon can be harvested and used to reconstruct the MPFL. The patella is approached through a 4 cm midline incision. The prepatellar fascia is elevated to allow the medial and lateral walls of the patella to be exposed. Two transverse tunnels are made in the upper third of the patella. The diameter of the tunnel depended on the diameter of the tendon and varies between 3.0 and 4.0 mm (Fig. 3). They are drilled parallel to one another and 1 cm apart. The graft is passed through the two transverse tunnels from medial to lateral and then from lateral to medial (Fig. 4), so that the graft forms a loop through the patella. The medial epicondyle is palpated through the skin and exposed using a 2 cm incision, and the graft is passed between the deep fascia and the capsule of the knee joint and out over the medial epicondyle. The two ends of the graft are secured into a 7 mm tunnel about 3 cm long, sited on the posterior aspect of the medial epicondyle, proximal to the medial collateral ligament and 1 cm distal to the adductor tubercle, guided by a transfemoral eyelet pin (Fig. 5). The knee is cycled several times from full flexion to full extension with the graft under tension. In this way, the graft tension is settled. The graft is then secured within the tunnel in the medial epicondyle using a 7 mm diameter and 30 mm long interference with the knee flexed to 20°. The wound is closed in layers, and routine dressings, bandages, and a straight knee splint are applied.

Postoperative mobilization consists of partial weight bearing in a straight knee splint. After 2 weeks, patients are allowed to progress from partial to full weight bearing. At 6 weeks, the straight knee splint is removed, and patients start gentle mobilization of the operated knee. For the first 3 weeks, they are encouraged to undertake cycling on an exercise bicycle, keeping the seat high. The height of the seat is lowered every second day, and normally patients are able to reach 90° of knee flexion by the seventh or eighth postoperative week. In addition, patients undertake gentle concentric training of their thigh muscles and proprioception training. At the eighth postoperative week, gentle on-the-spot jogging on a trampoline is started and gradually progressed over the next 4 weeks. At the 12th postoperative week, sports-specific rehabilitation

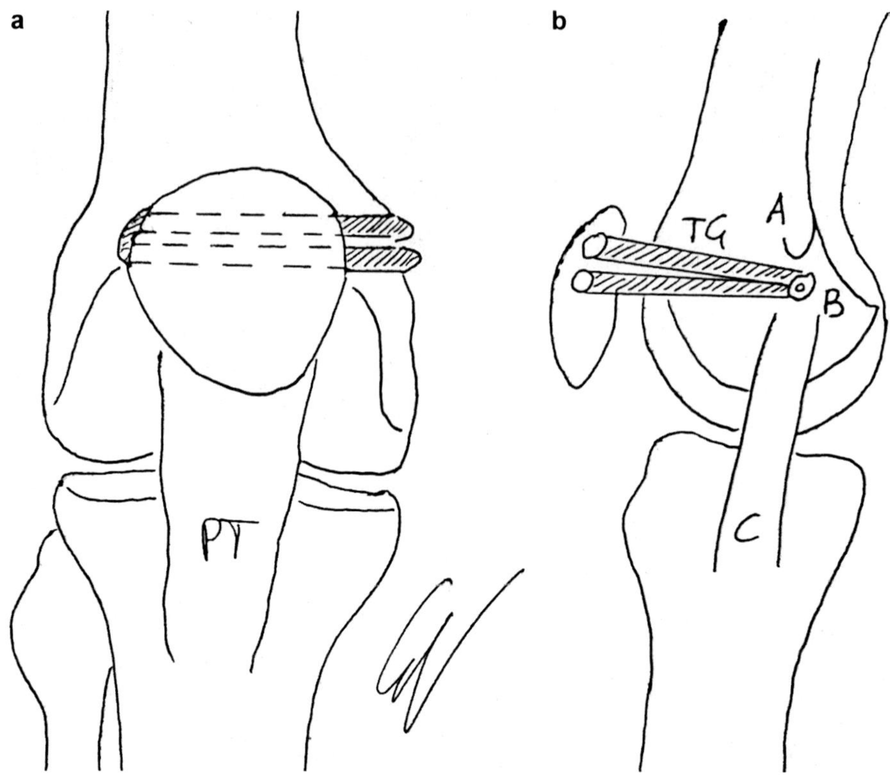

Fig. 2 Anatomical reconstruction of the MPFL with hamstring tendon. The graft is harvested in the usual fashion. It is passed through two transverse tunnels in the upper third of the patella. The graft is fixed with an absorbable 7 mm interference screw at the isometric point on the medial femoral epicondyle (B). The isometric femoral point is placed between the adductor tubercle (A) and the insertion of medial collateral ligament (C). PT: Patellar Tendon; TG: tendon graft (**Figure copyright © Alessio Giai Via**)

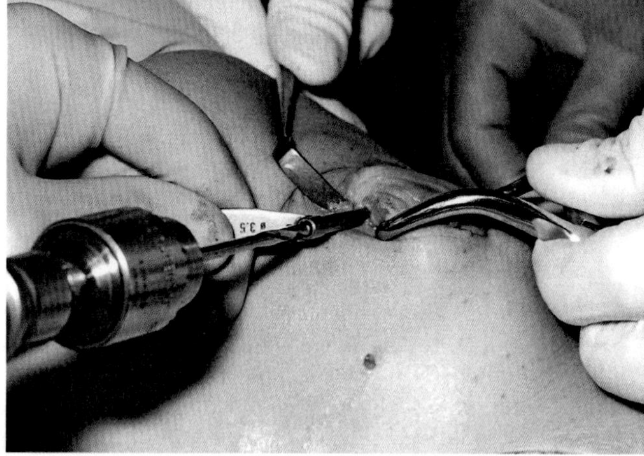

Fig. 3 Following medial and lateral parapatellar incisions, the patella is stabilized using a large clamp on the right of the figure. Tunnels are produced by sequential drill holes in the superior half of the patella, 1 cm apart

is started. Progressive return to normal daily activities occurs over the course of the next 3 months, with return to sport normally planned at the sixth postoperative month.

Discussion

When nonoperative management fails, surgical options can be considered to restore patellofemoral stability. Tears of the MPFL are the essential lesion of recurrent lateral patellar dislocation in patients without any predisposing factors (Amis et al. 2003). Many surgical techniques have been described to reconstruct this ligament, all showing good early to midterm results.

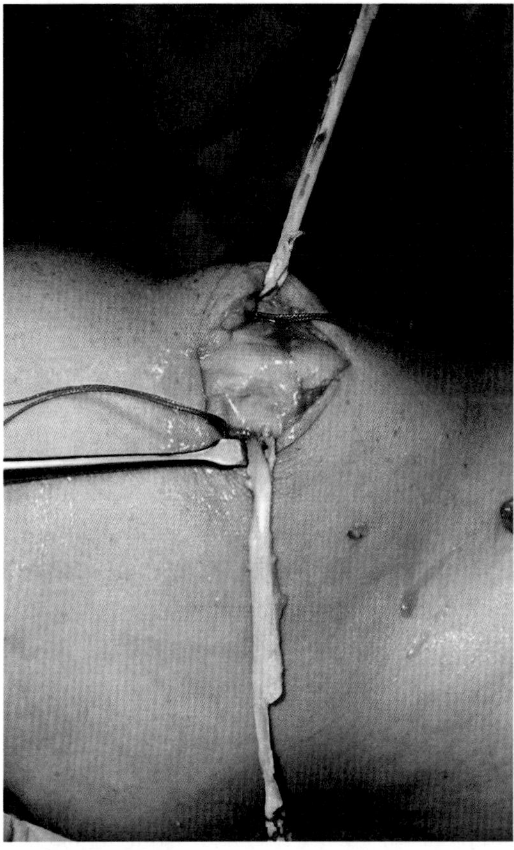

Fig. 4 A Beath pin is used to pass a Vicryl loop through the patella tunnels

Good results after isolated MPFL reconstruction have been reported in 28 patients with chronic patellar instability without any anatomic predisposing factors at an average follow-up of 3.1 years (Ronga et al. 2009). All patients continued to practice sports, and only four patients retired from their sport because of their age and because they were concerned about operated knee, but took part in low-impact recreational sports. Three patients (10.7 %) experienced a recurrent lateral patellar dislocation, and one of these did not return to sport. More recently, Schiavone et al. reviewed 48 active patients who underwent MPFL reconstruction using an autologous semitendinosus graft (Panni et al. 2011). They reported that 89 % were either satisfied or very satisfied with their functional result, and no patients experienced recurrent dislocations.

This technique is a safe and a reliable option for recurrent patellofemoral dislocation. It is technically demanding and requires meticulous positioning of bony tunnels, femoral insertion site, and accurate graft tensioning. Patellar tunnels are usually drilled parallel, but divergent tunnels have been described (Panni et al. 2011). Drilling two diverging bony tunnels may reproduce a more anatomic patellar insertion of the MPFL. But the possible advantages remain to be fully elucidated and significant differences in outcomes have yet to be reported. However, all authors agree to be careful during tunnels drilling to avoid breaching

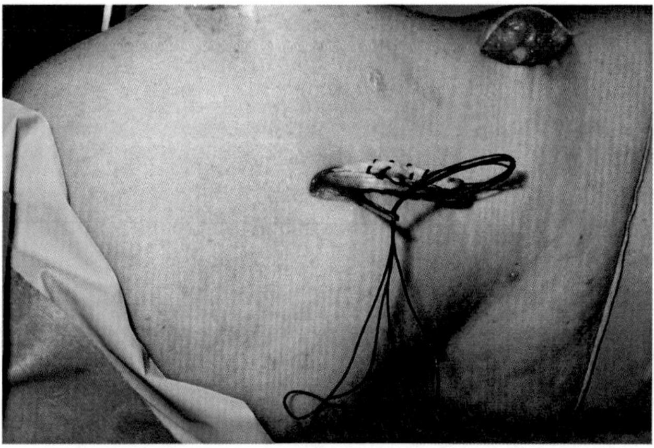

Fig. 5 The medial epicondyle is exposed, and the Beath pin is placed across the transepicondylar axis. A tunnel is drilled to accommodate and secure both ends of the graft. The graft is passed between the second and third layers of the knee. The graft is pulled into the tunnel using Vicryl through the eye of the Beath pin

either the chondral surface or the anterior cortex. In accordance with most anatomic studies, the femoral tunnel should be positioned on the posterior aspect of the medial epicondyle, proximal to the medial collateral ligament, and 1 cm distal to the adductor tubercle (Nomura et al. 2005). Although anatomic reconstruction of the MPFL is important, several studies showed that the femoral attachment of the MPFL is not clearly identifiable, and probably the convergence of various structures and layers toward the medial epicondyle makes it difficult to distinguish the MPFL origin (Elias and Cosgarea 2006). Recent biomechanical data showed significant increases in medial patellofemoral contact pressures when MPFL grafts were misplaced as little as 5 mm. Incorrect graft placement accompanied by a short graft increased medial patellofemoral contact pressures by over 50 % (Elias and Cosgarea 2006). Multiple MPFL reconstruction procedures have been described using semitendinosus, gracilis, or quadriceps tendon and synthetic grafts (Ellera 1992; Hamner et al. 1999), but there is no agreement regarding the best method. Although a semitendinosus tendon graft is stiffer and has a higher ultimate load than the gracilis tendon (Hamner et al. 1999), semitendinosus tendons require larger intraosseous patellar tunnels using a 5.0 mm drill. For this reason, gracilis tendon graft and smaller tunnels (3.0–4.0 mm of diameter) should be preferred to reduce the risks of patellar fractures. Another important aspect to take into account is the tension of the graft. Senavongse and Amis demonstrated that the patella is subluxed laterally most easily at 20° of flexion and that the contribution of the MPFL to resist lateral dislocation of the patella is maximal between 0 and 20°(Senavongse and Amis 2005). This supports the choice to fix the graft at 20° of the flexion. Tensioning and fixing the graft at 60–90° of knee flexion may produce overtightening of the graft and increased loads on the patellofemoral joint, which may result in degenerative joint disease at long-term follow-up.

This technique is not without complications. Recurrent patellar dislocation is a well-known complication. A rate of 10 % of patellar redislocations after MPFL reconstruction has been reported (Drez et al. 2001; Schottle et al. 2005). But one of the advantages of this technique is that it does not preclude further surgical procedures when failure occurs. Patellar fracture is another risk of this procedure. If the two tunnels converge at the lateral edge of the patella, they may produce a figure-of-8 appearance of the exit hole. In these cases, the graft can be sutured to the periosteum. Persistent postoperative anterior knee pain was also reported by some patients. It can be caused by overtightening of the graft or by degenerative disease of patellofemoral joint facet. In fact poorer outcomes have been reported in patients with concurrent patellofemoral chondral damage, particularly in relation to continuing pain and reduced sports participation (Ellera 1992; Christiansen et al. 2008; Panni et al. 2011). Hypoesthesia of the medial or lateral aspect of the knee has also been described, but patients do not report any inconvenience from it.

Conclusion

MPFL reconstruction using autogenous gracilis tendon through a double patellar bony tunnel is a safe and reliable technique for recurrent patellofemoral dislocation in patients without any predisposing anatomic factors. Correct indications, careful preoperative evaluation, and restoration of normal anatomy are the keys for successful long-term outcome. This technique does not preclude further surgical procedures when failure occurs. However, long-term evaluation is necessary, particularly to monitor the possible development of patellofemoral osteoarthritis and the long-term functional deficit that recurrent patellar dislocation may cause.

Cross-References

► Medial Patellofemoral Ligament Reconstruction: Current Concepts
► Patellar Dislocations: Overview
► Return to Play After Acute Patellar Dislocation

References

Abraham E, Washington E, Huang TL (1989) Insall proximal realignment for disorders of the patella. Clin Orthop Relat Res 248:61–65

Aglietti P, Buzzi R, De Biase P, Giron F (1994) Surgical treatment of recurrent dislocation of the patella. Clin Orthop Relat Res 308:8–17

Ahmad CS, Stein BE, Matuz D, Henry JH (2000) Immediate surgical repair of the medial patellar stabilizers for acute patellar dislocation: a review of eight cases. Am J Sports Med 28:804–810

Amis AA, Firer P, Mountney J, Senavongse W, Thomas NP (2003) Anatomy and biomechanics of the medial patellofemoral ligament. Knee 10:215–220

Christiansen SE, Jakobsen BW, Lund B, Lind M (2008) Isolated repair of the medial patellofemoral ligament in primary dislocation of the patella: a prospective randomized study. Arthroscopy 24:881–887

Conlan T, Garth WP Jr, Lemons JE (1993) Evaluation of the medial soft tissue restraints of the extensor mechanism of the knee. J Bone Joint Surg Am 75:682–693

Deie M, Ochi M, Sumen Y, Yasumoto M, Kobayashi K, Kimura H (2003) Reconstruction of the medial patellofemoral ligament for the treatment of habitual or recurrent dislocation of the patella in children. J Bone Joint Surg (Br) 85:887–890

Dejour H, Walch G, Nove-Josserand L, Guier C (1994) Factors of patellar instability: an anatomic radiographic study. Knee Surg Sports Traumatol Arthrosc 2:19–26

Drez D Jr, Edwards TB, Williams CS (2001) Results of medial patellofemoral ligament reconstruction in the treatment of patellar dislocation. Arthroscopy 17:298–306

Elias JJ, Cosgarea AJ (2006) Technical errors during medial patellofemoral ligament reconstruction could overload medial patellofemoral cartilage: a computational analysis. Am J Sports Med 34:1478–1485

Ellera Gomes JL (1992) Medial patellofemoral ligament reconstruction for recurrent dislocation of the patella: a preliminary report. Arthroscopy 8:335–340

Hamner DL, Brown CH Jr, Steiner ME, Hecker AT, Hayes WC (1999) Hamstring tendon grafts for reconstruction of the anterior cruciate ligament: biomechanical evaluation of the use of multiple strands and tensioning techniques. J Bone Joint Surg Am 81:549–557

Kang HJ, Wang F, Chen BC, Su YL, Zhang ZC, Yan CB (2010) Functional bundles of the medial patellofemoral ligament. Knee Surg Sports Traumatol Arthrosc 18:1511–1516

Maenpaa H, Lehto MU (1997) Patellar dislocation: the long-term results of nonoperative management in 100 patients. Am J Sports Med 25:213–217

Maffulli N, Leadbetter WB (2005) Free gracilis tendon graft in neglected tears of the Achilles tendon. Clin J Sport Med 15:56–61

Mountney J, Senavongse W, Amis A, Thomas NP (2005) Tensile strength of the medial patellofemoral ligament before and after repair or reconstruction. J Bone Joint Surg 87-B:36–40

Muneta T, Sekiya I, Tsuchiya M, Shinomiya K (1999) A technique for reconstruction of the medial patellofemoral ligament. Clin Orthop Relat Res 359:151–155

Nakagawa K, Wada Y, Minamide M, Tsuchiya A, Moriya H (2002) Deterioration of long-term clinical results after the Elmslie-Trillat procedure for dislocation of the patella. J Bone Joint Surg (Br) 84:861–864

Nomura E, Inoue M, Osada N (2005) Anatomical analysis of the medial patellofemoral ligament of the knee, especially the femoral attachment. Knee Surg Sports Traumatol Arthrosc 13:510–515

Ostemeier S, Stukenborg-Colsman C, Hurschler C, Wirth CJ (2006) In vitro investigation of the effect of medial patellofemoral ligament reconstruction and medial tibial tuberosity transfer on lateral patella stability. Arthroscopy 22:308–319

Palmu S, Kallio PE, Donell ST, Helenius I, Nietosvaara Y (2008) Acute patellar dislocation in children and adolescents: a randomized clinical trial. J Bone Joint Surg Am 90:463–470

Panni AS, Tartarone M, Patricola A, Paxton EW, Fithian DC (2005) Long-term results of lateral retinacular release. Arthroscopy 21:526–531

Panni AS, Alam M, Cerciello S, Vasso M, Maffulli N (2011) Medial patellofemoral ligament reconstruction with a divergent patellar transverse 2-tunnel technique. Am J Sports Med 39:2647–2655

Ronga M, Oliva F, Longo UG, Testa V, Capasso G, Maffulli N (2009) Isolated medial patellofemoral ligament reconstruction for recurrent patellar dislocation. Am J Sports Med 37:1735–42

Schottle PB, Fucentese SF, Romero J (2005) Clinical and radiological outcome of medial patellofemoral ligament reconstruction with a semitendinosus autograft for patella instability. Knee Surg Sports Traumatol Arthrosc 13:516–521

Senavongse W, Amis AA (2005) The effects of articular, retinacular, or muscular deficiencies on patellofemoral joint stability. J Bone Joint Surg (Br) 87:577–582

Sillanpaa P, Mattila VM, Iivonen T, Visuri T, Pihlajamaki H (2008) Incidence and risk factors of acute traumatic primary patellar dislocation. Med Sci Sports Exerc 40:606–611

Spritzer CE, Courneya DL, Burk DL Jr, Garrett WE, Strong JA (1997) Medial retinacular complex injury in acute patellar dislocation: MR findings and surgical implications. AJR Am J Roentgenol 168:117–122

Tsai CH, Hsu CJ, Hung CH, Hsu HC (2012) Primary traumatic patellar dislocation. J Orthop Surg Res 7:21, 6

Reconstruction of the Posterolateral Corner of the Knee

115

Colin J. Anderson, Nicholas I. Kennedy, and Robert F. LaPrade

Contents

C.J. Anderson
Department of Orthopedic Surgery, School of Medicine, University of Colorado, Aurora, CO, USA
e-mail: colin.anderson@ucdenver.edu

N.I. Kennedy
Steadman Philippon Research Institute, Vail, CO, USA
e-mail: nickkennedy2202@gmail.com

R.F. LaPrade (✉)
The Steadman Clinic and Steadman Philippon Research Institute, Vail, CO, USA
e-mail: drlaprade@sprivail.org; rlaprade@thesteadmanclinic.com

M.N. Doral, J. Karlsson (eds.), *Sports Injuries*,
DOI 10.1007/978-3-642-36569-0_116

Abstract

Injuries to the posterolateral corner of the knee present unique challenges to the orthopedic surgeon. In recent years, there has been an evolution in surgical techniques from nonanatomic sling procedures to anatomically based and biomechanically validated reconstructions. The purpose of this chapter is to review the clinically relevant anatomy and biomechanics of the posterolateral corner of the knee, to discuss the proper clinical evaluation to aid in diagnosis, and to describe anatomical reconstruction following these injuries.

Abbreviations

ACL Anterior cruciate ligament
FCL Fibular (lateral) collateral ligament
LGT Lateral gastrocnemius tendon
PFL Popliteofibular ligament
PCL Posterior cruciate ligament

Introduction

The evaluation and treatment of injuries to the posterolateral corner of the knee has evolved substantially over the past few decades. These injuries present unique challenges to the orthopedic surgeon because of their reported rare occurrence and their often-complicated nature. It is estimated that only a quarter of posterolateral corner injuries are isolated (Geeslin and LaPrade 2011). Unidentified posterolateral corner instability in the setting of cruciate ligament reconstructions provides a source for residual knee laxity and increases the risk of graft failure (LaPrade et al. 2002). The annual rate of posterolateral corner injury has been estimated to be 9.1 in 100,000 (Gianotti et al. 2009), although more recent studies suggest that the reported lower incidence in the past may have been due to a lack of recognition of this injury rather than a rarity of its occurrence (LaPrade et al. 2007). It has been estimated that the incidence of posterolateral corner injuries in patients with a hemarthrosis is 9.1 % (LaPrade et al. 2007). In recent years, improved biomechanical-based research has led to an evolution in surgical techniques from nonanatomic sling procedures to anatomically based and biomechanically validated reconstructions (LaPrade et al. 2004a). The purpose of this chapter is to review the clinically relevant anatomy and biomechanics of the posterolateral corner, to discuss the proper clinical evaluation to aid in diagnosis, and to describe anatomical reconstruction following these injuries.

Clinically Relevant Anatomy and Biomechanics

A thorough understanding of the anatomy of the posterolateral corner of the knee is not only necessary for surgical reconstruction but is also required for proper interpretation of physical examination and radiographic findings. The anatomy of the posterolateral corner of the knee has been described in intricate detail in recent years (LaPrade et al. 2003). Despite over 28 identified structures in the posterolateral knee (LaPrade and Terry 1997; LaPrade et al. 2003), biomechanical studies have demonstrated that the main stabilizers are the fibular (lateral) collateral ligament (FCL), the popliteus tendon, and the popliteofibular ligament (PFL) (LaPrade et al. 2003).

The structures of the posterolateral corner provide stability to the knee against varus angulation, tibial external rotation, and hyperextension, serving a more prominent role with the knee at flexion angles less than 45°. As a result of observations that patients with chronic posterolateral corner injuries often had failed anterior cruciate ligament (ACL) or posterior cruciate ligament (PCL) reconstructions, biomechanical studies were performed to evaluate the effect of posterolateral corner instability on cruciate ligament reconstruction grafts. Sectioning of the FCL, popliteus tendon, and PFL was found to significantly increase loads on ACL grafts at 0° and 30° of knee flexion under varus stresses (LaPrade et al. 1999). Furthermore, it has been reported that fixation of the ACL graft prior to the posterolateral corner structures in a combined reconstruction leads to a significant increase in external rotation of the tibia (Wentorf et al. 2002). Additionally, significant increases in the force on a PCL reconstruction graft with varus loads at all angles of knee flexion have also been reported with sectioning of the posterolateral structures (LaPrade et al. 2002). Thus, identification of concomitant posterolateral corner injuries is imperative with ACL or PCL reconstructions in order to avoid graft failure.

Fibular Collateral Ligament

The FCL (Fig. 1) is approximately 70 millimeters (mm) in length (LaPrade et al. 2003). The femoral attachment of the FCL is not located directly on the lateral epicondyle, as it is commonly depicted in anatomical textbooks. Rather, it is located in a sulcus 1.4 mm proximal and 3.1 mm posterior to the lateral epicondyle. The FCL courses distally to attach to the lateral aspect of the fibular head, 8.2 mm posterior to the anterior edge (LaPrade et al. 2003).

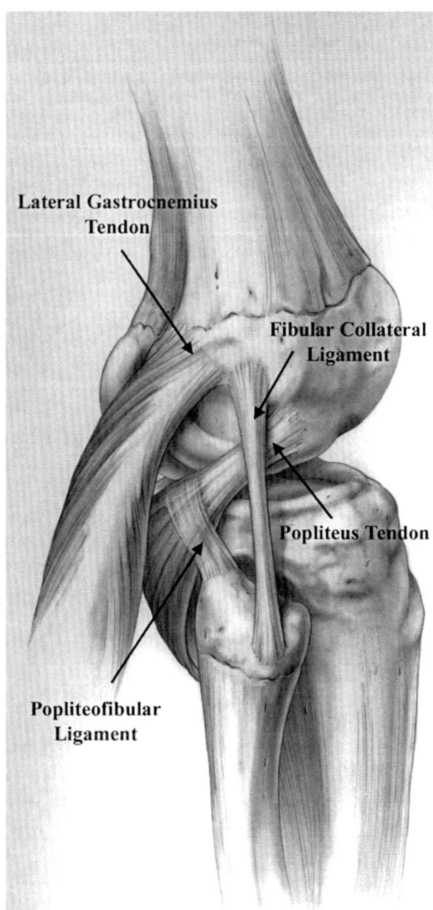

Fig. 1 Illustration of right knee demonstrating the anatomy of the fibular collateral ligament (*FCL*), popliteus tendon, and popliteofibular ligament (*PFL*) (Reprinted with permission from LaPrade et al. (2003))

Biomechanical studies of the posterolateral knee have reported that the FCL is the primary stabilizer to varus stresses (Gollehon et al. 1987; Grood et al., 1988; LaPrade et al. 2004b). While resisting varus angulation throughout the full range of motion of the knee, the FCL plays a more prominent role in extension. The PCL has been shown to provide a significant contribution to varus stability in the face of a combined grade III posterolateral knee injury (Grood et al. 1988; LaPrade et al. 2004b).

Popliteus Tendon

The popliteus tendon (Fig. 1), which arises from the popliteus muscle on the posterior aspect of the tibia, courses proximally around the posterolateral aspect of the knee joint, enters the joint capsule, and attaches to the anterior half of the proximal fifth of the popliteal sulcus intraarticularly (LaPrade et al. 2003). When measured from the musculotendinous junction, the average length of the popliteus tendon is 54.5 mm (LaPrade et al. 2003). The average distance between the femoral FCL and the popliteus tendon attachments has been reported to be 18.5 mm (Fig. 2; LaPrade et al. 2003). This distance is clinically important because it implies that reconstructions that use a single tunnel to combine the FCL and popliteus tendon attachments result in nonanatomic graft placement on the femur.

In addition to the FCL, the popliteus tendon also contributes to stability against external rotation. A reciprocal relationship has been demonstrated between the two structures, where the FCL resists a majority of external rotation loads with the knee in the extended position, while the popliteus tendon bears a larger portion of the load with the knee in the flexed position (Grood et al. 1988; LaPrade et al. 2004b). In conjunction with the posterior cruciate ligament, the popliteus tendon also

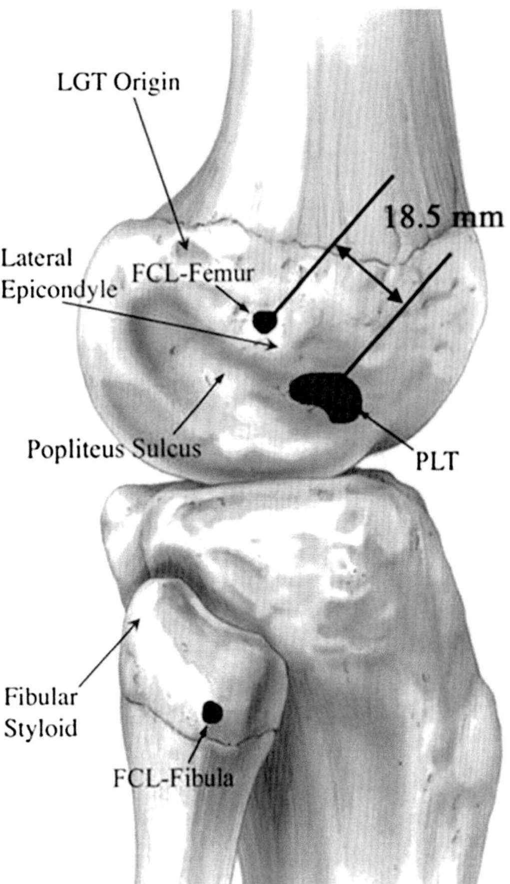

Fig. 2 Illustration of right knee demonstrating the average distance between the femoral attachment sites of the FCL and popliteus tendon. (*LGT* lateral gastrocnemius tendon) (Reprinted with permission from LaPrade et al. (2003))

contributes as a secondary stabilizer against posterior translation of the knee (Harner et al. 1998).

Popliteofibular Ligament

Termed the arcuate ligament in older literature, the PFL (Fig. 1) arises from the musculotendinous junction of the popliteus complex and courses disto-laterally to the fibular styloid. It has both an anterior and a posterior division, of which the posterior division is larger and stronger (LaPrade et al. 2003). The PFL has been reported to play an important secondary role in stabilization against varus and external rotation forces on the knee (Maynard et al. 1996; McCarthy et al. 2010).

Biceps Femoris

In addition to providing secondary and dynamic stabilization against varus forces to the knee, familiarity with the biceps femoris is important during surgical reconstruction of the posterolateral corner. The biceps femoris has two portions: the long and short heads. The long head of the biceps divides into a direct arm and an anterior arm approximately 1 centimeter (cm) proximal to its insertion on the fibular head (LaPrade et al. 2003). The direct arm attaches to the posterolateral aspect of the fibular head and provides a majority of the force transmission from the muscle body. The anterior arm passes superficial to the FCL to insert into a broad fascial aponeurosis on the anterolateral aspect of the proximal leg. As it passes the FCL, it forms an overlying bursa (biceps bursa) that serves as an important surgical landmark for identification of the distal portion of the FCL (LaPrade et al. 2003). Additionally, the common peroneal nerve can be easily identified with dissection just posterior to the posterior edge of the long head.

Iliotibial Band

The iliotibial band forms a broad fibrous layer on the lateral aspect of the thigh and knee as it travels from the tensor fascia lata muscle distally to attach to Gerdy's tubercle on the anterior aspect of the tibia. Because the iliotibial band has been reported to be injured in only 3 % of posterolateral knee injuries, it is an important surgical landmark for identification of both the FCL and popliteus tendon attachments on the femur (LaPrade and Terry 1997).

Clinical Evaluation

History

The clinical evaluation of the knee should begin with a thorough history including the mechanism, chronology, and nature of symptoms, presence of side-to-side instability, presence of catching or locking, previous knee injuries, and previous operations. When concern for a posterolateral corner injury exists, symptoms of paresthesias in the common peroneal nerve distribution or a foot drop should be assessed because common peroneal nerve injuries of some sort have been reported in up to one third of posterolateral corner injuries (LaPrade and Terry 1997). Standard assessment of pertinent past medical history, medications, allergies, tobacco use, and particularly goals of returning to sports activities should be included as well.

Physical Examination

While a complete knee physical examination needs to be performed, since 72 % of posterolateral knee injuries are associated with a concomitant ACL or PCL rupture (Geeslin and LaPrade 2011), physical examination maneuvers to assess for the posterolateral injuries include the external rotation recurvatum test, the varus stress test at both 0° and 30° of knee flexion, the dial test at both 30° and 90° of knee flexion, the posterolateral drawer test, and the reverse pivot shift test. Additionally, gait should be assessed to detect the presence of a varus thrust gait, particularly in patients with chronic posterolateral corner injuries. While originally reported to be pathognomonic for a posterolateral knee injury (Hughston and Norwood 1980), the external rotation recurvatum test was found to be positive in only 10 % of patients with an isolated posterolateral corner injury in a prospective study of 134 patients (LaPrade et al. 2008b). However, the test was found to be positive in all patients with a combined ACL and posterolateral corner injury (LaPrade et al. 2008b). Likewise, a positive dial test at both 30° and 90° of knee flexion indicates a probable combined PCL and posterolateral corner injury. Caution must be exercised, however, because chronic medial knee instability may result in a falsely positive dial test. In addition to the specific physical examination techniques used to examine for a posterolateral knee injury, it is important to recognize that these injuries most commonly occur in the presence of a concurrent cruciate ligament injury. In these circumstances, the posterolateral structures serve an important role to preventing additional increases in both anterior and posterior tibial translation. Thus, in the presence of excessive anterior laxity with an ACL tear or posterior laxity with a PCL tear, one must always be aware of the possibility of concurrent posterolateral knee injury.

Imaging

Imaging should include plain anterior-posterior and lateral radiographs to assess for the presence of bony Segond and arcuate avulsion fractures. Long leg alignment radiographs, especially important in patients with chronic posterolateral injuries, are recommended to assess for the presence of genu varus alignment and the need for corrective osteotomy. Varus stress radiographs serve as an important tool for the evaluation of posterolateral knee injuries. In all patients, bilateral varus stress radiographs should be obtained to objectively assess for the amount of lateral compartment gapping on the injured knee. It has been reported that increases of lateral compartment gapping of 2.7 mm are consistent with an FCL tear, while greater than 4.0 mm is consistent with a complete grade III posterolateral knee injury (LaPrade et al. 2008a). Additionally, high-resolution magnetic resonance imaging may be used in the identification of posterolateral knee injuries (LaPrade et al. 2000). The presence of an anteromedial bone bruise or a medial tibial plateau fracture has been reported to be concerning for a posterolateral knee injury (Geeslin and LaPrade 2011).

Treatment

While grade I and II posterolateral corner injuries can be treated nonoperatively in a hinged knee brace locked in extension for 3–6 weeks, surgical reconstruction is recommended for grade III injuries due to the significant risk for continued symptomatic instability (LaPrade and Terry 1997; LaPrade and Wentorf 2002). When concurrent

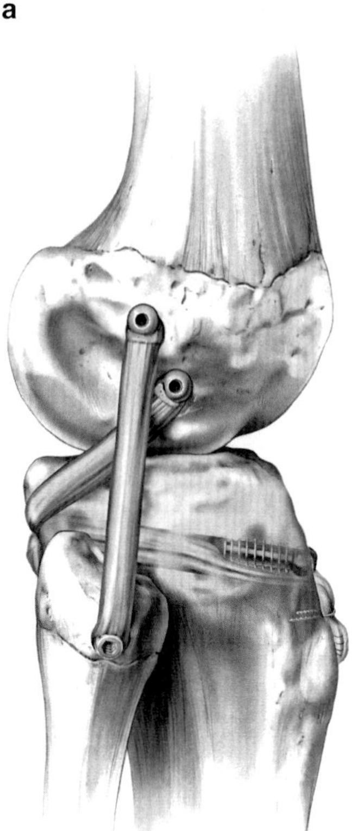

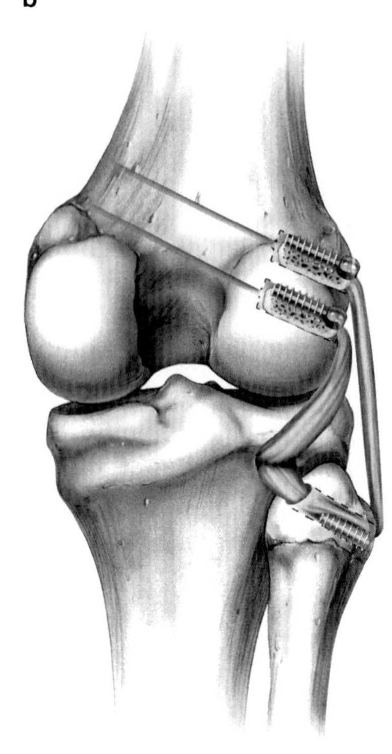

Fig. 3 Illustrations of lateral (**a**) and posterior (**b**) views of right knee anatomical posterolateral corner reconstruction (LaPrade et al. (2004a))

cruciate ligament rupture exists, combined repair is recommended to avoid the high risk of cruciate ligament graft failure with continuous posterolateral corner instability (LaPrade et al. 2002). While numerous reconstruction techniques for the posterolateral corner have been created, this section will focus on the author's preferred technique for anatomical posterolateral corner reconstruction (Fig. 3).

Surgical Approach

The patient is positioned supine on the operating table, and examination under anesthesia is performed to confirm suspected pathology. When concomitant intraarticular pathology exists, arthroscopy is delayed until after open dissection of the posterolateral corner to avoid anatomical distortion from fluid extravasation. The surgical approach begins with a hockey stick-shaped incision (Fig. 4) centered over the posterior aspect of the iliotibial band and coursed distally, slightly posterior to Gerdy's tubercle (Terry and LaPrade 1996). The dissection is carried down to the superficial layer of the iliotibial band and to the long and short heads of the biceps femoris. The common peroneal nerve is identified at the posterolateral edge of the long head of the biceps femoris, and neurolysis is performed. This starts approximately 6–8 cm proximal to the fibular head and extends distally to include release of the peroneus longus fascia distal to the fibular head. The nerve is retracted during the procedure to allow access to the interval between the lateral gastrocnemius tendon and the soleus muscle (LaPrade et al. 2004a).

Next, the distal aspect of the FCL is identified with a 2–3 cm horizontal incision through the biceps bursa, and a tag stitch is placed into the remnant ligament. Then, the anterior aspect of the long head of the biceps is dissected off the fibular head to isolate and identify the fibular collateral ligament attachment site on the lateral aspect of the fibular head. The proximal and distal

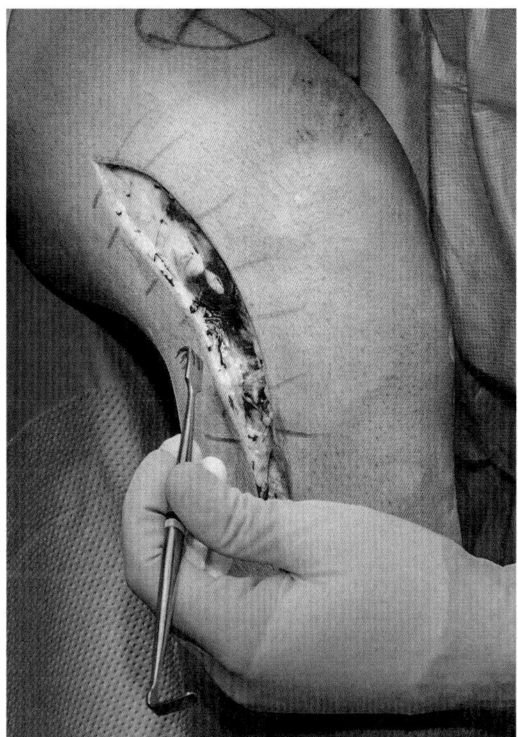

Fig. 4 Photo of lateral hockey stick incision used to approach posterolateral aspect of knee

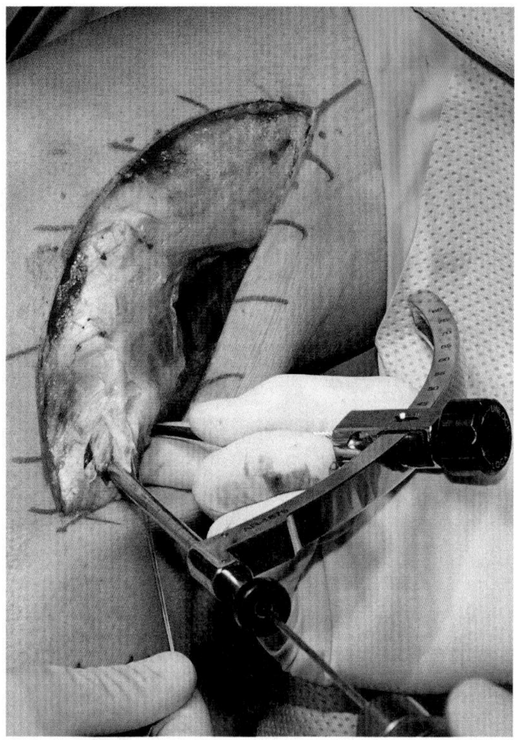

Fig. 5 Right knee photograph of guide pin placement for fibular tunnel starting at FCL attachment site on lateral fibula directed toward PFL attachment on posteromedial fibular styloid

attachments of the PFL – the musculotendinous junction of the popliteus muscle and the posteromedial aspect of the fibular styloid, respectively – are found with blunt dissection in the interval between the lateral gastrocnemius tendon and soleus muscle (LaPrade et al. 2004a).

The tibial and fibular bony reconstruction tunnels are reamed through the midpoints of the ligament attachment sites. A guide pin is drilled from the distal FCL attachment site on the lateral aspect of the fibular head toward the distal PFL attachment on the posteromedial aspect of the fibular styloid (Fig. 5). While protecting the tip of the guide pin with a large Chandler retractor, a 6 or 7 mm diameter acorn reamer is reamed over this guide pin to create the fibular head reconstruction tunnel. The tibial reconstruction tunnel is prepared by drilling a guide pin from anterior to posterior, starting at the flat spot just distal and medial to Gerdy's tubercle and through to the popliteal sulcus on the posterolateral tibia, which demarcates the musculotendinous junction of the popliteus (LaPrade et al. 2004a). Again, using a large Chandler for protection, the tunnel is reamed with a 9 mm acorn reamer over the guide pin (Fig. 6). A passing suture is placed through the tunnel from anterior to posterior to facilitate graft passage later in the case.

Next, attention is turned to the femoral attachments of the fibular collateral ligament and popliteus tendon. The traction stitch within the fibular collateral ligament remnant is used to help identify its femoral attachment. An iliotibial band splitting incision is then performed for approximately 8–10 cm in length (Fig. 7). The attachment site of the fibular collateral ligament, slightly proximal and posterior to the lateral epicondyle, is then identified (Fig. 2). A guide pin is then drilled through this attachment site (Fig. 8). It is important to aim this eyelet pin so that it exits the anteromedial thigh anterior and proximal to the adductor tubercle (LaPrade et al. 2004a).

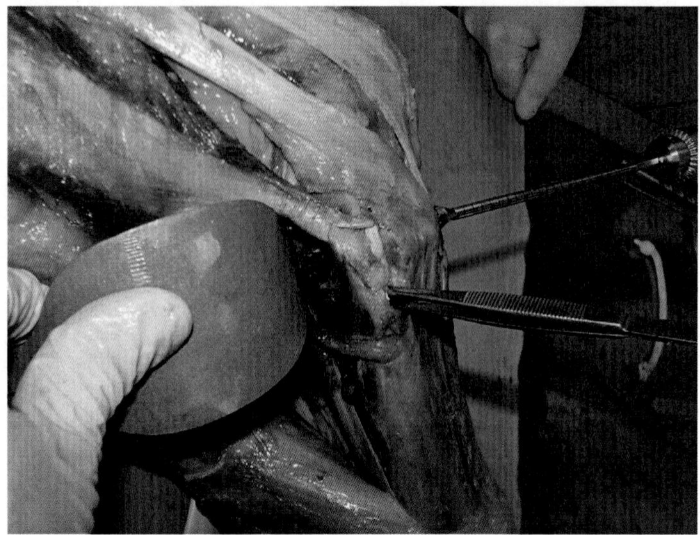

Fig. 6 Right knee photograph of anatomical specimen demonstrating reaming of tibial tunnel. Relationship of fibular tunnel (forceps) and tibial tunnel placement is shown posteriorly. A large Chandler retractor is protecting the common peroneal nerve

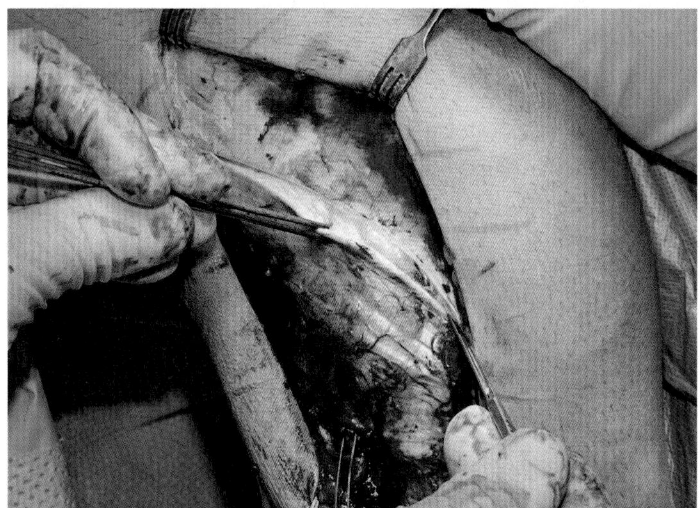

Fig. 7 Photo showing size and directionality of iliotibial band incision used to visualize the femoral attachments of posterolateral structures

This allows for placement of the tunnel such that it does not interfere or converge with any concurrent ACL graft reconstruction tunnels. Once the fibular collateral ligament pin is placed, the attachment site of the popliteus tendon is identified at the top fifth of the popliteal sulcus (Fig. 2). A small vertical incision is made through the joint capsule over the popliteal sulcus, which can usually be identified by palpation at this point in time. This popliteus guide pin should be drilled parallel to the FCL tunnel.

Once both pins are in place and prior to reaming, correct placement should be validated by measuring between the two attachment sites, for which the average distance is 18.5 mm (Fig. 2; LaPrade et al. 2003). After determined to be correctly placed, a 9 mm diameter acorn reamer is used to create closed socket tunnels to a depth of 20–25 mm. Individual passing sutures are then placed into the tunnels to facilitate graft passage later.

Reconstruction Graft Preparation

An Achilles tendon allograft is used with a minimum graft length of at least 23 cm to allow for

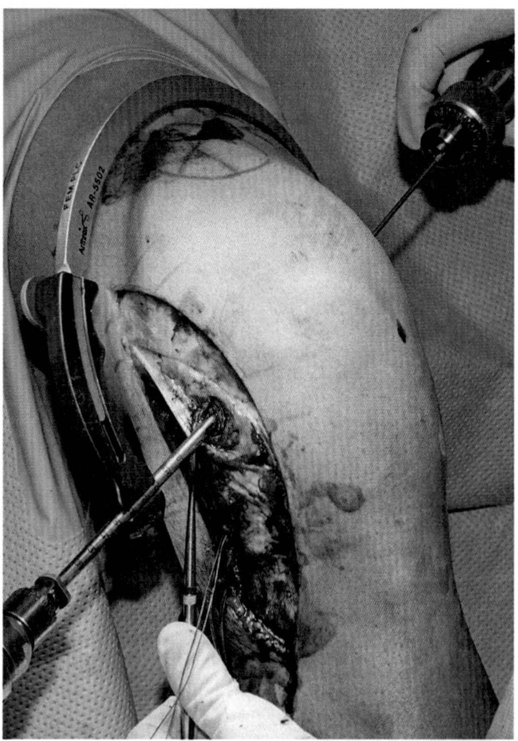

Fig. 8 Photo showing entrance and exit of guide pin for FCL femoral tunnel

adequate length of the reconstruction grafts. The calcaneal bone plug is split lengthwise to create two separate 9 mm diameter and 20 mm long bone plugs. The distal aspects of the grafts are then tubularized with nonabsorbable sutures so that they can fit through the reconstruction tunnels. It is important to ensure that the FCL/PFL graft is tubularized sufficiently enough so that it will fit through the fibular tunnel without bunching up.

Concurrent Intraarticular Procedures

At this point, any intra-articular arthroscopic work can be performed. Meniscal tears are repaired if possible. Cruciate ligament reconstruction tunnels are reamed and the cruciate reconstruction grafts are passed into their femoral tunnels and fixed with interference screws, but without fixation in the tibial tunnels.

Passing and Fixation of Reconstruction Grafts

The previously placed passing sutures are utilized to facilitate passage of the bone plugs into their femoral tunnels. The grafts are then secured in place with nonabsorbable interference screws. The grafts should be manually stressed laterally to ensure secure fixation. In addition, one should palpate over the screws to ensure that they are adequately positioned within the tunnel because proud screws can lead to iliotibial band irritation postoperatively.

The popliteus tendon graft is first passed down the popliteal hiatus along its anatomical path and then pulled out laterally between the lateral gastrocnemius tendon and soleus muscles, awaiting placement in the tibial tunnel until later in the procedure (LaPrade et al. 2004a). The fibular collateral ligament graft is then passed along its anatomical path deep to the superficial layer of the iliotibial band and the lateral aponeurosis of the long head of the biceps femoris. The graft is then placed into the previous reamed fibular head tunnel.

At this point in time, the fixation order of the reconstruction grafts is important to follow correctly. For a concurrent PCL reconstruction, the PCL graft should be fixed prior to fixation of the posterolateral reconstruction grafts. However, for a concurrent ACL reconstruction, fixation of the ACL graft should occur following fixation of the posterolateral grafts to avoid an external rotation deformity of the tibia (Wentorf et al. 2002).

For fixation of the posterolateral grafts, first traction is applied to the FCL graft, the knee is flexed to 20° with a slight valgus reduction force, the foot is held in neutral rotation, and the graft is secured with a bioabsorbable screw. Once this graft has been secured, an exam under anesthesia should verify that all varus instability has been eliminated prior to moving on to further graft fixation. Then, both the popliteus tendon graft and the remainder of the FCL graft are passed anteriorly through the tibial tunnel, thus recreating the PFL with the remainder of the FCL graft (Fig. 3). Tension is applied to each graft, the knee is held at 60° of flexion, the foot is held in neutral rotation, and the grafts are fixed with a

9 mm bioabsorbable screw into the anterior aspect of the tibial tunnel. Subsequently, it is important to validate that posterolateral drawer instability has been completely eliminated. Backup fixation of the grafts in the tibia with a staple may be utilized for patients with osteopenic bone.

A standard layered closure with a subcuticular stitch for the skin is performed with loosely applied Steri-Strips to assist with skin approximation. Then, a standard long leg knee immobilizer is placed, and the patient may be transferred to the recovery room.

Postoperative Rehabilitation

Postoperative rehabilitation is a crucial component in the treatment of posterolateral corner injuries (Lunden et al. 2010). A key principle in the rehabilitation of anatomical posterolateral corner reconstruction is that the reconstruction should not have any significant stress placed on it. For isolated posterolateral corner reconstructions, patients are kept non-weight-bearing in a knee immobilizer for the first 6 weeks. Physical therapy is initiated on postoperative day one with focus on quadriceps strengthening, edema control, and range of motion exercises, with the goal of a minimum of 0–90° of knee flexion within the first few days postoperatively. Patients are instructed to avoid isolated hamstring exercises for the first 4 months postoperatively as well as tibial external rotation to avoid placing extra stress on the reconstruction grafts (Lunden et al. 2010).

Further progression of the rehabilitation program involves initiation of weight-bearing at 6 weeks postoperatively, slowly weaning off crutches once the patient can ambulate without a limp, and the use of a stationary bike with no resistance. Leg presses may also be initiated at this point in time at one-quarter body weight with a maximum of 70° of knee flexion. Side-to-side and Bosu-ball or other types of balance exercises are avoided until 4–5 months postoperatively when varus stress radiographs have verified that there is sufficient healing of the posterolateral corner reconstruction grafts to initiate this program. Patients will then progress to agility and running exercises and will be allowed back to competition upon demonstration of sufficient agility, endurance, and strength at approximately 7–9 months postoperatively.

In the setting of concurrent PCL reconstruction, a more specific PCL protocol is utilized. Prone knee flexion exercises are initiated on postoperative day one. Progression to higher-level activities is delayed until between 9 and 12 months postoperatively, pending sufficient healing of the PCL reconstruction and demonstration of sufficient stability on PCL and varus stress radiographs at 6 months postoperatively.

Considerations for Acute Versus Chronic Injuries

There are important distinctions between the treatments for acute versus chronic posterolateral corner injuries. Outcomes for the treatment of chronic posterolateral knee injuries are inferior to those treated acutely. Thus, diagnosis and treatment of these pathologies early after the injury are optimal. In the setting of acute posterolateral corner injury, often defined as surgery within 3–6 weeks, treatment may be limited to specifically address the injured structures, as opposed to the entire anatomical reconstruction as described above. Furthermore, structures may be amenable to repair rather than reconstruction when there is soft tissue or bony avulsion, and the tissue quality remains adequate. Significant tissue retraction, midsubstance tears, or poor tissue quality are indications for reconstruction. For isolated FCL or popliteus tendon ruptures not amenable to repair, individual anatomical reconstructions have been described using an autogenous hamstring graft (Coobs et al. 2007; LaPrade et al. 2010). However, when both tendons are ruptured, a complete anatomical posterolateral corner reconstruction is recommended. Avulsions of the PFL may be treated with direct repair if the popliteus tendon remains intact and the soft tissues are not excessively damaged.

In patients with chronic posterolateral corner injuries, it is well recognized that genu varus malalignment substantially increases the risk for reconstruction failure if the alignment is not corrected preoperatively or concurrently (Arthur et al. 2007). Thus, in the evaluation of all patients with chronic posterolateral corner injuries, long leg standing films are necessary to evaluate alignment. If present, genu varus malalignment should be corrected with a proximal tibial opening wedge osteotomy. Interestingly, it has been reported that some patients experience resolution of their posterolateral instability following the corrective osteotomy, negating the need for second-stage or concomitant posterolateral corner reconstruction (Arthur et al. 2007).

Conclusions

Injuries to the posterolateral corner of the knee present unique challenges to the orthopedic surgeon. In recent years, improved biomechanical-based research has led to an evolution in surgical techniques from nonanatomic sling procedures to anatomically based and biomechanically validated reconstructions. Biomechanical studies demonstrate that the most important posterolateral stabilizing structures are the fibular (lateral) collateral ligament, the popliteus tendon, and the popliteofibular ligament. Physical examination to assess for the posterolateral corner injury should include the external rotation recurvatum test, varus stress at both 0° and 30°, the dial test at both 30° and 90°, the posterolateral drawer test, and the reverse pivot shift test. Posterolateral corner reconstructions in the acute setting may repair or reconstruct injured structures individually. However, in the setting of severe acute or chronic injuries, anatomical posterolateral corner reconstruction should be performed. In chronic injuries, it is imperative to assess for the presence of genu varus malalignment preoperatively due to the increased risk of reconstruction failure.

Cross-References

- ▶ Anatomy and Biomechanics of the Knee
- ▶ Combined Anterior and Posterior Cruciate Ligament Injuries
- ▶ Current Concepts in the Treatment of Posterior Cruciate Ligament Injuries
- ▶ Rehabilitation of Complex Knee Injuries and Key Points
- ▶ Role of Osteotomy for Knee Cartilage, Meniscus, and Ligament Injuries

References

Arthur A, LaPrade RF, Agel J (2007) Proximal tibial opening wedge osteotomy as the initial treatment for chronic posterolateral corner deficiency in the varus knee: a prospective clinical study. Am J Sports Med 35:1844–1850

Coobs BR, LaPrade RF, Griffith CJ, Nelson BJ (2007) Biomechanical analysis of an isolated fibular (lateral) collateral ligament reconstruction using an autogenous semitendinosus graft. Am J Sports Med 35:1521–1527

Geeslin AG, LaPrade RF (2011) Outcomes of treatment of acute grade-III isolated and combined posterolateral knee injuries: a prospective case series and surgical technique. J Bone Joint Surg Am 93:1672–1683

Gianotti SM, Marshall SW, Hume PA, Bunt L (2009) Incidence of anterior cruciate ligament injury and other knee ligament injuries: a national population-based study. J Sci Med Sport 12:622–627

Gollehon DL, Torzilli PA, Warren RF (1987) The role of the posterolateral and cruciate ligaments in the stability of the human knee. A biomechanical study. J Bone Joint Surg Am 69:233–242

Grood ES, Stowers SF, Noyes FR (1988) Limits of movement in the human knee. Effect of sectioning the posterior cruciate ligament and posterolateral structures. J Bone Joint Surg Am 70:88–97

Harner CD, Hoher J, Vogrin TM, Carlin GJ, Woo SL (1998) The effects of a popliteus muscle load on in situ forces in the posterior cruciate ligament and on knee kinematics. A human cadaveric study. Am J Sports Med 26:669–673

Hughston JC, Norwood LA Jr (1980) The posterolateral drawer test and external rotational recurvatum test for posterolateral rotatory instability of the knee. Clin Orthop Relat Res 147:82–87

LaPrade RF, Terry GC (1997) Injuries to the posterolateral aspect of the knee. Association of anatomic injury patterns with clinical instability. Am J Sports Med 25:433–438

LaPrade RF, Wentorf F (2002) Diagnosis and treatment of posterolateral knee injuries. Clin Orthop Relat Res 402:110–121

LaPrade RF, Resig S, Wentorf F, Lewis JL (1999) The effects of grade III posterolateral knee complex injuries on anterior cruciate ligament graft force. A biomechanical analysis. Am J Sports Med 27:469–475

LaPrade RF, Gilbert TJ, Bollom TS, Wentorf F, Chaljub G (2000) The magnetic resonance imaging appearance of individual structures of the posterolateral knee. A prospective study of normal knees and knees with surgically verified grade III injuries. Am J Sports Med 28:191–199

LaPrade RF, Muench C, Wentorf F, Lewis JL (2002) The effect of injury to the posterolateral structures of the knee on force in a posterior cruciate ligament graft: a biomechanical study. Am J Sports Med 30:233–238

LaPrade RF, Ly TV, Wentorf FA, Engebretsen L (2003) The posterolateral attachments of the knee: a qualitative and quantitative morphologic analysis of the fibular collateral ligament, popliteus tendon, popliteofibular ligament, and lateral gastrocnemius tendon. Am J Sports Med 31:854–860

LaPrade RF, Johansen S, Wentorf FA, Engebretsen L, Esterberg JL, Tso A (2004a) An analysis of an anatomical posterolateral knee reconstruction: an in vitro biomechanical study and development of a surgical technique. Am J Sports Med 32:1405–1414

LaPrade RF, Tso A, Wentorf FA (2004b) Force measurements on the fibular collateral ligament, popliteofibular ligament, and popliteus tendon to applied loads. Am J Sports Med 32:1695–1701

LaPrade RF, Wentorf FA, Fritts H, Gundry C, Hightower CD (2007) A prospective magnetic resonance imaging study of the incidence of posterolateral and multiple ligament injuries in acute knee injuries presenting with a hemarthrosis. Arthroscopy 23:1341–1347

LaPrade RF, Heikes C, Bakker AJ, Jakobsen RB (2008a) The reproducibility and repeatability of varus stress radiographs in the assessment of isolated fibular collateral ligament and grade-III posterolateral knee injuries. An in vitro biomechanical study. J Bone Joint Surg Am 90:2069–2076

LaPrade RF, Ly TV, Griffith C (2008b) The external rotation recurvatum test revisited: reevaluation of the sagittal plane tibiofemoral relationship. Am J Sports Med 36:709–712

LaPrade RF, Wozniczka JK, Stellmaker MP, Wijdicks CA (2010) Analysis of the static function of the popliteus tendon and evaluation of an anatomic reconstruction: the "fifth ligament" of the knee. Am J Sports Med 38:543–549

Lunden JB, Bzdusek PJ, Monson JK, Malcomson KW, Laprade RF (2010) Current concepts in the recognition and treatment of posterolateral corner injuries of the knee. J Orthop Sports Phys Ther 40:502–516

Maynard MJ, Deng X, Wickiewicz TL, Warren RF (1996) The popliteofibular ligament. Rediscovery of a key element in posterolateral stability. Am J Sports Med 24:311–316

McCarthy M, Camarda L, Wijdicks CA, Johansen S, Engebretsen L, Laprade RF (2010) Anatomic posterolateral knee reconstructions require a popliteofibular ligament reconstruction through a tibial tunnel. Am J Sports Med 38:1674–1681

Terry GC, LaPrade RF (1996) The posterolateral aspect of the knee. Anatomy and surgical approach. Am J Sports Med 24:732–739

Wentorf FA, LaPrade RF, Lewis JL, Resig S (2002) The influence of the integrity of posterolateral structures on tibiofemoral orientation when an anterior cruciate ligament graft is tensioned. Am J Sports Med 30:796–799

Reconstruction of the Posteromedial Corner of the Knee

116

Matthew T. Rasmussen, Christopher M. LaPrade, and Robert F. LaPrade

Contents

M.T. Rasmussen • C.M. LaPrade
Department of BioMedical Engineering, Steadman Philippon Research Institute, Vail, CO, USA
e-mail: mrasmus@purdue.edu; rasmussenmatt31@gmail.com; lapr0005@umn.edu

R.F. LaPrade (✉)
The Steadman Clinic and Steadman Philippon Research Institute, Vail, CO, USA
e-mail: drlaprade@sprivail.org; rlaprade@thesteadmanclinic.com

M.N. Doral, J. Karlsson (eds.), *Sports Injuries*,
DOI 10.1007/978-3-642-36569-0_117

Abstract

Within the past decade, an innovative surgical technique designed to restore the native characteristics of injured structures of the posteromedial corner (PMC) of the knee has emerged. This technique is anatomically based and has been validated through biomechanical testing. In this approach, two separate grafts are used to reconstruct the superficial medial collateral ligament (sMCL) and posterior oblique ligament (POL). Surgical complications are often avoided by ensuring that the reconstruction tunnels are placed accurately by the utilization of anatomic landmarks. It is recommended that an early range of motion program be used for the postoperative rehabilitation protocol to enable early restoration of knee flexion and decrease the incidence of arthrofibrosis. This chapter focuses on the surgical treatment recommended for complex acute and chronic injuries to the posteromedial corner of the knee.

Introduction

Even though the superficial medial collateral ligament (sMCL) has been the most commonly reported ligament injury, the majority of these injuries are isolated and can be treated nonsurgically (Bollen 2000; Pedowitz et al. 2003). While most studies have reported good results from nonsurgical treatment, there are certain subsets that progress to chronic sMCL instability

(Sandberg et al. 1987; Edson 2006). These include those associated with knee dislocations, meniscotibial-based avulsions where the distal attachment of the sMCL is pulled proximal to the pes tendons, and valgus gapping in full extension. It is reported in the literature that in these circumstances initial nonsurgical treatment – while it may be recommended by many centers – often results in continued instability and an ensuing surgical reconstruction (Lind et al. 2009).

Recently, an innovative surgical treatment of chronic posteromedial knee injuries has been proposed. This approach is based upon the principles of defining the anatomy both qualitatively and quantitatively, revisiting clinically based biomechanical studies and then performing biomechanical validation of anatomic-based reconstructions. From this, clinical outcome studies on patients were performed to evaluate the procedure. Thus, these surgical reconstruction recommendations for the posteromedial knee are based upon several peer-reviewed studies (LaPrade et al. 2007; Griffith et al. 2009a, b; Coobs et al. 2010), which have been built upon each other and evolved into the recommended surgical treatment technique (LaPrade and Wijdicks 2012a).

In addition, because the highest postoperative complication rate after medial knee injury treatment has been reported to be arthrofibrosis, an anatomic-based reconstruction method that can withstand the rigors of early mobilization has been developed (Lind et al. 2009; LaPrade and Wijdicks 2012a, b). The goal of this reconstruction is to start range of motion exercises on postoperative day 1 in order to minimize the risk of arthrofibrosis. Peer-reviewed publications have validated that these anatomic reconstructions do not stretch out and also have a very low risk of arthrofibrosis (LaPrade and Wijdicks 2012a).

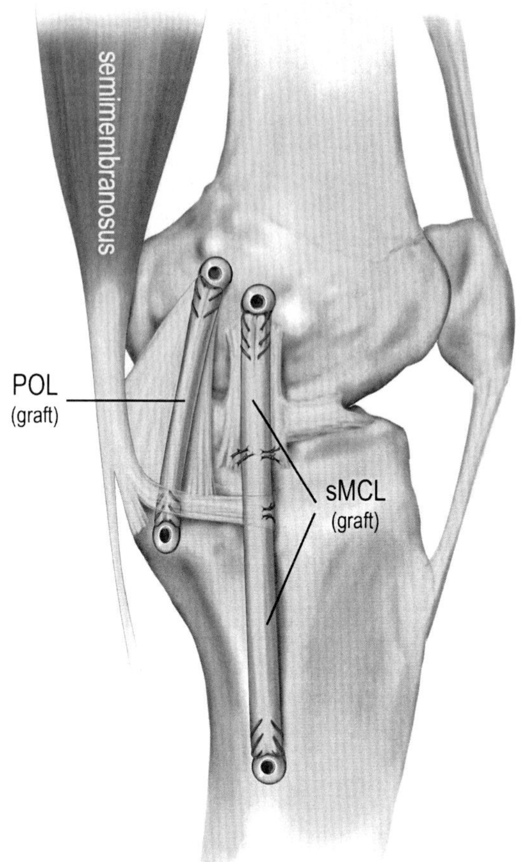

Fig. 1 A left medial knee reconstruction procedure demonstrating the reconstructed sMCL and POL. Note that the proximal tibial attachment point of the sMCL, which was primarily to soft tissues and located just distal to the joint line, was recreated by suturing the sMCL graft to the anterior arm of the semimembranosus (Reprinted with permission from Coobs BR, Wijdicks CA, Armitage BM, et al (2010) An in vitro analysis of an anatomic medial knee reconstruction. Am J Sports Med 38:339–347)

Anatomic Reconstruction for the Posteromedial Corner of the Knee

The preferred technique for the treatment of complete medial knee injuries is a biomechanically validated anatomic reconstruction of both the sMCL and the POL. In this technique, the two aforementioned ligaments are reconstructed by restoring their native attachment sites with two separate grafts (Fig. 1; Coobs et al. 2010).

Surgical Technique

All patients undergo an examination under anesthesia to confirm that they have both an increase in valgus gapping and external rotation in the affected knee. The increase in external rotation is validated both on the anteromedial drawer test at 90° of knee flexion and the dial test at 30° and 90° of knee flexion. The technique has evolved to the point where all operative knees are placed into a leg holder and the contralateral legs into a stirrup to prevent potential pressure areas. A leg holder is often used because a large percentage of the time either an arthroscopy or a concurrent cruciate ligament reconstruction is being performed on the affected knee.

It is recommended that the surgical approach be performed prior to the arthroscopy to prevent fluid extravasation, which makes it very difficult to visualize the medial and posteromedial knee structures. The authors have found it particularly more difficult to identify the femoral-based medial knee structures compared with the anatomic landmarks associated with other knee ligament injuries.

An anteromedial skin incision is made from the distal aspect of the vastus medialis oblique muscle, centered between the medial border of the patella and the adductor tubercle, and coursing over the midportion of the tibia. This incision should extend approximately 7–8 cm distal to the joint line. As part of the surgical approach, one should typically start distally after the initial skin incision, identify the pes anserine tendons, and then dissect along the sartorius fascia proximally. The first important anatomic attachment site to identify is the distal aspect of the sMCL. If one elects to harvest the semitendinosus tendon as the reconstruction graft, an open hamstring harvester is used to harvest this tendon at this point in time. Technically, it is very important to release all of the adhesions on this portion of the knee, which are often much more present in this situation than when the graft may be harvested for an ACL reconstruction, to ensure that the graft is not amputated and that at least 28–30 cm of overall graft length is obtained for the reconstruction. Once the pes anserine bursa is identified, the remnant of the distal attachment of the sMCL is identified. Based upon anatomic studies, the midportion of this attachment site is almost always 6 cm distal to the medial joint line (LaPrade et al. 2007). Thus, one can identify the medial joint line and use a surgical marker to outline this position. A reconstruction tunnel is then reamed for this portion of the reconstruction.

The distal tibial sMCL tunnel attachment location is important to locate as far posterior along the medial aspect of the proximal tibia as possible. An anteriorly placed tunnel can result in the graft stretching out with early knee motion. One should utilize an islet pin and a cruciate ligament aiming device to drill across the proximal tibia while aiming anterior to avoid the common peroneal nerve and enter exactly 6 cm distal to the medial joint line on the tibia. A 7-mm closed socket tunnel is then reamed directly over the islet pin. The more distal aspect of this tunnel should be notched to facilitate interference screw fixation later in the procedure. A passing stitch can then be placed using the islet pin at this point in time to allow for easier graft passing later in the case.

Next, one can dissect more proximal to identify the POL attachment site on the posteromedial aspect of the tibia. The sartorius fascia must be further incised to identify the anterior arm of the semimembranosus. The most important portion of the POL for knee stability is the central arm. The central arm attaches to the tibia and along the anterior arm of the semimembranosus (LaPrade et al. 2007). Identification of this structure, which is rarely injured, allows one to place the tibial tunnel for the POL reconstruction graft.

The tibial tunnel for the POL graft is slightly more distal and along the groove that the anterior arm of the semimembranosus forms (LaPrade et al. 2007). A guide pin is inserted here, using a cruciate ligament aiming device, and it exits the anterolateral aspect of the tibia slightly distal to Gerdy's tubercle. A 7-mm reamer is then used to drill a closed socket tunnel over the guide pin at this location. An additional passing stitch can also be placed at this point in time to allow for easier graft passage later in the case.

A more proximal dissection can now be carried out to identify the sMCL and POL femoral attachment sites. These attachment sites are much more difficult to identify, especially in chronic cases where there may be heterotopic ossification present and thickened medial knee tissue, which make it difficult to palpate the actual bony landmarks. In order to best identify these structures, it is important to identify the vastus medialis oblique attachment on the adductor magnus tendon. A curved hemostat is placed under the adductor magnus tendon, which allows a direct identification of the adductor tubercle. Once the adductor tubercle is identified, it is easier to identify the medial epicondyle and the gastrocnemius tubercle. It is especially important to identify these bony landmarks so that a precise anatomic restoration can be performed for the attachment sites of the POL and sMCL in the femur. It is well recognized that even a slight misplacement of 5 mm of these attachment sites can cause the graft to stretch out or have the knee become arthrofibrotic postoperatively.

Once the adductor tubercle has been located, the medial epicondyle can be identified. The sMCL femoral attachment site is 3.2 mm proximal and 4.8 mm posterior to the medial epicondyle in a bony depression in this area (LaPrade et al. 2007). A cruciate ligament aiming device is used to drill an islet pin across the anterolateral aspect of the distal thigh at this point in time. Next, the attachment site of the POL on the femur should be located, and this is done by identifying the gastrocnemius tubercle. The attachment site of the POL should be approximately 1.4 mm distal and 2.9 mm anterior to the gastrocnemius tubercle (LaPrade et al. 2007). An islet pin can then be placed using an aiming device, which is positioned parallel to the sMCL attachment site. Once the two guide pins are in place, one can measure between the two landmarks to verify that the normal relationship of 12.9 mm is maintained (LaPrade et al. 2007). If it appears that the relationship is off, one should further validate that the proper locations of the attachment sites have been identified by verifying that the medial epicondyle, adductor tubercle, and gastrocnemius tubercle have been correctly identified. Once it has been determined that these guide pins are in the desired locations, a 7-mm reamer is used to ream 25-mm deep closed sockets over both islet pins. Passing sutures are then pulled across the femur with the loops on the medial side to allow for graft passage later in the case.

It is preferable to identify these medial knee attachment sites, ream the tunnels, and place passing stitches prior to any intra-articular work. This allows one to identify them under the best circumstances, without fluid extravasation, and the passing stitches are used to easily pass the grafts later in the case, especially if the tourniquet has to be let down.

The arthroscopy can now be performed. The medial portals can often be placed through the skin incision that has been made as part of the posteromedial knee reconstruction approach. Any cruciate ligament reconstructions can be performed along with meniscal repairs, at this point in time. If the cruciate ligaments do need to be reconstructed, one can pass the grafts into the femur, fix them in place in the femur, and hold off fixing the tibial attachment sites until the medial knee reconstruction grafts have been placed into their respective femoral tunnels and secured.

The medial knee reconstruction grafts can be prepared from an autogenous semitendinosus graft or an allograft. Anatomic studies have verified that the length of the sMCL graft is almost always 16 cm, whereas the POL graft is almost always 12 cm (Coobs et al. 2010). Thus, an assistant can prepare the grafts ahead of time and be fairly certain that these grafts will be of the correct length at the time of surgical reconstruction (Fig. 2). This helps to ensure that the case can proceed in a timely fashion with minimal need to go over a 2-h tourniquet time.

Each graft is marked with a methylene blue marking pen 25 mm from each end to allow for more precise graft placement within the tunnels, especially as the case proceeds, and it is difficult to visualize the structures due to the use of arthroscopic fluid and potential bleeding after the tourniquet has been let down.

Next, both the sMCL and POL grafts can be passed into the femur. A bioabsorbable interference screw is placed anterior to the graft at both femoral locations. It is important to make sure that the screw is recessed down to the cortical level so it is not prominent since this can otherwise cause postoperative pain in these areas. A 7-mm cannulated bioabsorbable screw is used to fix each graft to the femur. After each graft is secured, it is

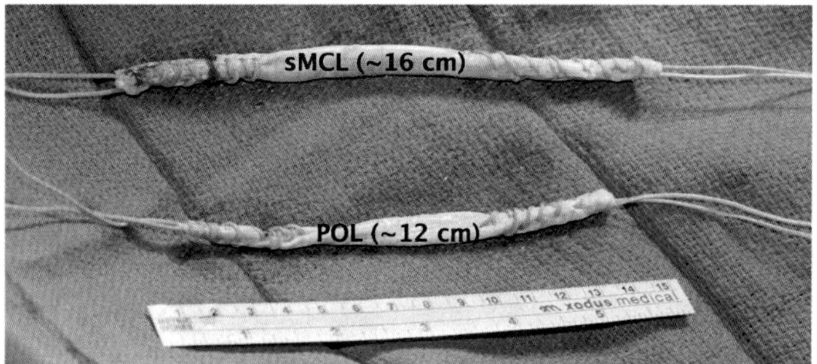

Fig. 2 The 16-cm superficial medial collateral ligament (*top*) and 12-cm posterior oblique ligament (*bottom*) grafts can be prepared preemptively

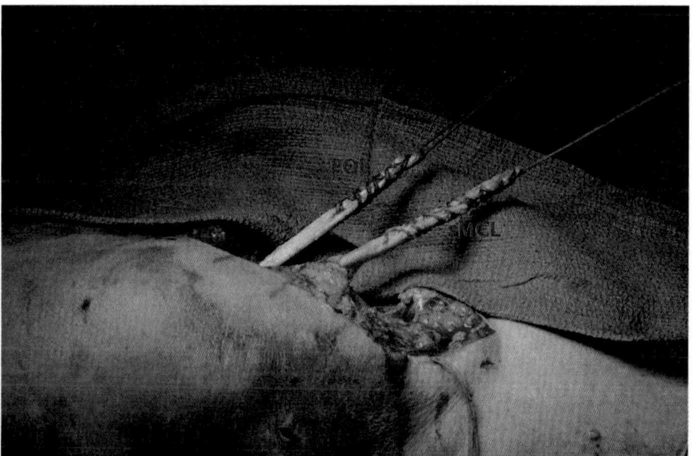

Fig. 3 Traction is applied to each graft to ensure secure fixation within each reconstruction tunnel

important to apply medial traction on the grafts to ensure that the grafts are well secured within each reconstruction tunnel (Fig. 3).

The sMCL graft is passed under the sartorius fascia and distally to the tibial reconstruction tunnel. The passing stitch can then be used to pull the graft into its respective tunnel (Fig. 4). Likewise, the POL graft is passed through the substance of the posteromedial capsule and into its reconstruction tunnel. At this point in time, the cruciate ligament grafts can be secured in their respective tibial tunnels. For posterior cruciate ligament reconstructions, the anterolateral bundle graft is fixed at 90° of knee flexion, whereas the posteromedial bundle graft is fixed in full extension (Girgis et al. 1975; Van Dommelen and Fowler 1989; Spiridonov et al. 2011). The ACL reconstruction graft is also fixed close to full extension.

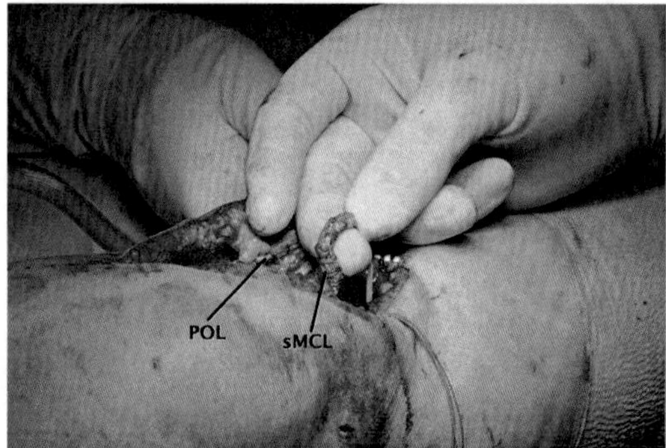

Fig. 4 A passing stitch is used to guide the superficial medial collateral ligament graft into its respective tibial tunnel

Once the cruciate ligament reconstruction grafts have been fixed, one should proceed with the stabilization and securing of the medial knee grafts into their respective tibial tunnels. The sMCL graft is fixed first with the knee in slight varus, to prevent any medial gapping, in neutral rotation and at 20° of knee flexion. Because the tibial bone can be quite hard at this location, sometimes a notching may be necessary of the reconstruction tunnel, or other means to increase the tunnel size, to allow for the bioabsorbable screw to be placed without damaging the sMCL graft (Fig. 5). Once this graft is placed using a screw inserted distally within the tunnel to secure the sMCL graft, one should verify that all of the valgus instability has been eliminated, that the graft is taut, and that one can flex from at least 0° to 105° of knee flexion on the table without having any significant tension on the reconstruction graft. Once this graft has been secured, the POL graft can be fixed (Fig. 6). It is important to recognize that the POL is tightest in full extension and it becomes loose with flexion (Griffith et al. 2009b). Thus, the graft must be secured in full extension, to avoid overconstraining the graft and risk having it stretch out or completely fail as when striving to achieve full knee extension. Taken together, the POL graft is fixed with the knee in full extension, in neutral rotation, and with traction on the graft.

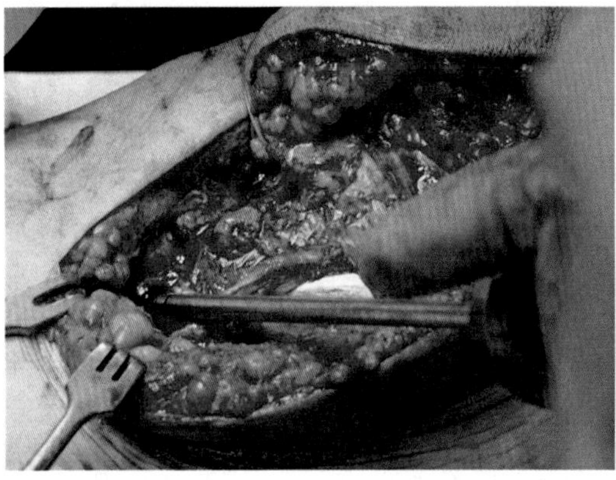

Fig. 5 The graft for the superficial medial collateral ligament is fixed at the distal tibial attachment site with the knee (*right* knee shown) at 20° of flexion, slight varus alignment, and in neutral rotation

In addition, the proximal tibial attachment of the sMCL must be secured at this point in time (Fig. 7). Wijdicks et al. validated that this attachment site strength is equivalent to a suture anchor, so it is advisable to use a suture anchor at this proximal tibial attachment site to reattach the sMCL graft to the tibia in order to encourage tissue integration and the return to full ligament functionality during load bearing (Wijdicks et al. 2010a). The attachment site is approximately 12–13 mm distal to the joint line and directly over the termination of the anterior arm of the semimembranosus and the tibia (LaPrade et al. 2007). When structures are completely blown apart, it is very rare that this portion of the medial knee is injured, and one can identify it to ensure that the correct attachment relationship can be restored.

A thorough exam under anesthesia should now be performed to verify that all associated instability has been eliminated. Internal rotation should be checked near full extension, valgus instability at 0° and 20°, and anteromedial rotation at 90° of flexion. It is important to verify that one can flex

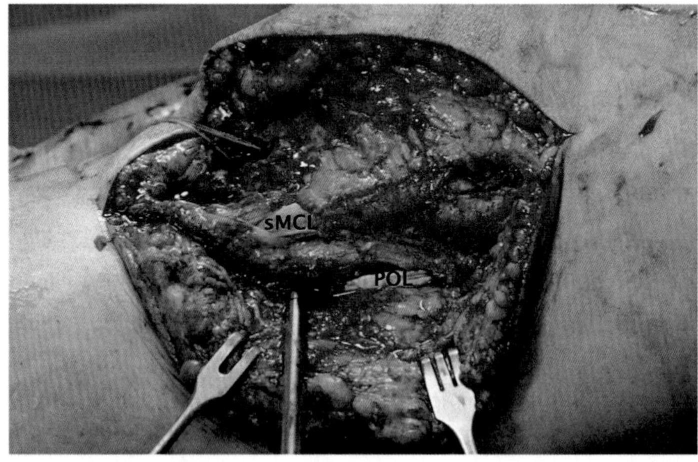

Fig. 6 The graft for the posterior oblique ligament is fixed at the tibial attachment site of the knee (*right* knee shown) at full extension, in neutral rotation, and with traction applied to the graft

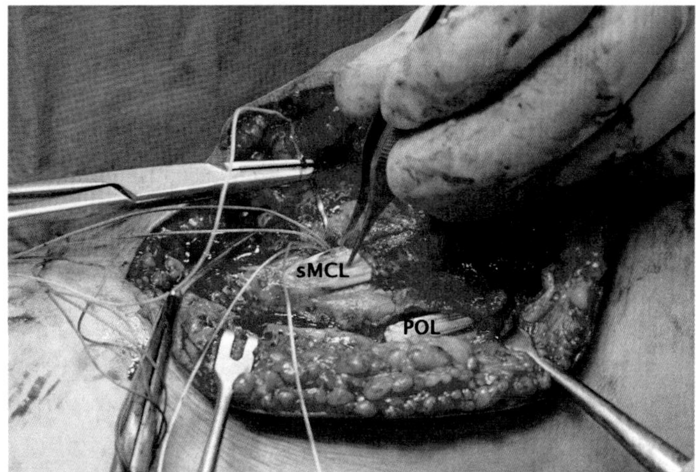

Fig. 7 The graft for the superficial medial collateral ligament is secured at the proximal tibial attachment site with suture anchors

the knee from at least 0 to 90° such that an early motion program can be initiated in physical therapy on the first postoperative day.

After the examination under anesthesia verifies restoration of valgus and rotatory stability, the closure is performed. Initially, the patient is placed into an immobilizer in full extension until his or her quadriceps control is sufficient.

Potential Surgical Complications

Intraoperative complications may arise from improper placement of the reconstruction tunnels. Therefore, a thorough knowledge of medial knee anatomy is required, especially in patients who have been recognized to have risk of heterotopic ossification or very thick medial knee structures. Placement of the sMCL femoral tunnel can easily be malpositioned. It is not uncommon for the authors to see reconstruction tunnels which are more than 1 cm from the anatomic attachment site in referral. In these circumstances, whereby identification of the normal and injured anatomy may be difficult, peer-reviewed publications that identify the attachment sites of these structures on radiographs should be reviewed and the use of intraoperative fluoroscopy would be advised (LaPrade et al. 2010). Intraoperative tunnel convergence is also potentially possible. Convergence can be avoided with the use of passing sutures to identify where these tunnels are located, and this is particularly helpful when one performs a PCL reconstruction. A concurrent double-bundle PCL reconstruction with a complete medial knee reconstruction needs to be carefully planned. One should not place the medial knee grafts directly transversely across the femur in the coronal plane, but should instead aim anterolateral to avoid the PCL reconstruction tunnels. When this is done, the risk of tunnel convergence is much lower. The final main intraoperative-based complication is a potential injury to the saphenous nerve. The sartorial branch of the saphenous nerve is located 4.8–5 cm perpendicularly from the anterior border of the sMCL, 2 cm distal to the joint line (Wijdicks et al. 2010b). Therefore, by sticking along the sartorius fascia and gently dissecting, the biggest risk of injury to this structure would be due to adhesions during graft harvest.

Postoperative Rehabilitation

The authors advocate an early motion program as part of the rehabilitation protocol. It is recommended that one determine the "safe zone" ranges of motion intraoperatively and utilize this in the first few postoperative days. The authors support having indwelling femoral nerve blocks to assist with pain control such that the physical therapist can work with the patient on knee motion prior to any stiffness developing. In general, one should strive for a range of motion of 0–90° on postoperative day 1, and after 2 weeks, range of motion is increased as tolerated. The patients are non-weight bearing for the first 6 weeks and strive to work on quadriceps activation, edema control, and knee motion during the first few weeks. As part of this, patellofemoral mobility should be aggressively pursued.

After 6 weeks postoperatively, the knee is placed into a hinged knee brace and patients are allowed to increase their weight bearing as tolerated. They may wean off crutches when they can ambulate without a limp. They may also start the use of a stationary bike once they have achieved 95–100° of knee flexion. The goal is to have them walking normally within 1 or 2 weeks after the initiation of ambulation. They may also start some simple leg presses, usually to a maximum of 70° of knee flexion, between weeks 6 and 12.

The goal is to obtain bilateral valgus stress radiographs to verify sufficient healing between 4 and 5 months postoperatively. If a concurrent cruciate ligament reconstruction is performed, this time frame may be pushed out to up to 6 months, especially for double-bundle PCL reconstructions. After verification of graft healing with valgus stress radiographs, patients are allowed to initiate agility exercises, perform side-to-side activities, and use a balance ball. Jogging in a brace may also be initiated at this point in time. Once the patient has appropriate endurance, strength, and agility, a functional sports test is performed to determine if they are able to return back to full activities. The patients should wear a knee brace for the first year postoperatively to protect their medial knee reconstruction graft (s) from stretching out.

Conclusions

In conclusion, an anatomic-based posteromedial knee reconstruction has been validated to improve patient function and restore knee stability. An early rehabilitation program can be performed to allow early motion and significantly decrease the risk of arthrofibrosis, and it has been validated that these reconstructions do not result in the graft stretching out. Thus, anatomic-based posteromedial knee reconstructions to restore complex acute and chronic medial knee injuries are recommended.

Cross-References

- ▶ Medial Collateral Ligament and Anterior Cruciate Ligament Synergy: Functional Interdependence
- ▶ Medial Side Instability and Reconstruction
- ▶ Rehabilitation of Complex Knee Injuries and Key Points
- ▶ Special Considerations for Multiple-Ligament Knee Injuries

References

Bollen S (2000) Epidemiology of knee injuries: diagnosis and triage. Br J Sports Med 34(3):227–228

Coobs BR, Wijdicks CA, Armitage BM et al (2010) An in vitro analysis of an anatomic medial knee reconstruction. Am J Sports Med 38:339–347

Edson CJ (2006) Conservative and postoperative rehabilitation of isolated and combined injuries of the medial collateral ligament. Sports Med Arthrosc 14:105–110

Girgis FG, Marshall JL, Al Monajem ARS (1975) The cruciate ligaments of the knee joint: anatomical, functional, and experimental analysis. Clin Orthop Relat Res 106:216–231

Griffith CJ, LaPrade RF, Johansen S et al (2009a) Medial knee injury: part 1, static function of the individual components of the main medial knee structures. Am J Sports Med 37:1762–1770

Griffith CJ, Wijdicks CA, LaPrade RF et al (2009b) Force measurements on the posterior oblique ligament and superficial medial collateral ligament proximal and distal divisions to applied loads. Am J Sports Med 37:140–148

LaPrade RF, Wijdicks CA (2012a) Surgical technique: development of an anatomic medial knee reconstruction. Clin Orthop Relat Res 470(3):806–814

LaPrade RF, Wijdicks CA (2012b) The management of injuries to the medial side of the knee. J Orthop Sports Phys Ther 42:221–233

LaPrade RF, Engebretsen AH, Ly TV et al (2007) The anatomy of the medial part of the knee. J Bone Joint Surg Am 89:2000–2010

LaPrade RF, Bernhardson AS, Griffith CJ et al (2010) Correlation of valgus stress radiographs with medial knee ligament injuries: an in vitro biomechanical study. Am J Sports Med 38:330–338

Lind M, Jakobsen BW, Lund B et al (2009) Anatomical reconstruction of the medial collateral ligament and posteromedial corner of the knee in patients with chronic medial collateral ligament instability. Am J Sports Med 37(6):1116–1122

Pedowitz RA, O'Connor JJ, Akeson WH (2003) Daniel's knee injuries: ligament and cartilage structure, function, injury, and repair, 2nd edn. Lippincott Williams & Wilkins, Philadelphia

Sandberg R, Balkfors B, Nilsson B et al (1987) Operative treatment of recent injuries to the ligaments of the knee: a prospective randomized study. J Bone Joint Surg Am 69:1120–1126

Spiridonov SI, Slinkard NJ, LaPrade RF (2011) Isolated and combined grade-III posterior cruciate ligament tears treated with double-bundle reconstruction with use of endoscopically placed femoral tunnels and grafts. J Bone Joint Surg Am 93:1773–1780

Van Dommelen BA, Fowler PJ (1989) Anatomy of the posterior cruciate ligament: a review. Am J Sports Med 17(1):24–29

Wijdicks CA, Ewart DT, Nuckley DJ et al (2010a) Structural properties of the primary medial knee ligaments. Am J Sports Med 38(8):1638–1646

Wijdicks CA, Westerhaus BD, Brand EJ et al (2010b) Sartorial branch of the saphenous nerve in relation to a medial knee ligament repair or reconstruction. Knee Surg Sports Traumatol Arthrosc 18:1105–1109

Structured Rehabilitation Model with Clinical Outcomes After Anterior Cruciate Ligament Reconstruction

117

Roland Thomeé and Joanna Kvist

Contents

R. Thomeé (✉)
Sahlgrenska Academy, Institute of Neuroscience and Physiology Section of Health and Rehabilitation, Unit of Physiotherapy, University of Gothenburg, Göteborg, Sweden
e-mail: roland.thomee@gu.se

J. Kvist
Division Physiotherapy, Department of Medical and Health Sciences, Linköping University, Linköping, Sweden
e-mail: joanna.kvist@liu.se

M.N. Doral, J. Karlsson (eds.), *Sports Injuries*,
DOI 10.1007/978-3-642-36569-0_104

Abstract
The goal of the rehabilitation after an anterior cruciate ligament reconstruction is to assure that the athlete can return to sports and avoid reinjury in the short term and that there is minimal risk for other injuries in the long term. The recommendation in the current literature is to implement a well-planned, individualized, and criteria-based rehabilitation program as soon as possible, preferably on the same day as surgery. The rehabilitation has to be based on knowledge about the healing process after reconstruction, about the effect of rehabilitation techniques and exercise on tissue, and about the short- and long-term consequences of the injury. It has also to be individualized to meet each athlete's personal physiological and psychological needs regarding the extent of the injury and sports-related demands on the knee. The structured rehabilitation model that is presented in this chapter consists of four rehab phases, which take the patient and the phases of the tissue healing process into consideration.

Introduction

A structured rehabilitation program should start immediately after an anterior cruciate ligament reconstruction (ACLR) for physiological and psychological reasons (Fig. 1). Rehabilitation before the reconstruction, in order to ensure good muscle function and information about the aim, content, and timeline of the postoperative rehabilitation, is crucial for a good outcome.

The goals of the rehabilitation program are to aid in, and not adventure, the healing process and improve tissue load tolerance and function so that the athlete can return to sports and avoid reinjury in the short term. In the long term, the goal is to secure that the injured athlete can be physically active to maintain good health in order to minimize the risk for knee osteoarthritis and other diseases pertaining to lifestyle.

A Structured Rehabilitation Model

A literature search yielded 66 systematic reviews and more than 118 randomized controlled trials (RCTs) on rehabilitation after ACLR. In addition, numerous papers presenting current concepts exist. A general consensus is that structured rehabilitation is needed after ACLR (Risberg et al. 2004; Myer et al. 2006; Wright et al. 2008a, b; Andersson et al. 2009; Coppola and Collins 2009; Glass et al. 2010; van Grinsven et al. 2010; Adams et al. 2012; Kruse et al. 2012; Lobb et al. 2012). The recommendation is to implement a well-planned, individualized, and criteria-based rehabilitation program as soon as possible, preferably on the same day as surgery. The rehabilitation has to be based on knowledge about the healing process after reconstruction, about the effect of rehabilitation techniques and exercise on tissue, and about the short- and long-term consequences of the injury. It has also to be individualized to meet each athlete's personal physiological and psychological needs regarding the extent of the injury and sports-related demands on the knee.

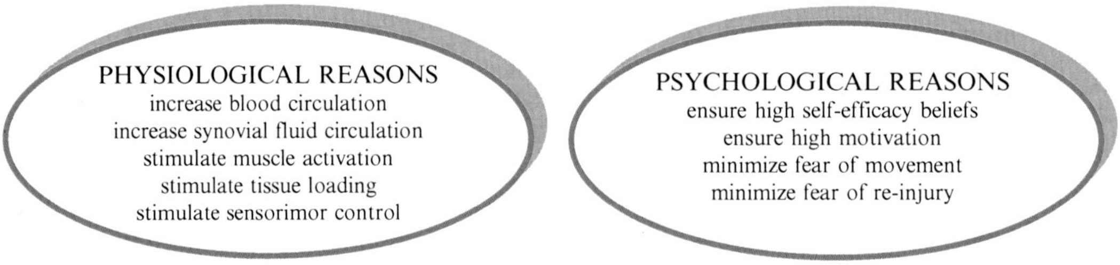

Fig. 1 Physiological and psychological reasons for a rehabilitation program after ACLR

Table 1 Phases during rehabilitation after ACLR

	Rehab phases	Patient phases	Healing phases
1	Initial	Understanding	Inflammation
2	Tolerance training	Conviction	Repair
3	Specific hard training	Fighting	Remodeling
4	Return to sports	High self-efficacy	Maturity

The structured rehabilitation model that is presented in this chapter consists of four rehab phases, which take the patient and the phases of the tissue healing process (Table 1) into consideration (Thomee et al. 2011b).

Requirements for a Successful Rehabilitation and a Good Outcome

In order to have a good effect of the treatment, the rehabilitation has to be individualized, be guided by a physiotherapist, and take in account the grade of the injury (associated injuries), type of surgery, sports demands, and the athlete's psychological status.

Individualized Rehabilitation

The individualized rehabilitation program has to take in account the specific needs for the athlete, concerning which activity or sport they want to return to, and also specific individual physiological and psychological factors that may influence the progress of the rehabilitation, the ability to return to specific activities and to sport, and the final outcome. The response to different exercises, both regarding inflammatory response and effect of the exercises, may differ between individuals. Associated injuries make the joint more vulnerable and may need more time before the joint can tolerate load. A well-trained athlete may have an advantage for the rehabilitation with fast recovery. The tissue is more accustomed to high load and will adapt faster to the progressed loading. A well-trained athlete may also be more motivated to return to sports.

Physiotherapist Supervision and Rehabilitation Confidence

The individualized rehabilitation program has to be planned and supervised by a physiotherapist, in close relation with the athlete. The athlete has to do the rehabilitation program often in the beginning of the rehab, i.e., exercise many times each day. Later on, the rehab should be reduced to once a day or three times a week. The rehab should be carefully supervised and controlled for adverse effects (inflammatory response) during progression. Some studies have pointed to the fact that supervised training not necessarily is superior to home-based training (Wright et al. 2008a, b; Kruse et al. 2012; Lobb et al. 2012). However, in these studies, the home-based program was supervised in terms of careful instructions by the physiotherapists, regular visits to the physiotherapist, and immediate contact if needed.

An experienced physiotherapist can together with the athlete plan for a detailed and individual rehabilitation, help the athlete to carry out rehab exercises with good quality, and inform about what to add as additional training. A proper treatment and a good start of the rehabilitation will give a good understanding of the injury and the rehabilitation that is needed. It is important that the physiotherapist in charge explains all details in the rehabilitation program carefully to strengthen the athlete's self-efficacy. The first weeks of rehab training serve as important "examinations" that give the athlete and the physiotherapist important information about the knee status, which structures are affected and to what extent. It is important, especially in the beginning but also later on, that the athlete have full control over the load/intensity of the exercises, range of motion, speed, and volume. The athlete should be able to control how heavy the load should be for the different exercises, or how much effort should be used, how much of the range of motion is performed and the speed at which exercises are performed, and how many repetitions the knee can tolerate. It is important that the athlete together with the physiotherapist decide when an exercise feels good, when it is too simple or too easy, which means that the athlete can move forward in the rehabilitation with more demanding exercises. Many athletes are very aware of symptoms from the body and can handle these either by themselves or by contact to professionals. The athlete has to understand that he or she has to take control over the rehabilitation and over the injured leg and the entire body and has to learn to listen and understand the signals from the body of when an overuse response is in progress (when the tissues do not tolerate the load) or when the exercises can be progressed to heavier loading. In the education of the patients, information about adverse effects and how they can handle them is included, for example, using the pain-monitoring model (Thomee 1997) and soreness rules (Adams et al. 2012). In the individualized structured rehabilitation, a discussion between the athlete and physiotherapist has to be made about where the training should be done. For many athletes, the environment where they are doing the training is crucial for the compliance. So, these athletes may prefer a gym with continuous contact with the physiotherapist.

Associated Injuries

An ACL injury almost always involves injuries of other structures such as other ligaments, menisci, cartilage and the underlying bone, joint capsule, or other knee joint structures. It is therefore important to individualize the rehabilitation program and allow for an individual progress of the program, as the time it takes for healing and improved tolerance in the damaged tissue can vary substantially. Preoperative meniscus injuries have a negative influence on the long-term postoperative function (Eitzen et al. 2009) and increase the risk for postoperative osteoarthritis (Andersson et al. 2009). For that reason, a more decelerated rehabilitation regime may be indicated for these patients, though scientific proof is lacking. After concurrent meniscal repair, cartilage repair intervention, or collateral ligament injuries, a more decelerated rehab is recommended (Adams et al. 2012).

Following a revision or a bilateral surgery, the athlete is more prepared for the rehabilitation period. Though, especially after revision surgery, the rehab may be decelerated. In both occasions, the outcome is usually worse compared to the primary reconstruction.

Graft Types

Most of the RCTs on rehabilitation are performed following ACL reconstruction with patella tendon graft. Donor-site morbidity on patellar tendon and anterior knee pain may occur. When hamstrings tendons are used, hamstrings muscle strengthening exercises may be done with reduced external load during the first 12 weeks after surgery (Adams et al. 2012; Escamilla et al. 2012a, b).

Loading of the Graft

The rehabilitation exercises should be planned so that they are effective to enhance neuromuscular control, muscle strength, and functional performance and not result in an overuse response or excessive load on the healing graft. Muscle contraction results in angular and linear translational motions between the bones. The role of the ACL is primarily to counteract an anterior translation of the tibia. Isolated activation of the quadriceps between 0° and 75° of knee flexion will result in anterior translation of the tibia and increased strain on the ACL. An isolated activation of the gastrocnemius muscle has the same effect. In contrast, isolated hamstrings activation in flexion angles greater than 20° will posteriorly translate the tibia and reduce the ACL strain (Kvist 2004; Escamilla et al. 2012a, b). Joint compression through weight bearing or muscle coactivation will stiffen the joint and reduce the translational movements. On the other hand, due to the posterior tilt of the tibial plateau, the tibia will translate to an anterior position (Kvist 2004). Experimental biomechanical studies and modeling have shown that non-weight-bearing exercises (open kinetic chain exercises, OKC) in flexion angles between 50° and 100° and weight-bearing exercises (i.e., closed kinetic chain exercises, CKC) in flexion angles between 0° and 45° result in low ACL loading (van Grinsven et al. 2010; Escamilla et al. 2012a, b).

Though most of these studies have been done on subjects without knee injuries or with ACL deficiency, studies on recently injured ACL subjects (Kvist et al. 2007) or soon after surgery (Kvist 2006; Tagesson et al. 2009) show that the translational movements are reduced, probably due to stiffening strategies.

Studies are inconclusive about the superiority of CKC or OKC exercises (Wright et al. 2008a, b; Andersson et al. 2009). CKC exercises load the graft less, but on the other hand, CKC exercises may not be sufficient for quadriceps strengthening (Mikkelsen et al. 2000; Tagesson et al. 2008). Only one study (Heijne and Werner 2007) indicates that early start of OKC exercises (4 weeks postoperatively) may increase knee laxity in patients reconstructed with hamstrings tendon.

A combination of CKC and OKC is recommended throughout the rehabilitation. Heavy loading exercises, aiming to strengthen the muscles, have to be done in OKC and are indicated at the late part of the rehabilitation, during the specific hard training phase.

Psychological Factors

Patients' perceived self-efficacy of knee function preoperatively is of predictive value for return to acceptable levels of physical activity, symptoms, and muscle function 1 year after ACLR (Thomee et al. 2008). Furthermore, psychological readiness to return to sport, fear of reinjury, sport locus of control, and the athlete's estimate of the number of months it would take to return to sport, all measured preoperatively, have been found to predict return to pre-injury level of sports performance (Ardern et al. 2012, 2013).

It has been shown that persons with high self-efficacy have better coping strategies to deal with pain, symptoms, and problems in general. These persons select more difficult goals, and, once selected, they have greater commitment to those goals. They also choose to perform more challenging tasks, and when setbacks occur, they recover more quickly and maintain their commitment to their goals. When negative discrepancies are experienced between aspirations and actual achievement level, performers with high self-efficacy will increase their level of effort and persistence, whereas low self-efficacy performers will give up (Locke et al. 1984; Bandura 1986, 1995; Thomee et al. 2008). A patient with high self-efficacy in his or her own ability and good experiences from previous injuries, and who uses positive strategies to cope with the injury and to complete the rehabilitation, is more motivated, diligent, and patient with the rehab program. A well-structured rehabilitation gradually strengthens the athlete's self-efficacy and ability to first cope with various daily activities and then with more demanding exercise and sports activities. This will reduce worries and the actual risk to get injured again. It is important to analyze all "weak links" carefully to prevent reinjury.

It can be speculated that if patients with less associated injury report also a higher self-efficacy due to the fact that they have fewer problems with their knee that may allow for a more effective preoperative as well as postoperative training but this perspective has not been studied.

Rehabilitation Before the Reconstruction

Patients who are prepared and well informed about the postoperative rehabilitation (Maddison et al. 2006) will do better during the rehabilitation period. In addition, patients with good knee function (Heijne et al. 2009), low levels of pain (Eitzen et al. 2009; Heijne et al. 2009), a good muscle strength (LSI > 90 %), and absence of meniscus injury (Eitzen et al. 2009) before the reconstruction will have better final outcome. Absent or minimal joint effusion preoperatively is also recommended (Adams et al. 2012).

Rehabilitation Phases

Timing and Progression of the Phases

Usually, rehabilitation after ACL reconstruction will last for 6–12 months. Successful return to sport may indicate the end of rehabilitation and is usually at least 6 months after the reconstruction

(Kvist 2004; Walden et al. 2011). However, not all athletes will return to sports (Ardern et al. 2011). The recommendation for return to sports is based on strict criteria about knee status and functional performance (Kvist 2004; Thomee et al. 2011a). In this chapter, time frames are presented as a guideline and may help the physiotherapist to plan the rehabilitation and to give realistic information and expectations to the athlete.

The time for each phase and for the entire rehabilitation may differ several days/weeks/months case by case. This is due to the fact that each injury can be more or less extensive and cause different symptoms, discomforts, and losses of function. It is often smart to make the exercises excessively easy in the beginning so that there is time to "check" that the injured tissue can tolerate the exercise and that the athlete does not get increased symptoms. If the athlete is too eager at first, before the athlete know how the knee will react, and train with too heavy exercises, there is a risk for setbacks and thus increased symptoms. The aim is to take bite-sized steps forward so that each step can be successfully completed. Then the athlete will feel more secure and more convinced to manage the rehab training. An experienced physiotherapist can help, support, and guide the athlete, but the athlete has to take responsibility for the fact that the exercises are carried out with good quality and that enough time is spent on rehab training.

In the case of acute tissue damage such as an ACL injury or a surgical procedure, the body reacts with inflammation for a few days. Parallel to the acute phase, the body's repair processes are gradually taking over, and damaged tissue is being repaired, which can last up to about 6 weeks (sometimes longer) depending on the extent of the injury. The repair is made largely with secondary tissue (scar tissue), which does not have the same quality and capacity as primary tissue. Then the remodeling and maturation phases take place, which can last very long (3–12 months, sometimes longer), where the secondary tissue is gradually replaced with "real" primary tissue. Both the repair, remodeling, and maturation are more effective and faster and lead to a better end result if the damaged tissue is loaded with a progressive and finally a relatively intense exercise program. With knowledge of these tissue healing phases, the rehabilitation phases can be planned.

Phase 1. The ***initial rehab phase*** is characterized by proper postoperative care and an early implementation of the proper treatment with low loading exercises. The most important is to control the inflammatory response, i.e., swelling, pain, heat, and redness, and keep a "clean" joint. The exercises should be progressed to increase ROM and weight-bearing ability. The neuromuscular training aims to give control of the limb during weight bearing and activities of daily living. At the same time, patient confidence to rehabilitation increases. This phase lasts usually during the first 2–3 weeks after reconstruction. Important milestones during the initial phase are low overuse response, normal gait pattern, range of motion with full extension and increased flexion (minimum 90°), and good patellar mobility during quadriceps activation.

Phase 2. Thereafter the ***phase for tolerance training*** can start with continued low loading exercises that gradually are progressed until the knee can tolerate the load necessary to induce improved muscle strength and volume. Tissue tolerance and neuromuscular control are in focus. This phase can last up to 2–3 months after the reconstruction. Important milestones during the tolerance phase are increased loading without overuse response, full active ROM, and good neuromuscular control with dynamic stability of the entire kinetic chain during activities of daily living.

Phase 3. This means that the ***specific hard training phase*** commences. This phase is characterized by a progressive and relatively heavy period of training with elements of training with high intensity including accelerations and decelerations and pivoting involving the stretch-shortening cycle in the end of the phase. During the ***specific hard training phase***, it is important to continually evaluate pain, symptoms, and function with different validated questionnaires on a regular basis and to evaluate muscle function with specific and reliable tests. This phase is usually between 3 and 5 months after the reconstruction. When knee status is normalized and muscle strength and functional performance are more

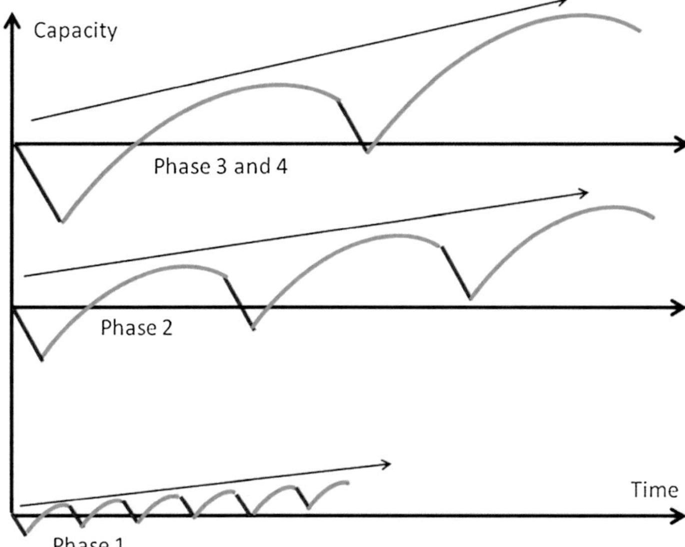

Fig. 2 It is important to ensure adequate recovery between the rehab sessions. In the initial phase (Phase 1), low loading circulation training can take place several times a day. In the tolerance phase (Phase 2), daily low loading rehab training continues, and in addition to that 2–3 tougher sessions per week. When weight training is heavy and when jumping and athletic training get intensified, the sessions must become more sparse, about 1–2 tough sessions per week (Phase 3 and 4)

than 60 % (Thomee et al. 2011a), the return to sports phase can be initiated.

Phase 4. The last and difficult ***phase for return to sports*** is characterized by rehab training that will restore the unique characters of all damaged tissue to withstand the often very intense loading during sports and to give the patient strong self-efficacy beliefs in his or her ability, without fear of injury.

It is not uncommon that athletes hurry through the ***tolerance training phase*** with too aggressive rehab training. This often results in setbacks and leads to frustration. It is often the case that the same athletes neglect to take enough time for the ***specific hard training phase*** as well and try to return to sports too soon. This results in an increased risk for sustaining a reinjury or a subsequent injury. These athletes do not have enough ***understanding*** about their injury and are not convinced about the rehabilitation that is required.

It is, however, not uncommon that some athletes get stuck in the ***tolerance training phase*** with rehab training that has too low intensity. They do not dare to move on because of fear of overuse or reinjury. These athletes often have low self-efficacy beliefs and therefore need support and guidance from an experienced physiotherapist.

The timing and progression during the phases are influenced by the severity of the injury. Some associated injuries in an ACL injured knee, for example, cartilage injuries, need a very long time (6–12 months or longer) to regain enough ***tolerance*** in the damaged tissue to allow for a more intense training to take place. Muscles do sometimes require a long ***specific hard training phase*** in order to fully restore muscle strength, volume, endurance, plyometric properties, and coordination. A tendon often requires an even longer ***specific hard training phase*** followed by a long period of training that involves the very high loading on the muscle/tendon complex during the stretch-shortening cycle in the end of the ***specific hard training phase*** and during the ***return to sports phase*** (Fig. 2).

Accelerated rehabilitation programs have not been found to be more effective than other protocols (Beynnon et al. 2005; Andersson et al. 2009; Kruse et al. 2012). The timing of the progression of the rehabilitation should always be individualized, and a variation of exercises aiming to address the specific impairments at each time should be used in the rehabilitation protocol.

In summary it seems important to address physiological as well as psychological factors in the rehabilitation program for a successful outcome and eventually a successful return to sports after ACLR.

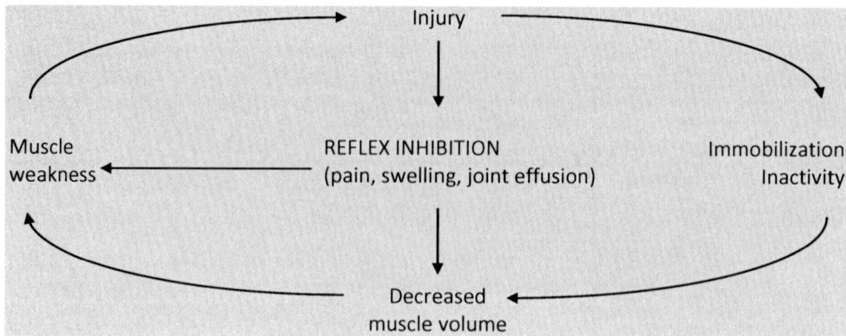

Fig. 3 A vicious cycle of injury, immobilization, inactivity, and inhibition causes decreased muscle volume and weakness, which in turn can cause further tissue damage. The immobilization, inactivity, and inhibition, which follow after an injury, result in deterioration of strength, flexibility, endurance, plyometric properties, elasticity, and strength in muscles and tendons, ligaments, cartilage and other joint structures, and the skeleton. Subsequently, the balance, coordination, and other nerve-muscle interaction are affected. This is the case of the damaged joint/muscle, in particular, and the rest of the body in general

The Four Rehab Phases

The Initial Phase

Rehab phase	Patient phase	Healing phase
Initial	Understanding	Inflammation

After an ACLR there is a long period of relatively high inactivity and low loading on several knee joint tissues and lower extremity structures. During this period there is therefore an increased risk of degradation of strength, endurance, and function, especially in and around the knee joint but also in the lower extremities and the rest of the body as well. This degradation can be minimized or avoided with a well-planned rehabilitation program under the supervision of an experienced physiotherapist.

Effects of Injury/Surgery, and Dosage and Progression During Rehabilitation

The immediate effects of immobilization, inactivity, pain, and swelling following an ACLR give a strong inhibition in muscle function, balance, and coordination. This inhibition produces a variety of disturbances that may be specific to certain muscles, muscle fiber types, and parts of joint range of motion. The inhibition may be significant even if the injured person experiences that the pain has diminished or disappeared. A vicious cycle that causes muscle weakness occurs, which in turn can lead to a worsening of the injury (Fig. 3). In the case of long-term problems, the consequence of the vicious cycle is already a fact.

The rehabilitation program should contain low loading knee exercises, progressed as tolerated, that means without symptoms of overuse, i.e., swelling, pain, heat, and redness. Postoperatively it is important to start with a structured rehabilitation program consisting of circulation training and range of motion training. The exercises are performed several times per day for the first 1–2 weeks after surgery. This way, adverse secondary effects and overuse response can be minimized. The healing process will be facilitated and the patient will have fewer symptoms and will not be as limited in their function.

During the initial phase, pain may be treated with analgesics, transcutaneous electrical stimulation (TENS), or acupuncture. Postoperatively cryotherapy can be used to lower pain (Raynor et al. 2005), though no positive effects on ROM have been found. Pain is however often most efficiently relieved with low loading exercises in a pain-free range of motion that increase blood circulation, or with repetitive pain-free isometric (static) muscular activations for 1–2 s.

Regaining of neuromuscular control needs to be started immediately after surgery in order for the patient to be able to control the lower extremity during activities of daily living. Pain and patella stiffness will result in quadriceps inhibition. Exercises for neuromuscular control during the initial phase are performed with low external load, as tolerated for the joint. The aim is not primarily to gain muscle strength but for neuromuscular reeducation and normalization of the sensorimotor function and to enhance the proprioception. Isolated isometric activations for quadriceps and hamstrings are performed without or with low external load in order to facilitate the muscle. Functional exercises in closed kinetic chain, involving lower limb muscles, are performed in order to increase the proprioception and gain control of the limb during ADL. There is moderate evidence for using neuromuscular electrical stimulation (NMES) together with voluntary muscle activation during early postoperative rehabilitation (Kruse et al. 2012).

No evidence can be found that support immobilization and non-weight bearing on injured leg after ACLR. Usually, crutches may be needed the first days after the reconstruction in order to control pain and swelling and also to ensure proper neuromuscular control. Loading is successively increased so that normal gait pattern without crutches can be achieved within approximately 10 days. Early weight bearing has no adverse effects on knee anterior laxity, decreases the risk of anterior knee pain and makes it possible for the patient to be more active, and minimizes the adverse effects of immobilization (Beynnon et al. 2005; van Grinsven et al. 2010).

Immediate knee motion and early training of passive and active ROM of the tibiofemoral and joint as patellofemoral joint can be beneficial for a fast recovery of ROM and reduce pain. Normalization of ROM is also suggested to be important for the progress of rehabilitation and regaining normal gait pattern (Beynnon et al. 2005). Full extension has to be reached during this phase, and aggressive ROM exercises may be added if full extension is not reached (Adams et al. 2012).

Rehabilitation braces that allow protected motion and aiming to prevent excessive loading on the knee have been used in the initial phase after reconstruction, but there are strong evidence for *no benefit by* using braces for the first 6 weeks after ACLR (Wright et al. 2008a, b; Andersson et al. 2009; Kruse et al. 2012).

An individual exercise program for the rest of the body is recommended in order to maintain/improve important physical qualities of strength, endurance, and function.

Examples of Exercises at the Initial Phase

Circulation, Range of Movement, and Joint Loading

Do two sets of 20–40 repetitions of ankle dorsi/plantar flexion and "glide-bicycling" in as large as possible range of movement. Keep a "bicycle tempo." Combine this with 3 × 5 s of passive knee flexion stretching. Repeat several times per day (every hour to every third hour) (Fig. 4).

Isometric Quadriceps Activation and Straight leg Raises

Activate the quadriceps isometrically with moderate force for 0.5 s and relax for 0.5 s. Aim at pressing the knee toward the underlying surface and lifting the heel from the surface.

If the heel cannot be lifted, use a roll under the knee. Repeat 10–20 times and combine with straight leg raises for a total of two sets. Repeat 3–5 times per day (Fig. 5).

Do 10–20 repetitions of straight leg raises lying on back, side, and stomach. Try to keep the knee as extended as possible and keep a "bicycling tempo." No rest in-between positions. Combine with isometric quadriceps activations for a total of two sets. Repeat 3–5 times per day (Fig. 6).

Loading of Knee with Body Weight

Gradually put more weight on the injured side for 3–5 s. Rest 1–2 s and do 20–40 repetitions several times per day (Fig. 7).

The Tolerance Training Phase

Rehab phase	Patient phase	Healing phase
Tolerance training	Conviction	Repair

During this phase circulatory exercises several times per day should be continued to minimize the inflammation response, i.e., swelling, stiffness,

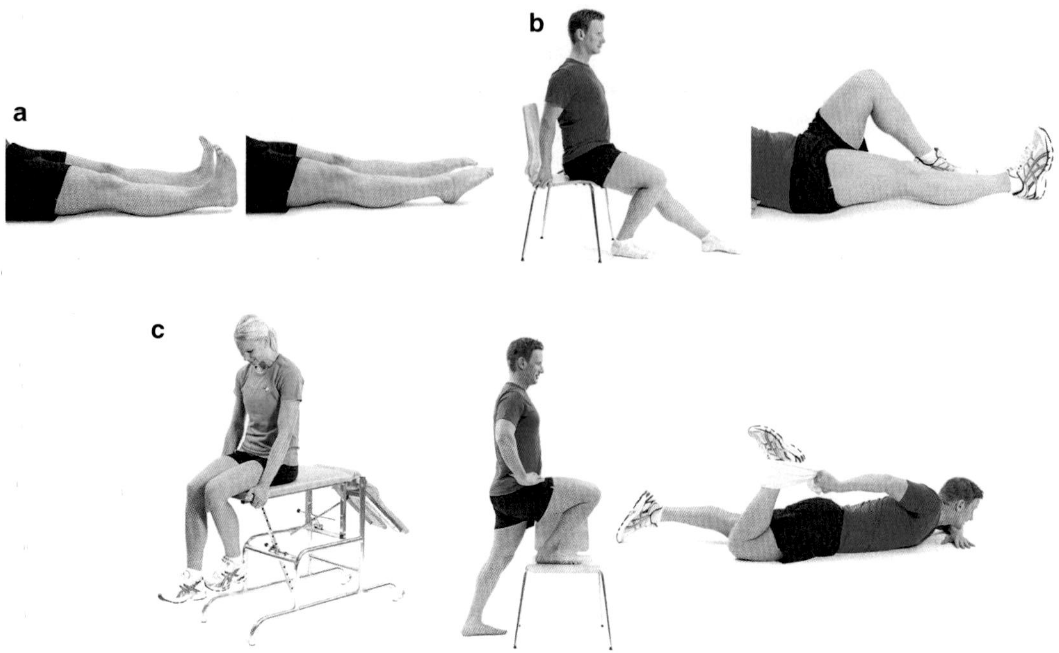

Fig. 4 Examples of exercises for circulation, range of movement, and joint loading. (**a**) Ankle dorsi/plantar flexion. (**b**) Glide-bicycling in sitting or lying down. Let the foot/heel glide back and forth in a "bicycling tempo." (**c**) Passive knee flexion

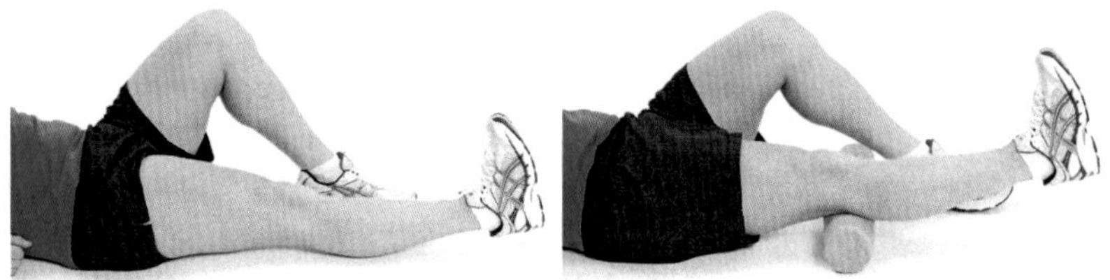

Fig. 5 Isometric quadriceps activation

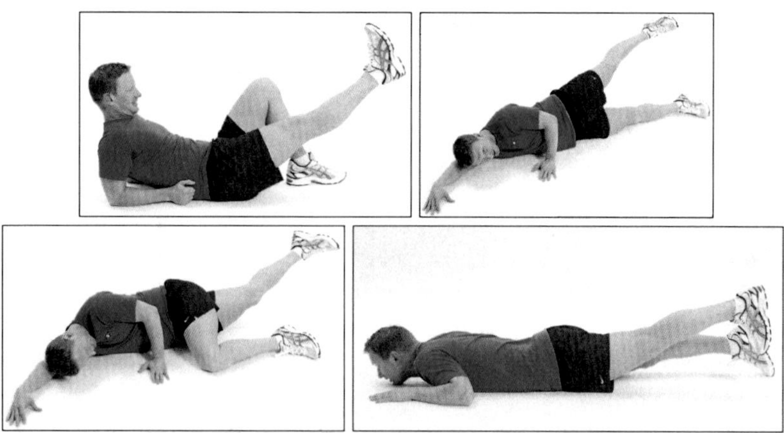

Fig. 6 Straight leg raises on back, side, and stomach

and pain, and increase the tissue tolerance to load. Improved circulation of synovial fluid and improved blood circulation contribute to faster and better healing by stimulation of the body processes for repair. A sufficient level of training gives pain relief due to the release of endorphins (the body's own "morphine"). To achieve this, the training session should make the athlete become "warm" and moderately tired in the muscles. A sign of pain relief is that it feels better during and after training. In addition, low loading circulatory exercises counteract the weakening of the tissues in the body that occur with inactivity and inability to load various body structures.

A combination of different exercises is used during this phase, with specific focus on increasing load, weight bearing, and neuromuscular control to enhance tolerance and sensorimotor function (Risberg et al. 2007). Additional therapeutic techniques such as manual therapy, taping, cryotherapy, etc., have not been shown to have any positive effect.

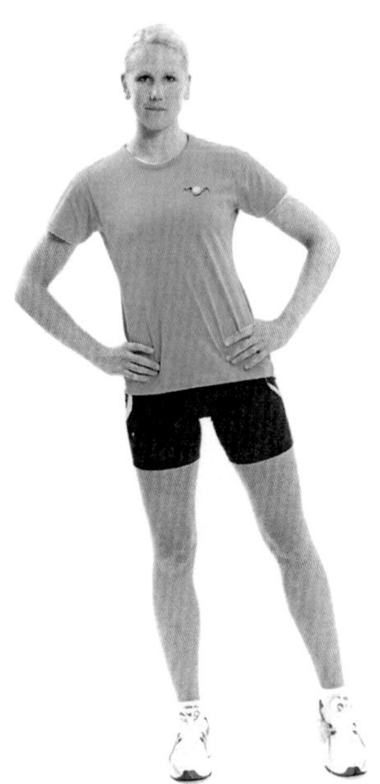

Fig. 7 Loading of knee with body weight

During this phase it is important to have a proper guidance from an experienced physiotherapist so that the athlete gains own tools to regulate the rehabilitation process and increase the self-efficacy. The load/intensity of the exercises increases so that the healing tissue can adapt and tolerate more loads. Too low load will not result in optimal healing and too much load may increase the overuse response and prolong the healing. Two useful tools that the athlete can use are the pain-monitoring model (Thomee 1997) and the soreness rules (Adams et al. 2012).

The pain-monitoring model is used to progress the training according to perceived pain during and after the exercise. The model uses a numerical pain rating where 0 is no pain at all and 10 is the highest pain one can tolerate. Usually it is acceptable to have pain up to 5 if the pain decreases to the normal level the day after the training. In the beginning of the tolerance phase, pain during exercises should be limited to the level of 2 in order to increase the tissue tolerance (Fig. 8).

The soreness rules are used to progress the training according to soreness felt during the warm-up or the day after training. For example, soreness during warm-up that continues indicates that the athlete needs to take 2 days off and drop down the training to level 1. Soreness the day after exercising (mot muscle soreness) indicates 1 day off and no advance of exercises to the next level (Adams et al. 2012).

Examples of Exercises at the Tolerance Phase

Continue with exercises from the initial phase as needed several times per day for circulation,

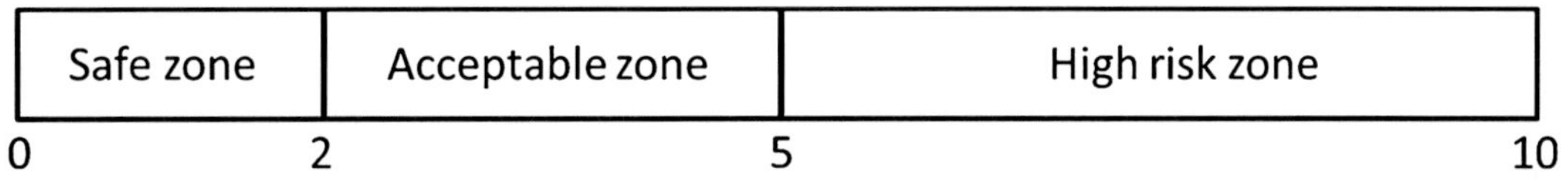

Safe zone	Acceptable zone	High risk zone

0 2 5 10

Fig. 8 Pain-monitoring model. Pain up to 2 during and after training is safe. Pain can be allowed up to 5 during the exercise if it decreases immediately after the end of the exercise. Pain up to 5 after the whole exercise program is allowed, if it disappears the following morning

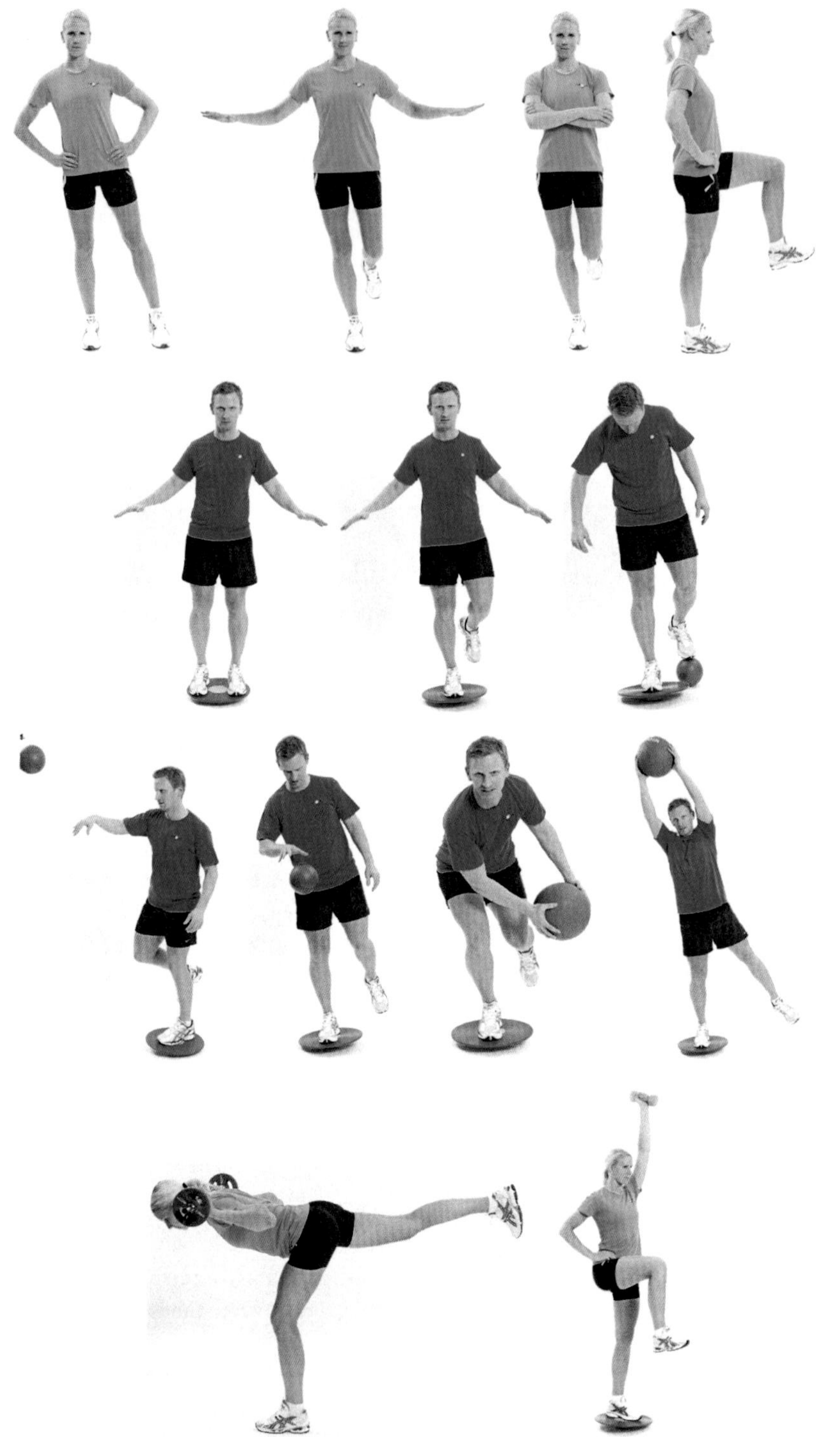

Fig. 9 Balance exercises

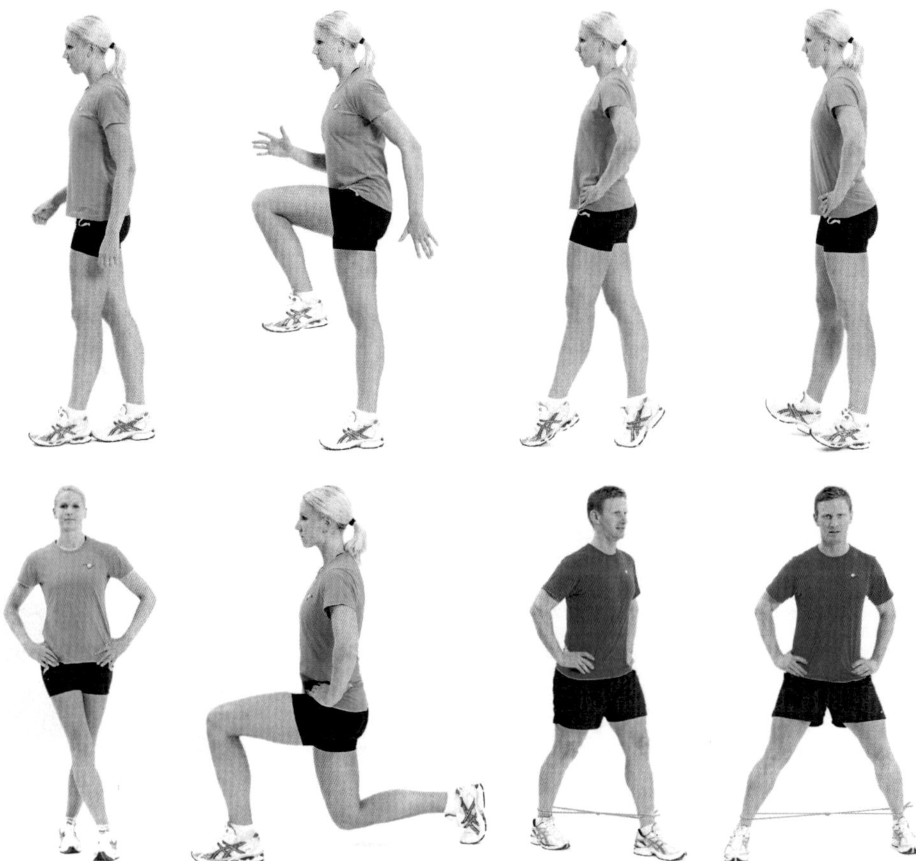

Fig. 10 Walking exercises

range of movement, and load tolerance to body weight. Progress to balance and walking.

Balance: 5 Min

As soon as full body weight is tolerated on the injured leg, balance exercises can start. Exercise for 30–60 s per leg. Progress gradually to more demanding exercises as your knee tolerates the rehab training. Compare with healthy side (Fig. 9).

Walking Exercises

Add walking exercises three to five times per day and 5–10 min per session (Fig. 10).

As soon as tolerated, add exercises on bicycle, rowing machine, and/or cross trainer. Start with 1–5 min a couple of times per day and increase 1–5 min per day up to 10–60 min. Gradually increase the load (Fig. 11).

Do somewhat more demanding rehab training for two to three times per week. Also do exercises for the rest of the body. Your physical therapist can help you with an individual and specific program and also support you in doing the exercises with good quality.

Warm-up – 5–10 min with bicycle, rowing machine, and/or cross trainer.

Balance training – 5 min. Progress to using an elastic cord with or without some balance support (Fig. 12).

Walking exercises – Progress to walking in a soft mattress, over boxes, or with various obstacles (Fig. 13).

Strength training – 10–20 min (Fig. 14).

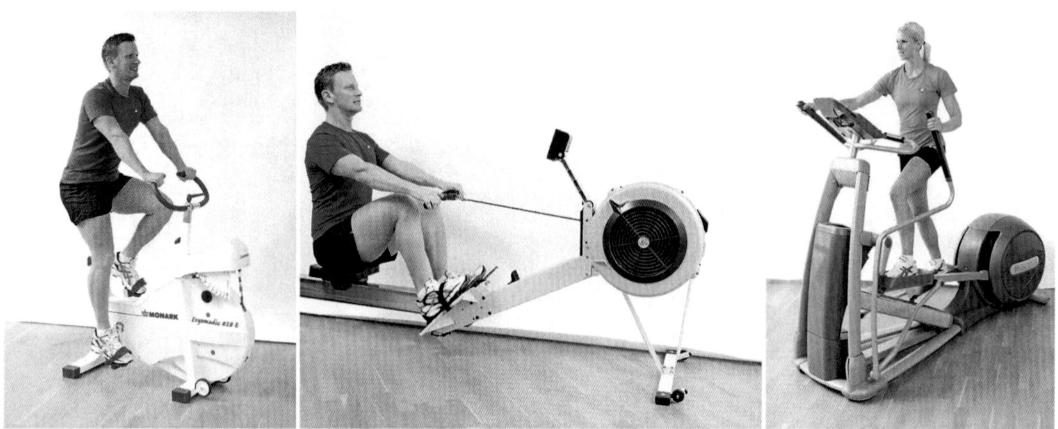

Fig. 11 Exercises on bicycle, rowing machine, and cross trainer

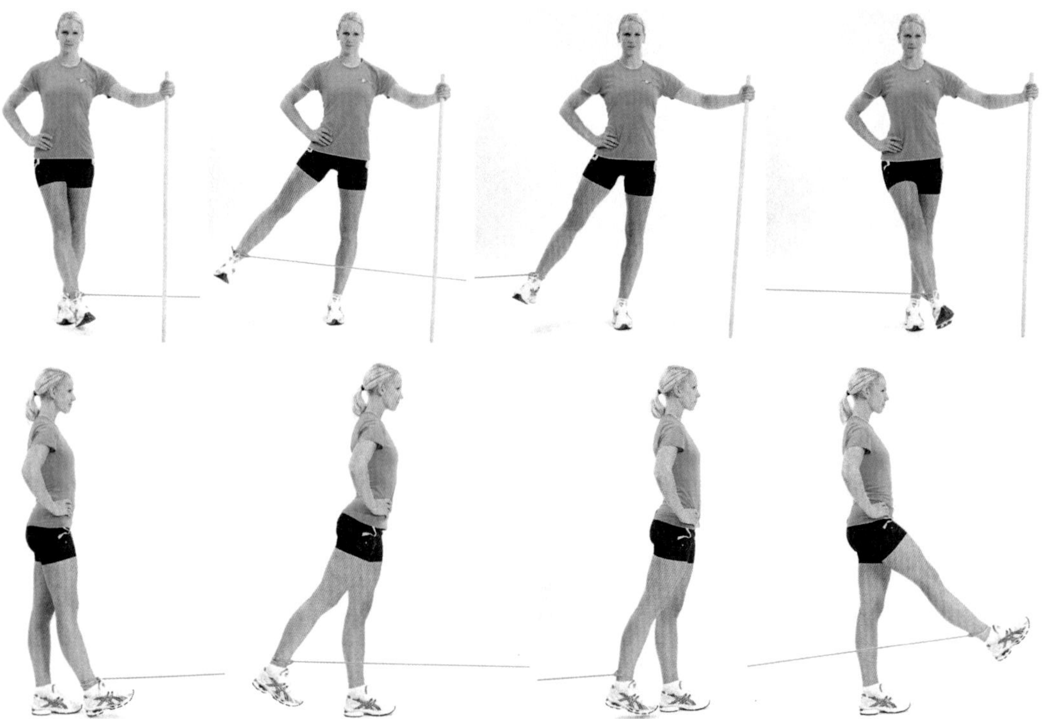

Fig. 12 Balance training

The Specific Hard Training Phase

Rehab phase	Patient phase	Healing phase
Specific hard training	Fighting	Remodeling

As the knee can tolerate more and is getting stronger, the rehab training should progress into ***specific hard training***, which means that the athlete has to fight with progressively heavier and more demanding exercises (heavy load and

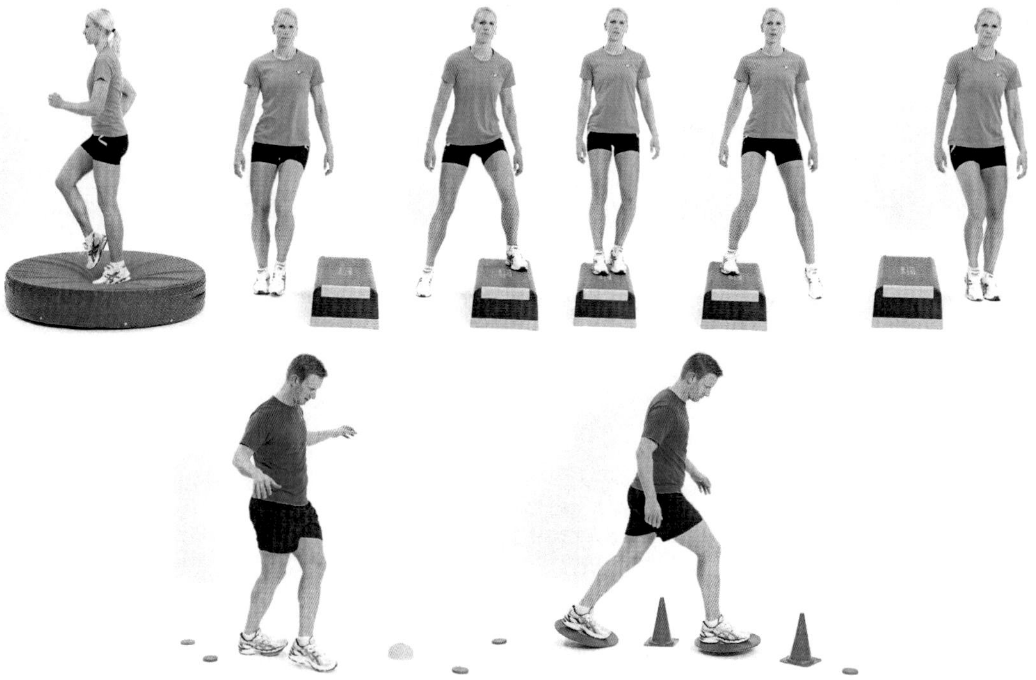

Fig. 13 Walking exercises

few repetitions) for a longer time. High loading on the body is first and foremost achieved by the explosive strength and technique exercises, running, jumping, and other activities involving the stretch-shortening cycle, where the loading on the various body tissues can momentarily reach 5–15 times the body weight. The rehab program has this far not included very high loading exercises, and the more time that has passed since the athlete last exposed the body for maximum training, the longer it takes for the body to withstand the high intensity again.

The specific hard training can gradually escalate to running, jumping, strength, endurance, exercises similar to sports, or various combinations thereof. The physiotherapist should arrange an individually tailored program. When the athlete's capacity begins to approach the pre-injury levels, or 90 % of the non-injured side, and the knee can withstand the heavy loading and intense training, the training can be intensified even more with exercises that involve the stretch-shortening cycle, such as faster running and more powerful jumps. The athlete should vary the specific hard training with sports-specific exercises before and after heavy weight training, so that everything works well even when the athlete is tired. It is also important to ensure adequate recovery (2–4 days, sometimes longer) between the heavy training sessions (Fig. 2).

The athlete can at this point to a large extent carry out the rehab training together with the team or training group. Though it is very common that patients resume their sport too soon, which means that they are exposed to a high risk of reinjury or a subsequent injury, it is very important to make sure that sufficient time for rehabilitation is provided. It is also important to continuously evaluate function with the help of a physiotherapist and test muscle function with reliable and valid tests.

The specific hard training phase must be managed carefully. Remember that daily activities and submaximal loading are often painless. Many moments in sport, however, are extremely stressful and require full strength, endurance, agility, and

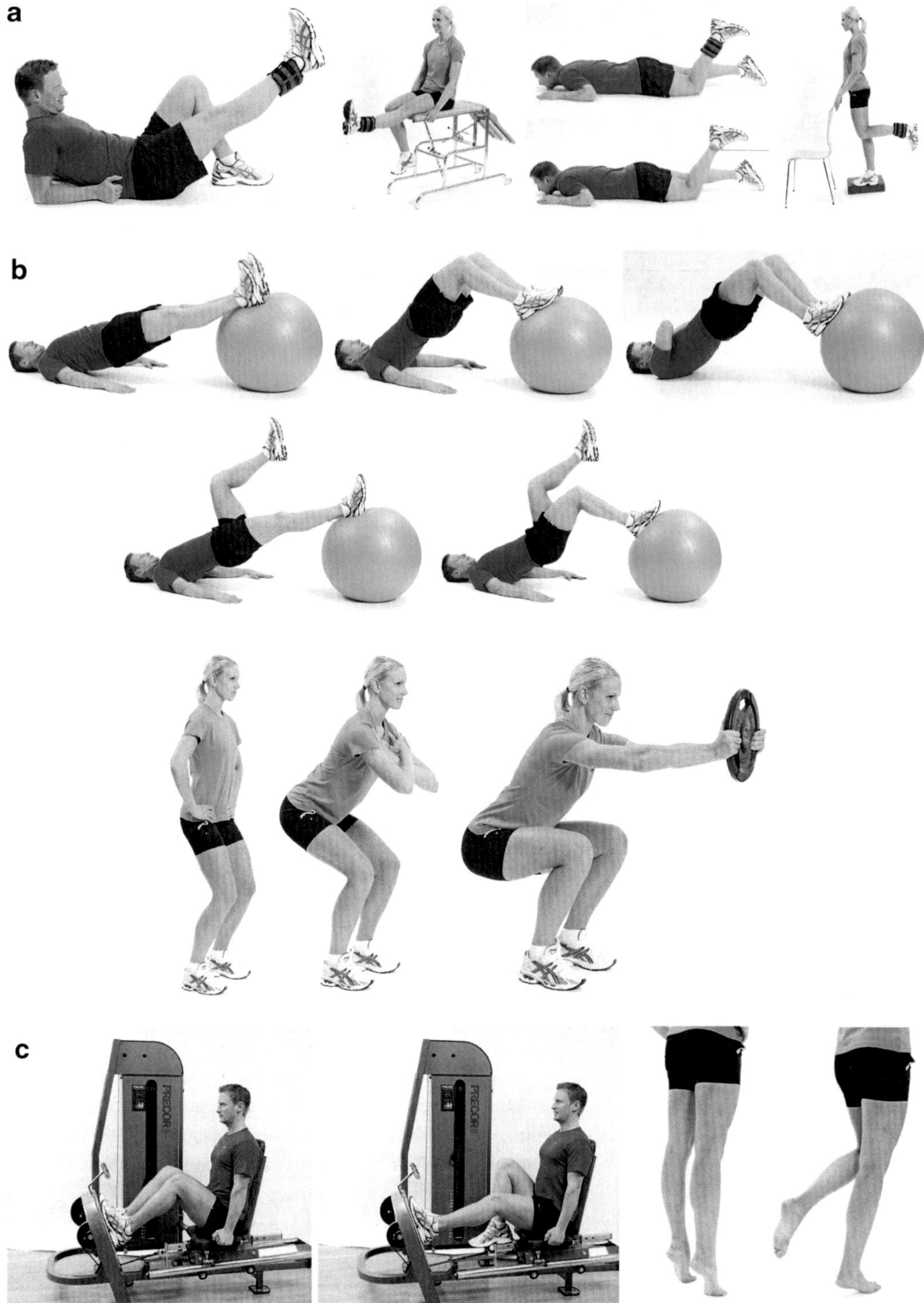

Fig. 14 Strengthening exercises. (**a**) Do 20 repetitions of each exercise and repeat one more time. (**b**) Do 20 repetitions of one of the hip raise exercises and one of the squat exercises. (**c**) Do two sets of 20 repetitions of two- or one-legged leg press and toe raises

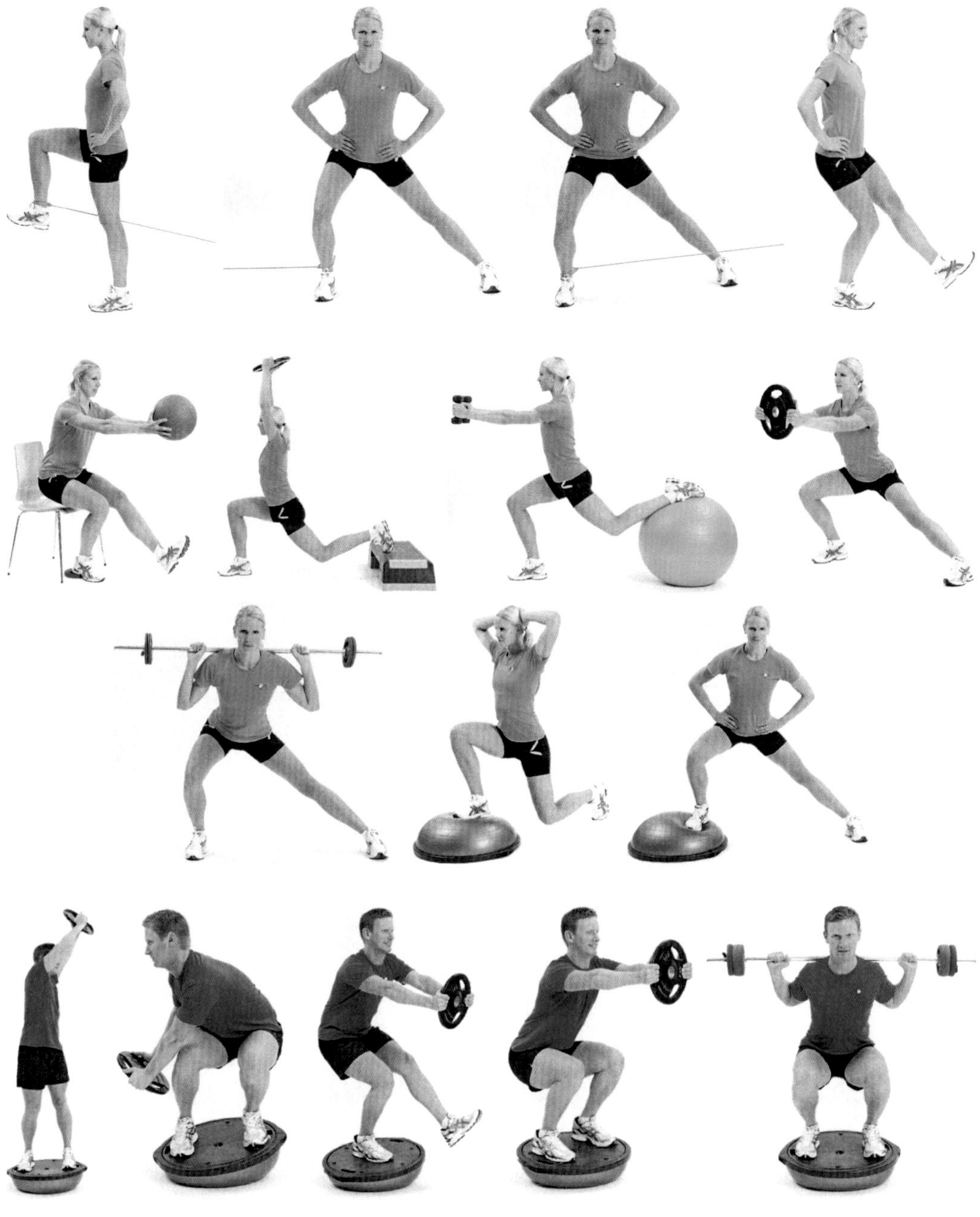

Fig. 15 Exercises for balance, stability, and coordination

coordination. Jumping, for example, stresses the knee joint with 5–15 times the body weight. The very high intensity in sports is often in effect during extremely short periods of time (a few tenths of a second) but also in repeated cycles during a full practice session or a competition and several times per week. Therefore, an optimally functioning joint and muscle/tendon complex with optimal balance and coordination is extremely important.

Relapse, causing reinjury or that a new injury occurs due to inadequate rehabilitation, is probably the most common cause of recreational and

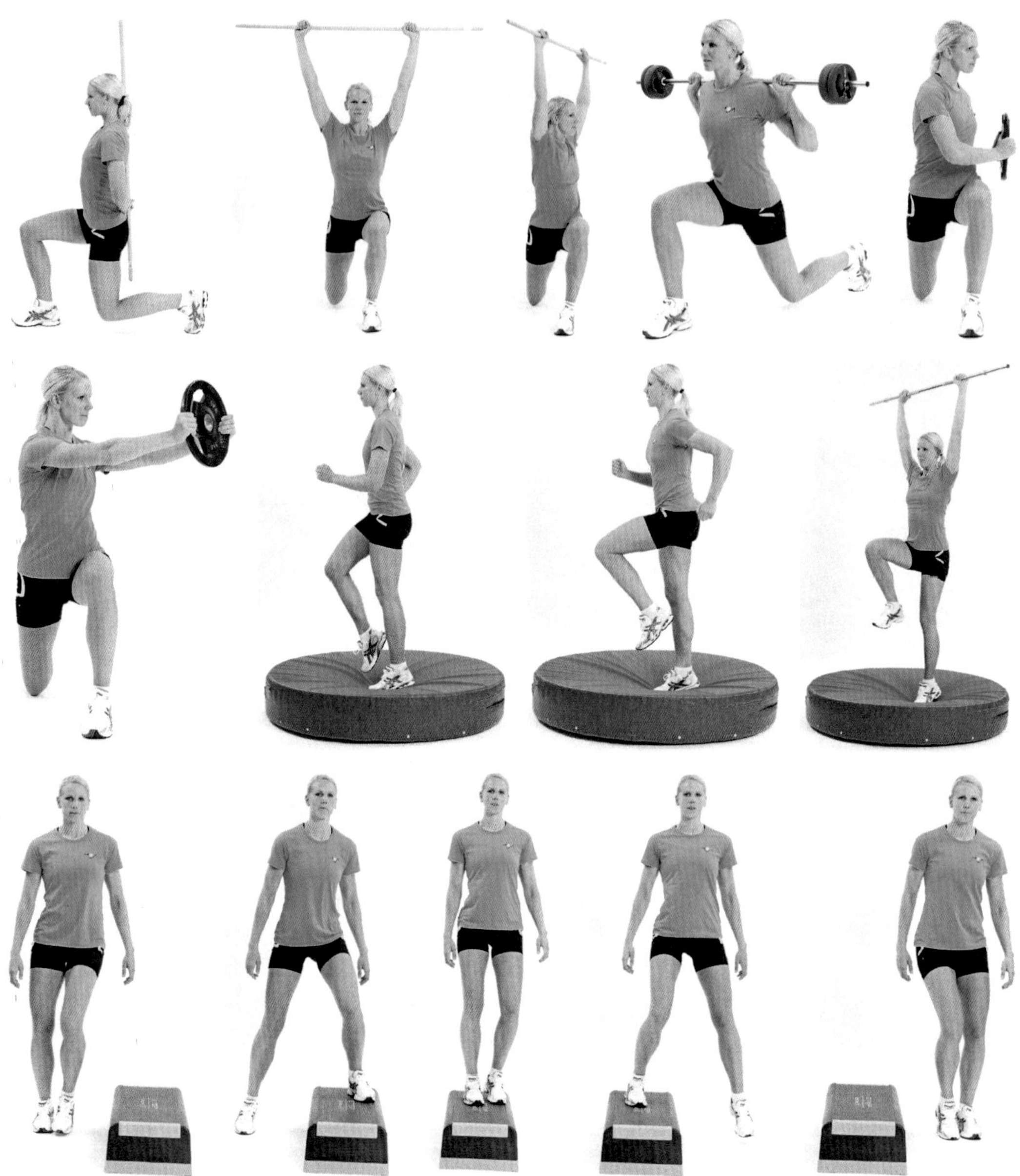

Fig. 16 Walking and jogging exercises

sports injuries. The gradual return to full sports activity must therefore be handled carefully and in full cooperation between the athlete and doctors, physiotherapists, coaches, leaders, and parents (in the case of young athletes).

Important milestones/aims during the specific hard training phase are increased muscle strength and neuromuscular control. The athlete should be able to load the knee more than during ACL, without any inflammation response. Muscle strength and functional performance should be greater than 90 % (Thomee et al. 2011a).

Examples of Exercises at the Specific Hard Training Phase

Keep suitable exercises from previous phases for daily training of balance, walking, and general conditioning.

Exercise 2–3 more demanding and gradually progressing knee sessions per week. Use 10–15 exercises for a total 35–55 min per session. Add 1–2 sessions with exercises for the rest of the body.

Warm-up – 10 min with bicycle, rowing machine, cross trainer, and low loading knee exercises.

Balance, stability, and coordination – 5–10 min. Do 2–3 sets of 10–20 repetitions with 3–5 exercises. Gradually progress the difficulty (Fig. 15).

Walking and jogging exercises – 5–10 min. Gradually progress to the exercise difficulty. Do 2–4 sets with 10–20 repetitions using 2–3 different exercises (Fig. 16).

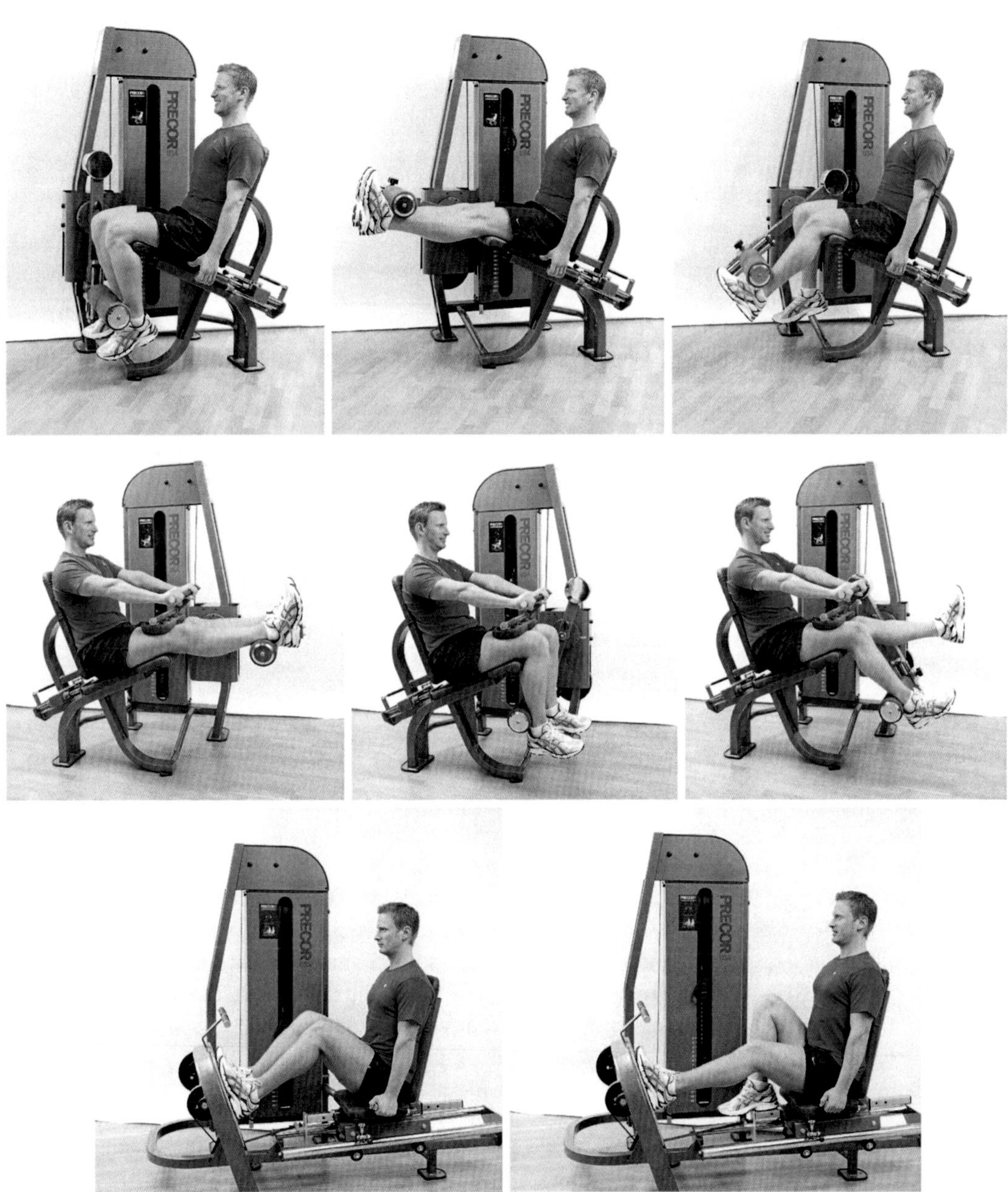

Fig. 17 (continued)

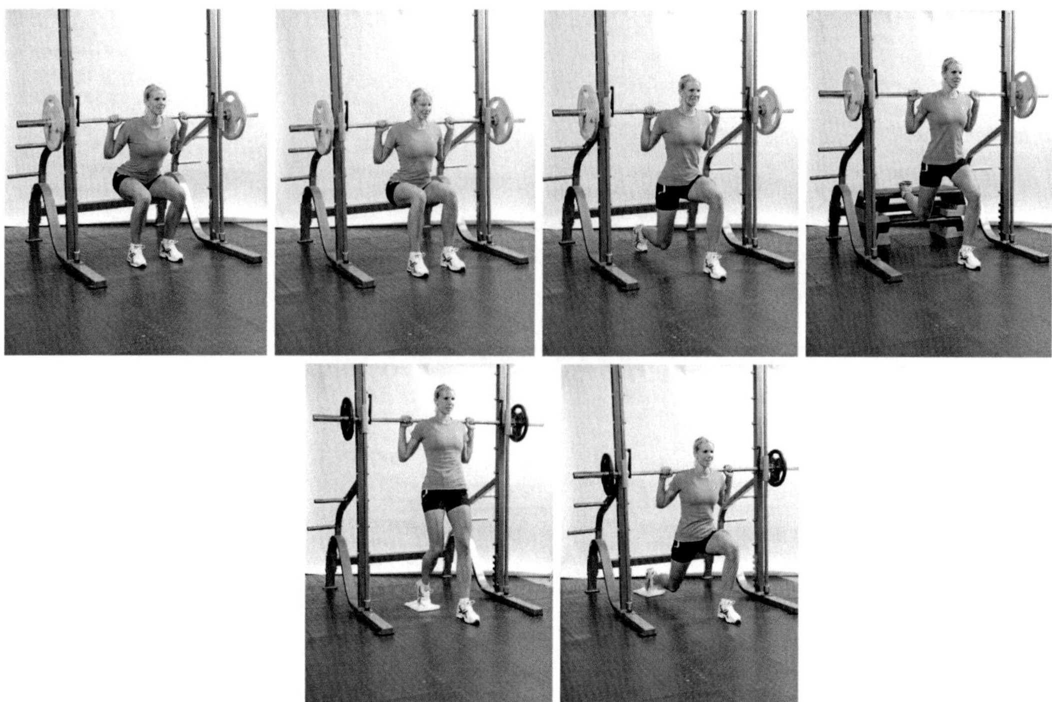

Fig. 17 Strength training exercises. (**a**) Add squats using a Smith machine. Do 2–4 sets using one of the exercises

Leg strength training Alt 1 – 10–20 min. Gradually increase load and lower repetitions from 20 to 15 to 10. Do 2–4 sets of seated two- or one-legged knee extension, knee flexion, and leg press (Fig. 17).

Leg strength training Alt 2 – 10–20 min. Do alternative 1 and 2 every other session in order to put greater demand on coordination during high knee loading. Do 2–4 sets with 2 of the exercises (Fig. 18).

Gradually add to your program high loading and demanding sports-specific exercises as well as specific jumping exercises 5–10 min.

Jumping exercises – Do a 5–10 min circuit program with 3–5 exercises with 10–20 repetitions or 30–60 s per exercise. Gradually increase the number/time and intensity as tolerated. Be aware of the very high knee loading forces (Fig. 19).

The Return-to-Sports Phase

Rehab phase	Patient phase	Healing phase
Return to sports	High self-efficacy	Maturity

The phase return to sports is the most difficult. When the symptoms are almost gone and the athlete is able to train hard with many different exercises, it is tempting to return to sports way too soon and too fast, with an increased risk of a reinjury or a subsequent injury.

It is therefore important for the athlete to continue to be diligent, consistent, and patient with all rehab exercises and the gradual progression of all high loading exercises. All tissues have to mature sufficiently so that the tissue's unique qualities can return to full function, sometimes even better than before the injury. The athlete should therefore continue with specific hard training, sports-specific training, and also heavy weight training

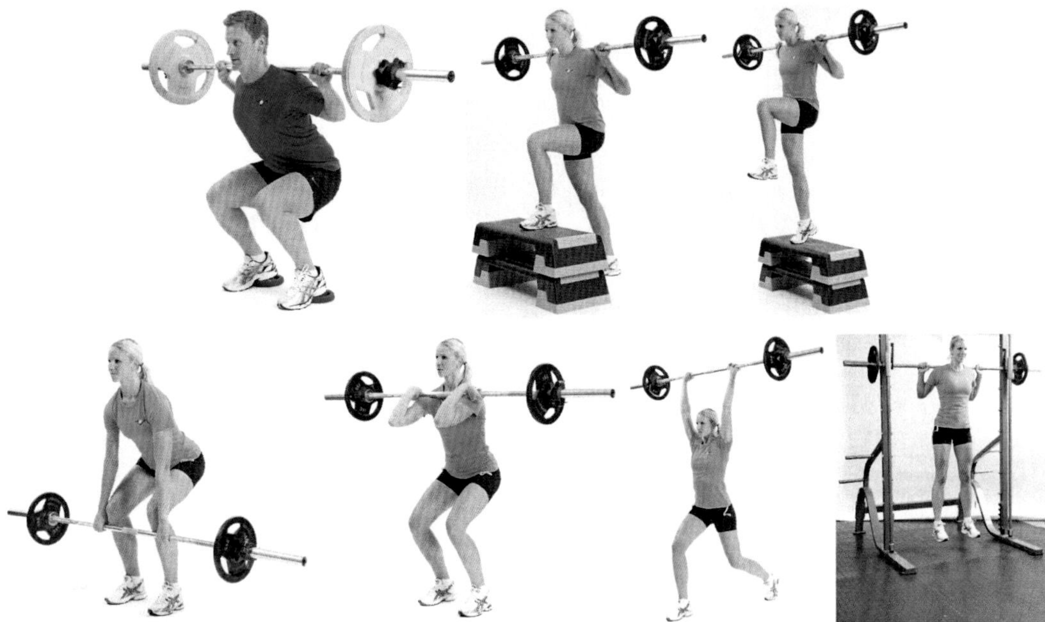

Fig. 18 Strength training exercises

and jumping and allow for sufficient time for recovery. In order to reach an optimal knee function for returning to sports, the athlete needs to complete the rehabilitation until full knee stability, balance and coordination, muscle strength, jumping ability, and endurance are reached in order to withstand the forces involved in sports. Specific strict criteria should be fulfilled in order to progress through the return-to-sports phase (Myer et al. 2006) and to be able to return to sports (Thomee et al. 2011a). High self-efficacy and no fear of reinjury are especially important when returning to: (1) activities that involve knee loading during pivoting and change in direction, (2) contact sports, (3) running forward/backward and sideways, (4) fast start/stop, change of direction activities, and (5) maximal jumping activities.

By regularly evaluating the athlete's symptoms and function with validated questionnaires and muscle function with reliable and valid tests, an updated status on the athlete's readiness can be achieved. Continued discussion, evaluation, and planning are important, in which the athlete, coach, doctor, and physiotherapist participate.

The sports-specific training must gradually progress toward various combinations of running, jumping, maximal strength, maximal explosive strength, maximal endurance, and sports-specific situations. During this phase, exercises used in ACL prevention protocols may be utilized. For example, plyometric exercises improve neuromuscular control. Control of proper landing techniques and control of dynamic valgus are enhanced by plyometrics (Myer et al. 2006) and may decrease the risk for injury (Walden et al. 2012). The aim is to let the athlete return to sports and to minimize the risk for new injuries.

Evaluation and Outcomes

The progression during the rehabilitation has to be assessed with outcome measures with good measurement properties (Shaw et al. 2004). Knee status, ROM, muscle strength, and functional performance need to be evaluated with objective measurements. The athlete's perceived function of the knee, as well as the psychological status

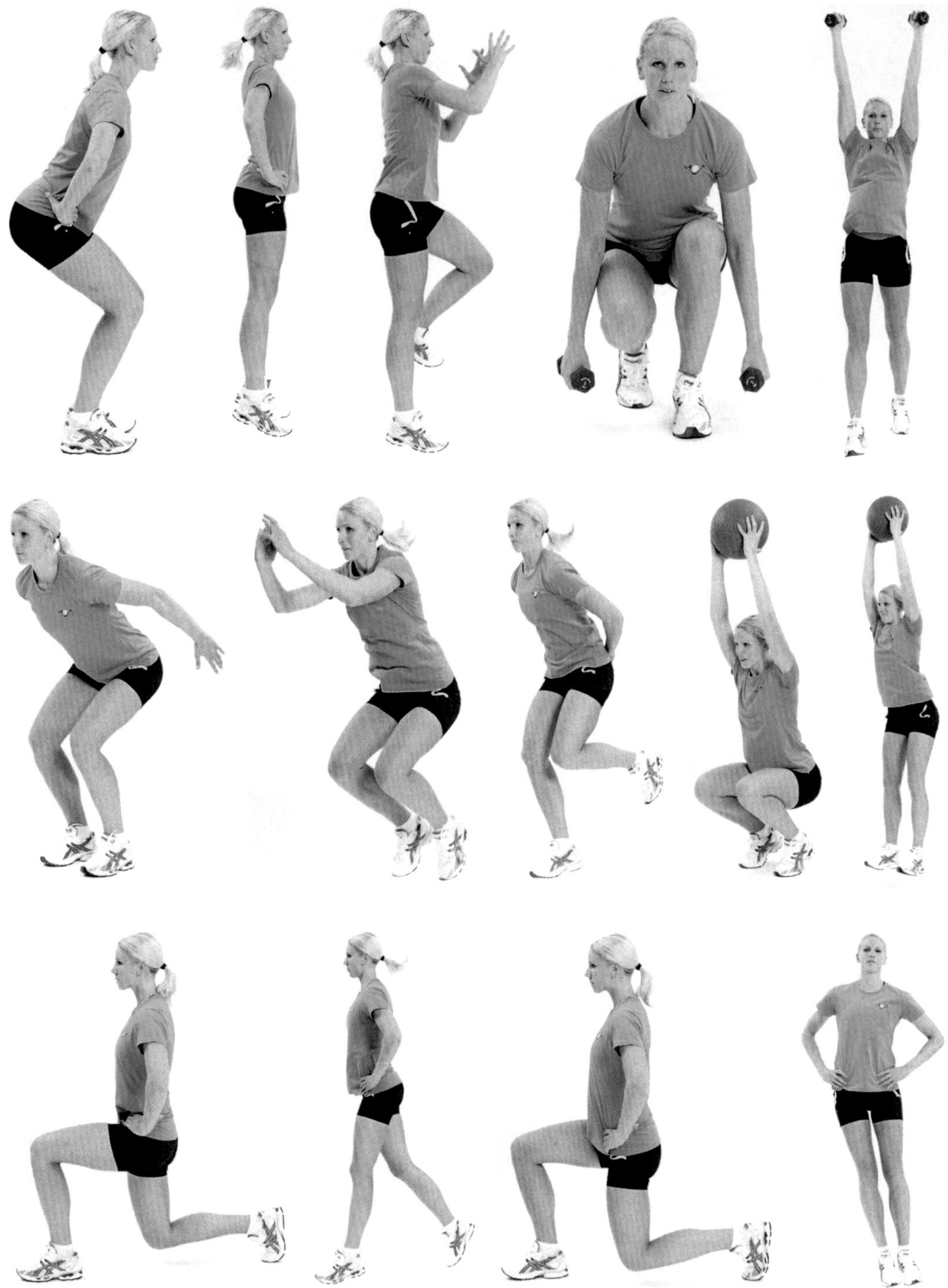

Fig. 19 (continued)

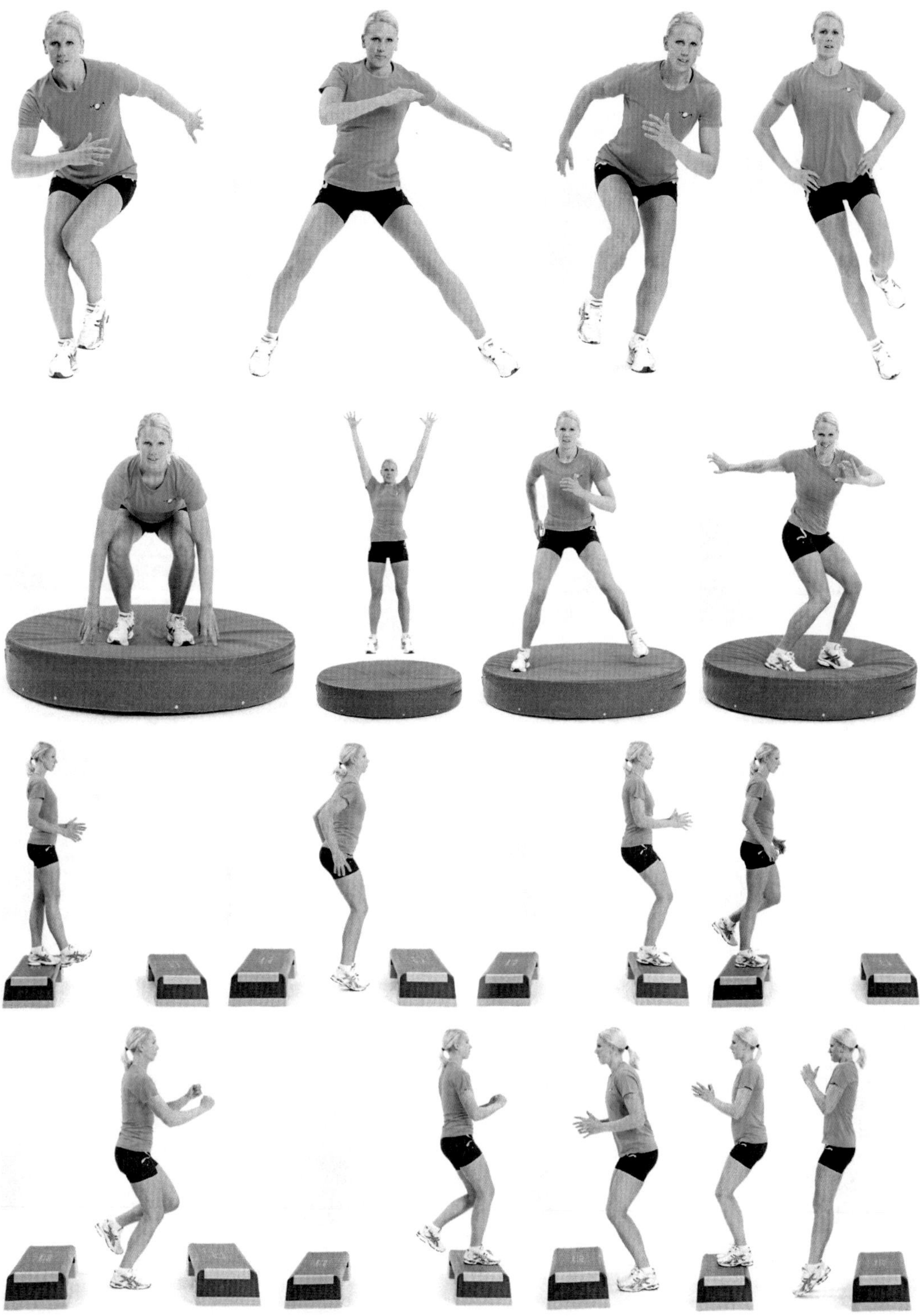

Fig. 19 (continued)

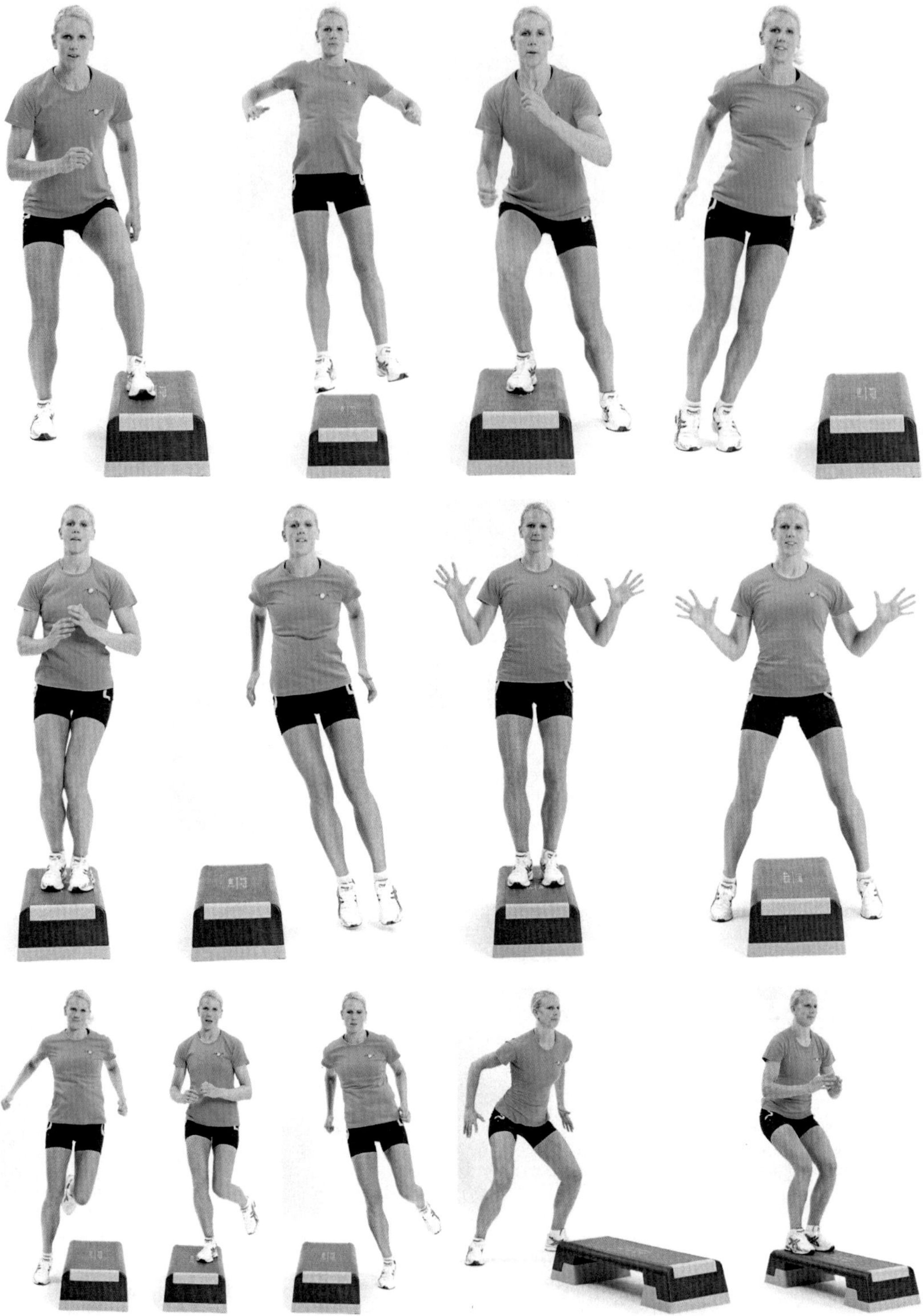

Fig. 19 (continued)

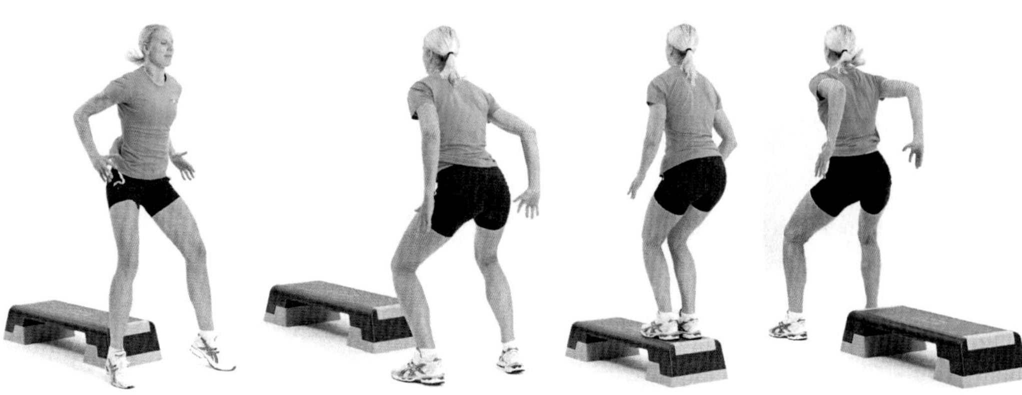

Fig. 19 Jumping exercises

for compliance to the rehabilitation and readiness for return to sports, is evaluated with patient-reported questionnaires.

Knee Status

ROM is reliably measured with goniometry. Joint effusion can be measured by circumference measure with a measuring tape, or the modified stroke test (Sturgill et al. 2009). The visual analogue scale is helpful for evaluating pain. Knee stability is evaluated with the Lachman test and pivot shift test. Neuromuscular control and dynamic control of the knee can be inspected visually or with video or other optoelectronic devices.

Muscle Strength and Functional Performance

Assessing muscle strength is important for the progression of the load during the rehabilitation and also for decision making about progression between phases and return to sports. Muscle strength can be evaluated in isolated motions, isotonic (one repetition maximum) or isokinetic.

Hop tests evaluate muscle strength, functional capacity (the ability to use the muscles to perform), and confidence in jumping and landing. It is recommended to combine different tests, i.e., to use batteries of tests, in order to evaluate different aspects of function (Thomee et al. 2011a).

Patient-Reported Outcomes: Questionnaires

Evaluating the patient's own perception of knee function is important. Patient-reported outcome measures (PROMs) are self-administrated questionnaires and represent the patient's perspective of their health. The most commonly used questionnaires to evaluate knee function are the International Knee Documentation Committee (IKDC) Subjective Knee Form and the Knee Injury and Osteoarthritis Outcome Score (KOOS).

In order to assess psychological factors related to rehabilitation, the Knee Self-Efficacy Scale (K-SES) can be recommended (Thomee et al. 2008). The ACL-Return to Sport after Injury (ACL-RSI) evaluates the athlete's psychological readiness (Webster et al. 2008).

Cross-References

- ▶ Anterior Cruciate Ligament Graft Selection and Fixation
- ▶ Anterior Cruciate Ligament Injuries and Surgery: Current Evidence and Modern Development
- ▶ Anterior Cruciate Ligament Injuries: Prevention Strategies
- ▶ Anterior Cruciate Ligament Reconstruction with Autologous Quadriceps Tendon

- ► Arthroscopic Repair of Partial Anterior Cruciate Ligament Tears: Perspective from an Orthopedics Surgeon
- ► Combined Anterior and Posterior Cruciate Ligament Injuries
- ► Different Techniques of Anterior Cruciate Ligament Reconstruction: Guidelines
- ► Factors Affecting Return to Sport After Anterior Cruciate Ligament Reconstruction
- ► Knee Dislocations
- ► Knee Ligament Surgery: Future Perspectives
- ► Medial Collateral Ligament and Anterior Cruciate Ligament Synergy: Functional Interdependence
- ► Partial Anterior Cruciate Ligament Ruptures: Knee Laxity Measurements and Pivot Shift
- ► Pediatric Anterior Cruciate Ligament Injuries and Combined Cartilage Problems: Current Concepts
- ► Perioperative and Postoperative Anterior Cruciate Ligament Rehabilitation Focused on Soft Tissue Grafts
- ► Rehabilitation of Complex Knee Injuries and Key Points
- ► Return to Play Decision-Making Following Anterior Cruciate Ligament Reconstruction: Multi-factor Considerations
- ► Revision Anterior Cruciate Ligament Reconstruction
- ► Single Versus Double Anterior Cruciate Ligament Reconstruction in Athletes
- ► State of the Art in Anterior Cruciate Ligament Surgery

References

Adams D, Logerstedt DS et al (2012) Current concepts for anterior cruciate ligament reconstruction: a criterion-based rehabilitation progression. J Orthop Sports Phys Ther 42(7):601–614

Andersson D, Samuelsson K et al (2009) Treatment of anterior cruciate ligament injuries with special reference to surgical technique and rehabilitation: an assessment of randomized controlled trials. Arthroscopy 25(6):653–685

Ardern CL, Webster KE et al (2011) Return to sport following anterior cruciate ligament reconstruction surgery: a systematic review and meta-analysis of the state of play. Br J Sports Med 45(7):596–606

Ardern CL, Taylor NF et al (2012) A systematic review of the psychological factors associated with returning to sport following injury. Br J Sports Med 47(17): 1120–1126

Ardern CL, Taylor NF et al (2013) Psychological responses matter in returning to preinjury level of sport after anterior cruciate ligament reconstruction surgery. Am J Sports Med 41(7):1549–1558

Bandura A (1986) The explanatory and predictive scope of self-efficacy theory. J Clin Soc Psychol 4:359–373

Bandura A (1995) Comments on the crusade against the causal efficacy of human thought. J Behav Ther Exp Psychiatry 26(3):179–190

Beynnon BD, Uh BS et al (2005) Rehabilitation after anterior cruciate ligament reconstruction: a prospective, randomized, double-blind comparison of programs administered over 2 different time intervals. Am J Sports Med 33(3):347–359

Coppola SM, Collins SM (2009) Is physical therapy more beneficial than unsupervised home exercise in treatment of post surgical knee disorders? A systematic review. Knee 16(3):171–175

Eitzen I, Holm I et al (2009) Preoperative quadriceps strength is a significant predictor of knee function two years after anterior cruciate ligament reconstruction. Br J Sports Med 43(5):371–376

Escamilla RF, Macleod TD et al (2012a) Anterior cruciate ligament strain and tensile forces for weight-bearing and non-weight-bearing exercises: a guide to exercise selection. J Orthop Sports Phys Ther 42(3):208–220

Escamilla RF, Macleod TD et al (2012b) Cruciate ligament loading during common knee rehabilitation exercises. Proc Inst Mech Eng H 226(9):670–680

Glass R, Waddell J et al (2010) The effects of open versus closed kinetic chain exercises on patients with ACL deficient or reconstructed knees: a systematic review. N Am J Sports Phys Ther 5(2):74–84

Heijne A, Werner S (2007) Early versus late start of open kinetic chain quadriceps exercises after ACL reconstruction with patellar tendon or hamstring grafts: a prospective randomized outcome study. Knee Surg Sports Traumatol Arthrosc 15(4):402–414

Heijne A, Ang BO et al (2009) Predictive factors for 12-month outcome after anterior cruciate ligament reconstruction. Scand J Med Sci Sports 19(6):842–849

Kruse LM, Gray B et al (2012) Rehabilitation after anterior cruciate ligament reconstruction: a systematic review. J Bone Joint Surg Am 94(19):1737–1748

Kvist J (2004) Rehabilitation following anterior cruciate ligament injury: current recommendations for sports participation. Sports Med 34(4):269–280

Kvist J (2006) Tibial translation in exercises used early in rehabilitation after anterior cruciate ligament reconstruction exercises to achieve weight-bearing. Knee 13(6):460–463

Kvist J, Good L et al (2007) Changes in knee motion pattern after anterior cruciate ligament injury – case report. Clin Biomech (Bristol, Avon) 22(5):551–556

Lobb R, Tumilty S et al (2012) A review of systematic reviews on anterior cruciate ligament reconstruction rehabilitation. Phys Ther Sport 13(4):270–278

Locke EA, Frederick E et al (1984) Effect of self-efficacy, goals and task strategies on task performance. J Appl Psychol 69:241–251

Maddison R, Prapavessis H et al (2006) Modeling and rehabilitation following anterior cruciate ligament reconstruction. Ann Behav Med 31(1):89–98

Mikkelsen C, Werner S et al (2000) Closed kinetic chain alone compared to combined open and closed kinetic chain exercises for quadriceps strengthening after anterior cruciate ligament reconstruction with respect to return to sports: a prospective matched follow-up study. Knee Surg Sports Traumatol Arthrosc 8(6):337–342

Myer GD, Paterno MV et al (2006) Rehabilitation after anterior cruciate ligament reconstruction: criteria-based progression through the return-to-sport phase. J Orthop Sports Phys Ther 36(6):385–402

Raynor MC, Pietrobon R et al (2005) Cryotherapy after ACL reconstruction: a meta-analysis. J Knee Surg 18(2):123–129

Risberg MA, Lewek M et al (2004) A systematic review of evidence for anterior cruciate ligament rehabilitation: how much and what type? Phys Ther Sport 5:125–145

Risberg MA, Holm I et al (2007) Neuromuscular training versus strength training during first 6 months after anterior cruciate ligament reconstruction: a randomized clinical trial. Phys Ther 87(6):737–750

Shaw T, Chipchase LS et al (2004) A users guide to outcome measurement following ACL reconstruction. Phys Ther Sport 5:57–67

Sturgill LP, Snyder-Mackler L et al (2009) Interrater reliability of a clinical scale to assess knee joint effusion. J Orthop Sports Phys Ther 39(12):845–849

Tagesson S, Oberg B et al (2008) A comprehensive rehabilitation program with quadriceps strengthening in closed versus open kinetic chain exercise in patients with anterior cruciate ligament deficiency: a randomized clinical trial evaluating dynamic tibial translation and muscle function. Am J Sports Med 36(2):298–307

Tagesson S, Oberg B et al (2009) Tibial translation and muscle activation during rehabilitation exercises 5 weeks after anterior cruciate ligament reconstruction. Scand J Med Sci Sports 20(1):154–64

Thomee R (1997) A comprehensive treatment approach for patellofemoral pain syndrome in young women. Phys Ther 77(12):1690–1703

Thomee P, Wahrborg P et al (2008) Self-efficacy of knee function as a pre-operative predictor of outcome 1 year after anterior cruciate ligament reconstruction. Knee Surg Sports Traumatol Arthrosc 16(2):118–127

Thomee R, Kaplan Y et al (2011a) Muscle strength and hop performance criteria prior to return to sports after ACL reconstruction. Knee Surg Sports Traumatol Arthrosc 19(11):1798–1805

Thomee R, Swärd L et al (2011b) Sports injuries and their rehabilitation. SISU, Stockholm

van Grinsven S, van Cingel RE et al (2010) Evidence-based rehabilitation following anterior cruciate ligament reconstruction. Knee Surg Sports Traumatol Arthrosc 18(8):1128–1144

Walden M, Hagglund M et al (2011) Anterior cruciate ligament injury in elite football: a prospective three-cohort study. Knee Surg Sports Traumatol Arthrosc 19(1):11–19

Walden M, Atroshi I et al (2012) Prevention of acute knee injuries in adolescent female football players: cluster randomised controlled trial. BMJ 344:e3042

Webster KE, Feller JA et al (2008) Development and preliminary validation of a scale to measure the psychological impact of returning to sport following anterior cruciate ligament reconstruction surgery. Phys Ther Sport 9(1):9–15

Wright RW, Preston E et al (2008a) A systematic review of anterior cruciate ligament reconstruction rehabilitation: part I: continuous passive motion, early weight bearing, postoperative bracing, and home-based rehabilitation. J Knee Surg 21(3):217–224

Wright RW, Preston E et al (2008b) A systematic review of anterior cruciate ligament reconstruction rehabilitation: part II: open versus closed kinetic chain exercises, neuromuscular electrical stimulation, accelerated rehabilitation, and miscellaneous topics. J Knee Surg 21(3):225–234

Rehabilitation of Complex Knee Injuries and Key Points

118

Andrew Ockuly, Luke O'Brien, and Robert F. LaPrade

Contents

A. Ockuly (✉)
Orthopaedic Surgery, St. Mary's Medical Center, Blue Springs, MO, USA
e-mail: ockuly@gmail.com

L. O'Brien
Howard Head Sports Medicine, Vail, CO, USA
e-mail: obrien@vvmc.com

R.F. LaPrade
The Steadman Clinic and Steadman Philippon Research Institute, Vail, CO, USA
e-mail: drlaprade@sprivail.org; rlaprade@thesteadmanclinic.com

M.N. Doral, J. Karlsson (eds.), *Sports Injuries*,
DOI 10.1007/978-3-642-36569-0_118

Abstract

A complex knee injury (CKI) is defined as an injury to two or more of the main ligament complexes of the knee: the anterior cruciate ligament, posterior cruciate ligaments, medial knee ligament complex, and ligament complex of the posterolateral corner (Goldblatt and Richmond 2003). The incidence and management of these injuries have not been well defined (Mook et al. 2009; Hirschmann et al. 2010), but this chapter applies current evidence to design appropriate postoperative rehabilitation protocols for CKIs. The stages of rehabilitation can be separated into acute, weight-bearing, and strengthening phases. The acute phase emphasizes protection of the reconstructed ligaments, preventing scar tissue formation within the joint (arthrofibrosis), minimizing hypotrophy of surrounding muscles and reducing inflammation. The weight-bearing and strengthening phases focus on exercises that achieve physiologic recuperation of the muscles acting across the knee.

Introduction

A complex knee injury (CKI) has historically been defined to occur from knee dislocation, resulting in multiligament injury. Knee dislocations are severe and rare injuries that result in disruption of more than one knee ligament (see "▸ Chap. 90, Knee Dislocations"). Dislocations, however, are not the only cause of multiligament injury (Brautigan and Johnson 2000; Hirschmann et al. 2010; Peskun and Whelan 2011). In fact, the incidence of non-dislocating injuries with two or more ligament tears is not uncommon. This chapter will cover the postoperative rehabilitation of knee injuries that result in two or more ligament tears, known hereafter as complex knee injuries (CKIs) (Liow et al. 2003). The anatomic classification system used for CKIs is shown in Table 1 (Schenck 2003). The four main ligament stabilizers of the knee are the anterior cruciate ligament (ACL), posterior cruciate ligaments (PCL), medial knee ligament complex, and ligament complex of the posterolateral corner (PLC) (Goldblatt and Richmond 2003). The medial ligament complex is comprised of the posterior oblique ligament and superficial and deep medial collateral ligaments. This complex is commonly referred to as the medial collateral ligament (MCL) (LaPrade and Wijdicks 2012). The main structures of the PLC are the fibular collateral ligament, popliteofibular ligament, and popliteus tendon. The tendon of the popliteus muscle has been considered the "fifth ligament" of the knee and has been incorporated into the anatomic PLC reconstruction (see "▶ Chap. 72, Anatomy and Biomechanics of the Knee") (LaPrade et al. 2004; McCarthy et al. 2010). The incidence and management of these injuries have not been well defined (Mook et al. 2009; Hirschmann et al. 2010).

Following surgery for a CKI, effective communication between the surgeon, physical therapist, and patient is essential to develop an appropriate rehabilitation plan. The variability of structures injured in CKIs dictates that no one protocol will suit all patients and injuries. One approach to rehabilitation planning is to develop a protocol based on the most vulnerable reconstructed or repaired anatomical structure. The protocol should involve range of motion (ROM), bracing, and weight-bearing limitations designed to protect that structure. The protocols for ACL tears/reconstructions (Table 1: KDI) have been studied at length and will not be focused on here (see "▶ Chap. 105, Perioperative and Postoperative Anterior Cruciate Ligament Rehabilitation Focused on Soft Tissue Grafts") (van Grinsven et al. 2010). The KDII through KDV (and KDI with PCL tear) injuries involve the PCL which requires the strictest protocol for rehabilitation (Schenck 2003). Therefore, the PCL protocol will determine the advancement for CKI postoperative therapy (Pierce et al. 2012).

Table 1 Anatomic knee dislocation classification (Schenck 2003)

Classification	Injury
KDI	Knee dislocation with one intact cruciate ligament
KDII	Bi-cruciate tear, collaterals intact
KDIII	Bi-cruciate tear, one collateral torn (KDIIIM for MCL tear, KDIIIL for PLC tear)
KDIV	All four main ligaments torn
KDV	Periarticular fracture/dislocation with all four ligaments torn
C	Arterial injury
N	Nerve injury

General Principles of Acute Phase (Week 0–6)

Ligament Healing Process

The healing of injured ligaments involves hemorrhage, inflammation, repair, and remodeling (DeLee et al. 2010). Injury to the cell matrix and adjacent blood vessels leads to hemorrhage which initiates inflammation. Inflammatory mediators are released from the damaged cells and vascular endothelium to promote vasodilatation, increased blood flow, migration of inflammatory cells, and vascular permeability. This presents clinically as swelling, erythema, increased temperature, pain, and impaired function, which lasts for 48–72 h. Blood continues to fill the injured site and forms a hematoma and clot that becomes the structure for vascular and fibroblast invasion. Cell debris and necrotic tissue are removed by macrophages, and the infiltrating fibroblasts initiate the repair stage. Repair is achieved by proliferation and synthesis of new matrix replacing the necrotic tissue. This also occurs within 48–72 h of injury and forms a soft, loose fibrous matrix. Vascular buds appear within 3–4 days, allowing blood flow to the new tissue. Repair continues for several weeks increasing density of type I collagen along lines of stress, strengthening the tissue. This matrix continues to change as the remodeling phase begins within several weeks of the injury, noted by decreasing numbers of fibroblasts and macrophages. Matrix orientation continues to align in response to loads applied to the tissue, achieving 50–70 % of normal tensile strength. This decrease in strength is due to the infiltration of type V collagen which is weaker than the normally present type I collage. However, there is little clinical effect due to the increased volume of the healing ligament. Most remodeling signs disappear within 4–6 months but may actually continue for years in some patients (DeLee et al. 2010).

Precautions

There are many precautions that must be considered during the initial phase of rehabilitation to maximize the healing process and minimize future complications. These principles should be initiated on the first postoperative day and followed throughout the acute phase to yield the best results. The goals are to protect the reconstructed ligaments, to restore symmetrical ROM, and to limit and manage inflammation.

Bracing

One potential complication following surgery for CKIs is residual joint laxity as a result of graft elongation. Frontal plane alignment can help clinicians determine a patient's potential susceptibility for graft elongation, especially for treatment of chronic knee ligament injuries, with valgus alignment related to residual medial knee instability and varus alignment with lateral instability. The effect of gravity is the largest risk factor in PCL graft elongation. In unsupported positions, gravity creates posterior tibial translation or "tibial sag," which increases the distance between the femoral and tibial attachment sites, straining the PCL graft and preventing healing at the correct length (Jung et al. 2008). Attempts to limit tibial sag have included cylindrical casting in full extension (Jung et al. 2008) and use of a knee immobilizer (Johnson 2009). These techniques use additional padding on the posterior tibia to supply an anterior force, but they have not been evaluated for biomechanical efficacy (Jansson et al. 2012). Additionally, immobilization is known to contribute to increased muscle hypotrophy and joint stiffness (D'Antona et al. 2007; Mook et al. 2009). More recently, the PCL Jack brace (Albrecht, Stephanskirchen, Germany) was developed to prevent tibial sag by directing a constant anterior force on the posterior aspect of the proximal tibia. Use of this brace has been reported to decrease PCL laxity at 12 and 24 month follow-up, with patients reporting good to excellent functional outcomes (Jacobi et al. 2010). Similar to other hinged braces, it prevents varus and valgus stress, which simultaneously protects the collateral ligaments. The brace itself has an upper thigh and leg component connected by the hinge component at the knee. The springs inside the brace, providing the anterior force, can be loaded in up to 15 positions. Each setting corresponds with an increasing translational force, allowing the practitioner to adjust the brace for the individual patient (Jansson et al. 2012). The hinge of the brace has two settings: unlocked and with limited ROM between 0° and 90°. The Jack brace is applied as soon as tolerated by the patient postsurgically, using the 0–90° setting, and should be worn at all times (including sleep) for the first 24 weeks. Removal of the brace is only allowed when the knee is in full extension and the quadriceps muscles are contracted (position used for showering) and while the patient is prone. The length of brace application is patient specific; however, it is recommended to use the brace for 24 weeks postoperatively to allow for graft maturation and an increase in ligament loading capacity (Lee et al. 2004; Spiridonov et al. 2011).

Prevention of Arthrofibrosis

Due to the typically extensive nature of CKI surgeries and the protective precautions postsurgically, the development of postsurgical arthrofibrosis may be higher in this population than other surgical groups (Steadman et al. 2008; Yenchak et al. 2011). Arthrofibrosis in the knee is primarily characterized by the abnormal proliferation of scar within the anterior interval and suprapatellar pouch. Scarring of these areas can be a significant source of knee pain and stiffness. The pain can be caused by an increase in patellofemoral and tibiofemoral joint contact pressures associated with limitations of patellar movement and is associated with a significant decrease in patient satisfaction (Kocher et al. 2002; Steadman et al. 2008). Stress on the ligaments and surrounding soft tissue from injury and consequent surgery leads to infiltration of fibroblasts and increase in extracellular matrix protein deposits (Murakami et al. 1995; Yenchak et al. 2011). This increase in scar tissue leads to joint stiffness, and as little as 3–5° of loss in extension can lead to the development of osteoarthritis (Shelbourne et al. 1991; Cosgarea et al. 1994; Yenchak et al. 2011). For this reason, prevention of arthrofibrosis is crucial for long-term patient satisfaction (see "▶ Chap. 74, Arthrofibrosis of the Knee).

Patellar mobilization and early postoperative passive ROM have been reported to counteract the development of arthrofibrosis (Noyes and Barber-Westin 1997; Noyes et al. 2000; Yenchak et al. 2011). Patellar mobilization should be performed 3–4 times a day by the patient and be reinforced by the treating therapist. Performance of isometric quadriceps sets has also been shown to mobilize the anterior interval (Wilkins 2011). Excessively aggressive rehabilitation should be avoided to prevent prolonging the initial inflammatory response (Murakami et al. 1997).

Passive ROM should be the mainstay of early rehabilitation following CKI, beginning on the first day following surgery (Shelbourne et al. 1999; Stannard et al. 2005; Steadman et al. 2008; Wijdicks et al. 2010; Spiridonov et al. 2011). Range of motion exercise has been associated with an increased speed of swelling resolution, a decrease in postoperative pain, and the maintenance of the spaces in the suprapatellar pouch and anterior intervals. Improvements in articular cartilage healing have also been attributed to range of motion exercise (Troyer 1975). Maintenance of full joint extension is essential to normal quadriceps function. It is also associated with higher levels of patient satisfaction (Kocher et al. 2002).

Early ROM decreases the incidence of arthrofibrosis and the need for additional arthrolysis or manipulation of the joint. Improved objective knee laxity has also been reported in several studies of patients who began early ROM versus patients who were immobilized postoperatively (Mook et al. 2009). Excessive ROM, however, can damage the newly reconstructed ligaments (LaPrade and Wijdicks 2012). Therefore, limiting the ROM of the knee may be necessary to protect the ligaments. One practice is to have the surgeon establish a restricted ROM for each patient intraoperatively (LaPrade and Wijdicks 2012). This restricted "safe zone" of knee motion must be communicated to the physical therapist and the patient. Biomechanical evidence suggests that this initial limitation of motion should be 0–90° to prevent shear stress on the PCL reconstruction while still allowing for the benefits of early ROM (Grood et al. 1988; Lutz et al. 1993; Pandy and Shelburne 1997; Fox et al. 1998; Pierce et al. 2012).

Prevention of Muscle Hypotrophy

Following CKIs a number of factors including pain inhibition and protected weight-bearing status lead to hypotrophy and weakening of muscles surrounding the knee (Jarvinen et al. 2005). However, hypotrophy does not affect all muscle groups equally. Postural muscles, such as the gluteals and quadriceps which have a predominance of slow twitch fibers, are more significantly affected than relative fast twitch fiber dense muscles such as the hamstrings which are involved in more dynamic activity (D'Antona et al. 2007). Therefore, resisting quadriceps hypotrophy and maintaining muscle function is imperative to produce better clinical outcomes (Snyder-Mackler et al. 1995). Function of these muscles can be maintained even while the knee is immobilized in a brace by using isometric muscle contraction exercises. Isometric exercises also activate the musculoskeletal pump which reduces swelling and mobilizes the patellofemoral joint (Wilkins 2011). Additional use of neuromuscular electrical stimulation (ES) and electromyographic biofeedback (EMB) has been reported to aid post-reconstruction recovery (Draper 1990; Ballard and Draper 1991; Snyder-Mackler et al. 1995).

Electromyographic biofeedback is the recording of electrical activity upon muscle contraction. In practice, patients are able to get immediate feedback upon muscle contraction, regardless of whether the patient sees or feels actual contraction. This feedback training has been reported to be beneficial following knee ligament reconstruction (Draper 1990). Isometric activation of the quadriceps muscles (quad sets), with or without EMB or electrical stimulation, may begin immediately after surgery and can be continued throughout the acute phase of rehabilitation (Wilkins 2011). A progression of quadriceps strengthening is accomplished with hip flexion straight leg raises (SLRs) in the supine position. These exercises should be initiated when 0° of active knee extension is present. Additional SLRs in hip extension and abduction maintain strength of the hamstrings and hip muscles (Wilkins 2011).

Weight-Bearing

Further protection of the reconstructed ligaments is achieved by restricting weight-bearing following surgery. There is an increase in inflammatory mediators in synovial fluid when full weight-bearing was initiated following osteochondral injury in animals (Green et al. 2006). Osteochondral injury is commonly seen following traumatic injury to the knee. Alternatively, interleukin-10 (an anti-inflammatory cytokine produced by chondrocytes) was more pronounced in minimal weight-bearing conditions (Green et al. 2006). Full weight-bearing following surgery strains reconstructed ligaments (Flemming et al. 2001) and can result in laxity or failure if adequate healing has not taken place. Wilkins has reported the various restrictions employed after surgery and recommended using non-weight-bearing for the first 6 weeks (Wilkins 2011). A progression to full weight-bearing and decreased reliance on crutches can then be pursued (Wilkins 2011) .

Controlling Inflammation

Inflammation and edema within the joint is reduced by the traditional regimens of rest, ice, compression, and elevation (Jarvinen et al. 2007). Ice or cold packs (cryotherapy) at 0–1 °C have been reported to alleviate pain and vasoconstrict vessels within the joint, limiting blood flow and inflammatory mediators (Ho et al. 1994; Schroder and Passler 1994). The optimal length of the "ice effect" is 25 min, applied every hour as needed for pain and swelling (Ho et al. 1994, 1995). The maximum length of application is recommended to be 30 min in order to avoid peroneal nerve palsy (Ho et al. 1995). Additional decrease in blood flow can be achieved with compression of the joint (Schroder and Passler 1994). Elastic wraps are an effective tool for applying compression. Used in concert with cryotherapy, compression has been reported to decrease edema, pain intensity, and use of pain medications and increase the muscle's activity leading to better rehabilitation outcomes (Schroder and Passler 1994). Elevation also aids in decreasing swelling and is commonly used but is less effective than compression (Schroder and Passler 1994).

Weight-Bearing Phase (Week 7–11)

Once weight-bearing restrictions are lifted, a gradual transition to full weight-bearing, while continuing to wear the PCL Jack brace, can be initiated. There is not a set time that a patient must spend weaning off crutches; however, a gradual increase in loading volume over a period of 2–4 weeks is recommended to limit the potential for overloading the joint. While the goal of this phase is to increase a patient's weight-bearing tolerance, treatment to restore symmetrical ROM and normal muscular function continues. A sample treatment plan for weeks 0–11 with restrictions is outlined in Table 2. After full weight-bearing is obtained, proprioception and balance (neuromuscular training) exercises can be integrated into the program, which have been reported to be helpful in improving knee stability after ACL reconstruction (Risberg et al. 2007). Exercises include tandem stance, heel-to-toe walking, single-leg standing, and backward walking.

Strengthening Phase (Week 12–30)

A transition in the rehabilitation program then progresses from the protection and range of motion emphasis, which dominates the initial phases, to the strengthening phase. The emphasis on strength development can occur once the patient has achieved full range of motion, possesses a joint that is not warm, and has no signs of joint effusion. For most, this transition can begin between 12 and 16 weeks.

One challenge facing physical therapists treating CKIs is developing long-term exercise programs that both respect the injured structures while providing adequate stimulus to generate gains in muscle function and strength. By defining the repetition and set parameters as well as the duration of each strength component (muscular endurance, strength, and power), the principles of periodization can be extremely useful in providing structure to and improving the outcomes of a rehabilitation program.

The use of periodized programs has been reported to be an effective method of improving strength and conditioning (Kraemer et al. 2000; Deschenes and Kraemer 2002) and has also been advocated for rehabilitation programs (Fees et al. 1998). It involves organizing exercises into cycles of training. These cycles typically have a duration of 4–8 weeks and focus on the development of a specific physiological response (e.g., muscular endurance) by varying training intensity and volume. The cycles of periodized program designed for CKI can look like the following:

1. Muscle retraining/activation – day 1 postsurgery (12 weeks)
2. Muscular endurance/stability – 12–18 weeks
3. Muscular strength – 19–24 weeks
4. Muscular power – 25–30 weeks

Table 2 Sample ROM and protection phase plan

Treatment	Restrictions
Patellar, patellar tendon, quadriceps tendon mobilization	ROM: 0–90 × 2 weeks then full range of motion
Prone passive ROM	non-weight-bearing × 6 weeks then full weight-bearing
Extension mobilization to 0	PCL Jack brace × 6 months
Quadriceps sets with progressions once no quad lag	No isolated hamstrings × 16 weeks
Stationary bike with no resistance at 6 weeks	–
Ice	–

The prolonged period of non-weight-bearing required to protect the reconstructed/repaired tissue in CKIs can cause inhibited muscular function and muscular hypotrophy in the muscle groups of the affected leg. These muscle changes provide the physiological rationale for structuring the first two cycles of training on establishing correct muscle firing patterns and rebuilding the muscular endurance and stability capability of the affected postural muscles.

Muscular Endurance Phase (Week 12–18)

Correct load prescription is important to stimulate the desired physiological response while limiting the risk of overload injury. Exercises during the muscular endurance phase are characterized by a low load, high repetition, and set structure that has been demonstrated to be effective in developing muscular endurance (Deschenes and Kraemer 2002). Exercise selection should focus on shallow range of motion, double-leg exercises, or static-hold single-leg positions (Table 3, Figs. 1, 2, 3, 4, and 5).

Muscular Strength Phase (Week 19–24)

A transition to developing muscular strength requires a manipulation of training variables to create the desired physiological change. This can be accomplished in many ways including adding

Table 3 Sample muscular endurance phase program

Exercise	Sets and repetitions
Double-leg press	1–6 sets × >20 reps
Squat progression (Figs. 1, 2, and 3)	1–6 sets × >20 reps
Static box hold with medicine ball press (Figs. 4–5)	1–6 sets × >20 reps
Single-leg dead lift	1–6 sets × >20 reps
Static lunge hold with chop	1–6 sets × >20 reps
Double-leg bridges	1–6 sets × >20 reps

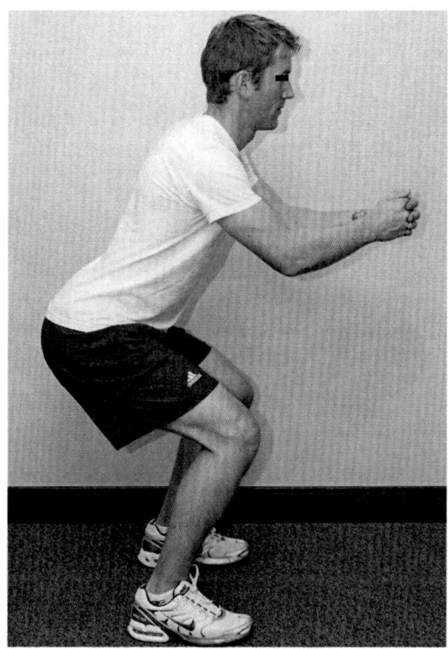

Fig. 1 Squat progression: regular squat

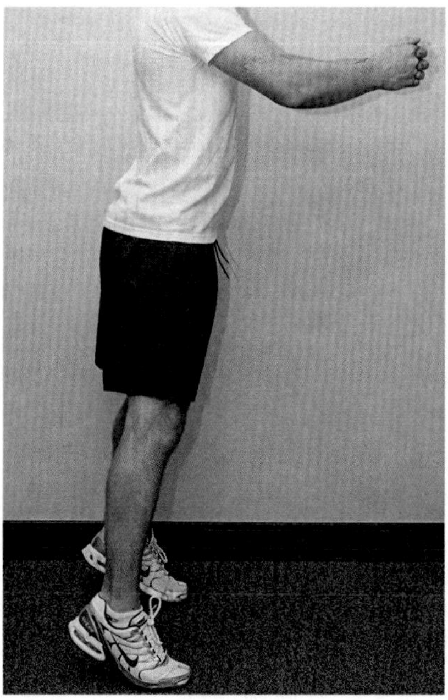

Fig. 2 Squat progression: squat to calf raise

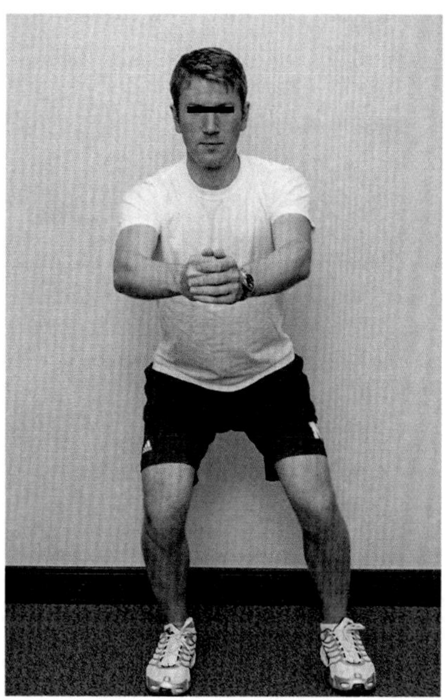

Fig. 3 Squat progression: squat to weight shift

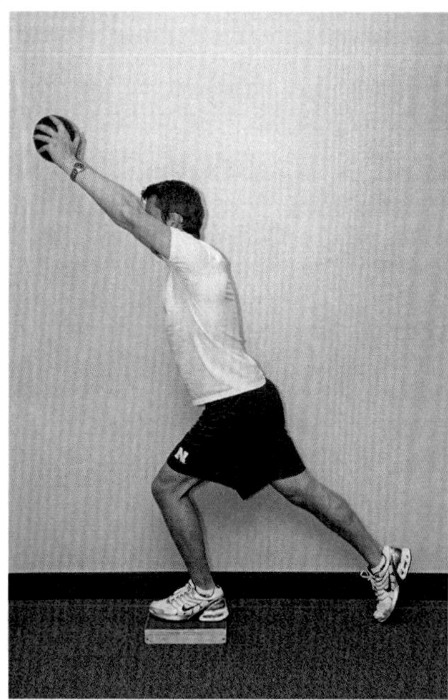

Fig. 4 Static box hold with medicine ball press: starting position

load, decreasing recovery time, and increasing the frequency of strength sessions. An effective way of increasing load in the CKI population is to add load to double-leg exercises and incorporate single-leg exercises (Table 4, Figs. 6 and 7). This manipulation of load should be such that the 8–12 repetitions of each exercise should be able to be completed with sound form.

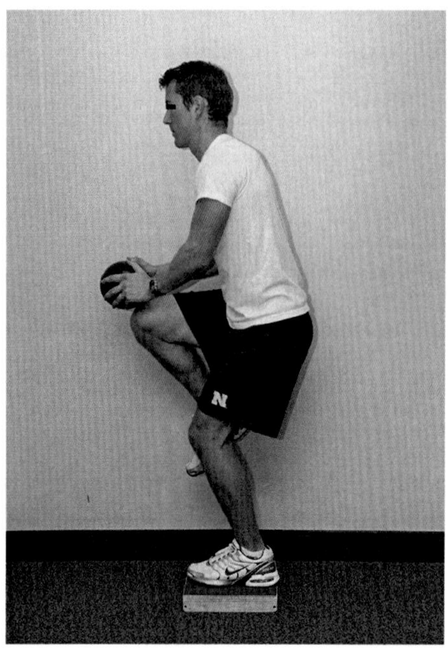

Fig. 5 Static box hold with medicine ball press: finishing position

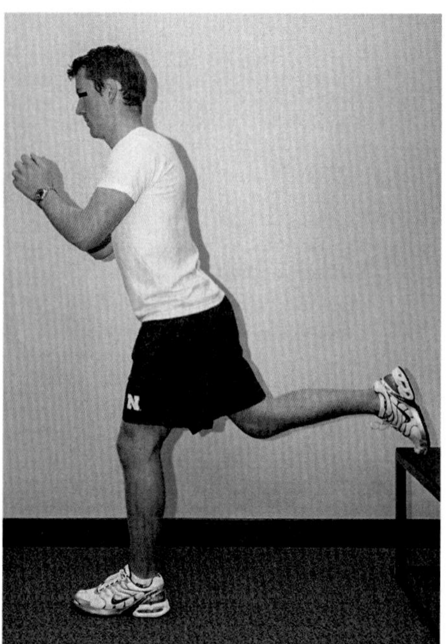

Fig. 6 Balance squat: starting position

Table 4 Sample muscular strength phase program

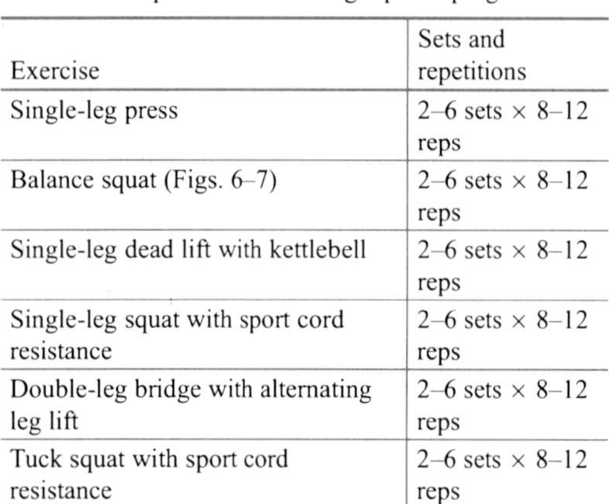

Exercise	Sets and repetitions
Single-leg press	2–6 sets × 8–12 reps
Balance squat (Figs. 6–7)	2–6 sets × 8–12 reps
Single-leg dead lift with kettlebell	2–6 sets × 8–12 reps
Single-leg squat with sport cord resistance	2–6 sets × 8–12 reps
Double-leg bridge with alternating leg lift	2–6 sets × 8–12 reps
Tuck squat with sport cord resistance	2–6 sets × 8–12 reps

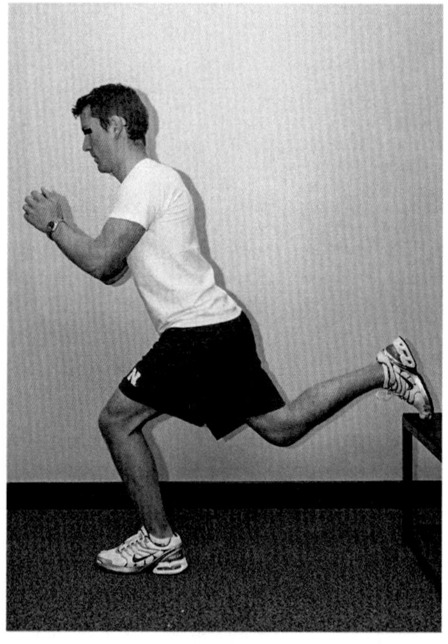

Fig. 7 Balance squat: finishing position

Muscular Power Phase (Week 25–30)

Development of muscular power requires the application of speed to the already developed strength base. Frequently, many clinicians have achieved this by incorporating jumping activity into a training program. This approach can be risky in the CKI population and may be unnecessary for patients not involved in jumping sports/activities. An alternate and perhaps safer approach is to keep the affected leg's foot on the ground while completing power-based exercises (Table 5, Figs. 8 and 9). Speed of

Table 5 Sample muscular power phase program

Exercise	Sets and repetitions
Single-leg press	3–6 sets × 1–6 reps
Prone press on shuttle	3–6 sets × 1–6 reps
High bench step-ups with leg drive	3–6 sets × 1–6 reps
Reverse lunge with leg drive (Figs. 8–9)	3–6 sets × 1–6 reps
Dead lift with Olympic bar	3–6 sets × 1–6 reps

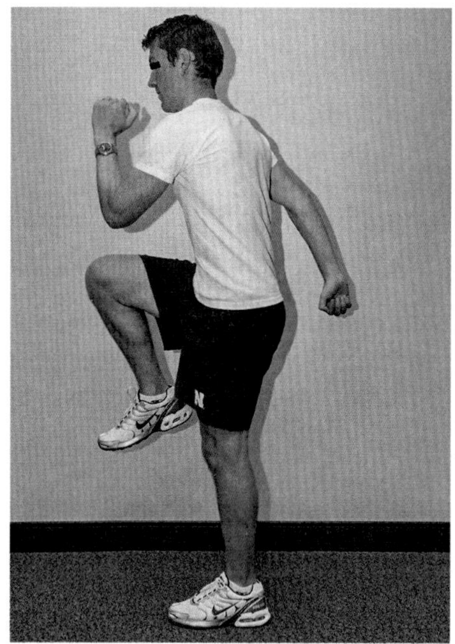

Fig. 9 Reverse lung with leg drive: finishing position

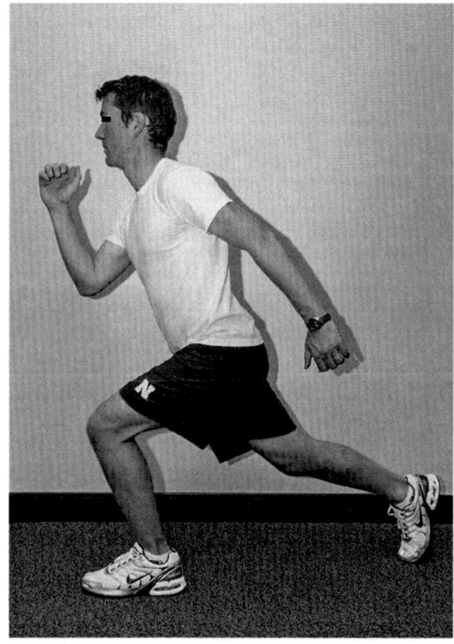

Fig. 8 Reverse lung with leg drive: starting position

Table 6 Running progression

Running progression week	Walk time (mins)	Run time (mins)	Total time (mins)
1	4	1	20
2	3	2	20
3	2	3	20
4	1	4	20
5	–	20	20

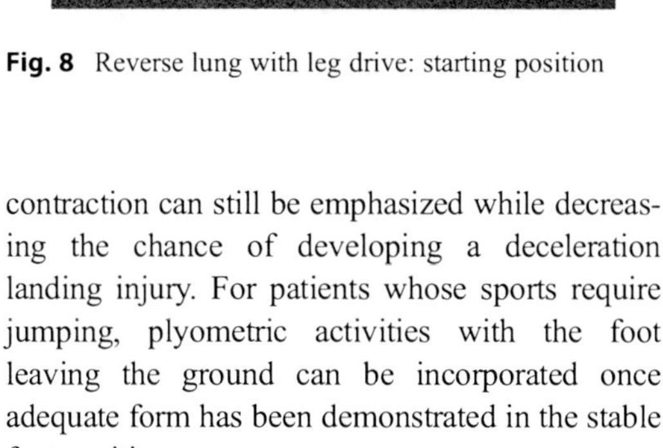

contraction can still be emphasized while decreasing the chance of developing a deceleration landing injury. For patients whose sports require jumping, plyometric activities with the foot leaving the ground can be incorporated once adequate form has been demonstrated in the stable foot positions.

For patients whose sports require running, a walk-jogging program can be started following the completion of the power program (Table 6). The volume and type of running are sport dependent and should be tailored to the patient's needs.

Conclusion

Recovery from complex knee injuries involves intensive postoperative rehabilitation. The rehabilitation sequence provided in this chapter is based on the underlying physiology of the healing process and muscle function. Although every patient should have a program tailored to their specific needs by an orthopedic surgeon and rehabilitation specialist, protocols following the evidence-based guidelines above will optimize ligament healing and knee function.

Cross-References

- ▶ Anatomy and Biomechanics of the Knee
- ▶ Arthrofibrosis of the Knee
- ▶ Knee Dislocations
- ▶ Perioperative and Postoperative Anterior Cruciate Ligament Rehabilitation Focused on Soft Tissue Grafts

References

Ballard L, Draper V (1991) Electrical stimulation versus electromyographic biofeedback in the recovery of quadriceps femoris muscle function following anterior cruciate ligament surgery. Phys Ther 71:455–461

Brautigan B, Johnson DL (2000) The epidemiology of knee dislocations. Clin Sports Med 19:387–397

Cosgarea AJ, DeHaven KE, Lovelock JE (1994) The surgical treatment of arthrofibrosis of the knee. Am J Sports Med 22:184–191

D'Antona G, Pellegrino MA, Carlizzi CN et al (2007) Deterioration of contractile properties of muscle fibres in elderly subjects is modulated by the level of physical activity. Euro J Appl Physiol 100:603–611

DeLee JC, Drez D, Miller MD (2010) DeLee and Drez's orthopaedic sports medicine: principles and practice. Sauders, Philadelphia

Deschenes MR, Kraemer WJ (2002) Performance and physiologic adaptations to resistance training. Am J Phys Med Rehabil 81:S3–16

Draper V (1990) Electromyographic biofeedback and recovery of quadriceps femoris muscle function following anterior cruciate ligament reconstruction. Phys Ther 70:11–17

Fees M, Decker T, Snyder-Mackler L et al (1998) Upper extremity weight-training modifications for the injured athlete: a clinical perspective. Am J Sports Med 26:732–742

Flemming BC, Renstrom PA, Beynnon BD et al (2001) The effect of weightbearing and external loading on anterior cruciate ligament strain. J Biomech 34:163–170

Fox RJ, Harner CD, Sakane M et al (1998) Determination of the in situ forces in the human posterior cruciate ligament using robotic technology: a cadaveric study. Am J Sports Med 26:395–401

Goldblatt JP, Richmond JC (2003) Anatomy and biomechanics of the knee. Oper Tech Sports Med 11:172–186

Green DM, Noble PC, Bocell JR et al (2006) Effect of early full weight-bearing after joint injury on inflammation and cartilage degradation. J Bone Joint Surg 88:2201–2209

Grood ES, Stowers SF, Noyes FR (1988) Limits of movement in the human knee: effect of sectioning the posterior cruciate ligament and posterolateral structures. J Bone Joint Surg Am 70:88–97

Hirschmann MT, Iranpour F, Muller W et al (2010) Surgical treatment of complex bicruciate knee ligament injuries in elite athletes: what long-term outcome can we expect? Am J Sports Med 38:1103–1109

Ho SS, Coel MN, Kagawa R et al (1994) The effects of ice on blood flow and bone metabolism in knees. Am J Sports Med 22:537–540

Ho SS, Illgen RL, Meyer RW et al (1995) Comparison of various icing times in decreasing bone metabolism and blood flow in the knee. Am J Sports Med 23:74–76

Jacobi M, Reischl N, Wahl P et al (2010) Acute isolated injury of the posterior cruciate ligament treated by a dynamic anterior drawer brace: a preliminary report. J Bone Joint Surg Br 92:1381–1384

Jansson KS, Costello KE, O'Brien L et al (2012) A historical perspective of PCL bracing. Knee Surg Sports Traumatol Arthrosc. 21:1064–1070 doi:10.1007/s00167-012-2048-9

Jarvinen TA, Jarvinen TL, Kaariainen M et al (2005) Muscle injuries: biology and treatment. Am J Sports Med 33:745–764

Jarvinen TAH, Jarvinen TLN, Kaariainen M et al (2007) Muscle injuries: optimizing recovery. Best Pract Res Clin Rheumatol 21:317–331

Johnson D (2009) Posterior cruciate ligament injuries: my approach. Oper Tech Sports Med 17:167–174

Jung YB, Tae SK, Lee YS et al (2008) Active non-operative treatment of acute isolated posterior cruciate ligament injury with cylinder cast immobilization. Knee Surg Sports Traumatol Arthrosc 16:729–733

Kocher MS, Steadman JR, Briggs K et al (2002) Determinants of patient satisfaction with outcome after anterior cruciate ligament reconstruction. J Bone Joint Surg Am 84:1560–1572

Kraemer WJ, Ratamess N, Fry AC et al (2000) Influence of resistance training volume and periodization on physiological and performance adaptations in collegiate women tennis players. Am J Sports Med 28:626–633

LaPrade RF, Wijdicks CA (2012) The management of injuries to the medial side of the knee. J Orthop Sports Phys Ther 42:221–233

LaPrade RF, Johansen S, Wentorf FA et al (2004) An analysis of an anatomical posterolateral knee reconstruction: an in vitro biomechanical study and development of a surgical technique. Am J Sports Med 32:1405–1414

Lee CA, Meyer JV, Shilt JS et al (2004) Allograft maturation in anterior cruciate ligament reconstruction. Arthrosc 20:46–49

Liow RY, McNicholas MJ, Keating JF et al (2003) Ligament repair and reconstruction in traumatic dislocation of the knee. J Bone Joint Surg Br 85:845–851

Lutz GE, Palmitier RA, An KN et al (1993) Comparison of tibiofemoral joint forces during open-kinetic-chain and closed-kinetic-chain exercises. J Bone Joint Surg Am 75:732–739

McCarthy M, Camarda L, Wijdicks CA et al (2010) Anatomic posterolateral knee reconstructions require a popliteofibular ligament reconstruction through a tibial tunnel. Am J Sports Med 38:1674–1681

Mook WR, Miller MD, Diduch DR et al (2009) Multiple-ligament knee injuries: a systematic review of the timing of operative intervention and postoperative rehabilitation. J Bone Joint Surg Am 91:2946–2957

Murakami S, Muneta T, Furuya K et al (1995) Immunohistologic analysis of synovium in infrapatellar fat pad after anterior cruciate ligament injury. Am J Sports Med 23:763–768

Murakami S, Muneta T, Ezura Y et al (1997) Quantitative analysis of synovial fibrosis in the infrapatellar fat pad before and after anterior cruciate ligament reconstruction. Am J Sports Med 25:29–34

Noyes FR, Barber-Westin SD (1997) Reconstruction of the anterior and posterior cruciate ligaments after knee dislocation: use of early protected postoperative motion to decrease arthrofibrosis. Am J Sports Med 25:769–778

Noyes FR, Berrios-Torres S, Barber-Westin SD et al (2000) Prevention of permanent arthrofibrosis after anterior cruciate ligament reconstruction alone or combined with associated procedures: a prospective study in 443 knees. Knee Surg Sports Traumatol Arthrosc 8:196–206

Pandy MG, Shelburne KB (1997) Dependence of cruciate-ligament loading on muscle forces and external load. J Biomech 30:1015–1024

Peskun CJ, Whelan DB (2011) Outcomes of operative and nonoperative treatment of multiligament knee injuries: an evidence based review. Sports Med Arthrosc Rev 19:167–173

Pierce CM, O'Brien L, Griffin LW et al. (2012) Posterior cruciate ligament tears: functional and postoperative rehabilitation. Knee Surg Sport Traumatol Arthrosc 20. doi: 10.1007/s00167-012-1970-1

Risberg MA, Holm I, Myklebust G et al (2007) Neuromuscular training versus strength training during first 6 months after anterior cruciate ligament reconstruction: a randomized clinical trial. Phys Ther 87:737–750

Schenck R (2003) Classification of knee dislocations. Oper Tech Sports Med 11:193–198

Schroder D, Passler HH (1994) Combination of cold and compression after knee surgery: a prospective randomized study. Knee Surg Sports Traumatol Arthrosc 2:158–165

Shelbourne KD, Wilckens JH, Mollabashy A et al (1991) Arthrofibrosis in acute anterior cruciate ligament reconstruction: the effect of timing of reconstruction and rehabilitation. Am J Sports Med 19:332–336

Shelbourne KD, Davis TJ, Patel DV (1999) The natural history of acute, isolated, nonoperatively treated posterior cruciate ligament injuries: a prospective study. Am J Sports Med 27:276–283

Snyder-Mackler L, Delitto A, Bailey SL et al (1995) Strength of the quadriceps femoris muscle and functional recovery after reconstruction of the anterior cruciate ligament. J Bone Joint Surg Am 77:1166–1173

Spiridonov SI, Slinkard NJ, LaPrade RF (2011) Isolated and combined grade-III posterior cruciate ligament tears treated with double-bundle reconstruction with use of endoscopically placed femoral tunnels and grafts: operative technique and clinical outcomes. J Bone Joint Surg Am 93:1773–1780

Stannard JP, Brown SL, Farris RC et al (2005) The posterolateral corner of the knee: repair versus reconstruction. Am J Sports Med 33:881–888

Steadman JR, Dragoo JL, Hines SL et al (2008) Arthroscopic release for symptomatic scarring of the anterior interval of the knee. Am J Sports Med 36:1763–1769

Troyer H (1975) The effect of short-term immobilization on the rabbit knee joint cartilage. Clin Orthop Relat Res 107:249–257

van Grinsven S, van Cingel REH, Holla CJM et al (2010) Evidence-based rehabilitation following anterior cruciate ligament reconstruction. Knee Surg Sports Traumatol Arthrosc 18:1128–1144

Wijdicks CA, Griffith CJ, Johansen S et al (2010) Injuries to the medial collateral ligament and associated medial structures of the knee. J Bone Joint Surg Am 92:1266–1280

Wilkins SA (2011) Rehabilitation of the multiple ligament injured knee. Tech Knee Surg 10:2–10

Yenchak AJ, Wilk KE, Arrigo CA et al (2011) Criteria-based management of an acute multistructure knee injury in a professional football player: a case report. J Orthop Sports Phys Ther 41:675–686

Return to Play After Acute Patellar Dislocation

119

J. Paul Schroeppel, Jill Monson, and Elizabeth A. Arendt

Contents

Abstract

Primary traumatic patellar dislocation is a knee injury primarily encountered among young active athletes. Over recent decades, the medial patellofemoral ligament (MPFL) has been identified as the primary soft tissue restraint to lateral patellar dislocation/instability. Although acute surgical management has been explored, physiotherapy and *nonsurgical management* remain the mainstay of treatment after primary lateral *patellar dislocation*. Questions persist regarding optimal immobilization, bracing, taping, and physiotherapy regimens. *Return to play* programs should involve an individualized progression through objective knee and functional limb variables, supervised by a trained professional. The ultimate goal of management is to minimize recurrence and return athletes to previous level of play.

Introduction

Primary traumatic patellar dislocation is a knee injury encountered among young active athletes (Fig. 1); it is the second most common cause of traumatic hemarthrosis of the knee (DeHaven 1980; Harilainen et al. 1988). Although once considered a condition associated with sedentary, overweight, adolescent females, the literature has reported that this injury occurs most commonly during sporting activities, with the knee in a position near terminal extension with an axial-valgus

J.P. Schroeppel (✉)
Department of Orthopedics and Sports Medicine, University of Kansas Medical Center, Kansas, KS, USA
e-mail: jschroeppel@kumc.edu

J. Monson
University Orthopaedic Therapy Center, Minneapolis, MN, USA
e-mail: jmonson1@fairview.org

E.A. Arendt
Department of Orthopaedic Surgery, University of Minnesota, Minneapolis, MN, USA
e-mail: arend001@umn.edu

M.N. Doral, J. Karlsson (eds.), *Sports Injuries*,
DOI 10.1007/978-3-642-36569-0_131

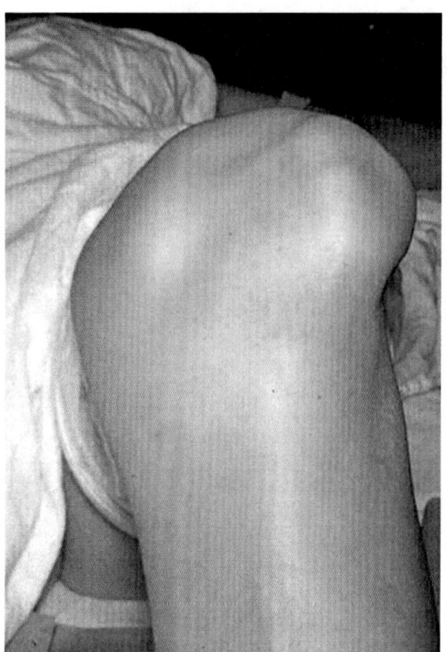

Fig. 1 Patient with a laterally displaced patella (Published with permission of © the Regents of the University of Minnesota (2013). All rights reserved)

stress on the knee during rotation (Fithian et al. 2004; Smith et al. 2011). The estimated per capita risk of first-time patellar dislocation among 10–17 year olds is reported to be between 24 and 43 per 100,000 (Nietosvaara et al. 1994; Fithian et al. 2004).

Historically these injuries have been treated with nonsurgical management, with the literature reporting a redislocation rate ranging from 13 % to 70 % (Hing et al. 2011). The high redislocation rate, combined with surgical techniques aimed at the primary ligament disruption (Feller et al. 2011), has prompted some surgeons to evaluate early operative intervention for primary traumatic dislocations. The topic of surgical versus nonsurgical acute management of primary patellar dislocations continues to be controversial. Current evidence is insufficient to confidently recommend one treatment modality over the other, and additional high-level studies are necessary to accurately identify who may specifically benefit from early surgical intervention.

Most clinicians agree, though, that nonsurgical management remains the standard of care for the treatment of most primary traumatic patellar dislocations. This chapter will discuss the biology of healing among extra-articular knee ligaments, review published nonoperative treatment regimens, and propose a preferred treatment protocol in an attempt to guide the clinician when choosing nonoperative management of this condition.

Biology of Healing

Recent years have improved physicians' understanding of the medial soft tissue restraints to lateral patellar dislocation (LPD), specifically the anatomy and injury-specific details of the medial patellofemoral ligament (MPFL). In 1948, Last described the medial anatomy of the knee joint, stating that strong retinacular fibers extend from the medial border of the patella "towards the medial collateral ligament" (Last 1948). The authors depict the MPFL, though not by name, as inserting distal to or underneath the femoral insertion of the medial collateral ligament (MCL). In Warren and Marshall's seminal 1979 anatomic work, a thorough qualitative description of the medial side of the knee was detailed (Warren and Marshall 1979). Their description was organized by a three-layer system. The MPFL and the medial retinaculum were described as within layer II, which was the same layer as the sMCL, making the MPFL an extracapsular structure. Despite these early literature reports, it was not until the 1990s that the medial patellofemoral ligament's important role in the biomechanics of the patellofemoral (PF) joint and PF joint injury came to be recognized (Conlan et al. 1993; Desio et al. 1998; Nomura et al. 2002).

The MPFL is a thin transverse band of retinacular tissue that extends from a point on the femur between the adductor tubercle and the medial epicondyle to the proximal two-thirds of the medial margin of the patella, deep to the vastus medialis oblique insertion (LaPrade et al. 2007; Kang et al. 2013). The MPFL provides 50–60 % of the resisting force against LPD, making it the primary ligamentous restraint (Conlan et al. 1993; Desio et al. 1998; Hautamaa et al. 1998).

Clinically, the MPFL is ruptured in 94–100 % of cases after acute patellar dislocation (Kang et al. 2013).

According to the information available, studies specific to the cellular and molecular basis of MPFL healing have not been performed. However, one can look to an analogous extra-articular medial knee structure to gain considerable insight into healing: the superficial medial collateral ligament (sMCL). Both the MPFL and the sMCL are found in the second soft tissue layer of the medial knee, as described by Warren and Marshall (1979), and because of this extra-articular location, both ligaments have a much greater propensity to heal than their intra-articular corollaries, the anterior and posterior cruciate ligaments (Woo et al. 2000; Creighton et al. 2005). Because the MCL is commonly injured, easily defined, and easily tested, it has become the prototypical extra-articular ligament for study purposes.

Animal models evaluating sMCL injury have reported that the ligament undergoes distinct phases during healing: hemorrhage, inflammation, repair (matrix and cellular proliferation), and remodeling and maturation (Frank et al. 1995; Woo et al. 2000; Creighton et al. 2005). Following a grade III injury (complete ligament disruption), the healing process initially involves retraction of the disrupted ligament ends and the formation of a blood clot in the ligament gap. This blood clot is resorbed and subsequently replaced with a heavy cellular infiltrate. A localized hypertrophic vascular response ensues, leading to the proliferative phase and the production of scar tissue by hypertrophic fibroblasts. Although initially disorganized, within weeks the collagen begins to align with the long axis of the ligament. Type III collagen is the first to return to the healing ligament, but this is slowly replaced with the type I collagen that is more characteristic of the native ligament. During the remodeling phase the ligaments gradually return to a near-normal state, but some differences will persist. Among the biomechanical differences of native and scarred ligaments are mildly decreased viscoelastic properties (80–90 % of normal), inferior creep properties, and inferior load to failure values (Frank et al. 1995).

Variables that impact healing appear to be the size of ligamentous disruption, location of injury, and relative motion. Loitz-Ramage et al. found injuries that created a larger ligament gap that had inferior biomechanical properties when compared to relatively smaller gaps and that these changes persisted long term, at 104 weeks after injury (Loitz-Ramage et al. 1997). When evaluating the location of injury in animal models, Frank et al. analyzed three areas of the MCL: femoral origin, tibial insertion, or mid-substance, and compared their healing response (Frank et al. 1995). This study suggested that rabbit MCLs, injured near either ends, healed more slowly than the mid-substance injury and often developed abnormal insertional morphology. Nakamura et al. prospectively studied the location of MCL injury among 17 patients with combined ACL injury (Nakamura et al. 2003). They found most proximal sMCL injuries went on to heal nonoperatively, but all five patients who demonstrated diffuse injury to the sMCL required surgical intervention. Isolated distal injury to the sMCL was not present in this cohort and was unable to be specifically analyzed.

If one were to correlate the known biology of MCL healing to the MPFL, one would need to consider whether the location of the lesion is associated with improved healing and whether the degree of knee motion in the early phase of healing is associated with improved healing.

Similarly, the location of injury has been frequently discussed as it relates to the MPFL. Studies of acute *MPFL injury* often divide the injury patterns into four types: femoral origin, mid-substance, patellar insertion, or combined injuries (Fig. 2). Authors have debated the most frequent location of MPFL injury, some citing the femoral origin as the most frequent and as many others citing the patellar insertion as most frequent (Kepler et al. 2011; Sillanpaa and Maenpaa 2012). After compiling the reported incidence of injury, Sillanpaa and Maenpaa calculated a mean reported incidence of injury location (Sillanpaa and Maenpaa 2012). The patellar insertion was implicated in 54 % of MPFL injuries, with the femoral origin identified in 34 % and a mid-substance injury in 12 %. More recently,

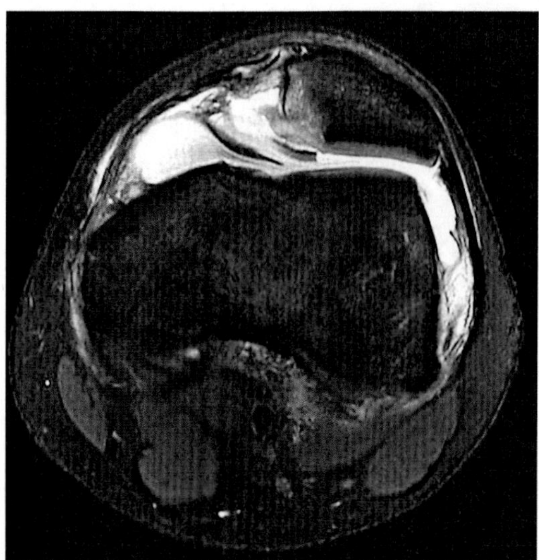

Fig. 2 Axial MRI of a recent patellar dislocation showing a tear of the medial patella femoral ligament off of the patella. An osteochondral fracture of the medial aspect of the patella is noted as well (Published with permission of © the Regents of the University of Minnesota (2013). All rights reserved)

Kang et al. proposed a new classification of MPFL injury based on the anatomic relationship to the vastus medialis oblique (VMO) (Kang et al. 2013). The authors reported that the MPFL was on average 58.8 mm in length, of which 20.3 mm was overlapped by the VMO insertion on the medial patella according to their dissection technique. These authors then divided the location of injury into three categories: the VMO overlap region, the non-overlap region, and combined injuries. They found that the recurrent instability rate of an injury to the non-overlap region was more than double that of an injury to the VMO overlap region (38.5 % vs. 15.2 %). However, this may simply represent VMO dysplasia (i.e., dysplasia of the soft tissue associated with trochlear dysplasia), both well-known risk factors associated with LPD (Dejour 1990; Nove-Josserand and Dejour 1995). Similarly, Sillanpaa et al. found that avulsion from the femoral origin predicted recurrent instability in their all-male cohort at 7-year follow-up (Sillanpaa et al. 2009).

Animal models of sMCL injury have also offered cellular and molecular information regarding immobilization. Historically, immobilization was believed to be necessary to protect ligaments, namely, the sMCL, from stress while healing. In 1946, Richman and Barnes advocated 6–10 weeks of immobilization to successfully treat sMCL injuries nonoperatively (Richman and Barnes 1946). More than three decades later, Indelicato (1983) and Fetto and Marshall (1978) recommended 2 and at least 4 weeks, respectively, for nonoperative management of a grade III isolated sMCL injury. It has been reported in the laboratory in animal models though that immobilization results in less organized collagen fibrils, decreases in structural properties of the bone-ligament-bone complex, and other detrimental effects to knee biomechanics (Woo et al. 2000). Noyes specifically analyzed the effects to the bone-ligament complex following 8 weeks of total-body plaster immobilization of the Rhesus monkey (Noyes 1977). Among his findings were a significant decrease in maximum load to failure, dramatic change to the ligament load-elongation behavior, and reduced bone density and mineralization which had a direct negative impact on the tibial insertion of the sMCL. Furthermore, clinical studies have demonstrated that even short periods of rigid immobilization are harmful to the bone, cartilage, ligaments, tendons, and muscles and cause substantial atrophy of affected tissues (Kannus et al. 1992). An improved understanding of immobilization has driven contemporary rehabilitation protocols to encourage immediate range-of-motion exercises and early weight bearing as pain and swelling will allow (Reider et al. 1994).

Despite the negative effects of immobilization, stability is important in creating an environment conducive to ligament healing. Anderson et al. compared isolated MCL injuries in rabbits to injuries of the sMCL, ACL, and medial meniscus (Anderson et al. 1992). They found that the additional instability of combined knee injury had deleterious effects on the ability of the MCL to heal and that the sMCL in this injury setting demonstrated a larger healing mass (scar) and inferior ligament mechanical properties. Clinical literature also supports the importance of identifying concomitant ligamentous injury and treating it appropriately. Multiple authors have demonstrated that restoring cruciate stability will facilitate satisfactory healing of most high-grade sMCL injuries without repair (Indelicato 1983; Noyes and Barber-Westin 1995; Millett et al. 2004).

As knowledge of ligament healing has grown, so too has the number of potential targets to stimulate a more "normal" healed ligament. Among those studied are controlled motion, hyperbaric oxygen, energy application, growth factors, tissue engineering, and gene therapy. These areas will continue to be a focus of further investigation and may offer promising adjuncts to conservative management in the future. These may be of value to augment what is fundamental to successful nonoperative management, that is, appropriate and directed rehabilitation following this injury.

Nonsurgical Management of Acute Patellar Dislocation

Nonoperative management has been the mainstay of treatment for the acute primary patellar dislocation. Despite this fact, very little literature exists to support an optimal rehabilitation method to treat this injury. In addition, few well-designed studies compare type or duration of immobilization or investigate optimal patellar bracing patterns during rehabilitation. Most studies do share similar characteristics among their rehabilitation protocols, but future study is required to determine the best management. No study to date has stratified ultimate outcomes with the patient profile and imaging characteristics that are known risk factors for recurrence (Maenpaa and Lehto 1995; Fithian et al. 2004; Fisher et al. 2010; Lewallen et al. 2013).

Rehabilitation protocols begin with the goals of controlling the effusion, limiting pain, and returning joint range of motion to its pre-injury state. The ultimate goal is to minimize the risk of recurrence. The literature cannot help in determining the best method to accomplish these goals. Some authors also advocate taping as a means of early swelling reduction, pain control, and patellar stabilization (McConnell 2007; Rood et al. 2012). The role of immobilization continues to be debated, with advocates for both immobilization and early motion. Significant heterogeneity exists between studies regarding the technique and duration of initial immobilization. The immobilization period has been reported to range from zero to 6 weeks, and has included splinting, bracing, and cylinder casting among other techniques. In 1977, Cofield and Bryan reported on their retrospective cohort of 48 acute patellar dislocations with a minimum of 5-year follow-up (Cofield and Bryan 1977). Although most patients were immobilized for 3–4 weeks, they found no identifiable difference between those not immobilized and those immobilized for up to 6 weeks. Larsen and Lauridsen treated the first episode of dislocation among their cohort of 79 knees with either elastic bandage or plaster cast. They found that clinical outcome and recurrent dislocation were independent of immobilization technique (Larsen and Lauridsen 1982).

In regard to the degree of knee motion in the early post-injury phase, one must consider the goal of immobilization. If the goal of immobilization is to help the MPFL heal in its most favorable (shortened) length, then it would logically follow that full extension be avoided, to limit superior movement of the patella associated with quadriceps contraction in extension. Flexion also helps to stabilize the patella within the trochlear groove, with confinement of the patella performed by the bony anatomy and not its soft tissue tethers, giving the soft tissue a less stressful healing environment. Indeed, the early studies of MCL nonoperative treatment immobilized the knee in 30° of knee flexion for 2 weeks and then limited knee flexion for 4 more weeks (Indelicato 1983). A key concern with immobilizing the knee in a fixed angle of flexion is patient compliance, as it relates to comfort and ease of motion with activities of daily living.

More recently, authors performed a meta-analysis of operative versus nonoperative management of patellar dislocation; 11 articles were deemed eligible for this analysis (Smith et al. 2011). Of those that reported on early treatment, 6 reported some period of immobilization for 2–4 weeks, and 3 allowed some motion with a limited arc. This meta-analysis suggested that

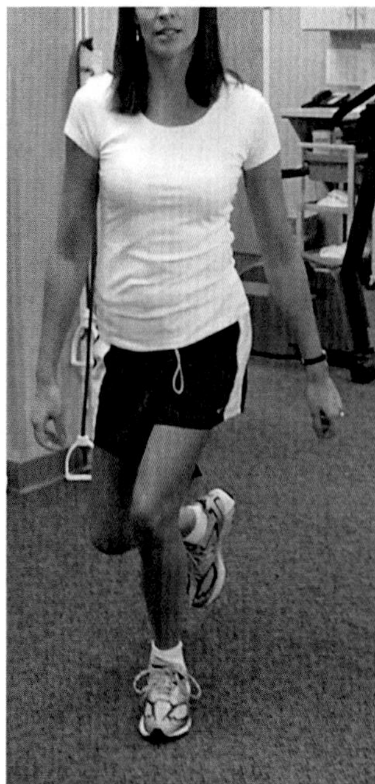

Fig. 3 Single-leg squat demonstrating functional valgus knee: hip substitution, excessive contralateral pelvic drop, femoral collapse into internal rotation (Published with permission of © the Regents of the University of Minnesota (2013). All rights reserved)

Table 1 Therapeutic treatment progression

Functional progression is used incorporating the following overlapping stages:
Patellar stability maintained
Taping, bracing
Effusion resolved
Full passive and active knee ROM
Adequate early quadriceps muscle activation
No pattern of hamstring/quadriceps cocontraction
Progression of quadriceps strength with "safe" PFJ activities
85 % LSI with quadriceps strength measures
Dynamometry
Circumferential thigh girth
Single-leg squat/step/hop activities
Restoration of normal gait pattern and speed (attention to sagittal plane knee control with loading response, frontal plane hip control)
Normal, symmetrical gluteal muscle strength
Repetitions to failure with leg lifting activities
Dynamometry
Core stability progressions
Postural limb stability/proprioceptive control
Squat retraining progression (per control and symptoms)
Static to dynamic
2 → 1 leg
Increasing squat depth
Increasing exercise intensity (per control and symptoms)
Increased external load (strength, power)
Increased speed of movement (agility, power)
Increased duration/repetitions (endurance)
Increased task complexity and directional challenge (coordination)
Sport-specific training

operative management of patellar dislocation (primary was not distinguished from recurrent) was associated with a significantly higher risk of patellofemoral joint osteoarthritis but reduced the risk of subsequent patellar dislocation compared to nonoperative management. The authors confirmed that there were significant methodological flaws including failure to differentiate between primary and recurrent dislocation, with virtually no study stratifying any outcomes according to patient- and injury-specific risk factors.

One randomized controlled trial studied patients with primary LPD utilized taping versus casting for 6 weeks followed by intense rehabilitation in both groups. This small cohort ($n = 12$) found greater activity level as judged by the Lysholm score in the taped group 5 years after index injury. There were no redislocations (Rood et al. 2012).

What is lacking in the literature is not that one *can* return an athlete to their sport after a LPD; it is rather a question of whether some period of immobilization is favored for decreasing one's risk of recurrence. Which patient benefits from immobilization, in what degree of knee flexion, and how long to immobilize continue to be an individual decision based on physician-, patient-, and injury-related factors.

During the period of joint protection following the injury, whether immobilization is employed or not, the patient will benefit from the use of a gait-assistive device to manage pain and swelling and to minimize gait pattern dysfunction. Most therapists agree that beyond the restoration of the

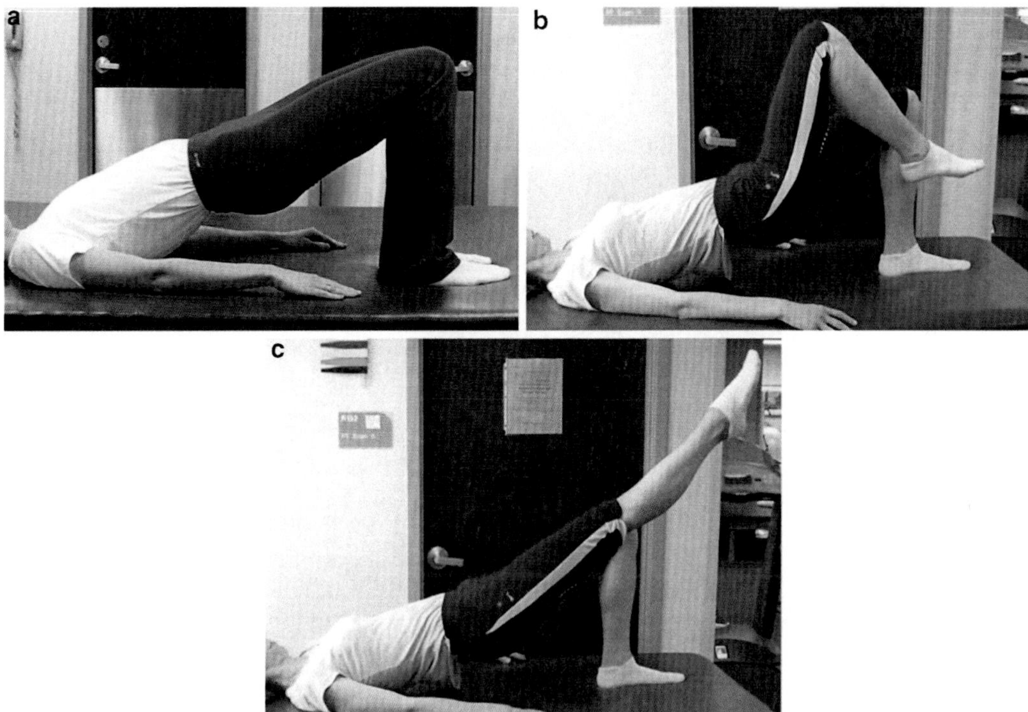

Fig. 4 Bridging exercises, commonly used to strengthen core musculature, of advancing levels of difficulty. This exercise may be performed either by repetitions or by holding the bridge position to the onset of fatigue. Image (**a**) basic. Image (**b**) intermediate. Image (**c**) advanced (Published with permission of © the Regents of the University of Minnesota (2013). All rights reserved)

fundamental impairments associated with the injury, other deficiencies should be concurrently addressed, such as gluteal weakness, quadriceps muscle dysfunction, poor core strength, abnormal lower extremity kinematics with functional tasks, hamstring tightness, or limited ankle dorsiflexion, to name a few (McConnell 2007; Prins and van der Wurff 2009; Monson and Arendt 2012).

Following patellar dislocation, several hallmark physical side effects are commonly observed. Initially, the dramatic hemarthrosis creates a significant shutdown of the quadriceps muscle (Fahrer et al. 1988; Hopkins et al. 2001). This is of significance, as contraction of the vastus medialis muscle has been proposed to "dynamize" the MPFL, reducing the extent of lateral patellar subluxation during the early angles of knee flexion through the intimate anatomic proximity of these structures (Goh et al. 1995; Panagiotopoulos et al. 2006). With the inhibition of the quadriceps muscle, it is perceivable that recurrent instability is more likely; therefore, early retraining of the quadriceps muscle in positions of enhanced patellar stability should be employed.

Another point of concern following dislocation is faulty kinematics contributing to increased lateral patellar translation. Increased lateral patellar translation is noted in the terminal degrees of knee extension in both weight-bearing and non-weight-bearing conditions. The underlying mechanism of the lateral translation differs between the two conditions, with internal rotation of the femur underneath the patella being responsible for subluxation in weight bearing. In non-weight bearing, it is the patella that is observed to translate laterally over the femur (Powers et al. 2003). Functionally, dislocation primarily occurs with weight-bearing activity, so observation of poor positional control of the femur with weight-bearing tasks should be addressed to reduce this contributor to increased lateral subluxation. In the patellofemoral pain

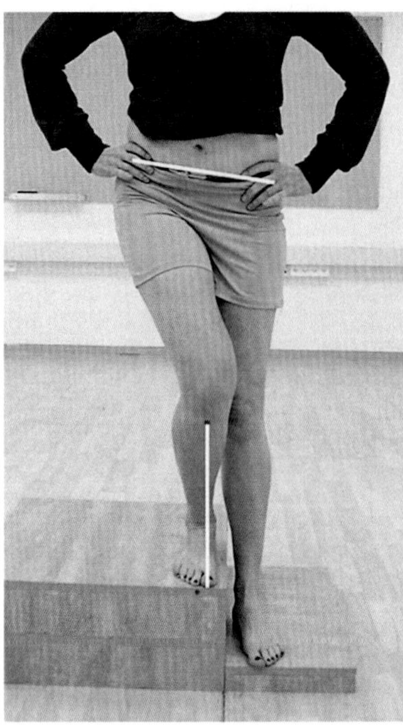

Fig. 5 Patient demonstrating contralateral pelvic drop and dynamic valgus knee, indicating lack of rotational control of the limb when performing a simple step-down task (Published with permission of © the Regents of the University of Minnesota (2013). All rights reserved)

Table 2 ISAKOS guidelines for return to sports after lateral patellar dislocation

No complaints of pain or knee instability
Full ROM/no new effusion
Test for CORE strength and endurance
Test for dynamic balance activities (e.g., SEBT)
LSI > 85 % on hop tests (+) pivoting/jumping sports
Adequate performance in physical therapy with sport-specific drills (simulate the intensity and body movement patterns of the athlete's given sport/activity)
Athlete demonstrates a psychological readiness

ISAKOS Orthopaedic Sports Medicine Committee – Almquist, F; Arendt E.A.; Coolican M.; Doral N.; and Ernlund L. Guidelines for the Evaluation, Management and Safe Return to Sport after Lateral Patellar Dislocation or Surgical Stabilization in the Athletic Population. ISAKOS Return to Play Consensus meeting, London, England, May 2012

population, increased femoral internal rotation and adduction is noted with a variety of tasks (e.g., walking, squatting, running, jumping) (Dierks et al. 2008; Souza and Powers 2009; Fig. 3). This movement pattern has been associated with gluteal muscle weakness (Prins and van der Wurff 2009). The correction of this faulty movement pattern has been associated with symptom reduction (Souza and Powers 2009; Monson and Arendt 2012).

The consideration of joint biomechanics, healing principles, and the patient's unique physical presentation minimizes a "cookbook" approach to post-injury patient care. Physical therapy should be customized to the patient's level of strength and fitness, with the exercises themselves increasing in intensity, complexity, and duration as the patient develops better strength and limb control in their activities.

The treatment progression is listed in Table 1. The challenge and complexity of therapy tasks are elevated as the patient demonstrates appropriate mastery of each component. Core exercises (Fig. 4) should be introduced early and are the base upon which other activities are built. Low-impact cardiovascular conditioning may be initiated once a baseline of adequate strength and kinematic control with closed kinetic chain activities is demonstrated. Regaining muscular strength, building muscular endurance, and restoring normal gait and daily functional movement patterns are critical during this phase. Continued pain and/or effusion control must also dictate activity progressions.

The advanced training phase involves examination of complex body movement patterns. This helps to reduce the risk of reinjury and minimize the chance of future pain in that joint. This phase is often left off or abbreviated within structured therapy settings. A foundation of basic function, with primary impairments resolved, is necessary for the mastery of more complex movement patterns. It is critical that patients receive instruction on normal and abnormal kinematics and ideally learn to detect and correct their own faulty movement patterns when present (i.e., dynamic valgus knee with partial squatting (Fig. 3)). Specific attention must be paid to not only the movement patterns and postures demonstrated with specific

Table 3 Physical performance testing elements

Domain tested	Test activity	Recorded value
Anthropometric data	Knee ROM	Degrees of motion
	Joint line circumference	Centimeters around the joint line
	Thigh circumference	Centimeters around the thigh (15 cm proximal to suprapatellar border)
Core stability	Prone plank timed hold	Seconds held, maintaining ideal alignment (out of maximum of 60 s)
	Side plank timed hold	Seconds held, maintaining ideal alignment (out of maximum of 60 s)
	Single-leg bridge repetitions to fatigue	Maximum repetitions to muscle fatigue
Balance	Single-limb balance with eyes closed	Seconds held (out of maximum of 60 s)
	Single-limb stand and reach	Centimeters reached with opposite arm of stance limb
	Star excursion balance test	Centimeters reached with opposite toe from stance limb
Lower extremity muscle strength	Single-limb maximum depth squat	Maximum knee flexion angle reached at depth of squat
	Retro step-up/step-down	Maximum step height successfully completed (inches)
Lower extremity muscle endurance	2 min single-leg repeated squat test	Maximum number of squats completed to 60° knee flexion at 60 bpm tempo × 2 min, preserving ideal trunk and limb alignment (max value = 60 squats)
Lower extremity power	Single-limb hop for distance	Maximum distance hopped in centimeters/meters
	6 m timed hop	Maximum speed recorded in seconds
	Triple crossover hop for distance	Maximum distance hopped in centimeters/meters

therapy exercises but also the patterns of muscular activation used to achieve the task. This is critical, as PF pain patients exhibit dysfunctional gluteal muscle activation and/or recruitment (Brindle et al. 2003; Cowan et al. 2009; Souza and Powers 2009; Fig. 5). The degree to which these observations are true for the patella instability group has not been studied.

The approval for clearance to return to sport is typically based on functional criteria. ISAKOS has recently produced guidelines for return to sports after a LPD (Table 2).

Although the use of functional tests is advocated in return to play after this injury, their use has been studied most as a testing tool after anterior cruciate ligament reconstruction (Fitzgerald et al. 2000; Thomeé et al. 2012). The applicability of functional testing as an assessment for return to sport after patellofemoral problems is less studied.

Summary

Nonoperative management of acute lateral patellar dislocation has the "best practice" on management. Its treatment continues to be highly individualized and varies with the patient's condition as well as physiotherapist's/surgeon's preference. Most programs advance with the monitoring of objective knee and functional limb variables by a trained professional, most often a physiotherapist. It is not clear whether there is any benefit from joint immobilization or restriction of joint motion, specifically full extension.

It is hoped that this chapter will provide the reader with the tools to fashion a safe return to activities after an acute lateral patellar dislocation. The program should incorporate at a minimum:

- Knee protection with crutches and/or limited motion until a normal gait pattern is restored
- A management scheme to restore the envelope of tissue function at each phase of rehabilitation
- Adequate performance in PT with sport-specific drills which simulate the intensity and body movement patterns of the athlete's given sport/activity prior to return to play
- Functional testing of knee muscle strength and endurance prior to return to play (Table 3)

Cross-References

▶ Patellar Dislocations: Overview

References

Anderson DR, Weiss JA, Takai S et al (1992) Healing of the medial collateral ligament following a triad injury: a biomechanical and histological study of the knee in rabbits. J Orthop Res 10(4):485–495

Brindle TJ, Mattacola C, McCrory J (2003) Electromyographic changes in the gluteus medius during stair ascent and descent in subjects with anterior knee pain. Knee Surg Sports Traumatol Arthrosc 11(4):244–251

Cofield RH, Bryan RS (1977) Acute dislocation of the patella: results of conservative treatment. J Trauma 17(7):526–531

Conlan T, Garth WP, Lemons JE (1993) Evaluation of the medial soft-tissue restraints of the extensor mechanism of the knee. J Bone Joint Surg Am 75A(5):682–693

Cowan SM, Crossley KM, Bennell KL (2009) Altered hip and trunk muscle function in individuals with patellofemoral pain. Br J Sports Med 43(8):584–588

Creighton RA, Spang JT, Dahners LE (2005) Basic science of ligament healing: medial collateral ligament healing with and without treatment. Sports Med Arthrosc 13(3):145–150

DeHaven KE (1980) Diagnosis of acute knee injuries with hemarthrosis. Am J Sports Med 8(1):9–14

Dejour H, Walch G, Neyret P et al (1990) La dysplasie de la trochlée fémorale. Rev Chir Orthop 76: 45–54

Dejour H (1990) La dysplasie de la trochlee femorale. Rev Chir Orthop 76:45

Desio SM, Burks RT, Bachus KN (1998) Soft tissue restraints to lateral patellar translation in the human knee. Am J Sports Med 26:59–65

Dierks TA, Manal KT, Hamill J et al (2008) Proximal and distal influences on hip and knee kinematics in runners with patellofemoral pain during a prolonged run. J Orthop Sports Phys Ther 38(8):448–456

Fahrer H, Rentsch HU, Gerber NJ et al (1988) Knee effusion and reflex inhibition of the quadriceps. A bar to effective retraining. J Bone Joint Surg Br 70(4):635–638

Feller JA, Lind M, Nelson J et al (2011) Repair and reconstruction of the medial patellofemoral ligament for treatment of lateral patellar dislocations: surgical techniques and clinical results. In: Scott WN (ed) Insall & scott – surgery of the knee, 5th edn. Churchill Livingstone, Philadelphia, pp 677–687

Fetto JF, Marshall JL (1978) Medial collateral ligament injuries of the knee: a rationale for treatment. Clin Orthop Relat Res 132:206–218

Fisher B, Nyland J, Brand E et al (2010) Medial patellofemoral ligament reconstruction for recurrent patellar dislocation: a systematic review including rehabilitation and return-to-sports efficacy. Arthroscopy 26(10):1384–1394

Fithian DC, Paxton EW, Stone ML et al (2004) Epidemiology and natural history of acute patellar dislocation. Am J Sports Med 32(5):1114–1121

Fitzgerald GK, Axe MJ, Synder-Mackler L (2000) A decision-making scheme for returning patients to high-level activity with nonoperative treatment after anterior cruciate ligament rupture. Knee Surg Sports Traumatol Arthrosc 8(2):76–82

Frank CB, Loitz BJ, Shrive NG (1995) Injury location affects ligament healing. A morphologic and mechanical study of the healing rabbit medial collateral ligament. Acta Orthop Scand 66(5):455–462

Goh JC, Lee PY, Bose K (1995) A cadaver study of the function of the oblique part of vastus medialis. J Bone Joint Surg (Br) 77(2):225–231

Harilainen A, Myllynen P, Antila H et al (1988) The significance of arthroscopy and examination under anaesthesia in the diagnosis of fresh injury haemarthrosis of the knee joint. Injury 19(1):21–24

Hautamaa PV, Fithian DC, Pohlmeyer AM et al (1998) The medial soft tissue restraints in lateral patellar instability and repair. Clin Orthop Relat Res (349):174–182

Hing CB, Smith TO, Donell S et al (2011) Surgical versus non-surgical interventions for treating patellar dislocation. Cochrane Database Syst Rev (11):CD008106

Hopkins JT, Ingersoll CD, Krause BA et al (2001) Effect of knee joint effusion on quadriceps and soleus motoneuron pool excitability. Med Sci Sports Exerc 33(1):123–126

Indelicato PA (1983) Non-operative treatment of complete tears of the medial collateral ligament of the knee. J Bone Joint Surg Am 65(3):323–329

Kang HJ, Wang F, Chen BC et al (2013) Non-surgical treatment for acute patellar dislocation with special emphasis on the MPFL injury patterns. Knee Surg Sports Traumatol Arthrosc 21(2):325–331

Kannus R, Jòzsa L, Renström R et al (1992) The effects of training, immobilization and remobilization on musculoskeletal tissue. Scand J Med Sci Sports 2(3):100–118

Kepler CK, Bogner EA, Hammoud S et al (2011) Zone of injury of the medial patellofemoral ligament after acute

patellar dislocation in children and adolescents. Am J Sports Med 39(7):1444–1449
LaPrade RF, Engebretsen AH, Ly TV et al (2007) The anatomy of the medial part of the knee. J Bone Joint Surg Am 89(9):2000–2010
Larsen E, Lauridsen F (1982) Conservative treatment of patellar dislocations. Influence of evident factors on the tendency to redislocation and the therapeutic result. Clin Orthop Relat Res (171):131–136
Last RJ (1948) Some anatomical details of the knee joint. J Bone Joint Surg (Br) 30B(4):683–688
Lewallen LW, McIntosh AL, Dahm DL (2013) Predictors of recurrent instability after acute patellofemoral dislocation in pediatric and adolescent patients. Am J Sports Med 41(3):575–581
Loitz-Ramage BJ, Frank CB, Shrive NG (1997) Injury size affects long-term strength of the rabbit medial collateral ligament. Clin Orthop Relat Res (337):272–280
Maenpaa H, Lehto MU (1995) Surgery in acute patellar dislocation – evaluation of the effect of injury mechanism and family occurrence on the outcome of treatment. Br J Sports Med 29(4):239–241
McConnell J (2007) Rehabilitation and nonoperative treatment of patellar instability. Sports Med Arthrosc 15(2):95–104
Millett PJ, Pennock AT, Sterett WI et al (2004) Early acl reconstruction in combined acl-mcl injuries. J Knee Surg 17(2):94–98
Monson J, Arendt EA (2012) Rehabilitative protocols for select patellofemoral procedures and nonoperative management schemes. Sports Med Arthrosc 20(3):136–144
Nakamura N, Horibe S, Toritsuka Y et al (2003) Acute grade iii medial collateral ligament injury of the knee associated with anterior cruciate ligament tear. The usefulness of magnetic resonance imaging in determining a treatment regimen. Am J Sports Med 31(2):261–267
Nietosvaara Y, Aalto K, Kallio PE (1994) Acute patellar dislocation in children: incidence and associated osteochondral fractures. J Pediatr Orthop 14(4):513–515
Nomura E, Horiuchi Y, Inoue M (2002) Correlation of mr imaging findings and open exploration of medial patellofemoral ligament injuries in acute patellar dislocations. Knee 9(2):139–143
Nove-Josserand L, Dejour D (1995) Quadriceps dysplasia and patellar tilt in objective patellar instability. Rev Chir Orthop Reparatrice Appar Mot 81(6):497–504
Noyes FR (1977) Functional properties of knee ligaments and alterations induced by immobilization: a correlative biomechanical and histological study in primates. Clin Orthop Relat Res (123):210–242
Noyes FR, Barber-Westin SD (1995) The treatment of acute combined ruptures of the anterior cruciate and medial ligaments of the knee. Am J Sports Med 23(4):380–389
Panagiotopoulos E, Strzelczyk P, Herrmann M et al (2006) Cadaveric study on static medial patellar stabilizers: the dynamizing role of the vastus medialis obliquus on medial patellofemoral ligament. Knee Surg Sports Traumatol Arthrosc 14(1):7–12
Powers CM, Ward SR, Fredericson M et al (2003) Patellofemoral kinematics during weight-bearing and non-weight-bearing knee extension in persons with lateral subluxation of the patella: a preliminary study. J Orthop Sports Phys Ther 33(11):677–685
Prins MR, van der Wurff P (2009) Females with patellofemoral pain syndrome have weak hip muscles: a systematic review. Aust J Physiother 55(1):9–15
Reider B, Sathy MR, Talkington J et al (1994) Treatment of isolated medial collateral ligament injuries in athletes with early functional rehabilitation. A five-year follow-up study. Am J Sports Med 22(4):470–477
Richman RM, Barnes KO (1946) Acute instability of the ligaments of the knee as a result of injuries to parachutists. J Bone Joint Surg Am 28:473–490
Rood A, Boons H, Ploegmakers J et al (2012) Tape versus cast for non-operative treatment of primary patellar dislocation: a randomized controlled trial. Arch Orthop Trauma Surg 132(8):1199–1203
Sillanpaa PJ, Maenpaa HM (2012) First-time patellar dislocation: surgery or conservative treatment? Sports Med Arthrosc 20(3):128–135
Sillanpaa PJ, Mattila VM, Maenpaa H et al (2009) Treatment with and without initial stabilizing surgery for primary traumatic patellar dislocation. A prospective randomized study. J Bone Joint Surg Am 91(2):263–273
Smith TO, Song F, Donell ST et al (2011) Operative versus non-operative management of patellar dislocation. A meta-analysis. Knee Surg Sports Traumatol Arthrosc 19(6):988–998
Souza RB, Powers CM (2009) Predictors of hip internal rotation during running: an evaluation of hip strength and femoral structure in women with and without patellofemoral pain. Am J Sports Med 37(3):579–587
Thomeé R, Neeter C, Gustavsson A et al (2012) Variability in leg muscle power and hop performance after anterior cruciate ligament reconstruction. Knee Surg Sports Traumatol Arthrosc 20(6):1143–1151
Warren RF, Marshall JL (1979) The supporting structures and layers on the medial side of the knee. J Bone Joint Surg Am 61(1):56–62
Woo SL, Vogrin TM, Abramowitch SD (2000) Healing and repair of ligament injuries in the knee. J Am Acad Orthop Surg 8(6):364–372

Return to Play Decision-Making Following Anterior Cruciate Ligament Reconstruction: Multi-factor Considerations

120

John Nyland, Kenneth G. W. MacKinlay, Jeff Wera, and Ryan J. Krupp

Contents

J. Nyland (✉)
Kosair Charities College of Health and Natural Sciences, Spalding University, Louisville, USA
e-mail: jnyland@spalding.edu

K.G.W. MacKinlay • J. Wera
Division of Sports Medicine, Department of Orthopaedic Surgery, University of Louisville, Louisville, KY, USA
e-mail: kgmack01@louisville.edu; jeff.c.wera@gmail.com

R.J. Krupp
Division of Sports Medicine, Department of Orthopaedic Surgery, University of Louisville, Louisville, KY, USA

SportsHealth Program, Norton Orthopaedic Specialists, Louisville, KY, USA
e-mail: ryan.krupp@nortonhealthcare.org

M.N. Doral, J. Karlsson (eds.), *Sports Injuries*,
DOI 10.1007/978-3-642-36569-0_107

Abstract

Determining the appropriate time to release an athlete that has sustained an ACL tear back to competition is not easy. The traditional focus on knee range of motion, laxity, and strength has been superseded by concerns related to the reestablishment of sufficient lower extremity power and neuromuscular control as well as more diverse factors such as reestablishing knee region tissue homeostasis, graft remodeling and ligamentization, and physiological system readiness. Overarching the biological, biomechanical, and physiological factors of return to competitive sports readiness is the patient-athlete's psychobehavioral status, which may be the most difficult component to accurately evaluate and treat. All too often, athletes are ill-pre pared for returning to competition following rehabilitation. Evidence-based criteria need to be established to better insure athlete safety when determining appropriate timing of release back to competitive play.

Introduction

Severe knee injuries during athletic play are common. The knowledge base regarding the most effective surgical, rehabilitative, and patient outcome assessment methods to treat these injuries is continually growing. Athletes often require a 6–12-month hiatus from sports for full recovery following an ACL tear, surgical reconstruction, and rehabilitation (Kvist 2004). Unfortunately, many patients never return to pre-injury sports activity levels (Biau et al. 2007). Patients often report a continued fear of knee reinjury for up to 4 years post-ACL reconstruction (Kvist et al. 2005). Athletes that successfully return to their pre-injury sports level at 12 months post-ACL reconstruction score higher on the ACL-Return to Sports After Injury Scale which assesses confidence, emotions, and risk appraisal (Webster et al. 2008).

Many patients do not return to the same sports post-ACL reconstruction despite being "physically" rehabilitated (Kvist 2004; Kvist et al. 2005), and many of those who resume pre-injury sports participate at a reduced level or with impaired function (Smith et al. 2004). In a meta-analysis of 48 studies representing 5,770 patients, Ardern et al. (2011a) reported a 63 % rate of return to pre-injury sports participation, and only 44 % returned to competitive sports by 36.7 months postsurgery. At 12 months post-ACL reconstruction, only 33 % of patients attempted competitive sports at their pre-injury level, and only 67 % returned to sports participation. A possible explanation for such a low return to competitive sports rate is the operational definition that was used. In this study, return to sports referred specifically to returning to the same level of competition in the primary sports that subjects had participated in prior to their ACL injury (Ardern et al. 2011a). Despite the same intentions to return, fewer women than men return to competitive sports by 12 months postsurgery, possibly because of greater neuromuscular and postural control deficits (Ardern et al. 2011a).

Determining what percentage of patients actually return to their full pre-injury sports participation is of greater importance than knee range of motion, isolated muscle strength, hop test, or perceived function measurements (Ardern et al. 2011a). While 90 % of patients achieve normal or nearly normal knee function based on postsurgery impairment-based measurements and 85 % based on IKDC self-reported knee function scores, it has been reported that approximately half do not return to competitive sports (Ardern et al. 2011b). No relationship was found between IKDC self-reported knee function score and patient return-to-sports rate (Ardern et al. 2011b). Athletically active patients may require a longer, more comprehensive rehabilitation progression to achieve a truly safe and successful return to competitive sports (Fig. 1).

The term "return to play" is a bit of a misnomer. Play can be defined as the engagement in activity for enjoyment and recreation. In contrast, competition represents striving to win something by defeating or establishing superiority over others who are trying to do the same. Therefore, one can assume, based on this comparison, that returning to play is less stressful and potentially less injurious than returning to competition. The surgeon, rehabilitation team, and athlete have different but equally important and overlapping roles in the

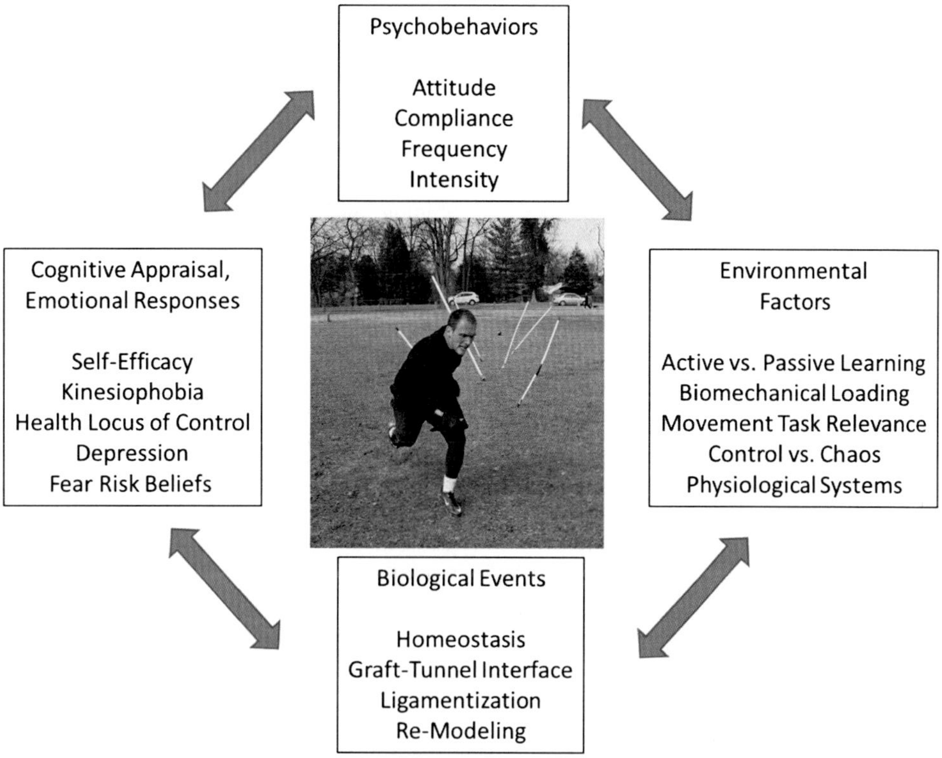

Psychobehaviors

Attitude
Compliance
Frequency
Intensity

Cognitive Appraisal, Emotional Responses

Self-Efficacy
Kinesiophobia
Health Locus of Control
Depression
Fear Risk Beliefs

Environmental Factors

Active vs. Passive Learning
Biomechanical Loading
Movement Task Relevance
Control vs. Chaos
Physiological Systems

Biological Events

Homeostasis
Graft-Tunnel Interface
Ligamentization
Re-Modeling

Fig. 1 The interrelationship between psychobehavioral and environmental factors, biological events, and cognitive appraisals strongly influences both the readiness for an athlete to return to competition following ACL reconstruction and long-term outcomes

recovery process following ACL reconstruction. The surgeon uses arthroscopy to meticulously reconstruct the injured ACL by attempting to securely place a tendon graft in the appropriate anatomical position and repair concomitant injuries to the meniscus or articular cartilage, generally in a single operative session. The rehabilitation process, however, is much longer, more arduous, more variable in problem-solving requirements, and more likely to directly influence the eventual patient outcome, assuming the surgical procedure was properly performed. The knee surgeon and rehabilitation team are concerned with the efficacy of safely returning an athlete to sports competition at their pre-injury performance level. Although surgical descriptions and acute care rehabilitation interventions are generally described in precise detail in the medical literature, intermediate to long-term rehabilitation program advancement criteria are, at best, poorly outlined, with increasing vagueness as the timetable for release to sports approaches (Wera et al. 2014). When described, decisions appear to be based primarily on time from surgery; however, this is a false assumption from a neuromuscular function standpoint (Myer et al. 2012). Recovery from an ACL tear and reconstruction involves a progression from more foundational elemental capabilities such as fully activating the quadriceps femoris muscle group during a straight leg raise movement to more functional, integrated, sport-relevant movements. To successfully integrate functional movements into the rehabilitation program, foundational elemental capabilities such as strength and knee range of motion should be well established. Reports regarding brain function (Valeriani et al. 1999), tibia and femur integrity (Nyland et al. 2010a), postural sway (Howells et al. 2011), quadriceps femoris fast-twitch muscle fiber activation (Angelozzi et al. 2012; Myer et al. 2012), vertical ground reaction force production (Myer et al. 2006, 2012), lower extremity neuromuscular responsiveness (Nyland et al. 2010b), tissue homeostasis (Dye 1996), graft remodeling and ligamentization (Claes et al. 2011; Xie et al. 2013), and psychobehavioral readiness (Brewer et al. 1993; Chmielewski et al. 2008; Langford et al. 2009; Ardern et al. 2013; Tjong et al. 2014) suggest compromised function for longer than the 6–12-month period routinely reported as the time of potential release back to athletic competition following ACL reconstruction.

Surgically reconstructing the ACL using an anatomically positioned tendon graft may resemble the native structure biomechanically; however, the neurosensory component has not been restored. No matter how innovative the surgical procedure or how carefully the ACL stump remnants are incorporated into the tendon graft, there is little evidence that supports full neurosensory restoration using existing ACL reconstruction methods. Beginning with the ACL injury and advancing through pre- and postsurgical time periods, there is a progressive erosion of athletic skills, conditioning, self-efficacy, and function. Although time postsurgery is not a valid indicator of neuromuscular control or functional readiness for returning to sports (Myer et al. 2012), it does provide reasonable insight as to the likelihood of complete graft-bone tunnel integration, ligamentization remodeling, and strength of fixation (Claes et al. 2011; Xie et al. 2013). However, current understanding of the human graft remodeling timetable is poor and is too often based on animal model studies which have limited relevance to the human condition (Claes et al. 2011). As with the able-bodied athlete, time away from sports tends to decrease performance capabilities across a broad continuum. Biomechanical, biological, physiological, and psychobehavioral factors must be considered prior to releasing an athlete back to competition.

Biological, Biomechanical, Physiological, and Psychobehavioral Considerations

Return-to-sports competition criteria need to consider more than knee joint-specific and whole-body biological, biomechanical, and physiological factors. It needs to delve into psychobehaviors, the athlete's cognitive appraisal of their situation (Walker et al. 2007), disparities between perceived and actual performance capabilities, and the linkage between biomechanical and physiological factors and psychobehaviors. The sport-specific training and release to sports phases of recovery post-ACL reconstruction represent a complicated crossroad between the patient and athlete roles (Fig. 2). In many ways, this represents poorly understood territory, likely correlating with the previously mentioned vagueness of return-to-play readiness decision-making in the medical literature. Although acute care rehabilitation following ACL reconstruction is well described, comparatively little evidence-based information exists regarding the decision-making criteria that lead to formal unrestricted release to competitive sports. The culmination of innovative and expensive surgical and rehabilitation progressions and return-to-play readiness decisions often seem to be largely left to chance. Despite advances in less invasive, more anatomical surgical approaches and early, innovative postoperative rehabilitation management, much work remains regarding the evidence basis for safely advancing patients from the end stages of rehabilitation through sport-specific training and conditioning and return to competitive sports. Many times the returning athlete has poor strength, poor fatigue resistance, and growing fear as the time to return to competition approaches (Fig. 3). This may be related to clinical testing that does not adequately stress recovering systems in a manner that can validly and accurately predict return-to-play readiness (Thomee et al. 2011).

Cognitive Appraisal Drives Psychobehaviors

Both personal and situational factors contribute to an athlete's cognitive appraisal of their injured condition. This appraisal has an ongoing influence on the athlete's psychobehavioral and emotional responses (Walker et al. 2007). In reviewing the literature, it is often difficult to firmly establish what "return to play" or

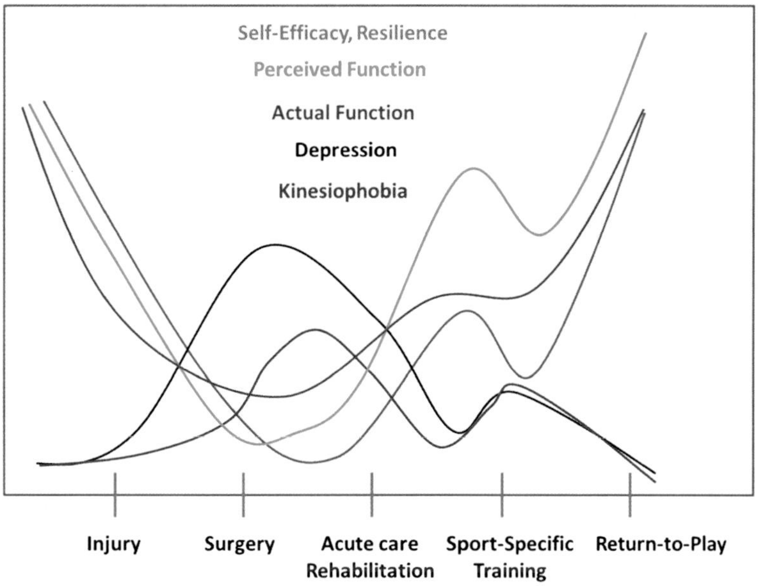

Self-Efficacy, Resilience
Perceived Function
Actual Function
Depression
Kinesiophobia

Injury
Surgery
Acute care Rehabilitation
Sport-Specific Training
Return-to-Play

Fig. 2 An example of how psychobehavioral factors such as self-efficacy and resilience, depression, and kinesiophobia may interact with actual and perceived function following ACL reconstruction. After acute or early rehabilitation, as the recovering athlete progresses through sport-specific training to return-to-play consideration, rapid changes may be observed for all factors. Of particular interest may be sudden changes in depression and kinesiophobia levels and perceived (subjective) knee function being substantially greater than actual (objective) knee function

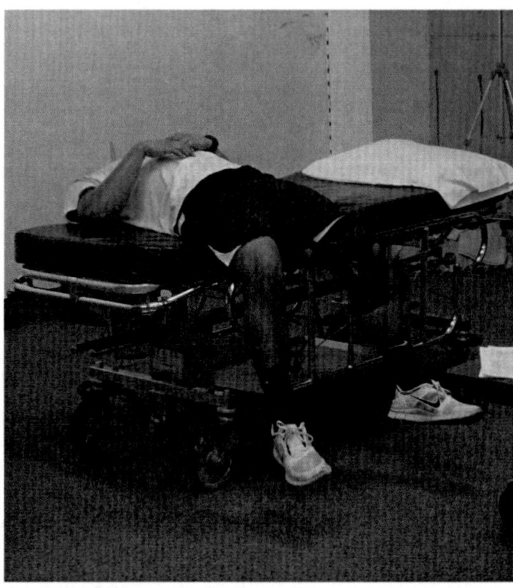

Fig. 3 The recovering athlete is often not ready for intense physical conditioning challenges. From a sport-specific training perspective, all too often, they appear to be weaker, less fatigue resistant, and more anxious regarding the return-to-play timeline than is desired

"return to activity" truly represents. Confusion often exists regarding recreational or vocational sporting activities, competitive or practice situations, sport-specific training, or routine activities of daily living. Similarly, it is often difficult to ascertain the true intensity, duration, frequency, and participation to which the athlete has returned. The athlete may have difficulty transitioning between the roles of patient and athlete at any time during the recovery process following ACL reconstruction. This is particularly true during end-stage rehabilitation. The question of when a given patient completely transitions from the patient role to the athlete role following ACL reconstruction and rehabilitation is a complicated one. Certainly if their attention is focused largely on their surgically reconstructed knee, they are not completely fulfilling the athlete role and are likely not ready for returning to sports participation (Brewer et al. 1993; Brewer and Cornelius 2010).

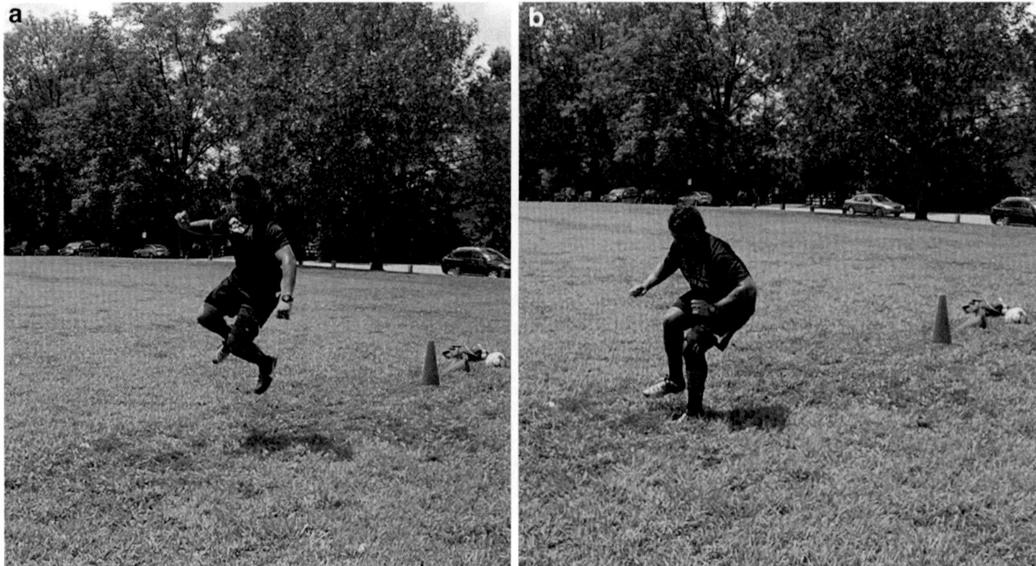

Fig. 4 Single-leg double hop for distance ("hop-go-stop") second hop mid-flight (**a**) and landing (**b**)

The "Moments of Truth"

Functionally the athlete should display comparable range of motion, strength, power, endurance, and single-leg postural control between the surgical and nonsurgical lower extremities as foundational requirements before return to sports can be considered (Paterno et al. 2007; Thomee et al. 2011; Angelozzi et al. 2012) (Figs. 4, 5, 6, and 7). During the sudden single-leg support associated with jump landings or high-speed running directional changes, the knee must be able to withstand the external flexion (sagittal plane), abduction-adduction (frontal plane), and internal-external rotation (transverse plane) "moments of truth." The external knee flexion "moment of truth" largely represents the neuromuscular integrity of the quadriceps femoris muscle group in controlling vertical deceleration of the body's center of mass during jump landings or high-speed running directional changes. These moments are largely influenced by the maintenance of proper whole-body postural alignment and coordination between the trunk, lumbopelvic, and hip regions (Paterno et al. 2010; Hewett and Myer 2011). Once equivalent bilateral lower extremity loading is consistently observed during sports movements, periodic assessment should be performed to verify long-term maintenance of this requirement. The external knee abduction-adduction "moment of truth" largely represents neuromuscular control of appropriate trunk

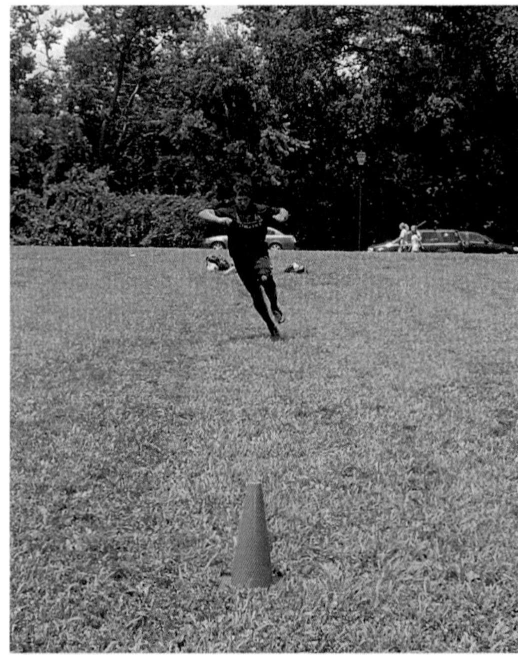

Fig. 5 Twenty meter timed single-leg crossover hop

alignment and frontal and transverse plane knee alignment during jump landings or high-speed running directional changes through pelvic deltoid (gluteus maximus, gluteus medius, tensor fasciae latae) and hamstring muscle group function (Hewett and Myer 2011).

Knee Homeostasis

Restoring knee tissue homeostasis post-ACL injury and reconstruction is a concept that has been gaining support in rehabilitation literature

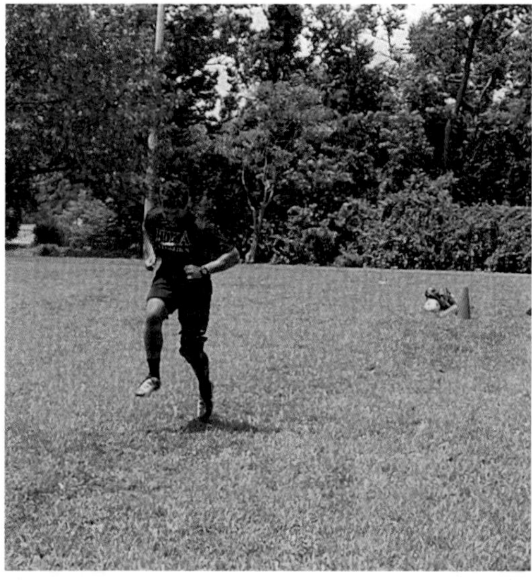

Fig. 6 Twenty meter timed single-leg hop

(Dye 1996; Nyland et al. 2010b). Based on our current understanding of tissue biology and biomechanics, rehabilitation clinicians attempt to apply the appropriate exercise dose to get the desired biological and physiological responses at differing recovery phases whether it is full knee range of motion, improved quadriceps femoris activation, or bilaterally equivalent single-leg hop test performance. To achieve this, therapeutic exercise variables such as exercise movement selection, resistance level, frequency, and total volume need to be regularly modified. In doing this, it is essential that the rehabilitation clinician and patient-athlete establish a regular, open, and honest dialogue regarding both the intensity and location of training-induced discomfort or pain experienced in the ACL reconstruction region of interest and throughout the body following each session. Quadriceps femoris and gluteus maximus muscular discomfort associated with progressive resistance exercises from a previous session may be a desired response. A lack of muscular discomfort in these areas, however, with increased discomfort at the patellofemoral joint, patellar tendon, tibiofemoral joint line, or femoral-tibial tunnel regions likely represents divergence from a homeostatic knee tissue environment. This requires rehabilitation program modification or increased recovery periods between intense training sessions. Furthermore, maintaining appropriate vitamin D (Bogunovic et al. 2010) and calcium levels and maintaining a

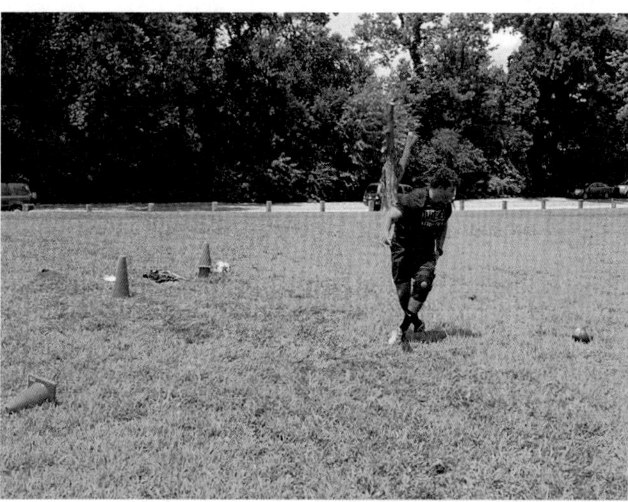

Fig. 7 "3-cone agility drill." Athlete begins in prone position. Upon cue such as "short ball tall," they move quickly to touch the "short" cone, medicine ball, and "tall" cone returning to the center of the triangle to position themselves in supine and await the next cue. Three 30 s interval test repetitions are generally performed

nutrient-rich diet and appropriate hydration in conjunction with adequate rest and recovery between training sessions help tissue healing and growth as well as restoration of knee homeostasis.

Evidence other than time from surgery is needed to determine when an athlete is ready to begin sport-specific training following ACL reconstruction. It is important to determine the time when the athlete consistently displays comparable postural stability and neuromuscular control during single-leg stance between the surgical and nonsurgical lower extremities. An example of this is the consistent display of bilaterally comparable vertical, mediolateral, and anteroposterior ground reaction forces when performing multidirectional single-leg jumps and jump landings. Restoration of tissue homeostasis as evidenced using bone scans of the tibia and femur in the ACL reconstruction region of interest, evidence of improved apparent bone mineral density throughout the surgical lower extremity, and absence of palpable discomfort in the ACL reconstruction region of interest are likewise important (Nyland et al. 2010b). Knowledge of the athlete's medication history regarding anti-inflammatory medication use or any other related or non-related medications, nutraceuticals, or supplements that might influence the rehabilitation progression is also important. These are important considerations before transitioning the recovering athlete from sport-specific rehabilitation and conditioning to intense daily sports practices (often including multiple practices/day during early preseason). The influence of added factors such as limited rest-recovery periods, possible influences of multiple sports or team participation (such as playing for both school and club teams during the same time period), and the seemingly "endless seasons" and minimal rest associated with many contemporary youth sports should also be considered.

The Rehabilitation Clinician as a Guide and Advocate

Psychobehavioral factors such as cognitive appraisal regarding injury, surgery and rehabilitation, fear of re-injury, depression, the need for self-protection, and transitioning between the patient-athlete role have the potential to strongly influence return to athletic competition success or failure (Ardern et al. 2013; Tjong et al. 2014). Therefore, the rehabilitation clinician needs to skillfully guide the patient through their transition back to competitive athletics and advocate on their behalf with coaches, parents, and other essential stakeholders for the athlete's well-being. Some type of long-term social support and advocacy is also helpful post-release to competitive sports, particularly if coaches, family, and friends are involved.

Layered Progressions, Short-Term Goals, and Performance Acuity Restoration

Safe athletic competition following ACL reconstruction and rehabilitation requires a performance acuity focus that is difficult to simulate in most rehabilitation settings. The return-to-sports decision-making process requires many layers of progressively more intense athletic movement challenges and progressively more independent task assignments, with numerous small goals. More layered, more comprehensive, and multifactor performance criteria need to be established to better guide the athlete toward a safe competitive sports return. Within each layer, many short-term goals should be established that are specific, measurable, attainable, realistic, and timely in their need to occur at a particular phase during the recovery process. Although side-to-side comparisons of lower extremity function are important, return-to-sports readiness decisions need to consider more than just the percentage of bilateral equivalence displayed by the surgical lower extremity in comparison to the nonsurgical lower extremity. Regarding intermediate to end-stage athletic movement task challenges, occasional mistakes by the athlete should be expected during their performance. If no mistakes are observed, the athlete is likely not performing at full intensity or the selected task is too easy. From the mentoring that occurs following movement challenge mistakes come motor learning insight, skill development, and confidence. Prior to return to athletic play, the athlete needs to refine their sports and position- specific skill set. After an athlete has undergone ACL reconstruction, they should understand that they require individual practice and game preparation in addition to team preparation. They also require long-term neuromuscular control maintenance training with regular follow-up. Embedded within these layers of care and multiple short-term goals is the opportunity for all stakeholders to share input during the return-to-sports decision-making process.

Subjective and Objective Patient Outcome Measurements

To achieve improved outcomes in athletes who have undergone ACL reconstruction and rehabilitation, surgeons and rehabilitation clinicians need to move beyond the current way of doing things. Traditionally, both objective and subjective criteria for return to play have focused primarily on musculoskeletal status with consideration of estimated graft and graft-bone socket or tunnel biomechanical integrity based largely on animal model study data. Little consideration has been placed on long-term knee homeostasis and even less on the psychobehavioral readiness of the athlete. Revolutionary changes are needed in the sports readiness determination process following ACL reconstruction. In our opinion, at some point, comparison with the pre-surgery level of function is not a realistic treatment goal. The low ceiling effect displayed by many self-reported function surveys that are currently used needs to be eliminated. Record-setting National Football League running back Adrian Peterson who returned to competition by 6 months postsurgery would have likely reached the ceiling of many perceived function surveys after only several weeks of rehabilitation. Care providers need to step back and reassess the validity, relevance, and effectiveness of each of the items that contribute to perceived function surveys. The "gray zone" regarding survey development, administration, interpretation regarding return-to-sports readiness, and relationships with objective functional performance testing requires more work.

As patients age, there is a natural tendency for expectations of sports activity intensity and frequency to decrease somewhat while still providing similar satisfaction levels. Clinicians need to better align and interpret end of surgical and rehabilitation care patient outcome measurements, as well as early and long-term outcome measurement timing with consideration for patient age. Too many failures post-ACL reconstruction, rehabilitation, and return-to-sports occur because essential factors such as psychobehavioral status or graft biomechanical integrity lie outside our current level of understanding and control. Multiple stakeholders are involved in the athlete's recovery, and perhaps more of them should participate in determining the return-to-play readiness of a given athlete. Perceived function surveys need to place greater consideration on psychobehavioral status and long-term quality of life considerations, in addition to age- and expectation-relevant patient satisfaction levels.

Patient outcomes at the end of surgical and rehabilitative care are not the same as return-to-sports outcome. Patient outcomes at the end of surgical and rehabilitative care merely represent the beginning of the journey for the athlete who has undergone ACL reconstruction and rehabilitation. Subjective or perceived knee function surveys often ask athletes many questions regarding their perceived sports function before they have had an opportunity to self-assess their performance capabilities based on actually attempting sport-specific performance skills. This practice has the potential to create an inaccurately high perceived function score that decreases the validity of this information and suggests that the athlete has greater functional capacity, self-efficacy, and confidence and less kinesiophobia than what truly exists. Numerous factors may influence patient outcomes. Conceivably, the timing of both objective and subjective outcome measurements should be obtained prior to surgery and rehabilitation, at the end of surgical and rehabilitative care, at the end of the initial athletic season (early), and at the end of each athletic season (intermediate) through 5 years postsurgery (long term). A better understanding of the validity of the interventions may be achieved by procuring the initial postsurgery outcome measurement with well-designed tools at the end of surgical and rehabilitation care, whether or not release to sports has been achieved at that point. The next outcome should be at the completion of the first return to sports year after release from care, approximately 2 years following surgery. Long-term outcomes should be considered at 5 years postsurgery after a multitude of potential confounding factors have had a reasonable chance to manifest. One of these factors is a change in patient expectation for sports activity satisfaction with aging. Although it may be unrealistic to believe that many patients will return for a standard 2- and 5-year reevaluation, information from these time periods is essential to answering important questions related to return-to-play decision-making. The need for longer-term, more comprehensive follow-up also supports the notion of having an extended network of stakeholders who provide input regarding functional recovery status.

Many factors such as going to college, getting a job, marriage, having children, maturing, and developing new interests may influence patient outcomes following release from surgical and rehabilitation care (Tjong et al. 2014). When an athlete undergoes successful ACL reconstruction and rehabilitation and chooses not to return to competitive sports at the same level, it should not be considered as an object failure on the part of the surgical and rehabilitation team. Therefore, an outcome following ACL reconstruction and rehabilitation that matches the natural pre-injury capabilities of the athlete and their knee should not always be expected. Clinicians need to improve existing patient outcome standards with respect to athletes who possess differing performance expectations, given the more comprehensive understanding of their injury, surgery, rehabilitation, and long-term prognosis developed over the course of recovery. Patients may become satisfied with modified sports activities through psychobehavioral adaptations. Clinicians may have helped them with cognitively appraising their injury, surgery, rehabilitation, and emotional responses. Patients such as these should also be considered as treatment successes. Return to play, sports, or competition at the same level in the same sports as prior to injury should not be the only acceptable outcome. Improvements in the expanse of an athlete's resilience and coping skills as taught by the rehabilitation team should also be factored into intervention success. When an athlete has returned successfully to their primary sports, clinicians need to have more detailed information regarding the actual intensity, frequency, and duration of play as well as their actual level of production as a player. If an athlete who has undergone ACL reconstruction and rehabilitation chooses to return to a lower level of sports participation intensity or frequency based on concerns about further traumatizing their knees, this should not necessarily be considered a failure by the surgical or rehabilitative teams.

At some level the criteria and responsibility for return to competitive sports should be shared by multiple stakeholders, and release from care timing should be related to the outcome expectation. The vigilance of care to successfully return an athlete to an occasional game of recreational basketball would likely be less than that needed to successfully return an athlete to professional basketball competition. The surgical and rehabilitation team need to have a complete understanding of the activity to which the athlete will be returning. With high-intensity, high-frequency contact sports, it behooves the athlete to be functioning optimally in each area and to continue specific therapeutic exercise interventions to maintain and further improve neuromuscular control, cognitive focus, and motor skill acuity. Competitive play, particularly in contact sports, represents chaotic events with sudden, often violent knee loading. Since ACL neurosensory function is not fully restored following injury and reconstruction, it is essential that neuromuscular control system capabilities be optimized before the athlete returns to sports (Valeriani et al. 1999; Nyland et al. 2010a, b). The longer the athlete is away from sports participation for any reason, the greater the potential for sports skill, physical conditioning, and mental focus erosion. This is compounded by ACL injury, surgery, and rehabilitation. Clinicians need to be especially vigilant to ensure sufficient neuromuscular control, lower extremity power, and performance conditioning recovery prior to advancing the recovering athlete to sport-specific training and eventual release to unrestricted sports participation.

Lower Extremity Orthoses and Footwear Interfaces

Beginning with a long-leg postsurgical brace, the athlete who is recovering from ACL reconstruction and rehabilitation may be initiating a long association with assorted orthoses and assistive devices. One of the primary reasons for undergoing ACL reconstruction is to eventually have no need to rely on a functional knee brace. However, once it is understood that existing surgical methods can effectively simulate ACL biomechanical function, but not complete neurosensory mechanoreceptor function, then prolonged use of some type of proprioception-enhancing garment makes sense. In combination with a collateral hinge, a well-designed simple sleeve-based brace can protect against sudden valgus loading. Although functional bracing may be deemed essential for preventing sudden "frontal plane" loading following the initial season after release to play, it is also important that the athlete train outside of the brace in a protected environment to maintain and improve somatosensory acuity, whole-body postural alignment, and neuromuscular control in the absence of the knee region stress shielding provided by the brace. Over time functional knee braces can adversely influence knee joint kinematics, kinetics, and lower extremity neuromuscular activation patterns. Tissues get stronger and the neuromuscular system becomes more functionally responsive when progressively greater loads are applied through non-impaired knee ranges of motion during sports movements. Care must be taken to carefully evaluate the appropriateness of other interfaces as well, including foot orthotics to control transverse plane tibial rotation (Jenkins et al. 2008), motion control, cushioning, or "gripping"-type footwear and bracing at adjacent joints such as the ankle. High stiffness and rigidity in ankle and foot orthoses have the potential to transfer injurious forces and torques proximally to the knee.

Summary

Much remains to be achieved to develop more effective evidence-based return-to-play criteria that better ensure athlete safety following ACL reconstruction and rehabilitation. More strenuous functional assessments of lower extremity neuromuscular strength, power, and endurance in addition to local (knee), regional (lower extremity), and global (whole-body) neuromuscular control of postural alignment need to occur earlier during the recovery timeframe. Prescriptive continued therapeutic exercise performance ensures that positive treatment effects continue long term. Further research is greatly needed to better understand human graft healing dynamics and the psychobehavioral status of the recovering athlete prior to release to competitive play.

Cross-References

- ▸ Factors Affecting Return to Sport After Anterior Cruciate Ligament Reconstruction
- ▸ Perioperative and Postoperative Anterior Cruciate Ligament Rehabilitation Focused on Soft Tissue Grafts
- ▸ Structured Rehabilitation Model with Clinical Outcomes After Anterior Cruciate Ligament Reconstruction
- ▸ Return to the Field for Football (Soccer) After Anterior Cruciate Ligament Reconstruction: Guidelines

References

Angelozzi M, Madama M, Corsica C et al (2012) Rate of force development as an adjunctive outcome measure for return-to-sport decisions after anterior cruciate ligament reconstruction. J Orthop Sports Phys Ther 42(9):772–780

Ardern CL, Taylor NF, Feller JA, Whitehead TS, Webster KE (2013) Psychological responses matter in returning to preinjury level of sport after anterior cruciate ligament reconstruction surgery. Am J Sports Med 41:1549–1558

Ardern CL, Webster KE, Taylor NF et al (2011a) Return to sport following anterior cruciate ligament reconstruction surgery: a systematic review and meta-analysis of the state of play. Br J Sports Med 45:596–606

Ardern CL, Webster KE, Taylor NF et al (2011b) Return to the preinjury level of competitive sport after anterior cruciate ligament reconstruction surgery. Two-thirds of patients have not returned by 12 months after surgery. Am J Sports Med 39:538–543

Biau DJ, Tournoux C, Katsahian S et al (2007) ACL reconstruction: a meta-analysis of functional scores. Clin Orthop Relat Res 458:180–187

Bogunovic L, Kim AD, Beamer BS et al (2010) Hypovitaminosis D in patients scheduled to undergo orthopaedic surgery: a single-center analysis. J Bone Joint Surg Am 92(13):2300–2304

Brewer BW, Cornelius AE (2010) Self-protective changes in athletic identity following anterior cruciate ligament reconstruction. Psychol Sport Exerc 11(1):1–5

Brewer BW, Van Raalte JL, Linder DE (1993) Athletic identity: Hercules' muscles or Achilles Heel? Int J Sport Psychol 24:237–254

Chmielewski TL, Jones D, Day T et al (2008) The association of pain and fear of movement/reinjury with function during anterior cruciate ligament reconstruction rehabilitation. J Orthop Sports Phys Ther 38(12):746–753

Claes S, Verdonk P, Forsyth R et al (2011) The "ligamentization" process in anterior cruciate ligament reconstruction: what happens to the human graft" a systematic review of the literature. Am J Sports Med 39(11):2476–2483

Dye SF (1996) The knee as a biological transmission with an envelope of function: a theory. Clin Orthop Relat Res 325:10–18

Hewett TE, Myer GD (2011) The mechanistic connection between the trunk, hip, knee, and anterior cruciate ligament injury. Exerc Sport Sci Rev 39(4):161–166

Howells BE, Ardern CL, Webster KE (2011) Is postural control restored following anterior cruciate ligament reconstruction? A systematic review. Knee Surg Sports Traumatol Arthrosc 19:1168–1177

Jenkins WL, Raedeke SG, Williams DS 3rd (2008) The relationship between the use of foot orthoses and knee ligament injury in female collegiate basketball players. J Am Podiatr Assoc 98(3):207–211

Kvist J (2004) Rehabilitation following anterior cruciate ligament injury: current recommendations for sports participation. Sports Med 34(4):269–280

Kvist J, Ek A, Sporrstedt K, Good L (2005) Fear of re-injury: a hindrance for returning to sports after anterior cruciate ligament reconstruction. Knee Surg Sports Traumatol Arthrosc 13:393–397

Langford JL, Webster KE, Feller JA (2009) A prospective longitudinal study to assess psychological changes following anterior cruciate ligament reconstruction surgery. Br J Sports Med 43(5):377–381

Myer GD, Paterno MV, Ford KR et al (2006) Rehabilitation after anterior cruciate ligament reconstruction: criteria-based progression through the return-to-sport phase. J Orthop Sports Phys Ther 36(6): 385–402

Myer GD, Martin L Jr, Ford KR et al (2012) No association of time from surgery with functional deficits in athletes after anterior cruciate ligament reconstruction: evidence for objective return-to-sport criteria. Am J Sports Med 40:2256–2263

Nyland J, Fisher B, Brand E et al (2010a) Osseous deficits after anterior cruciate ligament injury and reconstruction: a systematic review with suggestions to improve osseous homeostasis. Arthroscopy 26:1248–1257

Nyland J, Klein S, Caborn DN (2010b) Lower extremity compensatory neuromuscular and biomechanical adaptations 2 to 11 years after anterior cruciate ligament reconstruction. Arthroscopy 26:1212–1225

Paterno MV, Ford KR, Myer GD et al (2007) Limb asymmetries in landing and jumping 2 years following anterior cruciate ligament reconstruction. Clin J Sports Med 17(4):258–262

Paterno MV, Schmitt LC, Ford KR et al (2010) Biomechanical measures during landing and postural stability predict second anterior cruciate ligament injury after anterior cruciate ligament reconstruction and return to sport. Am J Sports Med 38:1968–1978

Smith FW, Rosenlund EA, Aune AK et al (2004) Subjective functional assessments and the return to competitive sport after anterior cruciate ligament reconstruction. Br J Sports Med 38:279–284

Thomee R, Kaplan Y, Kvist J et al (2011) Muscle strength and hop performance criteria prior to return to sports after ACL reconstruction. Knee Surg Sports Traumatol Arthrosc 19(11):1798–1805

Tjong VK, Murnaghan ML, Nyhof-Young JM, Ogilvie-Harris DJ (2014) A qualitative investigation of the decision to return to sport after anterior cruciate ligament reconstruction: to play or not to play. Am J Sports Med 42(2):336–342

Valeriani M, Restuccia D, Di Lazaro V et al (1999) Clinical and neurophysiological abnormalities before and after reconstruction of the anterior cruciate ligament of the knee. Acta Neurol Scand 99:303–307

Walker N, Thatcher J, Lavallee D (2007) Psychological responses to injury in competitive sport: a critical review. J R Soc Promot Health 127(4):174–180

Wera JC, Nyland J, Ghazi C et al (2014) International knee documentation committee knee survey use after anterior cruciate ligament reconstruction: A 2005–2012 systematic review and world region comparison. Arthroscopy 05–2. doi: 10.1016/j.arthro.2014.05.043. [Epub ahead of print]

Webster KE, Feller JA, Lambros C (2008) Development and preliminary validation of a scale to measure the psychological impact of returning to sport following anterior cruciate ligament surgery. Phys Ther Sport 9(1):9–15

Xie X, Zhao S, Wu H et al (2013) Platelet-rich plasma enhances autograft revascularization and reinnervation in a dog model of anterior cruciate ligament reconstruction. J Surg Res 183(1):214–222

Return to the Field for Football (Soccer) After Anterior Cruciate Ligament Reconstruction: Guidelines

121

Polyvios Kyritsis, Erik Witvrouw, and Philippe Landreau

Contents

P. Kyritsis (✉) • E. Witvrouw • P. Landreau
Orthopaedic and Sports Medicine Hospital, Aspetar, Doha, Qatar
e-mail: polyvios.kyritsis@aspetar.com; erik.witvrouw@aspetar.com; philippe.landreau@aspetar.com

M.N. Doral, J. Karlsson (eds.), *Sports Injuries*,
DOI 10.1007/978-3-642-36569-0_106

Abstract

Anterior cruciate ligament reconstruction in athletes is carried out to achieve a stable knee that can enable them to return to their desired activities. Unfortunately, today a successful return to sport cannot be guaranteed, and the criteria to return to sport are poorly investigated and poorly described. The purpose of this chapter is to describe the criteria used in Aspetar, based on the existing literature and the long experience of ACL treatments in Aspetar. Therefore, it is the aim of this chapter to deliver a very practical article which can be used by physiotherapists as a guideline in the enigmatic area of return to sport after an ACL reconstruction. The article describes the different phases of the rehabilitation, starting from the *running progression program*, going to the *on-field functional training*, and ending by the *on-field sports-specific training* before returning to team training. Each of these phases is clearly described and objective tests are given to progress from one phase to the other.

Introduction

The purpose of this chapter is to present "the Aspetar approach" of return to sport after anterior cruciate ligament (ACL) reconstruction.

The following section is a description of the return to sports program used in Aspetar Orthopedic and Sports Medicine Hospital, Doha, Qatar. This program is based on the existing body of evidence from the literature, combined with the clinical experience of the treatment of around 60 ACL athletes a day at Aspetar. This on-field rehabilitation can reduce the risk of reinjury, prepare the athlete to perform at the same pre-injury level (Wilk et al. 1999; Griffin et al. 2000; Cascio et al. 2004; Roi et al. 2005; Langford et al. 2009), and secure the safe transition of the player from physiotherapy to normal training (Myer et al. 2006).

Running Progression Program

Running progression which sets the beginning of the last phase of ACL rehabilitation should start before the on-field rehabilitation and when patients meet specific criteria. In Aspetar, a patient is allowed to start running if the bilateral muscle strength deficit for quadriceps and hamstrings is less or equal to 30 % and when he/she is able to perform a single leg squat with good knee control and has a good knee alignment on unstable surfaces.

The running progression program must be very progressive and should start with very easy exercises like ladder drills in order to reassure that patients have good knee control. On average, this running program starts around 3 months postoperation. Static running on soft surfaces, like trampoline or mats, will be the next step, and at this phase in-water running can be performed. Deepwater running is followed by shallow-water running until the athlete reaches the point to start normal running outside the swimming pool. At the beginning, running should be combined with walking where walking distance will be greater than running distance and this will be inverted with time. Figure 1 shows an example of a running progression program.

The whole running progression for an athlete is expected to last for almost 1 month, and when patients meet the following specific criteria, they can start the on-field functional rehabilitation program:

- Full knee ROM
- Pain-free
- Limited or no swelling
- Muscle strength deficit less than 25 %
- Run for 45–60 min with proper alignment
- Good knee control and alignment during balance exercises
- Good knee control during bilateral and unilateral jumps

1. 100m jog, 300m walk (up to 10 times)
2. 200m jog, 200m walk (up to 8 times)
3. 400m jog, 200m walk (up to 5 times)
4. 800m jog, 200m walk (up to 3 times)
5. Jog 4x5 minutes
6. Jog 3x8 minutes
7. Jog 3x10 minutes
8. Jog 4x10 minutes
9. Jog 3x15 minutes
10. Jog 3x20 minutes
11. Jog 2x30 minutes
12. Jog 1x60 minutes
13. Start interval running

Fig 1 Running progression: Patients should complete the running progression program before progress to the on-field functional rehabilitation

On-Field Rehabilitation Program

The duration of the on-field functional and sports-specific rehabilitation should be criteria based. On average, the patients start running at about 3 months postoperatively; then approximately 1 month later (4 months), they are expected to meet all the criteria in order to start the on-field functional rehabilitation. This phase will last about 1 month, and at approximately 5 months after surgery, the average athlete will be able to start the on-field sports-specific rehabilitation. By completion of the whole program (at around 6 months), athletes are highly advised to start training with their team, and only if they are able to train pain-free for 3–4 weeks, they can participate in official games.

All the above-suggested time frames are suggested to be used only for athletes, who will participate in a rehabilitation program on an everyday basis, for at least five times per week.

Fig. 2 Assessment/goal setting form: This form is completed during the first session of the on-field rehabilitation, where goals are also set

Injury mechanism			
Knee Rating Scale			
Running Duration			
FMS Tests	Bilateral Squats	One leg Squat	Norwegian Squat
		L R	L R
Ilinois test			
505 test			
Comments			
Goals			

Steps of the on-field rehabilitation program:

- Goal setting
- Evaluating psychological readiness
- Evaluating overall knee status

Step A: Goal Setting

The on-field functional rehabilitation program will start by setting personal goals for each patient. It will be performed by the patient and the treating therapist together. It will be written down on the initial assessment form (Fig. 2) like "player wants to return to competition level by March 2014." It has been suggested that there is a positive relation between goal setting and the positive outcome of the rehabilitation after ACL injury (Wierike et al. 2012). What does every specific patient want to do after completing his/her rehabilitation? Return to sport has to be defined very precisely for each individual athlete (Barber et al. 1990; Podlog et al. 2011; Ardern et al. 2012).

Step B: Evaluating Psychological Readiness

Another focus at the beginning of the on-field functional rehabilitation is to evaluate the psychological readiness of the player. Once this is evaluated, one of the aims of the on-field rehabilitation program is to increase the confidence of the patient and step-by-step prepare him/her to return to their desired level of activity.

This will be done by evaluating the different activities that may affect the psychological readiness of the patients. For this purpose the "patient-specific functional scale" (Fig. 3) is used (Chatman et al. 1997). The patient-specific functional scale lists different activities. Patients are asked to score these activities from 0 to 10. Scoring 0 means that

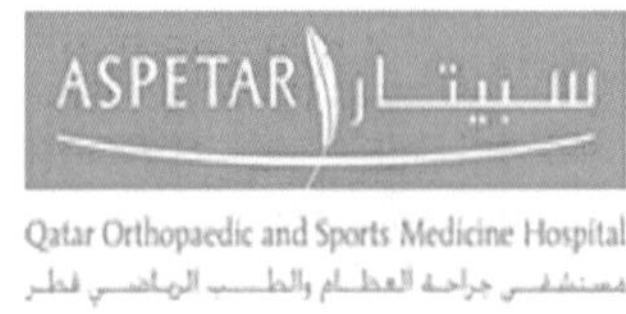

Patient Specific Functional Scale

Patient's Referral Diagnosis:

Therapist to read and fill in the table below at the completion of the subjective assessment.

Initial Assessment

"I want you to identify up to 3 activities that you are unable to do or are having difficulty with as a result of your .... problem. Today, are there any activities that you are unable to do or are having difficulty with as a result of your .... Problem?"

(Write the 3 activities, then show the patient the scale and ask them to rate each activity).

Follow Up Assessment

"When I saw you on (state previous assessment date), you told me you had difficulty with (read the activities from the list). Today, do you still have difficulty with ....?" (read and have the patient score each activity on the list).

Patient Specific Activity Scoring Scale (Select one number)

Unable to perform activity 0 1 2 3 4 5 6 7 8 9 10 Able to perform at same level as before injury

	Date 1	**Date 2**	**Date 3**	**Date 4**	**Date 5**	**Date 6**
Activity						
Total Score						

Total Score= sum of activity scores /number of activities

Minimal detectable change for average score= 2 points

Minimal detectable change for individual score= 3 points

Adapted from Stratford et al. (Physiotherapy Canada, 1995)

Fig. 3 Patient-specific functional scale: Different activities are recorded and reevaluated during the whole course of rehabilitation

they are unable to perform this specific activity, whereas 10 means that they can perform this activity at the same pre-injured level. Based upon this, the therapist knows on which activities he/she has to emphasize on. Later, the patient will be asked to fill in the questionnaire again in order to reevaluate and check for improvement. For example, if a patient reports difficulty on landing on one leg after a jump, the therapist will focus extra on this activity during the on-field rehabilitation program.

In addition to the patient-specific functional scale, patients are asked to rate their overall knee status from 0 to 100 %. Every 2 weeks these two questionnaires are reevaluated.

Step C: Evaluating Overall Knee Status

The patients' overall knee status will be evaluated by using the patients' ability to perform a bilateral squat (Fig. 4a, b), a single leg squat (Fig. 4c, d),

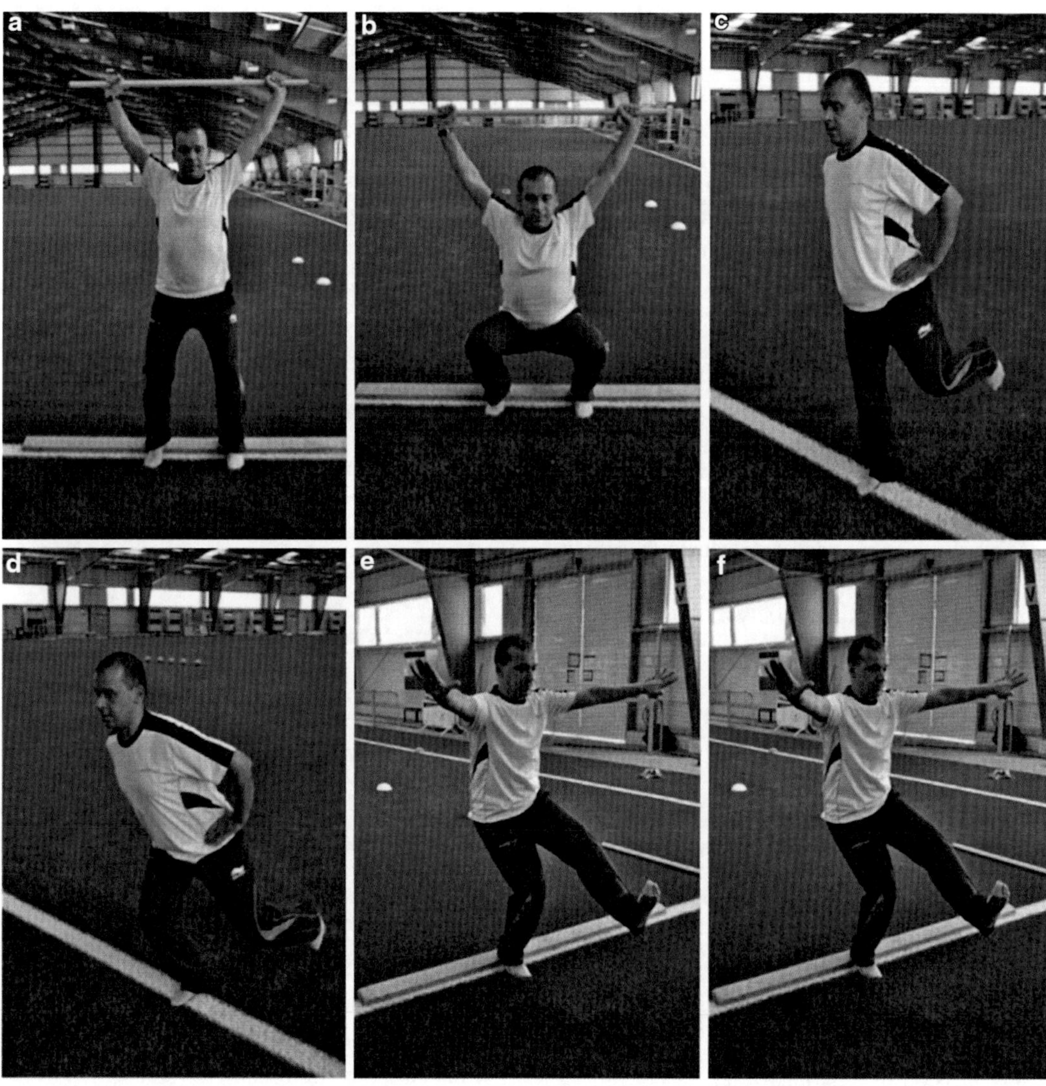

Fig. 4 (**a**) Double leg squat (starting position). (**b**) Double leg squat (final position). (**c**) Single leg squat (starting position). (**d**) Single leg squat (final position). (**e**) Norwegian squat (starting position). (**f**) Norwegian squat (final position)

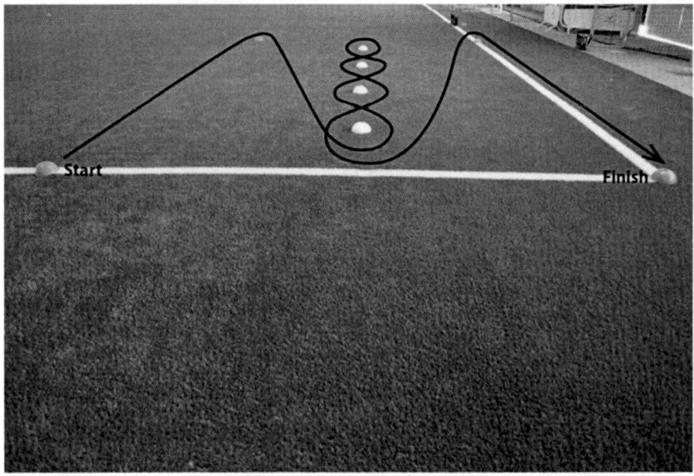

Fig. 5 Illinois test: Athletes have to perform the test at the maximum possible speed considering they feel fully confident

and a Norwegian squat (Fig. 4e, f). These movements are evaluated and scored according to the functional movement screening (FMS) method which evaluates the flexibility and strength of knee, ankle, lower back, and shoulder (Cook et al. 2006). The quality of exercise execution is scored from 0 to 3, where 0 means that there is pain and 3 that the exercise can be performed on the exact way described by the instructor.

Furthermore, some agility tests are performed: The Illinois test (Fig. 5), the 505 test (Fig. 6), and a *T*-test (Fig. 7) are used to evaluate the quality of movement during direction changes when running, as well as their ability to stop fast.

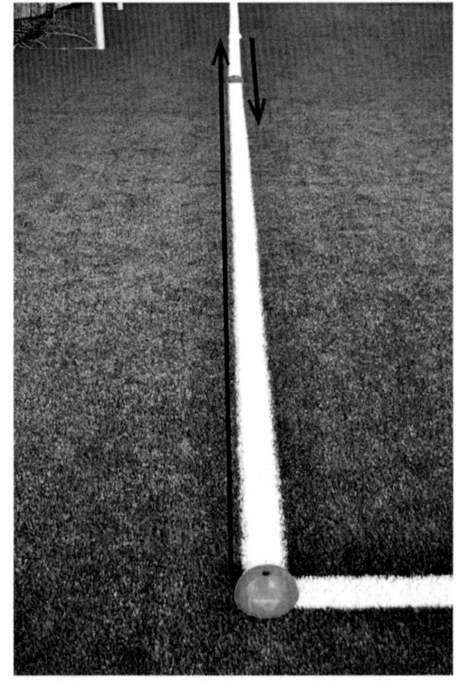

Fig. 6 505 test: Test must be performed at the maximum possible speed. Athletes should perform a side stop and change direction

On-Field Functional Rehabilitation Program

The on-field rehabilitation will start with the on-field functional rehabilitation (approximately 4 months postoperation) and will progress to the on-field sports-specific rehabilitation. The on-field rehabilitation is very important in order to achieve high levels of confidence, and all different exercises should be performed on a very progressive way.

Progression of functional exercises during the on-field functional rehabilitation:

- Zigzag running without and with ball (Fig. 8a)
- Side steps without and with ball (Fig. 8b)
- Front, side stops (Fig. 8c)
- Changing direction with ball
- 45° direction change without/with ball (Fig. 8d)
- 90° direction change without/with ball (Fig. 8d)
- 120° pivoting direction change without/with ball (Fig. 8d)

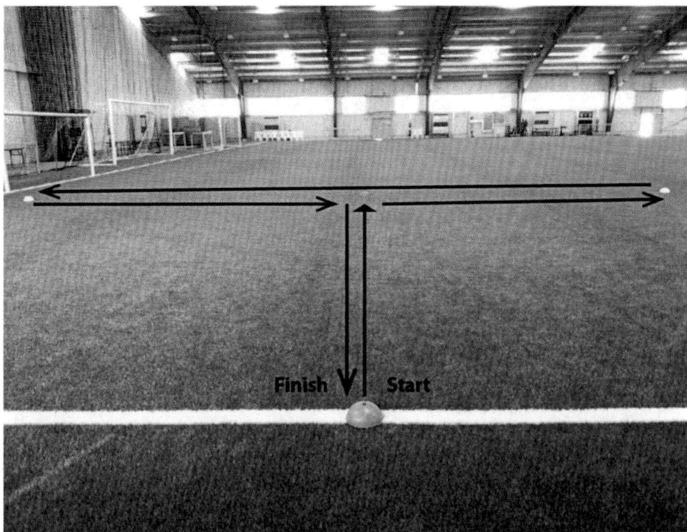

Fig. 7 *T*-test: Athletes must run front, side, and backwards at the maximum possible speed considering they feel fully confident

- Continuous figure of eight without/with ball (Fig. 8e)
- Bilateral/unilateral jumps (Fig. 8f)
- Short submaximum sprints
- Plyometric jumps (Fig. 8g,h)
- Long maximum sprints

It is of great importance for every different sport to analyze and break down all the possible multidirectional movements. Asking the patient at the beginning to perform simpler, unidirectional movements, which will progress to more advanced, multidirectional, pivoting, sports-specific movements, will increase the confidence level of the athlete and progressively load their knee with external forces.

Low-intensity, easy direction changes (e.g., front–back, side stops) are the first exercises suggested at this stage. Progression to a higher intensity level or more difficult exercises with the use of a ball can be done when exercises can be performed with a good quality of movement, with full knee control and pain-free.

Explosive movements are also very important in most sports. Jumps and sprints should also be progressed during the on-field functional rehabilitation. At this stage, patients can perform sports-specific jumps which are closer to a game situation. For example, a football player after jumping for a heading may land on one leg or two legs, he/she may be pushed in the air or may not. All these possible scenarios must be addressed and inside a controlled environment should be progressively performed.

Sprinting should also be progressively performed. Firstly, for sports that include long sprints, fast runs in short distance should be performed and then progress to maximum long-distance sprints. For sports like football, futsal, basketball, handball, etc., exercises can be further progressed to sprints with a ball that will create a more sports-specific and complex situation.

Criteria for Progression to On-Field Sports-Specific Rehabilitation Program

With the completion of all the above steps, an evaluation has to be performed, which will give the therapist an indication if the patient is ready to progress from the on-field functional rehabilitation to the on-field sports-specific rehabilitation.

Testing consists of three agility tests (Illinois test, the 505 test, and *T*-test) (Figs. 5, 6, 7), four hop tests (single hop, triple hop, triple crossover, and 6 m timed hop) from which a limb symmetry index (LSI) is calculated (Lephart et al. 1989; Barber et al. 1990; Lephart et al. 1993; Risberg et al. 1995; Bolgla and Keskula 1997;

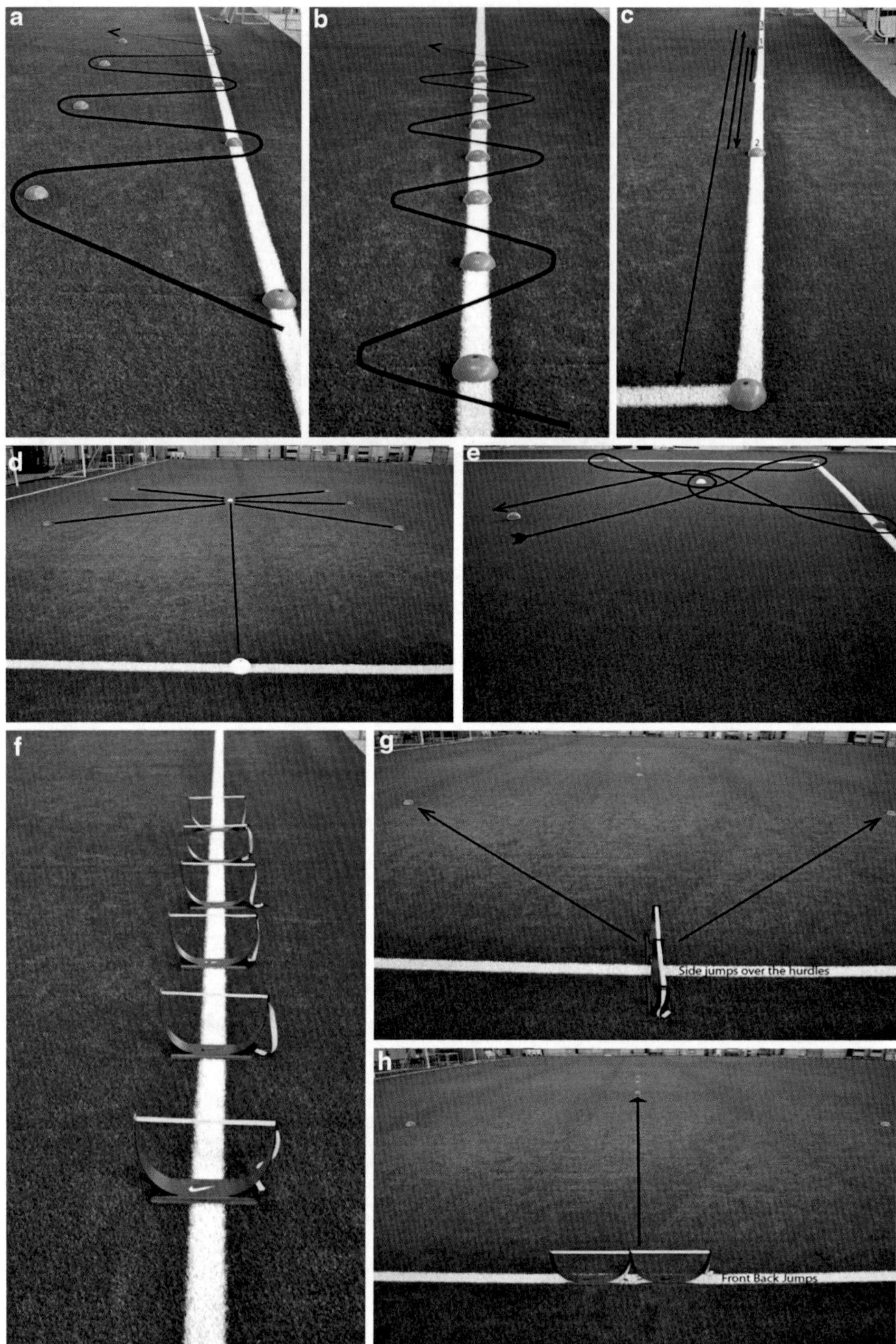

Fig. 8 (**a**) Zigzag direction changes: Athletes run through the cones with and without a ball. (**b**) Side steps: Athletes perform side steps through the cones going forward and backward, with and without the ball. (**c**) Front–side stops and change of direction with the ball: Athletes start from the white cone and perform side stops, front–back stops, and direction changes with the ball from cone to cone. (**d**) 45°, 90°, and 120° direction changes with/without ball: running straight and changing direction at 45°, 90°, and 120°. Athletes must reach the level of performing all

Rudolph et al. 2000; Wainner 2001; Reid et al. 2007; Van Grinsven et al. 2010; Ardern et al. 2011; Barber-Westin and Noyes 2011), and an isokinetic muscle strength evaluation (Table 1).

Patients can progress from the on-field functional rehabilitation to the on-field sports-specific rehabilitation when the following criteria are met:

The score on the Illinois test should be less than 16 s, the score on the 505 test should be less than 2.8 s, and at the *T*-test the athlete should have a time of 11 s or less. LSI values must be equal or greater than 80 % and muscle strength deficits for quadriceps and hamstrings less than 15 %. The criteria are set based upon the Aspetar experience, but are only for male patients.

On-Field Sports-Specific Rehabilitation Program

Once the athletes have reached the on-field sports-specific rehabilitation (approximately 5 months postoperation), the rehabilitation starts looking more and more like a normal team training. Here is an example of a football player with an ACL reconstruction on his right knee, who wants to return to his high pre-injury level of playing and fulfills all the criteria to start working on football-specific rehabilitation:

Progression of football-specific exercises:

- Passes progression
- Crosses (static) (Fig. 9a)
- Corner kicks
- Crosses (dynamic) (Fig. 9b)
- Shooting scenarios (no defense) (Fig. 9c)
- 1 vs. 1 (attack and/or defense)
- Shooting scenarios (with defense)
- Scoring
- Finishing scenarios
- Maximum shoots (Fig. 9d)

The main interest at the beginning is to make sure that he can pass the ball, so passes progression exercises will be performed. He will start passing on short distance and progress to long passes by using both legs. It is necessary to check how his injured leg may react when passing with the left leg (all the body weight is supported by the injured leg). It is important to perform the ball exercises with their injured as well as their noninjured leg.

The next set of exercises will be on crossing with nonmoving balls (static cross). The distance of the cross should be small at the beginning and then move further away. If the athlete feels confident and his technique is correct, then he can progress to corner kicks which are more technical crosses. After this, crosses with moving balls can be performed (dynamic cross). By the time the patient is able to perform all the above exercises, then shooting can be also performed, progressing from easy shoots close to the goal to stronger shoots from greater distance.

At that stage (approximately 6 months postoperation), the football (soccer) player has performed all possible football-specific movements, broken down, and it is now time to put everything together to game situation scenarios. These scenarios can combine direction changes, shoots, sprints, defending, and attacking exercises at the same time and be as much position-specific as possible. One against one (1 vs. 1) exercises, where the patient takes the role of the defender and/or striker, are very crucial for the confidence level of the athlete. This kind of exercises will make the athletes more confident and at the same time increase their fitness level. It is very important that when the patient returns back to normal training with the rest of his/her team, he/she will be as best prepared as possible in terms of fitness. It is highly recommended that fitness training starts in combination with the rehabilitation

Fig. 8 (continued) direction changes at maximum speed. (**e**) Continuous figure of 8: Change directions continuously left and right through the cones. (**f**) Jumps over hurdles bilateral and unilateral: Athletes jump over the hurdles with two legs, progressing to one leg jumping front and side. (**g**) Plyometric side jumps with short sprint: Athletes perform continuous side jumps with two legs and sprint for 10 m. (**h**) Plyometric front–back jumps with long sprint: Athletes perform continuous front–back jumps and sprint for longer distances, 20, 30, and 40 m

Table 1 Demonstrates all the suggested tests and questionnaires and the time that they should be performed during rehabilitation

Test	Start of on-field functional rehab	Start of on-field sports-specific rehab
Illinois	Performed at patient's own pace to evaluate movement quality	Less than 16 s
505	Performed at patient's own pace to evaluate movement quality	Less than 2.8 s
Patient-specific functional scale	Patient defines activities and reevaluated every 2 weeks	Patient defines activities and reevaluated every 2 weeks
Overall knee status	Patient rates his/her knee status and reevaluated every 2 weeks	Patient rates his/her knee status and reevaluated every 2 weeks
Isokinetic evaluation	Performed at 60,180,and 300 °/s. Deficits less than 25 % are accepted	Deficits less than 15 % are accepted
Hop tests	No	LSI values greater than 80 %
FMS	Bilateral squat, single leg squat, and Norwegian squat are evaluated	Bilateral squat, single leg squat, and Norwegian squat are evaluated
T-test	No	Less than 11 s
Yo-Yo intermittent	No	No

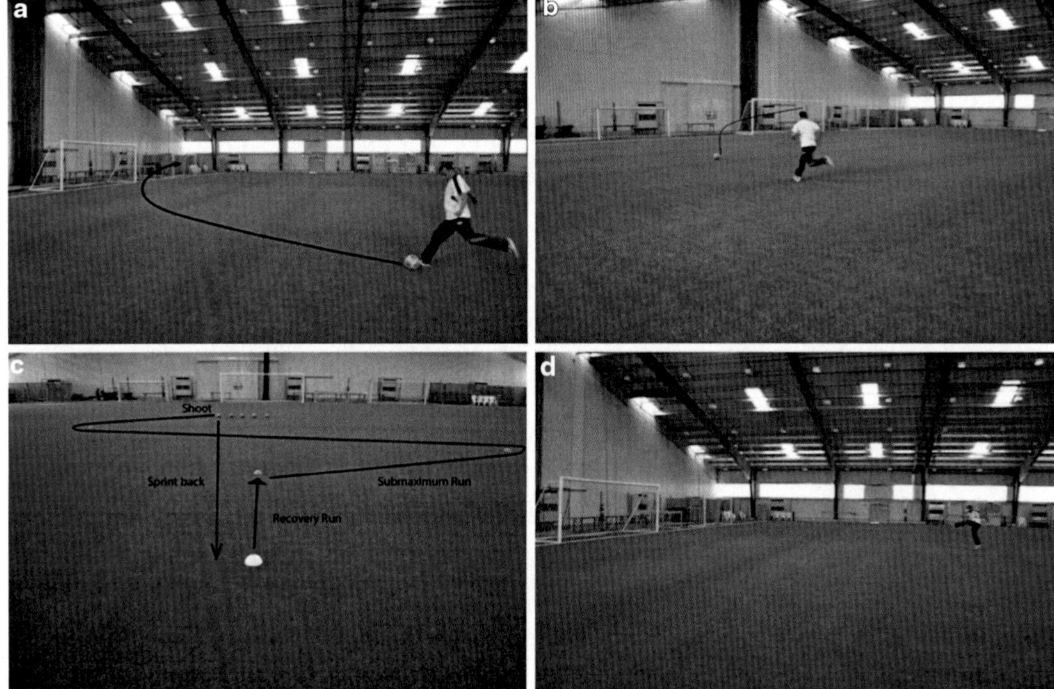

Fig. 9 (**a**) Static crosses: Athletes perform crosses while the ball is not moving. (**b**) Dynamic crosses: Athletes perform crosses while the ball is moving away from them. (**c**) Shooting scenarios: Athletes perform a zigzag direction change at submaximum speed, shoot the ball, and sprint back behind the starting point. (**d**) Maximum shoots: Athletes progress the strength of their shoot till they reach their maximum possible shoot

program, from the very early stages and lasts till full return to the team training; Yo-Yo intermittent 20 m IR1 and IR2 recovery tests (Bangsbo et al. 2008) are used at the end of Aspetar's ACL rehabilitation protocol in order to evaluate athletes' fitness level. Based upon these results, information can be given to the coach about the level of fitness they have achieved, since the better the

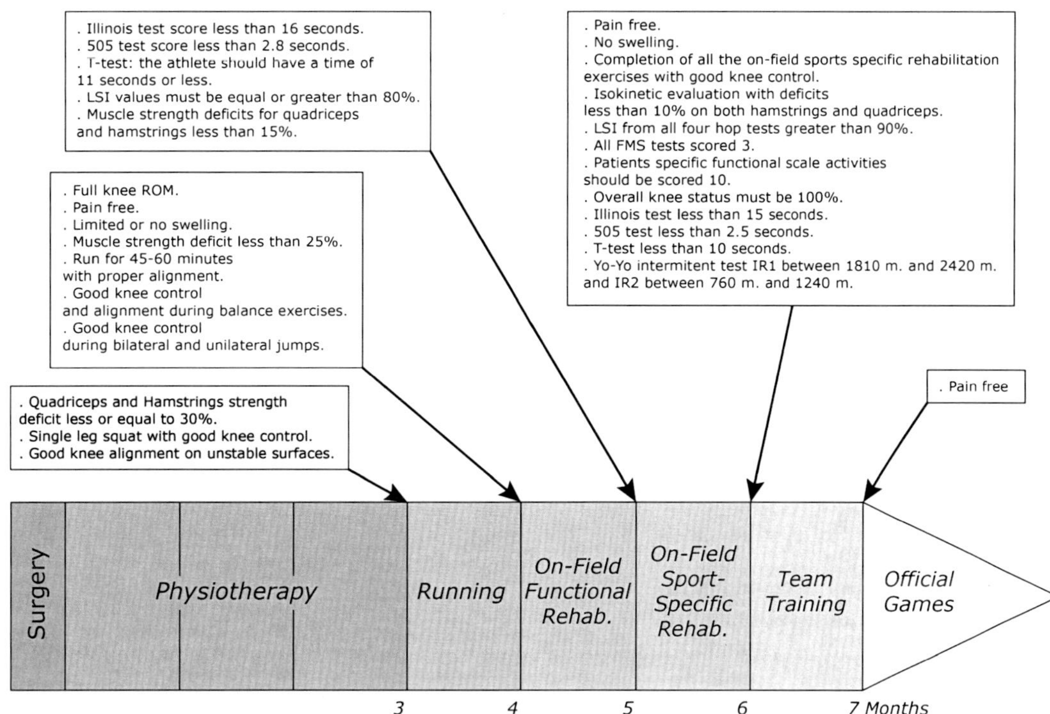

Fig. 10 Return to the field after ACL reconstruction: summary of Aspetar protocol

athlete performs on the test, the higher his/her competition level can be (Bangsbo et al. 2008). According to the level of participation (elite level or recreational) and activity (football, basketball, etc.) of each patient, different values are accepted. As the literature suggests (Bangsbo et al. 2008) for IR1 test, a result from 1,810 to 2,420 m is accepted, whereas for IR2 test from 760 to 1,240 m (Bangsbo et al. 2008) (Fig. 10).

Table 2 Tests performed on day 1 and day 2

Test	Day 1	Day 2
Isokinetic test	✓	
Patient-specific functional scale	✓	
Overall knee status	✓	
T-test	✓	
Yo-Yo intermittent		✓
FMS tests		✓
Hop tests		✓
Illinois test		✓
505 test		✓

Discharge Criteria before Return to Team Training

Today, many different criteria for discharge for ACL reconstruction are used. At Aspetar, a battery of different tests for discharge is used. This is divided into two different days as shown below (Table 2).

Discharge criteria to return to team training:

- Pain-free.
- No swelling.
- Completion of all the on-field sports-specific rehabilitation exercises with good knee control.
- Isokinetic evaluation (60°, 180°, 300° per second) with deficits less than 10 % on both hamstrings and quadriceps.
- LSI from all four hop tests greater than 90 %.
- All FMS tests scored 3.
- Patient-specific functional scale activities should be scored 10.

- Overall knee status must be 100 %.
- Illinois test less than 15 s.
- 505 test less than 2.5 s.
- *T*-test less than 10 s.
- Yo-Yo intermittent test IR1 between 1,810 and 2,420 m and IR2 between 760 and 1,240 m.

Hop tests, agility tests, and FMS tests are all performed under fatigue in order to make the procedure more demanding and reassure that there is a good knee control in fatigued situations. In order to bring the patients under fatigue, they are asked to perform first the Yo-Yo intermittent test and then all the other functional tests.

By setting all these demanding and difficult-to-achieve criteria (Fig. 10), the risk of reinjury remains low and return of the patients to their desired activity will be successful. Future studies should increase the knowledge in order to better define the ideal return to sports protocol after ACL injury.

Conclusion

An ACL injury is a very devastating injury which mostly requires an ACL reconstruction in order to achieve a stable knee that can enable athletes to return to their pre-injury level of sports activities.

However, today a successful return to sport cannot be guaranteed, and the criteria to return to sport are poorly investigated and poorly described. This chapter describes the on-field functional and sports-specific rehabilitation and its progression in a very practical way which can be used by physiotherapists as a guideline in the enigmatic area of return to sport after an ACL reconstruction.

The duration of the on-field functional and sports-specific rehabilitation should be criteria based, but on average the patients start running at about 3 months postoperatively; then approximately 1 month later (4 months), they are expected to meet all the criteria in order to start the on-field functional rehabilitation. This phase will last about 1 month, and at approximately 5 months after surgery, the average athlete will be able to start the on-field sports-specific rehabilitation. By completion of the whole program (at around 6 months), athletes are highly advised to start training with their team, and only if they are able to train pain-free for 3–4 weeks, they can participate in official games.

We have described the criteria to return to sport used in Aspetar, based on the existing literature and the long experience of ACL treatments in Aspetar, taking into account personal goals for each patient and the psychological readiness of the player.

References

Ardern CL, Webster KE, Taylor NF, Feller JA (2011) Return to the preinjury level of competitive sport after anterior cruciate ligament reconstruction surgery two-thirds of patients have not returned by 12 months after surgery. Am J Sports Med 39(3):538–543

Ardern CL, Taylor NF, Feller JA, Webster KE (2012) Return-to-sport outcomes at 2 to 7 years after anterior cruciate ligament reconstruction surgery. Am J Sports Med 40(1):41–48

Bangsbo J, Iaia FM, Krustrup P (2008) The Yo-Yo intermittent recovery test. Sports Med 38(1):37–51

Barber SD, Noyes FR, Mangine RE, Hartman W (1990) Quantitative assessment of functional limitations in normal and anterior cruciate ligament-deficient knees. Clin Orthop Relat Res 255:204–214

Barber-Westin SD, Noyes FR (2011) Factors used to determine return to unrestricted sports activities after anterior cruciate ligament reconstruction. Arthroscopy 27(12):1697–1705

Bolgla LA, Keskula DR (1997) Reliability of lower extremity functional performance tests. J Orthop Sports Phys Ther 26(3):138–142

Cascio BM, Culp L, Cosgarea AJ (2004) Return to play after anterior cruciate ligament reconstruction. Clin Sports Med 23(3):395–408

Chatman AB, Hyams SP, Neel JM, Binkley JM, Stratford PW, Schomberg A, Stabler M (1997) The patient-specific functional scale: measurement properties in patients with knee dysfunction. Phys Ther 77(8): 820–829

Cook G, Burton L, Hoogenboom B (2006) Pre-participation screening: the use of fundamental movements as an assessment of function–Part 1. N Am J Sports Phys Ther 1(2):62

Griffin LY, Agel J, Albohm MJ, Arendt EA, Dick RW, Garrett WE, Wojtys EM (2000) Noncontact anterior cruciate ligament injuries: risk factors and prevention strategies. J Am Acad Orthop Surg 8(3): 141–150

Langford JL, Webster KE, Feller JA (2009) A prospective longitudinal study to assess psychological changes following anterior cruciate ligament reconstruction surgery. Br J Sports Med 43(5):377–378

Lephart SM, Perrin DH, Fu FH, Gieck JH, McCue FC, Irrgang JJ (1989) Relationship between selected physical characteristics and functional capacity in the anterior cruciate ligament insufficient individual. Doctoral dissertation, University of Virginia

Lephart SM, Kocher MS, Harner CD, Fu FH (1993) Quadriceps strength and functional capacity after anterior cruciate ligament reconstruction patellar tendon autograft versus allograft. Am J Sports Med 21(5): 738–743

Myer GD, Paterno MV, Ford KR, Quatman CE, Hewett TE (2006) Rehabilitation after anterior cruciate ligament reconstruction: criteria-based progression through the return-to-sport phase. J Orthop Sports Phys Ther 36(6): 385–402

Podlog L, Dimmock J, Miller J (2011) A review of return to sport concerns following injury rehabilitation: practitioner strategies for enhancing recovery outcomes. Phys Ther Sport 12(1):36–42

Reid A, Birmingham TB, Stratford PW, Alcock GK, Giffin JR (2007) Hop testing provides a reliable and valid outcome measure during rehabilitation after anterior cruciate ligament reconstruction. Phys Ther 87(3): 337–349

Risberg MA, Holm I, Ekeland A (1995) Reliability of functional knee tests in normal athletes. Scand J Med Sci Sports 5(1):24–28

Roi GS, Creta D, Nanni G, Marcacci M, Zaffagnini S, Snyder-Mackler L, Fithian DC (2005) Return to official Italian First Division soccer games within 90 days after anterior cruciate ligament reconstruction: a case report. J Orthop Sports Phys Ther 35(2):52–66

Rudolph KS, Axe MJ, Snyder-Mackler L (2000) Dynamic stability after ACL injury: who can hop? Knee Surg Sports Traumatol Arthrosc 8(5):262–269

Van Grinsven S, Van Cingel REH, Holla CJM, Van Loon CJM (2010) Evidence-based rehabilitation following anterior cruciate ligament reconstruction. Knee Surg Sports Traumatol Arthrosc 18(8):1128–1144

Wainner MRS (2001) Hop tests as predictors of dynamic knee stability. J Orthop Sports Phys Ther 31(10): 588–597

Wierike SCM, Sluis A, Akker Scheek I, Elferink Gemser MT, Visscher C (2012) Psychosocial factors influencing the recovery of athletes with anterior cruciate ligament injury: a systematic review. Scand J Med Sci Sports 23(5):527–540

Wilk KE, Arrigo C, Andrews JR, Clancy WG Jr (1999) Rehabilitation after anterior cruciate ligament reconstruction in the female athlete. J Athl Train 34(2):177

Revision Anterior Cruciate Ligament Reconstruction

122

Demetris Delos and Robert G. Marx

Contents

Abstract

Anterior cruciate ligament (ACL) reconstruction surgery is common and clinical outcomes are typically good. However, a minority of patients develop recurrent instability, necessitating revision surgery.

Successful revision ACL reconstruction requires a thorough history and physical examination along with a careful review of imaging studies in order to determine the etiology of failure and identify appropriate surgical candidates. Once the decision to proceed with revision ACL reconstruction is made, a meticulous preoperative plan that takes into consideration graft selection, tunnel placement, residual hardware, bone stock, alignment, and skin integrity is critical. In this manner, outcomes after revision ACL reconstruction can be optimized.

Introduction

Definition of Failure

Although anterior cruciate ligament (ACL) reconstruction is a common procedure, less than satisfactory outcomes have been reported to occur in up to 25 % of patients (Bach et al. 2003; Spindler et al. 2004; Biau et al. 2006, 2007; Baer and Harner 2007). However, there is no universally applied definition for failure of ACL reconstruction, thereby making it difficult to quantify. For the purposes of this chapter, failure will be

D. Delos (✉)
Department of Orthopedic Surgery, Hospital for Special Surgery, New York, NY, USA
e-mail: delosd@hss.edu

R.G. Marx
Foster Center for Clinical Outcome Research, Hospital for Special Surgery, New York, NY, USA
e-mail: marxr@hss.edu

M.N. Doral, J. Karlsson (eds.), *Sports Injuries*,
DOI 10.1007/978-3-642-36569-0_101

Table 1 Causes of ACL reconstruction failure

Technical	Biologic	Mechanical
Poor tunnel placement	Infection	Overly aggressive physical therapy, too rapid rehabilitation
Inadequate graft/ poor graft selection	Arthrofibrosis	Typical ACL injury mechanism (noncontact, hyperextension, valgus, rotational load)
Inadequate fixation/graft tensioning	Poor graft incorporation	
Failure to address other significant knee pathology		

defined as recurrent knee instability after ACL reconstruction, as demonstrated by a positive Lachman exam and/or a positive pivot shift exam. According to the literature, recurrent instability rates after primary ACL reconstruction range from 1 % to 8 % (Harter et al. 1988; Howe et al. 1991; Kaplan et al. 1991).

The reasons for clinical failure after ACL reconstruction are numerous but can be broadly separated into three categories (Getelman and Friedman 1999; Battaglia et al. 2007; Marx 2014) (Table 1):

1. Technical: These can include incorrect or poor tunnel placement, poor graft selection or inadequate graft material, poor or insufficient fixation and graft tensioning, and failure to recognize and/or address other knee pathologies (Getelman and Friedman 1999; Kamath et al. 2011). Technical error has been reported to be the most common reason for failure and has been associated as a cause in as many as 79 % of cases (Fox et al. 2004; Garofalo et al. 2006). It is generally thought that poor tunnel positioning (especially femoral) is the most common technical error.
2. Biologic: These can include infection, stiffness due to arthrofibrosis, and poor graft incorporation (Marzo et al. 1992; Corsetti and Jackson 1996; Shelbourne et al. 1996; Shelbourne and Patel 1999; Kamath et al. 2011). Although rare (in one large retrospective series, the rate of infection after ACL reconstruction was determined to be 0.58 %) (Barker et al. 2010), infection can be a devastating complication and may require removal of all implants and/or graft. Stiffness due to arthrofibrosis typically affects extension more than flexion and has been associated with excessive postoperative immobilization, early ACL reconstruction prior to restoration of complete range of motion after injury, cyclops lesions, and technical error (inappropriate graft tensioning and poor graft placement) (Marzo et al. 1992; Shelbourne et al. 1996; Shelbourne and Patel 1999; Kamath et al. 2011). Poor graft incorporation has also been associated with failed ACL reconstruction. Poor local vascularity, failure of repopulation of the graft, inadequate remodeling, and excessive loads may all contribute to failed graft incorporation (Corsetti and Jackson 1996).
3. Mechanical: In those with early failure (i.e., those <6 months after surgery), mechanical causes of failure can include graft stretch due to overly aggressive physical therapy or too rapid rehabilitation (Graf and Uhr 1988). In those with late failure (i.e., >6 months after surgery), graft rupture is usually due to mechanisms similar to those involved in primary ACL injury (such as pivoting injury during sport). Younger age and return to competitive sports have been identified as possible risk factors for reinjury (Salmon et al. 2005; Wright et al. 2007; Lyman et al. 2009; Shelbourne et al. 2009). However, it is believed that patients who have undergone well-executed ACL reconstruction surgeries are at no higher risk of re-rupturing the reconstructed ACL compared to the contralateral side (Salmon et al. 2006; Wright et al. 2007; Shelbourne et al. 2009; Reinhardt et al. 2012).

It is critical to keep these various causes of failure in mind as one evaluates the patient for failed surgical reconstruction since the ability to pinpoint the exact cause(s) of failure can increase the likelihood of successful revision surgery.

Preoperative Workup

History

In patients who present with symptoms after previous ACL reconstruction, a careful and thorough history is necessary to help lead the clinician down the appropriate diagnostic path. It is important to first define the problem and genuinely understand the patients' signs and symptoms – whether they may be pain, stiffness, or instability. Pain may be due to any number of causes – either anatomic (articular wear, meniscal injury, etc.) or biologic (i.e., inflammation, infection, etc.) – while stiffness suggests that the patient may have progressed slower than expected after the initial procedure or may have never regained full motion prior to the reconstruction. Evaluation and treatment for these causes is beyond the scope of this chapter. Patient-reported instability, including the "double-fist sign" (clenched fists facing each other and rotating) and a sense of giving way or buckling, suggests ligamentous insufficiency.

An important clue to the underlying cause of ACL reconstruction failure is the timing of the signs and symptoms. Failures that occur within 6 months of the index procedure are usually due to technical reasons related to the surgery or noncompliance (i.e., return to sports too early). Failures after 6 months are more likely attributable to traumatic re-rupture or biologic failure (such as lack of graft incorporation), osteolysis, and degenerative joint disease. Therefore, it is important to obtain detailed information about the date of surgery and the onset of symptoms.

Knowledge of the surgical approach used in the index procedure, graft type, and method of graft fixation is also critically important for preoperative planning. Retrieval of previous operative reports, arthroscopic images, and both pre- and postoperative imaging studies is critical. The physician should also check for any concomitant procedures that were done (such as meniscal or cartilage procedures) at the time of the index procedure.

The examining physician should evaluate for any preoperative or postoperative issues relating to the prior operation. Specifically, it is important to determine whether full motion was regained prior to the index surgery, the postoperative rehabilitation program, and whether the patient was able to return to sports at the prior level of competition. Answers to these questions can provide insight into the degree of disability.

Finally, it is important to get a sense of the patient's current and future expectations, as these may require adjustment in the context of revision surgery.

Physical Examination

Lower extremity alignment should be evaluated first. Any signs of asymmetry and excessive valgus or varus deformity should be noted as these may require an alignment-correcting procedure (i.e., osteotomy). Gait should also be observed – a varus thrust may indicate posterolateral corner insufficiency. Next, inspection of the local skin, specifically looking for any previous incisions and scars will be helpful for better understanding the previous surgical approach and the type of graft utilized if the patient is unaware and prior documentation is unavailable. Muscle tone and thigh circumference should also be reviewed to determine whether the patient was able to regain their thigh musculature after surgery. Knee range of motion and strength testing should also be evaluated.

A complete and thorough ligamentous exam is critical, not only to assess the status of the previously reconstructed ACL but to look for any laxity in the collaterals, posterior cruciate ligament (PCL), or posterolateral corner (PLC). A complete ligamentous exam should include: the Lachman, anterior drawer and pivot shift tests for the ACL the posterior drawer, posterior sag sign, and quadriceps active test for the PCL; valgus stress testing at 0° and 30° of knee flexion for the MCL; varus stress testing at 0° and 30° of knee flexion for the LCL; the anteromedial drawer test for the posteromedial corner; and the dial test at 30° and 90° for the posterolateral corner (greater than 15° excessive external rotation compared to the contralateral) with the knee at 30° of flexion indicating possible posterolateral corner injury (greater than 15° excessive external rotation with the knee at 90° of flexion indicates possible concomitant PCL injury as well). The posterolateral spin test to detect posterolateral corner injury is also useful (Marx et al. 2009). With the patient supine and the knee flexed at 30° or 90°, the step-off of the lateral tibial plateau with regard to the lateral femoral condyle can be palpated with the examiner's thumb and compared with the contralateral side. This test also avoids error because of rotation of the ankle or foot, which may be associated with the dial test.

Finally, examination for patellar, meniscal, and articular cartilage pathology should be performed. The patella can be examined by evaluating its degree of mobility both in the medial and lateral direction, as well as its degree of eversion. Patellar apprehension may be elicited by applying a laterally directed force to the patella with the knee extended. A positive test is noted when the patient senses apprehension. Meniscal pathology can be detected by evaluating for joint line tenderness and by utilizing provocative maneuvers such as the McMurray, Apley compression/distraction, or Thessaly tests.

Imaging

In revision cases review of alignment is critical – therefore, obtaining a standing hip to ankle film to evaluate the mechanical axis is necessary. Weightbearing AP and PA flexed views should be obtained to examine the joint line both in extension (which can provide information on the status of the anterior joint surface) and in flexion (to evaluate the posterior joint surface). The AP view is particularly useful for evaluating tunnel positioning (especially coronal obliquity of the tunnels), hardware integrity and positioning, and tunnel diameter. Lateral knee X-rays are important to carefully review tunnel position on the tibia in the anteroposterior plane, sagittal obliquity of the graft, and femoral tunnel position. A merchant view is also important to better characterize the nature of the patellofemoral joint. For patients with possible tunnel widening, CT scan is the modality of choice. With CT, the clinician can measure the greatest dimension of both the tibial and femoral tunnels in multiple planes. Typically, excessive tunnel widening will require a staged ACL reconstruction with the first procedure dedicated to bone grafting of the tunnels. However, it depends on the position and orientation of the tunnels and each case should be individualized.

For patients that have previously undergone ACL reconstruction, it is generally recommended that an MRI with articular cartilage sequence be obtained to evaluate the key soft tissue structures, including the articular surfaces, the menisci, and of course the ligaments.

Indications/Contraindications

Laxity, demonstrated clinically with a positive Lachman exam and/or a positive pivot shift exam, that results in symptoms either with daily activities and/or athletic participation is the main indication for revision ACL reconstruction. Younger patients (i.e., 25 years and younger) in particular are at risk for articular cartilage and meniscal lesions with recurrent instability episodes and should be counseled as such. Older patients that are more sedentary and less likely to sustain repeat pivoting/instability episodes may benefit with an initial course of conservative therapy with a formal rehabilitation program and activity modification.

Absolute contraindications are few, but include concurrent septic arthritis or systemic infection. A relative contraindication includes advanced osteoarthrosis. Patients with diffuse degenerative joint disease may have minimal benefit with revision ACL reconstruction that will address the instability but not the arthritis.

Preoperative Planning

A preoperative plan is performed well before the day of surgery so that all necessary instruments and implants may be available. Key concepts to consider prior to surgery include the following:

Alignment

As with other knee procedures, critical review of the patient's alignment should be performed first. If excessive valgus or varus deformity is present, then an osteotomy may be indicated. If that is the case, then the procedures may either be staged (osteotomy first, followed by the soft tissue procedure) or performed concomitantly (osteotomy and ACL revision reconstruction at the same surgery). Osteotomy procedures are beyond the scope of this chapter. In some cases, instability may resolve after osteotomy and revision ACL reconstruction may not be necessary.

Tunnel Widening

If the ACL tunnels appear enlarged on plain X-ray (i.e., >15 mm in greatest dimension), then a CT scan to more accurately quantify the degree of tunnel widening may be indicated. CT scan is also helpful for identifying the precise location of hardware. Excessive tunnel widening (or expansion) may be an indication for staged ACL reconstruction with initial bone grafting of the tunnels performed prior to the definitive procedure (Maak et al. 2010). During the procedure the tunnels are gently re-reamed to remove sclerotic and fibrotic tissue and provide a bleeding surface, and then bone graft is inserted to fill the defects. There are several ways to do this, whether one hand makes dowels from allograft bone (femoral head for instance) or one uses commercial allograft bone dowels or bone chips. The dowels are then advanced into the tunnels either over a wire or passed in retrograde fashion with a suture.

The revision reconstruction is planned for 5–6 months after the grafting procedure, once healing and filling in of the defect is demonstrated (as observed on radiograph and/or CT scan). Other techniques to consider in the case of mild tunnel widening include: jumbo plugs, divergent tunnels, stacking screws, and matchstick or bullet grafting (Maak et al. 2010).

Skin Incision

The utilization of previous skin incisions should be considered as long as they allow for a safe and unhindered surgical approach. Should another incision be necessary, it is important to take into consideration the time from previous surgery (to account for revascularization) and the distance from prior incisions (to minimize the risk of skin necrosis, skin bridges should ideally be at least 7 cm). If there is any question regarding the viability of the local skin, or if the patient sustained a previous postoperative wound infection, a plastic surgery consultation should be considered.

Graft Selection

Typical graft options for revision ACL reconstruction include ipsilateral bone-patellar tendon-bone (BTB) autograft or contralateral BTB if the ipsilateral side was previously used. Other possible autologous graft options include ipsilateral (or contralateral) hamstring tendon (quadrupled gracilis and semitendinosus tendons), or quadriceps tendon (with or without a patellar bone block). Considering the higher rate of re-rupture with allograft compared to autograft (approximately four times higher in one study (Kaeding et al. 2011)), allograft tendon is typically reserved for multiligamentous knee injuries (where graft harvest can significantly increase morbidity), older patients (i.e., greater than 40 years of age), and low-demand patients. It is critical to review the previous graft type utilized and choose the graft option most appropriate for both the surgeon and patient.

Removal of Hardware

Removal of previously placed hardware is not always necessary, especially if the hardware does not interfere with tunnel placement during the revision procedure. However, metallic hardware, such as screws, often should be removed prior to tunnel creation if it precludes optimal tunnel placement. To remove a screw, it is useful to identify the manufacturer and size before the procedure and have the correct removal devices available. It is not uncommon for hardware to be enveloped in bone; thus, curettes, osteotomes, and burrs should be available as needed. Stripped metallic screws can usually be removed with either an oversized screwdriver impacted into the screw head, a reverse threaded screw removal instrument, or a coring reamer. Bioabsorbable-type hardware, on the other hand, can usually be reamed through without much difficulty since the screws are softer than the metallic drills/reamers. For removal of orthopedic staples, either an implant-specific staple removal device or an osteotome is adequate.

Tunnel Placement/Revision

Preoperative review of tunnel placement (as demonstrated on X-ray, CT, and/or MRI) in conjunction with diagnostic arthroscopy can help determine whether the previously placed tunnels will need revision. (It is generally preferred by the authors to place the tunnels at the center of anatomic footprint both on the femur and the tibia.) One of four scenarios may be present: (1) tibial tunnel placement is appropriate but femoral tunnel placement is not, (2) femoral tunnel placement is appropriate but tibial tunnel placement is not, (3) both tunnels are inappropriately placed, and (4) both tunnels are appropriately placed. In the latter scenario, both tunnels can simply be re-reamed and hardware can be removed as necessary, though one should always beware that redrilling and removing hardware can result in excessively large tunnels that may need to be grafted or addressed in some other manner (such as with divergent tunnel placement utilizing the same footprint for the femur or convergent tunnel placement for the tibia).

The virtue of the anteromedial portal technique and the two-incision (outside-in) technique as compared to the transtibial method is that femoral sockets/tunnels can be created independent of tibial tunnel positioning. If the transtibial method was used previously and femoral tunnel placement is the main issue, converting to the anteromedial portal method or the two-incision (outside-in) method may allow for more anatomic placement of the graft along the wall of the lateral condyle. If tibial tunnel placement is the main issue (i.e., too anterior or too posterior), it is usually not too difficult to reorient the tibial tunnel so that the aperture is at a more anatomic position.

If the posterior wall of the femoral tunnel was compromised (either at the index procedure or the revision surgery), then reorienting of the tunnel can be performed either with the anteromedial technique or the outside-in technique. Otherwise, the surgeon should be prepared to perform an "over-the-top" reconstruction with suspensory fixation.

If during surgery the newly prepared femoral tunnel "falls" into the previous one, then it may be necessary to "stack" screws in order to achieve an interference fit/aperture fixation or fill in the defect with graft (i.e., matchstick, dowel, etc.) at the time of the revision (Maak et al. 2010). If the defect is too large, then the reconstruction should be staged, and a formal bone grafting procedure as described in the above section should be performed.

Graft Fixation

The method of fixation will vary depending on the type of graft used. Typical fixation options include: aperture/interference fixation with screws and suspensory fixation with cortical ligament buttons and contemporary suture anchors, staples, or posts (screw and washer). For BTB grafts, metallic interference screws on both the femoral and tibial sides are usually recommended. For other types of grafts where one side has a bone block (i.e., Achilles, tibialis anterior, etc.), one may place metallic interference screws on the bone block side and either biodegradable screws or metallic soft tissue screws on the soft tissue sides. Other options on the soft tissue side include staple fixation or tensioning and fixation over a post and washer.

For hamstring tendons, suspensory fixation is performed on the femoral side using a cortical suture button (i.e., Endobutton, Smith and Nephew or TightRope, Arthrex). On the tibial side, interference screw fixation with a biointerference screw or a soft tissue metallic screw can be utilized, with or without additional fixation using a suture post or suture anchor.

Concomitant Procedures

Concomitant meniscal or cartilage procedures should be performed as indicated. These are beyond the scope of this chapter.

Pearls
1. It is critical to first identify the cause of failure. Simply indicating a patient for a revision reconstruction without a clear cause of failure is likely to result in less than optimal results
2. To be adept at revision reconstruction surgery, one must be comfortable with various graft choices. The ability to harvest hamstring, BTB, and quadriceps tendon autograft and use any number of allograft tendons increases the number of surgical options available
3. As in primary surgery, tunnel placement is critical. Creating a different tibial tunnel, if necessary, is usually not technically difficult; however, creating a new femoral tunnel/socket often requires creativity due to the more limited access arthroscopically. For the femoral side, utilizing the anteromedial portal can help to redirect the socket/tunnel placement in order to diverge from the original tunnel
4. Staged revision with an initial bone grafting procedure if the size of the tunnels is greater than 16 mm may be indicated
5. Add additional fixation with a post or an anchor if the fixation achieved intraoperatively is less than satisfactory
6. Have instrument removal sets ready for possible use
Pitfalls
1. Smaller-sized grafts (i.e., 7 mm or less) should not used be in the revision setting
2. Undiagnosed indolent infection or inflammatory disorder can be disastrous – one must always have a high level of suspicion for these causes of failure prior to indicating the patient for revision surgery
3. Rehabilitation should usually progress at a slower rate than in primary ACL reconstruction due to the more tenuous nature of the fixation and the soft tissues

Conclusions

The causes of failed primary ACL reconstruction are multiple but can typically be placed into three categories: technical, biologic, or mechanical. Some patients may have a combination of these factors. Technical causes of failure are the most common. Patients who present with recurrent instability that affects their activities of daily living and/or athletic participation may be indicated for revision ACL surgery.

Successful revision surgery depends on a careful review of the history, physical examination, and imaging studies. In addition, a well-thought out preoperative plan that incorporates the key elements outlined in this chapter can help optimize the possibility of successful outcomes.

Cross-References

- ▶ Allografts in Anterior Cruciate Ligament Reconstruction
- ▶ Anterior Cruciate Ligament Graft Selection and Fixation
- ▶ Anterior Cruciate Ligament Injuries and Surgery: Current Evidence and Modern Development
- ▶ Anterior Cruciate Ligament Reconstruction with Autologous Quadriceps Tendon
- ▶ Different Techniques of Anterior Cruciate Ligament Reconstruction: Guidelines
- ▶ State of the Art in Anterior Cruciate Ligament Surgery

References

Bach BR Jr, Mazzocca A, Fox JA (2003) Revision anterior cruciate ligament surgery. Arthroscopy 19:14–29

Baer GS, Harner CD (2007) Clinical outcomes of allograft versus autograft in anterior cruciate ligament reconstruction. Clin Sports Med 26:661–681. doi:10.1016/j.csm.2007.06.010

Barker JU, Drakos MC, Maak TG et al (2010) Effect of graft selection on the incidence of postoperative infection in anterior cruciate ligament reconstruction. Am J Sports Med 38:281–286. doi:10.1177/0363546509346414

Battaglia MJ, Cordasco FA, Hannafin JA et al (2007) Results of revision anterior cruciate ligament surgery. Am J Sports Med 35:2057–2066. doi:10.1177/0363546507307391

Biau DJ, Tournoux C, Katsahian S et al (2006) Bone-patellar tendon-bone autografts versus hamstring autografts for reconstruction of anterior cruciate ligament: meta-analysis. BMJ 332:995–1001. doi:10.1136/bmj.38784.384109.2F

Biau DJ, Tournoux C, Katsahian S et al (2007) ACL reconstruction: a meta-analysis of functional scores. Clin Orthop Relat Res 458:180–187. doi:10.1097/BLO.0b013e31803dcd6b

Corsetti JR, Jackson DW (1996) Failure of anterior cruciate ligament reconstruction: the biologic basis. Clin Orthop Relat Res 325:42–49

Fox JA, Pierce M, Bojchuk J et al (2004) Revision anterior cruciate ligament reconstruction with nonirradiated fresh-frozen patellar tendon allograft. Arthroscopy 20:787–794. doi:10.1016/j.arthro.2004.07.019

Garofalo R, Djahangiri A, Siegrist O (2006) Revision anterior cruciate ligament reconstruction with quadriceps tendon-patellar bone autograft. Arthroscopy 22:205–214. doi:10.1016/j.arthro.2005.08.045

Getelman MH, Friedman MJ (1999) Revision anterior cruciate ligament reconstruction surgery. J Am Acad Orthop Surg 7:189–198

Graf B, Uhr F (1988) Complications of intra-articular anterior cruciate reconstruction. Clin Sports Med 7:835–848

Harter RA, Osternig LR, Singer KM et al (1988) Long-term evaluation of knee stability and function following surgical reconstruction for anterior cruciate ligament insufficiency. Am J Sports Med 16:434–443

Howe JG, Johnson RJ, Kaplan MJ et al (1991) Anterior cruciate ligament reconstruction using quadriceps patellar tendon graft. Part I. Long-term followup. Am J Sports Med 19:447–457

Kaeding CC, Aros B, Pedroza A et al (2011) Allograft versus autograft anterior cruciate ligament reconstruction: predictors of failure from a moon prospective longitudinal cohort. Sports Health 3:73–81. doi:10.1177/1941738110386185

Kamath GV, Redfern JC, Greis PE, Burks RT (2011) Revision anterior cruciate ligament reconstruction. Am J Sports Med 39:199–217. doi:10.1177/0363546510370929

Kaplan MJ, Howe JG, Fleming B et al (1991) Anterior cruciate ligament reconstruction using quadriceps patellar tendon graft. Part II. A specific sport review. Am J Sports Med 19:458–462

Lyman S, Koulouvaris P, Sherman S et al (2009) Epidemiology of anterior cruciate ligament reconstruction: trends, readmissions, and subsequent knee surgery. J Bone Joint Surg Am 91:2321–2328. doi:10.2106/JBJS.H.00539

Maak TG, Voos JE, Wickiewicz TL, Warren RF (2010) Tunnel widening in revision anterior cruciate ligament reconstruction. J Am Acad Orthop Surg 18:695–706

Marx RG (ed) (2014) Revision ACL reconstruction: indications and techniques. Springer, New York

Marx RG, Shindle MK, Warren RF (2009) Management of posterior cruciate ligament injuries. Oper Tech Sports 7:162–166

Marzo JM, Bowen MK, Warren RF et al (1992) Intraarticular fibrous nodule as a cause of loss of extension following anterior cruciate ligament reconstruction. Arthroscopy 8:10–18

Reinhardt KR, Hammoud S, Bowers AL et al (2012) Revision ACL reconstruction in skeletally mature athletes younger than 18 years. Clin Orthop Relat Res 470:835–842. doi:10.1007/s11999-011-1956-1

Salmon L, Russell V, Musgrove T et al (2005) Incidence and risk factors for graft rupture and contralateral rupture after anterior cruciate ligament reconstruction. Arthroscopy 21:948–957. doi:10.1016/j.arthro.2005.04.110

Salmon LJ, Pinczewski LA, Russell VJ, Refshauge K (2006) Revision anterior cruciate ligament reconstruction with hamstring tendon autograft: 5- to 9-year follow-up. Am J Sports Med 34:1604–1614. doi:10.1177/0363546506288015

Shelbourne KD, Patel DV (1999) Treatment of limited motion after anterior cruciate ligament reconstruction. Knee Surg Sports Traumatol Arthrosc 7:85–92

Shelbourne KD, Patel DV, Martini DJ (1996) Classification and management of arthrofibrosis of the knee after anterior cruciate ligament reconstruction. Am J Sports Med 24:857–862

Shelbourne KD, Gray T, Haro M (2009) Incidence of subsequent injury to either knee within 5 years after anterior cruciate ligament reconstruction with patellar tendon autograft. Am J Sports Med 37:246–251. doi:10.1177/0363546508325665

Spindler KP, Kuhn JE, Freedman KB et al (2004) Anterior cruciate ligament reconstruction autograft choice: bone-tendon-bone versus hamstring: does it really matter? A systematic review. Am J Sports Med 32:1986–1995

Wright RW, Dunn WR, Amendola A et al (2007) Risk of tearing the intact anterior cruciate ligament in the contralateral knee and rupturing the anterior cruciate ligament graft during the first 2 years after anterior cruciate ligament reconstruction: a prospective MOON cohort study. Am J Sports Med 35:1131–1134. doi:10.1177/0363546507301318

Anterior Cruciate Ligament Injuries Identifiable for Pre-participation Imagiological Analysis: Risk Factors

123

Hélder Pereira, Margarida Fernandes, Rogério Pereira, Henrique Jones, J. C. Vasconcelos, Joaquim Miguel Oliveira, Rui Luís Reis, Volker Musahl, and João Espregueira-Mendes

Contents

H. Pereira (✉)
3B's Research Group – Biomaterials, Biodegradables and Biomimetics, Headquarters of the European Institute of Excellence on Tissue Engineering and Regenerative Medicine, University of Minho, Taipas, Guimarães, Portugal

ICVS/3B's – PT Government Associated Laboratory, Guimarães, Portugal

Clínica Espregueira–Mendes F.C. Porto Stadium – FIFA Medical Centre of Excellence, Porto, Portugal

Orthopedic Department, Centro Hospitalar Póvoa de Varzim, Vila do Conde, Portugal
e-mail: heldermdpereira@gmail.com

M. Fernandes • R. Pereira • J.C. Vasconcelos
FIFA Medical Centre of Excellence, Clínica Espregueira-Mendes F.C. Porto Stadium, Porto, Portugal
e-mail: margarida.mi@gmail.com; rp@espregueira.com; vaspor@sapo.pt

H. Jones
Department of Orthopedic Surgery, Knee and Sports Traumatology, Montijo Orthopaedic Clinic, Lusofona University, Lisbon, Portugal
e-mail: ortojones@gmail.com

J.M. Oliveira
3B's Research Group – Biomaterials, Biodegradables and Biomimetics, Headquarters of the European Institute of Excellence on Tissue Engineering and Regenerative Medicine, University of Minho, Taipas, Guimarães, Portugal

ICVS/3B's – PT Government Associated Laboratory, Braga/Guimarães, Portugal

FIFA Medical Centre of Excellence, Clínica Espregueira-Mendes F.C. Porto Stadium, Porto, Portugal
e-mail: miguel.oliveira@dep.uminho.pt

M.N. Doral, J. Karlsson (eds.), *Sports Injuries*,
DOI 10.1007/978-3-642-36569-0_80

Abstract

Identification of pre-participation risk factors for noncontact anterior cruciate ligament (ACL) injuries has been attracting a great deal of interest in the sports medicine and traumatology communities. Appropriate methods that enable predicting which patients could benefit from preventive strategies are most welcome. This would enable athlete-specific training and conditioning or tailored equipment in order to develop appropriate strategies to reduce incidence of injury. In order to accomplish these goals, the ideal system should be able to assess both anatomic and functional features. Complementarily, the screening method must be cost-effective and suited for widespread application. Anatomic study protocol requiring only standard X rays could answer some of such demands. Dynamic MRI/CT evaluation and electronically assisted pivot-shift evaluation can be powerful tools providing complementary information. These upcoming insights, when validated and properly combined, envision changing pre-participation knee examination in the near future. Herein different methods (validated or under research) aiming to improve the capacity to identify persons/athletes with higher risk for ACL injury are overviewed.

Introduction

Knee ligament reconstruction surgery is currently a common practice worldwide. In particular, anterior cruciate ligament (ACL) injury remains among the most common causes of orthopedic surgery (Griffin et al. 2000; Chadwick et al. 2008). Considering surgical reconstruction of ACL alone, it is estimated that more than 100,000 procedures are performed annually in the USA (Owings and Kozak 1998; Griffin et al. 2000), thus representing yearly costs that exceed 0.5 billion dollars. Such prevalence states the importance of knee surgeons to define strategies for early diagnosis and prevention based in detection of risk factors. Any action able to contribute for reducing the incidence of this injury, besides the personal and athletic benefit, would probably have a significant social and economic impact (Chadwick et al. 2008).

If it were possible to identify pre-participation athletes with increased risk of noncontact ACL injury based in a method suitable for widespread

R.L. Reis
Clínica Espregueira–Mendes F.C. Porto Stadium – FIFA Medical Centre of Excellence, Porto, Portugal

Orthopaedic Department, Hospital de S. Sebastião, Feira, Portugal

ICVS/3B's – PT Government Associated Laboratory, Braga/Guimarães, Portugal

3B's Research Group – Biomaterials, Biodegradables and Biomimetics, Headquarters of the European Institute of Excellence on Tissue Engineering and Regenerative Medicine, University of Minho, Taipas, Guimarães, Portugal
e-mail: rgreis@dep.uminho.pt

V. Musahl
Department of Orthopaedic Surgery, University of Pittsburgh Medical Center, Pittsburgh, PA, USA

Division of Sports Medicine, Orthopaedic Surgery, University of Pittsburgh, Pittsburgh, PA, USA
e-mail: musahlv@upmc.edu

J. Espregueira-Mendes
3B's Research Group – Biomaterials, Biodegradables and Biomimetics, Headquarters of the European Institute of Excellence on Tissue Engineering and Regenerative Medicine, University of Minho, Taipas, Guimarães, Portugal

Clínica Espregueira–Mendes F.C. Porto Stadium – FIFA Medical Centre of Excellence, Porto, Portugal

Orthopedic Department, Centro Hospitalar Póvoa de Varzim, Vila do Conde, Portugal

ICVS/3B's – PT Government Associated Laboratory, Braga/Guimarães, Portugal

Orthopaedic Department, Hospital de S. Sebastião, Feira, Portugal
e-mail: jem@espregueira.com; joaoespregueira@netcabo.pt

application, one could properly adjust their training methods.

Intensive research on ACL pathophysiology and surgery (anatomy, biology, physiopathology, and biomechanics) has been done, which contributed to important clinical improvements (e.g., graft selection, surgical techniques, tunnel placement, graft fixation, and rehabilitation protocols). Recently, new trends related to the biology of graft incorporation and "ligamentization" process have also improved the ability to prevent postoperative complications such as excessive graft elongation, pullout, or slippage (Menetrey et al. 2008).

Recognizing all the previous, it seems mandatory to put similar efforts focused on prevention strategies (Arendt and Brown 2012).

Athletes and general population have higher expectations concerning medical care. From the initial stand for prevention of arthritis following ACL rupture, nowadays people want to prevent injury by "working" in advance. Only if this is not possible, then the actual demand is complete repair of anatomy and functional recovery including highly demanding activities (Georgoulis et al. 2007; Tashman et al. 2007).

A group of ACL injury risk factors including neuromuscular, hormonal, genetic, cognitive, functional, and previous injury or a variety of extrinsic risk factors will be discussed separately (Sward et al. 2010; Smith et al. 2012a, b).

In the following sections, the identifiable risk factors for ACL rupture, with a particular emphasis in the morphologic/anatomic characteristics determined by clinical examination, conventional radiology or dynamic MRI/CT protocols, or technologically enhanced evaluation methods will be summarized.

Manual Instrumented Devices

Manual instrumented tests aim to enhance manual examination by providing more objective information which could be more easily transmitted and analyzed but still be suitable for use "in office."

However, most of such devices share some limitations with clinical examination such as: absence of bony landmarks, influenced by muscle guarding, or being operator dependent (Pereira et al. 2012).

Table 1 Currently available manual instrumented devices

Device	References
KT-1000 laximeter (Medmetric, San Diego, CA, USA)	Daniel et al. 1985
KT-2000 laximeter (Medmetric, San Diego, CA, USA)	Myrer et al. 1996
Stryker Knee Laxity Tester (Stryker, Kalamazoo, MI)	Boniface et al. 1986, Highgenboten et al. 1989
Genucom Knee Analysis System (FARO Medical Technologies, Montreal, Ontario Canada)	Oliver and Coughlin 1987
Kneelax 3 (Monitored Rehab Systems, Haarlem, The Netherlands)	Benvenuti et al. 1998
Rolimeter (Aircast Europa, Neubeuern, Germany)	Balasch et al. 1999
CA-4000 Electrogoniometer (OSI, Hayward, CA)	Kvist 2004

Several arthrometers have been presented through time. The KT-1000 laximeter (Medmetric, San Diego, CA, USA) (Daniel et al. 1985) is probably the most commonly used and is still the reference instrument to which new devices have been tested (Robert et al. 2009). However, KT-1000 has been considered as operator dependent with significant false-negative results and questionable reproducibility (Jardin et al. 1999; Boyer et al. 2004). The KT-2000 Ligament Arthrometer (KT-2000; Medmetric Corp) uses the same method as the KT-1000, and the main difference concerns the data output which includes a graphic presentation representing the amount of tibial displacement correlated to the amount of applied force via an X-Y plotter (Myrer et al. 1996). Neither of them is suitable for rotatory laxity assessment.

Several devices are currently accessible (see Table 1).

However, none of these systems have proved to be more effective than clinical examination alone (Myrer et al. 1996) and share comparable limitations (intraclass correlation coefficient [ICC], 0.6).

iPad Application

Methods for ACL injury prediction using clinic-based measurements and computer analyses that require only freely available public domain software have been envisioned (Myer et al. 2011).

Common electronic devices used in daily living such as the iPad (Apple Inc., Cupertino, CA, USA) by means of an adequate user-friendly application might enhance clinical analysis protocol in the near future. This could be true either for clinical testing or imaging study.

Manual examinations are influenced by surgeon's training and experience and currently rely in subjective impressions (Branch et al. 2010b). Pivot-shift test has been considered a better predictor of clinical outcomes than any other uniplanar maneuver (Katz and Fingeroth 1986; Citak et al. 2011). Nevertheless, the Lachman test has been considered as more sensitive (Prins 2006), and the limitations of the pivot-shift test, particularly in an awake patient, must be considered.

By providing a tool based in recorded motion images, it promises to improve objective assessment of clinical examination (Hoshino et al. 2013). The iPad app is currently under process of validation (PIVOT study; ISAKOS/OREF research grant) and it envisions creating new perspectives on detection of risk factors, preoperative evaluation, and clinical outcomes for patients. Possibly, in the future a similar computed analysis might combine clinical information with protocolled analysis of X-ray, CT, and MRI exams. Such electronic devices could ease the application of more complex analytic algorithms combining consideration of multiple factors but keeping it fast, easy to use, and affordable.

Robotic Systems

Robotic systems have promised to overcome bias inherent to manual force application by means of comprising mechanical methods to apply load or torque in a controlled mode (magnitude, direction, rate) (Lob et al. 2006; Park et al. 2008; Tsai et al. 2008; Robert et al. 2009; Woo and Fisher 2009; Branch et al. 2010a; Musahl et al. 2010; Citak et al. 2011; Mayr et al. 2011).

Using such approach, the Pittsburgh's study group has contributed great insights for understanding knee joint kinematics in multiple degree of freedom (Woo and Fisher 2009; Musahl et al. 2010).

The GNRB knee laxity testing device (Genurob, Montenay, France), provides an anteriorly directed force to the proximal tibia with the knee at 0° rotation and 20° flexion in a rigid leg support (Robert et al. 2009). The load is delivered gradually and the software compares side-to-side differences on the magnitude of anterior tibial translation but also a force-displacement curve whose slopes would reflect ACL elasticity.

It has been demonstrated in cadaveric hip-to-toe models that mechanized pivot-shift tests provide more reliable and consistent measurements of pivot-shift phenomenon (Musahl et al. 2010; Citak et al. 2011). Another device designed to assess knee rotation in non-injured knees has also been presented including its intra-tester, test-retest, and inter-tester reliability (Tsai et al. 2008). The authors concluded that such method presents acceptable reliability for clinical use.

Another study (Park et al. 2008) compared ten healthy men and ten healthy women with the knee at 60° of flexion and established that women had increased external rotation laxity. Branch et al. (2010a) also reported gender-related outcomes with implications on detection of risk factors for ACL injury. Assuming the hypothesis that the opposite knee of patients with a previous ACL reconstruction presents biomechanical characteristics of greater risk for ACL rupture, the authors could demonstrate that knees with greater tibial internal rotation have higher risk for ACL injury when compared with healthy volunteers' (Balasch et al. 1999).

Another method (Mayr et al. 2011) was tested in the awake and non-anesthetized patient measuring anteroposterior translation and rotation of the knee joint. Tibial external/internal rotation was imposed with a torque of 2 Nm on the footrest with the ankle locked in dorsiflexion. Anterior translation of the tibia in relation to the femur was measured in neutral position, internal and external rotation. Intra- and inter-rater reliability was validated in ten healthy volunteers. The authors concluded that the method enables to objectively discriminate isolated ACL rupture and ACL rupture combined with medial instability. The method demonstrated inter- and intra-observer reliability and reproducibility.

All these systems have not yet been included in routine clinical practice. They might be considered as somewhat expensive, time consuming, and/or requiring logistic demands which limit their "in office" application so far.

Stress Radiography/Radiostereometry

The combination of a stress device and radiography (stress radiography) has been proposed as a knee laxity measurement technique for ACL (Jonsson et al. 1992; Jardin et al. 1999; Isberg et al. 2006) and posterior cruciate ligament (PCL) assessment (Schulz et al. 2005; Jung et al. 2006).

The TELOS device (Telos GmbH, Laubscher, Hölstein, Switzerland) is the most common example of such a device. It permits to measure anterior and posterior drawer displacements controlling the magnitude of load transmission. The method considers the displacement of the midpoint between the tangents to the posterior contours of the tibial condyles drawn perpendicular to the tibial plateau and relative to the position of the corresponding midpoint between the two posterior aspects of the femoral condyles.

The reliability of TELOS device has been reported (Staubli et al. 1992).

These methods present the advantage over several others by considering bony landmarks to measure translation, thus avoiding issues related to soft-tissue artifact. However, no further information of knee joint soft-tissue, cartilage, or meniscus status is provided.

Radiostereometric analysis, originally presented by Selvik (1989), has been proposed as a method to enhance precision of translation measurement of the knee joint by stress radiography. This started as an invasive method that relies on implantation of tantalum beads and has high accuracy (within 0.1 mm), which has also been proposed to assess migration of arthroplasty components throughout time.

There are reports stating the advantage of TELOS method over KT-1000 (Jardin et al. 1999), but limitations have been recognized even combining radiostereometric analysis based on the absence of a stress device that can produce reliable joint translation (Sorensen et al. 2011).

Radiographic Assessment of Bone Morphology Risk Factors

Morphologic characteristics identified in conventional X-ray protocols can provide an inexpensive, effective, and feasible tool to identify individuals in higher risk for ACL lesion. Standard radiological evaluation should include: (i) full-leg standing anteroposterior view (mechanical axes), (ii) standing anteroposterior and schuss view (assessment of notch morphology, evaluation of arthritic changes), (iii) standing lateral view in full extension and 30° of flexion (tibial slope), and (iv) skyline view (30° or 45° of flexion) to evaluate patellofemoral articulation. The radiological protocols are a valuable, low-cost, accessible tool which helps gathering varied and fundamental information concerning bone morphology.

Femoral notch characteristics and tibial plateau slope and/or depth have been proposed as morphologic risk factors possible to identify from standard X-ray evaluation (Vyas et al. 2011; Smith et al. 2012b; Wordeman et al. 2012). Females are more likely than males to have a narrow A-shaped intercondylar notch which has been associated to gender-specific risk factor (Sutton and Bullock 2013). However, notch width index has not been considered a feasible method (Vyas et al. 2011).

There has been growing interest on study of tibial morphology by lateral X-ray or MRI (Wordeman et al. 2012). Dejour and Bonnin used lateral radiographs to demonstrate a mean 6 mm increase in anterior tibial translation (ATT) for each 10° increase in posterior tibial slope in ACL-deficient patients and healthy controls (Dejour and Bonnin 1994).

A recent meta-analysis proposed to assess in vivo studies reporting tibial plateau slope as a risk factor for anterior cruciate ligament (ACL) injury (Wordeman et al. 2012). Most radiographic studies reporting medial tibial plateau slope (MTPS) demonstrated significant differences between controls and ACL-injured groups (Wordeman et al. 2012). Lateral tibial plateau slope (LTPS) was reported to be significantly greater in ACL-injured. It has been recognized that characterizing the tibial plateau surface with a single slope measurement represents an insufficient approximation of its three-dimensionality, and the biomechanical impact of the tibial slope likely is more complex than previously appreciated (Feucht et al. 2013). Reported tibial slope values for control groups vary greatly between studies (Wordeman et al. 2012). A recent study proposed that the correlation between anteroposterior length of the external condyle and anteroposterior length of tibial plateau had stronger association to risk for ACL rupture (Fig. 1) (Pereira et al. 2013).

The clinical utility of imaging-based measurement methods for the determination of ACL injury risk requires more reliable techniques capable to demonstrate and preserve consistency between studies.

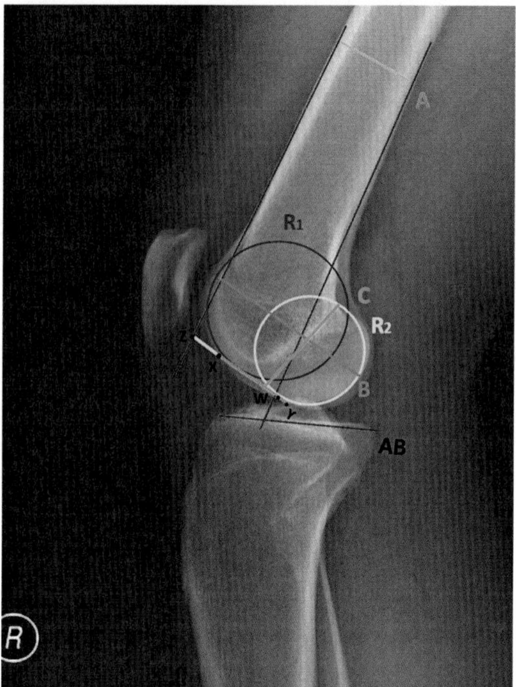

Fig. 1 Lateral X-ray view analysis: width of the femoral shaft (*E*), anteroposterior length of the external condyle (*C*), the proximal-distal height of external condyle (*D*). Two perfect *circles* were created to adapt to the greater extent of anterior and posterior contour of lateral condyle and their radius considered (*R1* and *R2*, respectively). A tangent to both circles is drawn and the points where it intersects circle 1 (*x*) and circle 2 (*y*) are considered. The points where this straight line intersects the line of anterior (*z*) and posterior (*w*) femoral cortex lines are also drawn

Morphologic and Functional MRI Assessment: PKTD®

It has been proposed that a narrow intercondylar notch assessed by intercondylar notch width index on MRI may increase the risk of ACL injury, but the data are somewhat conflicting (Alizadeh and Kiavash 2008). Females are more likely than males to have a narrow A-shaped intercondylar notch, and special surgical considerations are required in such cases (Fig. 2) (Sutton and Bullock 2013). Intercondylar notch stenosis and larger inner angle of lateral condyle of the femur are risk factors for ACL rupture by

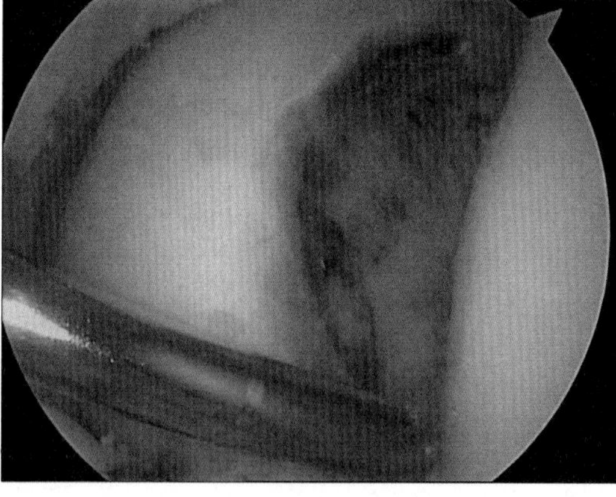

Fig. 2 Arthroscopic view of a type A intercondylar notch

Table 2 Studies assessing tibial slope by MRI imaging as risk factor for ACL injury

Author(s)	Study design (level of evidence)	N (patients enrolled)	MRI protocol	Conclusions
Stijak et al. 2008	Case-control study (level III)	Cases: $n = 33$ (21 ♂, 12 ♀)	Sagittal MRI	The greater tibial slope of the lateral tibial plateau may be the factor that leads to the injury of the anterior cruciate ligament. The tibial slope of the medial and lateral condyles should be compared separately
		Controls: $n = 33$ (21 ♂, 12 ♀)		
Bisson and Gurske-DePerio 2010	Retrospective case-control study (level III)	Cases: $n = 40$ (20 ♂, 20 ♀)	Axial and parasagittal MRI	Women's knees presented proportionally deeper medial and lateral femoral condyles, as well as deeper medial tibial plateaus. Men with ACL tears had deeper medial and lateral tibial plateaus, as well as an increased posterior slope of the lateral tibial plateau comparing to controls
		Controls: $n = 40$ (20 ♂, 20 ♀)		
Hashemi et al. 2010	Case-control study (level III)	Cases: $n = 49$ (22 ♂, 27 ♀)	Sagittal MRI	A combination of increased posterior tibial plateau slope and shallow medial tibial plateau depth could be a major risk factor in anterior cruciate ligament injury susceptibility regardless of gender. Men and women present different risk factors
		Controls: $n = 55$ (22 ♂, 33 ♀)		
Simon et al. 2010	Retrospective case-control study (level III)	Cases: $n = 27$ (17 ♂, 10 ♀)	3D-SPGR axial and sagittal MRI	The lateral tibial plateaus in the uninjured contralateral knees of the injured subjects had a significantly steeper posterior slope
		Controls: $n = 27$ (17 ♂, 10 ♀)		
Hudek et al. 2011	Prognostic study (level II)	Cases: $n = 55$ (24 ♂, 31 ♀)	Sagittal MRI	There is no obvious link between the medial or lateral posterior tibial slopes (PTS) and ACL injury. However, a greater lateral meniscus slope may indicate a greater risk of injury. The PTS can differ between the genders but the average difference is small
		Controls: $n = 55$ (24 ♂, 31 ♀)		
Khan et al. 2011	Retrospective case-control study (level III)	Cases: $n = 73$ (53 ♂, 20 ♀)	Sagittal MRI	Women with shallower medial tibial plateau depth and men with steeper lateral tibial plateau slope (LTPS) are at higher risk of sustaining ACL injury. Overall, steeper LTPS is a significant risk factor for sustaining ACL injury
		Controls: $n = 51$ (32 ♂, 19 ♀)		
Terauchi et al. 2011	Cross-sectional study (level III)	Cases: $n = 77$ (33 ♂, 40 ♀)	T2-weighted sagittal MRI	There were 2 types of large femoral plateau angles: one had its origin in an increasing tibial posterior slope and the other resulted from hyperextension of the knee. Large posterior tibial slope and hyperextension are both correlated with noncontact ACL injury in women
		Controls: $n = 58$ (28 ♂, 30 ♀)		

increasing the risk of ACL impingement in female athletes measured on coronal MR images (Miljko et al. 2012). The intercondylar notch dimensions were found to be smaller in the ACL-injured subjects, potentially putting the ACL at risk of impingement, and intercondylar notch volume was correlated to ACL volume ($r = 0.58$). Discriminant analysis showed that the notch width at the inlet could be a predictor of ACL injury (Simon et al. 2010). Enhanced height of the intercondylar notch and lesser value of the notch shape index were associated with rupture of the ACL in males but not in females (Stijak et al. 2012). It has been recently concluded that

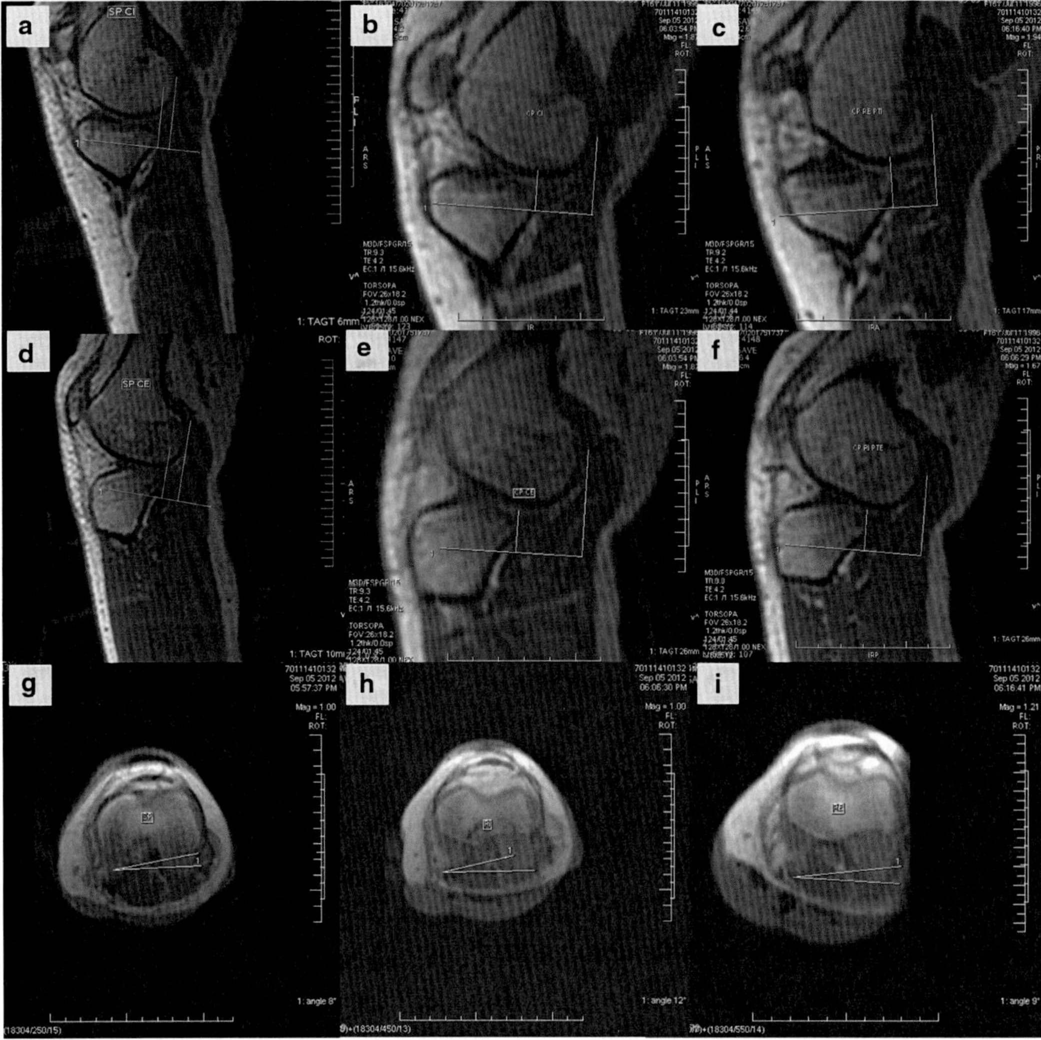

Fig. 3 Standard protocol evaluation with PKTD: Sagittal view with foot in neutral position without load application correspondent to medial (**a**) and lateral compartments (**c**). Result after load applications correspondent to medial (**b**) and lateral compartments (**d**). In this case, the differential would be respectively of 17 and 16 mm. Image correspondent to load after maximum internal foot rotation in lateral compartment (**e**) and after maximum external foot rotation in medial compartment (**f**). Evaluation of angular and linear tibial dislocation from axial views: without load (**g**) and with load after internal (**h**) and external foot rotation (**i**). Evaluation confirmed global ACL insufficiency

type A femoral notch appears to be a risk factor for ACL injury, whereas a reduced notch index has no significant correlation to ACL injury (Al-Saeed et al. 2013).

Proximal tibia morphologic study by MRI has generated increased interest through time (Table 2).

When compared with normal men, men with ACL tears had deeper medial and lateral tibial plateaus, as well as an increased posterior slope of the lateral tibial plateau (Bisson and Gurske-DePerio 2010). Women with shallower medial tibial plateau depth and men with steeper lateral tibial plateau slope (LTPS) are at higher risk of sustaining ACL injury. Overall, steeper LTPS might be considered a significant risk factor for sustaining ACL injury (Khan et al. 2011).

Besides morphologic assessment, nowadays it is possible to combine morphologic and functional assessment of the knee joint during

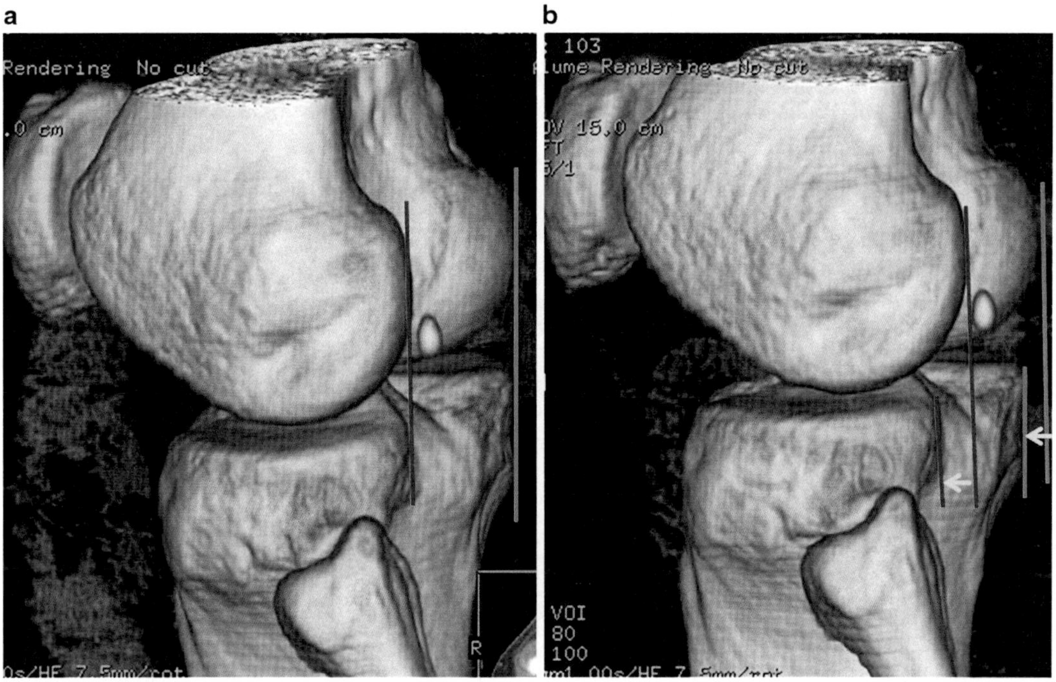

Fig. 4 CT 3D imaging reconstruction of PKTD examination. Initial position without load application (**a**). After load application notice *yellow arrows* representing anterior tibial displacement (**b**)

one single MRI or CT-based examination by means of using the Porto Knee Testing Device (PKTD) (Espregueira-Mendes et al. 2012; Pereira et al. 2012). In this way one might combine the study of morphologic bony parameters with evaluation of anteroposterior and rotational laxity (Fig. 3).

CT scan is many times useful particularly in patients submitted to previous primary ACL reconstruction to study tunnel placement as well as the surrounding bony structure. By combining CT with PKTD, we simultaneously can objective measure joint parameters concerning laxity (Fig. 4).

PKTD might play a role in prevention strategies by favoring detection of risk factors and/or identifying those patients presenting higher rotational instability and who may require an ACL reconstruction technique which provides higher rotational constraint (e.g., double-bundle) (Hemmerich et al. 2011).

These data provide one further step in understanding knee kinematics, but their functional implication and the way in which they might affect ACL reconstruction are not fully achieved. ACL research demands perseverance and patience (Lubowitz and Poehling 2010).

Summary

Ideal screening methods for risk factors need to be relatively low cost, noninvasive, and simple, with minimal time requirements.

Currently there is no effective "tool" nor even straightforward guidelines for how some of the identified risk factors can be used to assist the clinician.

The relevance of bone morphology as a possible risk factor for ACL rupture has been reinforced. Besides all the knowledge achieved by research using expensive technological devices such as robotics, gait analysis laboratories or navigation keeps being far from routine use aiming for detection of risk factors. New technological options such as the iPad app promise to provide significant progress in standardization and quantification of clinical examinations. Moreover, such devices could combine, in future, consideration of clinical and imaging findings in a user-friendly method while combining multiple factors in more complex algorithms. Dynamic MRI with PKTD has brought novel insights to more detailed anatomic and functional evaluation.

More important than "isolated" research lines, it would be necessary to combine all up-to-date insights and modern knowledge in a single and practical screening method.

Cross-References

- ▶ Anterior Cruciate Ligament Augmentation in Partial Ruptures
- ▶ Anterior Cruciate Ligament Injuries and Surgery: Current Evidence and Modern Development
- ▶ Anterior Cruciate Ligament Injuries in Children
- ▶ Partial Anterior Cruciate Ligament Ruptures: Knee Laxity Measurements and Pivot Shift

References

Alizadeh A, Kiavash V (2008) Mean intercondylar notch width index in cases with and without anterior cruciate ligament tears. Iran J Radiol 5:205–208

Al-Saeed O, Brown M, Athyal R, Sheikh M (2013) Association of femoral intercondylar notch morphology, width index and the risk of anterior cruciate ligament injury. Knee Surg Sports Traumatol Arthrosc 21:678–682

Arendt EA, Brown GA (2012) Non-contact ACL injury: can anatomic factors be used in screening at-risk athletes? Commentary on an article by Christopher J. Wahl, MD, et al.: "An association of lateral knee sagittal anatomic factors with non-contact ACL injury: sex or geometry?". J Bone Joint Surg Am 94:e20

Balasch H, Schiller M, Friebel H, Hoffmann F (1999) Evaluation of anterior knee joint instability with the Rolimeter. A test in comparison with manual assessment and measuring with the KT-1000 arthrometer. Knee Surg Sports Traumatol Arthrosc 7:204–208

Benvenuti JF, Vallotton JA, Meystre JL, Leyvraz PF (1998) Objective assessment of the anterior tibial translation in Lachman test position. Comparison between three types of measurement. Knee Surg Sports Traumatol Arthrosc 6:215–219

Bisson LJ, Gurske-DePerio J (2010) Axial and sagittal knee geometry as a risk factor for noncontact anterior cruciate ligament tear: a case-control study. Arthroscopy 26:901–906

Boniface RJ, Fu FH, Ilkhanipour K (1986) Objective anterior cruciate ligament testing. Orthopedics 9:391–393

Boyer P, Djian P, Christel P, Paoletti X, Degeorges R (2004) Reliability of the KT-1000 arthrometer (Medmetric) for measuring anterior knee laxity: comparison with Telos in 147 knees. Rev Chir Orthop Reparatrice Appar Mot 90:757–764

Branch TP, Browne JE, Campbell JD, Siebold R, Freedberg HI, Arendt EA et al (2010a) Rotational laxity greater in patients with contralateral anterior cruciate ligament injury than healthy volunteers. Knee Surg Sports Traumatol Arthrosc 18:1379–1384

Branch TP, Mayr HO, Browne JE, Campbell JC, Stoehr A, Jacobs CA (2010b) Instrumented examination of anterior cruciate ligament injuries: minimizing flaws of the manual clinical examination. Arthroscopy 26:997–1004

Chadwick CC, Rogowski J, Joyce BT (2008) The economics of anterior cruciate ligament reconstruction. In: Prodromos C, Brown C, F FH, Georgoulis AD, Gobbi A, Howell SM (eds) The anterior cruciate ligament: reconstruction and basic science. Saunders Elsevier, Philadelphia, pp 79–83

Citak M, Suero EM, Rozell JC, Bosscher MR, Kuestermeyer J, Pearle AD (2011) A mechanized and standardized pivot shifter: technical description and first evaluation. Knee Surg Sports Traumatol Arthrosc 19:707–711

Daniel DM, Stone ML, Sachs R, Malcom L (1985) Instrumented measurement of anterior knee laxity in patients with acute anterior cruciate ligament disruption. Am J Sports Med 13:401–407

Dejour H, Bonnin M (1994) Tibial translation after anterior cruciate ligament rupture. Two radiological tests compared. J Bone Joint Surg (Br) 76:745–749

Espregueira-Mendes J, Pereira H, Sevivas N, Passos C, Vasconcelos JC, Monteiro A et al (2012) Assessment of rotatory laxity in anterior cruciate ligament-deficient knees using magnetic resonance imaging with Porto-knee testing device. Knee Surg Sports Traumatol Arthrosc 20:671–678

Feucht MJ, Mauro CS, Brucker PU, Imhoff AB, Hinterwimmer S (2013) The role of the tibial slope in sustaining and treating anterior cruciate ligament injuries. Knee Surg Sports Traumatol Arthrosc 21:134–145

Georgoulis AD, Ristanis S, Chouliaras V, Moraiti C, Stergiou N (2007) Tibial rotation is not restored after ACL reconstruction with a hamstring graft. Clin Orthop Relat Res 454:89–94

Griffin LY, Agel J, Albohm MJ, Arendt EA, Dick RW, Garrett WE et al (2000) Noncontact anterior cruciate ligament injuries: risk factors and prevention strategies. J Am Acad Orthop Surg 8:141–150

Hashemi J, Chandrashekar N, Mansouri H, Gill B, Slauterbeck JR, Schutt RC Jr et al (2010) Shallow medial tibial plateau and steep medial and lateral tibial slopes: new risk factors for anterior cruciate ligament injuries. Am J Sports Med 38:54–62

Hemmerich A, van der Merwe W, Batterham M, Vaughan CL (2011) Knee rotational laxity in a randomized comparison of single- versus double-bundle anterior cruciate ligament reconstruction. Am J Sports Med 39:48–56

Highgenboten CL, Jackson A, Meske NB (1989) Genucom, KT-1000, and Stryker knee laxity measuring device comparisons. Am J Sports Med 17:743–746

Hoshino Y, Araujo P, Ahlden M, Samuelsson K, Muller B, Hofbauer M et al (2013) Quantitative evaluation of the pivot shift by image analysis using the iPad. Knee Surg Sports Traumatol Arthrosc 21:975–980

Hudek R, Fuchs B, Regenfelder F, Koch PP (2011) Is noncontact ACL injury associated with the posterior tibial and meniscal slope? Clin Orthop Relat Res 469:2377–2384

Isberg J, Faxen E, Brandsson S, Eriksson BI, Karrholm J, Karlsson J (2006) KT-1000 records smaller side-to-side differences than radiostereometric analysis before and after an ACL reconstruction. Knee Surg Sports Traumatol Arthrosc 14:529–535

Jardin C, Chantelot C, Migaud H, Gougeon F, Debroucker MJ, Duquennoy A (1999) Reliability of the KT-1000 arthrometer in measuring anterior laxity of the knee: comparative analysis with Telos of 48 reconstructions of the anterior cruciate ligament and intra- and interobserver reproducibility. Rev Chir Orthop Reparatrice Appar Mot 85:698–707

Jonsson H, Elmqvist LG, Karrholm J, Fugl-Meyer A (1992) Lengthening of anterior cruciate ligament graft. Roentgen stereophotogrammetry of 32 cases 2 years after repair. Acta Orthop Scand 63:587–592

Jung TM, Reinhardt C, Scheffler SU, Weiler A (2006) Stress radiography to measure posterior cruciate ligament insufficiency: a comparison of five different techniques. Knee Surg Sports Traumatol Arthrosc 14:1116–1121

Katz JW, Fingeroth RJ (1986) The diagnostic accuracy of ruptures of the anterior cruciate ligament comparing the Lachman test, the anterior drawer sign, and the pivot shift test in acute and chronic knee injuries. Am J Sports Med 14:88–91

Khan MS, Seon JK, Song EK (2011) Risk factors for anterior cruciate ligament injury: assessment of tibial plateau anatomic variables on conventional MRI using a new combined method. Int Orthop 35:1251–1256

Kvist J (2004) Sagittal plane translation during level walking in poor-functioning and well-functioning patients with anterior cruciate ligament deficiency. Am J Sports Med 32:1250–1255

Lob T, Verheyden AP, Josten Ch, (2006) The function of the ACL measured in an vertical opened MRI (0.5 Tesla). In: 12th F S ESSKA congress, Innsbruck

Lubowitz JH, Poehling GG (2010) Understanding ACL research requires patience and persistence. Arthroscopy 26:869–871

Mayr HO, Hoell A, Bernstein A, Hube R, Zeiler C, Kalteis T et al (2011) Validation of a measurement device for instrumented quantification of anterior translation and rotational assessment of the knee. Arthroscopy 27:1096–1104

Menetrey J, Duthon VB, Laumonier T, Fritschy D (2008) "Biological failure" of the anterior cruciate ligament graft. Knee Surg Sports Traumatol Arthrosc 16:224–231

Miljko M, Grle M, Kozul S, Kolobaric M, Djak I (2012) Intercondylar notch width and inner angle of lateral femoral condyle as the risk factors for anterior cruciate ligament injury in female handball players in Herzegovina. Coll Antropol 36:195–200

Musahl V, Voos J, O'Loughlin PF, Stueber V, Kendoff D, Pearle AD (2010) Mechanized pivot shift test achieves greater accuracy than manual pivot shift test. Knee Surg Sports Traumatol Arthrosc 18:1208–1213

Myer GD, Ford KR, Hewett TE (2011) New method to identify athletes at high risk of ACL injury using clinic-based measurements and freeware computer analysis. Br J Sports Med 45:238–244

Myrer JW, Schulthies SS, Fellingham GW (1996) Relative and absolute reliability of the KT-2000 arthrometer for uninjured knees. Am J Sports Med 24:104–108

Oliver JH, Coughlin LP (1987) Objective knee evaluation using the Genucom Knee Analysis System. Clinical implications. Am J Sports Med 15:571–578

Owings MF, Kozak LJ (1998) Ambulatory and inpatient procedures in the United States, 1996. Vital Health Stat 13:1–119

Park HS, Wilson NA, Zhang LQ (2008) Gender differences in passive knee biomechanical properties in tibial rotation. J Orthop Res 26:937–944

Pereira H, Sevivas N, Pereira R, Monteiro A, Oliveira JM, Reis RL et al (2012) New tools for diagnosis, assessment of surgical outcome and follow-up. In: Hernández J, Monllau JC (eds) Lesiones Ligamentosas de La Rodilla. Marge Books, Barcelona, pp 185–194

Pereira H, Silva-Correia J, Yan LP, Oliveira A, Oliveira JM, Espregueira-Mendes J et al (2013) Radiographic method to determine risk factors for ACL rupture in athletes based in bone morphology. In: French Arthroscopy Society meeting, Bordeaux

Prins M (2006) The Lachman test is the most sensitive and the pivot shift the most specific test for the diagnosis of ACL rupture. Aust J Physiother 52:66

Robert H, Nouveau S, Gageot S, Gagniere B (2009) A new knee arthrometer, the GNRB: experience in ACL complete and partial tears. Orthop Traumatol Surg Res 95:171–176

Schulz MS, Russe K, Lampakis G, Strobel MJ (2005) Reliability of stress radiography for evaluation of posterior knee laxity. Am J Sports Med 33:502–506

Selvik G (1989) Roentgen stereophotogrammetry. A method for the study of the kinematics of the skeletal system. Acta Orthop Scand Suppl 232:1–51

Simon RA, Everhart JS, Nagaraja HN, Chaudhari AM (2010) A case-control study of anterior cruciate ligament volume, tibial plateau slopes and intercondylar notch dimensions in ACL-injured knees. J Biomech 43:1702–1707

Smith HC, Vacek P, Johnson RJ, Slauterbeck JR, Hashemi J, Shultz S et al (2012a) Risk factors for anterior cruciate ligament injury: a review of the literature-part 2: hormonal, genetic, cognitive function, previous injury, and extrinsic risk factors. Sports Health 4:155–161

Smith HC, Vacek P, Johnson RJ, Slauterbeck JR, Hashemi J, Shultz S et al (2012b) Risk factors for anterior cruciate ligament injury: a review of the literature – part 1: neuromuscular and anatomic risk. Sports Health 4:69–78

Sorensen OG, Larsen K, Jakobsen BW, Kold S, Hansen TB, Lind M et al (2011) The combination of radiostereometric analysis and the telos stress device results in poor precision for knee laxity measurements after anterior cruciate ligament reconstruction. Knee Surg Sports Traumatol Arthrosc 19:355–362

Staubli HU, Noesberger B, Jakob RP (1992) Stress radiography of the knee. Cruciate ligament function studied in 138 patients. Acta Orthop Scand Suppl 249:1–27

Stijak L, Herzog RF, Schai P (2008) Is there an influence of the tibial slope of the lateral condyle on the ACL lesion? A case-control study. Knee Surg Sports Traumatol Arthrosc 16:112–117

Stijak L, Malis M, Maksimovic R, Aksic M, Filipovic B (2012) The influence of the morphometric parameters of the intercondylar notch on rupture of the anterior cruciate ligament. Vojnosanit Pregl 69:576–580

Sutton KM, Bullock JM (2013) Anterior cruciate ligament rupture: differences between males and females. J Am Acad Orthop Surg 21:41–50

Sward P, Kostogiannis I, Roos H (2010) Risk factors for a contralateral anterior cruciate ligament injury. Knee Surg Sports Traumatol Arthrosc 18:277–291

Tashman S, Kolowich P, Collon D, Anderson K, Anderst W (2007) Dynamic function of the ACL-reconstructed knee during running. Clin Orthop Relat Res 454:66–73

Terauchi M, Hatayama K, Yanagisawa S, Saito K, Takagishi K (2011) Sagittal alignment of the knee and its relationship to noncontact anterior cruciate ligament injuries. Am J Sports Med 39:1090–1094

Tsai AG, Musahl V, Steckel H, Bell KM, Zantop T, Irrgang JJ et al (2008) Rotational knee laxity: reliability of a simple measurement device in vivo. BMC Musculoskelet Disord 9:35

Vyas S, van Eck CF, Vyas N, Fu FH, Otsuka NY (2011) Increased medial tibial slope in teenage pediatric population with open physes and anterior cruciate ligament injuries. Knee Surg Sports Traumatol Arthrosc 19:372–377

Woo SLY, Fisher MB (2009) Evaluation of knee stability with use of a robotic system. J Bone Joint Surg (Am) 91:78–84

Wordeman SC, Quatman CE, Kaeding CC, Hewett TE (2012) In vivo evidence for tibial plateau slope as a risk factor for anterior cruciate ligament injury: a systematic review and meta-analysis. Am J Sports Med 40:1673–1681

Role of Osteotomy for Knee Cartilage, Meniscus, and Ligament Injuries

124

Joel Huleatt and Robert F. LaPrade

Contents

J. Huleatt (✉) • R.F. LaPrade
The Steadman Clinic and Steadman Philippon Research Institute, Vail, CO, USA
e-mail: joelhuleatt@gmail.com; drlaprade@sprivail.org; rlaprade@thesteadmanclinic.com

M.N. Doral, J. Karlsson (eds.), *Sports Injuries*,
DOI 10.1007/978-3-642-36569-0_130

Abstract
Knee cartilage, meniscus, and ligament injuries that are associated with malalignment can benefit from the redistribution of load and tibiofemoral repositioning provided by an osteotomy. A knee osteotomy as the first step or in combination with a ligament reconstruction improves outcomes in chronic anterior cruciate ligament and posterolateral corner instability, because it addresses the underlying mechanism for injury. For patients with malalignment receiving meniscal or osteochondral transplants, knee osteotomy can be expected to improve the survival of the grafts. However, careful patient selection and adequate biplanar angular correction are paramount to achieving durable success.

Introduction

Knee cartilage, meniscus, and ligament injuries are often associated with malalignment that excessively stresses the area of injury (Coventry 1973). In the aligned knee, roughly 60 % of the joint load is transferred through the medial compartment and 40 % through the lateral (Puddu and Franco 2009). The malaligned knee skews this ratio to overload either the medial or lateral compartment. In addition to excessive compressive forces, malalignment can also cause excessive tensile stress on ligaments due to a fulcrum effect. Degenerative cartilage changes can cause decreased joint space on the overloaded side, and medial or lateral ligamentous laxity can allow gapping of the joint on the unloaded side, both of which can lead to worsening malalignment and compounded stresses (Coventry 1973). Additionally, cruciate ligament injuries permit anteroposterior instability that can cause functional limitations and put other knee structures at greater risk of injury. The primary indication for a knee osteotomy is unicompartmental osteoarthritis in a young, active patient, with the goal to relieve pain and associated disability while retaining satisfactory range of motion, without precluding the possibility of future knee arthroplasty. However, this chapter will focus on the less prominent indications for knee osteotomy in treating ligament, meniscal, and osteochondral injuries of the knee.

Knee osteotomy involves altering the alignment of the proximal tibia, distal femur, or both, to change the geometry of the leg such that the loading forces through the knee are modified. This is accomplished through making either an opening wedge osteotomy, which is a single cut that is then wedged open, or a closing wedge osteotomy, which comprises cutting out a wedge of bone, and then stabilizing the bone in its revised angulation. Because this shifts the mechanical axis of the leg relative to the knee, one is able to direct the loading forces more medially or laterally in the joint to relieve unicompartmental overloading or reduce the stress on an injured ligament. Additionally, by concurrently introducing an anterior or posterior tilt to the osteotomy wedge, one can manipulate the posterior slope of the tibial plateaus to reduce anterior or posterior instability in cruciate ligament-deficient knees.

History

Osteotomy for Varus Malalignment

In the English literature, techniques for osteotomies around the knee for various bone deformities were described in the seventeenth century, but it was only in 1961 that Jackson and Waugh first published promising short-term results of performing tibial osteotomies for the treatment of knee osteoarthritis associated with valgus or varus malalignment. These "ball and socket"-shaped osteotomies distal to the tibial tubercle were based on the same principle as the intertrochanteric osteotomy, an established procedure at the time, to correct deformity for the relief of hip osteoarthritis. These authors commented on performing distal femoral osteotomies for valgus legs but found that they resulted in considerable restrictions in the range of motion (Jackson and Waugh 1961). Coventry is often credited for popularizing the high tibial osteotomy when in 1965 he described his technique of performing a lateral closing wedge valgus-producing osteotomy proximal to the tibial tubercle that became the standard surgical treatment for medial compartment osteoarthritis (Coventry 1965). The advantages of the more proximal osteotomy reportedly included a lower incidence of delayed unions or nonunions because the wedge was through the cancellous bone that healed promptly, and the contraction of the quadriceps compressed the osteotomy site (Coventry 1973). However, the satisfying results of knee osteotomies tended to regress within 10 years, and osteotomy began losing its appeal in the following decades with the advancement of knee arthroplasty and its more enduring relief of symptoms (Rönn et al. 2011). In 1987, Hernigou published promising long-term results of a proximal tibial osteotomy performed by creating a medial opening wedge that proved to be technically easier and more precise than the closing wedge techniques (Hernigou et al. 1987; Staubli et al. 2003; Puddu et al. 2007). This helped to maintain a role for knee osteotomies in treating young patients who wished to remain active and at least temporarily avoid arthroplasty. By the 1990s, the indications for knee osteotomies began expanding with increased recognition of varus alignment's negative influence on posterolateral corner and anterior cruciate ligament reconstructions, medial meniscal transplants, and medial osteochondral transplants (Allen et al. 1984; Oakeshott et al. 1988; Dugdale et al. 1992; van Arkel and de Boer 1995; Cameron and Saha 1997; Ghazavi et al. 1997; LaPrade et al. 1997; Verdonk et al. 2005, 2006). Additionally, the significance of the posterior tibial slope in contributing to anteroposterior instability and the benefits of adjusting it have become topics of recent scrutiny (Giffin et al. 2004, 2007; Brandon et al. 2006; Rodner et al. 2006; Van Raaij and De Waal 2006; Fening et al. 2008; Hohmann et al. 2010; LaPrade et al. 2010a; Todd et al. 2010; Kostogiannis et al. 2011; Feucht et al. 2012; Zeng et al. 2012).

Osteotomy for Valgus Malalignment

For valgus knee deformity, some early results with proximal tibial osteotomy published in the 1970s were discouraging (Shoji and Insall 1973). At this time distal femoral osteotomies were being described with enthusiasm in the French and Belgian literature, and Coventry commented on the indication for femoral osteotomy with severe valgus, yet favorable outcomes only became more broadly published in the English literature in the 1980s (Bouillet and Van Gaver 1961; Coventry 1973; Postel and Langlais 1977; Maquet 1985; Healy et al. 1988; McDermott et al. 1988). The distal femoral osteotomy has now become the standard method for addressing valgus malalignment, and the recent development of a locking plate for an opening wedge technique has the potential to provide more precise and durable results (Puddu et al. 2007).

Indications

Chronic Ligament Injuries Associated with Varus Malalignment

Proximal tibial osteotomy is indicated for certain chronic ligamentous injuries associated with knee malalignment. In general, patients with chronic posterolateral and anterior cruciate ligament injuries tend to have worse outcomes with recurrence of knee instability following ligament reconstruction compared to those with acute injuries (LaPrade et al. 1997; Noyes et al. 2000). When there is an underlying varus alignment in chronic ligament deficiencies, soft tissue reconstructions are at greater risk of stretching out if the malalignment is not addressed first with an osteotomy (Dugdale et al. 1992; LaPrade et al. 1997; Noyes et al. 2000; Badhe and Forster 2002; Arthur et al. 2007; Laprade et al. 2008; van de Pol et al. 2009). In fact, the instability associated with chronic posterolateral injuries is sometimes treated adequately by osteotomy alone, especially if they are isolated or low-velocity injuries, sparing the need for ligament reconstruction all together (Arthur et al. 2007). This clinical finding has been corroborated by biomechanical evidence that proximal tibial medial opening wedge osteotomy decreases the varus and external rotation laxity of posterolateral corner-deficient knees (Laprade et al. 2008). For patients with chronic anterior cruciate ligament injuries associated with double varus (lateral compartment gapping) or triple varus (lateral compartment gapping and varus recurvatum) malalignment, osteotomy followed by ligament reconstruction has been reported to improve pain and instability (Noyes et al. 2000). For patients with only primary varus malalignment (no lateral compartment gapping) and no medial compartment arthritis or varus thrust, no differences in stability or function were reported after anterior cruciate ligament construction based on the degree of malalignment at short-term follow-up (mean 45 months) (Kim et al. 2011). Therefore, varus alignment associated with lateral compartment gapping in conjunction with either chronic posterolateral or anterior cruciate ligament injuries is an indication for osteotomy prior to ligament reconstruction.

Chronic Ligament Injuries Associated with Valgus Malalignment

For patients with chronic medial collateral ligament injuries and valgus malalignment, or in the relatively unusual situation where chronic anterior cruciate ligament instability is associated with valgus malalignment, distal femoral osteotomy may be indicated prior to or in combination with ligament reconstructions to reduce graft strain (Puddu and Franco 2009; Laprade and Wijdicks 2012).

Posterior Tibial Slope and Anteroposterior Instability

Anteroposterior laxity is considered a risk for graft stretching or failure with cruciate ligament reconstructions (Feucht et al. 2012). During osteotomy, manipulation of the posterior tibial slope to establish more of a posterior tilt in posterior cruciate ligament-deficient knees, and less of a posterior tilt in anterior cruciate ligament-deficient knees, can help to stabilize the joint. Since an increased posterior tibial slope decreases posterior sag by shifting the tibia anterior relative to the femur, it stands to reason that this will be protective for knees with posterior instability (Giffin et al. 2004, 2007; LaPrade et al. 2010a). In a study of anteriorly painful knees with idiopathic genu recurvatum treated with an anterior opening wedge osteotomy of the proximal tibia, the posterior tibial slope was increased by 9.4°, and 83 % of patients were satisfied at a mean follow-up of 7 years (Van Raaij and De Waal 2006).

Likewise, it has been anticipated that decreasing the posterior tibial slope would reduce anterior cruciate ligament stress in knees with anterior instability or inherently steeper tibial slopes (Dejour and Bonnin 1994; Noyes et al. 2000; LaPrade et al. 2010a; Song et al. 2010). However, this has not been uniformly confirmed in outcome studies. With increasing posterior tibial slope, there is a correspondingly greater anterior laxity that permits increased anterior tibial translation (Dejour and Bonnin 1994; Shelburne et al. 2011). This is consistent with a significant correlation that exists between steeper tibial slopes and non-contact anterior cruciate ligament injuries (Brandon et al. 2006; Todd et al. 2010; Zeng et al. 2012). Additionally, a cadaveric study demonstrated that with increased posterior tibial slope, there was a posterior shift in weight-bearing on the tibial plateau in anterior cruciate ligament-deficient knees, indicating the potential for accelerated arthritis in this area (Rodner et al. 2006). However, cadaveric studies have reported no increase in anterior cruciate strain with increased posterior tibial slope and the application of anteroposterior and axially compressive loads (Giffin et al. 2004; Fening et al. 2008), and the only study so far to investigate the effect of tibial slope on anterior cruciate ligament reconstruction reported higher functional outcomes with steeper tibial slopes (Hohmann et al. 2010). Additionally, a study on the conservative management of anterior cruciate ligament injuries reported that a flatter tibial slope increased the odds ratio of requiring reconstruction by fourfold (Kostogiannis et al. 2011). Therefore, while it appears that a steeper posterior tibial slope contributes to anterior cruciate ligament rupture and anterior instability, it also appears to have no negative influence on either conservative management or reconstruction outcomes, and may even be beneficial.

Revision Anterior Cruciate Ligament Reconstruction

With failure of anterior cruciate ligament reconstruction, it is especially important to evaluate for malalignment and excessive tibial slope as causes for increased graft strain (George et al. 2006). When there is varus malalignment, Noyes recommends staging the osteotomy first if there is lateral gapping and a varus thrust gait; otherwise, the ligament reconstruction can be done concurrently (Noyes et al. 2000).

Malalignment and Meniscal Transplantation

Knee osteotomy is indicated as a prophylactic measure in young patients with malalignment undergoing meniscectomy or meniscal transplantation. When the knee is in extension, intact medial and lateral menisci carry approximately 50 % and 70 % of the respective compartmental loads (Seedhom et al. 1974). With total medial and lateral meniscectomies, biomechanical studies have reported increases in compartment pressures by 136 % and 235–335 %, respectively (Paletta et al. 1997; Alhalki et al. 2000). Biomechanical testing has also demonstrated that in medially meniscectomized knees, the medial compartment load drops significantly when the alignment is adjusted from neutral to 3° valgus (Van Thiel et al. 2011). It should not be surprising, then, that clinically, an increase in medial compartment osteoarthritis directly related to the degree of varus deformity has been observed following medial meniscectomy (Allen et al. 1984). Following meniscal transplantation, patients with untreated malalignment have had poorer results, while patients treated with osteotomy either prior to or concurrently have had comparable outcomes, and in some studies superior results, to patients without malalignment who had isolated meniscal transplantation (Van Arkel and De Boer 1995; Cameron and Saha 1997; Verdonk et al. 2005, 2006). For combined osteotomy and meniscal transplantation to be successful, it is important to perform before bone on bone (grade 4) joint degeneration occurs (Amendola 2007).

Malalignment and Osteochondral Allograft Transplantation

Knee osteotomy is also indicated as a precautionary measure at the time of fresh or refrigerated osteochondral allograft transplantation to treat large osteochondral defects of a malaligned knee joint (Noyes et al. 2000; Lee et al. 2012). Osteochondral defects greater than 3 cm in diameter or 1 cm in depth in the weight-bearing surface of the knee have significant functional and clinical improvements with fresh or refrigerated osteochondral allograft transplantations (Aubin et al. 2001; Gross et al. 2005; LaPrade et al. 2009). However, uncorrected malalignment was reported to have a deleterious effect on outcomes early in the development of osteochondral transplantation, and therefore staged or concurrent osteotomy has been recommended for the last two decades (Oakeshott et al. 1988; Ghazavi et al. 1997).

Preoperative Planning

General Considerations

The preoperative work-up for a proximal tibial osteotomy to treat articular cartilage, meniscal, and ligament-related pathology includes the standard history, physical examination, and imaging work-up. Special attention should be given to determining that there is not bi-compartmental disease, fully evaluating the state of all ligaments and menisci, obtaining stress radiographs if ligament injuries are suspected, and assessing the degree of malalignment. If there is any doubt regarding the utility of an osteotomy in a given situation, the patient can be placed in an unloader knee brace for 2 months to evaluate for alleviation of symptoms (Laprade et al. 2012).

Timing of Surgery

For chronic ligament, meniscus, and osteochondral injuries, addressing malalignment and deciding between concurrent or staged procedures are the key considerations. Varus knees with chronic posterolateral corner injuries should have the malalignment corrected first with a proximal tibial osteotomy before any ligament reconstruction is pursued to avoid stretching out of the grafts. Otherwise, these patients tend to have worse outcomes with recurrence of knee instability following ligament reconstruction compared to acute injuries (Noyes and Barber-Westin 1996; LaPrade et al. 1997). In patients who suffer from isolated chronic posterolateral ligament injuries due to low-energy mechanisms, the osteotomy alone may result in adequate knee stability, precluding the need for later ligament reconstruction (Arthur et al. 2007). For patients with combined cruciate ligament injuries and varus malalignment, reconstruction of the ligaments should be staged after the osteotomy if lateral gapping is present on arthroscopic inspection (Noyes et al. 2000).

In valgus malaligned knees with chronic medial collateral ligament and/or anterior cruciate ligament instability, distal femoral osteotomy may be performed prior to or in combination with cruciate reconstruction (Phisitkul et al. 2006; Puddu and Franco 2009). Because the need for medial ligament reconstruction may be obviated after osteotomy, staging the procedures may be optimal (Phisitkul et al. 2006).

For proximal tibial osteotomy and meniscal transplantation, either staged or concurrent procedures are viable options. Large varus and valgus stresses may need to be applied to place the meniscal graft, so an osteotomy at least 1.5 cm distal to the tibial slot or root attachment tunnels is recommended to be performed only following the transplantation if done concurrently (Lee et al. 2012). If a malaligned, meniscally deficient knee also demonstrates anterior cruciate ligament deficiency, staging the osteotomy at least 6 months prior to concurrent meniscal transplantation and anterior cruciate ligament reconstruction has been recommended (Amendola 2007).

For malaligned patients undergoing osteochondral allograft transplantation, improved outcomes have been reported when osteotomy is completed prior or concurrently to the transplant procedure compared to a later date. However, a delayed osteotomy may have a role as a salvage procedure in young patients because it may postpone the need for knee replacement (Gross et al. 2005).

Assessing the Degree of Malalignment

In determining and defining the alignment of the lower extremity, both anatomic and mechanical axes are used. The anatomic axes correspond to the diaphyseal midlines of the femur and tibia in the frontal plane, which are not in alignment, but normally form a tibiofemoral angle that is in 5–7° of valgus (Berman et al. 1991). The individual mechanical axes of the thigh and leg, which respectively comprise the lines from the center of the femoral head to the medial tibial spine and from the medial tibial spine to the center of the talar dome, normally form a 0° angle, and therefore, the anatomic axis of the knee is approximately 6° valgus to the mechanical axis (Dugdale et al. 1992; Hungerford 1995). The weight-bearing mechanical axis of the lower extremity refers to the line drawn from the center of the femoral head to the center of the talar dome. If the lower extremity is in malalignment, this weight-bearing mechanical axis can vary from the individual mechanical axes of the thigh and leg, and where it crosses the knee joint line can be expressed as a percentage of the tibial width (Fig. 1). A knee is considered in varus if the weight-bearing mechanical axis is medial to the apex of the medial tibial eminence (Dugdale et al. 1992). In the preoperative work-up, full-length weight-bearing anteroposterior radiographs of the legs are therefore necessary to assess angular deformity (Coventry 1973).

Alignment Goals and Determining the Wedge Size

There are a variety of alignment goals and an equal number of techniques described for

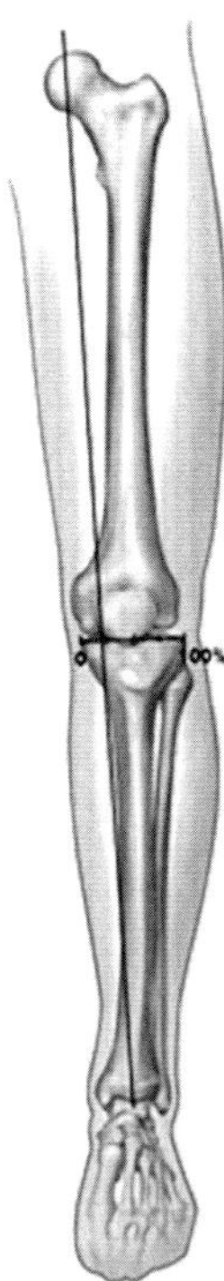

Fig. 1 Illustration of the weight-bearing mechanical axis of a left lower extremity in varus malalignment, demonstrating an intersection point at the knee that is medial to the center of the joint (Reprinted with permission from the American Journal of Sports Medicine, LaPrade et al. 2010a)

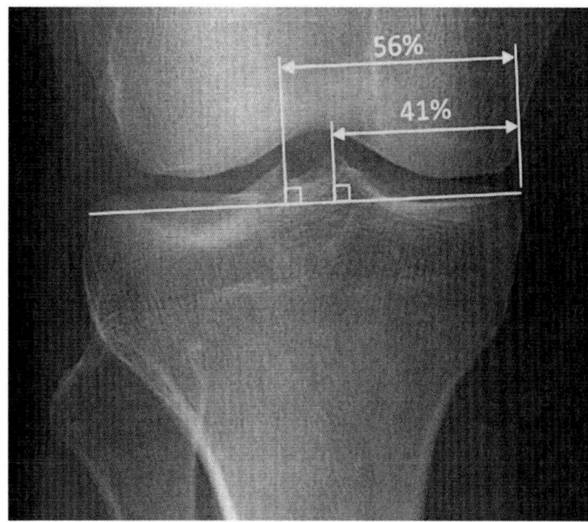

Fig. 2 Right knee anteroposterior radiograph demonstrating the apex of the lateral tibial eminence, 56 % of the way across the tibial plateau from medial to lateral. This is the intersection target for the mechanical weight-bearing axis in order to correct a varus deformity, which been found to produce an anatomic axis of approximately 10° valgus (Reprinted with permission from Arthroscopy: The Journal of Arthroscopic and Related Surgery, Laprade et al. 2012)

determining the size of the osteotomy wedge. One of the most recognized and straightforward methods of determining the appropriate wedge size was deduced through a series of rigorous algebraic formulas by Dugdale and coworkers (Dugdale et al. 1992). They proposed creating a 3–5° valgus mechanical axis at the knee by moving the lower extremity mechanical weight-bearing axis to intersect the tibial plateau at 62 % along the way from the medial to lateral edge. To determine the wedge size, lines from the center of the femoral head and talar dome to the 62 % lateral intersection point are plotted on a full-length standing leg film, and the angle formed by these lines makes up the wedge angle, which is then drawn onto the tibial silhouette in order to measure the size of the wedge (Dugdale et al. 1992). If there is lateral joint space opening evident on the radiograph due to ligament laxity, the joint line convergence angle formed by lines tangent to the distal femoral condyles and the tibial plateau needs to be subtracted from the wedge angle to account for the contribution of gapping to preoperative varus (Puddu et al. 2007). The senior author (R.F.L.) prefers a similar alignment goal and method but uses the midpoint of the downslope of the lateral tibial eminence (56 %) as the intersection target for the mechanical weight-bearing axis, which has been found to produce an anatomic axis of approximately 10° valgus (Figs. 2 and 3) (Arthur et al. 2007; LaPrade et al. 2010a; Laprade et al. 2012). Amendola recommends not overcorrecting but achieving a neutral alignment in cases of combined high tibial osteotomy and medial meniscal transplantation (Bonasia and Amendola 2010).

For the valgus knee, overcorrection past the normal tibiofemoral angle of 6° valgus to an angle of 0° is desired (Coventry 1987; McDermott et al. 1988). Overcorrection to varus leads to poor long-term results (Puddu and Franco 2009). In a severely valgus knee, the tibiofemoral joint line can have a significant medial tilt in the frontal plane. This can hinder the ability of a tibial osteotomy to transfer the load from the lateral to the medial compartment and can result in lateral tibial subluxation after tibial osteotomy (Coventry 1973; McDermott et al. 1988). Therefore, when the medial tilt is greater than 10° or valgus

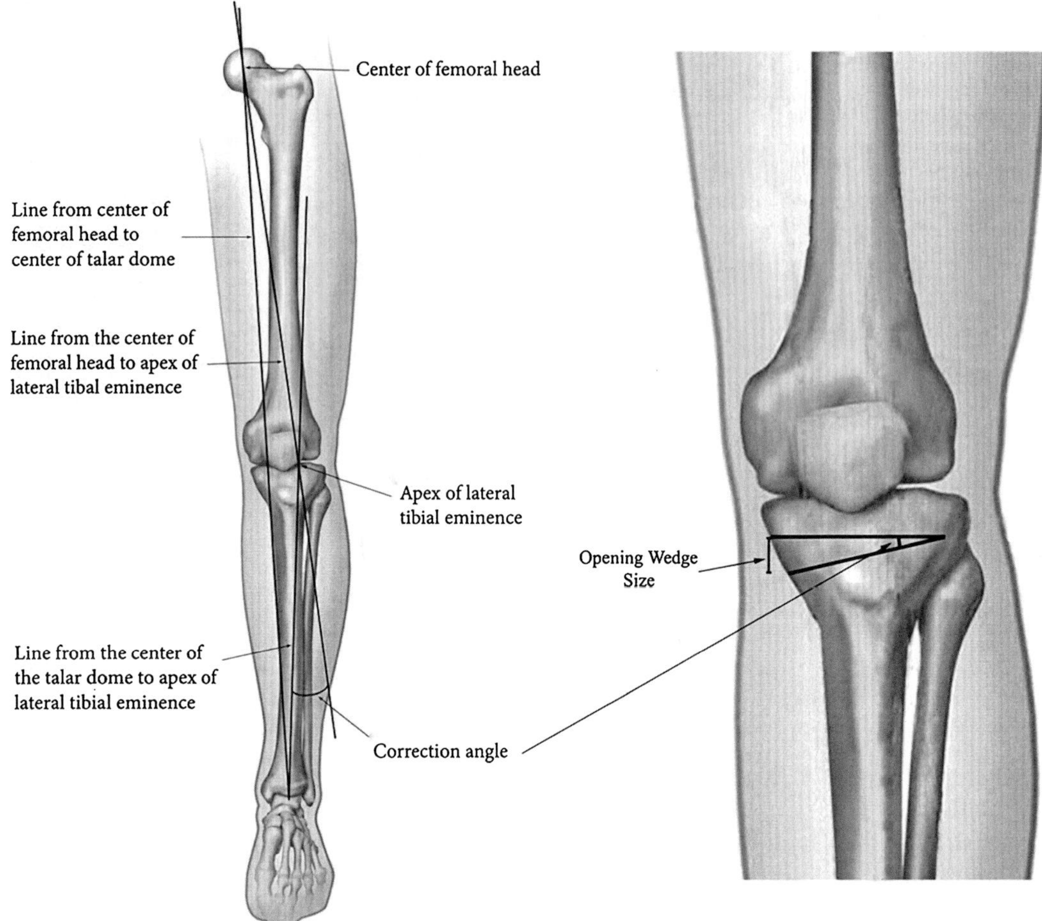

Fig. 3 Illustration of a method for determining the medial opening wedge size of a proximal tibial osteotomy in a left lower extremity. On a full-length standing leg radiograph, lines from the center of the femoral head and talar dome to the apex of the lateral tibial eminence (56 % lateral intersection point) are plotted on a full-length standing leg film. The angle formed by these lines makes up the wedge angle, which is then drawn onto the tibial silhouette so that the size of the wedge at the medial cortex can be measured (Reprinted with permission from Arthroscopy: The Journal of Arthroscopic and Related Surgery, Laprade et al. 2012)

malalignment exceeds 12°, a distal femoral osteotomy is indicated to improve stability by leveling the joint line (Coventry 1973, 1987). The degree of medial tilt appears to be less of an issue in the varus knee (Coventry 1973). The method of determining the wedge size is similar to that for a varus knee, with the use of full-length radiographs to determine the angle of correction needed and drawing the angle onto the silhouette of the proximal tibia or distal femur (Puddu and Franco 2009).

Assessing Posterior Tibial Slope and Planning Tilt Adjustments

It is also important to evaluate the posterior tibial slope with lateral radiographs, which is the angle formed by a line perpendicular to the tibial diaphysis and a line tangent to the tibial plateau (Fig. 4). The average posterior tibial slope has been found to be 10° ± 3° (Dejour and Bonnin 1994). A small inadvertent increase in the posterior tibial slope of around 1° can be expected in medial

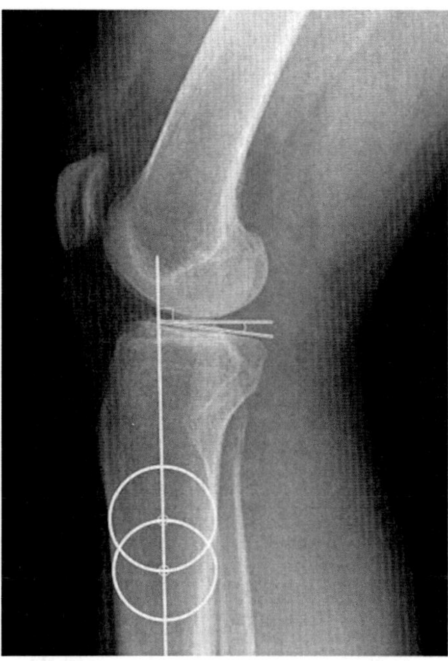

Fig. 4 Measurement of the posterior tibial slope on a lateral radiograph, which is the angle formed between a line perpendicular to the tibial diaphysis and a line tangent to the tibial plateau (Reprinted with permission from the American Journal of Sports Medicine, LaPrade et al. 2010a)

opening wedge tibial osteotomies, even with posteromedial plate positioning, which does not significantly increase knee instability or cruciate ligament stress (Giffin et al. 2004; LaPrade et al. 2010a; Song et al. 2010; Ducat et al. 2012). However, the tibial slope increases more with anteromedial plate positioning, and increased slope results in an increased horizontal sheer force and anterior translation of the tibia resting position relative to the femur in both anterior cruciate ligament competent and deficient knees (Giffin et al. 2004; LaPrade et al. 2010a). It has thus been hypothesized that an opening wedge technique with anteromedial plate positioning may decrease posterior sag and be protective for knees with posterior instability that do not already have an excessive tibial slope. Conversely, posteromedial plate positioning, or a lateral closing wedge osteotomy that can decrease tibial slope, is preferred in knees with anterior instability or inherently steeper tibial slopes (Dejour et al. 1994; Noyes et al. 2000; LaPrade et al. 2010a; Song et al. 2010). In addition, the results of Hernigou demonstrated that a preoperative posterior tibial slope greater than 15° may be associated with progressive posterior medial compartment degeneration despite corrective osteotomy (Hernigou et al. 1987). Therefore, measuring the posterior tibial slope assists in assessing both the candidacy of a patient for osteotomy and determining the operative plan.

Medial Opening Wedge Proximal Tibial Osteotomy to Treat the Varus Knee

Rationale for Use

In the treatment of the varus knee, the medial opening wedge technique has become the preferred choice because it offers a number of key advantages over the lateral closing wedge technique (Lobenhoffer et al. 2002; Stoffel et al. 2004; Song et al. 2010; Ducat et al. 2012). The medial approach avoids disrupting the proximal tibiofibular joint and causing laxity in the lateral ligaments, and minimizes the potential for anterior compartment syndrome and injury to the peroneal nerve, complications that occur with significant frequency with the lateral approach (Staubli et al. 2003; Noyes et al. 2006; Puddu et al. 2007; Song et al. 2010). The need to create only one cut of just the tibia for the opening wedge and the availability of internal plates that secure the new tibial alignment in both coronal and sagittal planes allow for a less technically demanding procedure that can more precisely achieve correction goals (Hernigou et al. 1987; Lobenhoffer et al. 2002; Staubli et al. 2003; Puddu et al. 2007; Laprade et al. 2012). However, the opening wedge technique also has its limitations, which include longer non-weight-bearing during recovery and greater risk of developing increased tibial slope, hardware failure, and delayed union or nonunion (Hernigou et al. 1987; Nagel et al. 1996; Noyes et al. 2006; Song et al. 2010; Laprade et al. 2012).

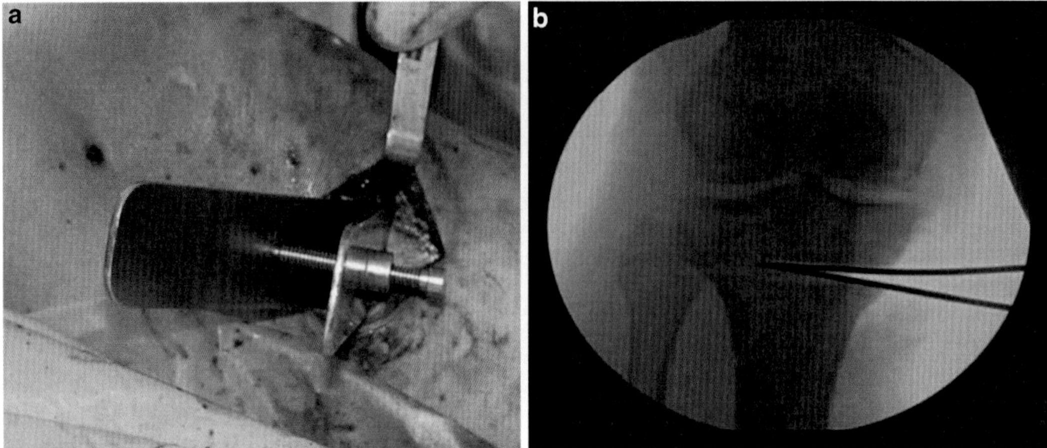

Fig. 5 (**a**) Left knee intraoperative photograph and (**b**) right knee fluoroscopic view of a spreader device being used to open the wedge in a proximal tibial osteotomy

Surgical Exposure

The anteromedial aspect of the proximal tibia is exposed through a vertical skin incision directly down to bone. Starting 1 cm distal to the medial joint line at the midpoint between the tibial tubercle and the posterior border of the tibia, the incision is carried 5 cm distally to just beyond the tibial tubercle. A subperiosteal dissection under the patellar tendon anteriorly and posteriorly deep to the pes anserine tendons, superficial medial collateral ligament, and popliteus musculature is performed to allow palpation along the intended tibial osteotomy site. This is facilitated by the release of the more anterior fibers of the superficial medial collateral ligament where they insert on the tibia.

Osteotomy

To perform the proximal tibial osteotomy parallel to the joint line at the level of the physeal scar, two guide pins are placed medially to laterally through the tibia under fluoroscopic guidance. When the osteotomy is being performed in conjunction with a meniscal transplantation, the guide pins should be placed at least 1.5 cm distal to the inferior aspect of the tibial root bone plug tunnels that have been made for the meniscal graft. The medial cortex is then scored with an oscillating saw on the distal side of the guide pins to avoid inadvertent deviation toward the joint. The osteotomy is carefully advanced laterally using osteotomes and frequent fluoroscopy until 1 cm of lateral cortex is left as an intact hinge, with complete division of the anterior and posterior cortices.

Opening the Wedge

A spreader device is inserted into the osteotomy site and slowly opened to the predetermined wedge size. The spreader device consists of two thin osteotomes that abut at the front tip with a screw mechanism at the back that can be turned to slowly increase the wedge angle of the osteotomes (Fig. 5). Increments of opening followed by periodic rest intervals allow for stress relaxation of the lateral hinge and help avoid fracture. A separate device with wedge-shaped tines is then placed in the osteotomy to keep it open at the desired angle, while the spreader is exchanged for the osteotomy plate (Fig. 6).

Fixation

Fixation may be obtained by using a specialized osteotomy plate, such as the standard Puddu plate

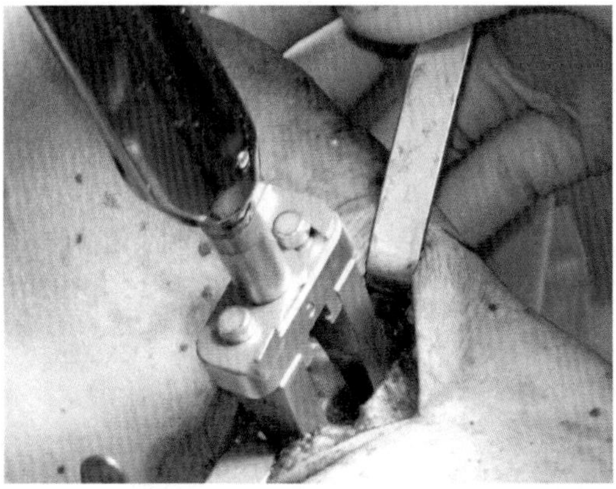

Fig. 6 Intraoperative photograph of graduated tines holding a left knee osteotomy open at the calculated wedge size while the spreader device is exchanged for a plate

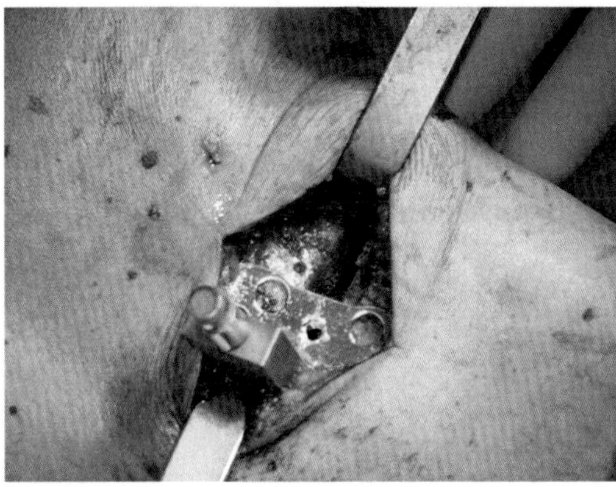

Fig. 7 Intraoperative photograph of a graduated tine and a Puddu plate in a left knee osteotomy prior to fixation

(Arthrex, Naples, FL), which has a block wedge that fits into the osteotomy site to hold the bone gap at the desired wedge size and resist compressive forces through the medial cortex (Fig. 7). To minimize increases in the tibial slope, the plate should be placed as far posteromedially as possible. Two 6.5 mm non-locking fully threaded cancellous screws are placed proximally, and two 4.5 mm non-locking self-tapping screws are placed distally to achieve bicortical fixation. It is recommended that when using the standard Puddu plate, the osteotomy void is packed with bone allograft to enhance union. Plates such as the modified Puddu locking plate (Arthrex, Naples, FL) and the TomoFix locking plate (Mathys Inc., Bettlach, Switzerland) may not require bone grafting (Staubli et al. 2003; Stoffel et al. 2004). A single staple that spans the anterior aspect of the osteotomy can be placed in cases where increases in the posterior tibial slope are undesirable (Fig. 8).

Lateral Cortex Fracture Fixation

A common intraoperative complication is the development of a cortex fracture through the lateral hinge due to a large correction angle, overly aggressive operative technique, or structural deficit, such as osteopenic bone or from previous surgery. To stabilize the lateral cortex, a small vertical incision can be made over Gerdy's tubercle and a single staple placed spanning the fracture.

Closure

A deep layer consisting of the pes anserine tendons and sartorius fascia is closed over the plate. The dermal layer is approximated with an absorbable monofilament suture.

Distal Femoral Osteotomy to Treat the Valgus Knee

Rationale for Use

Although proximal tibial osteotomy and distal femoral osteotomy are both techniques described for correcting valgus deformity of the knee, the femoral version has some distinct advantages. A valgus deformity of the knee is often associated with an increased superolateral joint line slope, which can cause lateral subluxation of the tibia (Puddu and Franco 2009). Because only a femoral osteotomy can correct this slope, when the superolateral tilt is greater than 10° or valgus malalignment exceeds 12°, a distal femoral osteotomy is indicated (Coventry 1973, 1987). Even in knees with less severe valgus deformity that are treated with proximal tibial osteotomy, biomechanical studies and long-term follow-up

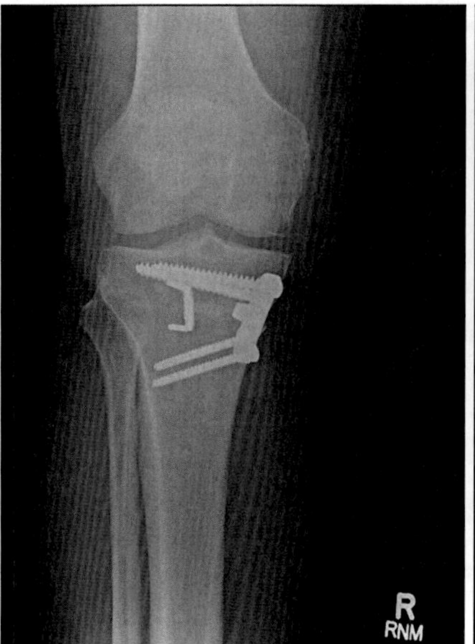

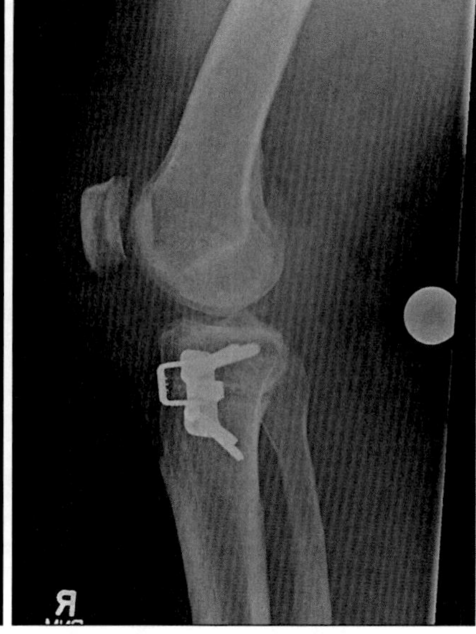

Fig. 8 Right knee postoperative anteroposterior and lateral radiographs 2 months after a concurrent proximal tibial osteotomy and fresh osteochondral allograft transplantation to the medial and lateral femoral condyles and trochlear groove

radiographs demonstrate that the load is not redistributed as well compared to a proximal tibial osteotomy, with increased load at the intercondylar area (Coventry 1987). Additionally, a distal femoral osteotomy's superior ability to reduce the Q-angle is advantageous considering the high association between valgus deformity and patellofemoral disorders (Puddu and Franco 2009). This may explain why multiple studies have reported poorer results with proximal tibial osteotomy for treating valgus deformity, whereas several studies of distal femoral osteotomy have yielded results comparable to the results of varus-correcting osteotomies (Shoji and Insall 1973; Healy et al. 1988; McDermott et al. 1988). Such factors have led Maquet, one of the pioneers of knee osteotomy, to report a clear preference for the femoral option for any degree of valgus malalignment (Maquet 1985).

Surgical Exposure

To expose the lateral aspect of the distal third of the femur, a vertical incision centered on the iliotibial band and beginning 4 cm distal to the lateral epicondyle is carried 15 cm proximally. The iliotibial band is split, the knee is then flexed, and the vastus lateralis is elevated anteriorly from the posterolateral intermuscular septum to visualize the lateral femur, with ligature or electrocautery of any perforating vessels. The posterior cortex of the femoral metaphysis is then exposed with blunt dissection, and the superficial femoral/popliteal artery and sciatic nerve are protected with a retractor (Puddu and Franco 2009).

Osteotomy

To create a superolateral oblique osteotomy just proximal to the trochlear groove, the knee is extended, and under fluoroscopic guidance, a guide wire is drilled at a 45° angle, aiming toward the adductor tubercle. A cutting guide should be used to ensure that the osteotomy does not develop an anterior-posterior slope. The lateral cortex is scored with an oscillating saw on the proximal side of the guide pins to avoid inadvertent distal deviation through the trochlear groove. The osteotomy is carefully advanced medially using osteotomes and frequent fluoroscopy until

1 cm of medial cortex is left intact as a hinge, with complete division of the anterior and posterior cortices (Puddu and Franco 2009).

Opening the Wedge

As with the proximal tibial opening wedge osteotomy, a spreader device is inserted into the osteotomy site and slowly opened to the predetermined wedge size. Increments of opening followed by periodic rest intervals allow for stress relaxation of the medial hinge and help avoid fracture. Wedge-shaped tines are then placed in the osteotomy to keep it open at the desired angle, while the spreader is exchanged for the osteotomy plate (Puddu and Franco 2009).

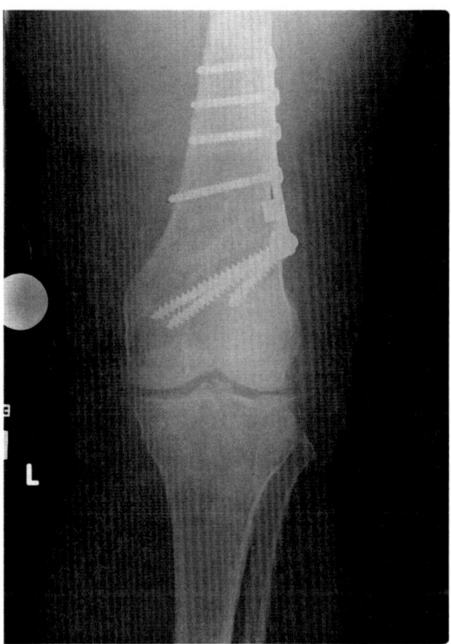

Fig. 9 Left knee postoperative anteroposterior radiograph 2 weeks after a concurrent distal femoral osteotomy and lateral meniscal transplantation

Fixation

The T-shaped plate designed by Puddu (Arthrex, Naples, FL) has a block wedge that fits into the osteotomy site to hold the bone gap at the desired wedge size and resist compressive forces through the lateral cortex (Fig. 9). The distal T-shape of the plate should be shaped to fit the contour of the distal femur to avoid hardware irritation. Puddu recommends using two cancellous screws distally and four cortical screws proximally, which can be locked into the second generation plate regardless of their orientation. The osteotomy void should be packed with bone graft to enhance union (Puddu and Franco 2009).

Rehabilitation

Following either proximal tibial or distal femoral osteotomy, the patient should be fitted with a knee immobilizer and remain non-weight-bearing for 8 weeks. During this time the rehabilitation protocol consists of isometric quadriceps sets, patellar mobilization, and straight-leg raises. To maintain knee range of motion, the immobilizer can be removed four times a day, and the knee flexed as tolerated with a goal of at least zero to 90° by 2 weeks. If radiographs demonstrate healing at the apex of the osteotomy after 8 weeks following surgery, partial weight-bearing up to 25 % of body weight is allowed, including exercise on a stationary bicycle. Patients then are allowed to increase weight-bearing by an additional 25 % of body weight each week until they are fully weight-bearing by 3 months, as long as they do not develop worsening pain or effusions with activities. Use of other plates such as the Block and Break locking plate (LIMMED, Nesles-la-Valée, France) may allow immediate full weight-bearing (Poignard et al. 2010). Patients who undergo posterolateral corner ligament reconstruction should avoid hyperextension and varus stresses for 6 months and can be fitted with a medial compartment unloader brace to protect the graft as they regain strength through weight-bearing (Noyes et al. 2000). For patients with concurrent meniscal transplants, squatting and pivoting should be avoided for at least 4 months (Lee et al. 2012). All osteotomy patients should refrain from high-impact knee activities until after 4–6 months, or until 12 months in the case of osteochondral allograft recipients, at which point such activities should still be cautioned against. Instead, patients should be encouraged to engage in low-impact recreational pursuits.

Clinical Outcomes

Osteotomy for Chronic Ligament Injury

No studies have prospectively evaluated the influence of osteotomies on the ligament reconstruction outcomes of malaligned, chronic knee ligament injury patients. However, experienced complex knee surgeons have realized the increased risk of failure with the added stresses of malalignment and have obtained improved results by treating these challenging injuries with the correction of malalignment prior to or concurrent with ligament reconstruction (LaPrade et al. 1997; Noyes et al. 2000; Badhe and Forster 2002). Additionally, in a study of chronic posterolateral corner injuries treated with osteotomy, at a mean follow-up of 3 years, 38 % of patients had sufficient improvement in knee function that a subsequent posterolateral corner reconstruction was not necessary (Arthur et al. 2007). In patients with chronic anterior cruciate ligament injuries with varus malalignment, high tibial osteotomy followed by ligament reconstruction 8 months later reduced pain, improved instability, and allowed patients to regain full range of motion (Noyes et al. 2000). Therefore, the logical conclusion is that an osteotomy can help return stability to a chronically unstable malaligned knee.

Osteotomy and Meniscal Transplantation

The synergistic benefit of osteotomy and meniscal transplantation has up to this point in time evaded quantification due to the small number of patients reported in studies as well as the lack of controls and randomization (Matava 2007; Elattar et al. 2011). However, studies have correlated malalignment with early failure of meniscal transplants (Van Arkel and De Boer 1995), while staged or concurrent osteotomies have been reported to provide comparable results to patients without malalignment (LaPrade et al. 2010b). Cameron reported that 85 % of patients had good to excellent results at an average follow-up of greater than 2 years following combined meniscal transplantation and osteotomy compared to 90 % good to excellent results following isolated meniscal transplantation (Cameron and Saha 1997). Verdonk and coworkers reported a greater mean survival time of 13 years and a greater improvement in pain for medial meniscal transplants combined with high tibial osteotomy compared to 11.6 years for both medial and lateral isolated meniscal transplants (Verdonk et al. 2005, 2006). Therefore, it would appear that correcting malalignment prior to meniscal transplantation is truly beneficial.

Osteotomy and Osteochondral Allograft Transplantation

In patients undergoing osteochondral allograft transplantation of the knee, osteotomy has proven to be an essential step for patients with malalignment. Whereas multiple studies have reported a significant association between early failure and uncorrected malalignment, a recent study of distal femur osteochondral transplant recipients reported that malaligned patients who also received a proximal tibial or distal femoral osteotomy had equally good results to those with initial normal alignment at a mean of 10 years follow-up (Aubin et al. 2001). In addition, the triple combination of meniscal transplantation, cartilage repair, and osteotomy has reportedly allowed young patients to return to unrestricted activities (Gomoll et al. 2009). Therefore, there seems to be a strong case for the incorporation of osteotomy in malaligned knees requiring osteochondral transplantation.

Summary

Knee cartilage, meniscus, and ligament injuries that are associated with malalignment can benefit from the redistribution of load and tibiofemoral repositioning provided by an osteotomy. A knee osteotomy as the first step or in combination with a ligament reconstruction improves outcomes in chronic anterior cruciate ligament and posterolateral corner instability, because it addresses the underlying mechanism for injury. For patients with malalignment receiving meniscal or osteochondral transplantation, knee osteotomy can be expected to improve the survival of the grafts. However, careful patient selection and adequate biplanar angular correction are paramount to achieving durable success.

Cross-References

- ► Meniscal Allografts: Indications and Results
- ► Second- and Third-Generation Cartilage Transplantation
- ► Special Considerations for Multiple-Ligament Knee Injuries

References

Alhalki MM, Hull ML, Howell SM (2000) Contact mechanics of the medial tibial plateau after implantation of a medial meniscal allograft. A human cadaveric study. Am J Sports Med 28:370–376

Allen PR, Denham RA, Swan AV (1984) Late degenerative changes after meniscectomy. Factors affecting the knee after operation. J Bone Joint Surg Br 66:666–671

Amendola A (2007) Knee osteotomy and meniscal transplantation: indications, technical considerations, and results. Sports Med Arthrosc 15:32–38. doi:10.1097/JSA.0b013e31802f997b

Arthur A, LaPrade RF, Agel J (2007) Proximal tibial opening wedge osteotomy as the initial treatment for chronic posterolateral corner deficiency in the varus knee: a prospective clinical study. Am J Sports Med 35:1844–1850. doi:10.1177/0363546507304717

Aubin PP, Cheah HK, Davis AM, Gross AE (2001) Long-term follow-up of fresh femoral osteochondral allografts for posttraumatic knee defects. Clin Orthop Relat Res 391(Suppl):S318–S327

Badhe NP, Forster IW (2002) High tibial osteotomy in knee instability: the rationale of treatment and early results. Knee Surg Sports Traumatol Arthrosc 10:38–43. doi:10.1007/s001670100244

Berman AT, Bosacco SJ, Kirshner S, Avolio A (1991) Factors influencing long-term results in high tibial osteotomy. Clin Orthop Relat Res 272:192–198

Bonasia DE, Amendola A (2010) Combined medial meniscal transplantation and high tibial osteotomy. Knee Surg Sports Traumatol Arthrosc 18:870–873. doi:10.1007/s00167-009-0999-2

Bouillet R, Van Gaver P (1961) L'arthrose du genou: etude pathogenique et traitement. Acta Orthop Belg 27:5–187

Brandon ML, Haynes PT, Bonamo JR et al (2006) The association between posterior-inferior tibial slope and anterior cruciate ligament insufficiency. Arthroscopy 22:894–899. doi:10.1016/j.arthro.2006.04.098

Cameron JC, Saha S (1997) Meniscal allograft transplantation for unicompartmental arthritis of the knee. Clin Orthop Relat Res 337:164–171

Coventry MB (1965) Osteotomy of the upper portion of the tibia for degenerative arthritis of the knee. A preliminary report. J Bone Joint Surg Am 47:984–990

Coventry MB (1973) Osteotomy about the knee for degenerative and rheumatoid arthritis. J Bone Joint Surg Am 55:23–48

Coventry MB (1987) Proximal tibial varus osteotomy for osteoarthritis of the lateral compartment of the knee. J Bone Joint Surg Am 69:32–38

Dejour H, Bonnin M (1994) Tibial translation after anterior cruciate ligament rupture. Two radiological tests compared. J Bone Joint Surg Br 76:745–749

Dejour H, Neyret P, Boileau P, Donell ST (1994) Anterior cruciate reconstruction combined with valgus tibial osteotomy. Clin Orthop Relat Res 299:220–228

Ducat A, Sariali E, Lebel B et al (2012) Posterior tibial slope changes after opening- and closing-wedge high tibial osteotomy: a comparative prospective multicenter study. Orthop Traumatol Surg Res 98(1):68–74. doi:10.1016/j.otsr.2011.08.013

Dugdale TW, Noyes FR, Styer D (1992) Preoperative planning for high tibial osteotomy. The effect of lateral tibiofemoral separation and tibiofemoral length. Clin Orthop Relat Res Jan(274):248–264

Elattar M, Dhollander A, Verdonk R et al (2011) Twenty-six years of meniscal allograft transplantation: is it still experimental? A meta-analysis of 44 trials. Knee Surg Sports Traumatol Arthrosc 19:147–157. doi:10.1007/s00167-010-1351-6

Fening SD, Kovacic J, Kambic H et al (2008) The effects of modified posterior tibial slope on anterior cruciate ligament strain and knee kinematics: a human cadaveric study. J Knee Surg 21:205–211

Feucht MJ, Mauro CS, Brucker PU et al (2012) The role of the tibial slope in sustaining and treating anterior cruciate ligament injuries. Knee Surg Sports Traumatol Arthrosc 21(1):134–145. doi:10.1007/s00167-012-1941-6

George MS, Dunn WR, Spindler KP (2006) Current concepts review: revision anterior cruciate ligament reconstruction. Am J Sports Med 34:2026–2037. doi:10.1177/0363546506295026

Ghazavi MT, Pritzker KP, Davis AM, Gross AE (1997) Fresh osteochondral allografts for post-traumatic osteochondral defects of the knee. J Bone Joint Surg Br 79:1008–1013

Giffin JR, Vogrin TM, Zantop T et al (2004) Effects of increasing tibial slope on the biomechanics of the knee. Am J Sports Med 32:376–382. doi:10.1177/0363546503258880

Giffin JR, Stabile KJ, Zantop T et al (2007) Importance of tibial slope for stability of the posterior cruciate ligament deficient knee. Am J Sports Med 35:1443–1449. doi:10.1177/0363546507304665

Gomoll AH, Kang RW, Chen AL, Cole BJ (2009) Triad of cartilage restoration for unicompartmental arthritis treatment in young patients: meniscus allograft transplantation, cartilage repair and osteotomy. J Knee Surg 22:137–141

Gross AE, Shasha N, Aubin P (2005) Long-term follow-up of the use of fresh osteochondral allografts for posttraumatic knee defects. Clin Orthop Relat Res 435:79–87. doi:10.1097/01.blo.0000165845.21735.05

Healy WL, Anglen JO, Wasilewski SA, Krackow KA (1988) Distal femoral varus osteotomy. J Bone Joint Surg Am 70:102–109

Hernigou P, Medevielle D, Debeyre J, Goutallier D (1987) Proximal tibial osteotomy for osteoarthritis with varus deformity. A ten to thirteen-year follow-up study. J Bone Joint Surg Am 69:332–354

Hohmann E, Bryant A, Reaburn P, Tetsworth K (2010) Does posterior tibial slope influence knee functionality in the anterior cruciate ligament-deficient and anterior cruciate ligament-reconstructed knee? Arthroscopy 26:1496–1502. doi:10.1016/j.arthro.2010.02.024

Hungerford DS (1995) Alignment in total knee replacement. Instruct Course Lect 44:455–468

Jackson JP, Waugh W (1961) Tibial osteotomy for osteoarthritis of the knee. J Bone Joint Surg Br 43-B:746–751

Kim S-J, Moon H-K, Chun Y-M et al (2011) Is correctional osteotomy crucial in primary varus knees undergoing anterior cruciate ligament reconstruction? Clinical Orthop Relat Res 469:1421–1426. doi:10.1007/s11999-010-1584-1

Kostogiannis I, Swärd P, Neuman P et al (2011) The influence of posterior-inferior tibial slope in ACL injury. Knee Surg Sports Traumatol Arthrosc 19:592–597. doi:10.1007/s00167-010-1295-x

Laprade RF, Wijdicks CA (2012) The management of injuries to the medial side of the knee. J Orthop Sports Phys Ther 42:221–233. doi:10.2519/jospt.2012.3624

LaPrade RF, Hamilton CD, Engebretsen L (1997) Treatment of acute and chronic combined anterior cruciate ligament and posterolateral knee ligament injuries. Sports Med Arthrosc Rev 5:91–99

Laprade RF, Engebretsen L, Johansen S et al (2008) The effect of a proximal tibial medial opening wedge osteotomy on posterolateral knee instability: a biomechanical study. Am J Sports Med 36:956–960. doi:10.1177/0363546507312380

LaPrade RF, Botker J, Herzog M, Agel J (2009) Refrigerated osteoarticular allografts to treat articular cartilage defects of the femoral condyles. A prospective outcomes study. J Bone Joint Surg Am Br 91:805–811. doi:10.2106/JBJS.H.00703

LaPrade RF, Oro FB, Ziegler CG et al (2010a) Patellar height and tibial slope after opening-wedge proximal tibial osteotomy: a prospective study. Am J Sports Med 38:160–170. doi:10.1177/0363546509342701

LaPrade RF, Wills NJ, Spiridonov SI, Perkinson S (2010b) A prospective outcomes study of meniscal allograft transplantation. Am J Sports Med 38:1804–1812. doi:10.1177/0363546510368133

Laprade RF, Spiridonov SI, Nystrom LM, Jansson KS (2012) Prospective outcomes of young and middle-aged adults with medial compartment osteoarthritis treated with a proximal tibial opening wedge osteotomy. Arthroscopy 28:354–364. doi:10.1016/j.arthro.2011.08.310

Lee AS, Kang RW, Kroin E et al (2012) Allograft meniscus transplantation. Sports Med Arthrosc 20:106–114. doi:10.1097/JSA.0b013e318246f005

Lobenhoffer P, De Simoni C, Staubli AE (2002) Open-wedge high-tibial osteotomy with rigid plate fixation. Techn Knee Surg 1:93–105

Maquet P (1985) The treatment of choice in osteoarthritis of the knee. Clin Orthop Relat Res 192:108–112

Matava MJ (2007) Meniscal allograft transplantation: a systematic review. Clin Orthop Relat Res 455:142–157. doi:10.1097/BLO.0b013e318030c24e

McDermott AG, Finklestein JA, Farine I et al (1988) Distal femoral varus osteotomy for valgus deformity of the knee. J Bone Joint Surg Am 70:110–116

Nagel A, Insall JN, Scuderi GR (1996) Proximal tibial osteotomy. A subjective outcome study. J Bone Joint Surg Am 78:1353–1358

Noyes FR, Barber-Westin SD (1996) Surgical restoration to treat chronic deficiency of the posterolateral complex and cruciate ligaments of the knee joint. Am J Sports Med 24:415–426

Noyes FR, Barber-Westin SD, Hewett TE (2000) High tibial osteotomy and ligament reconstruction for varus angulated anterior cruciate ligament-deficient knees. Am J Sports Med 28:282–296

Noyes FR, Mayfield W, Barber-Westin SD et al (2006) Opening wedge high tibial osteotomy: an operative technique and rehabilitation program to decrease complications and promote early union and function. Am J Sports Med 34:1262–1273. doi:10.1177/0363546505286144

Oakeshott RD, Farine I, Pritzker KP et al (1988) A clinical and histologic analysis of failed fresh osteochondral allografts. Clinl Orthop Relat Res 233:283–294

Paletta GA, Manning T, Snell E et al (1997) The effect of allograft meniscal replacement on intra-articular contact area and pressures in the human knee. A biomechanical study. Am J Sports Med 25:692–698

Phisitkul P, Wolf BR, Amendola A (2006) Role of high tibial and distal femoral osteotomies in the treatment of lateral-posterolateral and medial instabilities of the knee. Sports Med Arthrosc Rev 14:96–104. doi:10.1097/01.jsa.0000212306.47323.83

Poignard A, Flouzat Lachaniette CH, Amzallag J, Hernigou P (2010) Revisiting high tibial osteotomy: fifty years of experience with the opening-wedge technique. J Bone Joint Surg Am 92(2):187–195. doi:10.2106/JBJS.I.00771

Postel M, Langlais F (1977) Ostéotomies du genou pour gonarthrose. In: Encyclopédie médico-chirurgicale: techniques chirurgicales, orthopédie. Editions Techniques, Paris, pp 1–17

Puddu G, Franco V (2009) Distal femoral osteotomy for genu valgus correction. Techn Knee Surg 8:257–264

Puddu G, Cerullo G, Cipolla M et al (2007) Technique and outcomes of opening wedge high tibial osteotomy. Sem Arthroplasty 18:148–155. doi:10.1053/j.sart.2007.03.004

Rodner CM, Adams DJ, Diaz-Doran V et al (2006) Medial opening wedge tibial osteotomy and the sagittal plane: the effect of increasing tibial slope on tibiofemoral contact pressure. Am J Sports Med 34:1431–1441. doi:10.1177/0363546506287297

Rönn K, Reischl N, Gautier E, Jacobi M (2011) Current surgical treatment of knee osteoarthritis. Arthritis 2011:454873. doi:10.1155/2011/454873

Seedhom BB, Dowson D, Wright V (1974) Proceedings: functions of the menisci. A preliminary study. Ann Rheum Dis 33:111

Shelburne KB, Kim H-J, Sterett WI, Pandy MG (2011) Effect of posterior tibial slope on knee biomechanics during functional activity. J Orthop Res 29:223–231. doi:10.1002/jor.21242

Shoji H, Insall J (1973) High tibial osteotomy for osteoarthritis of the knee with valgus deformity. J Bone Joint Surg Am 55:963–973

Song EK, Seon JK, Park SJ, Jeong MS (2010) The complications of high tibial osteotomy: closing- versus opening-wedge methods. J Bone Joint Surg Br 92:1245–1252. doi:10.1302/0301-620X.92B9.23660

Staubli AE, De Simoni C, Babst R, Lobenhoffer P (2003) TomoFix: a new LCP-concept for open wedge osteotomy of the medial proximal tibia – early results in 92 cases. Injury 34:55–62. doi:10.1016/j.injury.2003.09.025

Stoffel K, Stachowiak G, Kuster M (2004) Open wedge high tibial osteotomy: biomechanical investigation of the modified Arthrex Osteotomy Plate (Puddu Plate) and the TomoFix Plate. Clin Biomech 19:944–950. doi:10.1016/j.clinbiomech.2004.06.007

Todd MS, Lalliss S, Garcia E et al (2010) The relationship between posterior tibial slope and anterior cruciate ligament injuries. Am J Sports Med 38:63–67. doi:10.1177/0363546509343198

Van Arkel ER, De Boer HH (1995) Human meniscal transplantation. Preliminary results at 2 to 5-year follow-up. J Bone Joint Surg Br 77:589–595

Van de Pol GJ, Arnold MP, Verdonschot N, Van Kampen A (2009) Varus alignment leads to increased forces in the anterior cruciate ligament. Am J Sports Med 37:481–487. doi:10.1177/0363546508326715

Van Raaij TM, De Waal MJ (2006) Anterior opening wedge osteotomy of the proximal tibia for anterior knee pain in idiopathic hyperextension knees. Int Orthop 30:248–252. doi:10.1007/s00264-005-0063-x

Van Thiel GS, Frank RM, Gupta A et al (2011) Biomechanical evaluation of a high tibial osteotomy with a meniscal transplant. J Knee Surg 24:45–53

Verdonk PCM, Demurie A, Almqvist KF et al (2005) Transplantation of viable meniscal allograft Survivorship analysis and clinical outcome of one hundred cases. J Bone Joint Surg Am 87:715–724. doi:10.2106/JBJS.C.01344

Verdonk PCM, Verstraete KL, Almqvist KF et al (2006) Meniscal allograft transplantation: long-term clinical results with radiological and magnetic resonance imaging correlations. Knee Surg Sports Traumatol Arthrosc 14:694–706. doi:10.1007/s00167-005-0033-2

Zeng C, Cheng L, Wei J et al (2012) The influence of the tibial plateau slopes on injury of the anterior cruciate ligament: a meta-analysis. Knee Surg Sports Traumatol Arthrosc 22(1):53–65. doi:10.1007/s00167-012-2277-y

Single Versus Double Anterior Cruciate Ligament Reconstruction in Athletes

125

Alberto Gobbi, Georgios Karnatzikos, and Dnyanesh G. Lad

Contents

Abstract

ACL reconstruction (ACLR) is the gold standard treatment for a complete ACL tear. Given the knowledge of the functional anatomy of the ACL, double-bundle reconstruction would appear to recreate a more natural situation within the knee. Controversy continues regarding the efficacy, safety, and true benefit of a double-bundle over a single-bundle ACLR. Very little has been described in the literature regarding the double-bundle surgical technique, and it has been agreed that there is a steep learning curve which coupled with the fact that not many studies have demonstrated significant difference in outcomes keeps the debate alive – to double bundle or not.

Introduction

The anterior cruciate ligament (ACL) consists of two functional bundles – the anteromedial (AM) and the posterolateral (PL) bundle, named in relation to their insertion on the tibial plateau (Radford and Amis 1990; Amis and Dawkins 1991; Ziegler et al. 2011). When the knee is flexed, the AM bundle tightens while the PL bundle slackens; while during knee extension, the PL bundle tightens and the AM bundle loosens (Mae et al. 2001).

Single-bundle (SB) ACL reconstruction has been the gold standard to treat ACL lesions (Freedman et al. 2003; Gobbi et al. 2003;

A. Gobbi (✉) • G. Karnatzikos • D.G. Lad
Orthopaedic Arthroscopic Surgery International (O.A.S.I.) Bioresearch Foundation, Gobbi Onlus, Milan, Italy
e-mail: gobbi@cartilagedoctor.it; info@oasibioresearchfoundation.org; giokarnes@gmail.com; dnyaneshlad@gmail.com

M.N. Doral, J. Karlsson (eds.), *Sports Injuries*,
DOI 10.1007/978-3-642-36569-0_263

Chen et al. 2006; Siebold et al. 2006). Good results have been demonstrated with respect to anteroposterior stability of the knee; however, doubts persist regarding its efficiency in restoring rotational stability which has led to an interest in anatomic reconstruction with double bundle (Yagi et al. 2002; Mae et al. 2006; Zelle et al. 2006; Crawford et al. 2007; Siebold et al. 2008; Gadikota et al. 2009; Kondo et al. 2010). Theoretically, the anatomic double-bundle ACL reconstruction should offer an improved pivot shift resistance and increase rotational knee control; furthermore, it should help in preserving menisci and limit progression toward arthritis. These theoretical advantages, however, could be negated by the complexity of the surgical procedure and the significant learning curve associated with it because there is very little mentioned in the literature regarding the operative technique (Van Eck et al. 2010). A review of most studies reveals no significant differences in outcomes between the two techniques with respect to objective and subjective IKDC scoring, anterior tibial translation, pivot shift, flexor-extensor deficit, proprioception, knee function, and return to sports (Calvisi et al. 2007; Lewis et al. 2008; Longo et al. 2008; Meredick et al. 2008; Kanaya et al. 2009; Song et al. 2009; Park et al. 2010).

At OASI Bioresearch Foundation, Milan, 60 randomly selected athletes were prospectively followed up for 3 years. All patients underwent anatomical ACL reconstruction (ACLR) with single- or double-bundle technique using the semitendinosus (ST) graft. The patients were randomly assigned to two treatment groups: ST single-bundle (SB group) and ST double-bundle (DB group) ACLR group, blinded as to the specific type of reconstruction they would undergo. The inclusion criteria were (1) ACL injury reported within 5 months; (2) normal opposite knee; (3) consent; (4) willingness to follow-up at 3, 6, 12, 24, and 36 months or when asked for; and (5) compliance to a specific rehabilitation program. Patients who had a previous knee surgery (except diagnostic arthroscopy or partial meniscectomy), associated grade three ligament injuries, grade III–IV chondral damage, and abnormal radiographs were excluded.

Table 1 Incidence of sport-specific injury

Sport	Incidence of ACL injury (%)
Soccer	38
Skiing	33
Motocross	16
Tennis	10
Karate	3

Table 2 Patient demographics

	Single bundle	Double bundle
No. of patients	30	30
Mean age (in years)	31.9 ± 1.92	28.9 ± 1.89
Male	15	18
Female	15	12

Patient demographics and incidence of injury are shown in Tables 1 and 2. Pivoting was the main mechanism of injury (82 %), while a fall during sport participation accounted for 18 %. Clinically presentation was of an ACL-deficient knee, with a positive Lachman and pivot shift test, confirmed with an MRI as having a completely torn ACL. Associated knee injuries included first- and second-degree MCL sprain in 11 %, meniscal lesions in 30 %, grade I or II chondropathy in 7 %, and a combined meniscal and chondropathy lesion in 15 %.

Surgical Technique

Under spinal or general anesthesia, a tourniquet is placed at the proximal aspect of the thigh with sufficient distance from the expected exit point of the Kirschner wire suture passer in the thigh's anterolateral aspect. A lateral post for thigh support and a foot bar are placed to enable the knee to be positioned to allow for full range of motion.

Graft Preparation

The preparation of the graft is similar for the single- and double-bundle techniques. After standard prepping and draping, the tourniquet is inflated only for graft harvest and is then deflated. A 3 cm vertical incision should be made centered

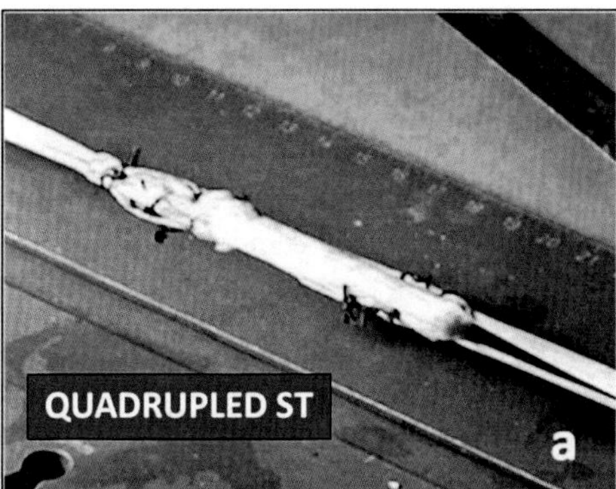

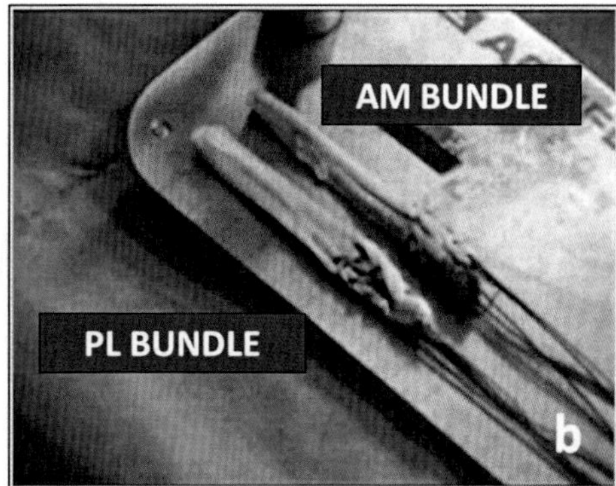

Fig. 1 Graft preparation for single-bundle (**a**) and double-bundle (**b**) ACLR using ST tendon

approximately 5 cm below the medial joint line and midway between the tibial tubercle and the posteromedial aspect of the tibia. The sartorial fascia is incised and the semitendinosus tendon dissected out. The tendon is completely detached from its proximal attachment with an open tendon stripper. On its tibial end, the tendon's length must be maximized preserving as much length as possible by detaching the ST close to the bone.

While the surgeon prepares the tunnels, the surgical assistant, if available, may prepare the graft, which is then cleaned and devoid of excess tissues. A length of 28 cm allows the possibility of cutting the graft in half with sufficient length to fold each half of the graft to a length of 7 cm. In this way, 2 cm graft length is available for the femoral and tibial tunnels and 3 cm intra-articularly. The ends of the grafts are then whip-stitched using permanent sutures (Fig. 1a, b).

Single-Bundle Technique

Using standard anterolateral and anteromedial arthroscopic portals, the knee joint is visualized and prepared for tunnel placements. The anatomic footprints of the native ACL on both the femoral and tibial sides are identified. The remnants of the torn ACL on the femoral and tibial sides may be used as landmarks for tunnel positioning. If only one ACL bundle is torn, it is a good idea to preserve the intact bundle. However, if both ACL bundles are torn, the center of ACL footprint on the femoral and tibial side is used as a landmark for placing tunnels for SB ACLR. The femoral tunnel position is first identified and drilled using a K-wire in an anatomic position through the anteromedial portal with the knee flexed at 110° of flexion. After checking the proper anatomical positioning, a 4.5 mm cannulated drill is used to create the femoral tunnel, and the length of the tunnel should be measured. The tunnel is prepared using a drill and dilators in order to obtain a tunnel 0.5 mm in diameter smaller than the graft in order to have a sufficient press fit and avoid possible graft movement. The tibial tunnel is then prepared in anatomical position at the ligament's footprint using an endoscopic aimer adjusted to a 45° position in the coronal plane. The alignment on the sagittal plane should be at 70° with respect to the medial plateau.

After selecting the appropriate size, the quadrupled semitendinosus tendon is inserted and fixed at the femoral end with EndoButton. At this point, it is appropriate to precondition the graft with cyclic flexion and extension of the knee, and finally, the two strands are fixed on the tibial side under maximum manual tension using a biocomposite screw, at 20° of flexion.

Double-Bundle Technique

The PL femoral tunnel is initially prepared using an "outside-in" technique. To properly achieve this step, a customized posterolateral (PL) tunnel guide (Smith & Nephew Anatomic ACLR PL femoral aimer) was utilized (Fig. 2). The arm of the PL guide is inserted in the anterolateral portal and positioned at the anatomical position on the medial wall of the lateral condyle, while the handle is maneuvered at the area of the junction of the distal femur and lateral condyle to fix the entry point for the tunnel. Use the lateral intercondylar ridge and lateral bifurcate ridge to indicate the superior border of the femoral ACL insertion site and the border between the AM and PL bundle, respectively, as bony landmarks for placement of tunnels (Fu and Karlsson 2010). A guide wire is inserted from outside-in, which is followed by a 4.5 mm cannulated drill to prepare the pilot hole. Once the length of this hole is measured, a 6 mm diameter PL tunnel of appropriate depth is drilled.

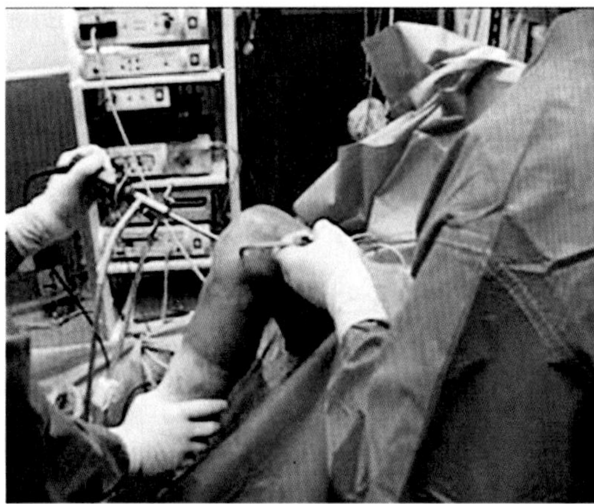

Fig. 2 Intraoperative use of the posterolateral tunnel guide in the "outside-in" technique of PL tunnel preparation

Preparation of the 7 mm AM tunnel is next, with the tunnel placed at either the 11 o'clock or 1 o'clock position. At the end of this step, there will be two divergent tunnels positioned anatomically. The tibial tunnels are prepared at an angle of 50°–60° with the entry point separated by a distance of 1–1.5 cm. These tunnels converge on the ACL ligament's tibial footprint intra-articularly (Fig. 3a).

With the tunnels ready, the PL bundle is positioned first followed by the AM bundle (Fig. 3b). Once in place, the femoral fixation should be double checked to determine if the EndoButton is securely anchored against the cortex. After pretensioning and preconditioning with cyclic flexion and extension, the tibial end of the graft maybe fixed using a single screw-post construct connected to the graft with new generation high-strength suture. The AM bundle is secured at 20° of flexion and the PL bundle fixed in full extension; check the graft for impingement and examine the knee for range of motion and stability with the Lachman test. Always obtain postoperative radiographs to ensure proper tunnel placement and hardware fixation (Fig. 4a, b).

Rehabilitation

The postoperative rehabilitation protocol was identical for both groups. Four weeks after surgery, patients returned to performing activities of

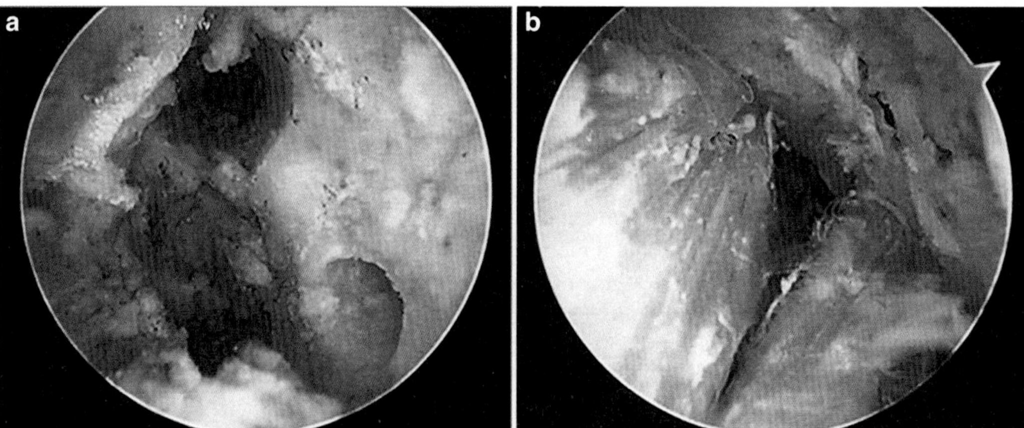

Fig. 3 Arthroscopic appearance after preparation of the tunnels (**a**) and after placement of both AM and PL bundles (**b**)

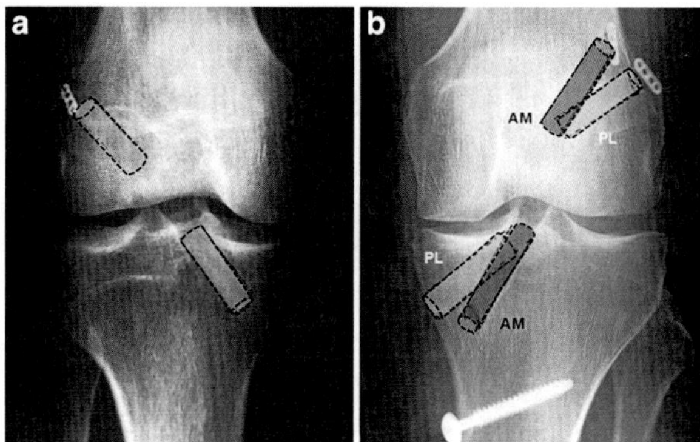

Fig. 4 (**a**, **b**) AP and lateral radiographs following double-bundle ACLR

daily living. Noncontact sports were permitted after 3 months, and contact sports were permitted 1 year after surgery (see Table 3).

Results

All the patients were followed up for a minimum of 3 years. Patients in both groups showed significant improvement in all scores (IKDC, Noyes, Lysholm, Tegner, and Marx) from preoperative to 6, 12- and 36-month follow-up ($P < 0.05$) (see Figs. 5a, b and 6a, b). The nonparametric Mann-Whitney *U* test showed no significant difference in improvement between the two groups at the prospective follow-up (Table 4). All the patients returned to previous sports activities. The rehabilitation time involved 10 % more sittings in the DB group than the SB group to regain the same range of motion. In the SB group, patients went back to competitive sports at an average of 7.4 months and in the DB group at an average of 8.2 months; however, there was no significant difference between pre-injury and final follow-up Tegner scores. Spearman's rho test showed significant correlation between preoperative psychovitality score and Tegner score at final follow-up for both groups (Fig. 7a, b).

Instability was described as a difference (ΔLaxity) in AP tibial translation compared with the contralateral healthy knee using a Rolimeter. There was a significant improvement in both knees from preoperative to postoperative follow-up. For postoperative range of joint motion, no statistically significant difference was found. The nonparametric Mann-Whitney *U* test on cross-comparisons showed no significant difference in improvement between the two groups (Table 4). Furthermore, Wilcoxon Ranks test showed no significant difference in measurements in laxity at 1- and 3-year follow-up, confirming that there was no difference between the two groups in maintaining postoperative stability. Additionally the lateral pivot shift test in SB group was negative in 83.3 % and 16.7 % patients and in DB group was negative in 87 % and grade one in 13 %, respectively, at 3 years postoperatively.

No major postoperative complications were noted and no re-ruptures observed. However, at follow-up of 1 year, one of the patients in the SB group while performing motocross sustained a high-energy trauma resulting in a fracture of the tibial plateau (Schatzker type I) and was managed conservatively with a brace; diagnostic arthroscopy showed that the ACL was intact and he went back to motocross again after 3 months. Another patient in the DB group after 4.5 years sustained a tibial plateau fracture (Schatzker type IV), involving medial femoral condyle, following a trauma while playing soccer (Gobbi et al. 2011). Previous to this injury at 4 years follow-up, the anteroposterior translation was 2 mm more when compared to the normal knee, International Knee Documentation Committee objective score was grade A, and radiographs showed intact tunnels and good bone quality without widening of tunnels. Radiographs and thin-slice computed tomography after injury showed that bone quality was good and there was no osteopenia or tunnel widening. The patient was managed operatively

Table 3 Rehabilitation protocol after ACL reconstruction

Month one	CPM: 8 h/day, 10°–60°, adding 5° per day until 90° is reached
1st week (From discharge until the 1st checkup)	At night, CPM at a slower speed
	Application of ice on the knee for 15 min every 2 h
	Partial weight-bearing crutch walking
	Isometric quadriceps exercises
	Active movement of the ankle
2nd week (After the 1st checkup)	Continue CPM 0° to 90°; ice packs on knee 2 hourly and partial weight-bearing crutch walking
	Start PT-assisted exercises
	Patellar mobilization
	Electrostimulation (low intensity)
	Isometric cocontraction on CPM
	Surgical wounds must be kept dry
3rd week (After the 2nd checkup)	Stop CPM 15 (should have achieved 110° of flexion)
	1 crutch outside the house for safety; full weight-bearing (except for other indications)
	Supervised PT as before, add the following
	Exercises in water-impermeable wound dressing
	Resisted flexion-extension exercises with TheraBand against manual resistance by the therapist at 10°–90°
	Proprioceptive exercises without loads
	Exercise other joints (no adduction)
4th week	Full weight-bearing – abandon crutches completely
	Achieve 120° of flexion
	Isometric contraction
	Careful leg presses, mini-squat (closed-chain exercises)
	Cycling and manually resisted flexion exercises

(*continued*)

Table 3 (continued)

Month two	Free full weight-bearing ambulation. Proprioceptive exercises with bipedal load
	Isotonic exercises with leg presses (closed-chain exercises)
	Exercise other joints (include adduction)
Month three	Free active extension
	Isokinetic work
	Swimming, controlled running exercises, road cycling
	1st knee laxity and isokinetic strength evaluation
Month four	Running on soft terrain, swimming
	Sport-specific drills
Month five	Return to individual low-risk sports
	Sport-specific drills
Month six	Return to team sports and higher-risk sports
	2nd knee laxity and isokinetic strength tests
One year	Strengthening and proprioceptive exercises
	3rd knee laxity and isokinetic strength tests

with opening reduction and fixation with LCP plate and screws; arthroscopic examination showed the integrity of the ACL reconstruction and meniscal structures. The authors speculated possible stress increase on the proximal tibia resulting from the two tunnels placed during primary anatomic DB ACLR. However, there is no study in literature comparing the stress over the bone resulting from tibial tunnels after SB or DB ACLR or calculating the volume of bone that is removed from the tibia from drilling.

Discussion

For a more successful reconstruction of the ACL, the ideal outcome would be restoration of the anatomy of the ACL which means functional restoration of the ACL to its native dimensions,

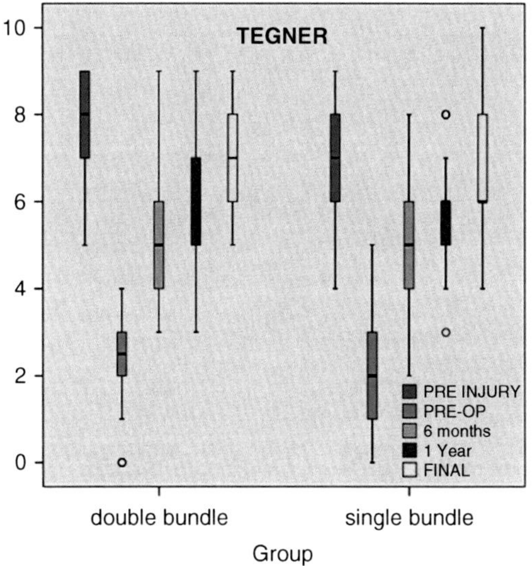

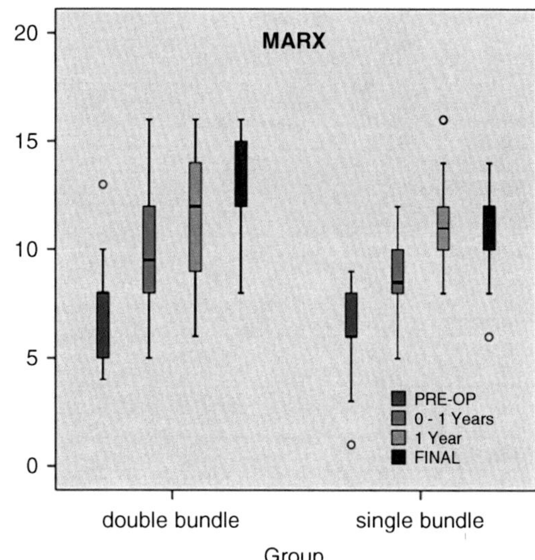

Fig. 5 Box plots showing improvement in Tegner (**a**) and Marx (**b**) scores from preoperative evaluation to 6 months, 1 year and final follow-up; Tegner score at final follow-up approached that of the pre-injury level in the single-bundle group

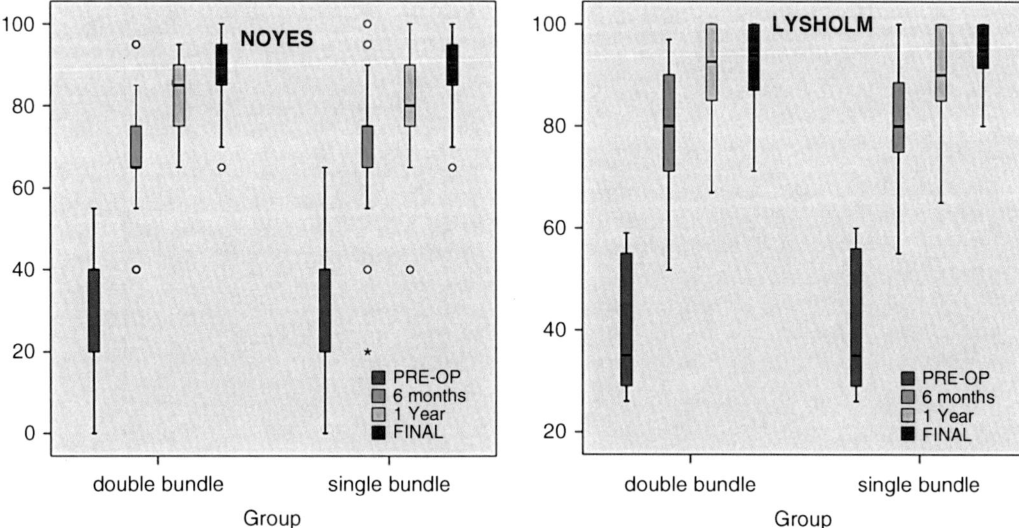

Fig. 6 Box plots showing improvement in Noyes (**a**) and Lysholm (**b**) scores from preoperative evaluation to 6 months, 1 year and final follow-up

collagen orientation, and insertion sites (Fu and Karlsson 2010). Many different techniques have been suggested for anatomical ACL reconstruction using different tunnels positions, fixation systems, and types of graft (Gobbi et al. 2002; Markolf et al. 2010; Reinhardt et al. 2010). Shino et al. (2008) developed a rectangular single femoral and tibial tunnel that would accommodate a bone-patellar tendon-bone inserted sideways. This orientation would span both the AM and PL footprints on the femur and tibia, and the anterior part of the tendon would function as the AM bundle and the posterior portion as part of the PL bundle. This is a very

Table 4 Clinical outcome at 3 years after ACL reconstruction

Parameter assessed	Surgical technique	Preoperative (mean ± SEM)	Three-year follow-up (mean ± SEM)	Improvement (*P*-value/Z-score)	Cross-comparison (*P*-value/Z-score)
IKDC subjective	**SB**	41.5 ± 4.21	89.4 ± 1.47	0.000/−4.798	0.690/−0.399
	DB	43 ± 3.98	88 ± 2.20	0.000/−4.782	
IKDC objective	**SB**	22C/8D	20A/10B	0.000/−4.788	0.411/−0.823
	DB	20C/10D	21A/9B	0.000/−4.808	
Tegner	**SB**	2.0 ± 0.37	6.73 ± 0.38	0.000/−4.804	0.874/−0.158
	DB	2.3 ± 0.32	7.10 ± 0.32	0.000/−4.811	
Marx	**SB**	6.4 ± 0.50	11.3 ± 0.47	0.000/−4.798	0.113/−1.584
	DB	7.1 ± 0.61	13.3 ± 0.56	0.000/−4.803	
Noyes	**SB**	29.5 ± 4.93	88.5 ± 2.01	0.000/−4.799	0.852/−0.187
	DB	30 ± 4.57	87.8 ± 2.37	0.000/−4.791	
Lysholm	**SB**	42.4 ± 3.30	93.3 ± 1.69	0.000/−4.779	0.784/−0.274
	DB	40.4 ± 3.11	92.8 ± 1.96	0.000/−4.785	
ΔLaxity (mm)	**SB**	7.7 ± 0.67	1.41 ± 0.26	0.000/−4.787	0.191/−1.307
Rolimeter	**DB**	8.6 ± 0.58	1.38 ± 0.21	0.000/−4.799	

The reported *p*-values are one tailed with an alpha level of 0.05 indicating significance. All the scores showed significant improvement from preoperative evaluation to 3 years follow-up. Mann-Whitney *U* test showed no significant difference in improvement between the two groups at the prospective follow-up

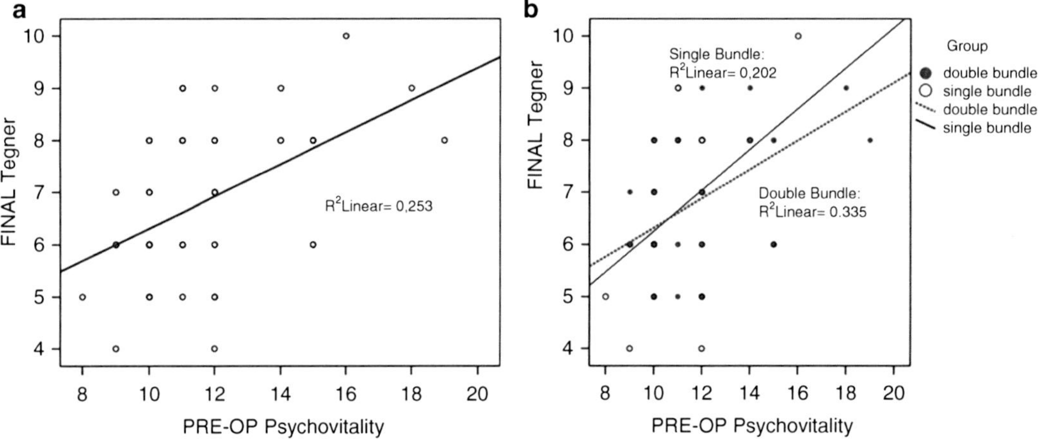

Fig. 7 Scatterplots showing a correlation between preoperative Psychovitality and Tegner score at last follow-up for all the patients (**a**) and each group separately (**b**)

simple innovative technique to reconstruct the anatomy of the double bundle.

Recent meta-analysis studies demonstrated that there is no difference between single- or double-bundle ACL reconstruction in regard to the odds of having a normal pivot shift (Song et al. 2009; Fu and Karlsson 2010; Park et al. 2010). However, the pivot shift test is a subjective test commonly used during clinical examination, while more sophisticated systems as well as gait analysis are not available in everyday practice to quantitatively measure rotational instability.

If carefully analyzed, it may be observed from the published studies that different groups of ACL-deficient patients have been studied, with no difference regarding associated or non-peripheral instability, as well as pivot shift grade, varus-valgus limb morphology, and type of sport. It has been recently reported that although double-bundle ACLR produces better intraoperative stability than single-bundle ACLR, the two modalities demonstrated similar clinical outcomes and postoperative stability at a 2-year follow-up (Markolf et al. 2010). Results from the study in Milan proved that stability was achieved and remained even after 3 years for both groups, in keeping with the findings of many recent studies (Gobbi et al. 2002; Markolf et al. 2010).

Surgery must always be individualized for a patient; considering the anthropometrical anatomy, for instance, a double-bundle ACLR may be more appropriate for an athlete of high contact or impact sport but not for a young ballet dancer, skeletally immature patient, or a patient with a significant lateral femoral condyle bone bruise (Gobbi et al. 2004). It is well known that there is a significant learning curve associated with double-bundle ACL reconstructions, and a study (Harner and Poehling 2004) suggested that most of the European and American surgeons individually perform less than ten cases per year, which raises the question whether they should be addressing the double-bundle ACL reconstruction technique at all, given the already high failure rate of approximately 10–20 % in all ACL reconstructions.

Complications

A recent study demonstrated a significantly higher number of patients operated with double bundle presenting with tibial and femoral bone tunnel enlargement and double tunnel communication (Siebold and Cafaltzis 2010). Performing an anatomic double-bundle reconstruction entails the use of both the semitendinosus (ST) and the gracilis autografts; requiring the use of independent femoral and tibial fixations and with the use of both tendons, hamstring strength deficits in deep flexion and internal rotation could represent a possible complication (Nakamura et al. 2002; Gobbi et al. 2005, 2012; Gobbi 2010).

Conclusions

With an increasing number of options in the sport surgeons arsenal, there should be an improved algorithm for the treatment of complete ACL tears, one which will answer questions regarding technique, graft type, and fixation. At present, the surgeon should use the most anatomic technique for ACL reconstruction with less complexity, easier fixation, least invasive revision technique, and minor graft harvesting morbidity. Both single- and double-bundle techniques could be used; however, double-bundle technique should be reserved for patients with complex instability and greater transverse plane rotational knee stress demands. Finally, surgeons contemplating the use of a double-bundle technique all have to answer the same question: Is double-bundle ACLR better than the conventional reconstruction techniques? At present, the answer remains a complicated one!

Cross-References

- ▶ Alternative Techniques for Double-Tunnel Anatomic Anterior Cruciate Ligament Reconstruction
- ▶ Anterior Cruciate Ligament Injuries and Surgery: Current Evidence and Modern Development
- ▶ Anterior Cruciate Ligament Reconstruction with Autologous Quadriceps Tendon
- ▶ Different Techniques of Anterior Cruciate Ligament Reconstruction: Guidelines
- ▶ Double-Tunnel Anatomic Anterior Cruciate Ligament Reconstruction

References

Amis AA, Dawkins GP (1991) Functional anatomy of the anterior cruciate ligament. Fibre bundle actions related to ligament replacements and injuries. J Bone Joint Surg (Br) 73:260–267

Calvisi V, Lupparelli S, Rinonapoli G et al (2007) Single-bundle versus double bundle arthroscopic reconstruction of the anterior cruciate ligament: what does the available evidence suggest? J Orthopaed Traumatol 8:95–100

Chen CH, Chuang TY, Wang KC et al (2006) Arthroscopic anterior cruciate ligament reconstruction with quadriceps tendon autograft: clinical outcome in 4–7 years. Knee Surg Sports Traumatol Arthrosc 14:1077–1085

Crawford C, Nyland J, Landes S et al (2007) Anatomic double bundle ACL reconstruction: a literature review. Knee Surg Sports Traumatol Arthrosc 15:946–964

Freedman KB, D'Amato MJ, Nedeff DD et al (2003) Arthroscopic anterior cruciate ligament reconstruction: a metaanalysis comparing patellar tendon and hamstring tendon autografts. Am J Sports Med 31:2–11

Fu FH, Karlsson J (2010) A long journey to be anatomic. Knee Surg Sports Traumatol Arthrosc 18:1151–1153

Gadikota HR, Seon JK, Kozanek M et al (2009) Biomechanical comparison of single-tunnel-double-bundle and single-bundle anterior cruciate ligament reconstructions. Am J Sports Med 37:962–969

Gobbi A (2010) Single versus double hamstring tendon harvest for ACL reconstruction. Sports Med Arthrosc 18:15–19

Gobbi A, Mahajan S, Tuy B, Panuncialman I (2002) Hamstring graft tibial fixation: biomechanical properties of different linkage systems. Knee Surg Sports Traumatol Arthrosc 10:330–334

Gobbi A, Mahajan S, Zanazzo M, Tuy B (2003) Patellar tendon versus quadrupled bone-semitendinosus anterior cruciate ligament reconstruction: a prospective clinical investigation in athletes. Arthroscopy 19:592–601

Gobbi A, Domzalski M, Pascual J (2004) Comparison of anterior cruciate ligament reconstruction in male and female athletes using the patellar tendon and hamstring autografts. Knee Surg Sports Traumatol Arthrosc 12:534–539

Gobbi A, Domzalski M, Pascual J, Zanazzo M (2005) Hamstring anterior cruciate ligament reconstruction: is it necessary to sacrifice the gracilis? Arthroscopy 21:275–280

Gobbi A, Mahajan V, Karnatzikos G (2011) Tibial plateau fracture after primary anatomic double-bundle anterior cruciate ligament reconstruction: a case report. Arthroscopy 27:735–740

Gobbi A, Mahajan V, Karnatzikos G, Nakamura N (2012) Single- versus double-bundle ACL reconstruction: is there any difference in stability and function at 3-year followup? Clin Orthop Relat Res 470:824–34

Harner CD, Poehling GG (2004) Double bundle or double trouble? Arthroscopy 20:1013–1014

Kanaya A, Ochi M, Deie M et al (2009) Intraoperative evaluation of anteroposterior and rotational stabilities in anterior cruciate ligament reconstruction: lower femoral tunnel placed single-bundle versus double-bundle reconstruction. Knee Surg Sports Traumatol Arthrosc 17:907–913

Kondo E, Merican AM, Yasuda K et al (2010) Biomechanical comparisons of knee stability after anterior cruciate ligament reconstruction between 2 clinically available transtibial procedures: anatomic double bundle versus single bundle. Am J Sports Med 38:1349–1358

Lewis PB, Parameswaran AD, Rue JP et al (2008) Systematic review of single-bundle anterior cruciate ligament reconstruction outcomes: a baseline assessment for consideration of double-bundle techniques. Am J Sports Med 36:2028–2036

Longo UG, King JB, Denaro V et al (2008) Double-bundle arthroscopic reconstruction of the anterior cruciate ligament: does the evidence add up? J Bone Joint Surg (Br) 90:995–999

Mae T, Shino K, Miyama T et al (2001) Single- versus two-femoral socket anterior cruciate ligament reconstruction technique: biomechanical analysis using a robotic simulator. Arthroscopy 17:708–716

Mae T, Shino K, Matsumoto N et al (2006) Force sharing between two grafts in the anatomical two-bundle anterior cruciate ligament reconstruction. Knee Surg Sports Traumatol Arthrosc 6:1–5

Markolf KL, Jackson SR, McAllister DR (2010) A comparison of 11 o'clock versus oblique femoral tunnels in the anterior cruciate ligament-reconstructed knee: knee kinematics during a simulated pivot test. Am J Sports Med 38:912–917

Meredick RB, Vance KJ, Appleby D et al (2008) Outcome of single-bundle versus double-bundle reconstruction of the anterior cruciate ligament: a meta-analysis. Am J Sports Med 36:1414–1421

Nakamura N, Horibe S, Sasaki S et al (2002) Evaluation of active knee flexion and hamstring strength after anterior cruciate ligament reconstruction using hamstring tendons. Arthroscopy 18:598–602

Park SJ, Jung YB, Jung HJ et al (2010) Outcome of arthroscopic single-bundle versus double-bundle reconstruction of the anterior cruciate ligament: a preliminary 2-year prospective study. Arthroscopy 26:630–636

Radford WJ, Amis AA (1990) Biomechanics of a double prosthetic ligament in the anterior cruciate ligament. J Bone Joint Surg (Br) 72:1038–1043

Reinhardt KR, Hetsroni I, Marx RG (2010) Graft selection for anterior cruciate ligament reconstruction: a level I systematic review comparing failure rates and functional outcomes. Orthop Clin N Am 41:249–262

Shino K, Nakata K, Nakamura N et al (2008) Rectangular tunnel double-bundle anterior cruciate ligament reconstruction with bone-patellar tendon-bone graft to mimic natural fiber arrangement. Arthroscopy 24:1178–1183

Siebold R, Cafaltzis K (2010) Differentiation between intraoperative and postoperative bone tunnel widening and communication in double-bundle anterior cruciate ligament reconstruction: a prospective study. Arthroscopy 26:1066–1073

Siebold R, Webster KE, Feller JA et al (2006) Anterior cruciate ligament reconstruction in females: a comparison of hamstring tendon and patellar tendon autografts. Knee Surg Sports Traumatol Arthrosc 14:1070–1076

Siebold R, Dehler C, Ellert T (2008) Prospective randomized comparison of double-bundle versus single-bundle anterior cruciate ligament reconstruction. Arthroscopy 24:137–145

Song EK, Oh LS, Gill TJ et al (2009) Prospective comparative study of anterior cruciate ligament reconstruction using the double-bundle and single-bundle techniques. Am J Sports Med 37:1705–1711

Van Eck CF, Schreiber VM, Mejia HA et al (2010) "Anatomic" anterior cruciate ligament reconstruction: a systematic review of surgical techniques and reporting of surgical data. Arthroscopy 26 (Suppl):S2–S12

Yagi M, Wong EK, Kanamori A et al (2002) Biomechanical analysis of an anatomic anterior cruciate ligament reconstruction. Am J Sports Med 30:660–666

Zelle BA, Brucker PU, Feng MT, Fu FH (2006) Anatomical double-bundle anterior cruciate ligament reconstruction. Sports Med 36(2):99–108

Ziegler CG, Pietrini SD, Westerhaus BD et al (2011) Arthroscopically pertinent landmarks for tunnel positioning in single-bundle and double-bundle anterior cruciate ligament reconstructions. Am J Sports Med 39:743–752

Special Considerations for Multiple-Ligament Knee Injuries

126

Joel Huleatt, Andrew Geeslin, and Robert F. LaPrade

Contents

J. Huleatt (✉) • R.F. LaPrade
The Steadman Clinic and Steadman Philippon Research Institute, Vail, CO, USA
e-mail: joelhuleatt@gmail.com; drlaprade@sprivail.org; rlaprade@thesteadmanclinic.com

A. Geeslin
School of Medicine, Western Michigan University, Kalamazoo, MI, USA
e-mail: andrew.geeslin@gmail.com

M.N. Doral, J. Karlsson (eds.), *Sports Injuries*,
DOI 10.1007/978-3-642-36569-0_112

Abstract

While high level of evidence studies on multiligament knee injuries are limited, a growing body of level III and IV clinical studies are available to guide treatment of these severe injuries. Early recognition and treatment is crucial for management of acute injuries, with immediate attention being directed toward ruling out or addressing vascular injuries. A thorough physical exam that delineates which structures are injured directs the need for more objective stress radiographs or other imaging modalities. The mechanical axis must be determined in patients with chronic injuries due to the high risk of failure of soft tissue grafts in patients with malalignment. An anatomic reconstruction of combined ligamentous injuries with early postoperative range of motion is recommended for best functional results. A multidisciplinary approach is necessary for the extensive rehabilitation following surgical treatment and should include the orthopedic surgeon, physical therapist, and athletic trainer if applicable.

Introduction

Although multiligament knee injuries are estimated to account for less than 1 % of orthopedic injuries, determining the optimal treatment strategies has been the focus of much research (Engebretsen et al. 2009). The complexity and heterogeneous nature of these injures presents a challenge both in diagnosis and treatment that warrants a systematic approach and attention to details. In all cases, fully appreciating the injury pattern and assessing all structures preoperatively is imperative for choosing the most suitable operative plan. In acute injuries, screening for chronic injuries, operating within 2–3 weeks, and attaining adequate range of motion preoperatively are important goals. In chronic injuries, addressing malalignment issues first and combining or staging surgeries in the optimal order can reduce the need for some reconstructions and improve outcomes. Although controversies exist regarding operative techniques, a great deal of effort has been spent precisely defining ligament anatomy and performing biomechanical tests on ligament-deficient and reconstructed knees, providing insight on how to create anatomically correct reconstructions that best restore stability and function.

Initial Assessment: Acute Versus Chronic Injuries

Vascular Status

The initial assessment of a patient with a suspected multiligament knee injury is based on the acuity of injury. In patients who have had a possible knee dislocation or been exposed to high-energy trauma, assessment of vascular status is the primary concern. Because the popliteal artery is tethered on both sides of the knee and is injured in approximately 25 % of high-velocity knee dislocations, an ankle-brachial index (ABI) should be obtained immediately if there is a chance of vascular injury (Green and Allen 1977; Treiman et al. 1992). In the absence of pulses or with an ABI of less than 0.9, which is highly specific and sensitive for arterial injury requiring surgical intervention, an emergent vascular service consultation and CT angiography or other rapid definitive vascular imaging modality are indicated (Mills et al. 2004). Due to the risk for delayed thrombus formation, patients who have experienced a knee dislocation, yet have an ABI greater than 0.9, should be monitored frequently (Fanelli et al. 2010).

Neurologic Status

Injury to the common peroneal nerve (Fig. 1) has been reported in 25–35 % of knee dislocations, so testing tibialis anterior and peroneus brevis and longus function (ankle dorsiflexion and eversion) and extensor hallucis longus and digitorum longus function (toe extension) is important (Johnson et al. 2008). Even an isolated posterolateral corner knee injury can present with full to partial peroneal nerve palsy due to tensile stress from a hyper-varus state (Johnson et al. 2008; Geeslin and LaPrade 2011). Tibial nerve injury may also occur with a knee dislocation, usually in concurrence with peroneal injury. Although less common, this is a devastating injury with characterized weakness of the tibialis posterior (foot inversion, arch support), flexor digitorum longus,

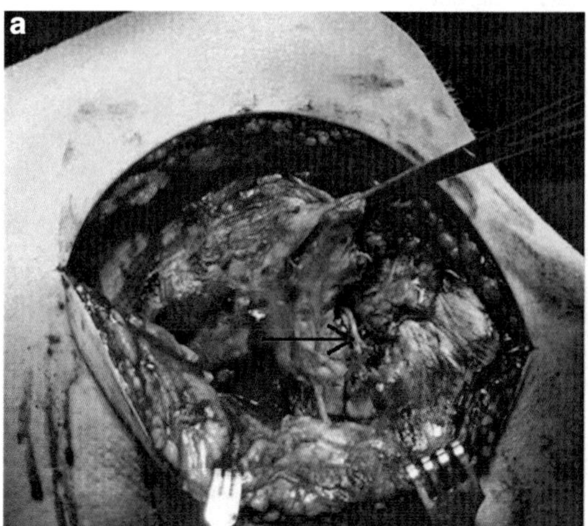

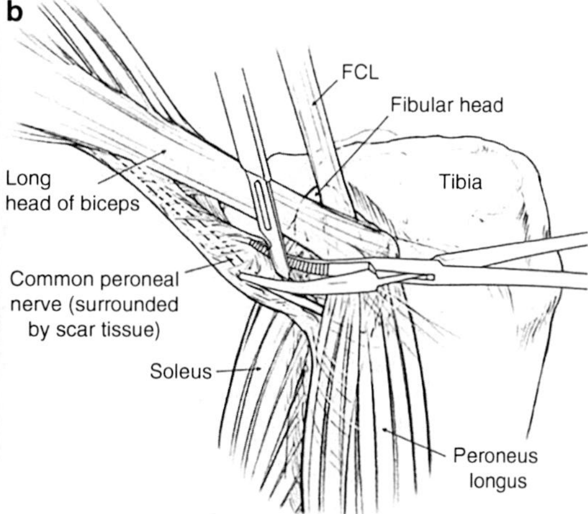

Fig. 1 (**a**) Intraoperative picture of the surgical approach to posterolateral corner of the right knee demonstrating a common peroneal nerve injury (*arrow*) in a patient with a concurrent avulsed biceps femoris tendon. (**b**) Illustration of a common peroneal neurolysis in a right knee that should be performed as a standard precaution when performing posterolateral corner reconstructions

and flexor hallucis longus and brevis (toe flexion) and loss of plantar sensation (Wascher et al. 1997). Testing for these nerve injuries at the initial assessment allows for documentation of the injury prior to surgery and for planning how to address the injury during surgery, such as whether intraoperative nerve conduction studies, nerve exploration, neurolysis, primary nerve repair, or nerve grafting may be indicated (Levy et al. 2010b). More rapid recognition and treatment of nerve injuries offers a better chance of avoiding permanent disability.

Alignment

In chronic multiligament injuries, long-leg standing radiographs should be obtained if malalignment is suspected. Chronic grade III posterolateral corner injuries are often associated with varus alignment, which should be corrected with a proximal tibial osteotomy prior to ligament reconstruction to avoid stretching out of the reconstruction grafts. Manipulation of the posterior tibial slope to establish more of a posterior tilt in combined PCL-deficient knees and less of a posterior tilt in combined ACL-deficient knees can also help stabilize the joint. For patients with chronic MCL injuries and valgus malalignment, distal femoral osteotomy may be beneficial. Patients with chronic ligament deficiencies that are exacerbated by malalignment will sometimes have sufficient return of joint stability following osteotomy to obviate the later need for ligament reconstruction (Arthur et al. 2007).

Combined Versus Isolated Ligament Injuries

When assessing a knee for ligamentous injury, it is important to appreciate the incidence of both isolated and combined injuries (Table 1). In patients with acute ACL injury, meniscal tears have been reported in approximately 50–80 %, concurrent MCL injuries in 17–41 %, posterior oblique ligament injuries in 31 %, articular surface lesions in 23 %, and only about 10 % were recorded as isolated injuries (Indelicato and Bittar 1985; Odensten et al. 1985; Shelbourne and Nitz 1991). In chronic ACL injuries, the percentage of meniscal tears and articular surface lesions is greater at 91 % and 54 %, respectively (Indelicato and Bittar 1985). In a study of PCL injuries, ligament deficiency was found in 38 % of 220 acute knee injuries identified by hemarthrosis of the knee, of which roughly one-third were sports related, and greater than 96 % were combined with other ligament injuries (Fanelli and Edson 1995). Of 173 patients in two studies of posterolateral corner injuries, 72 % had concurrent ligament injuries (Terry and LaPrade 1996; Geeslin and LaPrade 2010). Because the vast majority of knee ligament injuries occur in combination, it is important to pay close attention

Table 1 Combined knee ligament injury rates

Ligament injury	Concurrent injury	Rate
ACL (acute)	Medial meniscal tear	19–60 %[a,b,c]
	Lateral meniscal tear	32–48 %[a,b,c]
	MCL	17–41 %[b,c]
	Posterior oblique ligament	31 %[b]
	Articular surface lesion	23 %[a]
	Isolated	10 %[b]
ACL (chronic)	Medial meniscal tear	80 %[a]
	Lateral meniscal tear	36 %[a]
	Articular surface lesion	54 %[a]
PCL (acute)	Concurrent ligament injury	96 %[d]
Posterolateral corner (acute and chronic)	Concurrent ligament injury	72 %[e,f]

References: [a]Indelicato and Bittar (1985), [b]Odensten et al. (1985), [c]Shelbourne and Nitz (1991), [d] Fanelli and Edson (1995), [e]Geeslin and LaPrade (2010), [f]Terry and LaPrade (1996)

to the mechanism of injury while taking the history and to make sure each ligament is thoroughly evaluated on physical exam.

History

A proper history is essential for the efficient and accurate diagnosis of multiligament knee injuries because it focuses the exam and imaging strategy. Some important distinctions are whether the patient experienced a high- or low-energy impact, whether the injury was sustained by a contact or non-contact stress, and the type of instability that bothers the patient. Sports injuries to the knee are considered low-energy injuries and are typically localized, whereas high-energy events such as car accidents require examining for injuries elsewhere on the body. Meniscal tears and ACL injuries are often caused by non-contact cutting or twisting stresses. It is important to elicit the functional limitations of patients with chronic injuries, such as difficulty squatting or walking down stairs, giving way, pain with standing up, and snapping or catching, and to ask them what is hardest to do. Even in acutely injured patients, asking about chronic symptoms and instability may reveal an acute or chronic injury that would otherwise be missed. In all patients, it is useful to determine the patient's goals and expectations to plan the most beneficial treatment pathway.

Physical Exam

When examining a patient with a suspected multiligament knee injury, thoroughness and comparison to the uninjured side are invaluable. Multiligament injuries will inevitably present with conspicuous exam findings, yet performing a thorough exam with attention to subtle findings will delineate which ligaments are damaged and help to avoid overlooking additional injuries that can influence the treatment choice and outcomes (Table 2). To judge the significance of exam results, comparing the injured side to the

Table 2 Knee ligament examinations and utility

Exam	Utility
External rotation recurvatum test	100 % specificity, 30 % sensitivity for combined ACL and posterolateral ligament injuries (LaPrade et al. 2008c)
Valgus stress test	Gapping more than 1–2 mm in knee extension indicates combined MCL and cruciate ligament injury
	Gapping at 20° of knee flexion indicates sMCL injury (Griffith et al. 2009; LaPrade and Wijdicks 2012a)
Varus stress test	The FCL is the primary varus restraint at 20° of knee flexion, lateral gapping will sequentially increase with concurrent injuries to other posterolateral structures (LaPrade et al. 2008b)
Anterior translation (Lachman's) test	85 % sensitivity, 94 % specificity for ACL injury (Benjaminse et al. 2006)
	Anterior translation increases with concurrent posterolateral injuries; isolated posterolateral injuries have no impact (Nielsen and Helmig 1986)
Pivot shift test	98 % specificity, 24 % sensitivity for both acute and chronic ACL injuries (Benjaminse et al. 2006)
Posterior translation	A posterior sag sign or positive quadriceps active test indicates injury to the anterolateral bundle of the PCL (Spiridonov et al. 2011)
	With the posterior drawer test, 8 mm of posterior translation indicates isolated PCL injury, and more than 12 mm indicates concurrent posterolateral corner injury (Schulz et al. 2007)
Anteromedial drawer test	External rotation increases with injuries to the distal sMCL, posterior oblique ligament, and meniscotibial aspect of the deep MCL (Wijdicks et al. 2010)
Posterolateral drawer test	Posterior subluxation of the lateral tibial plateau indicates a popliteus tendon injury with an intact PCL (Hughston and Norwood 1980)

(*continued*)

Table 2 (continued)

Exam	Utility
Dial test	Greater than 10° of external rotation at 30° but not 90° of knee flexion indicates posterolateral ligament injury
	Greater than 10° of external rotation at both 30° and 90° of knee flexion indicates concurrent PCL injury (Grood et al. 1988)

uninjured side is of utmost importance, because there is a great physiologic variance in the laxity and flexibility between individuals. It is almost always beneficial to examine the most painful area last, because this will allow a less inhibited full exam and the development of patient trust.

External Rotation Recurvatum Test

The external rotation recurvatum test is used to identify posterolateral instability and anterior translation of the proximal tibia when the knee is placed in recurvatum, with external rotation and varus stress. With the patient in the supine position, the test is performed by gently pressing down on the distal thigh to keep it against the exam table while lifting the patient's great toe and measuring the relative knee hyperextension by a goniometer or heel height (Fig. 2). This test produces genu recurvatum in patients with posterolateral corner deficiency and has been reported to have near 100 % specificity for combined ACL and posterolateral knee injury, yet only a sensitivity of 30 % (LaPrade et al. 2008c).

Valgus Stress Test

A valgus stress test is performed at 0° and 20° of flexion to detect a subjective increase in valgus gapping that may indicate injury to the medial knee structures. To perform the test, the supine patient's leg can be cradled by grasping the proximal leg with both hands and applying a valgus stress. Medial gapping of more than 1–2 mm at full extension indicates a combined cruciate ligament injury and that the MCL will probably not heal without surgery. Gapping at 20° is indicative of injury to the superficial medial collateral ligament (sMCL) and possible posterior oblique or deep MCL injury (Griffith et al. 2009; LaPrade and Wijdicks 2012a). However, this assessment is limited by the patient's ability to relax and by the clinician's ability to detect an end point. If a positive result is found, valgus stress radiographs can be performed for more objective measurements (LaPrade et al. 2010).

Varus Stress Test

The varus stress test is another subjective test that can provide the clinician with an idea of the knee's laxity and prompt the acquisition of more objective stress radiographs if gapping is discernible (LaPrade et al. 2008a). The test is performed to the supine patient in 20° of knee flexion, with application of varus stress through the foot and ankle while creating a fulcrum at the medial knee and palpating for gapping by placing one's fingers over the lateral joint line. In larger patients, cradling the leg under one's arm can make the examination more feasible. The fibular collateral ligament (FCL) is the primary restraint to varus, but concurrent injuries to other posterolateral structures and the cruciate ligaments will sequentially increase lateral gapping with varus stress (LaPrade et al. 2008b). Of note, the commonly used grading scales published in the American Orthopaedic Society for Sports Medicine's *2000 IKDC Knee Form* and the American Medical Association's *Standard Nomenclature of Athletic Injuries* have not demonstrated utility in distinguishing which ligaments are injured in a recent biomechanical study (American Medical Association 1966; The International Knee Documentations Committee 2000; LaPrade et al. 2008b).

Anterior Translation (Lachman's Test)

The Lachman's test is the most effective exam for diagnosing injury to the ACL, with a sensitivity of

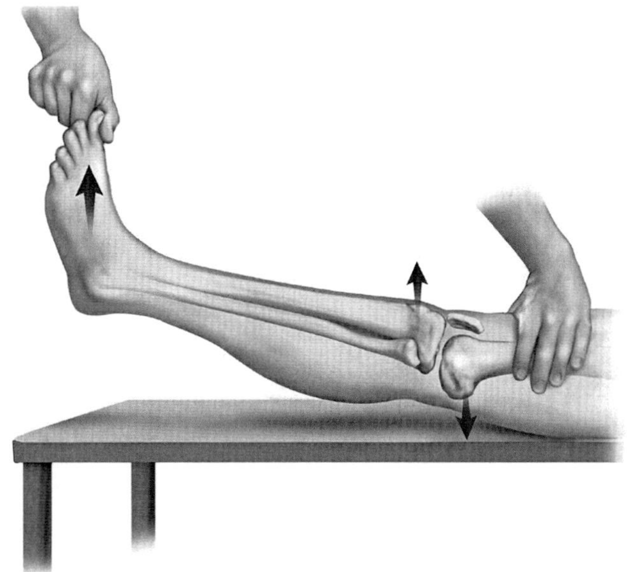

Fig. 2 Illustration of the anterior translation of the tibia relative to the femur at the tibiofemoral joint and the increased heel height in a patient with a posterolateral corner injury when examined with the external rotation recurvatum test (Reprinted with permission from the *American Journal of Sports Medicine* (LaPrade et al. 2008c))

85 % and a specificity of 94 % (Benjaminse et al. 2006). It is performed by testing for anterior translation of the tibia with the knee in 20–30° of flexion and is considered positive when there is a soft end point and greater than a 3 mm difference between knees. The KT-1000 arthrometer is a popular device to assist with diagnosing ACL injuries objectively, but it has been reported to be less reliable than the Lachman's test (Wiertsema et al. 2008). The Lachman's test can also help to diagnose combined ACL and posterolateral corner injuries. Isolated posterolateral corner injuries do not result in a positive Lachman's test, but in ACL-deficient knees, the addition of posterolateral corner injuries results in increased anterior translation (Nielsen and Helmig 1986; Wroble et al. 1993). The performance of the Lachman's test can be hampered in some clinical scenarios, such as with acute knee pain, guarding, and bucket-handle meniscus tears.

Pivot Shift Test

The pivot shift test is a confirmatory test of ACL injuries, because it has a high specificity of 98 % for both acute and chronic injuries, but has a poor sensitivity of 24 % (Benjaminse et al. 2006). Whereas the Lachman's test examines the static stability of ACL, the pivot shift test interrogates its dynamic stability, especially the competence of the posterolateral bundle that provides rotational restraint near full knee extension (Gabriel et al. 2004; Petersen and Zantop 2006). This test is accomplished by applying valgus and internal rotatory stresses to anterolaterally subluxate the tibia on the femur with the knee in extension and then flexing the knee; a tangible reduction of the knee at around 30° of flexion substantiates a positive result. However, a recent study reported that the clinical results of the pivot shift test correlate poorly with objective quantification (Kopf et al. 2012).

Posterior Translation

Assessment of tibial posterior translation is performed to examine the PCL, which is the primary restraint. The PCL is composed of two functional bundles; the larger anterolateral bundle is the greater stabilizer with the knee flexed to 90°, while the smaller posteromedial bundle contributes primarily at full extension and, in addition, acts as a secondary stabilizer to external rotation (Spiridonov et al. 2011). One way to evaluate posterior translation is to look for the posterior sag sign, which is a visible step-off from the patella to the proximal tibia with both knees flexed at 90°. The quadriceps active test, which demonstrates the reduction of a posteriorly subluxated tibia with quadriceps firing while the foot is secured and the knee at 90°, may be the most reliable exam. The posterior drawer test is also performed at 90° and requires complete relaxation while applying a posterior force. A posterior translation of 8 mm (grade 2) is indicative of an isolated PCL injury, while greater than 12 mm (grade 3+) is more consistent with a combined PCL and posterolateral or other ligamentous injury (Schulz et al. 2007).

Anteromedial Drawer Test

The anteromedial drawer test assesses for external rotatory instability permitted by deficiencies of medial knee structures, specifically the distal sMCL, the posterior oblique ligament, and the meniscotibial portion of the deep MCL. It is performed similar to the anterior drawer test with the knee flexed to 90°, but the foot is placed in 15° of external rotation, and the proximal tibia is pulled in an anteromedial direction with the application of an external rotatory force (Wijdicks et al. 2010).

Posterolateral Drawer Test

The posterolateral drawer test is performed to assess for posterolateral rotational instability due to posterolateral corner ligament injuries. With the patient supine and knee flexed at 80–90°, and with sequential stabilization of the foot in 15° of external rotation and then in 15–20° of internal rotation, the proximal tibia is grasped with the thumbs palpating the joint line similar to a posterior drawer test, and posterior stress is applied. If the PCL is intact and the popliteus tendon is injured, the lateral tibial plateau will sublux posteriorly, rotating externally around the PCL when the foot is in external rotation. However, in internal rotation, the PCL will be too taut to allow any posterior movement of the tibia (Hughston and Norwood 1980).

Dial Test

The dial test helps to diagnose and differentiate between isolated and combined posterolateral corner injuries. It is accomplished in the supine patient by hanging the leg off the side of the table, stabilizing the distal femur at the edge of the table with one hand, and then applying external rotatory stress through the foot and ankle while monitoring for external rotation of the tibial tubercle relative to the femur at both 30° and 90° of knee flexion. The test can also be performed with the patient prone, which allows easier comparison of bilateral rotation limits. With intact posterolateral ligaments, less than 2° of side-to-side difference of external rotation is found regardless of knee flexion or the status of the PCL. With deficiencies of just the posterolateral ligaments, the test reveals approximately 13° and 5° of external rotation at 30° and 90° of flexion, respectively, with increases in the respective external rotation to approximately 18° and 21° when the PCL is also injured (Grood et al. 1988). Therefore, a positive result at only 30° of knee flexion is consistent with an isolated posterolateral ligament injury, whereas the addition of a positive result at 90° indicates a combined PCL deficiency. With such a combined injury, performing the dial test with the patient in a prone position or the application of anterior traction on the proximal tibia helps to allow increased external rotation (Strauss et al. 2007). Of note, medial knee injuries can also result in increased external rotation and a positive dial test, so it is important to perform other tests that investigate both medial and lateral laxity.

Varus/Valgus Thrust Gait

Observing the patient walk is of great clinical value in gauging the extent of disability. In patients with lateral knee injuries, a varus thrust during the stance phase of gait with gapping of the lateral knee may be present. Additionally, lateral knee injuries place patients at risk for peroneal nerve injury and foot drop which can be observed during walking. Less commonly, a valgus thrust

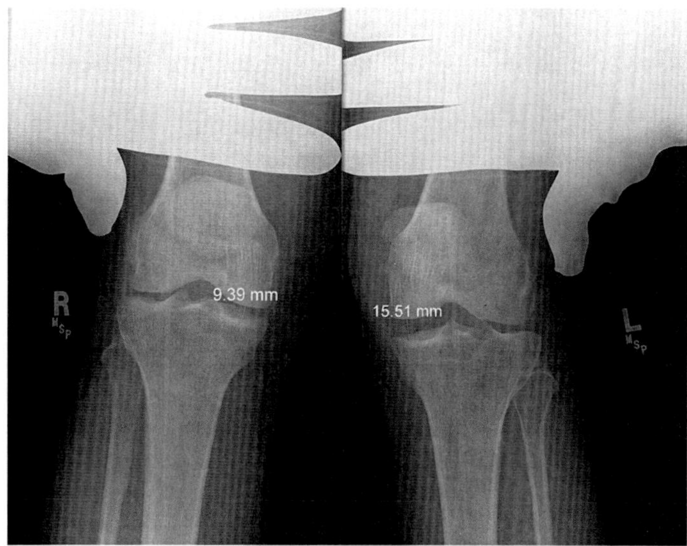

Fig. 3 Bilateral valgus stress radiographs demonstrating >4 mm of increased side-to-side medial gapping in the left knee

gait may be observed in patients with medial knee deficiencies, especially if they have genu valgus alignment. These sequelae can be extremely disabling and therefore influence the decision regarding surgical management.

Imaging

AP, Lateral, Rosenberg, and Long-Leg Standing Radiographs

The standard approach to imaging an injured knee almost universally begins with anteroposterior and lateral radiographs to rule out fractures. Tibial plateau and avulsion fractures of the femoral condyles, fibular head (arcuate fracture), and lateral tibial plateau (Segond fracture) should be evaluated for suspected multiligament injuries. Avulsion of the MCL from the medial femoral condyle can lead to the development of visible ossification in this area in chronic injuries (Pellegrini-Stieda lesion). A weight-bearing anteroposterior view with the knees in 45° of flexion (Rosenberg) allows visualization of posterior joint space narrowing, as this is where cartilage loss usually is most significant following a meniscectomy. Additionally, bilateral standing long-leg radiographs should be ordered in chronic ligament injury patients to assess for malalignment, which negatively impacts ligament reconstruction outcomes if not corrected (Noyes et al. 2000; Arthur et al. 2007).

Valgus and Varus Stress Radiographs

Valgus and varus stress radiographs can be used to objectively assess laxity patterns and operative outcomes (Figs. 3, 4). Because they are able to quantify and more objectively assess ligamentous laxity, they should be ordered preoperatively when there are exam findings of medial and lateral gapping, and should also be routinely ordered postoperatively after medial or posterolateral ligament reconstructions. In a radiographic study of cadaveric knees, sectioning of just the FCL (analogous to an isolated grade III FCL tear) resulted in a 2.7 mm increase in lateral gapping at 20° of flexion with a clinician-applied varus stress compared to the intact state, whereas sectioning of the FCL, popliteus, and popliteofibular ligaments (analogous to a grade III complete posterolateral tear) resulted in a 4 mm increase in gapping (LaPrade et al. 2008b). In a corresponding valgus stress radiograph study, sectioning of the proximal sMCL (analogous to an isolated grate III sMCL injury) resulted in a 3.2 mm increase in medial gapping at 20° of flexion with a clinician-applied valgus

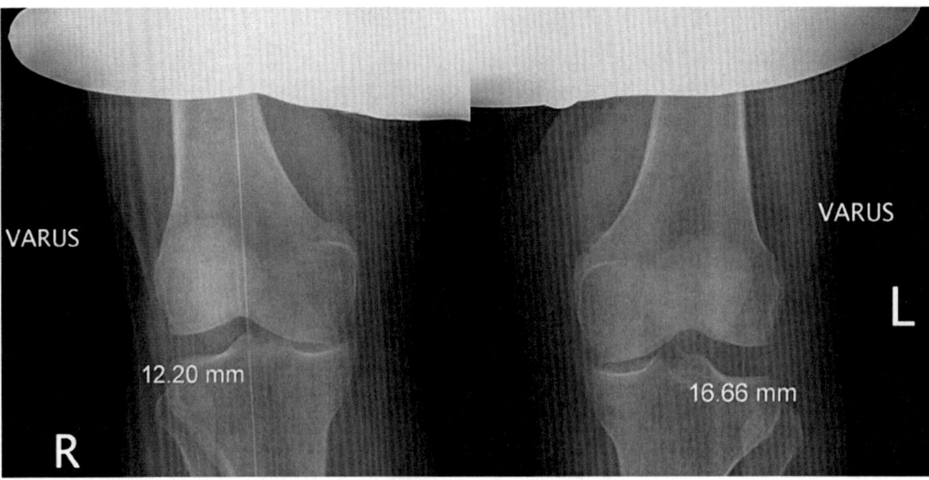

Fig. 4 Bilateral varus stress radiographs demonstrating >4 mm of increased lateral compartment gapping in the left knee

stress compared to the intact state, whereas sectioning of the proximal sMCL, meniscofemoral portion of the deep MCL, posterior oblique ligament, distal tibial attachment of the sMCL, and the meniscotibial ligament portion of the deep MCL (analogous to a complete grade III medial knee injury) resulted in a 9.8 mm increase in gapping (LaPrade et al. 2010). These values can be applied to clinical stress radiographs to assist with diagnosis, management, and postoperative evaluation of medial and posterolateral ligament injuries.

Kneeling PCL Stress Radiographs

Likewise, kneeling PCL stress radiographs can be used to quantitatively assess posterior laxity (Fig. 5). This is especially useful because the posterior drawer test can be highly inaccurate, and stress radiographs provide a reproducible, objective measurement that can be used to determine which posterior restraining ligaments are deficient (Jackman et al. 2008). Up to 7 mm of increased posterior translation is indicative of a partial PCL tear, 8–11 mm corresponds with an isolated but complete tear, and 12 mm or greater signifies combined PCL and posterolateral ligament tears (Schulz et al. 2007; Sekiya et al. 2008).

Magnetic Resonance Imaging

Magnetic resonance imaging (MRI) has become the standard of care for verifying the diagnosis of multiligament knee injuries and to assist with preoperative planning. It is especially useful in providing a highly sensitive, specific, and accurate diagnosis when the physical examination is impeded by pain and swelling in acute injuries (LaPrade et al. 2000). In addition to revealing the location of ligament tears and medial or lateral gapping, the imaged knee should be inspected for bone, cartilage, and meniscal damage. In knees with possible posterolateral corner injuries, it is important to check for lateral avulsion fractures such as arcuate and Segond fractures, biceps and PCL avulsions, and associated meniscal root avulsions and bone bruises. Anteromedial bone bruises should raise the suspicion for a posterolateral ligament tear. Posterolateral injury-associated bone bruises are mostly located on the anterior medial femoral condyle, but can also arise posteromedially when there is concurrent injury to the cruciate ligaments, and in rare cases, anterior medial tibial plateau fractures can occur (Geeslin and LaPrade 2010). For MCL injuries, MRI can help distinguish between meniscofemoral and meniscotibial lesions. Roughly half of MCL injuries are associated with bone bruises located on the lateral

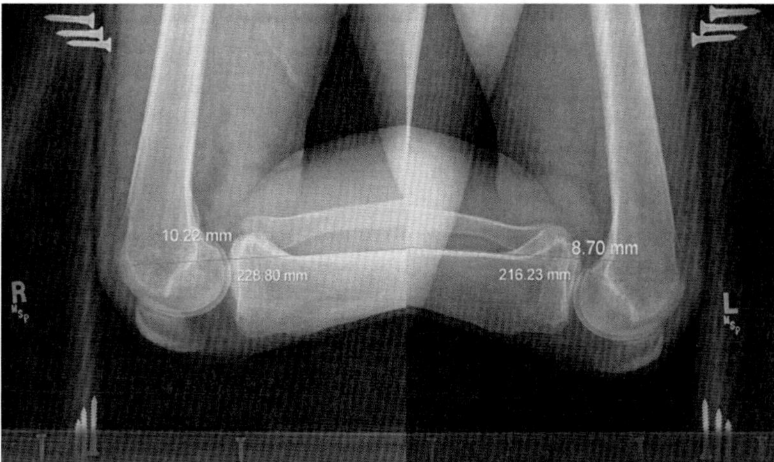

Fig. 5 Bilateral PCL stress radiographs demonstrating 19 mm of increased posterior tibial translation in the left compared to the right knee. To perform a stress radiograph, the patient kneels on a jig so as to put full body weight on the tibial tubercle of a single knee while a lateral radiograph is obtained. On the radiograph, a line can be drawn along the posterior tibial cortex that extends through the femoral condyles, and the perpendicular distance from this line to the most posterior point of the Blumensaat line may be measured. When calculating the difference in measurements between contralateral knees, it is important to take into consideration whether the posterior point of the Blumensaat line is anterior or posterior to the posterior tibial cortex line on each knee radiograph (Jackman et al. 2008)

femoral condyle and/or the lateral tibial plateau, which have been reported to resolve 2–4 months following the injury (Miller et al. 1998).

Preoperative Planning

Operative Versus Nonoperative Treatment

Quality evidence regarding operative versus nonoperative treatment of multiligament knee injuries is scarce due to the varying combination of ligaments involved in these relatively rare injury complexes. However, a meta-analysis performed in 2001 reported significant improvements in functional outcomes and range of motion as well as decreased flexion contractures with operative management of dislocated knees (Dedmond and Almekinders 2001). Two more recent systematic reviews reported significantly better knee stability, International Knee Documentation Committee (IKDC) scores, and levels of return to work and sport with surgical treatment (Levy et al. 2009; Peskun and Whelan 2011). Therefore, it would appear that operative management is often beneficial.

Other factors to consider include any associated injuries and the inherent stability of the involved side of the knee. Concurrent vascular injuries require rapid operative treatment, and the presence of fractures generally necessitates surgical fixation. It is important to identify peroneal and tibial nerve injuries during the initial assessment because they may benefit from repair or neurolysis. Because the lateral side of the knee is inherently unstable due to a convex femoral condyle articulating with a convex tibial plateau, posterolateral ligament injuries are less inclined to heal nonoperatively compared to the inherently stable medial side of the knee, where the tibial plateau is concave.

Timing of Surgery for Acute Injuries

For acute multiligament knee injuries, the general recommendation is to operate within 2–3 weeks before the scarring of injured structures obscures tissue planes. A systematic review of the literature by Levy et al. reported higher functional outcomes, a greater percentage of good/excellent IKDC scores, and better sports activity scores when surgery was performed within 3 weeks (Levy et al. 2009). However, preoperative range of motion deficits can also negatively affect rehabilitation and outcomes, so having patients enroll in physical therapy to obtain adequate motion preoperatively can be beneficial.

Order of Repair in Combined Ligament Injuries

For certain combinations of injuries, studies have been performed which guide the order of ligament repair. When both posterolateral structures and the ACL or PCL are torn, varus stress significantly loads the cruciate grafts. It is therefore logical to repair or reconstruct the posterolateral structures at the time of cruciate reconstruction to reduce the risk of failure (LaPrade et al. 1999, 2002). Additionally, since an external rotation deformity has been reported when the ACL graft is tightened first, the posterolateral grafts should be fixed in place before the ACL graft is tensioned and secured (Wentorf et al. 2002).

Addressing Malalignment and Staging of Surgeries for Chronic Injuries

For chronic injuries, addressing malalignment and deciding between combined and staged procedures are key considerations. Biomechanical testing has demonstrated that proximal tibial medial opening wedge osteotomy decreases the varus and external rotation laxity of posterolateral corner-deficient knees (LaPrade et al. 2008a). Varus knees with chronic posterolateral corner injuries should have the malalignment corrected first with a proximal tibial osteotomy before any ligament reconstruction is pursued to avoid stretching out the grafts. Otherwise, these patients tend to have worse outcomes with recurrence of knee instability following ligament reconstruction compared to acute injuries (Noyes and Barber-Westin 1996; LaPrade et al. 1997). In patients who suffer from isolated posterolateral ligament injuries due to low-energy mechanisms, the osteotomy alone may result in adequate knee stability, precluding the need for later ligament reconstruction (Arthur et al. 2007). Reconstruction of the cruciate ligaments should be staged after the osteotomy if lateral gapping is present on arthroscopic inspection (Noyes et al. 2000).

In valgus malaligned knees with chronic MCL and/or ACL laxity, a distal femoral osteotomy should be considered prior to or in combination with cruciate reconstruction (Phisitkul et al. 2006; Puddu and Franco 2009). Here as well, the stability gained by an osteotomy may obviate the need for a medial ligament reconstruction or repair (Phisitkul et al. 2006).

Ligamentous Repair Versus Reconstruction

A higher rate of failure has been reported with repair (37 %) compared to reconstruction (9 %) of multiligament knee injuries (Stannard et al. 2005). Looking at posterolateral corner midsubstance tears specifically, Levy found an even greater disparity of 40 % failure with repair versus a 6 % failure rate with reconstruction (Levy et al. 2010a). There does, however, appear to be a role for repair of avulsed posterolateral structures when combined with reconstruction of midsubstance tears of these structures, as patients treated with these "hybrid repairs" had similar IKDC stability scores to patients treated with complete reconstruction at two-year follow-up (Geeslin and LaPrade 2011).

Open Versus Arthroscopic and Arthroscopic-Assisted Surgery

Many factors play a role in the decision to perform multiligament reconstructions or repairs as an open procedure or as an arthroscopic or arthroscopic-assisted surgery. Presently there is limited evidence as to which techniques are safer or more effective, and with newly described techniques, it will be years if not decades before enough procedures will be performed with sufficient follow-up to produce more than anecdotal evidence of success (Salzler and Martin 2012). Training and experience, both of the surgeon and the surgical team, as well as the availability of special equipment, are often determinants of whether an arthroscopic procedure is feasible. On the other hand, the decision to harvest autografts around the knee may make an open procedure more favorable.

Allograft Versus Autograft

Injury pattern, availability of allografts, and surgeon and patient preference are the primary determinants in the choice between allograft and autograft, because no conclusive studies have been published to establish differences in performance for multiligament reconstructions. Due to the diverse allograft sizes available and the additional operative time and donor site morbidity associated with autograft harvesting, the use of allografts offers some distinct advantages in complex multiligament reconstructions.

Operative Technique

The following described operative technique encompasses the steps involved for a multiligament reconstruction of the knee that addresses posterolateral, medial, and cruciate ligament injuries as well as cartilaginous or meniscal pathology. It is the senior author's (R.F.L.) preference to begin with the posterolateral corner approach followed by medial exposure if these ligaments are involved, so that the extracapsular tissues can be fully identified and evaluated prior to arthroscopic fluid extravasation. The general rule of thumb is to perform the most difficult steps first, if possible, so that if tourniquet time becomes a concern, the least challenging steps can be performed in a surgical field obscured by bleeding. Peroneal nerve injuries should be identified, and all torn structures need to be systematically addressed.

Surgical Checklist, Patient Positioning, and Exam Under Anesthesia

Prior to incision, it is imperative to check that all required surgical equipment are available and functioning. This encompasses having the appropriate allografts or graft harvesting and preparation instruments, all arthroscopic tools including 30° and 70° arthroscopes, and cannulated interference screws. Preoperative imaging should be accessible for intraoperative review. The patient is placed in the supine position, and an examination under anesthesia allows a true sense of the patient's instability in a relaxed state. If a tourniquet is to be used, it should be well padded and placed on the proximal thigh. The operative leg is then placed in a leg holder that allows access to the medial and lateral knee, or positioned with a sandbag under the hip and taped to the operating table so the knee is able to be held at about 80° of flexion without additional support.

Posterolateral Corner Approach

To access the posterolateral structures, a hockey stick-shaped incision is made through the dermal layers, centered over the posterior border of the iliotibial band, and crossing the joint line at the level of Gerdy's tubercle (LaPrade et al. 2011). A posterior tissue flap is then meticulously developed with retraction of the superficial layer of the iliotibial band. If a patellar tendon autograft will be harvested, the lateral incision is shifted posteriorly to ensure a 6 cm skin bridge between incisions.

A common peroneal neurolysis is then performed to prevent damage from retraction and scar tissue entrapment. The common peroneal nerve is identified by palpation 2–3 cm distal to the long head of the biceps femoris, and approximately 8 cm is freed to allow gentle retraction away from the posterolateral structures (Fig. 1). A cautious, proximal-to-distal approach is advised in the presence of biceps avulsions in case the common peroneal nerve deviates from its normal course.

The presence of ligament injuries is best identified in a systematic approach, starting with

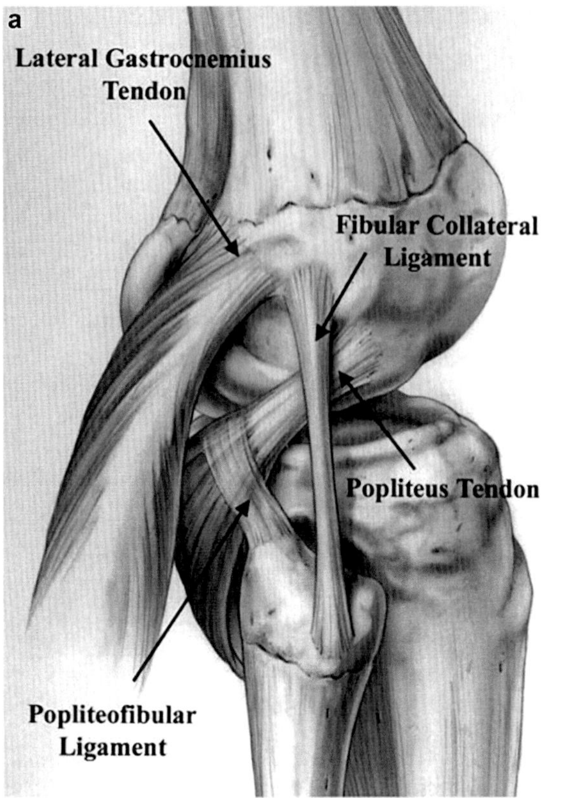

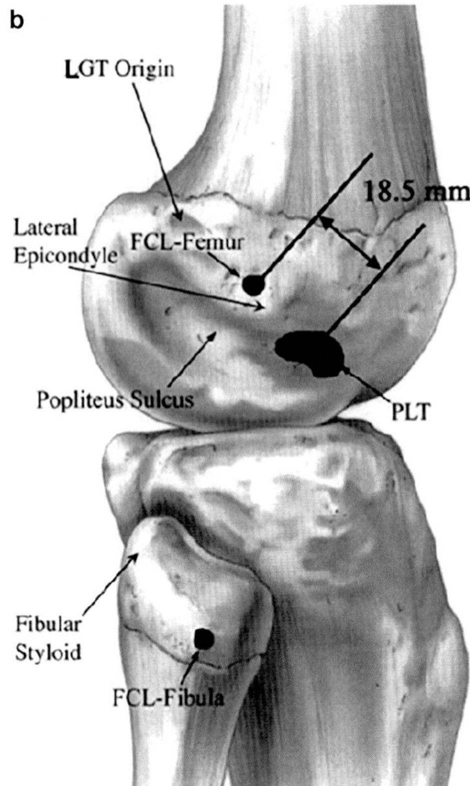

Fig. 6 Illustrations of (**a**) the posterolateral corner ligaments and of (**b**) posterolateral knee landmarks useful for identifying correct femoral reconstruction tunnel placement, including the lateral epicondyle, popliteus sulcus, and origin of the lateral gastrocnemius tendon (LGT). The average distance of 18.5 mm between the fibular collateral ligament (FCL) and popliteus tendon (PLT) femoral attachment sites is demonstrated (Both images are reprinted with permission from the *American Journal of Sports Medicine* (LaPrade et al. 2003))

fibular and tibial based lesions, then femoral attachments, and lastly lateral meniscal attachments. The interval between the lateral head of the gastrocnemius and soleus muscles is bluntly dissected in order to assess the popliteus musculotendinous junction and popliteofibular ligament for injuries and to access the posteromedial aspect of the fibular head for reconstruction tunnel placement. The origination of the popliteofibular ligament at the popliteal musculotendinous junction should be inspected, as well as the biceps and lateral capsule. The anterior arm of the long head of the biceps and biceps bursa is then incised 1 cm proximal to the fibular head, where the FCL's attachment site on the fibular head can be inspected. When a tear of the meniscotibial portion of the lateral capsular ligament has been identified on preoperative MRI, usually in conjunction with a tear of the anterior arm of the short head of the biceps femoris, an evaluation of these injuries can be accomplished by splitting the fascia at the interval between the posterior border of the iliotibial band and the short head of the biceps femoris. Next, an incision is made splitting the iliotibial band in line with its fibers, slightly anterior to the lateral epicondyle. The femoral attachment site of the FCL is then identified, in a mild depression approximately 3.2 mm proximal and posterior to the lateral epicondyle (Fig. 6). Placing a stitch through the FCL's distal remnant and exerting traction helps to identify the ligament's femoral attachment site. To expose the popliteus tendon's femoral attachment site in the anterior fifth of the popliteus sulcus, approximately 18.5 mm anterior and distal to the FCL attachment site, a vertical incision is made

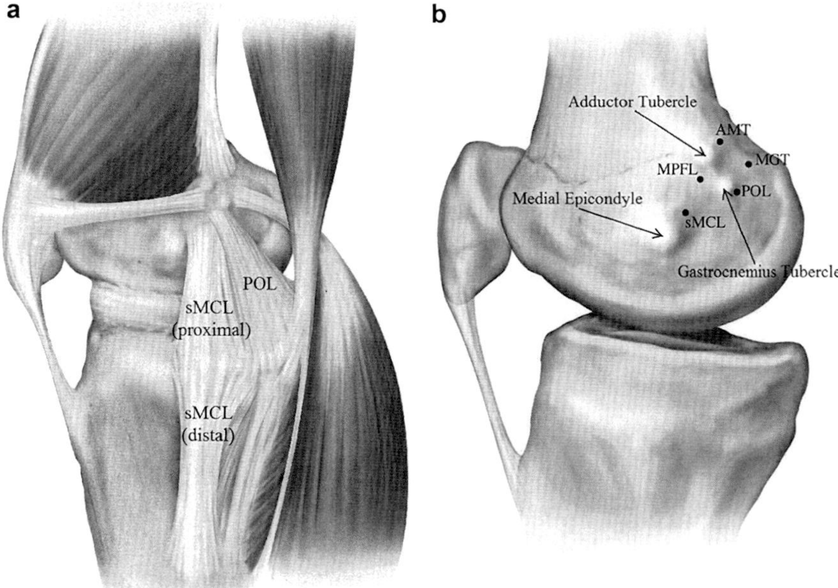

Fig. 7 (**a**) Illustration of the proximal and distal segments of the superficial medial collateral ligament (sMCL) and posterior oblique ligament (POL) on the medial side of a right knee. (**b**) Illustration of medial knee landmarks useful for identifying correct femoral reconstruction tunnel placement, namely, the adductor tubercle, gastrocnemius tubercle, and medial epicondyle on a right knee. Also demonstrated are the femoral attachment sites of the adductor magnus tendon (AMT), medial gastrocnemius tendon (MGT), sMCL, medial patellofemoral ligament (MPFL), and POL (Reprinted with permission from the *American Journal of Sports Medicine* (Coobs et al. 2010))

over this location in the lateral capsule. An arthroscopic assessment of the lateral compartment of the knee is the last step in the posterolateral evaluation, which is performed after a medial exposure in cases of medial ligament involvement.

Medial Approach

To expose the medial knee ligaments, an anteromedial dermal incision is carried from between the medial border of the patella and medial femoral epicondyle to the pes anserinus (LaPrade and Wijdicks 2012b). Incision of the sartorius fascia allows exposure of the gracilis and semitendinosus tendons and the distal tibial attachment site of the sMCL deep to the pes anserine bursa, 6 cm distal to the joint line. To assess the posterior oblique ligament, the sartorius tendon is retracted distally, and the tibial attachment site of the posterior oblique ligament's central arm can be identified on a bony ridge next to the insertion of the direct arm of the semimembranosus tendon. Identifying the femoral attachment sites of the medial ligaments is difficult, but facilitated by first finding the insertion site of the adductor magnus tendon. The adductor tubercle is just distal to this, and the medial epicondyle can then be more reliably identified as the bony prominence approximately 13 mm distal and 8 mm anterior to the adductor tubercle. The sMCL attachment site is approximately 6 mm posterosuperior to the medial epicondyle, and the posterior oblique ligament another 11 mm in the posterosuperior direction (Fig. 7). After assessing the medial ligaments and their bony attachment sites, attention is turned to evaluating the joint line for meniscofemoral and meniscotibial injuries, with repair or augmentation if needed.

Arthroscopic Evaluation

To perform the arthroscopic component of the surgery, vertical inferomedial and inferolateral parapatellar portals are incised to allow a standard arthroscopic evaluation of the knee. While observing for medial and lateral gapping, valgus and varus stresses are applied.

Meniscal Tears

The menisci are inspected for tears and repaired if possible, otherwise partial meniscectomy is performed. Popliteomeniscal fascicle tears are directly repaired if the lateral meniscus is unstable. Vertical tears are repaired preferentially using an inside-out vertical mattress. Medial and lateral meniscal root tears increase contact stress and decrease the contact area of articular surfaces, so an anatomic pull through repair is indicated.

Graft Harvest/Preparation

At this point, the necessary autografts are harvested and prepared. For medial ligament reconstructions, the semitendinosus tendon can be excised using a tendon harvester and divided into sMCL and posterior oblique ligament grafts that are 7 mm in diameter and 16 cm and 12 cm long, respectively (LaPrade et al. 2011). If an assistant is available, preparation of autografts or allografts can be done concurrently during the case. For posterolateral corner reconstruction grafts, an Achilles tendon allograft can be split down the middle to create two grafts with 9 mm diameter by 25 mm long calcaneal bone plugs and thicker ligament diameters with lengths of 70 mm for the FCL reconstruction and 60 mm for the popliteus tendon reconstruction. Tubularization and placement of passing sutures in both ends of the grafts are performed as part of the graft preparation.

PCL Reconstruction Tunnels

Fixing the cruciate grafts into the femur is the next step. In patients with multiligament injuries, an arthroscopic double-bundle PCL reconstruction using an Achilles tendon allograft for the anterolateral bundle and a semitendinosus allograft for the posteromedial bundle can be performed (Spiridonov et al. 2011). The first step is to identify and mark the femoral attachment sites. Then a posteromedial arthroscopic portal is established to allow identification of the tibial attachment site approximately 1 cm distal to the joint line, at which a drill pin is aimed and placed under fluoroscopic guidance, starting from approximately 6 cm distal to the joint line on the anteromedial tibia. The femoral tunnels (11 mm and 7 mm) are then reamed to a depth of 25 mm to created endoscopic closed tunnels that are separated by at least a 2 mm bone bridge. The tibial tunnel (12 mm) is reamed after all femoral cruciate tunnels have been reamed to minimize fluid extravasation during the critical reaming of the tibial tunnel.

ACL Reconstruction Tunnels

To reconstruct a torn ACL, a single-bundle anatomic reconstruction using bone-patellar tendon-bone autograft or allograft is a proven technique. Both the tibial and femoral attachment sites are identified and any residual ligament tissue is debrided. The femoral tunnel site is marked with a burr hole midway between the original anteromedial and posterolateral bundle attachment sites and posterior to the lateral intercondylar ridge. The medial portal is then used to ream a femoral closed tunnel. The tibial tunnel is created by placing a guide pin anteromedially into the joint, starting from a point 35 mm distal to the joint line and 10 mm anterior to the MCL insertion on the tibia, and aimed at the center of the native ligament attachment site, over which the tunnel is then reamed.

Cruciate Ligament Graft Fixation into Femur

The PCL grafts followed by the ACL graft are passed into the femoral tunnels and fixed with interference screws. The grafts are passed into the tibial tunnels, but tibial fixation is performed later: for the PCL, after the posterolateral corner reconstruction

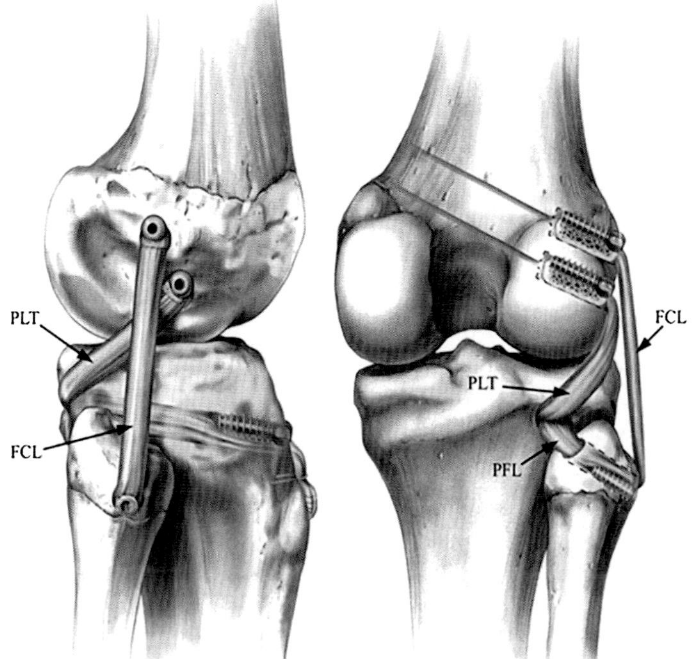

Fig. 8 Illustrations of a lateral and posterior view of an anatomic posterolateral corner knee reconstruction of the fibular collateral ligament (FCL), popliteus tendon (PLT), and popliteofibular ligament (PFL) in a right knee (Reprinted with permission from the *American Journal of Sports Medicine* (LaPrade et al. 2004))

grafts have been fixed in the femur and for the ACL, only after all posterolateral corner and medial ligaments have been fully reconstructed.

Posterolateral Corner Treatment Algorithm

In repairing and/or reconstructing the posterolateral structures, having a systematic approach improves efficiency and helps ensure all structures are addressed. The same stepwise treatment approach, starting with femoral attachments, then meniscal attachments, followed by tibial and then fibular attachments can be followed in almost every case. For a complete anatomic posterolateral corner reconstruction, two grafts are used to reconstruct the FCL, popliteus ligament, and popliteofibular ligament (Fig. 8).

Popliteus Avulsion Repair

There is a role for posterolateral ligament repair of avulsion injuries if the ligament can be fully reduced back to its anatomical attachment site with the knee in full extension (LaPrade et al. 1997; Geeslin and LaPrade 2011). For popliteus avulsions, a recess procedure can be utilized by placing an eyelet pin transfemorally that is centered on the popliteus attachment site and reaming a 5 mm tunnel to a depth of 1 cm over the pin. After the avulsed tendon is whipstitched, the suture ends are threaded through the eyelet pin and pulled out medially to bring the tendon into the tunnel, with fixation accomplished by tying the sutures over a button with the knee in full extension.

Popliteomeniscal Fascicle and Lateral Capsule Repairs

Tears of the popliteomeniscal fascicles and coronary ligament of the posterior horn of the lateral meniscus can be repaired with mattress sutures under direct visualization (Geeslin and LaPrade 2011). Avulsions of the lateral capsular ligament's tibial attachment can be repaired with suture anchors drilled at the joint line and the sutures placed into the undersurface of the lateral meniscus, with care to separate the capsule from the iliotibial band.

Fibular Head and Styloid Avulsion Repair

Popliteofibular ligament tears can be repaired with suture anchors if the popliteus and FCL are not both torn as well, which would make complete reconstruction the preferred choice (Geeslin and LaPrade 2011). Biceps femoris avulsions can be repaired with a whipstitch placed in the distal end of the avulsed tendon and suture anchors tightened with the knee in full extension. If there are adhesions restricting reduction of the tendon to its anatomical position, they are bluntly released. FCL avulsions can also be repaired with suture anchors that allow for early range of motion. Arcuate avulsion fractures of the fibular head can be repaired primarily by means of cerclage suture fixation. A cerclage suture is placed in the avulsed bone fragment, whipstitched into the distal aspect of the biceps femoris tendon, and then secured in fibular head drill holes 1 cm from the fracture line with the knee in extension.

Posterolateral Fibular Reconstruction Tunnel

For complete posterolateral corner reconstructions, the fibular tunnel is created with placement of a guide pin from the FCL attachment site on the lateral aspect of the fibular head to the popliteofibular ligament attachment site on the posteromedial downslope of the fibular styloid (LaPrade et al. 2011). Using a cruciate ligament-aiming device as a guide facilitates this step, and placing a retractor at the pin exit site before drilling protects the tissues from over-penetration of the pin. Once the pin is placed, the tip should be palpated to ensure correct positioning. If the popliteofibular ligament is not being reconstructed, the pin should be placed more posteriorly so the tunnel avoids disrupting this ligament, with care not to veer too far laterally and risk fracture of the lateral fibular head. A 7 mm tunnel is then reamed.

Posterolateral Tibial Reconstruction Tunnel

The tibial tunnel entry site for the guide pin placement is a flat region on the anterior tibia just distal and medial to Gerdy's tubercle, which requires release of superficial tissues from the distal iliotibial band and use of a rongeur or elevator to dissect through the overlying soft tissue and down to the bone (LaPrade et al. 2011). The exit site landmark is the popliteus musculotendinous junction on the posterolateral aspect of the lateral tibial plateau, approximately 1 cm medial and 1 cm proximal to the exit site of the fibular tunnel. Again, a cruciate ligament-aiming device and retractor are employed to aim the guide pin and protect posterior structures, and a correct pin exit site should be confirmed with fingertip palpation. A 9 mm tunnel is then reamed.

Posterolateral Femoral Reconstruction Tunnels

To create the femoral tunnels, parallel eyelet pins are placed from the previously identified attachment sites of the FCL (approximately 3.2 mm proximal and posterior to the lateral epicondyle) and popliteus ligament (in the anterior fifth of the popliteus sulcus, approximately 18.5 mm anterior and distal to the FCL site) through the femur transversely in a slightly anterior and proximal direction so as to avoid going through the intercondylar notch, the anterior collateral ligament tunnel, or saphenous nerve (LaPrade et al. 2011). A cruciate ligament-aiming device facilitates the placing of these pins. A 9 mm reamer is used to drill both closed tunnels to a depth of 25 mm.

Femoral Fixation of Posterolateral Grafts

Similar to ACL reconstruction graft passage, the FCL and popliteus tendon graft passing sutures are pulled through the femur with eyelet pins, and the bone plugs are pulled into the femoral tunnels, where they are secured with 7 mm by 20 mm cannulated interference screws (LaPrade et al. 2011). To verify sufficient graft purchase, lateral traction is applied.

Anatomic Layout of Posterolateral Grafts

Once femoral fixation is accomplished, the popliteus tendon graft is passed through the popliteal hiatus and out the surgical incision anterior to the lateral head of the gastrocnemius (LaPrade et al. 2011). The FCL graft is then passed under the distal superficial layer of the iliotibial band and long head of the biceps and through the fibular tunnel.

Tibial Fixation of PCL Graft

Next, the PCL graft is secured in the tibia to recreate the knee's native central pivot (Spiridonov et al. 2011). The anterolateral bundle graft is fixed with the knee flexed to 90°, and the posteromedial bundle is then fixed with the knee in extension. The surgeon should verify that normal tibiofemoral step-off is restored.

Fibular and Tibial Fixation of Posterolateral Grafts

Attention can then be turned to fixing the FCL within the fibular tunnel (LaPrade et al. 2011). The interference screw should be tightened with the knee in neutral rotation and 20° of flexion while applying a valgus force. An exam under anesthesia should be performed to ensure that the graft has restrained all lateral gapping under applied varus stress. The remaining FCL graft (now forming the popliteofibular ligament) and popliteus tendon graft can then be passed through the tibial tunnel together, and the knee cycled between flexion and extension a few times with the grafts under tension to remove any slack. They are then fixed with an anterior 9 mm by 23 mm interference screw with the knee in neutral rotation and flexed to 60°, and the knee then examined for a negative posterolateral drawer test and the normal amount of external rotation compared to the contralateral knee. The remaining graft ends can be secured to the anterior tibia with a small staple and then trimmed.

Medial Ligament Reconstructions

To perform reconstructions of the sMCL and posterior oblique ligament, guide pins are drilled through the tibia and femur at the previously identified attachment sites (LaPrade and Wijdicks 2012b). All tunnels are then reamed to 7 mm. Femoral fixation of both grafts is accomplished with 7 mm bio-absorbable interference screws. With the same type of screws used for femoral fixation, the posterior oblique ligament graft is then tensioned and secured with the knee in neutral rotation, 0° extension, and under varus stress, followed by tensioning and fixation of the sMCL with the knee in neutral rotation and at 20° of flexion. To recreate the proximal tibial sMCL insertion, a suture anchor is then placed, approximately 12 mm distal to the medial joint line (Fig. 9).

Tibial Fixation of the ACL Graft

After the PCL, posterolateral corner, and medial ligaments have been fully reconstructed, the ACL graft can be tensioned and fixed into the tibia with the knee in neutral rotation and near extension (Wentorf et al. 2002).

Determination of Knee Motion "Safe Zone"

At this point, it is imperative that the knee range of motion be checked to ensure full extension.

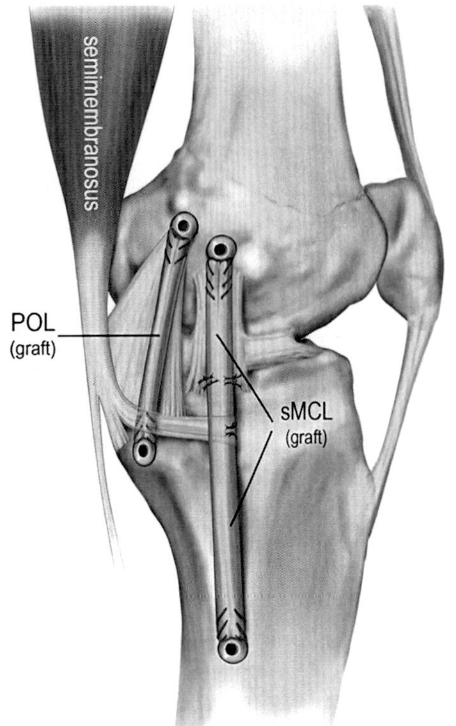

Fig. 9 Illustration of a medial view of an anatomic medial knee reconstruction demonstrating the reconstruction grafts of the superficial medial collateral ligament (sMCL) and posterior oblique ligament (POL) (Reprinted with permission from the *American Journal of Sports Medicine* (Coobs et al. 2010))

Additionally, the amount of safe flexion to allow the patient during initial recovery can be best gauged by examining the knee now while the patient is under anesthesia.

Postoperative Care and Rehabilitation

The postoperative management of patients with multiligament knee injuries requires a structured plan and close communication between surgeon, physical therapist, athletic trainer, and patient. Key principles for postoperative care include immediate postoperative range of motion, bracing, adequate pain control, and deep vein thrombosis (DVT) prophylaxis. A carefully monitored rehabilitation program, often lasting more than 6 months, focuses first on range of motion (ROM) with restrictions, followed by gradual strengthening, and then a progressive increase in intensity of activity, sport-specific therapy, and functional testing to assess feasibility of return to sport. An understanding of the phases of ligament healing and the biomechanics of open and closed kinetic chain exercises are crucial to the implementation of a rehabilitation plan and avoidance of complications and setbacks.

Patients are admitted to the hospital postoperatively for observation, pain control, and physical therapy. Generally, a combination of intravenous and oral pain medications is provided, often in combination with a femoral nerve block. Patients with a history of DVT are treated with subcutaneous enoxaparin sodium injections; the remainder are treated with aspirin. Management of swelling and inflammation is performed using cryotherapy. Early inpatient physical therapy includes early protected mobilization within the safe zone as determined intraoperatively (Medvecky et al. 2007; Wilkins 2011). Additionally, the patient is educated on limb positioning to avoid undue stress to the graft as well as activity modification to protect the surgical site.

A detailed two-phase rehabilitation program for patients following multiligament reconstructions of the knee has been developed by Wilkins, based on work by LaPrade et al.; an early phase (0–12 weeks) and late phase (4–12 months) are described (Wilkins 2011) (Table 3). Due to limited graft healing in the tunnels and potential graft necrosis, non-weight bearing is recommended for the first 6 weeks postoperatively with occasional toe-touch weight bearing during bathing and dressing activities. Weight bearing is then advanced according to the protocol, and crutches are gradually discontinued as gait normalizes and strength allows a gait without limping. At that point, patients may transition to a functional brace. Dynamic PCL braces are recommended through 6 months postoperatively to optimize PCL graft healing; this may be discontinued if examination and kneeling posterior stress radiographs demonstrate objective evidence of healing; otherwise patients are encouraged to continue wearing the brace at night until 1 year postoperatively (Jackman et al. 2008; Spiridonov et al. 2011; Jansson et al. 2012).

Table 3 Rehabilitation protocol for multiligament knee injuries, including variations based on PCL (PCL) or posterolateral corner (PLC) involvement

Rehabilitation	Weeks 1–2	Weeks 3–4	Weeks 5–6	Weeks 7–8	Months 3–4	Months 5+
Bracing	Hinged knee brace locked in full extension (except for ROM exercises)	Hinged knee brace, PCL brace for PCL reconstructions		Functional brace if no PCL reconstruction, otherwise PCL brace x 6 months		
Range of motion	Safe zone (goal of at least 0–90°)	Progressive ROM 4–5 times daily		Advance ROM to flexion goal of ≥125° Avoid active knee flexion/isolated hamstrings x 4 months with PCL or PLC reconstructions		Full ROM
Strengthening	Quad sets and straight leg raises in brace	Open kinetic chain exercises (30–60° arc with bicruciate injury, no flexion against resistance with PCL/PLC injury)		Add closed kinetic chain exercises		Non-impact aerobic activities
Weight bearing	NWB			WB with crutches until no limp		Full WB if normal gait

As described, a “safe zone” range of motion is determined intraoperatively, with a goal of allowing at least 0–90° without undue stress on the grafts. The postoperative brace is locked in full extension at 0° for the first 2 weeks; it is only unlocked during ROM exercises. A recent review evaluated patients with multiligament knee injuries that underwent ligament reconstruction within 3 weeks of injury and were treated with early ROM; it was found that they had a decreased risk of severe flexion loss, higher subjective outcomes, and decreased need for arthrolysis or manipulation (Mook et al. 2009). After 2 weeks, patients are allowed a progressive increase in ROM, outside their “safe zone,” 4–5 times daily. After 4 weeks, knee flexion is gradually advanced toward a goal of ≥125° over the following 8 weeks. Avoidance of active knee flexion is recommended, with no open-chain hamstring exercises until 4 months postoperatively, due to increased posterior tibial translation and potential deleterious effects on PCL or posterolateral corner reconstruction.

Strengthening via quadriceps sets and straight leg raises in a brace is advocated immediately postoperatively in order to minimize quadriceps atrophy due to immobilization. This activity also produces mobilization of the patellofemoral joint. In patients with bicruciate exercises, open kinetic chain exercises are limited to the 60° to 30° arc due to excessive anterior stresses from 90° to 60° and posterior stresses from 60° to 0°. No active open kinetic chain knee flexion exercises against resistance are allowed until 4 months postoperatively in patients with PCL or posterolateral corner involvement. Closed kinetic chain exercises are initiated at approximately 8 weeks, based on individual surgeon’s preference and the patient’s rehabilitation progress.

Late phase rehabilitation is initiated at approximately 4 months postoperatively. At this point, the patient should have achieved full active ROM, normal gait, and no signs of knee effusion. Full weight bearing in a functional brace is recommended during the late phase. Open- and closed kinetic chain exercises are gradually advanced, leading to sport-specific drills at 9 months. Quadriceps strengthening is a critical component of rehabilitation; quadriceps girth is compared to the contralateral side with a goal of 80 % circumference at 9 months. Non-impact aerobic activities are allowed from months 4 to 6; at 6 months a jogging program is initiated with gradual progression per physician discretion and tailored to the running requirements of the patient's sport. Special attention is paid to jumping techniques that avoid varus or valgus knee positioning and landing with an extended knee. At 9 months the patient is assessed via a functional test, which includes hop testing, isokinetic testing, and gait assessment during walking, running, and jumping. Clinical evaluation and stress radiographs are also performed for objective measurements of stability. At this point, athletes may return to noncompetitive practice if the injured extremity demonstrates 85 % of the strength of the uninjured extremity, followed by return to full-contact sports at 12 months if cleared by the surgeon.

Outcomes

Due to both the rarity and complexity of these injuries, there are no level I studies that address treatment and long-term outcomes. Most available studies on patients with multiligament knee injuries are level III or IV and are difficult to interpret due to the heterogeneity of injuries regarding timing of surgery, involved ligaments, and type of repair or reconstruction. On average, operative management of multiligament knee injuries results in a Lysholm score of around 85, an IKDC score of around 70, approximately 115° of knee ROM, return to employment in 80 %, and return to similar level of sport in 50 % (Peskun and Whelan 2011). Conversely, nonoperative treatment generally results in a Lysholm score of 70 or less, an IKDC score in the low 60s, approximately 115° of knee ROM, return to employment in 60 %, and return to similar level of sport in 20 % (Peskun and Whelan 2011).

Based on the Schenck classification, most reports of multiligament, or knee dislocation (KD) equivalent, injuries consist of patients with predominantly KD II–III injuries, with KD IV injuries being less common (Schenck 1994). In 2009, Engebretsen et al. reported outcomes on 85 injuries. Eighty-eight percent were KD II–III and the remainder were KD IV. Fifty were treated acutely and 35 treated chronically. The average Lysholm and IKDC subjective scores were 83 and 64, respectively; knee function was lower for patients with high-energy compared to low-energy injuries (Engebretsen et al. 2009). Harner et al. reported outcomes for 31 patients with knee dislocations. Nineteen patients were treated for acute injuries and 12 for chronic injuries; there were 9 patients with KD II, 12 with KD III-M, and 10 with KD III-L injuries. There was a trend toward higher subjective outcomes in patients treated acutely for their injuries; it is difficult to determine the impact of possible concomitant injuries in the chronically treated group that may contribute to their poorer average subjective outcomes (Harner et al. 2004). Fanelli reported outcomes for 35 patients treated for multiligament knee injuries; 19 patients were treated within 8 weeks and the remainder were treated for chronic injuries. There was 1 KD II injury, 19 KD III-L and 9 KD III-M injuries, and 6 KD IV injuries. The average Lysholm and HSS scores were 91.2 and 86.8, respectively (Fanelli and Edson 2002).

The majority of posterolateral corner injuries occur in combination with single or bicruciate ligament injuries (LaPrade 1997; Geeslin and LaPrade 2010; Geeslin and LaPrade 2011). Stannard et al. and Levy et al. reported on the outcomes of surgical treatment for grade II posterolateral corner injuries in a series of patients with isolated or multiligament injuries. In the study by Stannard et al., 44 patients had multiligament injuries and 13 were isolated posterolateral corner injuries; 13 of 35 repairs failed, whereas only two of the 22 reconstructions failed (Stannard et al. 2005). Levy et al. evaluated 28 multiligament injuries, all involving the posterolateral corner; 4 in 10 posterolateral corner repairs failed, whereas only one in 18 of the reconstructions failed (Levy et al. 2010a). The authors of both studies recommended reconstruction rather than repair for severe posterolateral corner injuries. In a study on the treatment of seven isolated and 19 multiligament grade III posterolateral knee injuries, Geeslin and LaPrade reported improvements in mean Cincinnati and IKDC subjective outcome scores from 21.9 to 81.4 points and from 29.1 to 81.5 points, respectively, with acute repair of avulsed structures, reconstruction of midsubstance tears, and concurrent reconstruction of any cruciate ligament tears (Geeslin and LaPrade 2011). Therefore, it appears that the best outcomes can be obtained by early repair of avulsed structures and reconstruction of midsubstance posterolateral corner structure tears.

Complications

Complications associated with multiligament knee injuries can be divided into those associated with the original injury, nonoperative treatment with immobilization, and surgical treatment. Neurovascular injuries are commonly associated with the initial trauma of the knee dislocation event that tears the ligaments. The incidence of popliteal artery injuries varies but is commonly reported to be 32 % (Green and Allen 1977). Urgent vascular consultation is required for suspected large vessel arterial injury as amputation may be necessary in patients with prolonged ischemia. Peroneal nerve injuries are common in patients with multiligament knee injuries, especially when associated with posterolateral corner injuries. The estimated rate of peroneal nerve injury is 25–35 % (Johnson et al. 2008); most incomplete palsies can be expected to recover, whereas a poor prognosis is associated with complete lesions. Patients with complete injuries have been treated with a variety of nonoperative and operative procedures including physical therapy with an ankle-foot orthosis, neurolysis, primary nerve repair, nerve grafting, and tendon transfers (Levy et al. 2010b). Tibial nerve injuries are much less common but have been reported.

Both nonoperative and operative treatments of multiligament knee injuries can be associated with persistent pain and functional deficits. Patients initially treated nonoperatively with immobilization may be deemed a failure due to persistent instability and may require surgical treatment for a chronic multiligament injury. A systematic review by Levy et al. reported better functional and clinical outcomes with early reconstruction compared to delayed reconstruction or nonoperative management (Levy et al. 2009). Another systematic review by Mook et al. reported that early operative treatment produced better subjective outcomes, but that early surgical treatment was associated with more range of motion deficits compared to delayed operative treatment. This underscores the importance of early mobilization following surgery, as Mook et al. also reported that doing so reduced the range of motion deficits in those reconstructed acutely (Mook et al. 2009).

Standard operative risks include infection, bleeding, and damage to deep structures. Infection may result from open injuries with poor soft tissue integrity or inadequate skin coverage. Bleeding can occur with difficult exposure of collateral structures. Iatrogenic injury to vascular structures, including the popliteal artery, may warrant emergent intraoperative vascular surgery consultation. Iatrogenic injury to the common peroneal nerve may occur during the exposure as a result of distorted anatomy in acute injuries or scarring in chronic injuries; excessive retraction during the procedure may also result in injury.

Commonly reported causes of ligament reconstruction failure include unrecognized or untreated ligament injuries, failure of allografts to fully incorporate, inadequate soft tissue integrity to support a repair, or technical concerns such as tunnel placement. A persistent effusion may complicate the postoperative course, possibly due to more extensive injuries or articular cartilage damage, and may delay the progression of rehabilitation.

Summary

While high level of evidence studies are limited, a growing body of level III and IV clinical studies are available to guide treatment of these severe injuries. Early recognition and treatment is crucial for management of acute injuries. The mechanical axis must be determined in patients with chronic injuries due to the high risk of failure of soft tissue grafts in patients with abnormal alignment. An anatomic reconstruction of ligamentous injuries with early postoperative range of motion is recommended for best functional results.

A multidisciplinary approach is necessary to ensure optimal treatment of these injuries and should include the orthopedic surgeon, physical therapist, and athletic trainer if applicable. Further investigations, likely multi-institutional, to determine the optimal surgical timing, surgical technique, and postoperative rehabilitation protocol are necessary.

Cross-References

- ► Combined Anterior and Posterior Cruciate Ligament Injuries
- ► Current Concepts in the Treatment of Posterior Cruciate Ligament Injuries
- ► Knee Dislocations
- ► Medial Collateral Ligament and Anterior Cruciate Ligament Synergy: Functional Interdependence
- ► Perioperative and Postoperative Anterior Cruciate Ligament Rehabilitation Focused on Soft Tissue Grafts
- ► Reconstruction of the Posterolateral Corner of the Knee
- ► Reconstruction of the Posteromedial Corner of the Knee
- ► Rehabilitation of Complex Knee Injuries and Key Points
- ► Role of Osteotomy for Knee Cartilage, Meniscus, and Ligament Injuries

References

American Medical Association (1966) Standard nomenclature of athletic injuries. American Medical Association, Chicago, pp 99–100

Arthur A, LaPrade RF, Agel J (2007) Proximal tibial opening wedge osteotomy as the initial treatment for chronic posterolateral corner deficiency in the varus knee: a prospective clinical study. Am J Sports Med 35:1844–1850. doi:10.1177/0363546507304717

Benjaminse A, Gokeler A, Van der Schans CP (2006) Clinical diagnosis of an anterior cruciate ligament rupture: a meta-analysis. J Orthop Sports Phys Ther 36:267–288. doi:10.2519/jospt.2006.2011

Coobs BR, Wijdicks CA, Armitage BM et al (2010) An in vitro analysis of an anatomical medial knee reconstruction. Am J Sports Med 38:339–347. doi:10.1177/0363546509347996

Dedmond BT, Almekinders LC (2001) Operative versus nonoperative treatment of knee dislocations: a meta-analysis. Am J Knee Surg 14:33–38

Engebretsen L, Risberg MA, Robertson B et al (2009) Outcome after knee dislocations: a 2–9 years follow-up of 85 consecutive patients. Knee Surg Sports Traumatol Arthrosc 17:1013–1026. doi:10.1007/s00167-009-0869-y

Fanelli GC, Edson CJ (1995) Posterior cruciate ligament injuries in trauma patients: Part II. Arthroscopy 11:526–529

Fanelli GC, Edson CJ (2002) Arthroscopically assisted combined anterior and posterior cruciate ligament reconstruction in the multiple ligament injured knee: 2- to 10-year follow-up. Arthroscopy 18:703–714. doi:10.1053/jars.2002.35142

Fanelli GC, Stannard JP, Stuart MJ et al (2010) Management of complex knee ligament injuries. J Bone Joint Surg Am 92:2235–2246

Gabriel MT, Wong EK, Woo SL-Y et al (2004) Distribution of in situ forces in the anterior cruciate ligament in response to rotatory loads. J Orthop Res 22:85–89. doi:10.1016/S0736-0266(03)00133-5

Geeslin AG, LaPrade RF (2010) Location of bone bruises and other osseous injuries associated with acute grade III isolated and combined posterolateral knee injuries. Am J Sports Med 38:2502–2508. doi:10.1177/0363546510376232

Geeslin AG, LaPrade RF (2011) Outcomes of treatment of acute grade-III isolated and combined posterolateral knee injuries: a prospective case series and surgical technique. J Bone Joint Surg Am 93:1672–1683. doi:10.2106/JBJS.J.01639

Green NE, Allen BL (1977) Vascular injuries associated with dislocation of the knee. J Bone Joint Surg Am 59:236–239

Griffith CJ, LaPrade RF, Johansen S et al (2009) Medial knee injury: Part 1, static function of the individual components of the main medial knee structures. Am J Sports Med 37:1762–1770. doi:10.1177/0363546509333852

Grood ES, Stowers SF, Noyes FR (1988) Limits of movement in the human knee. Effect of sectioning the posterior cruciate ligament and posterolateral structures. J Bone Joint Surg Am 70:88–97

Harner C, Waltrip R, Bennett C et al (2004) Surgical management of knee dislocations. J Bone Joint Surg Am 86:262–273

Hughston JC, Norwood LA (1980) The posterolateral drawer test and external rotational recurvatum test for posterolateral rotatory instability of the knee. Clin Orthop Relat Res 142:82–87

Indelicato PA, Bittar ES (1985) A perspective of lesions associated with ACL insufficiency of the knee. A review of 100 cases. Clin Orthop Relat Res 198:77–80

Jackman T, LaPrade RF, Pontinen T, Lender PA (2008) Intraobserver and interobserver reliability of the kneeling technique of stress radiography for the evaluation of posterior knee laxity. Am J Sports Med 36:1571–1576. doi:10.1177/0363546508315897

Jansson KS, Costello KE, O'Brien L et al (2012) A historical perspective of PCL bracing. Knee Surg Sports Traumatol Arthrosc 21:1064–1070. doi:10.1007/s00167-012-2048-9

Johnson ME, Foster L, DeLee JC (2008) Neurologic and vascular injuries associated with knee ligament injuries. Am J Sports Med 36:2448–2462. doi:10.1177/0363546508325669

Kopf S, Kauert R, Halfpaap J et al (2012) A new quantitative method for pivot shift grading. Knee Surg Sports Traumatol Arthrosc 20:718–723. doi:10.1007/s00167-012-1903-z

LaPrade RF (1997) Arthroscopic evaluation of the lateral compartment of knees with grade 3 posterolateral knee complex injuries. Am J Sports Med 25:596–602

LaPrade RF, Wijdicks CA (2012a) The management of injuries to the medial side of the knee. J Orthop Sports Phys Ther 42:221–233. doi:10.2519/jospt.2012.3624

LaPrade RF, Wijdicks CA (2012b) Surgical technique: development of an anatomic medial knee reconstruction. Clin Orthop Relat Res 470:806–814. doi:10.1007/s11999-011-2061-1

LaPrade RF, Hamilton CD, Engebretsen L (1997) Treatment of acute and chronic combined anterior cruciate ligament and posterolateral knee ligament injuries. Sports Med Arthrosc Rev 5:91–99

LaPrade RF, Resig S, Wentorf F, Lewis JL (1999) The effects of grade III posterolateral knee complex injuries on anterior cruciate ligament graft force. A biomechanical analysis. Am J Sports Med 27:469–475

LaPrade RF, Gilbert TJ, Bollom TS et al (2000) The magnetic resonance imaging appearance of individual structures of the posterolateral knee. A prospective study of normal knees and knees with surgically verified grade III injuries. Am J Sports Med 28:191–199

LaPrade RF, Muench C, Wentorf F, Lewis JL (2002) The effect of injury to the posterolateral structures of the knee on force in a posterior cruciate ligament graft: a biomechanical study. Am J Sports Med 30:233–238

LaPrade RF, Ly TV, Wentorf FA, Engebretsen L (2003) The posterolateral attachments of the knee: a qualitative and quantitative morphologic analysis of the fibular collateral ligament, popliteus tendon, popliteofibular ligament, and lateral gastrocnemius tendon. Am J Sports Med 31:854–860

LaPrade RF, Johansen S, Wentorf FA et al (2004) An analysis of an anatomical posterolateral knee reconstruction: an in vitro biomechanical study and development of a surgical technique. Am J Sports Med 32:1405–1414. doi:10.1177/0363546503262687

LaPrade RF, Engebretsen L, Johansen S et al (2008a) The effect of a proximal tibial medial opening wedge osteotomy on posterolateral knee instability: a biomechanical study. Am J Sports Med 36:956–960. doi:10.1177/0363546507312380

LaPrade RF, Heikes C, Bakker AJ, Jakobsen RB (2008b) The reproducibility and repeatability of varus stress radiographs in the assessment of isolated fibular collateral ligament and grade-III posterolateral knee injuries. An in vitro biomechanical study. J Bone Joint Surg Am 90:2069–2076. doi:10.2106/JBJS.G.00979

LaPrade RF, Ly TV, Griffith C (2008c) The external rotation recurvatum test revisited: reevaluation of the sagittal plane tibiofemoral relationship. Am J Sports Med 36:709–712. doi:10.1177/0363546507311096

LaPrade RF, Bernhardson AS, Griffith CJ et al (2010) Correlation of valgus stress radiographs with medial knee ligament injuries: an in vitro biomechanical study. Am J Sports Med 38:330–338. doi:10.1177/0363546509349347

LaPrade RF, Johansen S, Engebretsen L (2011) Outcomes of an anatomic posterolateral knee reconstruction: surgical technique. J Bone Joint Surg Am 93(Suppl 1):10–20. doi:10.2106/JBJS.J.01243

Levy BA, Dajani KA, Whelan DB et al (2009) Decision making in the multiligament-injured knee: an evidence-based systematic review. Arthroscopy 25:430–438. doi:10.1016/j.arthro.2009.01.008

Levy BA, Dajani KA, Morgan JA et al (2010a) Repair versus reconstruction of the fibular collateral ligament and posterolateral corner in the multiligament-injured knee. Am J Sports Med 38:804–809. doi:10.1177/0363546509352459

Levy BA, Giuseffi SA, Bishop AT et al (2010b) Surgical treatment of peroneal nerve palsy after knee dislocation. Knee Surg Sports Traumatol Arthrosc 18:1583–1586. doi:10.1007/s00167-010-1204-3

Medvecky MJ, Zazulak BT, Hewett TE (2007) A multidisciplinary approach to the evaluation, reconstruction and rehabilitation of the multi-ligament injured athlete. Sports Med 37:169–187

Miller MD, Osborne JR, Gordon WT et al (1998) The natural history of bone bruises. A prospective study of magnetic resonance imaging-detected trabecular microfractures in patients with isolated medial collateral ligament injuries. Am J Sports Med 26:15–19

Mills WJ, Barei DP, McNair P (2004) The value of the ankle-brachial index for diagnosing arterial injury after knee dislocation: a prospective study. J Trauma 56:1261–1265. doi:10.1097/01.TA.0000068995.63201.0B

Mook WR, Miller MD, Diduch DR et al (2009) Multiple-ligament knee injuries: a systematic review of the timing of operative intervention and postoperative rehabilitation. J Bone Joint Surg Am 91:2946–2957. doi:10.2106/JBJS.H.01328

Nielsen S, Helmig P (1986) The static stabilizing function of the popliteal tendon in the knee. An experimental study. Arch Orthop Trauma Surg 104:357–362. doi:10.1007/BF00454430

Noyes FR, Barber-Westin SD (1996) Surgical restoration to treat chronic deficiency of the posterolateral complex and cruciate ligaments of the knee joint. Am J Sports Med 24:415–426

Noyes FR, Barber-Westin SD, Hewett TE (2000) High tibial osteotomy and ligament reconstruction for varus angulated anterior cruciate ligament-deficient knees. Am J Sports Med 28:282–296

Odensten M, Hamberg P, Nordin M et al (1985) Surgical or conservative treatment of the acutely torn anterior cruciate ligament. A randomized study with short-term follow-up observations. Clin Orthop Relat Res 198:87–93

Peskun CJ, Whelan DB (2011) Outcomes of operative and nonoperative treatment of multiligament knee injuries: an evidence-based review. Sports Med Arthrosc Rev 19:167–173. doi:10.1097/JSA.0b013e3182107d5f

Petersen W, Zantop T (2006) Partial rupture of the anterior cruciate ligament. Arthroscopy 22:1143–1145. doi:10.1016/j.arthro.2006.08.017

Phisitkul P, Wolf BR, Amendola A (2006) Role of high tibial and distal femoral osteotomies in the treatment of lateral-posterolateral and medial instabilities of the knee. Sports Med Arthrosc Rev 14:96–104. doi:10.1097/01.jsa.0000212306.47323.83

Puddu G, Franco V (2009) Distal femoral osteotomy for genu valgus correction. Techn Knee Surg 8:257–264

Salzler MJ, Martin SD (2012) All-arthroscopic anatomic repair of an avulsed popliteus tendon in a multiple ligament-injured knee. Orthopedics 35:e973–e976. doi:10.3928/01477447-20120525-46

Schenck RC (1994) The dislocated knee. Instr Course Lect 43:127–136

Schulz MS, Steenlage ES, Russe K, Strobel MJ (2007) Distribution of posterior tibial displacement in knees with posterior cruciate ligament tears. J Bone Joint Surg Am 89:332–338. doi:10.2106/JBJS.C.00834

Sekiya JK, Whiddon DR, Zehms CT, Miller MD (2008) A clinically relevant assessment of posterior cruciate ligament and posterolateral corner injuries. Evaluation of isolated and combined deficiency. J Bone Joint Surg Am 90:1621–1627. doi:10.2106/JBJS.G.01365

Shelbourne KD, Nitz PA (1991) The O'Donoghue triad revisited. Combined knee injuries involving anterior cruciate and medial collateral ligament tears. Am J Sports Med 19:474–477

Spiridonov S, Slinkard N, LaPrade R (2011) Isolated and combined grade-III posterior cruciate ligament tears treated with double-bundle reconstruction with use of endoscopically placed femoral. J Bone Joint Surg Am 93:1773–1780

Stannard JP, Brown SL, Farris RC et al (2005) The posterolateral corner of the knee: repair versus reconstruction. Am J Sports Med 33:881–888. doi:10.1177/0363546504271208

Strauss EJ, Ishak C, Inzerillo C et al (2007) Effect of tibial positioning on the diagnosis of posterolateral rotatory instability in the posterior cruciate ligament-deficient knee. Br J Sports Med 41:481–485. doi:10.1136/bjsm.2006.030767 (discussion 485)

Terry GC, LaPrade RF (1996) The posterolateral aspect of the knee. Anatomy and surgical approach. Am J Sports Med 24:732–739

The International Knee Documentations Committee (2000) 2000 IKDC knee forms. In: The American Academy for Sports Medicine. http://www.sportsmed.org/uploadedFiles/Content/Medical_Professionals/Research/Grants/IKDC_Forms/IKDC 2000 - Revised Subjective Scoring.pdf. Accessed 22 Jan 2013

Treiman GS, Yellin AE, Weaver FA et al (1992) Examination of the patient with a knee dislocation. The case for selective arteriography. Arch Surg 127:1056–1062, discussion 1062–3

Wascher DC, Dvirnak PC, DeCoster TA (1997) Knee dislocation: initial assessment and implications for treatment. J Orthop Trauma 11:525–529

Wentorf FA, LaPrade RF, Lewis JL, Resig S (2002) The influence of the integrity of posterolateral structures on tibiofemoral orientation when an anterior cruciate ligament graft is tensioned. Am J Sports Med 30:796–799

Wiertsema SH, Van Hooff HJA, Migchelsen LAA, Steultjens MPM (2008) Reliability of the KT1000 arthrometer and the Lachman test in patients with an ACL rupture. Knee 15:107–110. doi:10.1016/j.knee.2008.01.003

Wijdicks CA, Griffith CJ, Johansen S et al (2010) Injuries to the medial collateral ligament and associated medial structures of the knee. J Bone Joint Surg Am 92:1266–1280. doi:10.2106/JBJS.I.01229

Wilkins SA (2011) Rehabilitation of the multiple ligament injured knee. Techn Knee Surg 10:2–10. doi:10.1097/BTK.0b013e31820d4a03

Wroble RR, Grood ES, Cummings JS et al (1993) The role of the lateral extraarticular restraints in the anterior cruciate ligament-deficient knee. Am J Sports Med 21:257–262 (discussion 263)

State of the Art in Anterior Cruciate Ligament Surgery

127

Takeshi Muneta and Hideyuki Koga

Contents

T. Muneta (✉) • H. Koga
Department of Joint Surgery and Sports Medicine, Graduate School of Medical Science, Tokyo Medical and Dental University, Bunkyo-ku, Tokyo, Japan

Department of Orthopaedic Surgery, Tokyo Medical and Dental University Hospital, Bunkyo-ku, Tokyo, Japan
e-mail: muneta.orj@tmd.ac.jp; koga.orj@tmd.ac.jp

M.N. Doral, J. Karlsson (eds.), *Sports Injuries*,
DOI 10.1007/978-3-642-36569-0_83

Abstract

The normal structure of the ACL (Anterior Cruciate Ligament) is different from the simple strands of a tendon. To consider graft harvest morbidity and surgical reproducibility with improved clinical stability, a double-bundle technique using semitendinosus tendon with a suspensory device for femoral fixation has been chosen as standard.

Tibial tunnel creation for both the anteromedial and posterolateral bundles should be created just lateral to the medial intercondylar eminence to avoid lateral wall impingement. The centers of the femoral tunnels are created on the posterior margin of the direct insertion of the normal attachment while avoiding merging of the two tunnels.

Remnant preservation is assured by the current procedure. A transtibial approach is simple but most difficult for controlling the tunnel placement. Each approach has its own advantages and disadvantages. It is necessary to accumulate evidence in consideration of a patient's needs and safety in order to take the next step forward in ACL reconstruction.

What Has Been Pursued to Accomplish State of Art in ACL Surgery

A superior ACL reconstruction should be patient oriented and friendly. The method should allow every experienced ACL surgeon to restore normal knee kinematics securely and reproducibly. Anatomic reconstruction is the way to be followed.

However, ACL reconstruction is tendon transplantation. The structure of the normal ACL anatomy is far more complex than a simple tendon structure (Hara et al. 2009; Mochizuki et al. 2014).

A double-bundle (DB) reconstructive procedure using a 4-strand semitendinosus (ST) tendon has been carried out over the past 20 years as a standard in Tokyo Medical and Dental University Hospital (Muneta et al. 1999). On the basis of the procedure, the pursuit of the state of the art in ACL surgery will be discussed in this chapter.

Normal ACL Anatomy and Function Related to Surgical Consideration

The normal ACL is comprised of 3-demensionally twisted small bundles (Hara et al. 2009), which allows control of normal knee kinematics throughout a wide range of motion. The tension of each small bundle is very low. Normal ACL is usually divided into two functional parts morphologically and functionally, that is, anteromedial (AM) and posterolateral (PL) bundles. The normal tension pattern of the AM bundle is a gradual decrease from full extension to flexion and increase again thereafter. The tension of the AM bundle in deep flexion is higher than that in full extension, while the tension of the PL bundle is highest in full extension and then decreases with knee flexion (Zavras et al. 2005).

The cross-sectional area of the midportion of the normal ACL is narrower than that of femoral and tibial attachments. This fact suggests that the graft tissue could be impinged upon by the bony structure of the femoral intercondylar notch, even if the graft is correctly placed in the normal footprint, because a transplanted tendon is a simple thick string. Each strand of a graft is compressed and slides against other strands.

The anterior half of the normal tibial attachment would be reportedly impinged if a straight tendon were inserted as a graft (Howell et al. 1991). The "physiological impingement" of tibial attachment would occur if a graft were inserted which covered the whole foot print, which might cause unknown effects on the knee joint (Zantop et al. 2008), or it could be at least said that impingement in extension would be a factor affecting full extension and possible control of anterior laxity.

The concept of the anatomic DB reconstruction, which was proposed by Yasuda et al. (2004), has opened a new field of ACL reconstruction, especially with regard to femoral tunnel creation. Nevertheless, controversies still exist regarding the normal femoral footprint and where to create the center of the AM and PL bundle tunnels. One of the reasons is that some researchers have

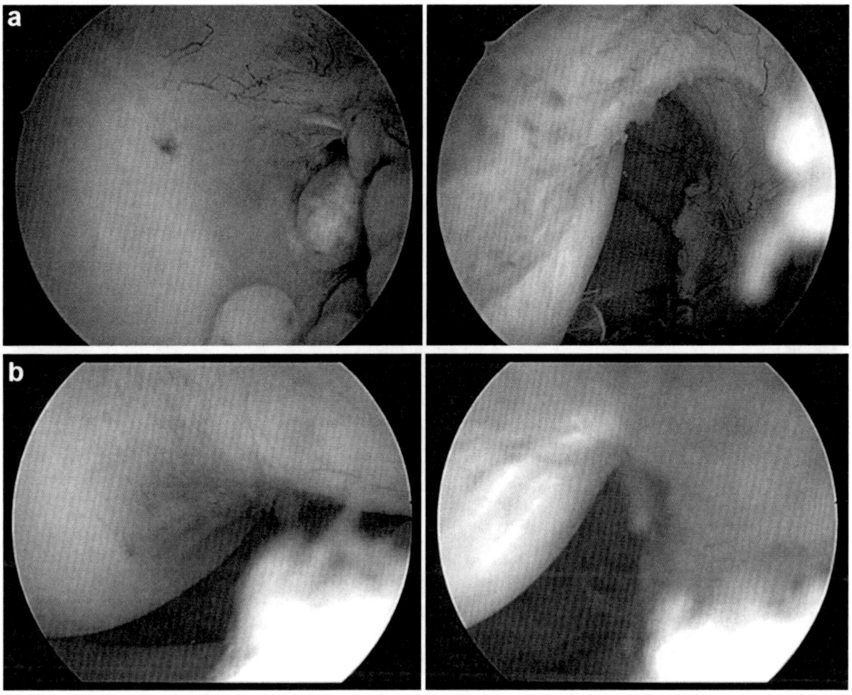

Fig. 1 (**a**) From arthroscopic observations, the majority of ACL injured knees show lack of integrity to the fanlike indirect insertion of the femoral attachment with some remnant of the direct insertion. (**b**) In a normal ACL, a well-tensioned fanlike insertion is observed through the anterior-posterior portion

considered only the direct insertion of the normal attachment as the attachment (Yasuda et al. 2004; Mochizuki et al. 2006), whereas others have considered the indirect insertion (in other words, fanlike extension portion) to be representative of the normal attachment in other studies (Colombet et al. 2006; Zantop et al. 2008). On the other hand, recent cadaveric studies have revealed that the combined portion of direct and indirect insertions is considered as a broad normal attachment (Ziegler et al. 2011; Sasaki et al. 2012; Mochizuki et al. 2014).

From arthroscopic observations, the majority of ACL injured knees demonstrate a lack of integrity of the indirect insertion to the femoral attachment, while the normal ACL maintains well-tensioned fanlike insertion (Fig. 1).

The normal tibial attachments of AM and PL bundles are still controversial with a variety of individual differences (Siebold et al. 2008; Zantop et al. 2008; Hara et al. 2009; Ziegler et al. 2011).

Tibial Tunnel Placement

The importance, problems, and achievability of anatomic tunnel placement of the tibia should be reconsidered. There are few studies examining the effects of selection of the tibial tunnel position on the clinical outcome.

The issues of tibial tunnel placement would involve notch impingement, posterior cruciate ligament (PCL) impingement, lateral wall impingement, and the possibility of 2-tunnel independence. The footprint covering the reconstruction seems to have difficulties due to such kinds of potential problems. The concept of notch impingement suggested by Howell (Howell et al. 1991) and physiological impingement (Zantop et al. 2008) would not be compatible.

Anterior placement of the tibial tunnel has advantages in terms of stability restoration; however, it more often causes notch impingement

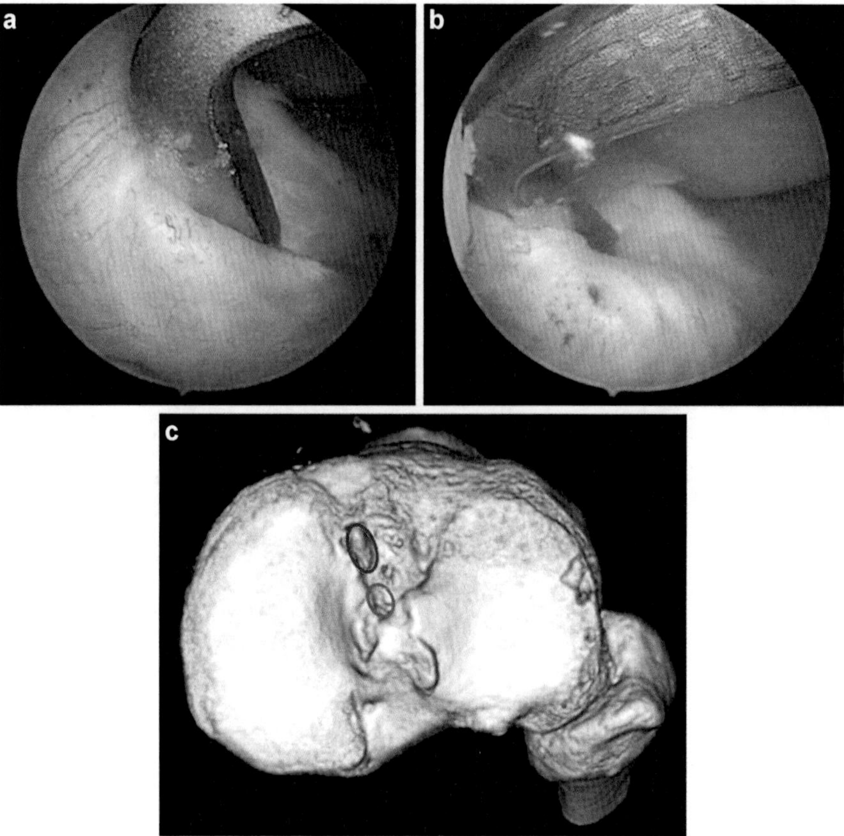

Fig. 2 (**a**) Drill guide position for the AM tibial tunnel created 3–5 mm posterior to the anterior margin of the normal footprint and just lateral to the medial intercondylar eminence in the normal footprint. (**b**) Drill guide position for the PL tibial tunnel created in the posterior end of the medial intercondylar eminence and just lateral to it. (**c**) A 3D CT shows two tibial tunnels of the AM and PL bundles just lateral to the medial intercondylar eminence

(Bedi et al. 2011) or an extension deficit. During the graft healing process under various biomechanical circumstances, the graft tissue will take the shortest route between the tibial and femoral tunnels; therefore, the graft tends to shift laterally in the tibial tunnel with more vulnerability to lateral wall impingement. If a PL tunnel is created laterally in the tibial attachment, it will have more risk of lateral wall impingement. Less than 65° from the joint line in the frontal plane has been recommended to avoid PCL impingement for tibial tunnel creation (Howell et al. 2001). More horizontal tibial tunnel placement would be necessary for creating the femoral PL tunnel if a transtibial technique was used for a DB reconstruction. Horizontal tunnel placement involves the risk of medial tibial plateau breakage. In the case series of Tokyo Medical and Dental University Hospital 2006–2007, there was no radiographic difference in the tibial tunnel position 1 year after surgery between cases with impingement-free tunnel placement and those with anatomic tunnel placement based on the normal footprint. This finding suggests the variation of the normal tibial footprint and the effects of tunnel widening in a hamstring tendon reconstruction.

In the current procedures of Tokyo Medical and Dental University Hospital, two tibial tunnels are created in the normal ACL footprint just lateral to the medial intercondylar eminence (Fig. 2). Using this method, the independence of the two tunnels is usually violated by a transtibial technique because of more horizontally made tunnels. To preserve the independence of the two tunnels and to avoid the risk of medial tibial plateau breakage, 20 mm-long drill holes with a diameter matching the graft diameter are first created in the anteromedial aspect of the tibia after guidewires for the AM and PL bundles were inserted. Thereafter, tibial tunnels for the AM and PL bundles are initially created by a 4.5 mm-wide drill, and then they are expanded to the AM and PL diameter, respectively, by a bony rasp. In that way, the two tunnels are created within the footprint without two-tunnel merging and medial tibial plateau breakage.

Femoral Tunnel Placement

There are a variety of clinical results related to femoral tunnel positioning in ACL reconstruction. Anatomic femoral tunnel placement has been found to be preferable to obtain better stability in an in vitro study (Yagi et al. 2002; Yamamoto et al. 2004; Kato et al. 2013). The importance of PL bundle positioning has been emphasized. The previous intraoperative measurements revealed that an overly deep tunnel position of the PL bundle would lead to significant tension reduction of the PLB near extension and thus insufficient tension in the PL bundle, resulting in a residual pivot shift (Koga et al. 2013).

The width of direct insertion of the normal ACL is approximately 5 mm (Mochizuki et al. 2006). The diameter of the graft is usually 6 mm or larger, even if a DB procedure is performed. If the center of the drill hole is set to the center of anatomic direct insertion, the margin of the femoral drill hole ends up more anteriorly placed to the normal attachment. With consideration of both the direct and indirect insertions together, it would be a practical choice for surgeons to set the center of the drill hole on the posterior margin rather than at the center of the normal direct insertion.

Tunnel expansion and graft deviation inside the tunnel after surgery should also be taken into account. If the posterior margin of the direct insertion is selected as the center of the drill hole, the femoral drill hole would be created more consistently in the normal attachment (Fig. 3).

In reality and more reproducibly, the femoral drill hole should be placed between the ACL remnant and the posterior articular cartilage margin based on arthroscopic observation during surgery (Fig. 4). To better refrain from merging the two femoral tunnels, a specially designed dilator with a fin is used. Two 4.5 mm tunnels can be enlarged to the desirable direction with this device (Fig. 5).

Healing Process, Length Change, and Tensile Pattern of an ACL Graft

A grafted tendon requires a long healing process. During the healing process, the graft sustains various loads of tension, twists, and pressure. The mechanical strength of the graft-bone complex is weak. As little as 50 % recovery of normal ACL strength has been reported in many animal studies. Clinically, the amount of recovery of mechanical strength of the ACL graft-bone complex still remains unknown in each case.

Considering such circumstances around the graft, too much of a load on the graft should be avoided in the early phase of the healing process. Higher loads in full extension and in deep flexion should be avoided as a graft tension as well. Therefore, during ACL reconstruction, a typical tension pattern of the AM bundle compared to a normal ACL may not be desirable. Too much tension in extension on the PL graft should also be avoided. An animal study suggested that high tension on the graft should be prevented for achieving better graft healing (Yoshiya et al. 1987). The concept of the anatomic DB reconstruction involves some caution in terms of the graft tension pattern of the AM bundle (Yasuda et al. 2008). Moreover, the concept of load sharing between two bundles might sometimes be risky. The two grafts have to be compatible to bear the load between extension and the midrange of flexion.

From the recent intraoperative measurements of each graft tension, the femoral tunnel of the AM bundle had better to be placed in the posterior portion to the direct insertion on the lateral wall of the intercondylar notch to avoid higher tension in

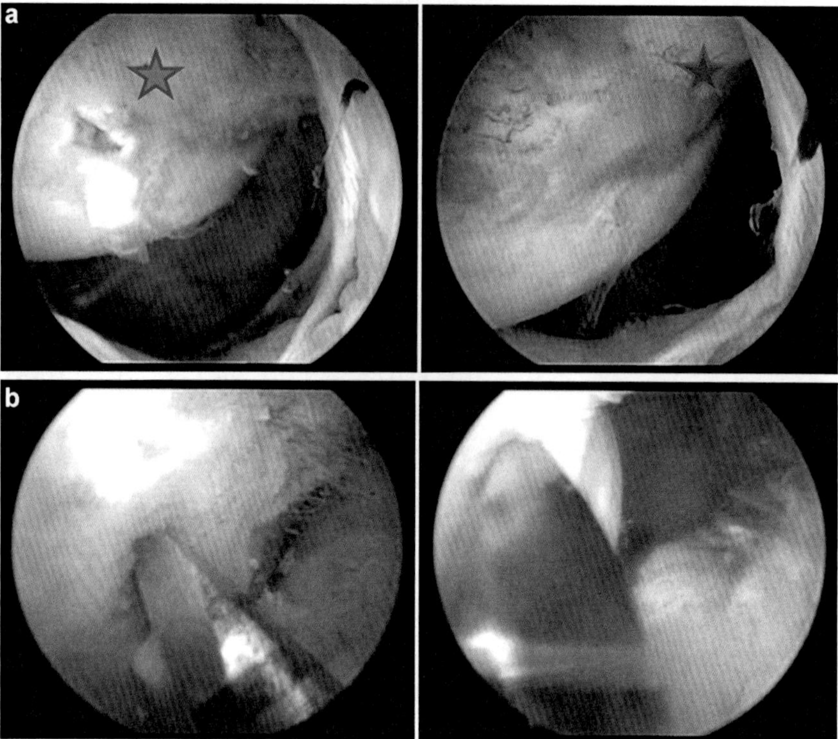

Fig. 3 (**a**) A *blue star* indicates the aiming point of the center of the PL femoral tunnel, which is on the posterior margin of the distal end of the scarred direct insertion of the ACL remnant. A *red star* indicates the aiming point of the center of AM femoral tunnel, which is on the posterior margin of the proximal end of the scarred direct insertion of the ACL remnant. (**b**) An example of the tip of the guidewires is shown (*left*, PL bundle; *right*, AM bundle)

deep flexion (unpublished data). Also, the femoral tunnel of the PL bundle should not be placed in an overly deep position in flexion to avoid too much tension in extension. For better rotational instability control, the femoral PL tunnel should not be created proximally (Koga et al. KSSTA 2013).

Initial Tensioning and Fixation Angle of a Graft

A porcine ACL reconstruction model using a tendon graft showed that the method of femoral graft fixation significantly influenced tension degradation during dynamic flexion-extension loading. In respect to bearing tension for a long time, a BTB (Bone-patellar Tendon-Bone) graft has advantages shown in an in vitro study.

A systematic review suggested that there is a trend toward an initial graft tension of 78.5–90 N resulting in a reduced side-to-side difference in anterior laxity in a single-bundle (SB) reconstruction with hamstring tendon or BTB (Kirwan et al. 2013). On the other hand, initial graft tension protocols produced predictable changes in the tibiofemoral compressive forces and joint positions (Brady et al. 2007). Larger initial tension caused mucoid degenerative change in a graft in a dog ACL reconstruction model (Yoshiya et al. 1987). Recently, as low as a 20 N initial load for a BTB graft was reportedly high enough to achieve good postoperative stability (Mae et al. 2010). Besides, an initial load of equalized anterior stability as the contralateral uninjured knee under anesthesia resulted in 3 mm more laxity than the normal knee after surgery (Bastian et al. 2014). There is little consensus regarding the ideal initial load condition exerted on the graft, in which better postoperative stability is achieved during DB reconstruction. From the previous

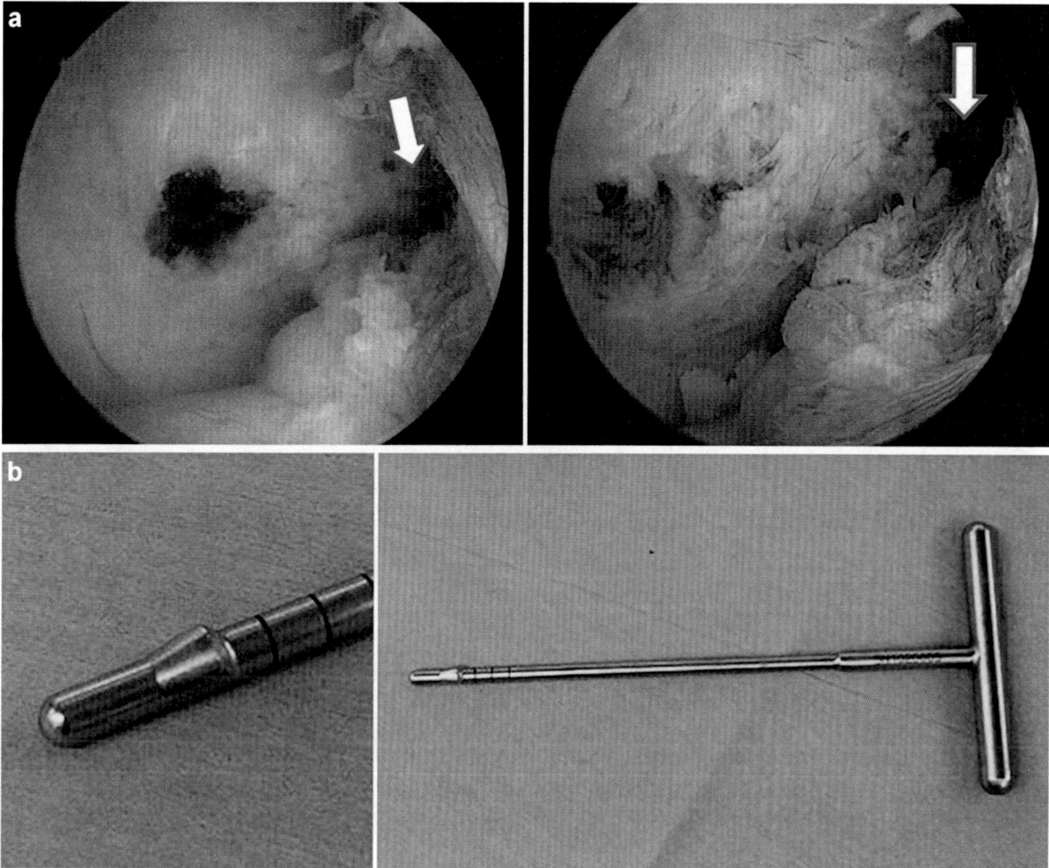

Fig. 4 (**a**) An example of two 4.5 mm-wide femoral drill holes is shown (*left*, PL tunnel; *right*, AM tunnel (*white arrow*)). (**b**) A specially designed dilator with a fin (*left*, magnified tip portion; *right*, whole shape)

intraoperative measurements, PL graft fixation at 0° of flexion would lead to significantly lower tension on the PL graft, which resulted in a significant number of positive pivot-shift tests (Koga et al. 2013).

Taking these results together into consideration, having the initial tension apply slightly more constraint than that of the contralateral uninjured knee would be realistic as a recommended practical initial loading. However, controlling anterior-posterior stability is not the same as rotational stability, and in such a condition, an appropriate investigation is lacking.

From the past clinical experience of DB ACL reconstructions, balancing of the initial load between the AM and PL bundles was more important than its magnitude on each bundle to obtain better stability (Muneta et al. 2011).

Fixation Methods

Hamstring tendon grafts with short fixation distances have been reported to be more advantageous than long fixation distance to control knee kinematics in in vitro cadaveric knee studies. Also, more prominent bone tunnel expansion has been reported when the fixation distance was longer. However, clinical outcome studies could not conclude the advantage of the shorter distance fixation methods (Harilainen and Sandelin 2009). Clinical disadvantages of bone tunnel expansion have not been clearly demonstrated either (Wilson et al. 2004).

Suspensory fixation by an EndoButton (Smith & Nephew, Andover, MA) is practical and safe and is still the first choice for a hamstring graft.

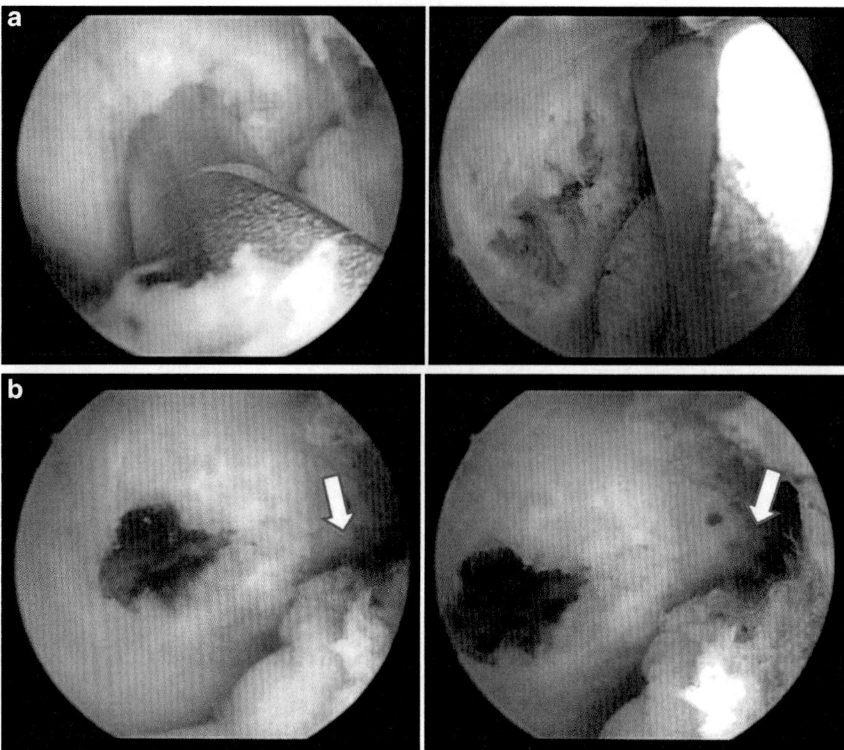

Fig. 5 (**a**) A PL tunnel is enlarged with the special dilator (*left*). An AM tunnel is enlarged with the dilator (*right*). (**b**) Two enlarged tunnels are observed (*left*, PL tunnel; *right*, AM tunnel (*white arrow*))

For the tibial end, two anchor staples are used for pullout fixations which are not strong but practical and useful.

Graft Selection

There is no consensus regarding the optimal graft tissue between BTB and hamstring tendon. A systematic review shows no clinical difference between them (Drogset et al. 2010). Flexion strength in deep knee flexion is weaker when a hamstring autograft tendon is used. Also, a higher re-tear rate of hamstring grafts has been reported. BTB grafts show slow recovery of knee extension strength and kneeling pain for a long time. A quadriceps tendon is an attractive graft choice; however, its strength as a graft tissue has not been well documented. Allograft reconstruction showed worse performance and higher revision rates. Infections and immune reactions are also a concern; however, the selection rate of the allograft has been increased. The ability to avoid graft harvest morbidity and shorter operation time can sometimes be attractive to patients and surgeons.

Graft size is one of the issues to be discussed for achieving better outcomes. Smaller-size grafts would be inferior in respect to controlling stability, while larger-size grafts would tend to be more impinged by intercondylar structures, which might cause extension loss and pain. If a harvested ST shows sufficient thickness, that is, if both bundles are 6 mm or more in diameter, it would not be necessary for a surgeon to harvest the gracilis (GR) tendon.

So far, no difference has been found in the clinical outcome between only ST and STGR tendon surgeries. Four-strand ST tendon graft is the authors' standard choice at Tokyo Medical and Dental University Hospital, also taking flexion strength into account.

Single-, Double-, and Triple-Bundle Surgeries

For tunnel placement in the normal ACL footprint, an SB procedure would involve more risk in violating normal anatomy because its usual diameter of 8 mm or more is too large for fitting in the normal direct insertion of the femoral footprint. Also, a greater interface area between the tendon and bone would be produced by multi-tunnel procedures and would better facilitate the healing process. A larger number of bundles would be more advantageous for graft healing, but more difficulties would result in terms of preserving tunnel independence and fixing the bundles securely. Thinner grafts might cause damage more easily during the postoperative period. DB reconstruction has been shown to have biomechanical advantages over SB reconstruction in in vitro cadaveric studies (Tsai et al. 2010).

These advantages have also been shown in an intraoperative kinematic study.

Clinically, DB reconstruction elucidated its superiority over SB reconstruction with regard to knee stability recovery in the majority of randomized comparative studies (Xu et al. 2013). A 3-dimensional kinematic analysis demonstrated that DB reconstructed knees had significantly better control of tibial rotation when fatigued in comparison to those of SB reconstruction.

Remnant Preservation

Remnant-preserving procedures could be recommended for every ACL surgery. Remnant preservation has several theoretical advantages in terms of proprioceptive function, stability, graft healing, and anatomic positioning. On the other hand, remnant volume may just reflect the integrity of knee structure, that is, meniscus preservation, preoperative stability, and so forth (Muneta et al. 2013). The actual advantages of remnant-preserving reconstruction have not been clarified (Papalia et al. 2012).

The backside approach aiming at the posterior margin of the direct insertion of the femoral attachment makes the remnant-preserving reconstruction easy and reproducible for experienced surgeons (Fig. 6).

Approach: Transtibial, Trans-portal, and Outside-In

Each individual approach of transtibial, trans-portal, and outside-in techniques has advantages and disadvantages (Takeda et al. 2013). If the desirable procedures were accomplished, every approach should be justified even if it is for DB reconstruction. A transtibial approach cannot accomplish anatomic reconstruction easily.

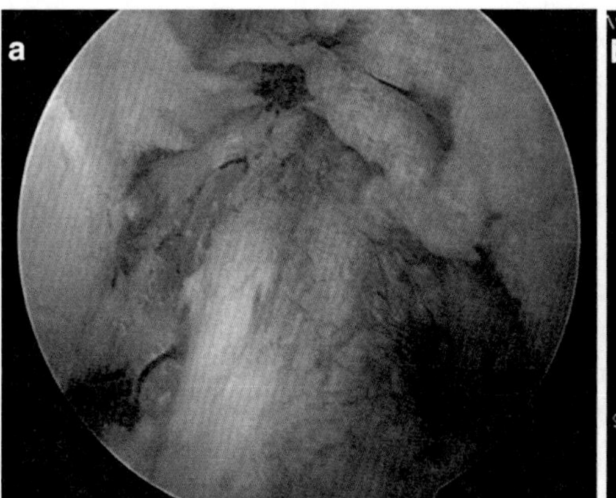

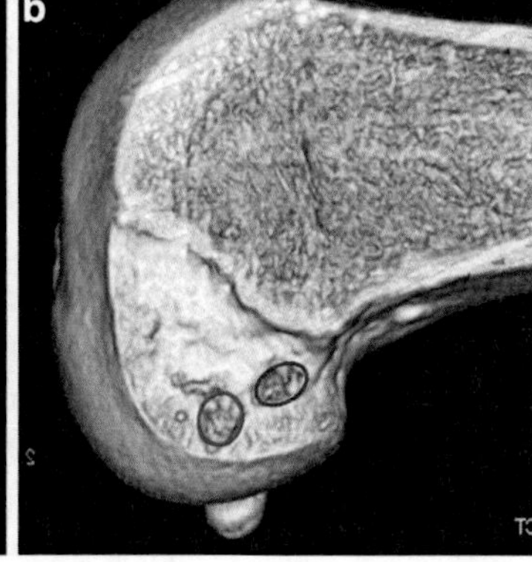

Fig. 6 (**a**) An arthroscopic view of the two grafts shows that the anteromedial part is covered with the ACL remnant. (**b**) A 3D CT shows two femoral tunnels of AM and PL bundles. The two tunnels are oval and aligned to the bony landmarks of the normal ACL

A transtibial approach is simplest for creating two independent tunnels, but it is most difficult for controlling anatomic tunnel positioning for a surgeon. Graft tissue passing is easiest by a transtibial procedure among the three approaches.

A trans-portal technique is easier and more reproducible to make two independent femoral anatomic tunnels, whereas the procedure requires deep knee flexion; otherwise, it is subject to likely break the posterior wall of the lateral femoral condyle during femoral tunnel creation. Also, the tunnel sometimes violates the lateral and posterolateral structures.

An outside-in technique might be the most reproducible and safest way to make two anatomic femoral tunnels, although positioning of the two separate tunnels is not easy and two additional small incisions are necessary.

These three approaches have their merits and defects, so that every surgeon should be skillful and familiar with each approach and had better select one of them case by case.

Preservation of Normal Knee Structures and Function and Various Augmentation Methods

In the knees with well-preserved native ACL remnant, meniscus damages were less frequently observed, and good stability was obtained postoperatively. That kind of observation indicates that it is not easy to recover the whole knee joint structures as a normal joint just by ACL reconstruction. It is necessary to restore the meniscus function and to repair the articular cartilage. Various injuries in every part of the knee joint progress along with time after an ACL injury. Each "giving-way" episode results in additional damage to knee structures. Recovery of anterior and rotational instability demands ACL reconstruction; however, is ACL graft alone sufficient for restoring knee stability in every knee with ACL insufficiency?

In such a case with meniscus damages and a long period after injury, lateral tenodesis may be a kind of necessary evil to eliminate pivot-shift phenomenon. Lateral tenodesis is a nonanatomic augmentation forcing external rotation of the tibia. The proper indication for such augmentation needs further investigation.

Many studies have been carried out to promote the healing process in various ways in ACL reconstruction. Attempts promoting the healing process in bone-tendon junction have been carried out with the application of bone morphologic protein-2, followed by other cytokines, platelet-rich proteins (PRPs), and mesenchymal stem cells (Muller et al. 2013). Promoting bone tunnel junction healing is important in terms of safer and faster return to sports after ACL reconstruction; however, to determine how much more it has been promoted and how much safer it is for each patient is too difficult to answer accurately. A more complex situation exists in terms of promotion of midsubstance graft healing.

Healing promotion does not always mean that the graft becomes stronger; rather it causes rapid decrease of graft strength. As clinicians, a more conservative and careful attitude is required for the application of those agents. PRP requires a guarantee of quality with content certification. Clinical application of cytokines requires a higher hurdle of safety.

Steady steps and consideration are required for surgeons to advance surgeries better without any thoughtless application of such augmentations from the stand point of a patient's benefit.

Conclusion

The anatomic ACL reconstruction is the way to be followed by every ligament surgeon. The remnant tissue is the better anatomic marker when the femoral tunnel creation approach is done from the backside of the remnant.

Cross-References

- ▶ Allografts in Anterior Cruciate Ligament Reconstruction
- ▶ Alternative Techniques for Double-Tunnel Anatomic Anterior Cruciate Ligament Reconstruction

- ▶ Anatomic Double-Tunnel Anterior Cruciate Ligament Reconstruction: Evolution and Principles
- ▶ Anterior Cruciate Ligament Graft Selection and Fixation
- ▶ Anterior Cruciate Ligament Injuries and Surgery: Current Evidence and Modern Development
- ▶ Anterior Cruciate Ligament Reconstruction with Autologous Quadriceps Tendon
- ▶ Different Techniques of Anterior Cruciate Ligament Reconstruction: Guidelines
- ▶ Double-Tunnel Anatomic Anterior Cruciate Ligament Reconstruction

References

Bastian JD, Tomagra S, Schuster AJ et al (2014) ACL reconstruction with physiological graft tension by intraoperative adjustment of the anteroposterior translation to the uninjured contralateral knee. Knee Surg Sports Traumatol Arthrosc 22:1055–1060

Bedi A, Maak T, Musahl V et al (2011) Effect of tibial tunnel position on stability of the knee after anterior cruciate ligament reconstruction: is the tibial tunnel position most important? Am J Sports Med 39:366–373

Brady MF, Bradley MP, Fleming BC et al (2007) Effects of initial graft tension on the tibiofemoral compressive forces and joint position after anterior cruciate ligament reconstruction. Am J Sports Med 35:395–403

Colombet P, Robinson J, Christel P et al (2006) Morphology of anterior cruciate ligament attachments for anatomic reconstruction: a cadaveric dissection and radiographic study. Arthroscopy 22:984–992

Drogset JO, Strand T, Uppheim G et al (2010) Autologous patellar tendon and quadrupled hamstring grafts in anterior cruciate ligament reconstruction: a prospective randomized multicenter review of different fixation methods. Knee Surg Sports Traumatol Arthrosc 18:1085–1093

Hara K, Mochizuki T, Sekiya I et al (2009) Anatomy of normal human anterior cruciate ligament attachments evaluated by divided small bundles. Am J Sports Med 37:2386–2391

Harilainen A, Sandelin J (2009) A prospective comparison of 3 hamstring ACL fixation devices–Rigidfix, BioScrew, and Intrafix–randomized into 4 groups with 2 years of follow-up. Am J Sports Med 37:699–706

Howell SM, Clark JA, Farley TE (1991) A rationale for predicting anterior cruciate graft impingement by the intercondylar roof. A magnetic resonance imaging study. Am J Sports Med 19:276–282

Howell SM, Gittins ME, Gottlieb JE et al (2001) The relationship between the angle of the tibial tunnel in the coronal plane and loss of flexion and anterior laxity after anterior cruciate ligament reconstruction. Am J Sports Med 29:567–574

Kato Y, Maeyama A, Lertwanich P et al (2013) Biomechanical comparison of different graft positions for single-bundle anterior cruciate ligament reconstruction. Knee Surg Sports Traumatol Arthrosc 21:816–823

Kirwan GW, Bourke MG, Chipchase L et al (2013) Initial graft tension and the effect on postoperative patient functional outcomes in anterior cruciate ligament reconstruction. Arthroscopy 29:934–941

Koga H, Muneta T, Yagishita K et al (2013) Effect of posterolateral bundle graft fixation angles on graft tension curves and load sharing in double-bundle anterior cruciate ligament reconstruction using a transtibial drilling technique. Arthroscopy 29:529–538

Mae T, Shino K, Matsumoto N et al (2010) Anatomic double-bundle anterior cruciate ligament reconstruction using hamstring tendons with minimally required initial tension. Arthroscopy 26:1289–1295

Mochizuki T, Muneta T, Nagase T et al (2006) Cadaveric knee observation study for describing anatomic femoral tunnel placement for two-bundle anterior cruciate ligament reconstruction. Arthroscopy 22:356–361

Mochizuki T, Fujishiro H, Nimura A et al (2014) Anatomic and histologic analysis of the mid-substance and fan-like extension fibres of the anterior cruciate ligament during knee motion, with special reference to the femoral attachment. Knee Surg Sports Traumatol Arthrosc 22:336–344

Muller B, Bowman KF Jr, Bedi A (2013) ACL graft healing and biologics. Clin Sports Med 32:93–109. doi:10.1016/j.csm.2012.08.010

Muneta T, Sekiya I, Yagishita K et al (1999) Two-bundle reconstruction of the anterior cruciate ligament using semitendinosus tendon with endobuttons: operative technique and preliminary results. Arthroscopy 15:618–624

Muneta T, Koga H, Ju YJ et al (2011) Effects of different initial bundle tensioning strategies on the outcome of double-bundle ACL reconstruction: a cohort study. Sports Med Arthrosc Rehabil Ther Technol 3:15

Muneta T, Koga H, Ju YJ et al (2013) Remnant volume of anterior cruciate ligament correlates preoperative patients' status and postoperative outcome. Knee Surg Sports Traumatol Arthrosc 21:906–913

Papalia R, Franceschi F, Vasta S et al (2012) Sparing the anterior cruciate ligament remnant: is it worth the hassle? Br Med Bull 104:91–111

Sasaki N, Ishibashi Y, Tsuda E et al (2012) The femoral insertion of the anterior cruciate ligament: discrepancy between macroscopic and histological observations. Arthroscopy 28:1135–1146

Siebold R, Ellert T, Metz S et al (2008) Tibial insertions of the anteromedial and posterolateral bundles of the anterior cruciate ligament: morphometry, arthroscopic landmarks, and orientation model for bone tunnel placement. Arthroscopy 24:154–161

Takeda Y, Iwame T, Takasago T et al (2013) Comparison of tunnel orientation between transtibial and portal techniques for anatomic double-bundle anterior cruciate ligament reconstruction using 3-dimensional computed tomography. Arthroscopy 29:195–204

Tsai AG, Wijdicks CA, Walsh MP et al (2010) Comparative kinematic evaluation of all-inside single-bundle and double-bundle anterior cruciate ligament reconstruction: a biomechanical study. Am J Sports Med 38:263–272

Wilson TC, Kantaras A, Atay A et al (2004) Tunnel enlargement after anterior cruciate ligament surgery. Am J Sports Med 32:543–549. Review

Xu M, Gao S, Zeng C et al (2013) Outcomes of anterior cruciate ligament reconstruction using single-bundle versus double-bundle technique: meta-analysis of 19 randomized controlled trials. Arthroscopy 29:357–365

Yagi M, Wong EK, Kanamori A et al (2002) Biomechanical analysis of an anatomic anterior cruciate ligament reconstruction. Am J Sports Med 30:660–666

Yamamoto Y, Hsu WH, Woo SL-Y et al (2004) Comparison of a lateral and an anatomical femoral tunnel placement. Am J Sports Med 32:1825–1832

Yasuda K, Kondo E, Ichiyama H et al (2004) Anatomic reconstruction of the anteromedial and posterolateral bundles of the anterior cruciate ligament using hamstring tendon grafts. Arthroscopy 20:1015–1025

Yasuda K, Ichiyama H, Kondo E et al (2008) An in vivo biomechanical study on the tension-versus-knee flexion angle curves of 2 grafts in anatomic double-bundle anterior cruciate ligament reconstruction: effects of initial tension and internal tibial rotation. Arthroscopy 24:276–284

Yoshiya S, Andrish JT, Manley MT et al (1987) Graft tension in anterior cruciate ligament reconstruction. An in vivo study in dogs. Am J Sports Med 15:464–470

Zantop T, Diermann N, Schumacher T et al (2008) Anatomical and nonanatomical double-bundle anterior cruciate ligament reconstruction: importance of femoral tunnel location on knee kinematics. Am J Sports Med 38:678–685

Zavras TD, Race A, Amis AA (2005) The effect of femoral attachment location on anterior cruciate ligament reconstruction: graft tension patterns and restoration of normal anterior-posterior laxity patterns. Knee Surg Sports Traumatol Arthrosc 13:92–100

Ziegler CG, Pietrini SD, Westerhaus BD et al (2011) Arthroscopically pertinent landmarks for tunnel positioning in single-bundle and double-bundle anterior cruciate ligament reconstructions. Am J Sports Med 39:743–752

128 Structured Rehabilitation Model for Patients with Patellofemoral Pain Syndrome

Thomas Rogers, Rumeal Whaley, Emily Monroe, Defne Kaya, and John Nyland

Contents

T. Rogers (✉) • R. Whaley
Department of Orthopaedic Surgery, Division of Sports Medicine, University of Louisville, Louisville, KY, USA
e-mail: throge2@gmail.com; rdwhal01@louisville.edu; rumeal@me.com

E. Monroe
Department of Orthopaedic Surgery, Northwestern University, Chicago, IL, USA
e-mail: bran0569@gmail.com

D. Kaya
Department of Physical Therapy and Rehabilitation, Faculty of Health Science, Biruni University, İstanbul, Turkey
e-mail: defne@hacettepe.edu.tr

J. Nyland
Kosair Charities College of Health and Natural Sciences, Spalding University, Louisville, USA
e-mail: john.nyland@louisville.edu; jnyland@spalding.edu

M.N. Doral, J. Karlsson (eds.), *Sports Injuries*,
DOI 10.1007/978-3-642-36569-0_286

Abstract

Treatments for patellofemoral pain syndrome (PFPS) are as numerous as its potential causes. This is most likely, in part, due to its multifactorial and complex nature.

Patellofemoral pain syndrome represents retropatellar and/or peripatellar pain that is usually exacerbated by activities such as sitting, kneeling, squatting, and stair climbing. The PFPS diagnosis is largely one of exclusion because many other conditions need to be ruled out first. In addition to providing an operational definition for PFPS, this chapter presents a structured rehabilitation model for its treatment based on regional symptom categorization. This categorization will enable rehabilitation clinicians to group patients with similar PFPS etiologies into the same treatment group, thereby helping develop more standardized care and stronger research evidence supporting treatment efficacy.

Introduction

Patellofemoral pain syndrome (PFPS) is a ubiquitous condition commonly encountered in sports medicine. Although the overall incidence of PFPS is about 22/1,000 men and women per year, women are more than twice as likely as men to be diagnosed with this condition (Boling et al. 2010). In the context of sports medicine, the negative impact of PFPS becomes even more evident. Of all injuries sustained due to running, PFPS is the most prevalent (Taunton et al. 2002). While numerous PFPS treatments generally provide some knee pain relief and improved function, long-term outcomes are not as encouraging. As many as 73 % of athletically active men and women with PFPS continue to experience knee pain at almost 6 years following initial diagnosis, 74 % display decreased athletic activity, and 6 % report a negative influence on employment status (Blond and Hansen 1998).

Numerous studies have evaluated widely varying PFPS treatment; however, consensus regarding its operational definition is still lacking. It is difficult to treat a phenomenon that one does not understand. This chapter describes a structured rehabilitation model that logically organizes the possible causes of PFPS by the primary region of influence. Regional categorization will better enable rehabilitation clinicians to perform clinical evaluations that more effectively translate into treatment plans, develop evidence-based treatments, and interpret the efficacy of differing treatment strategies. After describing PFPS as inclusively as possible to avoid missing any potentially relevant factors, the next step is to logically organize possible causes and relationships to facilitate clinical evaluations that better translate into standardized treatment planning.

Causes and Conditions

Although PFPS is classically expressed as retropatellar, or peripatellar pain exacerbated by repetitive squatting, kneeling, running, and stair climbing (Blond and Hansen 1998; Khayambashi et al. 2012), it may also be associated with joint crepitus, effusion, a sense of insecurity during ambulation, giving way, buckling, and/or a feeling of intermittent "knee catching" during active extension (Blond and Hansen 1998). Since a multitude of other conditions must be eliminated from consideration prior to selecting the PFPS diagnosis, it largely represents a diagnosis of exclusion. Trauma, prior knee surgery, intra-articular knee pathology, patellar tendinopathy, peripatellar bursitis, plica syndrome, Sinding-Larsen-Johansson syndrome, Osgood-Schlatter disease, Hoffa's disease, meniscal injury, and iliotibial band syndrome, all represent associated conditions that need to be ruled out (Witvrouw et al. 2005; Khayambashi et al. 2012).

The precise mechanism by which patellar malalignment or maltracking contribute to PFPS is poorly understood. Theories include increased patellofemoral subchondral bone pressure, neurosensory irritation associated with lateral retinaculum pathology, and loss of knee extensor mechanism tissue homeostasis (Powers et al. 2012). Patients who present with PFPS from lateral patellar tracking exhibit greater lateral translation and patellar tilt during weight-bearing conditions compared to non-weight-bearing conditions (Draper et al. 2010). One biomechanical explanation has attributed lateral patellar maltracking to excessive dynamic knee valgus associated with weak hip abductor muscle strength (Powers 2010). This commentary suggested that ipsilateral hip abductor muscle weakness leads to compensatory elevation at the contralateral pelvis. As this happens when viewed in the frontal plane, the ground reaction force vector moves closer to the ipsilateral hip joint center, creating an external knee valgus movement during single-leg support.

Model Rationale

Patellofemoral pain syndrome can be multifactorial and often has no clear etiology (Petersen et al. 2013). Some have proposed organizing PFPS causes based on lower extremity alignment and neuromuscular dysfunction (Witvrouw et al. 2005). Factors originating proximally through the hip, locally at the knee, and/or distally through the foot/ankle often contribute to patellofemoral joint malalignment and maltracking; others have proposed categorizing patients into treatment groups based on their primary region of PFPS origin (Powers et al. 2012).

Proximal Relationships

Proximal factors associated with PFPS include hip weakness and lumbopelvic instability, composite quadriceps femoris weakness, vastus medialis oblique (VMO) and vastus lateralis (VL) neuromotor activation coordination abnormalities, and hamstring muscle group tightness. Systematic reviews have reported a direct relationship between hip abductor and external rotator weakness and PFPS during single-leg support (Prins and van der Wurff 2009; Meira and Brumitt 2011). A case-control study reported that females with PFPS who also had reduced hip abductor strength displayed impaired medial-lateral lumbopelvic stability compared to a healthy control group with normal hip abductor strength (Lee et al. 2012). In women, it has been shown that PFPS is directly related to reduced total quadriceps femoris muscle volume and cross-sectional area on magnetic resonance imaging examination, and impaired isokinetic knee extensor strength compared to the unaffected lower extremity (Kaya et al. 2011).

Vastus medialis oblique and VL neuromotor activation irregularities, strength imbalances, and coordination deficiencies have also been associated with PFPS (Witvrouw et al. 2005). A prospective case-control study revealed that patients with PFPS displayed a target-trajectory neuromuscular coordination deficit during multi-joint lower limb tracking-trajectory testing (Yosmaoglu et al. 2013). The final proximal factor shown to be associated with PFPS is hamstring muscle group tightness (White et al. 2009).

Local Relationships

Local factors associated with PFPS include abnormal patellofemoral joint mechanics associated with maltracking, articular surface incongruency, retinacular dysfunction, excessive and/or highly repetitive loading, and psychological factors. Patellofemoral joint malalignment may be associated with abnormal quadriceps femoris neuromuscular activation, an underlying bony abnormality, or both (Witvrouw et al. 2005). An excessively tight retinaculum may contribute to patellar hypomobility, while a loose retinaculum may contribute to hypermobility (Witvrouw et al. 2005). Even in the absence of patellofemoral joint malalignment or articular incongruency, high-intensity training can create supraphysiologic overload at patellofemoral joint structures, leading to increased pain and decrease function (Witvrouw et al. 2005; Petersen et al. 2013).

While not always included in the discussion of PFPS, there is little doubt that there may be an association between patients who describe PFPS symptoms and psychological factors (Mann et al. 2007; Powers et al. 2012). In a study of 20 symptomatic patients, anterior knee pain was described as being a largely psychosomatic syndrome (Witonski 1999). Higher mental distress, lower self-perceived health (Jensen et al. 2005), and higher catastrophic thinking levels (Domenech et al. 2013) have been reported among patients with PFPS. Catastrophic thought may be a pivotal precursor to the development of movement-related fear and anxiety and its resultant disability among patients with PFPS (Domenech et al. 2013). These studies suggest that having a clear understanding of potential psychobehavioral attributes of patient's with PFPS may be important to treatment success.

Distal Relationships

Distally, the factors most commonly involved in PFPS are primarily associated with the foot and subtalar joint. A systematic review concluded that patients with PFPS exhibit differences in foot kinematics during walking and running compared to healthy subjects (Barton et al. 2009). While walking, patients with PFPS demonstrated delayed peak rear-foot eversion and increased rear-foot eversion at heel strike transient. While running, patients with PFPS displayed delayed peak rear-foot eversion timing, increased rear-foot eversion at heel strike, and reduced rear-foot eversion displacement. Patients with PFPS have also been reported to display increased foot pronation and foot hypermobility compared to asymptomatic patients (Barton et al. 2010).

Clinical Evaluation, Diagnosis, and Model Predictors

Understanding which factors best predict PFPS is important to the development of a structured rehabilitation model. With this information, the rehabilitation clinician will be more likely to include these predictors in their clinical evaluation. Independent systematic reviews with meta-analyses have concluded that knee extension strength is the only consistently reliable predictor for PFPS (Lankhorst et al. 2012; Pappas and Wong-Tom 2012).

Diagnostic modalities for PFPS have also been researched extensively. To properly treat the patient, one must be sure of the condition they are treating. In a systematic review of 22 different clinical tests, it was reported that the "best" diagnostic tests for PFPS could not be identified due to the wide variety of reference standards, diverse study methodologies, and diverse methods of diagnosis statistical analysis (Cook et al. 2011). The best method for diagnosing PFPS remains the identification of anterior knee pain in combination with decreased function that also excludes all other competing pathologies (Cook et al. 2011). In essence, PFPS remains a diagnosis of exclusion.

Many PFPS studies have focused on female subjects (Witonski 1999; Kaya et al. 2011; Khayambashi et al. 2012; Lee et al. 2012; Yosmaoglu et al. 2013). However, males are also greatly affected by PFPS, and they may display different lower extremity kinematic findings. A cross-sectional study examining male and female runners with PFPS revealed that males had increased knee adduction during running and squatting, while females squatted with increased hip adduction and decreased knee adduction (Willy et al. 2012). Key clinical evaluation components in relationship to their potential influence on proximal, local, and distal factors that are known to influence PFPS are displayed in Fig. 1.

Treatment

Most medical literature related to managing PFPS addresses overall treatment efficacy without consideration for regional influences. This tendency greatly contributes to the lack of robust evidence that currently exists regarding PFPS treatment efficacy. The structured rehabilitation model we propose (Fig. 2) enables the clinician to better tailor rehabilitation program planning to the primary region associated with PFPS causation.

Proximal Focus

Proximal PFPS treatments primarily involve hip abductor-external rotator strengthening, knee extensor strengthening, VMO/VL activation coordination exercises, and lower extremity musculotendinous stretching. A randomized controlled trial reported that hip abductor

- Pain
  - Location and type?
  - Exacerbated by sitting, kneeling, squatting, climbing stairs?
  - Instability?
  - Duration of pain (chronicity)?
- Proximal factors
  - Hip weakness or malalignment?
    - Dynamic knee valgus/varus?
  - Quadriceps weakness?
  - VMO/VL abnormalities?
    - VMO hypotrophy?
    - Altered VMO/VL contraction rate?
  - Target-trajectory muscular coordination deficit?
  - Hamstring tightness?
- Distal factors
  - Gait analysis abnormalities?
    - Rear-foot eversion?
    - Foot pronation?
- Local factors
  - Patellofemoral joint mechanical abnormalities?
    - Due to abnormal quadriceps contraction?
    - Underlying bony abnormality?
  - Retinaculum dysfunction?
    - Hypermobile patella?
    - Hypomobile patella?
  - Recent excessive loading on patellofemoral joint?
  - Psychological contributions?
    - Decreased self-perceived health? (Coop-Wonca Chart) (Jensen, Hystad, Baerheim, 2005)
    - Increased mental distress? (Hopkins Symptoms Checklist) (Jensen, Hystad, Baerheim, 2005)
    - Anxiety and/or depression? (Hospital Anxiety/Depression Subscale) (Jensen, Hystad, Baerheim, 2005)
    - Catastrophic thinking? (Pain Catastrophizing Scale) (Domenech J, Sanchis-Alfonso V, López L, Espejo B, 2013)
    - Kinesiophobia? (Tampa Scale for Kinesiophobia) (Domenech J, Sanchis-Alfonso V, López L, Espejo B, 2013)

Fig. 1 Clinical evaluation of patellofemoral pain syndrome

strengthening combined with knee extensor strengthening decreased PFPS more than knee extensor strengthening alone (Fukuda et al. 2010). A randomized controlled trial concluded that hip abductor and external rotator strengthening was also effective in reducing PFPS and improving self-reported health status as it relates to pain, stiffness, and physical function (Khayambashi et al. 2012). Other systematic reviews have also supported the efficacy of hip muscle strengthening

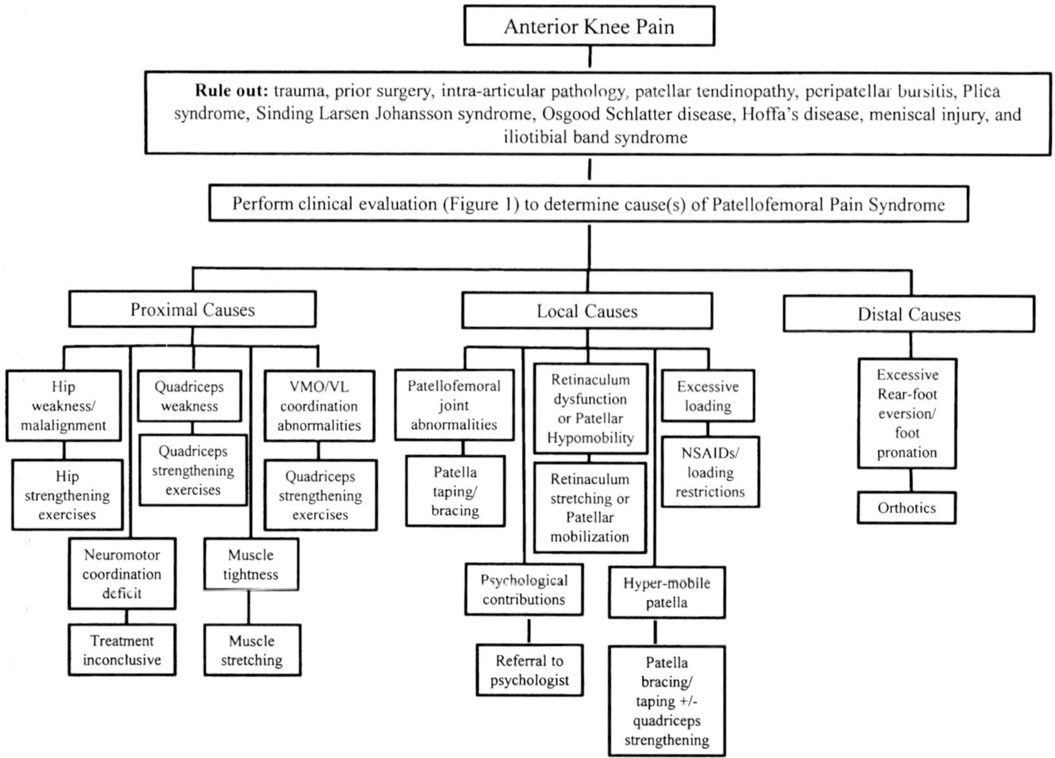

Fig. 2 Structured rehabilitation model for patellofemoral pain syndrome treatment

for patients with PFPS (Bolgla and Boling 2011; Harvie et al. 2011; Meira and Brumitt 2011). The efficacy of knee extensor strengthening has also been reported with patellofemoral pain reductions in patients who perform both non-weight-bearing and weight-bearing kinetic chain exercises (Bolgla and Boling 2011; Harvie et al. 2011). It is clear that hip and knee muscle strengthening is beneficial for patients with PFPS and knee extensor strengthening exercises are more effective when hip muscle strengthening is also addressed.

The treatment for PFPS is sometimes directed specifically at VMO and VL activation coordination. Electrical muscle stimulation to treat a hypotrophic VMO or to correct VMO/VL muscle activation coordination has been recommended (Witvrouw et al. 2005). Systematic reviews however have refuted this by concluding that there is no benefit to selective VMO/VL activation coordination exercises (Bolgla and Boling 2011; Harvie et al. 2011). Systematic reviews have also shown that no added benefit has been identified for including biofeedback or neuromuscular electrical stimulation to a knee extensor strengthening program designed to reduce patellofemoral pain (Bolgla and Boling 2011; Lake and Wofford 2011). Another controversial treatment modality is hamstring and adjacent muscle group stretching. Some have suggested the inclusion of stretching in rehabilitation programs for patients with PFPS (Witvrouw et al. 2005; Harvie et al. 2011). However, a study of women with PFPS concluded that the addition of static passive stretching to the muscle strengthening program had no additional benefit for pain reduction or function improvement (Bryk et al. 2013). The medical literature currently suggests that there is no benefit in having a patient with PFPS perform selective VMO or VL activation coordination exercises, knee extensor electrical muscle stimulation, or knee extensor biofeedback. While stretching cannot be recommended as firmly as hip and knee strengthening exercises, it should still be considered by rehabilitation clinicians when knee or hip range of motion restrictions are evident.

Local Focus

Local PFPS treatments include patellar taping and bracing, retinaculum stretching, patella mobilization, nonsteroidal anti-inflammatory drugs (NSAIDs), restricted weight-bearing or loading restrictions, and psychological intervention. A systematic review with meta-analysis reported that medially directed patella taping decreased PFPS symptoms in patients with chronic knee osteoarthritis (Warden et al. 2008). Their findings were inconclusive however as to whether medially or laterally directed taping was superior. The same authors determined that patella bracing efficacy could not be established due to inconclusive evidence. This study only evaluated one type of patellar brace, and although it may help reduce patellofemoral pain, more research is needed to recommend it conclusively. Another study reported that patella taping in conjunction with quadriceps femoris strengthening exercises was beneficial for alleviating PFPS symptoms at least in the short term (Bolgla and Boling 2011). While the aforementioned studies support the use of patella taping for patients with PFPS, a systematic review with meta-analysis reported that it is not possible to establish patella taping efficacy for patients with PFPS due to a lack of evidence in the medical literature (Callaghan and Selfe 2012). Patella taping and bracing seems to confer some benefit for patients with PFPS, at least in the short term, but studies with stronger designs, larger subject numbers, and greater use of control group comparisons are needed.

If a tight retinaculum is suspected to be the PFPS cause, some have advocated retinacular stretching either by the clinician or by the patient (Witvrouw et al. 2005). However, no evidence from systematic reviews currently supports this treatment approach (Bolgla and Boling 2011; Harvie et al. 2011). When patients with PFPS display no underlying anatomical or biomechanical abnormalities, but do present a history of excessive patellofemoral joint loading, NSAIDs, loading restrictions, and a gradual return to loading activity are recommended (Witvrouw et al. 2005). The use of NSAIDs remains controversial. A Cochrane review reported limited evidence supporting NSAIDs use for patients with PFPS (Heintjes et al. 2004). This study supported short-term NSAID use for patients with PFPS that is associated with excessive loading, provided that loading is reduced over the treatment period and other treatments with a stronger evidence base are also initiated. While much focus in this chapter has been placed on physical PFPS factors, psychological influences may also exist (Witonski 1999; Jensen et al. 2005; Mann et al. 2007; Domenech et al. 2013). If the confluence of clinical evaluation findings, patient history, impairments, and functional limitation observations provides conflicting evidence, referral to and clearance from a psychologist may be useful among this patient population.

Distal Focus

Distal treatment interventions focus primarily on the foot and subtalar joint. Orthotics with rear-foot posting and medial longitudinal arch support may decrease patellofemoral pain in some patients, but evidence is still lacking to confirm its efficacy (Bolgla and Boling 2011). The precise mechanism by which orthotics alleviate patellofemoral pain remains to be elucidated (Powers et al. 2012). Orthotic use in combination with prescriptive exercises in patients with PFPS may have an added beneficial effect (Bolgla and Boling 2011).

Additional Treatment Considerations

There have been many other treatment modalities used to treat patients with PFPS. For the sake of thoroughness, commonly used modalities will be discussed. A systematic review of studies that treated patients with PFPS has reported no evidence to support the benefit of cryotherapy, ultrasound, iontophoresis, phonophoresis, neuromuscular electrical stimulation, electromyographic biofeedback, electrical stimulation for pain control, or laser therapy for patients with PFPS (Lake and Wofford 2011).

Determining Treatment Intervention Efficacy

Although they have only been reported as providing relatively short-term PFPS treatment effectiveness, positive treatment outcomes are more likely among patients who possess less pre-rehabilitation program anterior knee pain, who have greater quadriceps femoris muscle group volume, and who have greater eccentric knee extensor torque capability (Pattyn et al. 2012). One review suggested that the optimum treatment plan for patients with patellofemoral pain should include both non-weight-bearing and weight-bearing exercises, have a duration of 6 weeks or more, use principles of progressive resistance overload and frequency, and include 20–40 repetitions per exercise to encourage muscle endurance development (Harvie et al. 2011).

There are three basic outcome measurement categories that should be considered by rehabilitation clinicians to evaluate intervention success when treating patients with PFPS. These include subjective symptom and perceived function testing, objective function testing, and objective strength testing. For subjective symptom testing, task-specific 10-cm visual analog scale (VAS) use with end-range descriptors of "no pain" and "extreme or severe pain" is recommended. For subjective perceived function testing, the Kujala Anterior Knee Pain Scale (AKPS) is recommended (Crossley et al. 2004). The minimum change necessary, from initial evaluation to follow-up, for the patient to consider their condition improved is 2 cm on the VAS and ten points on the AKPS (Crossley et al. 2004). Due to measurement efficacy, low cost, and ease of use, the VAS and AKPS should be administered to all patients with PFPS at baseline and during follow-up sessions to determine treatment success. Recommended objective function tests include the single-leg hop for distance test (Fukuda et al. 2010; Pattyn et al. 2012) and the triple-hop for distance test (Pattyn et al. 2012). For the single-leg hop for distance test, the patient hops as far as possible and lands on the affected lower extremity, and the distance from start to finish is recorded. The triple-hop for distance test represents the total distance covered as the patient uses the affected lower extremity for three consecutive hops. Due to the simplicity and cost-effectiveness of objective function testing, these tests should also be administered to all patients with PFPS at baseline (if possible, when pain is not too severe) and follow-up. The final category of objective strength testing applies only to patients with PFPS who initially present with hip and/or quadriceps muscle weakness. The medical literature describes isokinetic knee extensor strength testing (Lake and Wofford 2011) and hip strength testing using handheld dynamometry (Maffiuletti 2010; Khayambashi et al. 2012) as methods to evaluate PFPS treatment success. Therefore, if the patient is being treated for hip and/or quadriceps muscle weakness as contributing factors for PFPS, their hip and quadriceps strength should be individually evaluated with both isokinetic strength testing and handheld dynamometry if possible. The use of these three basic outcome measure categories will not only benefit the patient by identifying condition improvement or lack thereof, it will also solidify a system for validating specific treatment efficacy. Armed with data such as this, rehabilitation clinicians will be able to improve the evidence basis of PFPS treatment.

Structured Rehabilitation Model Application

After proper identification of PFPS causes and conditions, key clinical evaluation components based on the primary region of influence (Fig. 1), and evidence-based treatment approaches, using a structured rehabilitation model algorithm can be implemented (Fig. 2). This section illustrates how the model should be applied. Three representative patients are discussed. While the following discussion focuses on patients with PFPS that originate primarily from one region, it does not eliminate the likelihood that some patients may present significant contributions from more than one region (proximal, local, and/or distal). In cases such as this, the rehabilitation clinician needs to combine key strategies from the contributing regions to provide comprehensive care. For example, if the patient has proximal and distal contributing factors, the corresponding proximal and distal treatments should be implemented.

Patient A: Proximal Factors

Patient A is a 48-year-old woman who presented with 6 weeks of sharp, peripatellar pain at her left knee. The pain had been gradual in onset and she noted that it is exacerbated with stair climbing. This pain was particularly frightening as it limited her from "getting around as she used to." Clinical evaluation identified left hip abductor and external rotator weakness and left knee extensor weakness. During observational gait analysis, it was also noted that she displayed severe dynamic left knee valgus. While the rehabilitation clinician was suspicious of psychological contributions to her symptom complaints, the psychological assessment was negative for catastrophizing. In response to her left hip and knee muscle weakness, hip abductor, hip external rotator, and knee extensor strengthening exercises were initiated. These exercises combined weight-bearing and non-weight-bearing movements performed for a minimum of 6 weeks with 20–40 repetitions per set. The number of exercise sets/workout was determined by her tolerance. At 1-week following program initiation, a follow-up session was scheduled to make any necessary plan adjustments. At 6 weeks posttreatment initiation, her VAS score improved from seven at baseline to three and her AKPS score over the same time period improved from 47 to 84. Over the same time periods, her left side single-leg hop for distance test improved from 98 to 121 cm and right side single-leg hop for distance test improved from 124 to 128 cm. Over the same time periods, her left side triple-hop for distance test improved from 290 to 358 cm, while her right side triple-hop for distance test improved from 364 to 379 cm. Bilateral knee extensor and hip abductor strength testing was also performed over the same time periods using an isokinetic strength testing device and handheld dynamometer, respectively. Left knee extensor strength improved from 89 to 112 N•m after 6 weeks, while the right knee extensors remained steady at 117 and 120 N•m. Left hip abductor strength over the same time period improved from 170 to 191 N, while the right side was virtually unchanged at 197 and 199 N. The patient's left hip and knee strength improved significantly over the course of the initial 6 weeks treatment period. The VAS and AKPS score changes exceeded the minimum change needed to suggest successful condition improvement.

Patient B: Distal Factors

Patient B is a 31-year-old male automobile mechanic who presented with a 3-year history of bilateral retropatellar pain. He described the pain as "stabbing, coming, and going without ever lasting longer than a couple of hours." The pain is at its worst when he "squatted down to check tire pressures." He used to enjoy running but is no longer able to perform this activity secondary to PFPS. Upon observational gait evaluation, he presented with excessive bilateral rear-foot eversion at heel strike and excessive foot pronation. During clinical examination, he was also found to have slightly impaired right knee extensor strength. By following the structured rehabilitation model, the clinician's primary recommendation was orthotic use to control rear-foot eversion and pronation. Additionally, patient B began an 8-week duration rehabilitation program to strengthen his right knee extensors. Outcome measures were performed at baseline, 4 weeks after program initiation (when the patient was able to work without significant pain) and 8 weeks after program initiation (when he was able to begin running again). At baseline, 4 weeks, and 8 weeks, his VAS and AKPS scores were 5, 3, and 2 and 62, 81, and 89, respectively. His single-leg hop for distance test results at baseline, 4 weeks after program initiation, and 8 weeks after program initiation were 131 cm, 141 cm, and 146 cm for the right lower extremity and 128 cm, 140 cm, and 144 cm for the left lower extremity.

Triple-hop for distance test results revealed distances of 373 cm, 401 cm, and 412 cm for the right lower extremity, compared to 378 cm, 400 cm, and 418 cm for the left lower extremity. Bilateral isokinetic knee extensor strength testing (60°/s) performed at baseline, 4 weeks after program initiation, and 8 weeks after program initiation revealed right knee peak torque values of 184, 205, and 213 N•m and left knee values of 210, 217, and 211 N•m, respectively. This patient's VAS and AKPS score improvements over the course of rehabilitation, returning to work, and returning to running indicate significant subjective clinical improvement since his initial presentation with PFPS. Single-leg hop for distance test and triple-hop for distance test improvements suggest improved function. Right knee extensor strength improvements demonstrate objective evidence of improved quadriceps femoris strength.

Patient C: Local Factors

Patient C is a 23-year-old woman who presented with right peripatellar pain which had been present for approximately 2 weeks. The pain was acute in onset after beginning Zumba classes five times per week as part of a New Year's resolution. She stated that stair climbing, sitting, kneeling, and squatting exacerbated right knee pain. She also appeared to be somewhat distressed admitting that she thinks about the pain all the time and is beginning to "feel as though I will always have this pain." Her clinical evaluation was negative for any anatomical or biomechanical abnormalities. However, she has experienced recent excessive patellofemoral joint loading secondary to high-volume Zumba class participation without lead up. Also, her psychological assessment was positive for catastrophic thinking and increased mental distress. In relationship to this excessive loading, the rehabilitation clinician recommended NSAIDs for short-term pain and inflammation relief, no Zumba classes until the pain subsided, and an eventual slow return to Zumba to avoid recurrence. Since this patient had catastrophic thoughts, she was referred to a psychologist to better manage this mental distress. The rehabilitation clinician performed outcome measures at baseline and 4 weeks (when she was able to return to Zumba classes). Her VAS score improved from 6 at baseline to 2 at 4 weeks following program initiation. Her AKPS score improved from 55 at baseline to 92 at 4 weeks following program initiation. Right lower extremity single-leg hop for distance test improved from 119 cm at baseline to 127 cm at 4 weeks, while the left lower extremity remained steady at 136 cm and 135 cm, respectively. Her triple-hop for distance test distances over the same time period improved from 321 to 357 cm at the right lower extremity and from 394 to 398 cm at the left lower extremity. This patient demonstrated significant VAS and AKPS score improvements in addition to objective functional test score improvements. The relatively quick, condition improvement, particularly regarding subjective symptom testing, likely represents the amelioration of psychological factors that were initially contributing to her high pain level perception.

Summary

Treatment interventions for PFPS are as numerous as its potential causes. There is currently no consensus on relating particular etiologies to the treatments that address them in the most efficacious way. This is most likely, in part, due to the multifactorial and complex nature of PFPS. In the structured rehabilitation model we have described, patients are grouped by the region of likely PFPS cause and are then treated with associated evidence-based treatment modalities. This process enables rehabilitation clinicians to group patients with similar PFPS etiologies, thereby helping develop the more standardized care needed to increase the evidence basis of treatment interventions. Combined hip and knee musculature strengthening exercises display the greatest evidence-based treatment efficacy. Research designed to decrease pain and improve function among patients with PFPS should also implement this regional grouping approach to increase the evidence basis of treatment interventions.

Cross-References

- Patellar Dislocations: Overview
- Patellofemoral Problems in Adolescent Athletes
- Physiotherapy in Patellofemoral Pain Syndrome
- Return to Play after Acute Patellar Dislocation

References

Barton CJ, Levinger P, Menz HB et al (2009) Kinematic gait characteristics associated with patellofemoral pain syndrome: a systematic review. Gait Posture 30:405–416

Barton CJ, Bonanno D, Levinger P et al (2010) Foot and ankle characteristics in patellofemoral pain syndrome: a case control and reliability study. J Orthop Sports Phys Ther 40:286–296

Blond L, Hansen L (1998) Patellofemoral pain syndrome in athletes: a 5.7-year retrospective follow-up study of 250 athletes. Acta Orthop Belg 64:393–400

Bolgla LA, Boling MC (2011) An update for the conservative management of patellofemoral pain syndrome: a systematic review of the literature from 2000 to 2010. Int J Sports Phys Ther 6:112–125

Boling M, Padua D, Marshall S et al (2010) Gender differences in the incidence and prevalence of patellofemoral pain syndrome. Scand J Med Sci Sports 20:725–730

Bryk FF, Ruggerro AG, Lodovichi SS et al (2013) The influence of static passive stretching in sedentary women with patellofemoral pain syndrome: a randomized controlled trial. Proceedings of the Meeting Internacional Científico IBRAMED 2013 Oct 4–6; Amparo, São Paulo, Brazil. J Orthop Sports Phys Ther 43:A1–A2

Callaghan MJ, Selfe J (2012) Patellar taping for patellofemoral pain syndrome in adults. Cochrane Database Syst Rev 4:CD006717

Cook C, Mabry L, Reiman MP et al (2011) Best tests/clinical findings for screening and diagnosis of patellofemoral pain syndrome: a systematic review. Physiotherapy 98:93–100

Crossley KM, Bennell KL, Cowan SM et al (2004) Analysis of outcome measures for persons with patellofemoral pain: which are reliable and valid? Arch Phys Med Rehabil 85:815–822

Domenech J, Sanchis-Alfonso V, López L et al (2013) Influence of kinesiophobia and catastrophizing on pain and disability in anterior knee pain patients. Knee Surg Sports Traumatol Arthrosc 21:1562–1568

Draper CE, Besier TF, Fredericson M et al (2010) Differences in patellofemoral kinematics between weight-bearing and non-weight-bearing conditions in patients with patellofemoral pain. J Orthop Res 29:312–317

Fukuda TY, Rossetto FM, Magalhaes E et al (2010) Short-term effects of hip abductors and lateral rotators strengthening in females with patellofemoral pain syndrome: a randomized controlled clinical trial. J Orthop Sports Phys Ther 40:736–742

Harvie D, O'Leary T, Kumar S (2011) A systematic review of randomized controlled trials on exercise parameters in the treatment of patellofemoral pain: what works? J Multidiscip Healthc 4:383–392

Heintjes E, Berger MY, Bierma-Zeinstra SM et al (2004) Pharmacotherapy for patellofemoral pain syndrome. Cochrane Database Syst Rev 3:CD003470

Jensen R, Hystad T, Baerheim A (2005) Knee function and pain related to psychological variables in patients with long-term patellofemoral pain syndrome. J Orthop Sports Phys Ther 35:594–600

Kaya D, Citaker S, Kerimoglu U et al (2011) Women with patellofemoral pain syndrome have quadriceps femoris volume and strength deficiency. Knee Surg Sports Traumatol Arthrosc 19:242–247

Khayambashi K, Mohammadkhani Z, Ghaznavi K et al (2012) The effects of isolated hip abductor and external rotator muscle strengthening on pain, health status, and hip strength in females with patellofemoral pain: a randomized controlled trial. J Orthop Sports Phys Ther 42:22–29

Lake DA, Wofford NH (2011) Effect of therapeutic modalities on patients with patellofemoral pain syndrome: a systematic review. Sports Health 3:182–189

Lankhorst NE, Bierma-Zeinstra SM, Van Middelkoop M (2012) Risk factors for patellofemoral pain syndrome: a systematic review. J Orthop Sports Phys Ther 42(81–94):A1–A12

Lee S, Souza RB, Powers CM (2012) The influence of hip abductor muscle performance on dynamic postural stability in females with patellofemoral pain. Gait Posture 36:425–429

Maffiuletti NA (2010) Assessment of hip and knee muscle function in orthopaedic practice and research. J Bone Joint Surg Am 92(1):220–229

Mann G, Constantini N, Hetsroni I et al (2007) Anterior knee-pain syndrome. Adolesc Med State Art Rev 18:192–220

Meira EP, Brumitt J (2011) Influence of the hip on patients with patellofemoral pain syndrome: a systematic review. Sports Health 3:455–465

Pappas E, Wong-Tom WM (2012) Prospective predictors of patellofemoral pain syndrome: a systematic review with meta-analysis. Sports Health 4:115–120

Pattyn E, Mahieu N, Selfe J et al (2012) What predicts functional outcome after treatment for patellofemoral pain? Med Sci Sports Exerc 44:1827–1833

Petersen W, Ellermann A, Gösele-Koppenburg A et al (2013) Patellofemoral pain syndrome. Knee Surg Sports Traumatol Arthrosc [Epub ahead of print]

Powers CM (2010) The influence of abnormal hip mechanics on knee injury: a biomechanical perspective. J Orthop Sports Phys Ther 40:42–51

Powers CM, Bolgla LA, Callaghan MJ et al (2012) Patellofemoral pain: proximal, local, and distal factors. J Orthop Sports Phys Ther 42:A1–A18

Prins MR, van der Wurff P (2009) Females with patellofemoral pain syndrome have weak hip muscles: a systematic review. Aust J Physiother 55:9–15

Taunton JE, Ryan MB, Clement DB et al (2002) A retrospective case-control analysis of 2002 running injuries. Br J Sports Med 36:95–101

Warden SJ, Hinman RS, Watson MA et al (2008) Patellar taping and bracing for the treatment of chronic knee pain: a systematic review and meta-analysis. Arthritis Rheum 59:73–83

White LC, Dolphin P, Dixon J (2009) Hamstring length in patellofemoral pain syndrome. Physiotherapy 95:24–28

Willy RW, Manal KT, Witvrouw EE et al (2012) Are mechanics different between male and female runners with patellofemoral pain? Med Sci Sports Exerc 44:2165–2171

Witonski D (1999) Anterior knee pain syndrome. Int Orthop 23:341–344

Witvrouw E, Werner S, Mikkelsen C et al (2005) Clinical classification of patellofemoral pain syndrome: guidelines for non-operative treatment. Knee Surg Sports Traumatol Arthrosc 13:122–130

Yosmaoglu HB, Kaya D, Guney H et al (2013) Is there a relationship between tracking ability, joint position sense, and functional level in patellofemoral pain syndrome. Knee Surg Sports Traumatol Arthrosc 21:2564–2571

Anatomic Double-Tunnel Anterior Cruciate Ligament Reconstruction: Evolution and Principles

129

Garth N. Walker, Anne L. Versteeg, Liang R. Cui, Carola F. van Eck, and Freddie H. Fu

Contents

G.N. Walker
University of Pittsburgh Medical Center, Pittsburgh, PA, USA
e-mail: garth.walkerfu@gmail.com

A.L. Versteeg
Department of Orthopaedics Surgery, University Medical Center Utrecht, Utrecht, The Netherlands
e-mail: annelversteeg@gmail.com

L.R. Cui • C.F. van Eck
Department of Orthopaedic Surgery, University of Pittsburgh Medical Center, Pittsburgh, PA, USA
e-mail: richardbien@gmail.com; vaneckf@upmc.edu

F.H. Fu (✉)
Department of Orthopaedic Surgery, University of Pittsburgh School of Medicine, Pittsburgh, PA, USA
e-mail: ffu@msx.upmc.edu

M.N. Doral, J. Karlsson (eds.), *Sports Injuries*,
DOI 10.1007/978-3-642-36569-0_91

Abstract

Anterior cruciate ligament (ACL) rupture is a common sports injury, especially in young individuals involved in cutting, pivoting, and contact sports. Although treatment options include conservative management as well as surgical intervention, most active individuals will require surgical reconstruction of the ACL in order to be able to return to their pre-injury activity level. Individualized anatomic ACL reconstruction is a surgical technique which tailors the ACL surgery to the individual patient. It uses preoperative measurements on plain radiographs and MRI as well as intraoperative measurement of the patients' native ACL and knee anatomy in order to replicate it as closely as possible. The goal of anatomic ACL reconstruction is to restore the ACL to its native dimensions, collagen orientation, and insertion site. This chapter will address all the steps involved in individualized anatomic ACL reconstruction.

Historic Review

Anterior cruciate ligament (ACL) ruptures are one of the most common sports injuries nationwide, affecting roughly 30 out of every 100,000 people each year (Gianotti et al. 2009). Injury to the ACL is potentially devastating for the patient and can result in both acute and long-term clinical problems. Consequently, the ACL has always been and continues to be of great interest to orthopedic scientists and clinicians worldwide. Major advancements in ACL surgery have been made in the past few years. ACL reconstruction has shifted from an open to arthroscopic procedure, in which a two- and later one-incision technique was applied. However, although these new techniques were fast and efficient; identical reproduction of native ACL anatomy was not obtained. Studies have shown, for example, that the transtibial arthroscopic single-bundle ACL reconstruction does not fully restore rotational stability of the knee joint (Debandi et al. 2013). In addition, several studies show that up to 50 % of patients developed osteoarthritis within 12 years after this procedure (Lohmander et al. 2004; Li et al. 2011). As such, a more anatomic approach to ACL reconstruction has emerged. Individualized anatomic ACL reconstruction aims to restore the ACL to its native dimensions, collagen orientation, and insertion site. It is a concept that can be applied to single-bundle and double-bundle reconstruction, augmentation, and revision surgery (Fu et al. 2014).

Anatomy

The anatomy of the ACL has been described in detail as early as 1836 by Weber and Weber (1836). It consists of two functional bundles, the anteromedial (AM) and the posterolateral (PL) bundle named according to their tibial insertion site. The origin of the AM bundle is at the superior-posterior site of the femoral origin; it inserts at the anteromedial site of the tibial ACL insertion and has a close relationship with the anterior horn of the lateral meniscus. On the contrary, the PL bundle originates more distally at the femoral origin, inserts at the posterolateral site of the tibial insertion, and has a close relationship with the posterior horn of the lateral meniscus. The two bundles are separated by a distinct septum, containing vascular-derived stem cells, and are covered by a thin membrane (Matsumoto et al. 2012).

Two bony ridges define the femoral attachment site, the lateral intercondylar ridge and the lateral bifurcate ridge. The lateral intercondylar ridge, also called the resident's ridge, was first described by Dr. Clancy (Hutchinson and Ash 2003). It is an important landmark during ACL reconstruction as the femoral insertion of the native ACL always inserts inferior to this ridge. Another important landmark is the lateral bifurcate ridge; this ridge runs perpendicular to the lateral intercondylar ridge and separates the AM and PL bundles (Ferretti et al. 2007). The size of the femoral insertion site is reported to vary from 12 to 20 mm, with 66.3 % of the insertions between 16 and 18 mm. The width of the insertion site of the AM bundle is between 8 and 10 mm and the PL bundle between 6 and 8 mm (Kopf et al. 2011).

Many different anatomical landmarks have been described in the literature to identify the tibial insertion site, most often the anterior horn of the lateral meniscus and the anterior edge of the posterior cruciate ligament. However, these are soft tissue structures and therefore may have a varying anatomical relation with the ACL (Ferretti et al. 2012). A recent study tried therefore to identify bony landmarks for the tibial insertion site. The medial eminence and the intermeniscal ligament demonstrated to be the most reliable to identify the tibial insertion site of the ACL (Ferretti et al. 2012).

Biomechanics

Biomechanically, the AM and PL bundle function together to provide stability throughout knee range of motion. The AM bundle length stays constant during knee range of motion, showing the highest tension between 45° and 60° degrees of knee flexion. The PL bundle has its highest tension in full extension and decreases tension during knee flexion. The bundles are parallel in extension and cross each other during flexion. The AM bundle is primarily responsible for stabilization of the knee in the anterior-posterior direction, whereas the PL bundle allows knee rotation (Yagi et al. 2002).

The AM and PL bundle exposure to in situ forces is different. The forces experienced by each bundle are complementary in nature, with the AM bundle experiencing a majority of the load across all flexion angles and PL at lower flexion angles, most specifically 0–30° (Wu et al. 2010). Knowledge of the biomechanical relationship of the two bundles is important in anatomic ACL reconstruction. If the AM and PL bundle are restored anatomically, the grafts should experience the same forces as the native ACL. If the grafts are placed in a nonanatomic position, the graft will see lower than normal forces (Yagi et al. 2002; Kato et al. 2013). This may lead to a lower chance of graft failure, but these forces can be distributed through the joint, increasing the contact pressure of the cartilage, which may predispose to early osteoarthritis (Chu et al. 2014).

History and Physical Examination

A comprehensive history is a fundamental part of the patient evaluation. It can reveal the injury mechanism, the activity level of the patient, and their desire to return to their pre-injury sport. This is followed by a detailed physical examination which must include the Lachman test, pivot shift test, and anterior drawer test. Using these specific tests, it can be determined if the ACL is completely ruptured or if a partial ACL injury is present. For example, a positive Lachman test in the setting of a normal pivot shift test could point toward an isolated AM bundle injury. The KT arthrometer can be used to quantify the anterior tibial translation of the injured knee and compare this to the contralateral non-injured knee (van Eck et al. 2013b, c). Of course a full examination of the knee should be performed to evaluate for concomitant injuries.

Preoperative Imaging

Plain Radiographs

Patients evaluated for an ACL injury should have a complete knee series done. This should include an AP and lateral of the knee, as well as a sunrise view. In addition, flexion weight-bearing radiographs of the bilateral knee should be done. Preoperative radiographs can provide useful information about the bony morphology of the knee, the alignment, arthritic changes, bone quality, and the status of the physes.

Magnetic Resonance Imaging (MRI)

MRI imaging of the affected knee is routinely performed. MRI is useful in providing the conclusive diagnosis of ACL rupture but also helps to determine if there is partial versus complete injury and whether concomitant injuries are present. A 1.5 tesla magnet and scan of the knee can be used according to a specifically designed ACL protocol. This scans the knee in line with the fibers of the ACL, allowing evaluation of the AM and PL bundle individually (Casagranda et al. 2009).

However, MRI is also essential in preoperative planning. The size of the native ACL insertion site, ACL length, and inclination angle can be measured on the sagittal MRI. The normal range for the insertion site size is 12–22 mm for the tibial side and 12–20 mm femoral side. The normal length of the ACL is between 25 and 45 mm. The inclination angle of the native ACL varies from 43° to 57°. The inclination angle is determined by the position of the femoral ACL insertion site on the medial wall of the lateral femoral condyle. A higher position will result in a more vertical ACL and a higher angle. The goal of individualized anatomic ACL reconstruction is to place the ACL graft in such a way as to restore the native ACL's inclination angle. On postoperative MRI the inclination angle can be compared before and after ACL reconstruction to ensure the graft was not placed too vertically (high) in the notch, which can lead to impingement and graft failure (Illingworth et al. 2011).

Lastly, the size of available tendons for possible graft options can be measured. The size of the quadriceps and patellar tendons can be measured on the sagittal MRI. This also allows the surgeon to measure the patella itself to determine how large of a bone block can be harvested without risking postoperative patella fractures. The size of the hamstring tendon can be measured on the axial MRI sequence. These measurements will allow the surgeon to determine what graft options are available for a specific patient and if allograft tissue needs to be considered.

Graft Choices

Despite the generally good outcomes after ACL reconstruction, there is still an ongoing debate about the best graft option. The optimal graft would display some specific characteristics; it can closely reproduce the histology and kinematics of the native ACL, is of sufficient length and width, is easily available, is low in costs, and has minor or none donor site morbidity (Bonasia et al. 2012). Over the past decades many different graft types have been used in ACL reconstruction, such hamstring or patella tendon autograft, synthetic grafts, Achilles tendon allograft, and tibialis anterior or posterior allograft. Choice for a specific graft is made up on patient demands, the preference of the surgeon, and the patient.

Each graft type has benefits and limitations. Bone-patellar tendon-bone (BPTB) autograft has bone-to-bone healing in the tunnels, which can lead to faster healing and return to sports (Bartlett et al. 2001). Disadvantages of using the patella tendon autograft are the risk on patella fracture during or after surgery, anterior knee pain, weakness of the extensor mechanism, and paresthesia

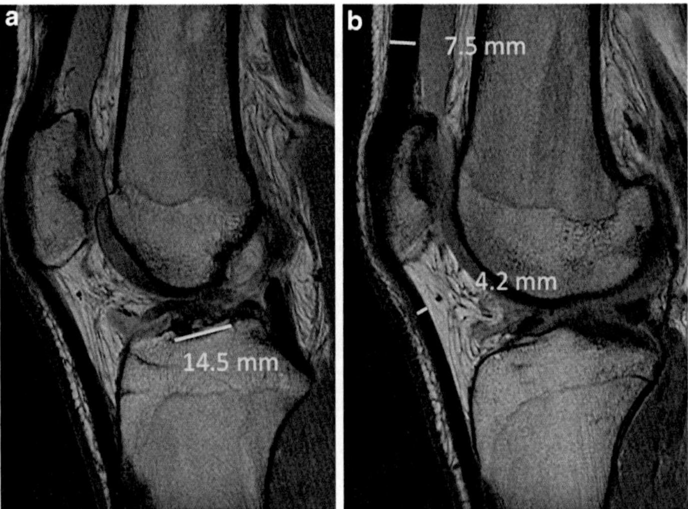

Fig. 1 (**a**) Sagittal MRI of the knee showing measurement of the tibial insertion site of the ACL. (**b**) Measurement of quadriceps and patellar tendon thickness

due to damages of the infrapatellar branch of the saphenous nerve (Bartlett et al. 2001).

Hamstring autograft has gained widespread popularity over the last decades and is by far the most used graft for ACL reconstruction in Europe (Persson et al. 2014). The hamstring graft is an all soft tissue graft and therefore requires bone-to-tendon healing which takes significantly longer compared to the bone-to-bone healing of the BPTB (Bartlett et al. 2001). However, the quadrupled hamstring autograft can resist increased tensile load and appears to be stiffer compared to a BPTB and even compared to the native ACL (Brown et al. 1993). A recent meta-analysis comparing hamstring and BPTB autograft showed no differences in outcomes in terms of restoring knee function (Li et al. 2012). Disadvantages of the hamstring autograft are a knee flexion deficit and paresthesia due to damage of the saphenous nerve (Bartlett et al. 2001). In addition, a hamstring autograft may not be the graft of first choice in patients having a concurrent MCL injury, as the hamstrings may also serve as stabilizers of the medial side of the knee.

The quadriceps tendon can be used as an autograft. The graft consists of the central third of the quadriceps tendon and can include a bone block from the upper pole of the patella, or it can be soft tissue only. The quadriceps tendon is the thickest graft for ACL reconstruction with an average of 8 mm, more closely replicating the dimensions of the native ACL. Another, advantage of the quadriceps tendon is the ability to use it for single- and double-bundle ACL reconstruction by splitting the graft if necessary. For double-bundle reconstruction, one option is a single tunnel on the femoral side for the end of the graft with the bone block, while the soft tissue end splits allowing for a separate AM and PL tunnel on the tibial side. This has the advantage of having bone-to-bone healing on the femoral side while allowing separate tensioning of the bundles on the tibial side. The quadriceps tendon autograft also has less anterior knee pain compared to the BPTB graft. Potential disadvantages are a decrease in strength of the extensor apparatus and a patella fracture as with the BPTB (Rabuck et al. 2013).

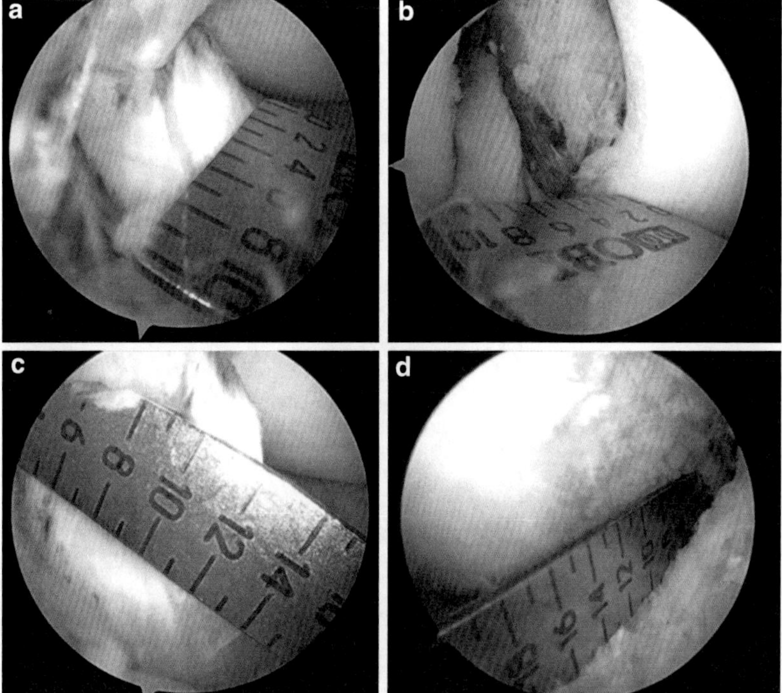

Fig. 2 (**a**) Intraoperative arthroscopic measurement of the tibial insertion site length (14 mm) using a ruler for calculating PRA. (**b**) Tibial med width (9 mm). (**c**) A relatively narrow notch width (9 mm). (**d**) Femoral insertion site length (14 mm)

Allografts have the advantage of improved cosmetics and absence of donor site morbidity. Inherent to the use of allografts is the risks on disease transmission and immune reactions compromising graft healing and graft incorporation. Various studies, however, have reported a higher failure rate in ACL reconstructions using allografts (van Eck et al. 2012). A failure rate of 13 % in recent publications has been found. Factors associated with an increased risk of graft failure were earlier return to sport, younger age, and increased body weight. The association of earlier return to sport participation may be explained by the delayed ligamentization process of an allograft compared to an autograft (van Eck et al. 2012).

Rupture Pattern

The etiology of ACL ruptures is still poorly understood. Different injury mechanisms such as hyperextension, hyperflexion, or a valgus-external rotation injury are known to cause ACL rupture. Schenck et al. already demonstrated a different rupture pattern in low- versus high-energy traumas in a biomechanical hyperextension model (Schenck et al. 1999). Zantop et al. were the first to conduct a prospective study to observe ACL rupture pattern during arthroscopy in 121 patients. Patients who only experienced one episode of instability were selected and were operated within 120 days of original trauma. Most of these patients (75 %) demonstrated a combined tear of the AM and PL bundle, and only in 12 % of the cases the PL bundle was intact.

It is important to understand the concept of variation in the rupture pattern of the ACL when examining a patient and preparing for ACL reconstruction. In the case of a single-bundle tear, preservation of the remaining bundle has the potential to facilitate improved vascularization, improved healing, as well as improved proprioception because of the remaining neuroreceptors. Additionally, the remnant serves as a landmark during surgery for tunnel positioning for the graft (Dejour et al. 2013).

Surgical Technique

Next, we will describe preferred surgical techniques for individualized anatomic ACL reconstruction (van Eck et al. 2013a). The patient is placed supine on the operating table. The injured knee is placed in a leg holder with an unsterile tourniquet around the upper thigh and enabling 120° of knee flexion. A three-portal technique is used with a high anterolateral portal, central portal, and accessory medial portal (Araujo et al. 2011). This approach allows visualization of all the structures within the knee, as well as precise placement of the femoral and tibial tunnels

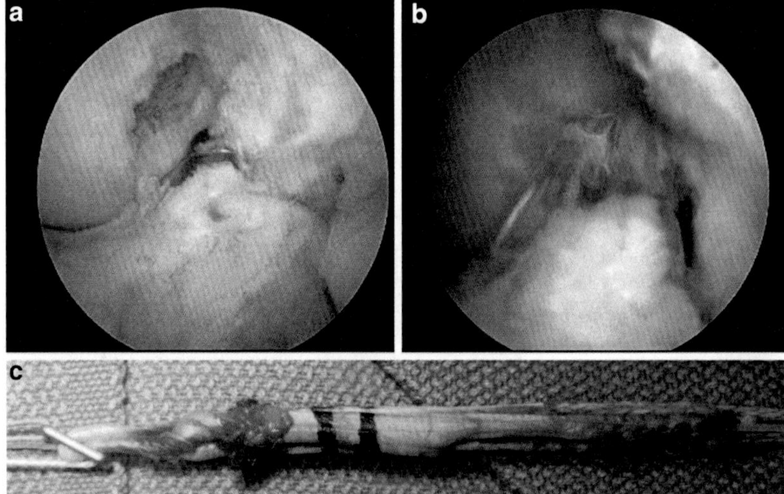

Fig. 3 (**a**) Arthroscopic view of drilled single tibial and femoral tunnel. (**b**) Graft in place. (**c**) Hamstring tendon autograft

Table 1 Percentage area reconstruction derived from measurements performed in Fig. 2

	Native ACL dimensions	Tunnel dimensions	
	Area (mm^2)	Area (mm^2)	Percent area reconstructed (PRA)
Tibial	14 mm × 10 mm	8 mm at 55°	56 %
	109.96	61.32	
Femoral	14 × 7 mm	8 mm × 8 mm	65 %
	76.97	50.26	

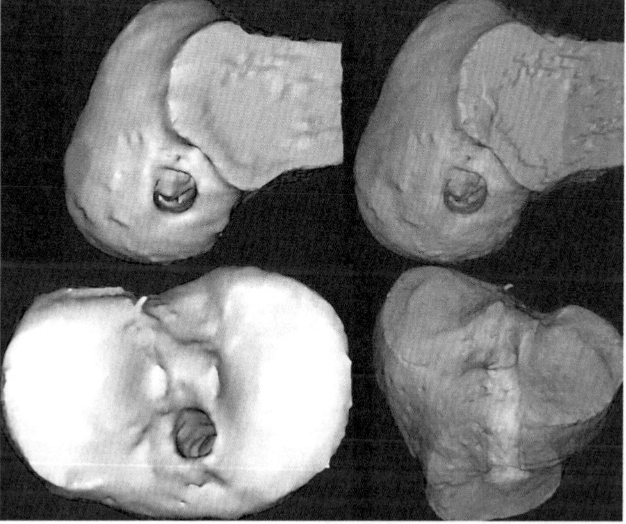

Fig. 4 Six-month postoperative 3D CT reconstruction showing locations of the tibial and femoral tunnels

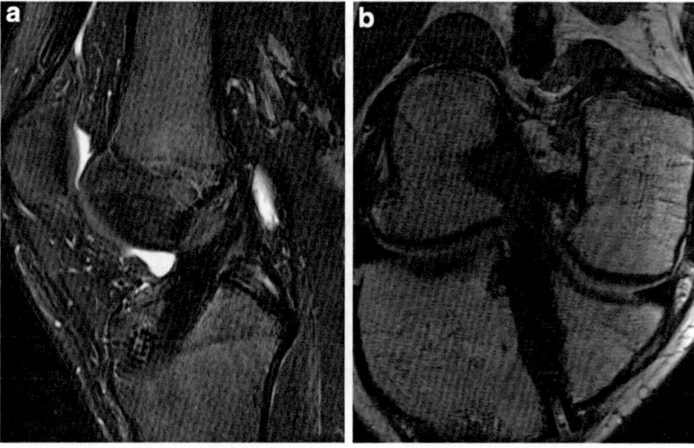

Fig. 5 (**a**) Six-month postoperative sagittal MRI after single-bundle ACL reconstruction with a hamstring tendon autograft. (**b**) Coronal oblique

The concept of individualized anatomical ACL reconstruction includes four principles. The first principle is to restore the two functional bundles of the ACL. The second principle is the ACL insertion sites on the tibia and femur should be restored by placing the tunnels in the native ACL footprint. The third principle is the correct tensioning pattern of each bundle. The fourth and final principle is individualized surgery for each patient (Shen et al. 2008).

After establishing the arthroscopic portals, a diagnostic arthroscopy is performed. This is to determine the extent of the ACL injury and the rupture pattern as well as to evaluate for possible concomitant injuries. The ACL remnant is then debrided to reveal the native insertion site location. The tibial and femoral insertion sites are marked and measured with an arthroscopic ruler. After this the size of the notch is measured. Similar to the preoperative MRI measurements, these intraoperative measurements will influence the decision for single- or double-bundle reconstruction. Single-bundle ACL reconstruction is generally considered if the tibial insertion site is smaller than 14 mm in length, if the width of the notch is smaller than 12 mm, if there is a multiple ligamentous knee injury, and when open physes are present in the knee with severe arthritis changes. Double-bundle ACL reconstruction is generally performed in patients with an insertion site larger than 14 mm in length and a notch width larger than 12 mm, especially in young athletes involved in cutting- or pivoting-type sports.

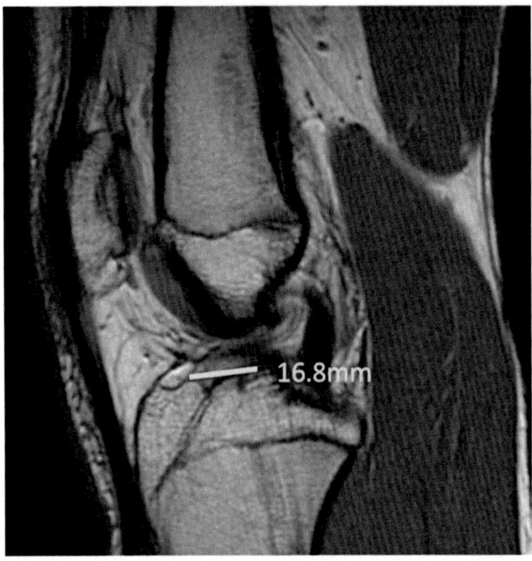

Fig. 6 Sagittal MRI of the knee showing the measurement of the tibial insertion site of the ACL. The insertion site is large enough for double-bundle ACL reconstruction

If single-bundle reconstruction is performed, the tibial and femoral tunnels are placed in the center of the tibial and femoral insertion site. If double-bundle reconstruction is performed, the tibial and femoral tunnels are placed in the center of the tibial and femoral AM and PL bundle insertion sites. The size of the tunnels is based on the size of the native ACL insertion site. After the tunnels are drilled, the graft is passed and routinely fixed on the femoral side with suspensory fixation and on the tibial side with interference fixation. For single-bundle reconstruction, the graft is fixed close to extension. For double-bundle reconstruction, the AM graft is fixed in 45° of flexion and the PL graft close to extension.

Postoperative evaluation is important to objectively evaluate surgical characteristics of anatomic ACL reconstruction. Middleton et al. used

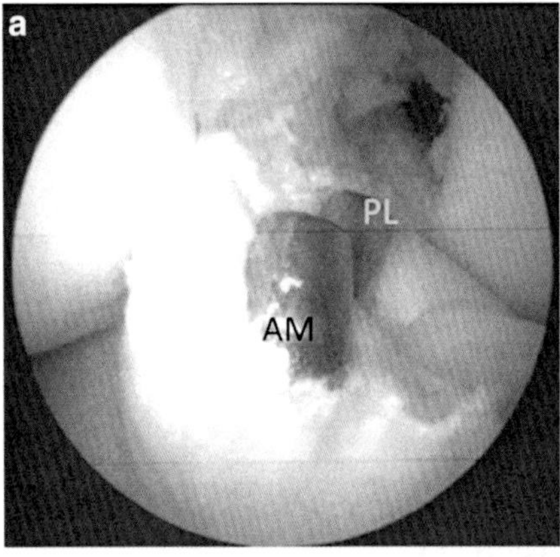

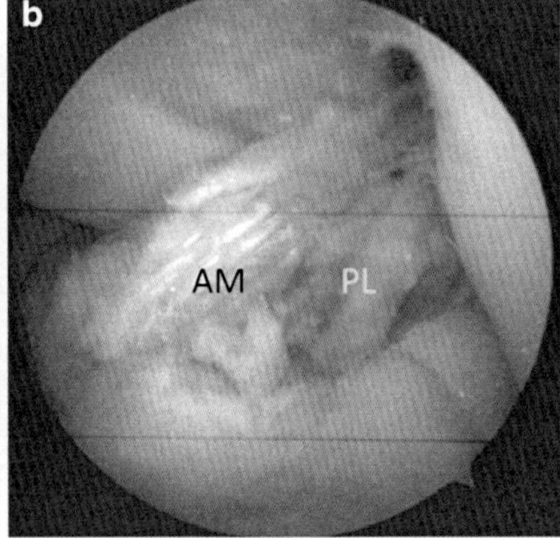

Fig. 7 (**a**) One tunnel is drilled on the femoral side for the quadriceps autograft bone block and a separate *AM* and *PL* tunnel on the tibial side for the split soft tissue end of the graft. (**b**) Graft in place with *PL* graft in *blue*

Table 2 Percentage area reconstruction (*PRA*) calculated from each patient's individual native insertion site dimensions and reconstructed tunnel dimensions based on the area of an ellipse. Tibial tunnel area also accounts for the oblique angle of the drill

	Native ACL dimensions	Tunnel dimensions	
	Area (mm^2)	Area (mm^2)	Percent area reconstructed (PRA)
Tibial	17 × 10 mm	AM: 7 mm at 55°	69 %
	125.651	46.98	
		PL: 6 mm at 55°	
		39.99	
		Total reconstructed AM + PL	
		86.97	
Femoral	12 × 7 mm	8 × 8 mm	76 %
	65.97	50.26	

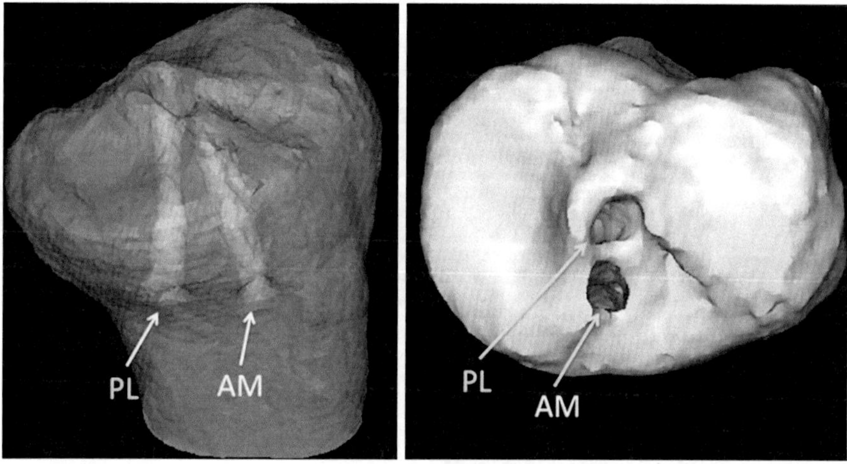

Fig. 8 3D CT reconstruction showing individual *AM* and *PL* tunnel in the tibia

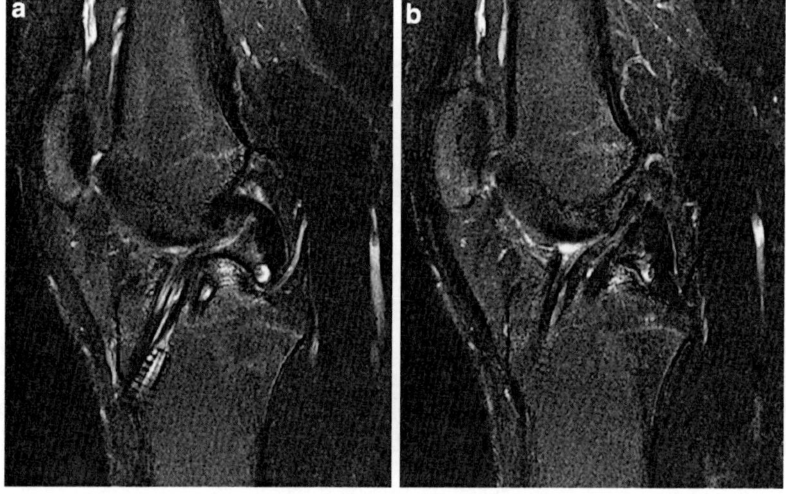

Fig. 9 Postoperative MRI after double-bundle ACL reconstruction using quadriceps tendon autograft with a single bone block on the femoral side and split soft tissue end for a separate AM and PL bundle graft on the tibial side

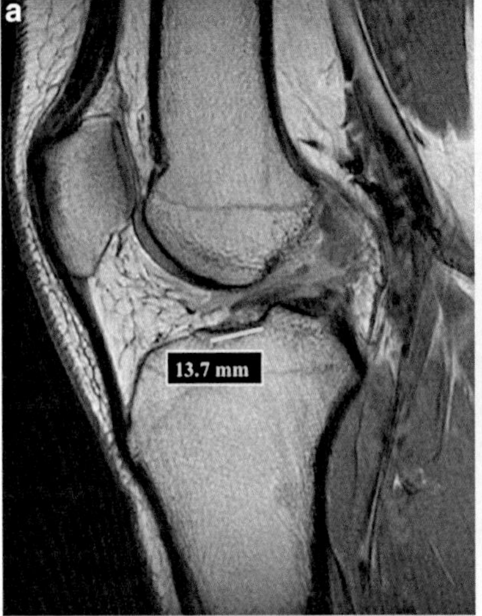

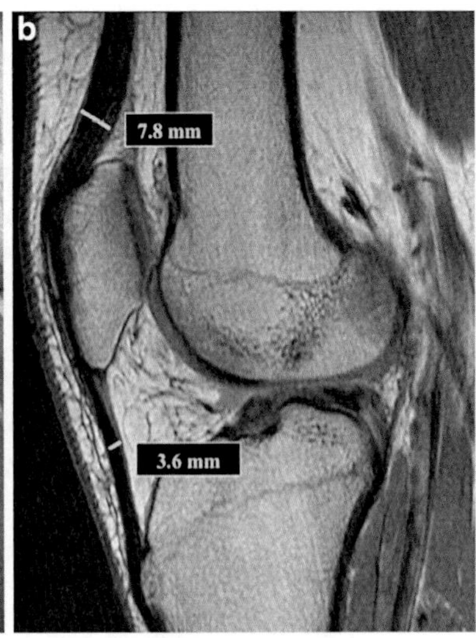

Fig. 10 (**a**) Sagittal MRI of the knee showing measurement of the tibial insertion site of the ACL. (**b**) Measurement of thickness of quadriceps and patellar tendon

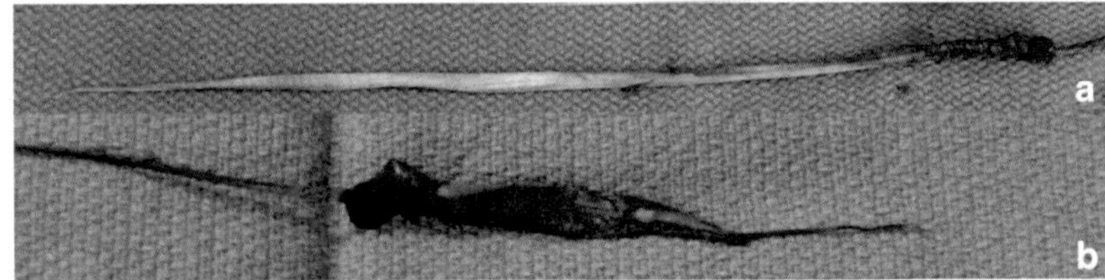

Fig. 11 (**a**) Very small gracilis tendon autograft. (**b**) Semitendinosus tendon autograft at 2.5 mm diameter and 5 mm in a double loop

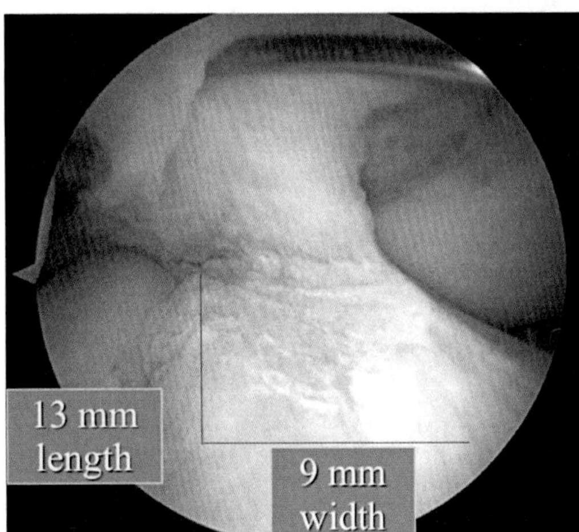

Fig. 12 Arthroscopic view of the tibial insertion site of the ACL

the area of an ellipse to calculate the percentage reconstruction of the native insertion site by collecting dimensions of each patient's native insertion site and the graft intraoperatively. This percentage reconstructed area (PRA) can be calculated to aid the physician in how successful that surgeon was in providing adequate graft for the reconstruction to be as close as possible to native dimensions (Middleton et al. 2014). At our institution, we aim for 60–80 % restoration with the graft of choice in DB and SB surgery.

Rehabilitation and Return to Sports

Rehabilitation after anatomic ACL reconstruction follows rehabilitation guidelines that are similar to those after traditional non-anatomic single-bundle ACL reconstruction. Initially thoughts concerning that anatomic double-bundle ACL reconstruction might interfere with restoration of range of motion; however, clinically, this has not been the case. In fact, earlier and fuller return of the range of both extension and flexion of the knee after anatomic ACL reconstruction has been documented (Fu et al. 2008). Another concern is that based on biomechanical studies, graft forces are higher when the graft is positioned

Table 3 Percentage reconstruction of this patient's tibial insertion site varying with graft diameter. With and without allograft augmentation is shown in underline and bold, respectively

Graft diameter (mm)	Percentage reconstructed area of tibial insertion site
4	17 %
5	*26 %*
6	38 %
7	51 %
8	68 %
9	**84 %**

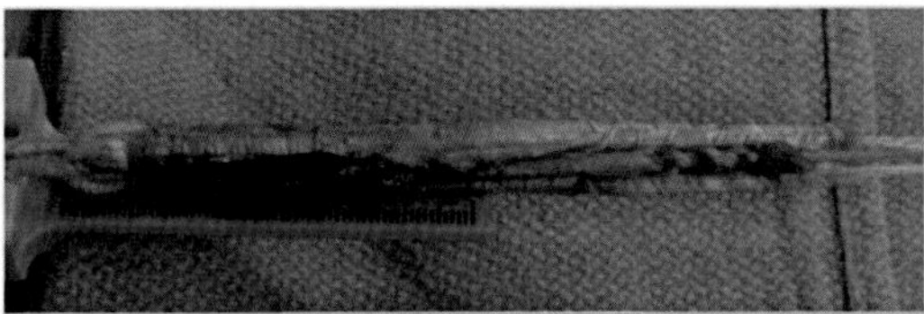

Fig. 13 Hybrid graft with semitendinosus autograft augmented with allograft

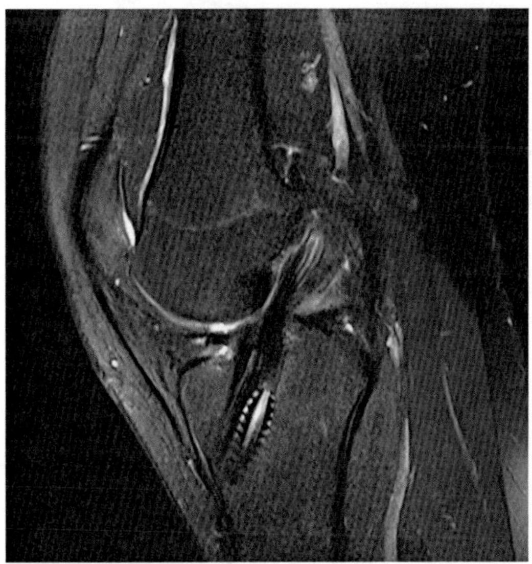

Fig. 14 Postoperative MRI after ACL reconstruction with an autograft-allograft hybrid

anatomically (Kato et al. 2013). For this reason initiation of functional activities that place a high load on the graft, such as jumping, cutting, pivoting, and return to sport, is progressed somewhat slower after anatomic ACL reconstruction.

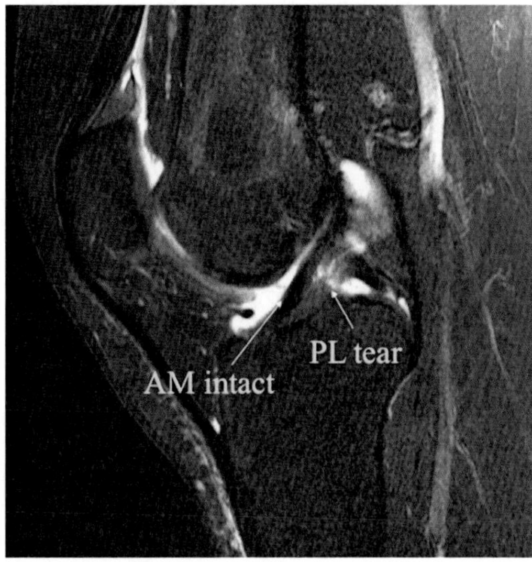

Fig. 15 Sagittal MRI with increased signal in the *PL* bundle consistent with rupture while the *AM* bundle appears intact

Immediately after surgery, the focus of postoperative rehabilitation is to minimize pain and swelling, restore full passive extension symmetrical to the non-involved knee, achieve 90–100° of knee flexion, restore the ability to perform a straight leg raise without a quadriceps lag, and progress to full weight bearing so that the individual can walk without assistive devices or a gait deviations.

During the first 4–6 weeks after surgery, the rehabilitation program is gradually progressed to involve active and active-assisted range of motion exercises in order to restore range of motion as tolerated. Gait training is also initiated.

Three to four months after surgery, the patient can be progressed to running on a treadmill or over the ground at a slow pace for 5–10 min every other day. The running program is gradually increased as long as the patient does not develop pain, swelling, or gait asymmetries.

Because of the individual variation, progression through the functional training and return to sports phases should be based on progression of the patient and the absence of symptoms.

During the functional training and return to sport phases of rehabilitation after ACL reconstruction, emphasis is placed on strengthening

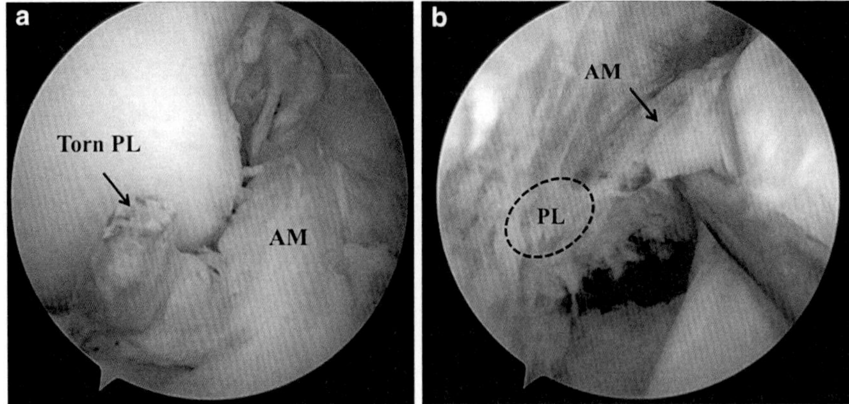

Fig. 16 (**a**) The *right* knee viewed from the central portal shows torn *PL* and intact *AM* bundle. (**b**) The *AM* bundle is being tested for integrity using a probe

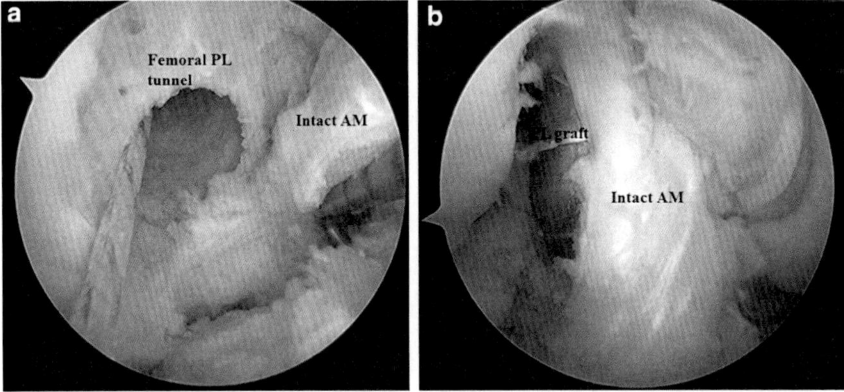

Fig. 17 (**a**) Tunnel for the PL tunnel is drilled in the native PL bundle insertion site, while care is taken not to injure the intact AM bundle. (**b**) PL augmentation graft in place next to the intact AM bundle

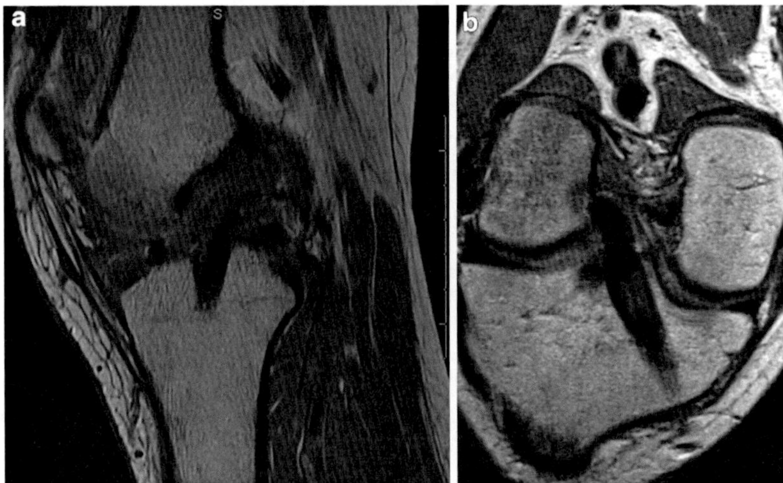

Fig. 18 Postoperative MRI at 6 months showing excellent graft healing of the PL graft and the intact AM bundle. (**a**) Sagittal sequence. (**b**) Coronal oblique sequence

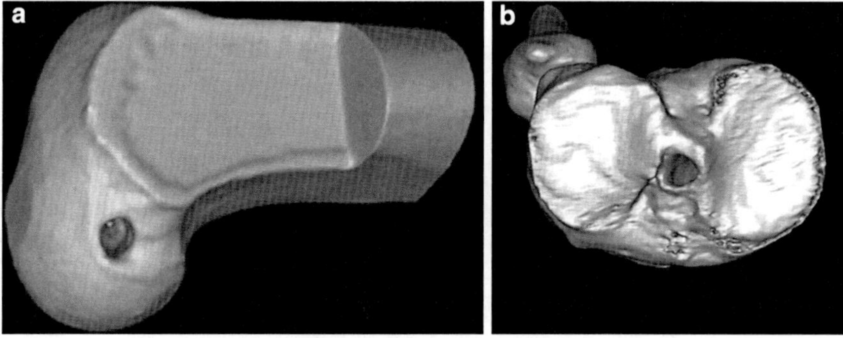

Fig. 19 3D reconstructed CT of the knee postoperatively showing the PL tunnel location. (**a**) Femur. (**b**) Tibia

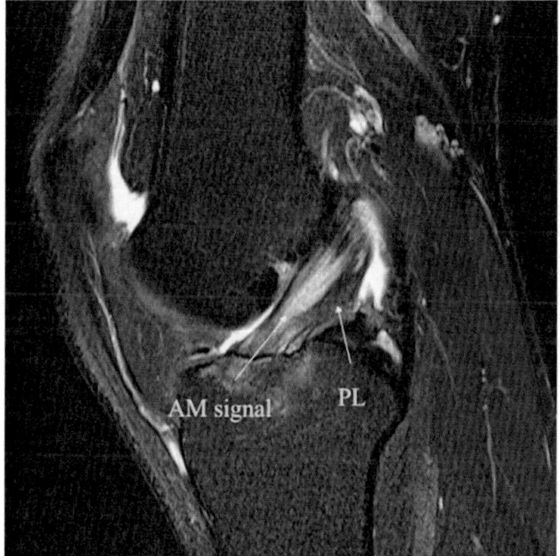

Fig. 20 Sagittal MRI with increased signal in the *AM* bundle and an intact *PL* bundle

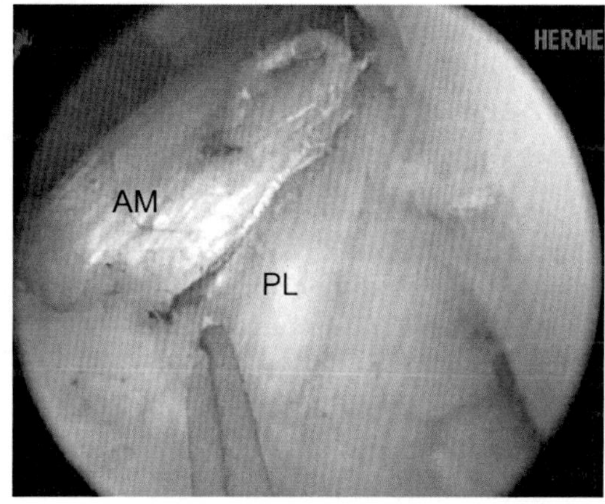

Fig. 21 Lateral portal view after *AM* augmentation with the *AM* graft in place passing anterior and medially to the native *PL* bundle

through the full range of motion, improving neuromuscular control, and a gradual increase in function that culminates with return to sports.

Once the patient is tolerating full-effort running, jumping, and agility drills, return to sports can be considered. The time frame for return to sport following anatomic ACL reconstruction is variable, but generally occurs 9–12 months after surgery.

If an athlete wants to return to sports sooner than the surgeon's postoperative protocol would permit, an MRI can be considered to evaluate the signal intensity of the graft to evaluate graft healing (Miyawaki et al. 2014).

Clinical Outcomes

Many studies have demonstrated superior clinical outcomes using anatomic ACL reconstruction techniques as compared to traditional non-anatomic ACL reconstruction. One example is a randomized clinical trial where three different techniques of ACL reconstruction was evaluated; conventional transtibial single-bundle, anatomic single-bundle, and anatomic double-bundle ACL reconrtuction. Three hundred and twenty patients were included and at the final follow-up, 281 patients were available. In all groups hamstring tendons were used with suspensory fixation on the femoral side, and bioabsorbable interference screw fixation on the tibial side.

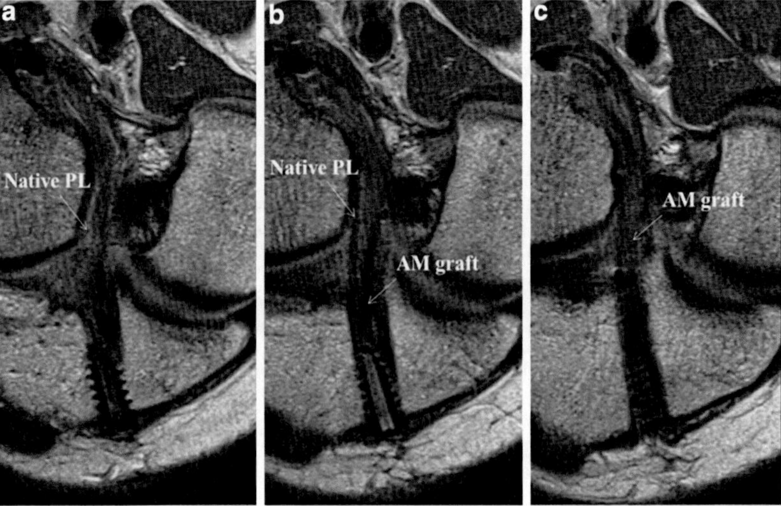

Fig. 22 Coronal oblique MRI postoperatively showing the AM augmentation graft and the native PL bundle in three subsequent cuts (**a**–**c**)

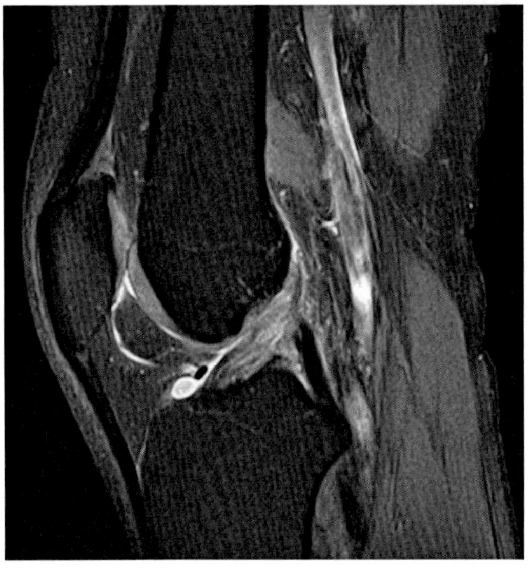

Fig. 23 Sagittal MRI with increased intensity in the proximal ACL

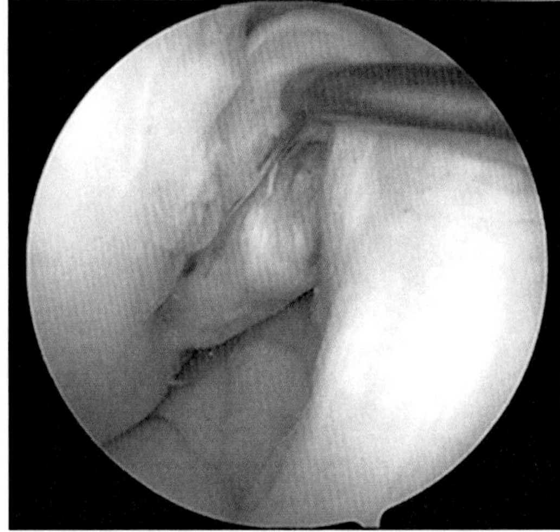

Fig. 24 Arthroscopic picture showing hemorrhage in the proximal ACL

The outcomes were evaluated by independent blinded observers using Lysholm score and subjective IKDC form. KT-1000 was used to evaluate anteroposterior stability and pivot shift was used for rotation stability. Average follow-up was 51.15 months (range 39–63). Anatomic single bundle resulted in superior anteroposterior and rotational stability than conventional single-bundle reconstruction. In addition, the results of anatomic double-bundle reconstruction were superior to the anatomic single-bundle reconstruction for anteroposterior and rotation stability (Hussein et al. 2012b).

A second study aimed to compare the results of single and double-bundle ACL reconstruction using an anatomic technique, individualized patients according to ACL anatomy as oppose to randomizing patients. The hypothesis stated that there would be no difference between the results of anatomic single-bundle and anatomic double-bundle reconstruction as long as the surgical technique is individualized. Depending on

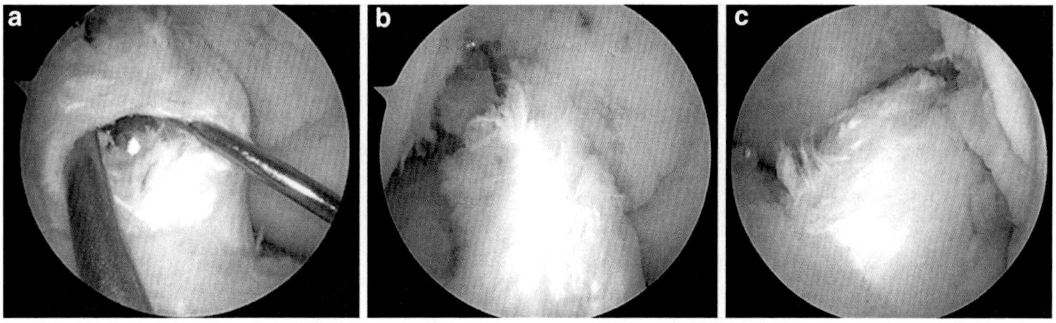

Fig. 25 (**a**–**c**) Sequence of remnant-preserving ACL reconstruction. A single soft tissue graft is passed amidst the remnant, while care is taken to leave as much of the remnant in place

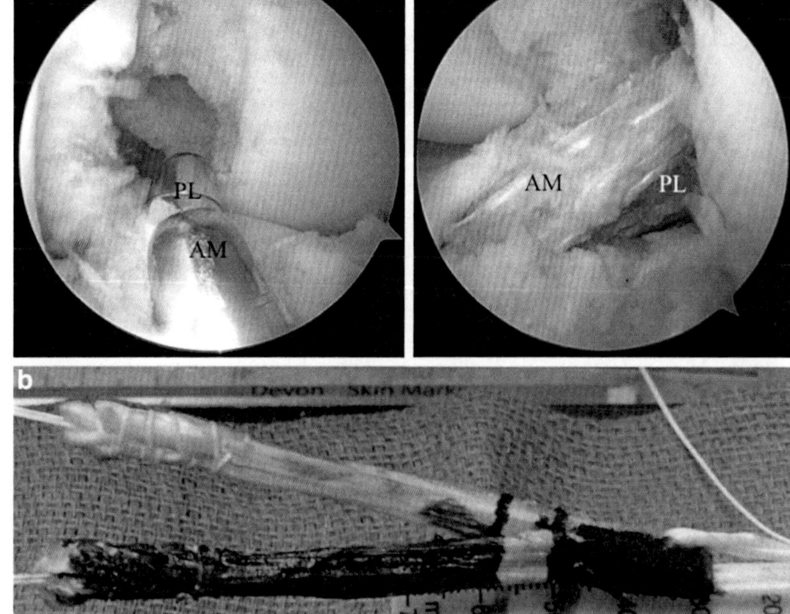

Fig. 26 Double-bundle reconstruction using quadriceps tendon autograft. (**a**) *AM* and *PL* tunnels are drilled. (**b**) Quadriceps tendon autograft with *PL* graft in *blue*. (**c**) End result

intraoperative measurements of the ACL insertion site size, patients were selected for either anatomic single- or double-bundle ACL reconstruction. There was no significant difference between the groups for Lysholm score (93.9 vs. 93.5), subjective IKDC (93.3 vs. 93.1), anterior tibial translation (1.5 vs. 1.6 mm side-to-side difference), and pivot shift (92 % vs. 90 % with negative pivot shift exam). This implies that anatomic double-bundle reconstruction is not superior to anatomic single-bundle reconstruction when an individualized ACL reconstruction technique is used (Hussein et al. 2012a).

Conclusion

In conclusion, individualized anatomic ACL reconstruction aims to restore the ACL to its native dimensions, collagen orientation, and insertion sites, with the aim to provide the patient with the best potential for a successful outcome. It is a concept rather than a technique and can be applied to single-bundle, double-bundle, augmentation, and revision surgery. Although this concept is new and long-term outcome studies are not yet available, biomechanical, kinematic, and

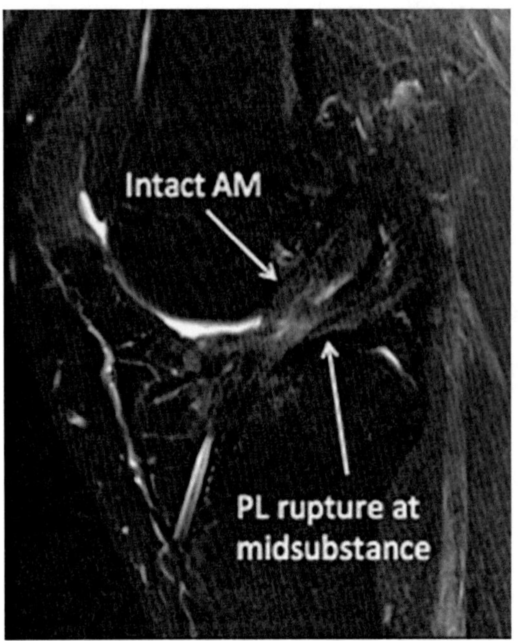

Fig. 27 Sagittal MRI demonstrates increased signal in the PL bundle consistent with mid-substance tear

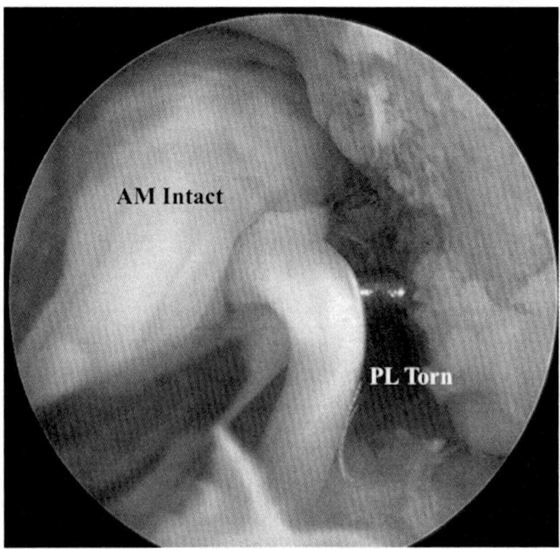

Fig. 28 Arthroscopic evaluation demonstrates increased laxity of the PL bundle consistent with rupture

short-term clinical studies show superior outcomes of anatomic ACL reconstruction over traditional ACL reconstruction techniques. The DB concept is a standard that can be mastered by all surgeons to achieve optimal, clinical, and kinematic outcomes. This translates to a decrease in the rate of early osteoarthritis after ACL reconstruction and that it will improve long-term knee health. The DB is an important concept to understand in order to be 100 % ACL surgeon to cover all presentations of ACL rupture.

Cases *Of note all cases presented below completed by one surgeon

Case 1

A 17-year-old female sustained a non-contact injury to her right knee while playing flag football. MRI demonstrated a complete ACL rupture. The tibial insertion site length measured 14.5 mm on sagittal MRI (Fig. 1). Native femoral and tibial insertion site dimensions as well as notch width were measured intraoperatively using a ruler and found to be small. A single-bundle ACL reconstruction using hamstring tendon autograft was performed (Figs. 2 and 3). The percentage of reconstructed ACL was calculated in Table 1. A 3D CT reconstruction and MRI were performed at 6 months postoperatively and shown in Figs. 4 and 5.

Case 2

A 17-year-old male sustained a knee injury after falling down a flight of stairs and complains of instability. MRI demonstrated a complete ACL rupture. His tibial insertion site length measured on sagittal MRI (16.8 mm) was amenable for a double-bundle reconstruction (Figs. 6 and 7). A quadriceps tendon autograft was used with a bone block on the femoral side and splitting the soft tissue end into a separate AM and PL bundle on the tibial side. The native ACL tibial and femoral insertion site dimensions were measured intraoperatively with a ruler, and percentage reconstructed areas were calculated (Table 2). MRI and 3D CT reconstructions were performed at 1.5 years postoperatively and shown in Figs. 8 and 9.

Case 3

A 16-year-old female sustained a knee injury while cheerleading and complains of instability. MRI shows ACL rupture. The tibial insertion site length is 13.7 mm measured on sagittal MRI. Quadriceps tendon and patellar tendon thickness measured on sagittal MRI were both relatively small, 7.8 and 3.6 mm, respectively (Fig. 10). The decision was made to harvest hamstring autograft. However, the semitendinosus was 2.5 mm in diameter and 5 mm in a double loop. The gracilis was unusable (Fig. 11). The native ACL tibial insertion site was measured with a ruler intraoperatively and found to be 13 mm in length and 9 mm in width (Fig. 12). The native tibia insertion site area was calculated using the formula of an ellipse. Using a 5 mm hamstring graft, only 26 % of the insertion site area would be restored (Table 3). An option is to supplement the harvested autograft with allograft. This patient received a hybrid semitendinosus allograft (9 mm diameter). This percentage reconstructed area was increased to 84 % using this method (Fig. 13).

MRI at follow-up showed a good graft position and size (Fig. 14).

Case 4

A 26-year-old male sustained a right knee injury during basketball. He presented 2 months after the initial injury. The exam revealed a 1B Lachman, +1 pivot shift, and 2 mm KT-1000 side-to-side difference. The sagittal MRI showed an isolated PL bundle tear (Fig. 15). Arthroscopy demonstrated a torn PL and intact AM (Fig. 16). A PL augmentation was performed using quadriceps tendon soft tissue autograft (Fig. 17). MRI and CT scan were done also and are shown in Figs. 18 and 19.

Case 5

A 37-year-old female sustained a twisting injury to her left knee. On exam there is a 2A Lachman, negative pivot shift, and 2 mm side-to-side difference on KT-1000 arthrometer testing.

The sagittal MRI demonstrates increased signal in the AM bundle (Fig. 20). Arthroscopy confirmed a ruptured AM bundle. An AM augmentation was performed (Fig. 21). MRI done postoperatively showed excellent graft healing of the AM graft with an intact PL bundle (Fig. 22).

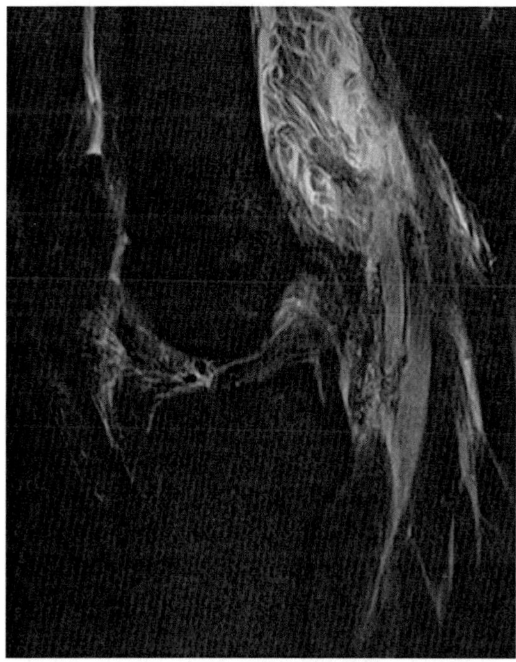

Fig. 29 Sagittal MRI demonstrates a complete ACL tear

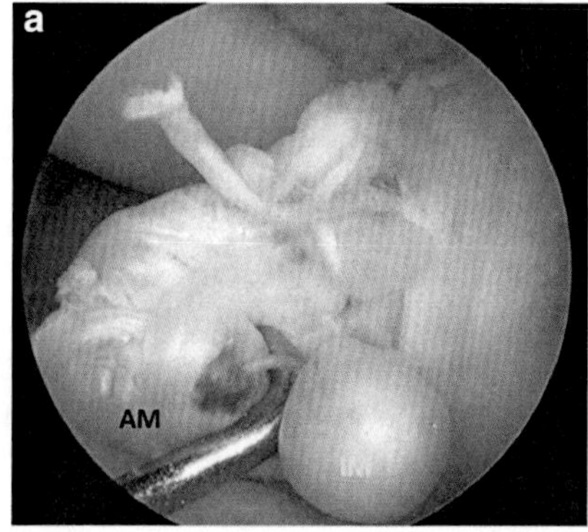

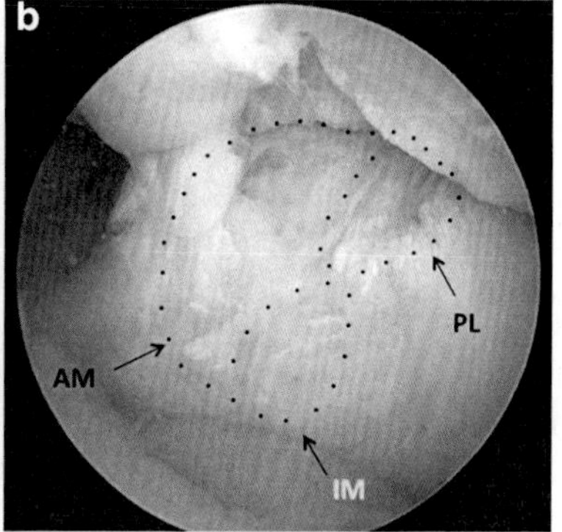

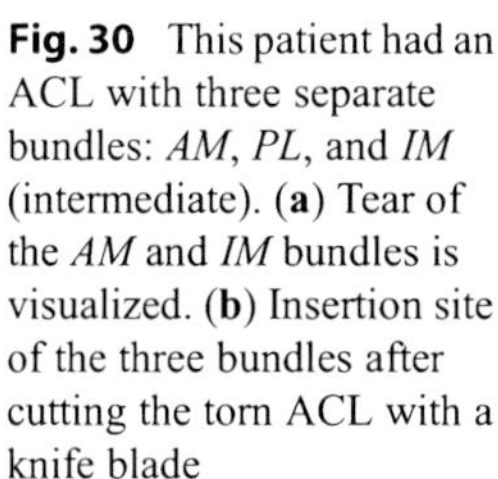

Fig. 30 This patient had an ACL with three separate bundles: *AM*, *PL*, and *IM* (intermediate). (**a**) Tear of the *AM* and *IM* bundles is visualized. (**b**) Insertion site of the three bundles after cutting the torn ACL with a knife blade

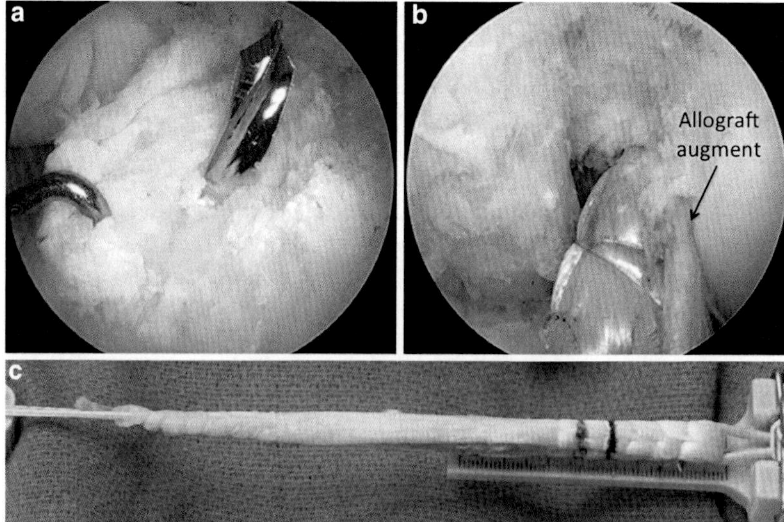

Fig. 31 Single-bundle ACL reconstruction with autograft/allograft hybrid. (**a**) Tibial tunnel position in the *center* of the tibial footprint. (**b**) End result after individualized anatomic single-bundle ACL reconstruction. (**c**) Hybrid graft consisting of hamstring autograft and semitendinosus allograft

Case 6

A 37-year-old male sustained a twisting injury to his right knee playing ice hockey. On exam there was a 2B Lachman, grade 1 pivot shift, and 3 mm difference on KT-1000 arthrometer testing. MRI demonstrated increased intensity of proximal ACL (Fig. 23). Arthroscopy revealed a complete proximal ACL tear (Fig. 24). A single-bundle ACL reconstruction was performed with a remnant-preserving technique (Fig. 25).

Case 7

A 23-year-old male sustained a left knee injury during soccer. His MRI revealed a complete ACL tear. He proceeded to undergo double-bundle ACL reconstruction with quadriceps tendon autograft (Fig. 26). At 13 months post-op, he sustained a contact reinjury. MRI obtained at an outside hospital was read as a complete ACL re-rupture. This did not fit with the patient's examination in the office which revealed a 1A Lachman and a negative pivot shift. So a new MRI was ordered with special coronal oblique cuts. The new MRI indicated a mid-substance re-rupture of the PL graft with the AM graft intact (Fig. 27). This was confirmed arthroscopically (Fig. 28).

Case 8

A 21-year-old female sustained a contact injury to her left knee during soccer. On exam, there was a 2B Lachman, grade 2+ pivot shift, and 4 mm difference on KT-1000 arthrometer. Her MRI revealed a complete ACL tear (Fig. 29). Arthroscopy revealed she had a three-bundle ACL (Fig. 30) The footprint of the AM, IM, and PL bundles was visualized after cutting the ACL remnant with blade (Fig. 30). She proceeded to undergo single-bundle ACL reconstruction with hybrid graft using hamstring autograft and semitendinosus allograft (Fig. 31).

Cross-References

- ▶ Anterior Cruciate Ligament Augmentation in Partial Ruptures
- ▶ Anterior Cruciate Ligament Graft Selection and Fixation
- ▶ Anterior Cruciate Ligament Reconstruction with Autologous Quadriceps Tendon
- ▶ Allografts in Anterior Cruciate Ligament Reconstruction
- ▶ Alternative Techniques for Double-Tunnel Anatomic Anterior Cruciate Ligament Reconstruction
- ▶ Anatomy and Biomechanics of the Knee
- ▶ Arthroscopic Repair of Partial Anterior Cruciate Ligament Tears: Perspective from an Orthopedics Surgeon

- ► Double-Tunnel Anatomic Anterior Cruciate Ligament Reconstruction
- ► Partial Anterior Cruciate Ligament Ruptures: Knee Laxity Measurements and Pivot Shift
- ► Return to Play Decision-Making Following Anterior Cruciate Ligament Reconstruction: Multi-factor Considerations

References

Araujo PH, van Eck CF, Macalena JA, Fu FH (2011) Advances in the three-portal technique for anatomical single- or double-bundle ACL reconstruction. Knee Surg Sports Traumatol Arthrosc 19(8):1239–1242

Bartlett RJ, Clatworthy MG, Nguyen TN (2001) Graft selection in reconstruction of the anterior cruciate ligament. J Bone Joint Surg Br 83(5):625–634

Bonasia DE, Amendola A, Graft Choice in ACL reconstruction. The Knee Joint 2012, pp 173–181. Springer Paris. ISBN 978-2-287-99352-7

Brown CH Jr, Steiner ME, Carson EW (1993) The use of hamstring tendons for anterior cruciate ligament reconstruction. Technique and results. Clin Sports Med 12(4):723–756

Casagranda BU, Maxwell NJ, Kavanagh EC, Towers JD, Shen W, Fu FH (2009) Normal appearance and complications of double-bundle and selective-bundle anterior cruciate ligament reconstructions using optimal MRI techniques. AJR Am J Roentgenol 192(5): 1407–1415

Chu CR, Williams AA, West RV, Qian Y, Fu FH, Do BH, Bruno S (2014) Quantitative magnetic resonance imaging UTE-T2* mapping of cartilage and meniscus healing after anatomic anterior cruciate ligament reconstruction. Am J Sports Med 42(8):1847–1856

Debandi A, Maeyama A, Hoshino Y, Asai S, Goto B, Smolinski P, Fu FH (2013) The effect of tunnel placement on rotational stability after ACL reconstruction: evaluation with use of triaxial accelerometry in a porcine model. Knee Surg Sports Traumatol Arthrosc 21(3):589–595

Dejour D, Ntagiopoulos PG, Saggin PR, Panisset JC (2013) The diagnostic value of clinical tests, magnetic resonance imaging, and instrumented laxity in the differentiation of complete versus partial anterior cruciate ligament tears. Arthroscopy 29(3):491–499

Ferretti M, Ekdahl M, Shen W, Fu FH (2007) Osseous landmarks of the femoral attachment of the anterior cruciate ligament: an anatomic study. Arthroscopy 23(11):1218–1225

Ferretti M, Doca D, Ingham SM, Cohen M, Fu FH (2012) Bony and soft tissue landmarks of the ACL tibial insertion site: an anatomical study. Knee Surg Sports Traumatol Arthrosc 20(1):62–68

Fu FH, Shen W, Starman JS, Okeke N, Irrgang JJ (2008) Primary anatomic double-bundle anterior cruciate ligament reconstruction: a preliminary 2-year prospective study. Am J Sports Med 36(7):1263–1274

Fu FH, van Eck CF, Tashman S, Irrgang JJ, Moreland MS (2014) Anatomic anterior cruciate ligament reconstruction: a changing paradigm. Knee Surg Sports Traumatol Arthrosc

Gianotti SM, Marshall SW, Hume PA, Bunt L (2009) Incidence of anterior cruciate ligament injury and other knee ligament injuries: a national population-based study. J Sci Med Sport 12(6):622–627

Hussein M, van Eck CF, Cretnik A, Dinevski D, Fu FH (2012a) Individualized anterior cruciate ligament surgery: a prospective study comparing anatomic single- and double-bundle reconstruction. Am J Sports Med 40(8):1781–1788

Hussein M, van Eck CF, Cretnik A, Dinevski D, Fu FH (2012b) Prospective randomized clinical evaluation of conventional single-bundle, anatomic single-bundle, and anatomic double-bundle anterior cruciate ligament reconstruction: 281 cases with 3- to 5-year follow-up. Am J Sports Med 40(3):512–520

Hutchinson MR, Ash SA (2003) Resident's ridge: assessing the cortical thickness of the lateral wall and roof of the intercondylar notch. Arthroscopy 19(9):931–935

Illingworth KD, Hensler D, Working ZM, Macalena JA, Tashman S, Fu FH (2011) A simple evaluation of anterior cruciate ligament femoral tunnel position: the inclination angle and femoral tunnel angle. Am J Sports Med 39(12):2611–2618

Kato Y, Maeyama A, Lertwanich P, Wang JH, Ingham SJ, Kramer S, Martins CQ, Smolinski P, Fu FH (2013) Biomechanical comparison of different graft positions for single-bundle anterior cruciate ligament reconstruction. Knee Surg Sports Traumatol Arthrosc 21(4): 816–823

Kopf S, Pombo MW, Szczodry M, Irrgang JJ, Fu FH (2011) Size variability of the human anterior cruciate ligament insertion sites. Am J Sports Med 39(1): 108–113

Li RT, Lorenz S, Xu Y, Harner CD, Fu FH, Irrgang JJ (2011) Predictors of radiographic knee osteoarthritis after anterior cruciate ligament reconstruction. Am J Sports Med 39(12):2595–2603

Li S, Chen Y, Lin Z, Cui W, Zhao J, Su W (2012) A systematic review of randomized controlled clinical trials comparing hamstring autografts versus bone-patellar tendon-bone autografts for the reconstruction of the anterior cruciate ligament. Arch Orthop Trauma Surg 132(9):1287–1297

Lohmander LS, Ostenberg A, Englund M, Roos H (2004) High prevalence of knee osteoarthritis, pain, and functional limitations in female soccer players twelve years after anterior cruciate ligament injury. Arthritis Rheum 50(10):3145–3152

Matsumoto T, Ingham SM, Mifune Y, Osawa A, Logar A, Usas A, Kuroda R, Kurosaka M, Fu FH, Huard J (2012) Isolation and characterization of human anterior cruciate ligament-derived vascular stem cells. Stem Cells Dev 21(6):859–872

Middleton KK, Muller B, Araujo PH, Fujimaki Y, Rabuck SJ, Irrgang JJ, Tashman S, Fu FH (2014) Is the native ACL insertion site "completely restored" using an individualized approach to single-bundle ACL-R? Knee Surg Sports Traumatol Arthrosc ISSN 1433-7347 (Electronic) 0942-2056 (Linking). Available at: http://www.ncbi.nlm.nih.gov/pubmed/24825174

Miyawaki M, Hensler D, Illingworth KD, Irrgang JJ, Fu FH (2014) Signal intensity on magnetic resonance imaging after allograft double-bundle anterior cruciate ligament reconstruction. Knee Surg Sports Traumatol Arthrosc 22(5):1002–1008

Persson A, Fjeldsgaard K, Gjertsen JE, Kjellsen AB, Engebretsen L, Hole RM, Fevang JM (2014) Increased risk of revision with hamstring tendon grafts compared with patellar tendon grafts after anterior cruciate ligament reconstruction: a study of 12,643 patients from the Norwegian Cruciate Ligament Registry, 2004–2012. Am J Sports Med 42(2):285–291

Rabuck SJ, Musahl V, Fu FH, West RV (2013) Anatomic anterior cruciate ligament reconstruction with quadriceps tendon autograft. Clin Sports Med 32(1):155–164

Schenck RC Jr, Kovach IS, Agarwal A, Brummett R, Ward RA, Lanctot D, Athanasiou KA (1999) Cruciate injury patterns in knee hyperextension: a cadaveric model. Arthroscopy 15(5):489–495

Shen W, Forsythe B, Ingham SM, Honkamp NJ, Fu FH (2008) Application of the anatomic double-bundle reconstruction concept to revision and augmentation anterior cruciate ligament surgeries. J Bone Joint Surg Am 90(Suppl 4):20–34

van Eck CF, Schkrohowsky JG, Working ZM, Irrgang JJ, Fu FH (2012) Prospective analysis of failure rate and predictors of failure after anatomic anterior cruciate ligament reconstruction with allograft. Am J Sports Med 40(4):800–807

van Eck CF, Gravare-Silbernagel K, Samuelsson K, Musahl V, van Dijk CN, Karlsson J, Irrgang JJ, Fu FH (2013a) Evidence to support the interpretation and use of the anatomic anterior cruciate ligament reconstruction checklist. J Bone Joint Surg Am 95(20):e153

van Eck CF, Loopik M, van den Bekerom MP, Fu FH, Kerkhoffs GM (2013b) Methods to diagnose acute anterior cruciate ligament rupture: a meta-analysis of instrumented knee laxity tests. Knee Surg Sports Traumatol Arthrosc 21(9):1989–1997

van Eck CF, van den Bekerom MP, Fu FH, Poolman RW, Kerkhoffs GM (2013c) Methods to diagnose acute anterior cruciate ligament rupture: a meta-analysis of physical examinations with and without anaesthesia. Knee Surg Sports Traumatol Arthrosc 21(8):1895–1903

Weber W, Weber E (1836) Mechanik der Menschlichen Gehwerkzeuge. Göttingen

Wu JL, Seon JK, Gadikota HR, Hosseini A, Sutton KM, Gill TJ, Li G (2010) In situ forces in the anteromedial and posterolateral bundles of the anterior cruciate ligament under simulated functional loading conditions. Am J Sports Med 38(3):558–563

Yagi M, Wong EK, Kanamori A, Debski RE, Fu FH, Woo SL (2002) Biomechanical analysis of an anatomic anterior cruciate ligament reconstruction. Am J Sports Med 30(5):660–666

Role of Biologicals in Meniscus Surgery

130

Sebastian Kopf and Roland Becker

Contents

S. Kopf (✉)
Section Sports Traumatology & Arthroscopy, Center for Musculoskeletal Surgery, Charité – University Medicine Berlin, Berlin, Germany
e-mail: Sebastian.Kopf@KSSTA.org; sebastian.kopf@charite.de; mail@koepfchen.org

R. Becker
Klinik für Orthopädie und Unfallchirurgie, Städtische Klinikum Brandenburg, Hochstrasse, Brandenburg an der Havel, Germany
e-mail: Roland.Becker@KSSTA.org; roland_becker@yahoo.de

M.N. Doral, J. Karlsson (eds.), *Sports Injuries*,
DOI 10.1007/978-3-642-36569-0_77

Abstract

Meniscus healing in the avascular, central zone, which includes more than two-thirds of the meniscus from the central region to the periphery, is strongly impaired, mainly because of the diminished blood supply but due to intrinsic factors. Over the last 30 years, an increasing number of research studies have focused on the enhancement of meniscus healing utilizing biologicals such blood products, growth factors, and certain types of cells including progenitor cells or surgical techniques such as synovial and meniscus rasping, needling, and trephination aiming to enhance biologically healing. The results varied significantly. Furthermore, most of these studies were in vitro or animal trials. Thus far, there has been no clear evidence to support the use of any of these biologicals. However, because of the ease of its usage and its low costs, many surgeons perform meniscus needling as well as synovial and meniscus rasping.

Introduction

Meniscus tears are known for their inferior healing potential. To improve the healing capacity of meniscus tears, several methods have been introduced including trephination or needling of the meniscus, rasping of the synovial membrane and the meniscus surface, opening of the medullary cavity to induce an intra-articular influx of

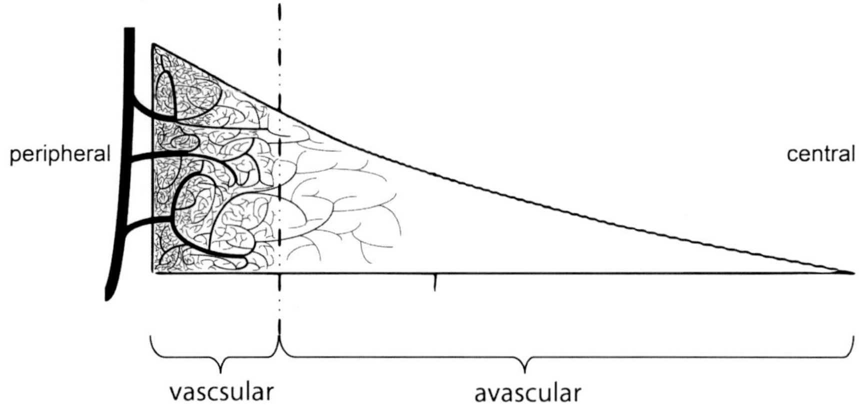

Fig. 1 Schematic figure of radial cut through a meniscus demonstrating schematically the vascularity

progenitor cells, as well as locally applying fibrin clots, platelet-rich plasma (PrP), growth factors, or progenitor cells into the meniscus lesion. The following chapter will introduce you to these methods presenting the literature and its clinical application.

Meniscus lesions are one of the most common sports injuries of the knee, and meniscus surgery is one of the most common knee surgeries (Burks 1997). In the USA about one million meniscus surgeries are performed per year. Until the 1970s meniscal tears were commonly treated by complete meniscectomy. Complete meniscectomy led to short-term pain release, but to a long-term degeneration of the knee and osteoarthritis (AnderssonMolina 2002). Roos et al. reported a sixfold increase of osteoarthritis after 21 years of follow-up of 107 patients after complete meniscectomy (Roos 1998). However, partial meniscectomy and untreated meniscus lesions lead, even though slower as with total meniscectomy, to a degeneration and finally osteoarthritis of the knee with all its consequences including pain, immobility, and finally knee arthroplasty (Chatain 2001; Englund 2001; Bonneux 2002; Cicuttini 2002; VanTienen 2003). The amount of resected meniscal tissue is inversely correlated with the onset and the degree of osteoarthritis (Englund 2001). Despite early reports of the healing potential of menisci, it remained contentious for a long time (Dieterich 1931; Webber 1985). Meniscus repair has been shown to be superior regarding onset of osteoarthritis and return to sports compared to partial meniscectomy (Stein 2010). Meniscus repair should be performed when feasible with good prospects. If partial meniscectomy is not avoidable, as much as possible meniscus tissue should be preserved.

The success of meniscus repair depends on the location of the tear. The more central the tear, the worse are the healing chances, which is presumed to be caused by the reduction or complete absence of blood supply. The meniscus is classified into a vascular, peripheral zone (=red zone) including 20–30 % of the medial and 10–25 % of the lateral meniscus with good healing capacity and an avascular zone, which can be subdivided roughly into a middle third (=intermediate zone = red-white zone) with some outspreading vessels and limited healing capacity as well as a central third without any vascularity (=central zone = white zone) (Fig. 1) and with no healing capacity.

The healing potential of the meniscus inner two-thirds is low. It is presumed that this is mainly because of insufficient blood supply (Arnoczky 1983a; Petersen 1995). Additionally, there is also a discussion about a lower intrinsic healing potential of the avascular region compared to the vascular region (Kobayashi 2004; Hennerbichler 2007).

Though, meniscus repair is mainly performed in longitudinal vertical or radial lesions of the vascular meniscus region. Meniscus repair is done to approximate the wound edges and provide a stable situation. In humans, a cutoff of 4 mm peripheral rim was found to be necessary for good healing chances of repairable meniscus lesions (Tenuta 1994). The failure rate of meniscus repair including sutures and all-inside devices has also been reported to be between 12 % and 48 % (Konan 2010; Tengrootenhuysen 2010) and is often followed by partial meniscectomy. Therefore, there has been an effort to improve healing of meniscal lesions utilizing biological methods such as rasping of the synovial membrane and meniscus to stimulate growth factors, creating vascular channels from the periphery to the lesion, and applying local adjuncts including fibrin and blood clots, platelet-rich plasma (PrP), growth factors, and different types of cells, e.g., progenitor cells (Arnoczky 1988a; Fox 1993; Becker 2004; Ishida 2007; Kopf 2010a; Dutton 2010). Tissue engineering of meniscus has been also an inspiring field of research over the last years and is extensively discussed in "▸ Chap. 89, Human Meniscus: From Biology to Tissue Engineering Strategies."

Creating Vascular Channels

The creation of vascular channels from the periphery to the meniscus lesion is intended to improve the vascular supply around the repaired meniscus lesion and thus to improve meniscus healing (Fig. 2). This can be done by utilizing cannulas and spinal needles or even through meniscus core removals. One of the first attempts to increase vascularity next to the sutured lesion was to cut off the peripheral white rim until the bleeding vascular region (Henning 1987). This open surgical technique showed good healing but created also an earlier onset of osteoarthritic changes compared to partial meniscectomy (Henning 1987). Furthermore, the reported failure rate of 22 % was clearly higher compared to 9 % with meniscal rasping. In an animal trial, a full-thickness cut from the well-vascularized peripheral attachment to the midpoint of the longitudinal lesion in the avascular meniscus region was created to improve the vascularity (Arnoczky 1983a). After 10 weeks, all canine menisci were healed completely, and the lesions were filled with fibrovascular tissue. In the control group without the cut, no healing was seen (Arnoczky 1983a). In contrast to the aforementioned human trial (Henning 1987), in this short-term canine study, menisci did not appear to be unstable, and no degenerative changes were seen at the tibial cartilage below the menisci.

To decrease the amount of injured meniscus tissue, the usefulness of cannulas was evaluated to improve vascularity and therefore meniscus healing. In a canine study, longitudinal meniscus lesions were created in the avascular region

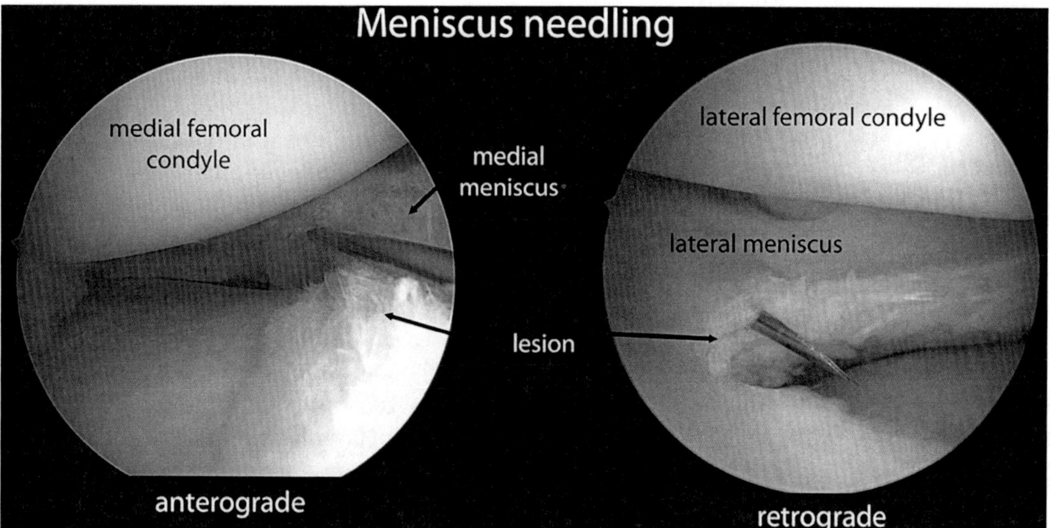

Fig. 2 Needling (=trephination) of the peripheral part of the meniscus lesion using a cannula

(Zhongnan 1988). In one group meniscus lesions were left untreated, and one group meniscus lesions were trephined from the periphery to the lesion using cannulas with a diameter of 1.5 mm. After 8 weeks, all trephined menisci healed partially. Around the trephination hole, about 1–2 mm of the meniscus lesions was filled with collagen. In the untreated group, no meniscus healed. Interestingly, there was no further progress in healing from the 8th to the 24th week (Zhongnan 1988). The authors of both studies (Henning 1987; Zhongnan 1988) noticed that the creation of a sufficient canal by using a usual biopsy needles failed, because the canal closes immediately after pulling out the needle. Due to this fact, they used cannulas with a larger diameter. In a goat study comparing the healing effect of a meniscus repair and an additional trephination to only a meniscus repair, trephined menisci healed better (Zhang 1995). Repair was performed with one horizontal suture, and one vascular channel was created using a 2.0 mm trephine in outside-in technique. In contrast to the aforementioned results of Zhongnan et al. (Zhongnan 1988), healing continued from the 8th to the 25th week (Zhang 1995). Despite the superiority of meniscus repair and trephination compared to meniscus repair, the detailed results are worthwhile further interpretation. Based on the authors' own healing classification system, in the suture plus trephination group, four menisci healed completely and 16 healed partially. In the suture group, three menisci healed partially. However, as mentioned in the discussion of the paper, if classic criteria of meniscus healing (Henning 1990a) based on the healing of the vertical *height* were applied, 80 % of the repairs failed, because the mean healing *length* was 69 % at 25 weeks (Zhang 1995). Thus, the short-term results of this meniscus tissue-damaging technique without any knowledge about long-term degenerative consequences are not convincing.

The next step was the development of a bioabsorbable conduit (poly-L-lactic acid = PLLA) (Cook 2007). In a canine study a 5 mm longitudinal meniscus lesion was created in the avascular region. In 21 lesions, trephination was performed with a 1.8 mm pin from the lesion into the periphery, and in 29 lesions the conduit with a diameter of 1.5 mm and a length of 4 mm was placed into the created vascular channel. Additionally, all lesions were sutured horizontally. After 12 and 24 weeks, four out five meniscus lesions treated with the conduit and a horizontal suture were healed, in contrast to the trephination group (trephination with a horizontal suture) that showed no complete healing. The biomechanical testing revealed significant stronger normal meniscus compared to the conduit and trephinations lesions. Interestingly, there was no significant difference between meniscus lesions with the conduit and with only the trephination. In four lesions out of 29 the conduit displaced, and despite the fact that no cartilage defect was seen in this study, there are reports in the literature about bioresorbable meniscus anchors that showed chondral damage (Sarimo 2005; Järvelä 2010). The disappointing results of the trephination group in this trial might be explained by the fact that a pin was used, which just pushed the meniscus tissue aside by advancing from the lesion to the periphery, in contrast to the cannulas (=hollow needle) that were used in the previous trials, which cut meniscus tissue out and leave a tunnel after being pulled out of the meniscus.

The effect of trephination was also evaluated in human trials. In a case series of 30 patients, 18 gauge (=1.024 mm) spinal needles were used for *incomplete* longitudinal tears. The needles were advanced from inside out until multiple bleeding areas occurred (Fox 1993). The lesions were not sutured, but the edges of the meniscus lesions were additionally abraded. A 90 % success rate of good and excellent results based on the Lysholm Score was found after a mean follow-up of 20 months (range, 12–27 months) (Fox 1993). One of the major concerns of this and many other studies evaluating meniscus repair is the inclusion of concomitant ACL injuries and reconstructions. Five anterior cruciate ligament reconstructions (ACL-R) out of seven complete and three partial ACL tears were performed at the same time, and it is well known that meniscus repair in conjunction with ACL reconstruction improves meniscus healing (Cannon 1992; Tenuta 1994; Haas 2005; Krych 2010; Kraus 2012). Another human trial compared the healing effect of meniscus repair and meniscus repair with trephination in 64 consecutive patients. Only longitudinal lesions in the avascular region of the posterior part of the medial menisci were included. Trephination was performed inside out with a motorized trephine with a diameter of 2.2 mm each 4–5 mm of the lesion. After in mean 47 months (range, 25–78), the trephined menisci had a lower retear rate (25 % vs. 6 %) (Zhang 1996). Retears were assessed by clinical symptoms in patients complaining of recurrence of knee swelling and episodes of locking or catching. In both groups, suture and suture plus trephination and concomitant ACL reconstruction were performed (93 % vs. 97 %), which also restricts the conclusion of the study. In a prospective, randomized study evaluating symptomatic grade 2 lesion, which are in general treated conservatively, partial meniscectomy (IKDC 100 %) was clinically superior to suture repair with trephination (IKDC 90 %), conservative treatment (IKDC 75 %), and minimal resection with fibrin clot and suture repair (IKDC 43 %) after on average 27 months (range, 12–38 months) (Biedert 2000).

The orientation of the cannula or trephine influences tremendously the amount of tissue damage (Staerke 2008). A cannula of 1.5 mm advanced twice perpendicular through the circumferential meniscus fibers creates a defect of 1.1 mm, thus cuts about 25 % of the meniscus tissue, as well as decreases the biomechanical stability by about 25 %. Interestingly, a cannula advanced in line with circumferential meniscus splits the fibers and creates almost no structural defect and, thus, does not almost compromise the biomechanical stability of the meniscus tissue. None of the mentioned study in this book chapter provided information about the orientation of the used cannulas, needles, or trephines.

In summary, core removal (Henning 1987), full-thickness cuts (Arnoczky 1983a), and trephination with bigger diameters (Zhang 1996) revealed good results, but this success was gained with considerable iatrogenic meniscus damage that may result in an earlier onset of osteoarthritis (Henning 1987). Smaller cannulas hollow needles as well as pins (Zhongnan 1988; Biedert 2000; Cook 2007) showed unconvincing results.

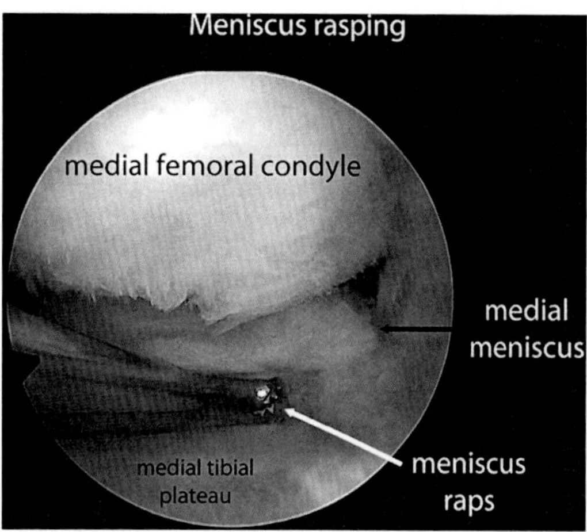

Fig. 3 Abrasion of the inferior meniscus area and the inferior parameniscal synovial membrane

Trephination with the installment of a bioresorbable conduit improved complete healing rates up to 80 %, but these devices tended to displace.

Rasping

Rasping or abrasion of the meniscus surface and the vascularized synovial membrane has been performed to improve the healing rate of repaired meniscus lesions by an increase of growth factors (Fig. 3) (Arnoczky 1982; Ochi 2001). One of the first clinical studies found superior results of rasping (91 % healed) compared to cutting the peripheral white rim until the vascular region (78 % healed) (Henning 1987) including 68 patients and 240 patients, respectively, in two case series. Again, it should be considered that 71 % of the included patients had a concomitant ACL-R. In contrast to these results, no improved healing was seen 3 months after rasping of the inferior and superior surface of the meniscus as well as the parameniscal synovial membrane in a sheep study, where longitudinal lesions of the anterior horn of the lateral meniscus were treated (Nakhostine 1990). In a goat study, after 6 months meniscal abrasion (87.5 % healed) was superior compared to fibrin clot treatment (17 %) in sutured medial meniscus lesions of the red-white and white region (Ritchie 1998). The edges of the meniscus lesions as well as the parameniscal synovial membrane were rasped. In a rabbit study, rasping of the medial meniscus lesion in the avascular region of the anterior was superior (four out of five menisci healed) compared to no treatment (one out of four menisci healed) after 16 weeks (Okuda 1999). Rasping was performed on the superior meniscus surface, on the parameniscal synovial membrane, and additionally at the edges of the meniscus lesion. After 2–4 weeks a hypertrophy of the synovial membrane occurred that migrated into the lesion. Unfortunately, menisci were not sutured as done in humans. The authors found also an increased level of growth factors and cytokines at the superior surface of the meniscus after rasping over the first 7 days including platelet derived growth factor (PDGF), interleukin-1α (IL-1α), transforming growth factor beta 1 (TGF-β1), and proliferating cell nuclear antigen (PCNA) (Ochi 2001). The study group evaluated their technique in a retrospective human study including 48 menisci with 26 full-thickness and 22 partial-thickness tears using second-look arthroscopy (Uchio 2003). Tears were in the vascular and avascular region. Ninety-two percent of the patients had a concomitant ACL-R. Second-look arthroscopy was performed in mean 21 months (range, 2–31 months) after the initial surgery. Complete healing was assessed in 71 % of the menisci, 21 % healed partially, and 8 % did not heal: whereby partial healing was classified as shortening of the tear length, which is in contrast to most of the studies that classify partial healing as closing the tear in its entire length but not in the vertical height. However, 71 % are slightly below the average healing rate of the four published studies (74 %) that evaluated the outcome of their meniscal sutures with second-look arthroscopy (Morgan 1991; Horibe 1996; Tachibana 2010; Ahn 2010; Kopf 2011a).

Thus, rasping of the meniscus surfaces, the parameniscal synovial membrane, and the edges of the lesion is quickly performed at low cost, and no negative side effects were reported. It elevates the number of growth factors, but published studies demonstrate controversial results.

Synovial Flap

A further surgical technique invented to improve meniscal healing is the transposition of a flap of the synovial membrane directly into the lesion (Gershuni 1989). This technique has been performed in an open fashion. At first, this technique was evaluated in a canine study. The synovial flap was placed from the superior parameniscal synovial membrane through the meniscus lesion onto the inferior parameniscal membrane and fixed with sutures. This treatment was compared with two groups: a removed cylindrical core and no treatment (Gershuni 1989). Treatment with synovial flap transposition and core removal were equally superior to the untreated group after 12 weeks. The good results were confirmed in a further canine trial comparing a transposed synovial flap (90 % healing) with sutured meniscus lesions (no healing) of the avascular medial meniscus after 3 months (Kobuna 1995).

In a human organ-culture model using a *free* synovial flap, an improved histologic repair including increased cell proliferation and newly formed collagen was found compared to locally applied fibrin glue and no treatment (Ochi 1996). This in vitro trial was transferred into a canine study transplanting a free synovial flap into a meniscus lesion (Shirakura 1997). The results of this study were sobering. Only 11 of 25 menisci were healed after 12 weeks; however, the healing rate was still better than the comparison groups including inserted mesh grafts, muscle grafts, and controls, which did not show any healing.

Therefore, attached (transposed) synovial flaps had a good healing potential in animal trials in contrast to free synovial flaps; but both techniques need open surgeries and have not yet been evaluated in humans.

Opening of the Medullary Cavity in the Notch

Meniscus lesions repaired concomitant with ACL-R achieve superior results compared to meniscus lesions repaired without ACL-R

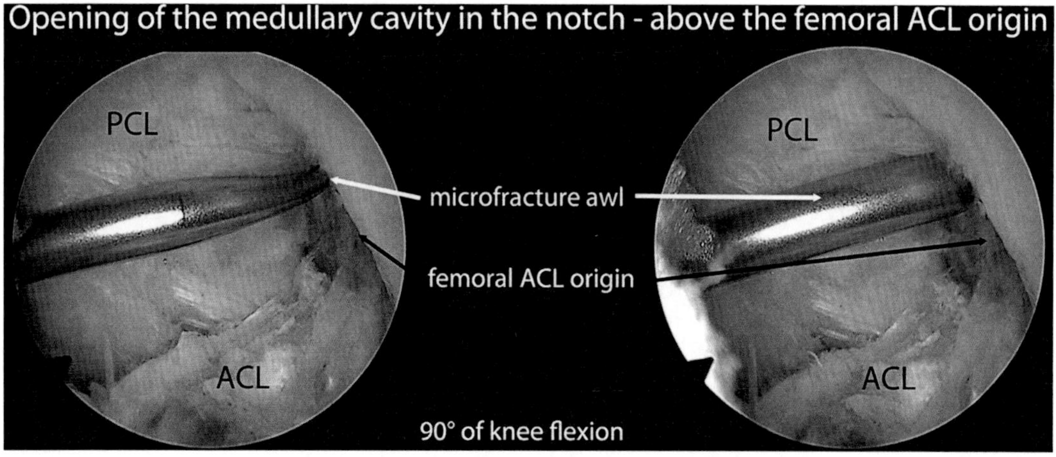

Fig. 4 Opening of the intramedullary cavity in the intercondylar notch (above the ACL origin) using a microfracture awl

(Cannon 1992; Tenuta 1994; Haas 2005; Krych 2010; Kraus 2012). It was hypothesized that the reason for this improved healing potential of meniscus repair plus ACL-R might be the opening of the medullary cavity. This opening leads to (i) an influx of progenitor cells into the knee, which might play a positive role for meniscus healing, (ii) longer rehabilitation time, and (iii) a prolonged hemarthrosis with blood clot formations in and around the meniscus lesion (Freedman 2003; Duygulu 2012). A recent study described a higher PDGF concentration after ACL reconstruction compared to partial meniscectomy (DeGirolamo 2013). The original operative technical note described an opening of the medullary cavity in the intercondylar notch using a microfracture awl (Fig. 4) (Freedman 2003).

To evaluate the abovementioned progenitor cell theory, in a sheep study autologous bone marrow cells from the femur were placed into longitudinal meniscus lesions of the red-white region (Duygulu 2012). After 16 weeks, which is already a long follow-up for animal trials to evaluate meniscus healing, only adhesions and loose connective tissue was found in the bone marrow group compared to untreated control group. Unfortunately, the authors described neither the macroscopic stability nor the amount of healing based on classical criteria by Henning et al. (Henning 1990a). However, more neovascularization and a higher cell count were found in the group with bone marrow treated menisci compared to the untreated menisci. In a further rabbit trial, a cylindrical lesion was created into the avascular meniscus region, and bone marrow from the femoral intercondylar notch was spilled into the knee (Driscoll 2013). The healing was compared to knees with untreated cylindrical meniscus lesions. After 12 weeks, the bone marrow treated lesions did not show a significantly improved repair tissue. However, at 1 week, increased staining of insulin-like growth factor 1 (IGF-1), TGF-β, and PDGF was observed in the repair tissue of the treated knees compared to the untreated lesions (Driscoll 2013).

Therefore, opening of the medullary cavity seems to have only a minor effect on meniscus healing, but it is a safe, quick, and cheap technique. The theory that an increased influx of progenitor cells improves meniscus healing, as seen in ACL-R, can be thus far neglected.

Growth Factors

Growth factors play an important role for tissue healing. In meniscus healing, growth factors such as TGFβ, IL1, PDGF, PCNA, and vascular endothelial growth factor (VEGF) are increased (Ochi 2001; Becker 2004). Several studies have shown positive effects of the addition of growth factors on meniscus cell proliferation, survival, and extracellular matrix synthesis, whereby TGFβ1 was in vitro one of the most potent anabolic growth factor (Imler 2004; Pangborn 2005a; Esparza 2012). The effects of growth factors differ in the avascular and vascular meniscus regions as well as in the surrounding *membrana synovialis* (Collier 1995; Esparza 2012). Additionally, the effect of growth factors differs dependent on the mechanical load (Agarwal 2001; Imler 2004; Ferretti 2006; Deschner 2006), whereby low magnitudes of cyclic loading seem to suppress the effects of catabolic cytokines (Agarwal 2001; Ferretti 2006; Deschner 2006) and static compression seems to suppress the effects of anabolic cytokines (Imler 2004).

In vitro studies using **TGF-β1**-transfected human and canine meniscus cells or applying TGF-β1 on sheep meniscus cells showed increases of proteoglycan and collagen synthesis of up to 100 % (Collier 1995; Goto 2000; Riera 2011; Esparza 2012). This also resulted in improved biomechanical properties (Huey 2011). These in vitro results were confirmed in an ex vivo model showing improved healing rates of TGF-β1-transfected bovine meniscus and mesenchymal stem cells (MSC) compared to controls including empty defects and unseeded scaffolds (Steinert 2007). It would be of interest to see a comparison between these transfected cells and non-transfected meniscus and MSC to further judge the effect of TGF-β1.

Similar positive effects have been reported for **PDGF-AB**, **IGF-1**, and **bFGF**, which increased in vitro fibrochondrocyte proliferation and matrix formation (Lietman 2003; Tumia 2004a, b; Izal 2008; Narita 2009; Tumia 2009; Esparza 2012). Of note, regarding the positive effect of bFGF on the in vitro synthesis of extracellular matrix, there exists some controversy in the literature (Tumia 2004a; Narita 2009; Cucchiarini 2009). These findings are in line with in vivo results of a rabbit trial, where locally applied bFGF incorporated in gelatin hydrogel improved meniscus healing in a horizontal tear of the vascular region (Narita 2011). Interestingly, the sole application of bFGF without the gel did not improve healing. This might be due to the prolonged release time of bFGF with the gel. PDGF, similar to hepatocyte growth factor/scatter factor (**HGF**) and bone morphogenetic protein-2 (**BMP-2**), stimulated in vitro DNA synthesis (Bhargava 1999). PDGF, as shown in an organ-culture model, also increased cellularity of the vascular region but not of the avascular region (Spindler 1995).

Tumor necrosis factor alpha (**TNF-α**) and **IL-1** are proinflammatory cytokines, which can lead to catabolic reactions and play an important role for osteoarthritis (Bian 2012). Their role in meniscus healing is still not completely understood. In vitro (cell culture and organ-culture models) IL-1 and TNF-α decreased cell proliferation, extracellular matrix production, and shear strength of the repairs (Mcnulty 2007; Hennerbichler 2007a; Wilusz 2008; Riera 2011). Bhargava et al. (Bhargava 1999) found that in vitro IL-1 stimulated selectively the migration of meniscus cells of the peripheral region. Furthermore, IL-1 induces amongst others matrix metalloproteinases (MMP). MMP are zinc-dependent endopeptidases responsible for the degradation of extracellular matrix. An inhibition of MMPs in existence of IL-1 improved the shear strength at the repair (Mcnulty 2009). MMP (MMP-13, MMP-1, MMP-2, MMP-3, and MMP-9) activity induced through IL-1 was negatively correlated with shear strength (Wilusz 2008). Contrary, anabolic growth factors such as TGF-β, FGF, IGF, and VEGF increased considerably the MMP-13 concentration. Interestingly, IL-1 is increased after rasping, and rasping is presumed to have a beneficial effect on meniscal healing. Interestingly from a clinical aspect, e.g., for physiotherapy, the catabolic effect of IL-1 can be suppressed with low magnitudes of cyclic tensile strain (Agarwal 2001; Ferretti 2006; Deschner 2006), which might be induced by partial weight-bearing.

Besides trying to enhance directly the healing capacity of meniscus cells, the improvement of vascularity especially for lesions in the avascular meniscus region has been investigated. In a rabbit model, it was shown that the **VEGF** concentration was elevated around meniscus lesions, but it did not improve vascularity and meniscus healing (Becker 2004). Thus, in a following study, VEGF was locally applied using coated sutures into an avascular longitudinal lesion of ovine menisci (Kopf 2010a). This elevated VEGF concentration did not also improve meniscus healing and did not increase vascularity compared to the control groups with uncoated sutures. Instead a gelatinous tissue was found around the VEGF-coated sutures after 8 weeks. Several explanations are possible. The initial supraphysiological concentration of VEGF might have induced an overweight of antiangiogenic factors such as MMP-2 (StetlerStevenson 1999; Brown 2003), TIMP-2 (Seo 2003), angiostatin (Oreilly 1999a), endostatin (Abdollahi 2004; Hoberg 2009), and soluble VEGF receptor 1 (Barleon 1997). Furthermore, these high levels of VEGF might have induced inflammation (Barleon 1996).

In general, the in vitro results of the evaluated growth factors are very promising. The effects depend on mechanical loading and maybe depend on time of application. The results of the animal trial were bipolar, VEGF failed, and bFGF in combination with gelatin hydrogel improved meniscus healing. Thus far, human trials have not been reported. Recent research in this field has focused more on natural combination of growth factors such as in PrP or produced by progenitor cells with its promising paracrine effects on wound healing. The effect of both PrP and progenitor cell application on meniscus healing will be discussed in the following subchapters.

Blood Products

To improve meniscus healing, several surgical techniques applying locally blood products were introduced including blood and fibrin clots as well as platelet-rich plasma. The terms *exogenous blood* or *fibrin clot* are often used as synonyms in the literature (Henning 1990a; Port 1996), but some authors also used fibrin glue and called it fibrin clot.

The idea of using blood products to improve meniscus healing is based on the observation that blood products improve the proliferation and stimulate fibrochondrocytes (Webber 1985). Fibrochondrocyte migrate from the wound edges of the meniscus to the **fibrin clot** in the lesion (Webber 1989). Thus, it was postulated that the fibrin clot works chemotactic and mitogenic, and it provides a scaffold for the ingrowing cells (Arnoczky 1985, 1988). As a result of these findings, a canine trial was conducted comparing avascular, cylindrical meniscus lesions treated with an autologous fibrin clot to untreated lesions (Arnoczky 1988). After 3 and 6 months, all lesions treated with a fibrin clot were filled with repair tissue, which was however different from original meniscus tissue. In contrast, all untreated lesions were not filled or only minor filled (below 5 %). These promising results could not be confirmed by two further goat studies (Port 1996; Ritchie 1998). The first one compared (1) sutured, fibrin clot-treated lesions, with (2) sutured, fibrin clot and bone marrow stem cell treated lesions, (3) sutured lesions, and (4) untreated lesions of the avascular region (Port 1996). After 4 months, the addition of both fibrin clot and fibrin clot with stem cells did not improve meniscus healing. The second study compared (1) sutured, fibrin clot-treated lesions with (2) sutured, abraded lesions, and (3) sutured lesions (Ritchie 1998). Of note, meniscus lesions of the (1) suture group were created in the vascular region, whereas lesions of the (2) fibrin clot group and the (3) abrasion group were created in the avascular meniscus region. After 6 months, the fibrin clot-treated lesions showed the worst healing results (17 %) compared to the abraded lesion (87.5 %) and solely sutured lesions (100 %).

The application of fibrin clots was also evaluated in humans (Henning 1990a, 1991). The first published human study, where a fibrin clot was placed into a meniscus lesion, showed good short-term results (Henning 1990a). After 4 months, the healing rate was 92 % in the group with isolated menisci compared to an unknown, previously treated patient group with a failure rate of 41 %. Unfortunately, a variety of further meniscus healing-enhancing techniques such as rasping and fascia sheets for complex tears were additionally applied. In addition, most of the included patients had a concomitant ACL-R (92 %). Two promising small cases series of radial splits of the lateral meniscus treated with sutures and fibrin clot including five and 12 patients were also published (VanTrommel 1998; Ra 20123). Both case series showed complete healing in almost all cases evaluated by second-look arthroscopy or

MRI. Another case series reported promising results for a sub-entity of meniscus lesions: horizontal cleavage tears. After 12 months all nine sutured and with an exogenous fibrin clot-treated menisci showed good healing during re-arthroscopy (Kamimura 2011).

In a prospective, randomized (by birthday) study evaluating the treatment of isolated, symptomatic grade two lesions, partial meniscectomy (IKDC 100 %) was clinically superior to suture repair with trephination (IKDC 90 %), conservative treatment (IKDC 75 %), and minimal resection with fibrin clot and suture repair (IKDC 43 %) after on average 27 months (range, 12–38 months) (Biedert 2000). These results are interesting, because in general grade two lesions are treated conservatively. Long-term analysis would be much appreciated, because partial meniscectomy is known to be a pre-osteoarthritic stage.

Besides using an exogenous fibrin clot, the usage of commercially available **fibrin glue** has been reported to improve meniscus healing (Ishimura 1991, 1997a), whereby all three reports were published by the same first and senior author. In a rabbit study, cylindrical 1.5 mm lesions were created in the avascular region of the medial meniscus. The menisci treated with fibrin glue or bone marrow cells were completely filled with reparative tissue after 6 weeks compared to the untreated lesions (Ishimura 1997). After 12 weeks, the treated defects were filled with cartilaginous or fibrocartilage tissue, respectively. In a human case series including 32 patients with 40 longitudinal tears, fibrin glue was locally applied, and only three menisci were sutured (Ishimura 1991). Only two patients had re-complained regarding their menisci after a follow-up of on average 3 years and 8 months (range, 10 months to 6.5 years). Concomitant ACL-R was performed in 77 % of the patients. These results are in line with a later published study including already 40 patients with 61 meniscus repairs (Ishimura 1997a). Again, only four menisci were additionally sutured to the fibrin glue treatment. After in mean 8 years (range, 5–11 years), six patients (15 %) complained after 2–4 years postsurgery, and menisci were partially resected. Twenty-seven patients (35 repairs) underwent second-look arthroscopy between 2 and 35 months after surgery. They showed in 77 % good results (firm adhesion even under traction), 11.5 % fair (soft adhesion and unstable under traction), and 11.5 % poor (not healed).

Another promising tool to enhance healing that has caught a lot of attention in the Orthopedic world over the last years is **platelet-rich plasma** (PrP) (Mishra 2006; Hammond 2009; Lippross 2011). Its promising effects in ACL repair and cartilage repair are discussed in "▶ Chaps. 110, Primary Anterior Cruciate Ligament Repair in Athletes with Mesenchymal Stem Cells and Platelet-Rich Plasma" and "▶ 151, Platelet-Rich Plasma in the Treatment of Cartilage Defects and Early Osteoarthritis of the Knee". Platelets have been well known to seal damaged vessel walls (Ruggeri 2007; Jackson 2007), but recently there has been growing evidence that they also play an important role for tissue healing (Lesurtel 2006; Myronovych 2008; Stellos 2010) and angiogenesis (Kisucka 2006; Klement 2009; Blair 2009). Especially their α-granulas contain a plethora of growth factors (Blair 2009) including important growth factors for meniscus healing such as FGF (Brunner 1993), PDGF (Kaplan 1979), IGF (Karey 1989), TGF-β1 (Castillo 2010), and VEGF (Möhle 1997; Wartiovaara 1998). Several different kinds and preparation techniques of PrP have been described and are in detail discussed in "▶ Chap. 261, Platelet-Rich Plasma: From Laboratory to the Clinic" (DohanEhrenfest 2009; Mazzocca 2012). In an in vitro leporine study, the addition of PrP to meniscus cells from the avascular region upregulated cell viability and promoted cell proliferation and the synthesis of extracellular matrix (ECM) (Ishida 2007). These results were only partially confirmed by the in vivo part of the study, where a 1.5 mm diameter full-thickness circular defect was created in the avascular region of the medial meniscus (Ishida 2007). Defects were filled with (1) hydrogel with PRP, (2) hydrogel, or (3) hydrogel with platelet-poor plasma (PPP). No difference in regenerated tissue quality was seen using hematoxylin and eosin staining. The ECM synthesis evaluated by Safranin-O staining was statistically higher in the PrP-treated group after 12 weeks. A further in vivo leporine study did not show an improved healing using a hyaluronan-collagen composite matrix loaded with PrP compared to an implantation of a cell-free scaffold in a circular defect of the avascular region after 6 and 12 weeks (Zellner 2010). These results were confirmed by a similar trial just using a longitudinal lesion instead of a circular defect, no significant healing improvement was achieved in the PrP group compared to the repair with cell-free scaffolds (Zellner 2013).

In conclusion, the in vitro results of locally applied blood products on meniscus cells were promising. The animal and human trials for the application of fibrin clots remain controversial. The results of the animal trials using PrP are also not convincing. The three studies, animal and human, by one study group regarding the use of commercially available fibrin glue were promising.

Application of Cells

An interesting treatment approach to enhance meniscus healing is the local application of cells. Several cell types have been investigated including chondrocytes, bone marrow-derived cells, and autogenous as well as allogenic stem cells (AbdelHamid 2005; Weinand 2006a; Angele 2008; Moriguchi 2013).

The ability of autogenous **chondrocytes** seeded in allogenic meniscus samples was evaluated in a porcine study (Peretti 2004). The cells were placed into a sutured, longitudinal medial meniscus lesion of the avascular region. They were superior compared to sutured lesions treated with unseeded allogenic meniscus samples, solely sutured lesions, and non-treated lesions. Three out of four menisci in the chondrocyte-treated group showed partial bonding of the lesion, whereas only one meniscus in the allogenic meniscus sample group showed partial bonding, and all other menisci did not heal (Peretti 2004; Weinand 2006a). This technique was advanced developing a new seeding technique [dynamic oscillating seeding (Weinand 2009)] with a Vicryl mesh. In a further trial, the effect of allogenic articular, auricular, and costal chondrocytes (each one animal) was evaluated for seeding. Again, a longitudinal medial meniscus lesion of the avascular region was created. After 12 weeks, the seeded Vicryl meshes showed in two animals complete (auricular and costal chondrocytes) and in one animal partial healing (articular chondrocytes) compared to no healing in the control groups with Vicryl mesh, solely suture, or without treatment (Weinand 2006a). In a similar trial, the study group showed that there was no statistical difference regarding healing capacity between allogenic and autogenous chondrocytes. However, in this study 3 out of 17 menisci healed completely, whereas the other menisci healed partially (Weinand 2006).

Stem cells are another promising tool to enhance tissue healing and have thus attracted a lot of attention over the last decade. Stem cells are known for their pluripotency, high regeneration potential, and stimulating paracrine effects; thus, these kinds of cells seem to be an ideal cell source to enhance tissue healing (Gharaibeh 2011). Previous in vitro and in vivo *animal studies* have evaluated this effect on meniscus tissue. Using an organ-culture model of rat menisci, MSC applied in fibrin glue improved extracellular matrix production compared to simple fibrin glue application (Izuta 2005a). In another organ-culture model (Pabbruwe 2010), a collagen scaffold was implanted between two tailored meniscus discs from the avascular zone (sandwich construct). In the first group, the collagen scaffold was seeded with MSC, and in the second group only the scaffold was implanted. The MSC group demonstrated superior integration and superior biomechanical strength. In an in vivo leporine study, the *complete pars intermedia* of the medial meniscus was removed. A collagen scaffold with MSC was delivered into the meniscus lesion (Angele 2008). Lesions treated with the MSC collagen scaffold demonstrated a significantly higher healing area compared to lesions treated with cell free collagen scaffolds and to untreated lesions. This study group showed in two further laporine and one porcine trials creating either a *punch defect* or a *longitudinal meniscus lesion* in the avascular region the superiority of locally applied allogenic and autogenous MSCs compared to bone marrow cells, PrP, and no treatment

(Zellner 2010, 2013; Moriguchi 2013). This positive healing effect of stem cells was confirmed in further leporine study using adipose MSCs (RuizIbán 2011). However, complete healing was still rare ranging between 12.5 % and 25 %. The stem cells were applied at the same time when the lesion was created or 3 weeks later; however, no difference was seen in regards to healing. A recent in vivo pig study demonstrated the influence of MSC on meniscal healing on *radial tears* (Dutton 2010). Two groups were established: (1) sutured menisci with MSC and (2) solely sutured menisci. MSC treatment led histologically to superior healing. However, still 25 % of menisci in the MSC group did not heal completely. Furthermore, biomechanical testing did not show an advantage of the MSC treatment compared to solely sutured menisci. Similar findings were reported in a canine trial evaluating the effect of *autologous bone marrow* and *bone marrow stem cells* (centrifugated) on a *longitudinal meniscus lesion* (AbdelHamid 2005). Of note, meniscus lesions were not sutured. Twenty-five percent of the menisci treated with bone marrow cells did not heal completely, and 63 % of the untreated menisci did not heal completely. No difference was observed regarding the healing rate of bone marrow and bone marrow stem cells.

In *humans,* the first reports using progenitor cells including MSC have been reported (Mazzocca 2011; Piontek 2012; Beitzel 2012, 2013). Cells used for knee surgery were harvested during surgery from either the distal femur or proximal tibia. Thus far, there has been one case series published describing a 10 % failure rate after in mean 2.5 years (Piontek 2012). Meniscal lesions were sutured, wrapped with a collagen membrane and bone marrow cells from the tibial head were locally applied. The authors reported a high complication rate in their 30 patients: one tibial compartment, two cases of arthrofibrosis, and one lesion of the saphenous nerve. Another report comparing the complication rate of arthroscopies with and without bone marrow harvesting from the distal femur did not find a statistical difference (Beitzel 2012). However, in the harvesting group 36 % and the control group 25 % of complications happened. Of note, no treatment with the harvested cells was performed, and all included patients achieved an ACL reconstruction, where the medullary cavity was open anyway.

Finally, chondrocytes seem to be not the ideal cell source to enhance meniscal repair, in contrast to MSC, which seem to be a promising tool. Most animal trials found in general positive results. The negative results have to be explained in the future, e.g., insufficient animal or healing model, cell type, etc. In humans, the high rate of complications has to be overcome, and the positive results known from animal trials have to be confirmed.

Conclusion

Given the low healing rate of meniscus repair of the avascular zone and the just acceptable healing rates of the vascular zone (Stärke 2009a; Konan 2010; Tengrootenhuysen 2010), there is a strong need for improvement of meniscus repair, especially by taking into account the long-term outcome of failed repairs that induce an early onset of osteoarthritis ending often in a knee arthroplasty with enormous consequences for the patient and the economy (Englund 2004) Up to now, there is no biological that has proven its clear benefit for daily routine usage.

References

Abdel-Hamid M, Hussein MR, Ahmad AF, Elgezawi EM (2005) Enhancement of the repair of meniscal wounds in the red-white zone (middle third) by the injection of bone marrow cells in canine animal model. Int J Exp Pathol 86:117–23

Andersson-Molina H, Karlsson H, Rockborn P (2002) Arthroscopic partial and total meniscectomy: A long-term follow-up study with matched controls. Arthroscopy 18:183–189

Angele P, Johnstone B, Kujat R, Zellner J, Nerlich M, Goldberg V, Yoo J (2008) Stem cell based tissue engineering for meniscus repair. J Biomed Mater Res A 85:445–455

Arnoczky SP, Warren RF (1983) The microvasculature of the meniscus and its response to injury. An experimental study in the dog. Am J Sports Med 11:131–141

Arnoczky SP, Warren RF, Spivak JM (1988) Meniscal repair using an exogenous fibrin clot. An experimental study in dogs. J Bone Joint Surg Am 70:1209–1217

Barleon B, Siemeister G, Martiny-Baron G, Weindel K, Herzog C, Marmé D (1997) Vascular endothelial growth factor up-regulates its receptor fms-like tyrosine kinase 1 (FLT-1) and a soluble variant of FLT-1 in human vascular endothelial cells. Cancer Res 57:5421–5425

Barleon B, Sozzani S, Zhou D, Weich HA, Mantovani A, Marme D (1996) Migration of human monocytes in response to vascular endothelial growth factor (VEGF) is mediated via the VEGF receptor flt-1. Blood 87:3336–3343

Becker R, Pufe T, Kulow S, Giessmann N, Neumann W, Mentlein R, Petersen W (2004) Expression of vascular endothelial growth factor during healing of the meniscus in a rabbit model. J Bone Joint Surg Br 86:1082–1087

Beitzel K, McCarthy MB, Cote MP, Chowaniec D, Falcone LM, Falcone JA, Dugdale EM, Deberardino TM, Arciero RA, Mazzocca AD (2012) Rapid isolation of human stem cells (connective progenitor cells) from the distal femur during arthroscopic knee surgery. Arthroscopy 28:74–84

Bhargava MM, Attia ET, Murrell GA, Dolan MM, Warren RF, Hannafin JA (1999) The effect of cytokines on the proliferation and migration of bovine meniscal cells. Am J Sports Med 27:636–643

Bian Q, Wang YJ, Liu SF, Li YP (2012) Osteoarthritis: genetic factors, animal models, mechanisms, and therapies. Front Biosci (Elite Ed) 4:74–100

Biedert RM (2000) Treatment of intrasubstance meniscal lesions: a randomized prospective study of four different methods. Knee Surg Sports Traumatol Arthrosc 8:104–108

Blair P, Flaumenhaft R (2009) Platelet alpha-granules: basic biology and clinical correlates. Blood Rev 23:177–189

Brunner G, Nguyen H, Gabrilove J, Rifkin DB, Wilson EL (1993) Basic fibroblast growth factor expression in human bone marrow and peripheral blood cells. Blood 81:631–638

Burks RT, Metcalf MH, Metcalf RW (1997) Fifteen-year follow-up of arthroscopic partial meniscectomy. Arthroscopy 13:673–679

Cannon WD, Vittori JM (1992) The incidence of healing in arthroscopic meniscal repairs in anterior cruciate ligament-reconstructed knees versus stable knees. Am J Sports Med 20:176–181

Castillo TN, Pouliot MA, Kim HJ, Dragoo JL (2010) Comparison of growth factor and platelet concentration from commercial platelet-rich plasma separation systems. Am J Sports Med

Collier S, Ghosh P (1995) Effects of transforming growth factor beta on proteoglycan synthesis by cell and explant cultures derived from the knee joint meniscus. Osteoarthritis Cartilage 3:127–138

Cook JL, Fox DB (2007) A novel bioabsorbable conduit augments healing of avascular meniscal tears in a dog model. Am J Sports Med 35:1877–1887

Cucchiarini M, Schetting S, Terwilliger EF, Kohn D, Madry H (2009) rAAV-mediated overexpression of FGF-2 promotes cell proliferation, survival, and alpha-SMA expression in human meniscal lesions. Gene Ther 16:1363–1372

Deschner J, Wypasek E, Ferretti M, Rath B, Anghelina M, Agarwal S (2006) Regulation of RANKL by biomechanical loading in fibrochondrocytes of meniscus. J Biomech 39:1796–1803

Dieterich H (1931) Die Regeneration des Meniscus Deutsche Zeitschrift f Chirurgie 230:251–260

Driscoll MD, Robin BN, Horie M, Hubert ZT, Sampson HW, Jupiter DC, Tharakan B, Reeve RE (2013) Marrow stimulation improves meniscal healing at early endpoints in a rabbit meniscal injury model. Arthroscopy 29:113–121

Dutton AQ, Choong PF, Goh JC, Lee EH, Hui JH (2010) Enhancement of meniscal repair in the avascular zone using mesenchymal stem cells in a porcine model. J Bone Joint Surg Br 92:169–175

Duygulu F, Demirel M, Atalan G, Kaymaz FF, Kocabey Y, Dülgeroğlu TC, Candemir H (2012) Effects of intra-articular administration of autologous bone marrow aspirate on healing of full-thickness meniscal tear: an experimental study on sheep. Acta Orthop Traumatol Turc 46:61–67

Englund M, Lohmander LS (2004) Risk factors for symptomatic knee osteoarthritis fifteen to twenty-two years after meniscectomy. Arthritis Rheum 50:2811–2819

Englund M, Roos EM, Roos HP, Lohmander LS (2001) Patient-relevant outcomes fourteen years after meniscectomy: influence of type of meniscal tear and size of resection. Rheumatology (Oxford) 40:631–639

Esparza R, Gortazar AR, Forriol F (2012) Cell study of the three areas of the meniscus: Effect of growth factors in an experimental model in sheep. J Orthop Res 30:1647–1651

Fox JM, Rintz KG, Ferkel RD (1993) Trephination of incomplete meniscal tears. Arthroscopy 9:451–455

Freedman KB, Nho SJ, Cole BJ (2003) Marrow stimulating technique to augment meniscus repair. Arthroscopy 19:794–798

Gershuni DH, Skyhar MJ, Danzig LA, Camp J, Hargens AR, Akeson WH (1989) Experimental models to promote healing of tears in the avascular segment of canine knee menisci. J Bone Joint Surg Am 71:1363–1370

Gharaibeh B, Lavasani M, Cummins JH, Huard J (2011) Terminal differentiation is not a major determinant for the success of stem cell therapy - cross-talk between muscle-derived stem cells and host cells. Stem Cell Res Ther 2:31

de Girolamo L, Galliera E, Volpi P, Denti M, Dogliotti G, Quaglia A, Cabitza P, Corsi Romanelli MM, Randelli P (2013) Why menisci show higher healing rate when repaired during ACL reconstruction? Growth factors release can be the explanation. Knee Surg Sports Traumatol Arthrosc

Hennerbichler A, Moutos FT, Hennerbichler D, Weinberg JB, Guilak F (2007) Interleukin-1 and tumor necrosis factor alpha inhibit repair of the porcine meniscus in vitro. Osteoarthritis Cartilage 15:1053–1060

Hennerbichler A, Moutos FT, Hennerbichler D, Weinberg JB, Guilak F (2007) Repair response of the inner and outer regions of the porcine meniscus in vitro. Am J Sports Med 35:754–762

Henning CE, Lynch MA, Clark JR (1987) Vascularity for healing of meniscus repairs. Arthroscopy 3:13–18

Henning CE, Lynch MA, Yearout KM, Vequist SW, Stallbaumer RJ, Decker KA (1990) Arthroscopic meniscal repair using an exogenous fibrin clot. Clin Orthop Relat Res 64–72

Henning CE, Yearout KM, Vequist SW, Stallbaumer RJ, Decker KA (1991) Use of the fascia sheath coverage and exogenous fibrin clot in the treatment of complex meniscal tears. Am J Sports Med 19:626–631

Hoberg M, Schmidt EL, Tuerk M, Stark V, Aicher WK, Rudert M (2009) Induction of endostatin expression in meniscal fibrochondrocytes by co-culture with endothelial cells. Arch Orthop Trauma Surg 129:1137–1143

Huey DJ, Athanasiou KA (2011) Maturational growth of self-assembled, functional menisci as a result of TGF-β1 and enzymatic chondroitinase-ABC stimulation. Biomaterials 32:2052–2058

Imler SM, Doshi AN, Levenston ME (2004) Combined effects of growth factors and static mechanical compression on meniscus explant biosynthesis. Osteoarthritis Cartilage 12:736–744

Ishida K, Kuroda R, Miwa M, Tabata Y, Hokugo A, Kawamoto T, Sasaki K, Doita M, Kurosaka M (2007) The regenerative effects of platelet-rich plasma on meniscal cells in vitro and its in vivo application with biodegradable gelatin hydrogel. Tissue Eng 13:1103–1112

Ishimura M, Ohgushi H, Habata T, Tamai S, Fujisawa Y (1997) Arthroscopic meniscal repair using fibrin glue. Part I: experimental study. Arthroscopy 13:551–557

Ishimura M, Ohgushi H, Habata T, Tamai S, Fujisawa Y (1997) Arthroscopic meniscal repair using fibrin glue. Part II: clinical applications. Arthroscopy 13:558–563

Ishimura M, Tamai S, Fujisawa Y (1991) Arthroscopic meniscal repair with fibrin glue. Arthroscopy 7:177–181

Izuta Y, Ochi M, Adachi N, Deie M, Yamasaki T, Shinomiya R (2005) Meniscal repair using bone marrow-derived mesenchymal stem cells: experimental study using green fluorescent protein transgenic rats. Knee 12:217–223

Järvelä S, Sihvonen R, Sirkeoja H, Järvelä T (2010) All-inside meniscal repair with bioabsorbable meniscal screws or with bioabsorbable meniscus arrows: a prospective, randomized clinical study with 2-year results. Am J Sports Med 38:2211–227

Kamimura T, Kimura M (2011) Repair of horizontal meniscal cleavage tears with exogenous fibrin clots. Knee Surg Sports Traumatol Arthrosc 19:1154–1157

Kaplan DR, Chao FC, Stiles CD, Antoniades HN, Scher CD (1979) Platelet alpha granules contain a growth factor for fibroblasts. Blood 53:1043–1052

Karey KP, Sirbasku DA (1989) Human platelet-derived mitogens. II. Subcellular localization of insulinlike growth factor I to the alpha-granule and release in response to thrombin. Blood 74:1093–1100

Kobayashi K, Fujimoto E, Deie M, Sumen Y, Ikuta Y, Ochi M (2004) Regional differences in the healing potential of the meniscus-an organ culture model to eliminate the influence of microvasculature and the synovium. Knee 11:271–278

Kobuna Y, Shirakura K, Niijima M (1995) Meniscal repair using a flap of synovium. An experimental study in the dog. Am J Knee Surg 8:52–55

Konan S, Haddad FS (2010) Outcomes of meniscal preservation using all-inside meniscus repair devices. Clin Orthop Relat Res 468:1209–1213

Kopf S, Birkenfeld F, Becker R, Petersen W, Stärke C, Wruck CJ, Tohidnezhad M, Varoga D, Pufe T (2010) Local treatment of meniscal lesions with vascular endothelial growth factor. J Bone Joint Surg Am 92:2682–2691

Kopf S, Stärke C, Becker R (2011) Klinische Ergebnisse nach Meniskusnaht Arthroskopie 24:30–35

Kraus T, Heidari N, Švehlík M, Schneider F, Sperl M, Linhart W (2012) Outcome of repaired unstable meniscal tears in children and adolescents. Acta Orthop 83:261–226

McNulty AL, Moutos FT, Weinberg JB, Guilak F (2007) Enhanced integrative repair of the porcine meniscus in vitro by inhibition of interleukin-1 or tumor necrosis factor alpha. Arthritis Rheum 56:3033–3043

McNulty AL, Weinberg JB, Guilak F (2009) Inhibition of matrix metalloproteinases enhances in vitro repair of the meniscus. Clin Orthop Relat Res 467:1557–1567

Mishra A, Pavelko T (2006) Treatment of chronic elbow tendinosis with buffered platelet-rich plasma. Am J Sports Med 34:1774–1778

Möhle R, Green D, Moore MA, Nachman RL, Rafii S (1997) Constitutive production and thrombin-induced release of vascular endothelial growth factor by human megakaryocytes and platelets. Proc Natl Acad Sci U S A 94:663–668

Nakhostine M, Gershuni DH, Anderson R, Danzig LA, Weiner GM (1990) Effects of abrasion therapy on tears in the avascular region of sheep menisci. Arthroscopy 6:280–287

Narita A, Takahara M, Ogino T, Fukushima S, Kimura Y, Tabata Y (2009) Effect of gelatin hydrogel incorporating fibroblast growth factor 2 on human meniscal cells in an organ culture model. Knee 16:285–289

Narita A, Takahara M, Sato D, Ogino T, Fukushima S, Kimura Y, Tabata Y (2012) Biodegradable gelatin hydrogels incorporating fibroblast growth factor 2 promote healing of horizontal tears in rabbit meniscus. Arthroscopy 28:255–263

Ochi M, Mochizuki Y, Deie M, Ikuta Y (1996) Augmented meniscal healing with free synovial autografts: an organ culture model. Arch Orthop Trauma Surg 115:123–126

Ochi M, Uchio Y, Okuda K, Shu N, Yamaguchi H, Sakai Y (2001) Expression of cytokines after meniscal rasping to promote meniscal healing. Arthroscopy 17:724–731

Okuda K, Ochi M, Shu N, Uchio Y (1999) Meniscal rasping for repair of meniscal tear in the avascular zone. Arthroscopy 15:281–286

O'Reilly MS, Wiederschain D, Stetler-Stevenson WG, Folkman J, Moses MA (1999) Regulation of angiostatin production by matrix metalloproteinase-2 in a model of concomitant resistance. J Biol Chem 274:29568-29571

Pabbruwe MB, Kafienah W, Tarlton JF, Mistry S, Fox DJ, Hollander AP (2010) Repair of meniscal cartilage white zone tears using a stem cell/collagen-scaffold implant. Biomaterials 31:2583–2591

Pangborn CA, Athanasiou KA (2005) Effects of growth factors on meniscal fibrochondrocytes. Tissue Eng 11:1141–1148

Peretti GM, Gill TJ, Xu JW, Randolph MA, Morse KR, Zaleske DJ (2004) Cell-based therapy for meniscal repair: a large animal study. Am J Sports Med 32:146–158

Piontek T, Ciemniewska-Gorzela K, Szulc A, Słomczykowski M, Jakob R (2012) All-arthroscopic technique of biological meniscal tear therapy with collagen matrix. Pol Orthop Traumatol 77:39–45

Port J, Jackson DW, Lee TQ, Simon TM (1996) Meniscal repair supplemented with exogenous fibrin clot and autogenous cultured marrow cells in the goat model. Am J Sports Med 24:547–555

Ra HJ, Ha JK, Jang SH, Lee DW, Kim JG (2013) Arthroscopic inside-out repair of complete radial tears of the meniscus with a fibrin clot. Knee Surg Sports Traumatol Arthrosc 21:2126–2130

Riera KM, Rothfusz NE, Wilusz RE, Weinberg JB, Guilak F, McNulty AL (2011) Interleukin-1, tumor necrosis factor-alpha, and transforming growth factor-beta 1 and integrative meniscal repair: influences on meniscal cell proliferation and migration. Arthritis Res Ther 13:R187

Ritchie JR, Miller MD, Bents RT, Smith DK (1998) Meniscal repair in the goat model. The use of healing adjuncts on central tears and the role of magnetic resonance arthrography in repair evaluation. Am J Sports Med 26:278–284

Roos H, Laurén M, Adalberth T, Roos EM, Jonsson K, Lohmander LS (1998) Knee osteoarthritis after meniscectomy: prevalence of radiographic changes after twenty-one years, compared with matched controls. Arthritis Rheum 41:687–693

Ruggeri ZM, Mendolicchio GL (2007) Adhesion mechanisms in platelet function. Circ Res 100:1673–1685

Ruiz-Ibán MA, Díaz-Heredia J, García-Gómez I, Gonzalez-Lizán F, Elías-Martín E, Abraira V (2011) The effect of the addition of adipose-derived mesenchymal stem cells to a meniscal repair in the avascular zone: an experimental study in rabbits. Arthroscopy 27:1688–1696

Sarimo J, Rantanen J, Tarvainen T, Härkönen M, Orava S (2005) Evaluation of the second-generation meniscus arrow in the fixation of bucket-handle tears in the vascular area of the meniscus. A prospective study of 20 patients with a mean follow-up of 26 months. Knee Surg Sports Traumatol Arthrosc 13:614–618

Seo DW, Li H, Guedez L, Wingfield PT, Diaz T, Salloum R, Wei BY, Stetler-Stevenson WG (2003) TIMP-2 mediated inhibition of angiogenesis: an MMP-independent mechanism. Cell 114:171–180

Shirakura K, Niijima M, Kobuna Y, Kizuki S (1997) Free synovium promotes meniscal healing. Synovium, muscle and synthetic mesh compared in dogs. Acta Orthop Scand 68:51–54

Spindler KP, Mayes CE, Miller RR, Imro AK, Davidson JM (1995) Regional mitogenic response of the meniscus to platelet-derived growth factor (PDGF-AB). J Orthop Res 13:201–207

Staerke C, Kopf S, Becker R (2008) The extent of laceration of circumferential fibers with suture repair of the knee meniscus. Winner of the AGA-DonJoy Award 2006. Arch Orthop Trauma Surg 128:525–530

Stärke C, Kopf S, Petersen W, Becker R (2009) Meniscal repair. Arthroscopy 25:1033–1044

Stein T, Mehling AP, Welsch F, von Eisenhart-Rothe R, Jäger A (2010) Long-term outcome after arthroscopic meniscal repair versus arthroscopic partial meniscectomy for traumatic meniscal tears. Am J Sports Med 38:1542–1548

Steinert AF, Palmer GD, Capito R, Hofstaetter JG, Pilapil C, Ghivizzani SC, Spector M, Evans CH (2007) Genetically enhanced engineering of meniscus tissue using ex vivo delivery of transforming growth factor-beta 1 complementary deoxyribonucleic acid. Tissue Eng 13:2227–2237

Stellos K, Kopf S, Paul A, Marquardt JU, Gawaz M, Huard J, Langer HF (2010) Platelets in regeneration. Semin Thromb Hemost 36:175–184

Stetler-Stevenson WG (1999) Matrix metalloproteinases in angiogenesis: a moving target for therapeutic intervention. J Clin Invest 103:1237–1241

Tengrootenhuysen M, Meermans G, Pittoors K, van Riet R, Victor J (2011) Long-term outcome after meniscal repair. Knee Surg Sports Traumatol Arthrosc 19:236–241

Tenuta JJ, Arciero RA (1994) Arthroscopic evaluation of meniscal repairs. Factors that effect healing. Am J Sports Med 22:797–802

Tumia NS, Johnstone AJ (2004) Promoting the proliferative and synthetic activity of knee meniscal fibrochondrocytes using basic fibroblast growth factor in vitro. Am J Sports Med 32:915–920

Tumia NS, Johnstone AJ (2004) Regional regenerative potential of meniscal cartilage exposed to recombinant insulin-like growth factor-I in vitro. J Bone Joint Surg Br 86:1077–1081

Tumia NS, Johnstone AJ (2009) Platelet derived growth factor-AB enhances knee meniscal cell activity in vitro. Knee 16:73–76

Uchio Y, Ochi M, Adachi N, Kawasaki K, Iwasa J (2003) Results of rasping of meniscal tears with and without anterior cruciate ligament injury as evaluated by second-look arthroscopy. Arthroscopy 19:463–469 van Trommel MF, Simonian PT, Potter HG, Wickiewicz TL (1998) Arthroscopic meniscal repair with fibrin clot of complete radial tears of the lateral meniscus in the avascular zone. Arthroscopy 14:360–365

Webber RJ, Harris MG, Hough AJ (1985) Cell culture of rabbit meniscal fibrochondrocytes: proliferative and synthetic response to growth factors and ascorbate. J Orthop Res 3:36–42

Webber RJ, York JL, Vanderschilden JL, Hough AJ (1989) An organ culture model for assaying wound repair of the fibrocartilaginous knee joint meniscus. Am J Sports Med 17:393–400

Weinand C, Peretti GM, Adams SB, Bonassar LJ, Randolph MA, Gill TJ (2006) An allogenic cell-based implant for meniscal lesions. Am J Sports Med 34:1779–1789

Weinand C, Peretti GM, Adams SB, Randolph MA, Savvidis E, Gill TJ (2006) Healing potential of transplanted allogeneic chondrocytes of three different sources in lesions of the avascular zone of the meniscus: a pilot study. Arch Orthop Trauma Surg 126:599–605

Weinand C, Xu JW, Peretti GM, Bonassar LJ, Gill TJ (2009) Conditions affecting cell seeding onto three-dimensional scaffolds for cellular-based biodegradable implants. J Biomed Mater Res B Appl Biomater

Wilusz RE, Weinberg JB, Guilak F, McNulty AL (2008) Inhibition of integrative repair of the meniscus following acute exposure to interleukin-1 in vitro. J Orthop Res 26:504–512

Zellner J, Hierl K, Mueller M, Pfeifer C, Berner A, Dienstknecht T, Krutsch W, Geis S, Gehmert S, Kujat R, Dendorfer S, Prantl L, Nerlich M, Angele P (2013) Stem cell-based tissue-engineering for treatment of meniscal tears in the avascular zone. J Biomed Mater Res B Appl Biomater 101:1133–1142

Zellner J, Mueller M, Berner A, Dienstknecht T, Kujat R, Nerlich M, Hennemann B, Koller M, Prantl L, Angele M, Angele P (2010) Role of mesenchymal stem cells in tissue engineering of meniscus. J Biomed Mater Res A 94:1150–1161

Zhang Z, Arnold JA (1996) Trephination and suturing of avascular meniscal tears: a clinical study of the trephination procedure. Arthroscopy 12:726–731

Zhang Z, Arnold JA, Williams T, McCann B (1995) Repairs by trephination and suturing of longitudinal injuries in the avascular area of the meniscus in goats. Am J Sports Med 23:35–41

Zhang ZN, Tu KY, Xu YK, Zhang WM, Liu ZT, Ou SH (1988) Treatment of longitudinal injuries in avascular area of meniscus in dogs by trephination. Arthroscopy 4:151–159

Role of Growth Factors in Anterior Cruciate Ligament Surgery

131

Roberto Seijas, Pedro Álvarez, and Ramón Cugat

Contents

Abstract

Biological treatments to complement surgery have been shown to improve surgical outcomes. These improvements have been appreciated as a potential acceleration in tendon maturation. Numerous studies on anterior cruciate ligament grafts have shown accelerated maturation or ligamentization with the help of biological treatments such as plasma rich in growth factors.

R. Seijas (✉)
Chair of Medicine and Regenerative Surgery, Garcia Cugat Foundation & CEU Cardenal Herrera University, Alfara del Patriarca, Valencia, Spain

Department of Orthopaedic Surgery, Sports Medicine and Trauma, Hospital Quiron Barcelona, Barcelona, Spain

Facultad de Medicina y Ciencias de la Salud, Universitat Internacional de Catalunya, Barcelona, Spain
e-mail: roberto6jas@gmail.com

P. Álvarez
Chair of Medicine and Regenerative Surgery, Garcia Cugat Foundation & CEU Cardenal Herrera University, Alfara del Patriarca, Valencia, Spain

Facultad de Medicina y Ciencias de la Salud, Universitat Internacional de Catalunya, Barcelona, Spain

Mutualidad de Futbolistas, Real Federacion Espanola de Futbol, Barcelona, Spain

Department of Orthopaedic Surgery, Sports Medicine and Trauma, Hospital Quiron Barcelona, Artroscopia gc, S.L., Barcelona, Spain

Facultad de Medicina, Universitat Internacional de Catalunya, Barcelona, Spain
e-mail: dr.pedroalvarezdiaz@gmail.com

R. Cugat
Mutualidad de Futbolistas, Real Federacion Espanola de Futbol, Barcelona, Spain

Garcia Cugat Foundation & CEU Cardenal Herrera University, Alfara del Patriarca, Valencia, Spain

Department of Orthopaedic Surgery, Sports Medicine and Trauma, Hospital Quiron Barcelona, Artroscopia gc, S.L., Barcelona, Spain

Facultad de Medicina, Universitat Internacional de Catalunya, Barcelona, Spain
e-mail: ramon.cugat@sportrauma.com

M.N. Doral, J. Karlsson (eds.), *Sports Injuries*,
DOI 10.1007/978-3-642-36569-0_97

Studies both in vitro and in animals, including human studies, have reported improved results in ligament structure and strength and earlier ACL graft maturation, with the use of growth factors.

Introduction

Anterior cruciate ligament (ACL) injuries are frequent, with an incidence of 300,000 annual ACL ruptures in the USA (Goldstein and Bosco 2001; Cohen and Sekiya 2007; Stergiou et al. 2007; Cimino et al. 2010). The majority of these injuries are sports related and affect patients between 15 and 45 years old (Smith et al. 1993). The ACL is the most frequently injured ligament in the knee and in 70 % the injury is produced during sports activity, typically with an indirect injury mechanism of deceleration-rotation without contact (Griffin et al. 2000; Goldstein and Bosco 2001). The majority of ACL tears occur in patients between 15 and 45 years old, with 47 % taking place during the decade from 30 to 40 years old (Griffin et al. 2000). It is estimated that one ACL tear occurs every 1,500 h of sports practice, including sports such as soccer, basketball, rugby, and skiing, which is equivalent to one injury for every 1,750 citizens of the USA (Griffin et al. 2000). Finally, the overall costs of sport-related injuries in the USA in 2002 were estimated at about 15.8 billion dollars (Taylor et al. 2011). The cost of an ACL reconstruction surgery in the USA is an estimated $ 17,000 to which one can add an additional $ 2,000 for the cost of the initial care of all ACL injuries and/or the conservative treatment of the patients who do not undergo ACL reconstruction. The annual cost of treating only ACL injuries is an estimated 1 billion dollars (Griffin et al. 2000). In over 80 % of cases, ACL tears are associated with injuries to other structures in the knee, including meniscal tears, collateral ligament tears, and articular cartilage damage (Gillquist and Messner 1999; Lohmander et al. 2007). The pattern of these depends on the mechanism and force of the traumatic event (Lohmander et al. 2007).

Works, such as that by von Porat, show the relationship between osteoarthritis and anterior cruciate ligament injury, postulating in their study that both the group of patients that underwent surgery and the group that did not were associated with 78 % radiographic osteoarthritis at 14 years of follow-up (von Porat et al. 2004). Recovery from joint injuries in active athletes is increasingly faster due in part to the progress and improvement of surgical techniques and the application of biological elements that promote rapid tissue regeneration (Foster et al. 2009). Anterior cruciate ligament (ACL) tears are usually treated surgically if the rupture is complete or causes instability of the knee. Graft selection has been extensively debated, and yet there still remains no clear consensus, although the use of the patient's autologous patellar tendon graft is clearly considered an eligible treatment in athletes (Magnussen et al. 2011).

In recent years the application of platelet-rich plasma (PRP) or plasma rich in growth factors (PRGF) has been linked to faster tissue regeneration in bone, cartilage, ligaments, and tendons, for studies in vitro, in vivo, and in humans (Kondo et al. 2005; Sanchez et al. 2007; Randelli et al. 2008; Foster et al. 2009). There are different ways to obtain PRP. The PRGF system has reportedly been used as the longest used technique, and the Food and Drug Administration (FDA) in the USA and Conformité Européenne (CE) in the European community have approved the system. The maturation of the graft used for the ACL has been correlated with the homogeneous image by magnetic resonance and the tension of the graft once placed (Weiler et al. 2004). Several studies assess the maturation of these grafts histologically, finding different stages of maturation (Aim et al. 1979; Falconiero et al. 1998). Additionally, changes in ligament maturation have been evaluated using magnetic resonance, separating different stages and finding complete maturation a year after surgery (Howell et al. 1991). Radice (Radice et al. 2010) suggest that the application of growth factors could accelerate the maturation process and by doing so develop protocols with earlier functional recovery.

Discussion

Anterior cruciate ligament reconstruction has the task of trying to restore knee functional stability. Due to this, different grafts have been used, such as the patellar tendon, hamstrings, iliotibial band, meniscus, allograft, synthetic tendons, and combinations thereof (Falconiero et al. 1998). Although reconstructive surgery aims to restore function to the prelesional condition, the question that arises about ligamentoplasty is the time required for graft maturation. Animal studies have shown a series of stages in the revascularization of the patellar graft used to reconstruct the anterior cruciate ligament. After a phase of graft avascular necrosis, with hypocellularity and collagen fragmentation, revascularization is produced through a synovial cover which originates from both the distal and proximal insertions of the graft that starts covering it and promotes intratendinous vascular growth up to complete coverage and cellularization at 1 year postsurgery (Arnoczky and Tarvin 1982).

PRGF Basics

It is known that in order for the tissue repair-regeneration process to take place, a multitude of elements must interact, from various cellular components to proteins, metabolites, and electrolytes, all encompassed within an appropriate environment. During this process, both in the acute inflammatory phase and in the cellular proliferation and remodeling phase (Bennett and Schultz 1993a, b), platelets play an important role, not only based on hemostatic capacity but also on their chemotactic activity and on growth, morphogenesis, and cell differentiation (Anitua et al. 2004). From the 1990s onward, several studies began to emerge which were aimed at taking advantage of the benefits offered by this cell type in tissue repair, stimulating research and development in the field of regenerative medicine (Tayapongsak et al. 1994; Ledent et al. 1995; Anitua et al. 2007; Sanchez et al. 2007; Ekdahl et al. 2008; Wang-Saegusa et al. 2011).

The tissue repair process involves several phases including angiogenesis, tissue proliferation, and extracellular matrix deposition. The remodeling and maturation processes are combined with the mechanical stresses to which the tissue in question is subjected (Sanchez et al. 2007). The tissue repair process is based on a complex cascade of biological events controlled by a long list of growth factors and proteins with biological activity. The spatiotemporal action of this group of mediators at the area of damaged tissue regulates the mechanisms and phases that govern tissue repair and regeneration. Throughout this process, another set of factors regulates the dynamic balance between stimulation and inhibition of cell proliferation, angiogenesis, and the formation of extracellular matrix (Anitua et al. 2007).

Growth factors are substances of polypeptide nature, soluble and diffusible regulating growth, differentiation, and phenotype of many cell types (Vega et al. 2000). These provide the initial signals for the activation of the cells in surrounding tissue. In response to signals provided by these molecules, local cells and those infiltrated undergo changes in proliferation, differentiation, and protein synthesis with different biological functions.

All these phenomena, together, define the process known as cell activation (Reed et al. 2000). These proteins act in an autocrine and/or paracrine manner. They affect cell behavior, binding to specific receptors located in cell membranes. Not all cell phenotypes have the same receptors; therefore, the effect of the growth factors will not be the same in all tissues and in all situations (Stone 1998). Platelet-rich plasma is obtained from small volumes of the patient's blood (20 cc). It is not a platelet concentrate and is obtained after single-stage centrifugation. It does not contain leukocytes and is simply platelet-rich plasma. White cells, and especially leukocytes, contain proinflammatory cytokines and express metalloproteinases (MMP-8 and 9) capable of degrading the extracellular matrix. PRGF is 100 % autologous and biocompatible (Anitua et al. 2007).

PRGF activation is performed with a standard dosage of calcium chloride, taking advantage of the patient's own thrombin and not using bovine thrombin; hence biosecurity risks are avoided. By using the technique described by the Biotechnology Institute (BTI Biotechnology Institute, Jacinto Quincoces Kalea, 39, 01007 Vitoria-Gasteiz, Araba) to obtain PRGF, a platelet concentration of two to three times higher than the physiological concentration is obtained, which has shown good results. Lower doses would be sub therapeutic and superior concentrations do not induce superior effects, they can even exert inhibitory actions (Anitua et al. 2007).

PRGF Studies

Culture studies with the use of PRGF have shown a cellular increase in tendon tissues and especially an increase in collagen levels (Yasuda et al. 2004; Anitua et al. 2007; De Mos et al. 2008; Kajikawa et al. 2008). Animal studies also show increases in cell density, neovascularization, and resistance force between 30 % and 65 % according to studies (Anderson et al. 2001; Aspenberg and Virchenko 2004; Anitua et al. 2006) with an improvement within biomechanical properties in the medial collateral ligament in its early stages. The study by Xie et al. suggested a role of PRGF in promoting synthesis of extracellular matrix after ACL reconstruction, in a study performed with dogs (Xie et al. 2013). Along the same lines, the study by Fernandez-Sarmiento et al. showed histological changes at 8 weeks, consistent with an accelerated early healing process in repaired Achilles tendons in sheep after surgical disruption and repair treated with PRGF (Fernandez-Sarmiento et al. 2013).

PRGF was associated with histological changes consistent with an accelerated early healing process in repaired Achilles tendons in sheep after experimental surgical disruption. PRGF-treated tendons showed improvements in the morphometric features of fibroblast nuclei, suggesting a more advanced stage of healing. At 8 weeks, histological examination revealed more mature organization of collagen bundles. Studies by Kondo et al. also demonstrated that the application of growth factors in ACL elongations achieved improved tension compared with patients where growth factors were not applied (Kondo et al. 2005).

Studies have shown growth factors to be useful in achieving early mobility and earlier return to sports in Achilles tendons and rotator cuff repair (Sanchez et al. 2007; Kovacevic and Rodeo 2008). Meanwhile Foster et al. published the series on medial collateral ligament injuries in soccer players with reductions of 27 % in recovery times (Foster et al. 2009). Studies show maturation of patellar graft evolution in terms of vascularization, cellularity, and collagen fiber pattern, and the presence of metaplasia with a high correlation (Falconiero et al. 1998) showed maturity with a peak at just after 1-year postsurgery but with vascularity and fiber pattern similar to normal in a period of 6–12 months.

Aim (Aim et al. 1979) studied the patellar graft viability by microangiography and histology showing revascularization at 8 weeks with tissues rich in collagen and a similar structure to the original ligament at 4–5 months.

In the first months the graft is in the process of maturation, a fact that has left ACL surgeons reluctant to carry out aggressive rehabilitation in the initial period for fear of graft failure (Rougraff and Shelbourne 1999). Rougraff in his study of graft biopsies in patellar ligamentoplasties reported tissue obtained in the early postoperative period (3–8 weeks post-op) show no more than 30 % tissue necrosis, in contrast to animal studies where the percentage is much higher. Therefore, he concluded that postoperative rehabilitation programs proposing an acceleration of physical therapy, not only do not have detrimental outcomes, but if not followed could lead to worse outcomes (Rougraff and Shelbourne 1999). MRI is the most accurate method of diagnosis for acute anterior cruciate ligament injury (Grøntvedt et al. 1996). Howell (Howell et al. 1991) illustrated how different grades in the maturation stages can be assessed using MRI. The system differentiates four levels based on the signal provided by different regions of the graft. These five categories could better show the different stages of ligament maturation.

The use of biological techniques for tissue repair has increased in recent years with the emergence of numerous articles on the application of autologous plasma rich in growth factors (Sanchez et al. 2007; Lopez-Vidriero et al. 2010; Radice et al. 2010; Wang-Saegusa et al. 2011). The tissue repair process involves various intervals including angiogenesis, tissue proliferation, and extracellular matrix. The remodeling and maturation processes are combined with the mechanical stresses to which the tendon or ligament in question are subjected (Sanchez et al. 2007, 2010). The preparation of plasma rich in growth factors contains a mixture of mediators that are involved in the natural repair process and include transforming growth factor-1 (TGF-1), platelet-derived growth factor (PDGF), vascular endothelial growth factor (VEGF), epithelial growth factor (EGF), hepatocyte growth factor (HGF), and insulin-like growth factor (IGF-I) (Sanchez et al. 2007).

These and many other factors have been identified as partakers in the processes of tendon healing, giving rise to motive for the use of PRP as a proposed approach to improve the cellular response to tendon injuries and in particular the quality of such repair (Sanchez et al. 2007). The system for obtaining plasma rich in growth factors is not always uniform, with different techniques being followed by various authors, making the resultant products significantly different without reaching any conclusion about the degree of effectiveness from one to the other (Weibrich and Kleis 2002). With specific reference to the ACL graft, PDGF, FGF-1, and some TGF subtypes are responsible for the acceleration of tissue healing and increased graft tension (Radice et al. 2010). Studies showed that platelet-rich plasma stimulated the proliferation and collagen production in cultured human tenocytes, and increase of collagen types I and III in flexor tendons in equine model with the use of plasma rich in growth factors and the presence of TGF-1, TGF-2, and TGF-3 have a direct influence on the graft, increasing tensile force resistance by 65 % (Schnabel et al. 2007).

In vivo studies in animals have shown a 30 % increase in Achilles tendon tensile strength or repair strength of the rotator cuff tendons. The effect of growth factors applied in the canine model indicating that TGF and EGF acted by increasing the collagen and fibroblast synthesis by 40 % in the graft and the usefulness of growth factors (PDGF-BB) in in vivo studies, improving the biomechanical properties in the healing process of the medial collateral ligament in early stages of ligament repair (Kovacevic and Rodeo 2008).

In 2005 Kondo demonstrated how the application of growth factors in ACL elongation achieved greater mean area tensioning with clearly superior biomechanical properties compared to cases without the application of growth factors (Kondo et al. 2005). In 2007 Sanchez published the use of PRP in Achilles tendon injury, achieving recovery in less time than the control (Sanchez et al. 2007). Randelli published results on the use of PRP in cuff repair surgery finding significant differences at a 2-year follow-up in pain and function (Randelli et al. 2008). Foster presented a series at ISAKOS 2009 on the application of PRP on the medial collateral ligament in soccer players with a 27 % time reduction (Foster et al. 2009). This paper did not report better results in the PRP group in terms of biomechanical properties, but demonstrated a clear time reduction to obtain the complete maturation process in accordance with works of Sanchez and Foster (Sanchez et al. 2007; Foster et al. 2009).

Weiler showed how the application of autologous PRP into the graft during surgery was able to alter natural maturation, improving tension and resistance, increasing the rate of maturation, and improving collagen quality (Weiler et al. 2004). Orrego showed greater maturation for the patellar graft assessed by MRI at 6 months without an increased tibial tunnel diameter (Orrego et al. 2008). The study by Nin (Nin et al. 2009) reported no significant differences with the application of plasma rich in growth factors in ligament grafts. The results obtained with the assessment carried out at 2-year postsurgery are concurrent with those obtained in the study by Seijas et al. showing equal numbers of completely mature ligaments in both groups with no differences between the two groups. The main difference between the authors' study (Seijas et al. 2013) and that of Nin is that the authors assessed the grade of maturity at earlier intervals, noting that although the two groups (PRP and control) reach maturity at 1 year at similar rates, the speed at which they do so is different.

In 2010, Radice published graft maturation rates, assessed by MRI, which showed figures 48 % faster for grafts treated with growth factors with respect to the speed of maturity (Radice et al. 2010). Sanchez for his part showed how the use of PRGF also accelerated the maturation process in hamstring grafts (Sánchez et al. 2010). In 2013 Seijas published a similar study with increased maturation at 4 and 6 months in a group of soccer players with the use of PRGF in BTB graft (Seijas et al. 2013).

Conclusion

Based on the studies reviewed, one can conclude that the use of PRGF, or different variants of PRP, accelerates the healing and regeneration processes of different tissues. PRGF is a biological treatment that can improve traditional treatments in the field of sport.

Cross-References

▶ Anterior Cruciate Ligament Injuries and Surgery: Current Evidence and Modern Development
▶ Clinical Relevance of Gene Therapy and Growth Factors in Sports Injuries
▶ Different Techniques of Anterior Cruciate Ligament Reconstruction: Guidelines
▶ Factors Affecting Return to Sport After Anterior Cruciate Ligament Reconstruction
▶ Graft Remodeling and Bony Ingrowth After Anterior Cruciate Ligament Reconstruction
▶ Knee Ligament Surgery: Future Perspectives
▶ Platelet-Rich Plasma: From Laboratory to the Clinic
▶ Primary Anterior Cruciate Ligament Repair in Athletes with Mesenchymal Stem Cells and Platelet-Rich Plasma
▶ State of the Art in Anterior Cruciate Ligament Surgery

References

Aim A, Liljedahl SO, Stromberg B (1979) Clinical and experimental experience in the reconstruction of the anterior cruciate ligament. Orthop Clin North Am 7:181–189

Anderson K, Seneviratne AM, Izawa K, Atkinson BL, Potter HG, Rodeo SA (2001) Augmentation of tendon healing in an intraarticular bone tunnel with use of a bone growth factor. Am J Sports Med 29:689–698

Anitua E, Andia I, Ardanza B, Nurden P, Nurden AT (2004) Autologous platelets as a source of proteins for healing and tissue regeneration. Thromb Haemost 91(1):4–15

Anitua E, Sanchez M, Nurden AT, Zalduendo M, de la Fuente M, Orive G et al (2006) Autologous fibrin matrices: a potential source of biological mediators that modulate tendon cell activities. J Biomed Mater Res A 77(2):285–293

Anitua E, Sanchez M, Orivea G, Andía I (2007) The potential impact of the preparation rich in growth factors (PRGF) in different medical fields. Biomaterials 28:4551–4560

Arnoczky SP, Tarvin GB (1982) Anterior cruciate ligament replacement using patellar tendon: an evaluation of graft revascularization in the dog. J Bone Joint Surg Am 64:217–224

Aspenberg P, Virchenko O (2004) Platelet concentrate injection improves Achilles tendon repair in rats. Acta Orthop Scand 75:93–99

Bennett NT, Schultz GS (1993a) Growth factors and wound healing: biochemical properties of growth factors and their receptors. Am J Surg 165(6):728–737

Bennett NT, Schultz GS (1993b) Growth factors and wound healing: part II Role in normal and chronic wound healing. Am J Surg 166(1):74–81

Cimino F, Volk BS, Setter D (2010) Anterior cruciate ligament injury: diagnosis, management and prevention. Am Fam Physician 82(8):917–922

Cohen SB, Sekiya JK (2007) Allograft safety in anterior cruciate ligament reconstruction. Clin Sports Med 26:597–605

De Mos M, van der Windt A, Jahr H et al (2008) Can platelet-rich plasma enhance tendon repair? A cell culture study. Am J Sports Med 36:1171–1178

Ekdahl M, Wang JH, Ronga M, Fu FH (2008) Graft healing in anterior cruciate ligament reconstruction. Knee Surg Sports Traumatol Arthrosc 16(10):935–947

Falconiero RP, DiStefano VJ, Cook TM (1998) Revascularization and ligamentization of autogenous anterior cruciate ligament grafts in humans. Arthroscopy 14:197–205

Fernandez-Sarmiento JA, Dominguez JM, Granados MM, Morgaz J, Navarrete J, Carrillo JM et al (2013) Histological study of the influence of plasma rich in growth factors (ORGF) on the healing of divided Achilles tendons in sheep. J Bone Joint Surg Am 95(3):246–255

Foster TE, Puskas BL, Mandelbaum BR et al (2009) Platelet-rich plasma. From basic science to clinical applications. Am J Sports Med 37:2259–2272

Gillquist J, Messner K (1999) Anterior cruciate ligament reconstruction and the long-term incidence of gonarthrosis. Sports Med 27(3):143–156

Goldstein J, Bosco JA 3rd (2001) The ACL-deficient knee: natural history and treatment options. Bull Hosp Jt Dis 60:173–178

Griffin LY, Agel J, Albohm MJ et al (2000) Noncontact anterior cruciate ligament injuries: risk factors and prevention strategies. J Am Acad Orthop Surg 8(3): 141–150

Grøntvedt T, Engebretsen L, Rossvoll I et al (1996) Comparison between magnetic resonance imaging findings and knee stability: measurements after anterior cruciate ligament repair with and without augmentation. A five- to seven year follow-up of 52 patients. Am J Sports Med 23:729–735

Howell SM, Clark JA, Blasier RD (1991) Serial magnetic resonance imaging of hamstring anterior cruciate ligament autografts during the first year of implantation. Am J Sports Med 19:42–47

Kajikawa Y, Morihara T, Sakamoto H et al (2008) Platelet-rich plasma enhances the initial mobilization of circulation-derived cells for tendon healing. J Cell Physiol 215:837–845

Kondo E, Yasuda K, Yamanaka M et al (2005) Effects of administration of exogenous growth factors on biomechanical properties of the elongation-type anterior cruciate ligament injury with partial laceration. Am J Sports Med 33:188–196

Kovacevic D, Rodeo SA (2008) Biological augmentation of rotator cuff tendon repair. Clin Orthop 466:622–633

Ledent E, Wasteson A, Berlin G (1995) Growth factor release during preparation and storage of platelet concentrates. Vox Sang 68(4):205–209

Lohmander LS, Englund PM, Dahl LL, Roos EM (2007) The long-term consequence of anterior cruciate ligament and meniscus injuries: osteoarthritis. Am J Sports Med 35(10):1756–1769

Lopez-Vidriero E, Goulding KA, Simon DA, Sanchez M, Johnson DH (2010) The use of platelet rich plasma in arthroscopy and sports medicine: optimizing the healing environment. Arthroscopy 26(2):269–278

Magnussen RA, Carey JL, Spindler KP (2011) Does autograft choice determine intermediate-term outcome of ACL reconstruction? Knee Surg Sports Traumatol Arthrosc 19(3):462–472

Nin JR, Gasque GM, Azcárate AV et al (2009) Has platelet-rich plasma any role in anterior cruciate ligament allograft healing? Arthroscopy 25(11):1206–1213

Orrego M, Larrain C, Rosales J et al (2008) Effects of platelet concentrate and bone plug on the healing of hamstring tendons in bone tunnel. Arthroscopy 24:1373–1380

Radice F, Yánez R, Gutiérrez V et al (2010) Comparison of magnetic resonance imaging findings in anterior cruciate ligament grafts with and without autologous platelet-derived growth factors. Arthroscopy 26(1): 50–57

Randelli PS, Arrigoni P, Cabitza P, Volpi P, Maffulli N (2008) Autologous platelet rich plasma for arthroscopic rotator cuff repair: a pilot study. Disabil Rehabil 30 (20-22):1584–1589

Reed GL, Fitzgerald ML, Polgár J (2000) Molecular mechanisms of platelet exocytosis: insights into the "secrete" life of thrombocytes. Blood 96(10):3334–3342

Rougraff BT, Shelbourne KD (1999) Early histologic appearance of human patellar tendon autografts used for anterior cruciate ligament reconstruction. Knee Surg Sports Traumatol Arthrosc 7:9–14

Sanchez M, Anitua E, Azofra J et al (2007) Comparison of surgically repaired Achilles tendon tears using platelet-rich fibrin matrices. Am J Sports Med 35:245–251

Sánchez M, Anitua E, Azofra J, Prado R, Muruzabal F, Andia I (2010) Ligamentization of tendon grafts treated with an endogenous preparation rich in growth factors: gross morphology and histology. Arthroscopy 26(4): 470–480

Seijas R, Ares O, Catala J, Alvarez-Diaz P, Cusco X, Cugat R (2013) Magnetic resonance imaging evaluation of patellar tendon graft remodeling after anterior cruciate ligament reconstruction with or without platelet-rich plasma. J Orthop Surg (Hong Kong) 21(1):10–14

Schnabel LV, Mohammed HO, Miller BJ et al (2007) Platelet rich plasma (PRP) enhances anabolic gene expression patterns in flexor digitorum superficialis tendons. J Orthop Res 25(2):230–240

Smith BA, Livesay GA, Woo SL (1993) Biology and biomechanics of the anterior cruciate ligament. Clin Sports Med 12:637–670

Stergiou N, Ristanis S, Morati C, Georgoulis AD (2007) Tibial rotation in anterior cruciate ligament (ACL) deficient and ACL-reconstructed knees: a theoretical proposition for the development of osteoarthritis. Sports Med 37:601–613

Stone DK (1998) Receptors: structure and function. Am J Med 105(3):244–250

Tayapongsak P, O'Brien DA, Monteiro CB, Arceo-Diaz LY (1994) Autologous fibrin adhesive in mandibular reconstruction with particulate cancellous bone and marrow. J Oral Maxillofac Surg 52(2):161–165

Taylor DW, Petrera M, Hendry M, Theodoropoulos JS (2011) A systematic review of the use of platelet-rich plasma in sports medicine as a new treatment for tendon and ligament injuries. Clin J Sport Med 21(4): 344–352

Vega JA, García-Suárez O, Martínez AA (2000) Cartílago articular y factores de crecimiento (primera parte). Mapfre Medicina 11:212–225

Von Porat A, Roos EM, Roos H (2004) High prevalence of osteoarthritis 14 years after an anterior cruciate ligament tear in male soccer players: a study of radiographic and patient relevant outcomes. Ann Rheum Dis 63(3):269–273

Wang-Saegusa A, Cugat R, Ares O et al (2011) Infiltration of plasma rich in growth factors for osteoarthritis of the knee short-term effects on function and quality of life. Arch Orthop Trauma Surg 131(3):311–317

Weibrich G, Kleis WK (2002) Curasan PRP kit vs PCCS PRP system: collection efficiency and platelets counts of two different methods for the preparation of platelet rich plasma. Clin Oral Implants 13:437–443

Weiler A, Förster C, Hunt P et al (2004) The influence of locally applied platelet-derived growth factor–BB on free tendon graft remodeling after anterior cruciate ligament reconstruction. Am J Sports Med 32:881–891

Xie X, Wu H, Zhao S, Xie G, Huangfu X, Zhao J (2013) The effect of platelet-rich plasma on patterns of gene expression in a dog model of anterior cruciate ligament reconstruction. J Surg Res 180(1):80–88

Yasuda K, Tomita F, Yamazaki S, Minami A, Tohyama H (2004) The effect of growth factors on biomechanical properties of the bone–patellar tendon–bone graft after anterior cruciate ligament reconstruction: a canine model study. Am J Sports Med 32:870–880